FUNCTIONAL NEUROANATOMY

FUNCTIONAL NEUROANATOMY

Text and Atlas

Adel K. Afifi, M.D., M.S.
Professor of Pediatrics, Neurology,
Anatomy and Cell Biology
University of Iowa College of Medicine
Iowa City, Iowa

Ronald A. Bergman, Ph.D.
Professor of Anatomy and Cell Biology
University of Iowa College of Medicine
Iowa City, Iowa

McGraw-Hill
HEALTH PROFESSIONS DIVISION

New York St. Louis San Francisco Auckland Bogotá Caracas Lisbon
London Madrid Mexico City Milan Montreal New Delhi
San Juan Singapore Sydney Tokyo Toronto

McGraw-Hill
A Division of The ***McGraw-Hill*** *Companies*

FUNCTIONAL NEUROANATOMY: Text and Atlas

1234567890 QPKQPK 9987

ISBN 0-07-001589-0

This book was set in Times Roman by Bi-Comp, Inc. The editors were Joseph Hefta and Steven Melvin; the production supervisor was Richard Ruzycka. Quebecor Printing/Kingsport, was the printer and binder.

Library of Congress Cataloging-in-Publication Data

To our families

and

to the memory of

Mohammed A. Soweid

and

Samih Y. Alami

C O N T E N T S

CONTENTS

PREFACE

Writing an integrated textbook in the field of neuroscience can be likened to walking a tightrope. All of the books in this area can be appreciated for trying to fill one or more needs of the student who is beginning to explore this fascinating and complex subject. The emphasis of a textbook may be toward research and the unknown or toward the clinic where the student will put into practice the facts he has learned. The most difficult problem for textbook authors is to provide a balanced and judicious product that stimulates the student to reach beyond the core text, that uses appropriately the time allotted for the subject, that avoids confusion by stating clearly what is known or thought to be known, and that course-sequences the subject matter without dependence on supporting prerequisites. No book can hope to fulfill all of these goals. We have tried to reach some of these objectives; only through use by students and teachers will we know how many we have achieved.

We believe that a textbook should be complete and balanced, but not exhaustive; it should stimulate the search for knowledge beyond its pages; and it should be relevant to the stage of development of the student. The text should be such that it can be assimilated by the student in the time usually allotted for such course work and it should be well illustrated. This is the tightrope we have tried to walk. The content is forward-looking and provides a base on which new and essential information can be added by students as they continue their studies and develop their expertise and experiences in this or in related fields of biomedical science.

To help the student reader navigate the material, we have included some special features. Each chapter opens with a brief content outline and closes with a list of suggested readings. At first mention, glossary terms are set in boldface type with definitions in the margins. In some cases, we chose these words for emphasis. Other words were chosen for clarification or expansion where more detail seemed unwarranted in the main body of the text. Accordingly, we caution the reader who is looking for a condensed review of the most important topics to focus instead on the Key Concepts: brief summaries of the ideas which we feel deserve the greatest attention.

We are indebted to many people who allowed us the luxury of time for this effort; most importantly, our families carried much of our personal daily workload with understanding and our colleagues encouraged and supported us. Numerous colleagues and friends helped produce this work. The manuscript was typed by Mrs. Melanie DeVore. The illustrations were prepared by Mr. John Woolsey, Mr. Gary Welch, and Mr. Greg Gambino. Mr. Paul Reimann photographed brain sections in the atlas and in the chapter on gross topography. The Armed Forces Institute of Pathology (AFIP) and Dr. Edward R. White, Associate Director of AFIP, gave us permission to photograph human brain sections from the Paul Yakovlev Collection. The late Mr. Mohamad Haleem, ex-curator of the Medical Museum of AFIP, assisted in the selection of material from the Yakovlev Collection. This collection is supported by Grant Y01-NS-7-0032-00 from the National Institute of Neurological Disorders and Stroke (NINDS) to the AFIP.

Dr. Jean Jew reviewed Chap. 3 and advised in selection of atlas illustrations. Dr. Gary Van Hoesen reviewed Chaps. 21 and 22 and provided photographs of the brain in Alzheimer's disease. Dr. Steven Moore provided the illustrations on Huntington's chorea and Parkinson's disease. Dr. Harold Adams provided the neuroimages of thalamic infarcts. Drs. William Yuh and Yutaka Sato provided the 3D computerized image of cerebral aneurysm. Drs. Terence Williams and Nedzad Gluhbegovic gave us permission to use several illustrations from their book *The Human Brain, a Photographic Guide.* The staff of Medical Photography and Medical Graphics at The University of Iowa provided assistance in printing and designing some of the text and atlas illustrations.

We are grateful to the staff of McGraw-Hill's Health Professions Division, and especially Mr. Joseph Hefta, Medical Editor, and Mr. Steven Melvin, Editing Supervisor, for their interest in this book.

We are solely responsible for errors of fact and expression and we invite suggestions and criticisms by students and teachers to be forwarded to us.

FUNCTIONAL NEUROANATOMY

PART ONE

TEXT

CHAPTER 1

NEURO-HISTOLOGY

The cells that form the nervous system are great in number and complexity. These cells, or neurons, may be divided into two systems as a descriptive convenience: the peripheral and central nervous systems. Neurons are distributed throughout the body, for they are required to a greater or lesser degree for all bodily functions.

Some of these remarkable cells in the skin and internal organs receive stimuli from both the external and the internal environments and transmit the information they receive as electrochemical impulses to cells within the central nervous system that can modify, coordinate, and integrate those impulses. Their final action is to deliver new electrochemical impulses to effector neurons that make muscles contract or glands function, in other words, to provide meaningful conscious experiences and/or coordinated motor activity. All manifestations of life are expressed as forms of muscular contraction and glandular secretion. The attention of the nervous system to muscle function can hardly be overestimated; it is best appreciated when control systems fail or begin to fail (e.g., in stroke patients and patients with neuromuscular defects).

The cells of the nervous system can be divided into two groups: nerve cells (neurons) and supporting cells (glia). Nerve cells are all associated with each other as a functional syncitium, a complex network somewhat like that found in a telephone company. In the case of the nervous system, neurons touch each other through specialized areas of neuronal contact called synapses. The complexity of the synaptic relationships among billions of neurons forms the basis for the behavioral complexity of humans.

Students of the nervous system have uncovered many facets of the structure and function of neurons and the fibrous extensions of the cells (pathways) that emanate from or project on them. To study the nervous system, a wide variety of methods and instrumentation had to be developed to demonstrate the structural components of the nervous system and their interrelationships in normal and disease states.

This chapter is concerned with the structural components of the nervous system.

THE CELLS AND THEIR UNIQUE CHARACTERISTICS

Overview of Neurons

Purkinje cells. Flask-shaped large cells in the cerebellum. Described by Johannes Purkinje, a Bohemian physiologist, in 1837.

A neuron, or nerve cell (the terms may be used interchangeably), has a cell body, or perikaryon (the part containing the nucleus), and all its processes (axon and dendrites). The names given to neurons were suggested by their size, shape, appearance, functional role, or presumed discoverer [e.g., **Purkinje cell** (neuron) of the cerebellum]. The size and shape of neuronal cell bodies are remarkably variable. The diameter of the cell body may be as small as 4 μm (a so-called granule cell of the cerebellum) or as large as 125 μm (a "motor" neuron of the spinal cord). Nerve cells may have a pyramidal, flask, stellate, or granular shape (Fig. 1-1). An additional feature of these perikarya is the number and organization of their processes. Some neurons have few dendrites, while others have numerous dendritic projections. With two known exceptions (the axonless amacrine cell of the retina and the granule cells of the olfactory bulb), all neurons have at least one axon and one or more dendrites.

In general, three basic types of neurons are recognized:

1. Unipolar or pseudounipolar neurons [e.g., sensory (or dorsal root) ganglion cells] have a spherical cell body with single process that bifurcates.
2. Bipolar neurons (e.g., cochlear and vestibular peripheral ganglia and olfactory and retinal receptor cells) are spindle-shaped, with one process at each end of the cell.
3. Multipolar neurons (e.g., autonomic ganglia and the enormous population of cells in the central nervous system).

The most interesting feature of the neurons is their processes. In humans, the axon of a neuron, the effector part of the cell, may be a meter or more in length, extending from the spinal cord to the fingers or toes or from the neurons of the cerebral cortex to the distal extent of the spinal cord. The dendrites, the primary receptor area of the cell, are variable in number and in branching pattern, which in some cases enormously increases a neuron's surface area to receive intput (synapses) from other neurons in diverse locations.

KEY CONCEPTS

- The cellular elements of the nervous system consist of neurons and glia.
- A neuron consists of a perikaryon (cell body) and its processes (axon and dendrites).
- Neurons vary in size and shape, and each neuron has one axon and many dendrites.

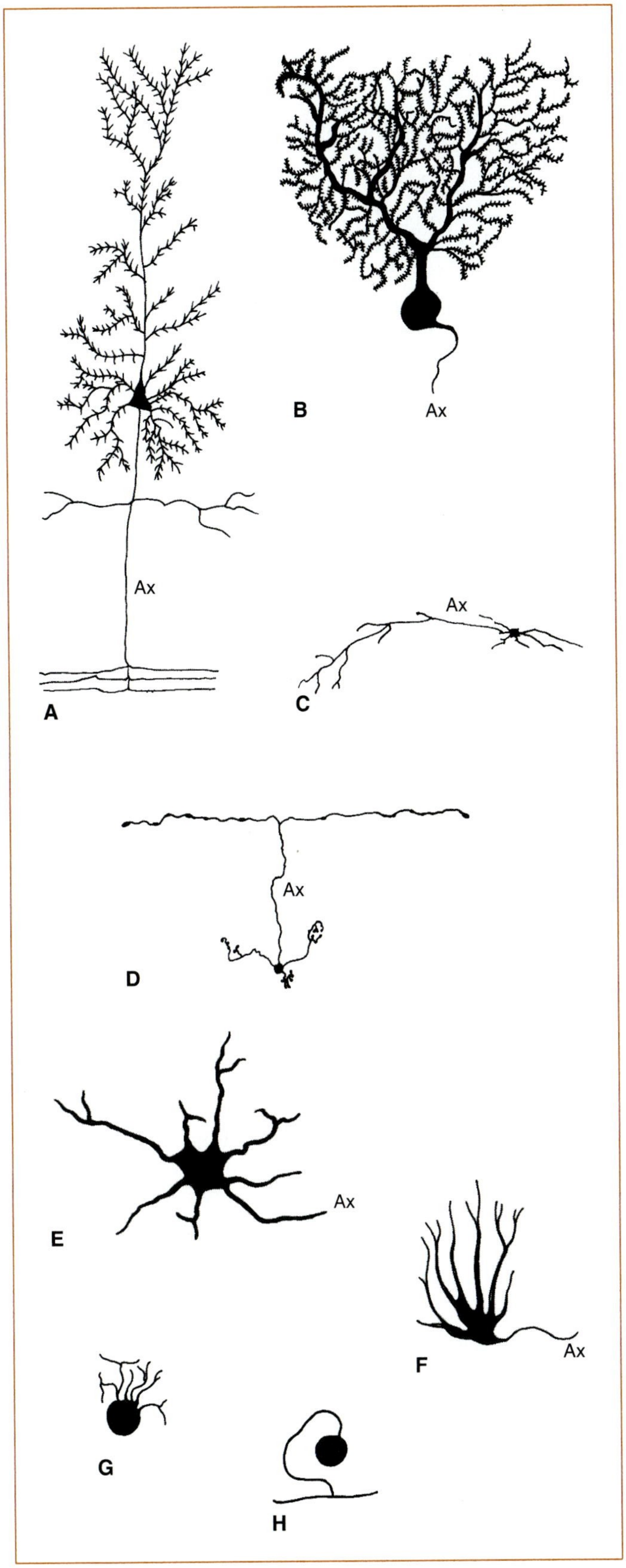

FIGURE 1-1

Schematic diagram illustrating variations in neuronal size, shape, and processes. *A*, pyramidal neuron; *B*, flask-shaped Purkinje neuron; *C*, stellate neuron; *D*, granular neuron; *E*, multipolar anterior horn neuron; *F*, multipolar sympathetic ganglion neuron; *G*, multipolar parasympathetic ganglion neuron; *H*, pseudounipolar dorsal root ganglion neuron; ax, axon.

Perikaryon

The perikaryon, or cell body, contains the nucleus and a number of organelles (Fig. 1-2).

The nucleus is usually round and centrally located. The nucleoplasm is typically homogeneous and stains poorly with basic dyes (nuclear stains). This indicates that the deoxyribonucleic acid (DNA) is dispersed and is in its functionally active form. The nucleoplasm is said to be in its euchromatic form. In stark contrast, each nucleus contains one deeply stainable (with basic dyes) nucleolus, composed in part of ribonucleic acid (RNA), which normally is present within the nucleus. The nuclear contents are enclosed in a distinct nuclear membrane.

The cytoplasm surrounding the nucleus is filled with a variety of organelles and inclusions.

Nissl substance. Granular endoplasmic reticulum of neurons. Named after Franz Nissl, a German neurologist, who described it in 1884.

The most dramatic organelle is the so-called chromophil substance (because of its affinity for basic dyes), or Nissl bodies (after its discoverer). Nissl bodies are particularly prominent in somatic motor neurons, such as those found in the anterior horn of the spinal cord or in some motor cranial nerve nuclei (in this case, the term *nuclei* refers to a cluster of cell bodies in the central nervous system rather than the nuclei of neurons). Nissl bodies, which are distinctive in shape and abundant, are composed of membrane-bound ribonucleoproteins (also known as granular endoplasmic reticulum). The role of the nucleus, nucleolus, and cytoplasmic RNA in protein synthesis is well established. Thus, the cell body synthesizes cytoplasmic proteins and other essential constituents, which are distributed throughout the neuron for maintenance and the functional activities that will be discussed below.

Nissl bodies are found not only in the cell body but also in dendrites. Hence, they too are involved in synthetic activity. The presence of Nissl bodies in dendrites confirms their identity as dendrites, something that otherwise would be impossible in the study of the dense mix of dendrites and axons in the neuropil.

Nissl bodies are absent from the axon hillock (part of the perikaryon from which the axon arises). Nissl bodies undergo characteristic changes in response to axonal injury (see below).

Numerous mitochondria dispersed throughout the cytoplasm play a vital role in the metabolic activity of the neuron.

Golgi apparatus. A perinuclear accumulation of smooth membrane vesicles and cisternae that are well developed in cells engaged in protein synthesis and secretion. Described by Camillo Golgi, an Italian anatomist, in 1896.

The **Golgi apparatus** (Fig. 1-2), which originally was discovered in neurons, is a highly developed system of flattened vesicles and small oval and/or round agranular vesicles. The Golgi apparatus is thought to be the region of the cell that receives the synthetic products of the Nissl substance to allow additional synthetic activity. It is thought that the Golgi area is the site where carbohydrates are linked to protein in the synthesis of glycoproteins. The small vesicles arising from this organelle may be the source of synaptic vesicles and their contents, which are found in axon terminals.

Neurofibrils (Fig. 1-2) are found in all neurons and are continuous throughout all their processes. They are composed of subunits (neurofilaments) that are 7.5 to 10 nm in diameter and thus are below the limit of resolution of the light microscope. In addition to neurofilaments, there are neurotubules with an external diameter of about 25 nm; these structures are similar to those found in cells that are not neuronal. Neurotubules are concerned with the rapid transport of protein molecules synthesized in the cell body, which are carried through the dendrites and axon.

Most large nerve cells contain lipochrome pigment granules (Fig. 1-2). These granules apparently accumulate with age and are more evident during the advancing

KEY CONCEPTS

- Nissl bodies are found in the perikaryon and dendrites but not in axons.
- Neurofibrils are found in perikarya and in all their processes (axon and dendrites).

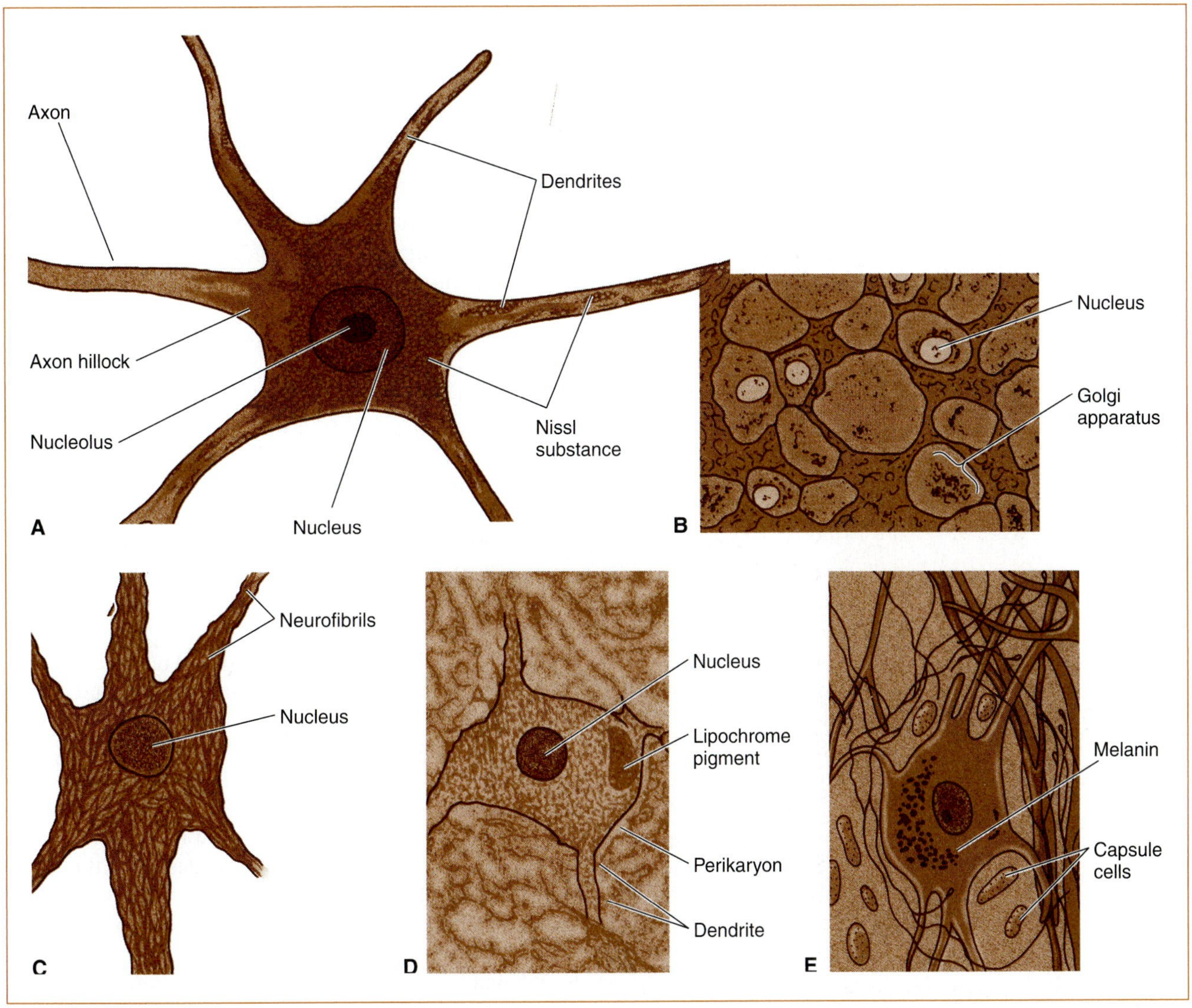

FIGURE 1-2

Schematic diagram of motor neuron and its organelles. *A*, Neuronal cell body and its processes; *B*, Golgi apparatus; *C*, neurofilaments; *D*, lipochrome pigment; *E*, melanin pigment.

age of the organism. In addition, certain nerve cells found in specific locations of the brain contain black (melanin pigment) granules (Fig. 1-2).

All these organelles and inclusions are features of the perikaryon, marking it as the neuron's trophic center. The separation of a process (axon or dendrite) from the perikaryon results in the disintegration of the process.

Axon

A single axon arises from the cell body. The point of departure of the axon is known as the axon hillock. The axon may be very long (120 cm or more) and is uniformly cylindrical. The diameter of axons is also variable and is related to their function. The diameter of specific types of neurons is discussed later in this chapter.

Axon (Greek *axon*, "axis"). The process of a neuron by which impulses are conducted. The axon, passing through its tubular sheaths, forms the axis of the nerve. Purkinje used the term *axis cylinder*. The term *axon* was used to conform with the term *neuron.*

KEY CONCEPTS

- Axons arise from neuronal perikarya at the axon hillock.

Axon hillock. The part of a neuron perikaryon that gives rise to the axon.

The origin of the axon is the **axon hillock,** a small projection of the cell body that is devoid of Nissl substance. Beneath the neuronal membrane at the axon hillock is a dense layer of granular material about 200 Å thick. In addition, there is a confluence of microtubules that exhibit clustering and cross-linkage. The area between the perikaryon (and axon hillock) and the axon is called the initial segment. This segment is short, narrow, and devoid of myelin, which covers some axons. It is at this segment that the nerve impulse or action potential is initiated. Just beyond the initial segment, many axons become myelinated; this increases their diameter in a uniform manner until an axon terminates at its end organ. The axoplasm contains many organelles, such as mitochondria, microtubules, microfilaments, neurofilaments, neurotubules, smooth endoplasmic reticulum, lysosomes, and vesicles of various sizes (Fig. 1-3). The axon, unlike the cell body, does not have any structures associated with protein synthesis or assembly [ribosomes, rough endoplasmic reticulum (Nissl substance), and the Golgi complex]. The smallest axoplasmic components are the microfilaments, which are paired helical chains of actin. The microfilaments usually are located in the cortical zone near the axolemma; their protein, actin (associated with the contractile process), may play a role in intraaxonal transport.

Neurofilaments are larger than microfilaments (7.5 to 10 nm in diameter) and more prevalent. They are scattered throughout the axoplasm, but not in a recognizable pattern. Neurofilaments are composed of three proteins with a molecular mass of 68 to 200 kDa, subunits of the protein tubulin. They are readily disassembled by intrinsic proteases and disappear rapidly in damaged axons. Microtubules are axially arranged hollow cylinders that measure 23 to 25 nm in diameter and are of indefinite length. The number of microtubules within an axon varies in direct relation to axonal mass and the type of nerve; they are more numerous in unmyelinated axons.

Mitochondria vary in number in an inverse ratio to axonal cross-sectional area. They are often topographically related to one or more microtubules.

Smooth endoplasmic reticulum (SER) provides secretory vesicles along the axon. SER is functionally concerned with axonal transport. Secretory vesicles range in size from 40 to 100 μm. Concentrations of vesicles are found in association with nodes of Ranvier (see below) and within nerve terminals.

Lysosomes usually are found near nodes of Ranvier and accumulate rapidly during the degeneration of nerves after an injury.

Axons retain a uniform diameter throughout their length. Axons may have collateral branches proximally and usually branch extensively at their distal ends (telodendria) before terminating by synaptic contact with dendrites and cell bodies of other neurons or on effector organs (muscles and glands).

Schwann cell. A myelin-forming cell in the peripheral nervous system. Named after Theordor Schwann, a German anatomist, who described them in 1838.

Axons may be myelinated or unmyelinated (Fig. 1-4). In both cases, however, the axons are ensheathed by supporting cells: **Schwann cells** in the peripheral nervous system and oligodendroglia cells in the central nervous system.

KEY CONCEPTS

- The initial segment is the segment of neuron between the perikaryon and axon hillock and the axon proper.
- The initial segment is the site of initiation of nerve impulses.
- Perikaryal organelles that are found in axons include mitochondria, microtubules, microfilaments, neurofilaments, neurotubules, smooth endoplasmic reticulum, lysosomes, and vesicles.
- The following perikaryal organelles are not found in axons: ribosomes, rough endoplasmic reticulum, and the Golgi complex.
- Axons may be myelinated or unmyelinated.

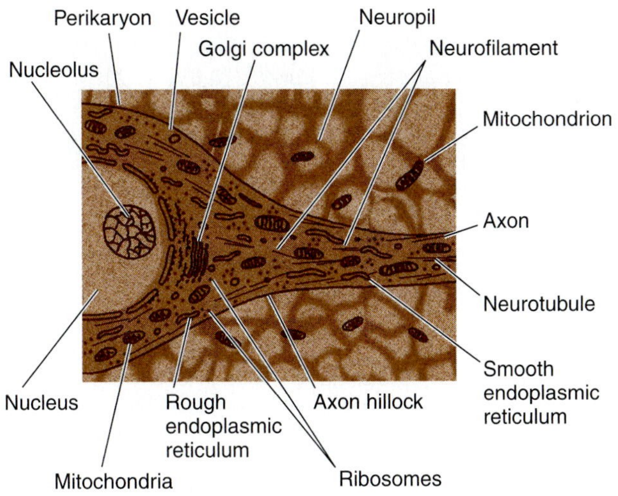

FIGURE 1-3

Schematic diagram showing part of neuronal perikaryon, its axon hillock, and axon.

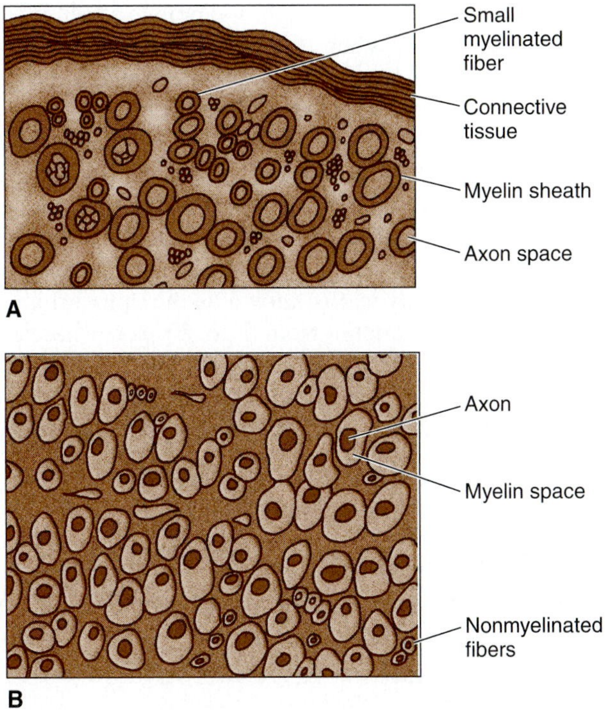

FIGURE 1-4

Schematic diagram of cross sections of a peripheral nerve stained to show myelin sheaths in *A*, and axons in *B*.

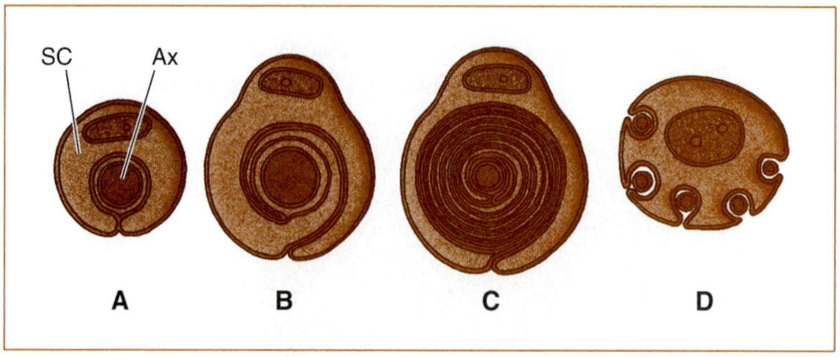

FIGURE 1-5

Schematic diagram of the process of formation of myelin sheaths. *A* and *B* show formation of myelin sheath by concentric double layers of Schwann cell (SC) membranes wrapping themselves around the axon (Ax). *C* shows how protoplasmic surfaces of the membrane become fused together to form the major dense lines. *D* shows how several unmyelinated axons are contained within the infoldings of a single Schwann cell.

Myelinated axons are formed when they become wrapped (Fig. 1-5) in multiple layers of Schwann or oligodendroglia plasmalemma (cell membrane). The process of myelination is discussed later in this chapter.

The myelin sheath is discontinuous at the distal ends of each cell (Schwann or oligodendroglia) involved in the ensheathing process. The area of discontinuity between cells is known as a **node of Ranvier** (Fig. 1-6) and is the site of voltage-gated sodium channels and other ionic displacements involved in impulse conduction (action potentials). The electric impulse flows across a myelinated axon by jumping from node to node. This type of impulse conduction is known as saltatory conduction; it tends to increase the conduction speed of the action potential. The nodes of Ranvier are not lined up with those of adjacent axons, and the myelin sheaths serve as electric insulation; hence, there is little if any spurious activation of axons.

Nodes of Ranvier. Interruptions in a myelin sheath along the axon at which Schwann cell cytoplasm comes in contact with the axon. Described by Louis Antoine Ranvier, a French histologist, in 1878.

Myelin, which is composed of variable tight wrappings of cell membrane around axons, is a lipid-protein complex. When it is prepared for light microscopy, lipid is extracted or lost during tissue preparation, leaving behind in the sectioned tissue a resistant proteolipid artifact known as neurokeratin.

In addition to myelin sheaths, peripheral nerve fibers are surrounded by connective tissue, the endoneurium. Connective tissues are continuous with each other throughout the nerve, but they are named differently according to their locations. The tissue covering individual axons is known as endoneurium, that surrounding a grouping of axons is known as perineurium, and that covering the entire nerve (a recognizable multibundle of axons) is known as the epineurium.

Myelinated axons vary in diameter from 1 to 20 μm, whereas unmyelinated axons are not larger than 2 μm. The size of the nerve fiber (the axon plus its myelin) has a direct relationship to the rate of impulse conduction; large myelinated fibers conduct nerve impulses at a faster rate than do small unmeylinated axons.

KEY CONCEPTS

- Myelin in the peripheral nervous system is made by Schwann cells; in the central nervous system, it is made by oligodendroglia
- A myelin sheath is discontinuous. The gaps between adjacent segments constitute the nodes of Ranvier.
- The nodes of Ranvier are sites of saltatory conduction of nerve impulses.

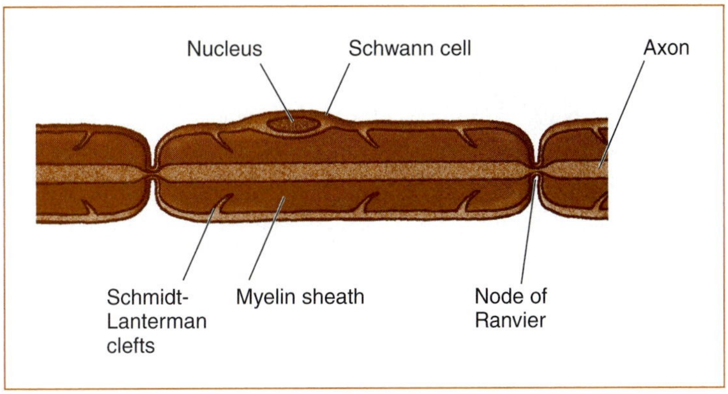

FIGURE 1-6

Schematic diagram of the structure of a myelinated peripheral nerve.

Dendrites

Dendrite (Greek *dendron*, "tree"). Processes of neurons may branch in a tree-like fashion. This term was introduced by Camillo Golgi, an Italian anatomist, in about 1870.

Neurons possess a single axon but usually have more than one dendrite, although there are exceptions (see below). Dendrites may increase the receptive surface area of the cell body enormously. Another method of increasing the receptive surface area of dendrites involves numerous projections from the dendrites known as spines or gemmules, which represent sites of synaptic contact by axon terminals from other neurons.

Dendrites contain all the organelles found in the neuroplasm of the perikaryon except the Golgi apparatus. Neurons that receive axon terminal or synaptic contacts from a variety of central nervous system sources may have an extremely complex dendritic organization. An outstanding example of this complexity is found in Purkinje cells in the cerebellum. Cells of the central nervous system and autonomic ganglia have dendrites extending from their perikarya. Cells with multiple dendrites are called multipolar; those which possess only axonlike processes extending from each end of the cell are named bipolar neurons. Bipolar neurons are found only in the retina of the eye, olfactory receptors, and the peripheral ganglia of the vestibulocochlear nerve (cranial nerve VIII). Sensory neurons in the dorsal root ganglia of spinal neurons are referred to as pseudounipolar because only a single process leaves the cell body before bifurcating to form proximal and distal segments.

The processes of bipolar and pseudounipolar neurons are axonlike in structure; they have a limited or specific receptive capacity. These neurons of the peripheral nervous system usually retain the diversified terminal axonal branching when they enter the central nervous system (brain and spinal cord).

A unique and unusual cell found in the retina, the amacrine cell, is regarded as an axonless neuron.

Neuroglia

The supporting cells between the neurons of the central nervous system are referred to as neuroglia (Fig. 1-7). There are several varieties, which may be organized as follows:

KEY CONCEPTS

- Nerve fibers in the peripheral nervous system are surrounded by connective tissue.
- Dendrites contain all the perikaryal organelles except the Golgi complex.

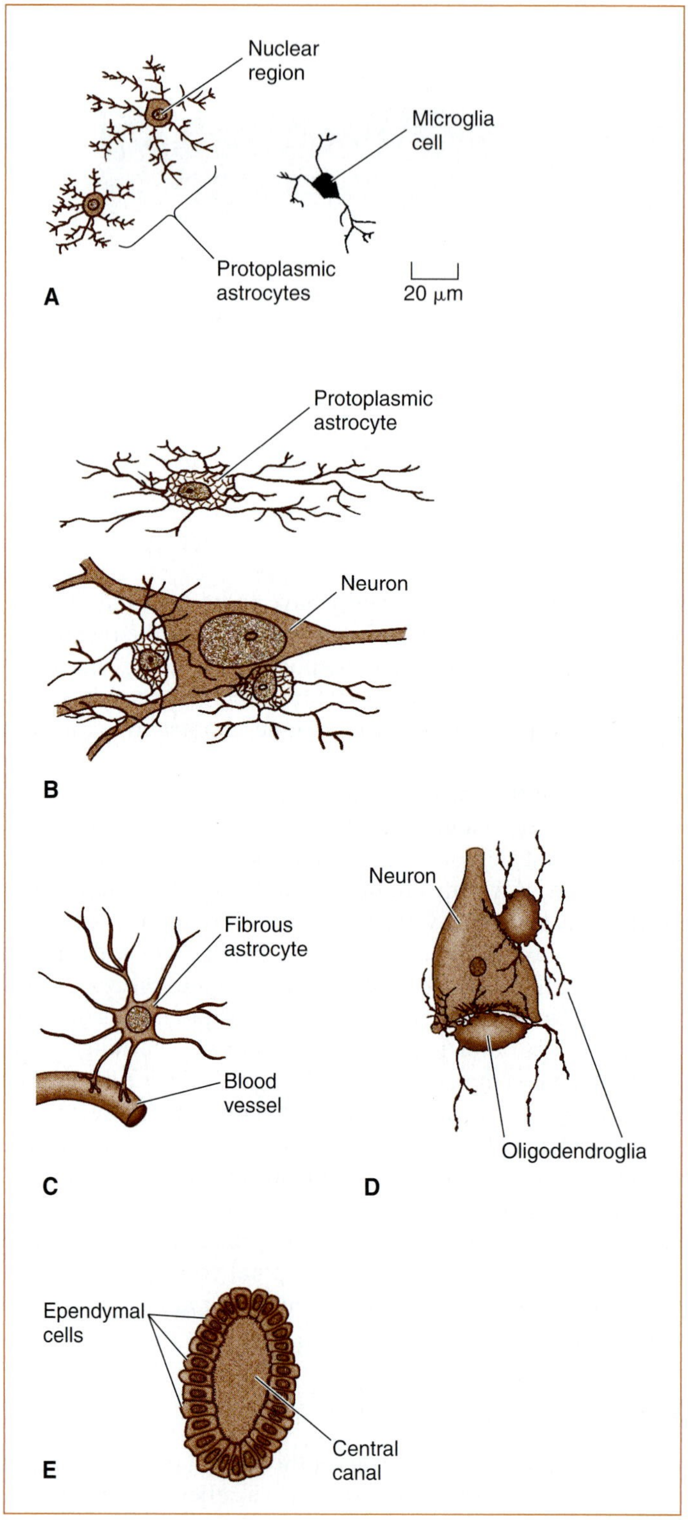

FIGURE 1-7

Schematic diagram of types of neuroglia showing, in *A*, the thick and numerous processes of protoplasmic astrocytes, and the slender and few processes of microglia; *B*, protoplasmic astrocytes in close proximity to neurons; *C*, fibrous astrocyte with processes in contact with a blood vessel; *D*, oligodendroglia in close proximity to a neuron; *E*, ependymal cells lining central canal of the spinal cord.

1. Astrocytes
   a. Fibrous
   b. Protoplasmic
2. Oligodendroglia
3. Ependymal cells
4. Microglia

Astrocytes and oligodendroglia are also known as the macroglia.

Astrocytes (Astroglia)
Astrocytes are the largest of the neuroglia. They are branched stellate cells. The nuclei of these cells are ovoid, are centrally located, and stain poorly because they lack significant amounts of heterochromatin and have no nucleoli. The nuclei do contain euchromatin, which does not stain with typical nuclear stains and is characteristic of active nuclear activity in its cellular function.

Astrocyte (Greek *astron*, "star"; *kytos*, "hollow vessel"). A starlike cell. The processes of astrocytes give them a starlike shape.

The cytoplasm of astrocytes may contain small round granules and glial filaments composed of glial fibrillary acidic protein (GFAP).

The processes of astroglia attach to and completely cover the outer surface of capillaries (perivascular end feet or footplates) as well as the pia mater.

Fibrous Astrocytes Fibrous astrocytes (Fig. 1-7) have thin, spindly processes that radiate from the cell body and terminate with distal expansions or footplates, which are also in contact with the external walls of blood vessels within the central nervous system. The foot processes form a continuous glial sheath, the so-called perivascular limiting membrane, surrounding blood vessels.

The cytoplasm of fibrous astrocytes contains filaments that extend throughout the cell as well as the usual (the generic group of) cytoplasmic organelles.

Fibrous astrocytes, which are found primarily within the white matter, are believed to be concerned with metabolite transference and the repair of damaged tissue (scarring).

Protoplasmic Astrocytes Protoplasmic astrocytes (Fig. 1-7) have thicker and more numerous branches. They are in close association with neurons and may partially envelop them; thus, they are known as satellite cells. Since they have a close relationship to neurons, they are located primarily in the gray matter, where the cell bodies are found, of the brain and spinal cord. Their function is not entirely clear, but they serve as a metabolic intermediary for nerve cells.

Oligodendroglia
Oligodendroglia (Fig. 1-7), which appear small, have fewer and shorter branches than do astrocytes. Their nuclei are round and have condensed, stainable (heterochromatin) nucleoplasm. The cytoplasm is densely filled with mitochondria, microtubules, and ribosomes but is devoid of neurofilaments. Oligodendroglia cells are found in both gray and white matter. They usually are seen lying in rows among axons in the white matter. Electron microscopic studies have implicated the oligo-

KEY CONCEPTS

- Neuroglia are the supporting elements of the central nervous system. They include macroglia (astrocytes and oligodendroglia), microglia, and ependymal cells.
- Astrocytes are of two types: fibrous and protoplasmic.
- Astrocytes are metabolic intermediaries for nerve cells. Fibrous astrocytes also serve a repair function after neural injury.
- Oligodendroglia elaborate central nervous system myelin.

dendroglia in myelination within the central nervous system in a manner similar to that of Schwann cells in the peripheral nervous system. Within the gray matter, these cells are closely associated with neurons, as are the protoplasmic astrocytes (perineuronal satellite cells).

Ependyma (Greek, upper "garment"). The lining cells of the brain ventricles and the central canal of the spinal cord. The term was introduced by Rudolph Ludwig Karl Virchow, a German pathologist.

Microglia (Greek *mikros*, "small"; *glia*, "glue"). Small interstitial, nonneural supporting cells in the central nervous system. Also known as Hortega cells after del Rio Hortega, who described them in 1921.

Ependymal Cells

Ependymal cells (Fig. 1-7) line the central canal of the spinal cord and the ventricles of the brain. They vary from cuboidal to columnar in shape and may possess cilia. Their cytoplasm contains mitochondria, a Golgi complex, and small granules. These cells are involved in the formation of cerebrospinal fluid. A specialized form of ependymal cell is seen in some areas of the nervous system, such as the subcommissural organ.

Microglia

The microglia (Fig. 1-7), unlike other nerve and glial cells, are of mesodermal origin and enter the central nervous system early in its development. Their cell bodies are small, usually with little cytoplasm, but are densely staining and have somewhat flattened and elongated nuclei. These cells have few processes, occasionally two, at either end. The processes are spindly and bear small thorny spines. Normally, the function of the microglia is uncertain, but when destructive lesions occur in the central nervous system, these cells enlarge and become mobile and phagocytic. Thus, they become the macrophages, or scavenger cells, of the central nervous sytem.

Glial cells have been described as the electrically passive elements of the central nervous system. However, it has been shown that glial cells in culture can express a variety of ligand- and voltage-gated ion channels that previously were believed to be properties of neurons. Although numerous ion channels have been described—sodium, calcium, chloride, and potassium—their full functional significance is uncertain. Oligodendrocytes have been shown to quickly change the potassium gradient across their cell membranes, giving rise to a potential change; thus, they serve as highly efficient potassium buffers.

Receptors for numerous neurotransmitters and neuromodulators, such as gamma-aminobutyric acid (GABA), glutamate, noradrenaline, and substance P, have been demonstrated on glia cells, particularly astrocytes. Patch clamp studies have revealed that these glial receptors are similar in many respects to those on neurons.

GANGLIA

Ganglia are defined as collections of nerve cell bodies located outside the central nervous system. There are two types of ganglia: craniospinal and autonomic.

Craniospinal Ganglia

The craniospinal ganglia (Fig. 1-1) are located in the dorsal roots of the 31 pairs of spinal nerves and in the sensory roots of the trigeminal (cranial nerve V), facial (cranial nerve VII), vestibulocochlear (cranial nerve VIII), glossopharyngeal

KEY CONCEPTS

- Microglia play a role in repair of the central nervous system.
- Ependymal cells line ventricular cavities and elaborate cerebrospinal fluid.
- Peripheral ganglia are craniospinal and autonomic.
- Craniospinal ganglia include the dorsal root ganglia and the ganglia of cranial nerves V, VII, VIII, IX, and X.

(cranial nerve IX), and vagus (cranial nerve X) nerves. The dorsal root ganglia and the cranial nerve ganglia are concerned with sensory reception and distribution. They receive stimulation from the external and internal environments at their distal ends and transmit nerve impulses to the central nervous system. The ganglion cells of the spinal group are classified as pseudounipolar neurons, whereas the ganglion cells of the vestibular and cochlear nerves are bipolar neurons.

Craniospinal ganglion cells vary in size from 15 to 100 μm. In general, these cells fall into two size groups. The smaller neurons have unmyelinated axons, whereas the larger cells have myelinated axons. Each ganglion cell is surrounded by connective tissue and supporting cells (the perineuronal satellite cells or capsule cells). From each cell, a single process arises to bifurcate and by doing so forms an inverted T or Y shape (Fig. 1-1). This axonlike structure extends to appropriate proximal and distal locations. The intracapsular process may be coiled (so-called glomerulus) or relatively straight. The bipolar ganglion cells of the vestibular and cochlear cranial nerves are not, however, encapsulated by satellite cells.

Autonomic Ganglia

Autonomic ganglia (Fig. 1-1) are clusters of neurons found from the base of the skull to the pelvis, in close association with and bilaterally arranged adjacent to vertebral bodies (sympathetic ganglia), or located within the organ they innervate (parasympathetic ganglia).

In contrast to cranial-spinal ganglia, the ganglion cells of the autonomic nervous system (sympathetic and parasympathetic) are multipolar and receive synaptic input from various areas of the nervous system. Autonomic ganglion cells are surrounded by connective tissue and small perineuronal satellite cells that are located between the dendrites and are in close association with the cell body.

Autonomic cells range in diameter from 20 to 60 μm and have clear (euchromatic) spherical or oval nuclei, with some cells being binucleate. The cytoplasm contains neurofibrils and small aggregates of RNA, a Golgi apparatus, small vesicles, and the ubiquitous mitochondria.

The dendritic processes of two or more adjacent cells often appear tangled and may form dendritic glomeruli; such cells usually are enclosed in a single capsule. The terminal arborizations of the ganglionic axons synapse on these dendritic glomeruli as well as on the dendrites of individual ganglion cells. In general, the preganglionic arborization of a single axon brings that axon into synaptic contact with numerous ganglion cells. The axons of these ganglion cells are small in diameter (0.3 to 1.3 μm). Autonomic ganglion cells within the viscera (intramural, parasympathetic ganglia) may be few in number and widely distributed. They are not encapsulated but are contained within connective tissue septa in the organ that is innervated. The cells of the autonomic ganglia innervate visceral effectors such as smooth muscle, cardiac muscle, and glandular epithelium.

NERVE FIBERS

A peripheral nerve is composed of nerve fibers (axons) that may vary in size, are myelinated or unmyelinated, and transmit nerve impulses either to or from the central nervous system. Peripheral nerves are often referred to as mixed nerves because they usually are composed of both motor and sensory fibers. Nerves con-

KEY CONCEPTS

- Autonomic ganglia are sympathetic when they are close to vertebral bodies or parasympathetic when they are within peripheral organs.

TABLE 1-1

Some Properties of Mammalian Peripheral Nerve Fibers

Nerve Fiber Type	Number Designation	Function and/or Source	Fiber Size, μm	Myelination	Conduction Velocity, ms
A alpha (α)	Ia	Proprioception, stretch (muscle spindle, annulospiral receptor), and motor to skeletal muscle fibers (extrafusal)	12–22	+	70–120
	Ib	Contractile force (Golgi tendon organ)	12–22	+	70–120
A beta (β)	II	Pressure, stretch (muscle spindle, flower spray receptor), touch, and vibratory sense	5–12	+	30–70
A gamma (γ)	II	Motor to muscle spindle (intrafusal muscle fibers)	2–8	+	15–30
A delta (δ)	III	Some nerve endings serving pain, temperature, and touch	1–5	+	5–30
B	—	Sympathetic preganglionic axons	<3	+	3–15
C	IV	Other pain, temperature, and mechanical receptors; sympathetic, postganglionic axons (motor to smooth muscle and glands)	0.1–1.3	−	0.6–2.0

NOTE: +, present; −, absent.

taining only sensory fibers are called sensory nerves; those which contain only motor fibers are called motor nerves. The structural organization changes along the length of the nerve because of the repeated division and union of different nerve fascicles, resulting in complex fascicular formations.

The nerve fibers that make up a peripheral nerve have been classified according to size and other functional characteristics (Table 1-1). Axons designated as A alpha axons range in size from 12 to 22 μm; A beta, from 5 to 12 μm; A gamma, from 2 to 8 μm; and A delta, from 1 to 5 μm. Preganglionic sympathetic fibers that are less than 3 μm in diameter are designated as B fibers. All these structures are myelinated nerve fibers. The smallest axons (0.1 to 3 μm in diameter) are designated C fibers and are unmyelinated.

A peripheral nerve may be composed of thousands of axons, but the number of axons in each peripheral nerve is variable. Some axons supply many end structures; others, a few.

An examination of nerve cross sections reveals that the amount of connective tissue varies from 25 to 85 percent. This value also varies from place to place and from nerve to nerve. For example, connective tissue is increased at points where nerves cross joints or where there are relatively greater numbers of smaller nerve fascicles or bundles within the peripheral nerve. The connective tissue elements provide the great tensile strength of peripheral nerves; because connective tissue ensheathes the axons, it prevents injury or damage caused by stretching.

Three parts of the connective tissue sheath are recognized (Fig. 1-8). The outer sheath, the epineurium, is relatively thick and is partially composed of loose (areolar) connective tissue. It contains blood and lymphatic vessels. It is also contiguous with

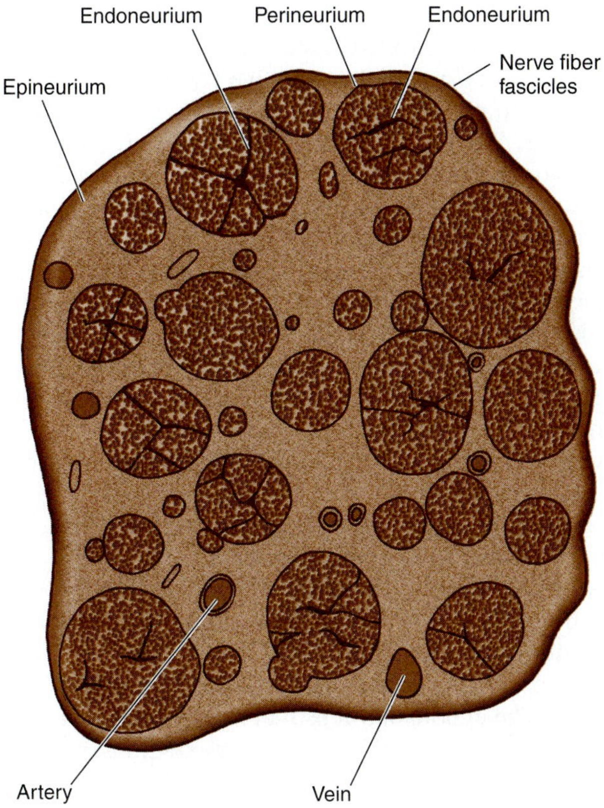
Endoneurium
Perineurium
Endoneurium
Nerve fiber fascicles
Epineurium
Artery
Vein

FIGURE 1-8

Schematic diagram of a cross section of a peripheral nerve showing the formation of three connective tissue septae: endoneurium, epineurium, and perineurium.

the dura mater where a peripheral nerve leaves the central nervous system. The epineurium gives the nerve its cordlike appearance and consistency and separates it from the surrounding tissues. The epineurium acts as a "shock absorber" that dissipates stresses set up in a nerve when that nerve is subjected to pressure or trauma. Nerves composed of closely packed fasciculi with little supporting epineurial tissue are more vulnerable to mechanical injury than are nerves in which fasciculi are more widely separated by a greater amount of epineurial tissue. Epineurial collagenous fibers are continuous with the dense perineurium, which separates and encompasses groups of axons into fascicles of different sizes. The perineurium also partitions the fascicles and follows nerve branches to the periphery, where they terminate on each individual axon (so-called sheath of Henle). These partitions, or septa, may be traversed by small blood vessels, and the perineurium is continuous with the pia-arachnoid membrane. The perineurium also gives tensile strength and some elasticity to the nerve.

The perineurium is also considered a specialized structure that provides active transport of selected materials across the perineural cells from and into the nerve

KEY CONCEPTS

- Peripheral nerves are surrounded by three connective tissue sheaths. Endoneurium invests individual axons, perineurium invests groups of axons in fascicles, and epineurium invests the whole nerve.

fascicles. It also acts as a diffusion (blood-nerve) barrier similar to the pia-arachnoid, with which it is continuous.

The innermost sheath of connective tissue, the endoneurium, invests each individual axon and is continuous with the connective tissue that forms the perineurium and epineurium. This connective tissue provides a tough, protective tubular sheath for the delicate axons. Within the endoneurium and surrounding each myelinated or unmyelinated axon are Schwann cells. Schwann cells produce the myelin sheath (Fig. 1-6). This nucleated sheath of peripheral nerve fibers is also known as the neurolemma or the sheath of Schwann.

In general, large axons are myelinated and small axons are unmyelinated. It is not known which factors determine the selection of fibers for myelination, but axon caliber and trophic influences on Schwann cells by the axon have been implicated. The conduction velocity of axons is directly related to axon diameter and the thickness of the myelin sheath. Conduction velocity rises with increasing axon diameter and increasing thickness of the myelin sheath.

Nerves are well supplied by a longitudinally arranged anastomosing system of blood vessels that originate from larger arteries and veins, perforating muscular vessels, and periosteal vessels. These vessels ramify within the epineurium and extend to reach the perineurium and endoneurium.

Anastomoses between arterioles, between venules, and between arterioles and venules are common. There are numerous anastomoses between epineurial and perineurial arterioles and endoneurial capillaries.

Electron microscopy has revealed structural differences between epineurial and endoneurial vessels. The endothelial cells that make up epineurial vessels have cell junctions of the "open" variety, which allow extravasation of protein macromolecules. Small amounts of serum proteins can diffuse into the epineurium but cannot pass through the perineurium. Endoneurial vessels, in contrast, have endothelial cells with tight junctions, which prevent the extravasation of proteins within the endoneurial space. These vessels, along with the perineurium, constitute the blood-nerve barrier.

Myelinated Nerve Fibers

Electron microscopic studies have demonstrated that most axons greater than 1 μm in diameter are myelinated. The myelin sheath, a proteophospholipid complex, is formed by many concentric double layers of Schwann cell membrane. The double layer of cell membrane is tightly wound, expressing the neuroplasm between the layers, and the inner or protoplasmic surfaces of the cell membrane become fused, forming the dense, thicker lamellae of the myelin sheath (so-called major dense lines) seen on electron microscopy. The inner, less dense lamellae (so-called intraperiod lines) are formed by the outer surfaces of the cell membrane.

The myelin sheath is not continuous over the entire length of the axon but is interrupted at either end because Schwann cells are much shorter than axons. Therefore, a gap always exists between adjacent Schwann cells; this gap is referred to as a node of Ranvier. Many Schwann cells are needed to myelinate a single axon. Sodium channels are known to be clustered at nodes of Ranvier, but they are also present in lower numbers in the internodal axonal membrane. The electron microscope has revealed that interdigitating processes of Schwann cells partially cover the node.

KEY CONCEPTS

- The conduction of nerve impulses is directly related to their size and myelin content.
- The blood-nerve barrier is composed of endothelial cells with tight junctions of endoneurial vessels and the perineurium.

The internodal distance is inconstant because of variations in the size of Schwann cells, differences in fiber diameter, and differences between animal species; it ranges between 400 and 1500 μm. The axon at the node of Ranvier also shows variations unique to this region. For example, the number of mitochondria at the node is fivefold that found in other areas. Lamellated autophagic vesicles, smooth endoplasmic profiles, glycogen granules, and lysosomelike granules are also more numerous at this site. There is also a relative swelling of the axon at the node.

The remarkable ultrastructural organization of the node of Ranvier suggests that the entire paranodal region, the adjacent Schwann cell membranes, and the nodal region of the axon may constitute or be thought of as a single functional unit.

Occasionally, myelin shows localized incomplete fusion of Schwann cell membrane, and small amounts of Schwann cell protoplasm may be found trapped between the membranes. These areas of incomplete fusion are called **Schmidt-Lanterman clefts** (Fig. 1-6). Their significance is not understood, but they may be an artifact or represent a shearing deficit in the formation of myelin or may merely represent a distension of areas of the myelin sheath in which Schwann cell cytoplasm was inadvertently left behind as the cell wound around the axon in the process of forming the myelin sheath. Once trapped, it is probably unremovable but produces no demonstrable change in function.

Schmidt-Lanterman clefts. Areas of incomplete fusion of Schwann cell membranes around the axon. Named after Henry D. Schmidt, an American pathologist who described them in 1874, 3 years before A. J. Lanterman, a German anatomist, described them.

Axonal myelin ends near the terminal arborization of the axon.

Research has established the fact that the axon provides the "signal" for myelination to take place. This signal probably is carried by molecules on the axonal membrane.

Myelination within the central nervous system is accomplished by oligodendroglia cells in a manner similar to that described above for the peripheral nervous system. The major difference in the central nervous system myelin is that the internodal distance and the gap of the node of Ranvier are smaller. In addition, in the peripheral nervous system one Schwann cell produces myelin for a part of a single axon, whereas in the central nervous system one oligodendroglia cell produces the myelin sheath segment for an entire group of axons in its vicinity, with the number ranging from 3 to 200 axons.

Unmyelinated Nerve Fibers

Unlike their larger counterparts, several (8 to 15) small axons may be contained within the infolding of a single Schwann cell (Fig. 1-5), from which they are separated by a constant periaxonal space. The invested axon appears in cross section to be suspended in the cytoplasm by a short segment of the invaginated outer membrane, which, after surrounding the axon, is directed back to the surface in close approximation to the incoming membrane. The similarity in appearance of this arrangement to a cross-sectional intestine with its supporting mesentery has prompted the use of the term *mesaxon* for nonmyelinated axons suspended by the cell membrane and located below the cell's outer surface (and surrounded by neuroplasm). Unmyelinated axons do not have nodes of Ranvier. Within the central nervous system, glia cells have the same function as Schwann cells in that they ensheath the nonmyelinated axons.

Conduction of Nerve Impulses

The cell membrane plays a key role in nerve transmission. In unmyelinated fibers the electric impulse is conducted via ion movement across an ionic destabilized cell membrane. The change in permeability of the membrane allows the influx of sodium ions and the efflux of potassium ions, resulting in a localized reversal of charge of the cell membrane; this is followed by a destabilization of adjacent membrane segments, resulting in a propagated action potential. This is followed by the restoration of the resting potential difference between the inside and the outside of the

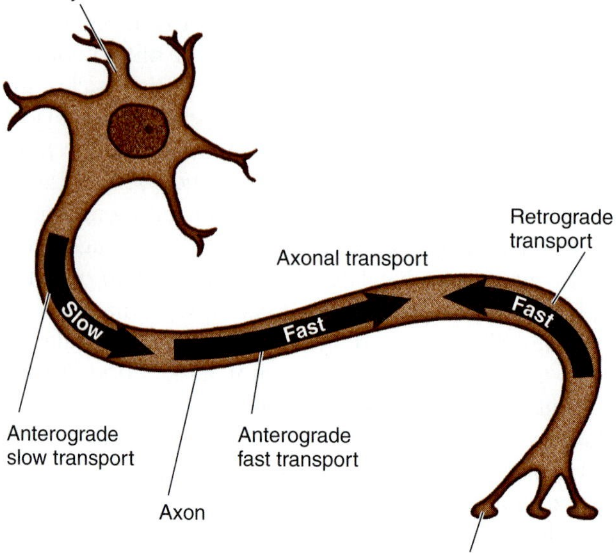

FIGURE 1-9

Schematic diagram of anterograde and retrograde axonal transport.

axon of the previously freely permeable membrane. Sodium and potassium levels inside and outside the axon are restored to their resting values.

In myelinated fibers, permeability changes occur only at the nodes of Ranvier. The insulating effect of the myelin between the nodes prevents propagation of the action potential along the axon; instead, the impulse jumps fron node to node. This type of conduction is known as saltatory conduction and is considerably faster than the process of continuous conduction found in nonmyelinated nerve fibers. Loss of the myelin sheath, known as demyelination, can disrupt conduction. Diseases in which this is known to occur (e.g., multiple sclerosis) produce profound neurologic deficits.

Axonal Transport

Proteins synthesized in the perikaryon are transported throughout the cell and through the axon to its terminal. Axonal transport flows in two directions: anterograde, or toward the axon terminal, and retrograde, or from the axon terminal to the cell body (Fig. 1-9). Anterograde transport flows primarily at two rates: a fast rate (100 to 400 mm/day) and a slow rate (0.25 to 3 mm/day).

The retrograde transport system is very important for recycling intraaxonal proteins and neurotransmitters and for the movement of extraneural substances from nerve endings to the neuron, providing a mechanism that allows trophic influences from end organs to have an effect on neurons. Retrograde axoplasmic transport is

KEY CONCEPTS

- Two types of axonal transport occur in axons: anterograde and retrograde.
- Two types of anterograde transport occur: fast and slow. Retrograde transport is fast.

fast and occurs at about half the velocity of the fast anterograde component. There is no slow retrograde transport component. There is also no rate difference of material transport between sensory and motor axons.

Microtubules are involved in fast anterograde and retrograde transport; thus, microtubule-disrupting drugs such as colchicine and vinblastine prevent fast axonal transport. In fast anterograde transport, a characteristic protein called kinesin is known to provide the motive force to drive organelles along microtubules. A different protein, dynein, may be involved in fast retrograde transport.

Substances that are moved are carried in the mitochondria or small vesicles of SER. The substances that are transported include enzymes of neurotransmitter metabolism and peptide neurotransmitters and neuromodulators. Fast axonal transport requires energy in the form of high-energy phosphate compounds [adenosine triphosphate (ATP)]; therefore, it is necessary for the neuron to be oxygenated adequately. Any interruption of mitochondrial oxidative phosphorylation causes the cessation of axoplasmic flow and transport.

Substances transported by the slow component include structural proteins such as tubulin, actin, and neurofilamentous proteins. The underlying mechanism of motility for slow transport is unclear.

Based on the concept of anterograde and retrograde axonal transport, neuroanatomic tracing methods have been developed to study neural connectivity. A radioactively labeled amino acid injected into a region of neuronal perikarya is incorporated into proteins and is transported anterogradely to the axon terminal. Alternatively, a histochemically demonstrable enzyme such as horseradish peroxidase travels retrogradely from the axonal terminals to the soma, or cell body. Different fluorescent dyes injected at different sites travel retrogradely to the neuron or neurons that project on those sites. Cell bodies sending axons to the two injected sites fluoresce in different colors. A neuron whose axon branches end in both injected areas will be labeled in two colors.

SYNAPSE

The simplest unit of segmental nerve function requires two neurons: a sensory receptor neuron and a motor or effector, neuron. This arrangement is found in the simplest reflexes, for example, the patellar tendon reflex (knee jerk). The structural-functional coupling of these two neurons occurs through what is termed a synapse. The terminal arborizations of the sensory neuron (axons) are dilated into small knobs or boutons (so-called **boutons terminaux,** a term coined by a French investigator), which lie in contact with the dendrites, cell bodies, and/or axons of effector neurons (Fig. 1-10). These small bulbs contain synaptic vesicles that range in size from 300 to 600 nm and may be round or flattened on two sides. The vesicles appear empty but actually contain in life the neurotransmitter acetylcholine. In other kinds of synapses, the vesicles may contain an electron-dense dark particle termed a core or a dark core vesicle that is presumed to be catecholamine. Acetylcholine and catecholamine are only two of several chemical transmitter substances that facilitate the transfer of nerve impulses from one neuron to another, at and across the synapse, or to a nonneuronal effector organ such as a gland or muscle.

Electron microscopy has revealed the specialized structure of the synapse, which consists of thickened pre- and/or postsynaptic membranes separated by a synaptic gap (or cleft) of about 20 nm. Although not all synapses are structurally identical, they are recognizably related. The membrane thickenings of the pre- and postsynaptic membranes represent accumulations of cytoplasmic proteins beneath the plasmalemma (cell membrane). In addition to synaptic vesicles, the synaptic terminal contains a collection of mitochondria and some neurofilaments.

When an action potential arrives at an axon terminal (end bulb or bouton terminaux), the membrane of the terminal is depolarized and Ca^{2+} ions enter the permeable terminal and promote the fusion of synaptic vesicles with the presynaptic

Synapse (Greek *synapsis*, "a conjunction, connection, clasp"). A term introduced by Foster and Sherrington in 1897 to describe the junction between two or more neurons. Sherrington had considered the term *syndesm* but changed to *synapse* at the suggestion of the Greek scholar Verrall.

Boutons terminaux. A French term for what Cajal in 1903 called terminal buttons to describe axon terminations in a synapse.

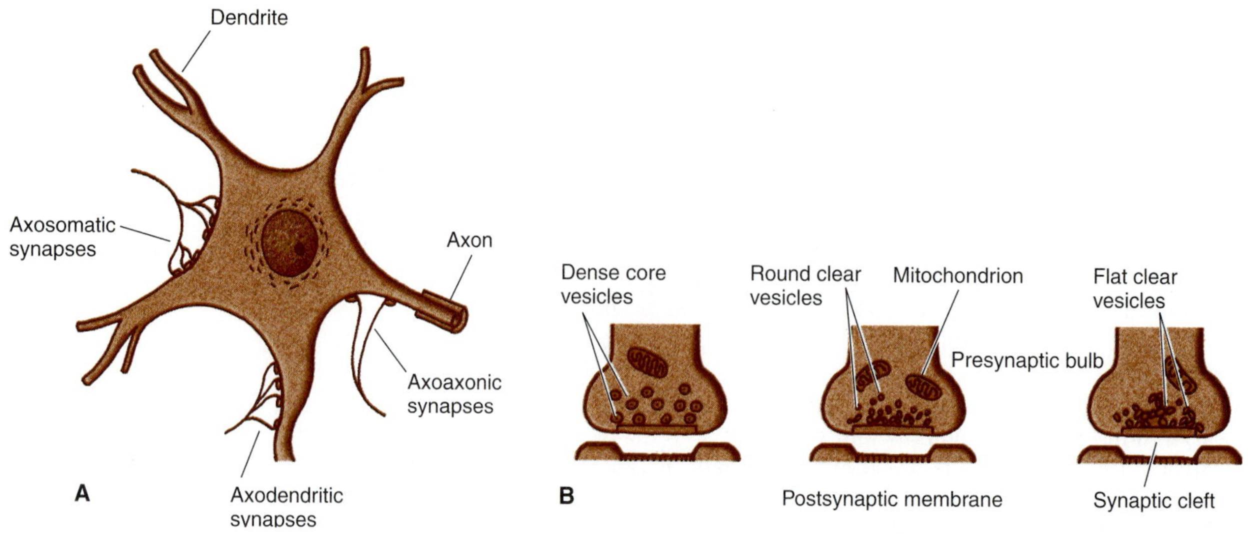

FIGURE 1-10

Schematic diagram showing, in *A*, axosomatic, axodendritic, and axoaxonic synapses, and, in *B*, ultrastructural components of the synapse.

membrane (membrane of the terminal bulb). The neurotransmitter, for example, acetylcholine, contained within the synaptic vesicles is released by exocytosis into the synaptic gap, or cleft (a space of 20 nm), where it diffuses out and binds to receptors on the postsynaptic membrane and promotes increased permeability of the postsynaptic membrane. The ionic permeability of the postsynaptic membrane is increased, leading to the membrane's depolarization and the generation of an action potential in the target postsynaptic cell (gland, muscle, or nerve) membrane.

Increasing evidence indicates the importance of protein phosphorylation in the regulation of the function of a presynaptic nerve terminal. Major synaptic vesicle–associated proteins include the synapsins (Ia and Ib, IIa and IIb), synaptophysin, and synaptobrevin. The precise physiologic functions of these phosphoproteins are unknown, but that of synapsin I is becoming increasingly apparent. Phosphorylation of synapsin I occurs in response to nerve impulses and to a variety of neurotransmitters acting at presynaptic receptors. Dephosphosynapsin I binds to vesicles and inhibits their availability for release.

Phosphorylation of synapsin I decreases its affinity for synaptic vesicles, which then become available for release. In addition to their role in neurotransmitter release, proteins of the synapsin family may regulate the formation of presynaptic nerve terminals. Synapsin expression has been shown to correlate temporally with synapse formation during development and to play a causal role in synaptogenesis.

Functionally, synapses may be excitatory or inhibitory; transmission usually is unidirectional and not obligatory, except at the neuromuscular junction. Electron microscopy, however, has shown a wide variety of structural arrangements in synapses; this suggests that transmission may in some cases be bidirectional.

Some synapses, termed electric, have no synaptic vesicles, and the adjacent cell membranes (pre- and postsynaptic) are fused. The fused membranes of electric synapses are called tight junctions or gap junctions. The transmission at these junctions occurs by electrotonic depolarization; it may be bidirectional, and this type of synapse is considered obligatory. These synapses are not common in the mammalian nervous system.

Synapses have been classified by their structural associations as follows:

1. Axoaxonic: axon to axon
2. Axodendritic: axon to dendrite
3. Axosomatic: axon to cell body
4. Dendrodendritic: dendrite to dendrite
5. Neuromuscular: axon to muscle fiber

In chemical synapses, the following substances have been identified as transmitters:

1. Acetylcholine
2. Monoamines (noradrenaline, adrenaline, dopamine, serotonin)
3. Glycine
4. GABA
5. Glutamic acid

Two natural brain peptide neurotransmitters—endorphins and enkephalins—have been shown to be potent inhibitors of pain receptors. They exhibit a morphinelike analgesic effect.

Other peptide hormones, such as substance P, cholecystokinin, vasopressin, oxytocin, vasoactive intestinal peptides (VIP), and bombesin, have been described in different regions of the brain, where they act as modulators of transmitter action.

The available data assign a role for peptides in chemical transmission that is auxiliary to that of classical neurotransmitters, but in some neuronal systems peptides play the main role. This is especially apparent in hypothalamic neurosecretory cells that produce and release the posterior pituitary hormones vasopressin and oxytocin.

Besides their role in transmission, peptides seem to have a trophic function. Tachykinins have been shown to stimulate the growth of fibroblasts and smooth muscle fibers; VIPs affect bone mineralization and stimulate the growth of human keratinocytes.

Recently, increasing evidence has suggested a messenger role for peptides in the nervous system. Peptides have their own receptors in the nervous system, and receptors for tachykinins, substance P, neurokinin A (substance K), and neurotensin have been cloned.

Neuromuscular Junction

The neuromuscular junction (also called the myoneural junction or motor end plate) is a synapse between a motor nerve terminal and the subjacent part of the muscle fiber. Motor neurons branch variably and extensively near their termination at the muscle fiber that is supplied. One neuron may innervate as few as 10 or as many as 500 or more skeletal muscle fibers. A motor neuron and the muscle fibers that it innervates constitute a motor unit. The motor unit, not the individual muscle fiber, is the basic unit of function.

As a nerve fiber approaches a muscle fiber, it loses its myelin sheath and forms a bulbous expansion that occupies a trough on the muscle fiber surface (Fig. 1-11). The trough is variable in its complexity, and no two subneural troughs appear exactly alike. There is no evidence that this variability has functional significance.

KEY CONCEPTS

- Synapses are classified according to their structural association into axodendritic, axosomatic, axoaxonic, dendrodendritic, and neuromuscular.
- On the basis of their function, synapses are classified into excitatory and inhibitory.

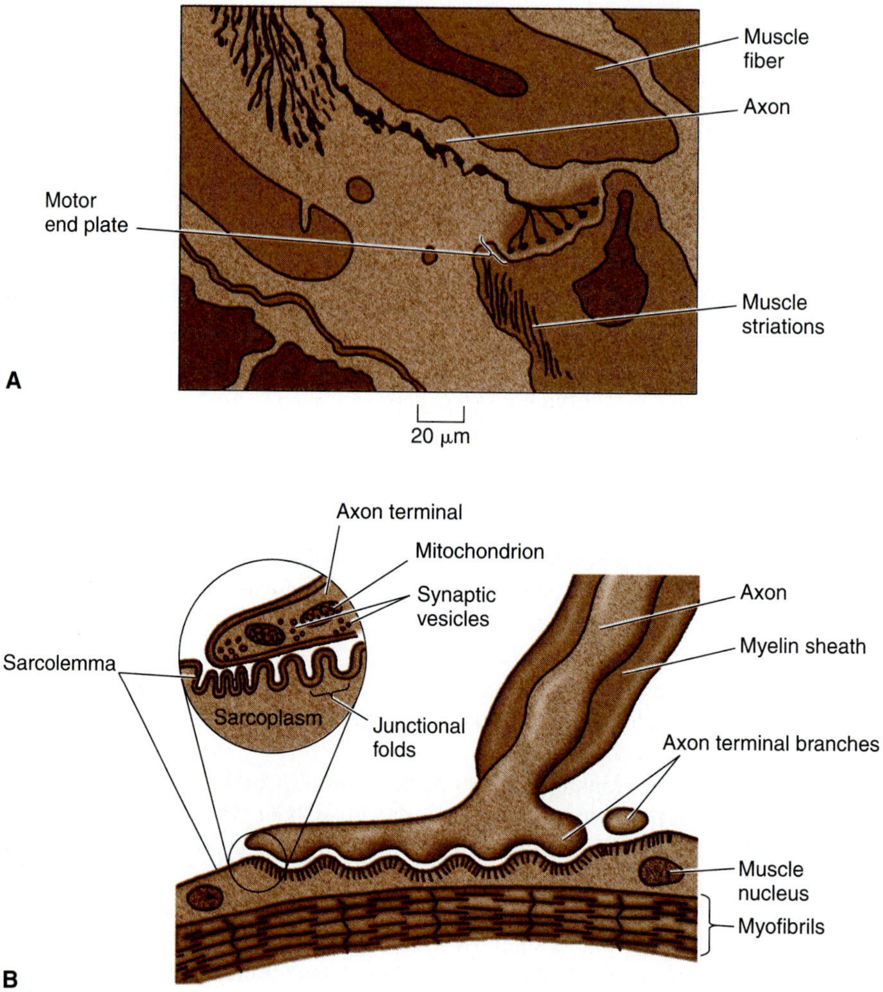

FIGURE 1-11

Schematic diagram of the motor end plate. *A*, light microscopic appearance; *B*, ultrastructural appearance.

The terminal expansion of the nerve fiber is covered by a cytoplasmic layer of Schwann cells, the neurilemmal sheath. The endoneurial sheath of connective tissue that surrounds the nerve fiber outside the neurilemmal sheath is, however, continuous with the connective tissue sheath of the muscle fiber.

The motor end plate (or end plate) is 40 to 60 μm in diameter, although these structures are not always round. They are typically located near the midpoint of the muscle fiber or are somewhat more proximal.

The axonal terminal contains synaptic vesicles (filled with acetycholine) and mitochondria. The synaptic gap between the nerve and muscle is about 50 μm. The postsynaptic membrane of the muscle has numerous infoldings called junctional folds. When a motor neuron is activated (fired), the nerve impulse reaches the axon terminal and the contents of the synaptic vesicle (acetylcholine) in the terminal are discharged into the gap or cleft between the pre- and postsynaptic membranes. Once the acetylcholine is released into the cleft, it diffuses very quickly to combine with acetylcholine receptors in the muscle membrane. The binding of acetylcholine to the receptor makes the muscle membrane more permeable to sodium. This in turn depolarizes the muscle cell membrane, leading to the appearance of a propagated muscle action potential and muscular contraction. This synaptic activity is always excitatory and is normally obligatory, that is, all or none.

The subneural sarcolemma or postsynaptic membrane contains the enzyme acetylcholinesterase, which breaks down the depolarizing transmitter. This allows the muscle membrane to reestablish its resting condition.

The most common disorder of the neuromuscular junction is a disease known as myasthenia gravis, which is characterized by the onset of muscular weakness after muscle use and the improvement of muscular strength with rest. In this disease, antibodies bind to acetylcholine receptors and render them less accessible to released acetylcholine. In addition, many commercial pesticides and nerve gases interfere with neuromuscular transmission by inhibiting the hydrolysis (destruction) of acetylcholine, thus prolonging its effect on the muscle and thereby inactivating the muscle. Botulinum toxin, however, interferes with neuromuscular transmission by blocking the release of acetylcholine from the presynaptic membrane.

RECEPTOR ORGANS OF SENSORY NEURONS

The peripheral termination of a sensory neuron is differentiated into specialized dendrites. These specialized dendrites are designed to change (transduce) one kind of energy to another (i.e., touch to electrochemical nerve impulses).

Sensory receptors may be classified by function, for example, nociceptor (pain) or mechanoreceptor; by structure, for example, encapsulated or nonencapsulated (so-called free); by a combination of both structure and function; or by anatomic location, for example, skin, joints.

Each receptor possesses a different sensitivity and different adaptive properties based on its response to continuous monotonic stimulation. Receptors may adapt quickly or slowly. Quickly adapting receptors produce impulses that gradually decrease in strength in response to constant and unvarying stimuli. Slowly adapting receptors continue their response level throughout their activation and the duration of stimulation.

Slowly adapting receptors are of two types. Type I receptors have no spontaneous discharge at rest and are more sensitive to vertical displacement. Type II receptors maintain a slow regular discharge at rest and are more sensitive to stretch. A more detailed discussion of specific receptor types appears in Chap. 23.

Free (Nonencapsulated) Nerve Endings

The receptors known as free nerve endings are the axonal endings designed for sensory reception. Their name arose not in a functional sense but rather in a structural one.

This type of receptor has the widest distribution throughout the body and is most numerous in the skin. Additional locations include the mucous membranes, deep fascia, muscles, and visceral organs; these receptors are ubiquitous. The distal arborizations are located in the epithelium between the cells, the epithelium of the

KEY CONCEPTS

- Synaptic activity at the neuromuscular junction is always excitatory and obligatory.
- Sensory receptor organs are classified according to their location (skin or joints), structure (encapsulated or free), function (nociceptor or mechanoreceptor), adaptive properties (slowly or quickly adapting), or a combination of these categories.
- Free nerve endings are the most widely distributed receptors but are most numerous in the skin.

skin (Fig. 1-12), the cornea, and the mucous membranes lining the digestive and urinary tracts, as well as in all the visceral organs and blood vessels. In addition, they are associated with hair follicles and respond to the movement of hair. Certain specialized epithelial cells (neuroepithelium), such as those found in taste buds (Fig. 1-12), olfactory epithelium, and the cochlear and vestibular organs (hair cells), receive free (receptor) endings. Tendons, joint capsules, periosteum, and deep fascia also may have this type of ending. Endings of this kind probably respond directly to a wide variety of stimuli, including pain, touch, pressure, and tension, and respond indirectly through so-called neuroepithelia to sound, smell, taste, and position sense. The axons of these sensory receptors may be myelinated or unmyelinated.

Merkel's corpuscles. Free nerve endings distributed in the germinal layer of the epidermis. They convey touch sensation. Described by Friedrich Sigmund Merkel, a German anatomist, in 1880.

Merkel's corpuscles are slowly adapting type I mechanoreceptors that are distributed in the germinal layer (stratum basale) of the epidermis. Groups of 5 or 10 of these corpuscles are interspersed among the basal layer cells. Unmyelinated free nerve endings form an axonal expansion (e.g., Merkel's disk) that is closely applied to a modified epidermal cell (Merkel's cell). Merkel's cells are found in glabrous skin and in the outer sheaths of hairs in hairy skin. These endings are also found in areas of transition between hairy skin and mucous membrane. Synapselike junctions have been observed between Merkel's disks and Merkel's cells; their functional significance is uncertain. This receptor subserves the sensory modality of constant touch or pressure and is responsible for the tactile gnosis of static objects. The discharge frequency of Merkel's corpuscles is temperature-dependent. Cooling the skin increases the discharge frequency, and warming inhibits the discharge rate.

Encapsulated Nerve Endings

This group of receptors includes the corpuscles of Meissner, Vater-Pacini, Golgi-Mazzoni, and Ruffini; the so-called end bulbs; the neuromuscular spindles; and the tendon organ of Golgi.

Meissner's Tactile Corpuscles

Meissner's corpuscles. Encapsulated nerve endings found in the greatest numbers in the hairless skin of the fingers, palm of the hand, plantar surface of the foot, toes, nipples, and lips. They convey flutter-vibration and moving touch. They were described by George Meissner, a German anatomist, in 1853.

Meissner's corpuscles are elongated, rounded bodies of spirals of receptor endings (Fig. 1-12) that are fitted into dermal papillae beneath the epidermis; they are about 100 μm in diameter. A Meissner's corpuscle possesses a connective tissue sheath that encloses the spiral stacks of horizontally arranged epitheloid cells. The endoneurium is continuous with the capsule. When the myelin sheath terminates, the axon (A beta fiber) arborizes among the epithelial cells. From one to four myelinated axons, as well as unmyelinated axons, enter the capsule. Meissner's corpuscles are distributed widely in the skin but are found in the greatest numbers in the hairless (glaborous) skin of the finger, palm of the hand, plantar surface of the foot, toes, nipples, and lips. These corpuscles are rapidly adapting mechanoreceptors.

The sensory modality subserved by Meissner's corpuscles is low-frequency (30 to 40 Hz) flutter-vibration and moving touch. Under sustained pressure, an impulse is produced at the onset, removal, or change of magnitude of the stimulus.

Vater-Pacini Corpuscles

Vater-Pacini, more commonly known as pacinian, corpuscles (Fig. 1-12) are the largest and most widely distributed encapsulated receptor organs. They range up

KEY CONCEPTS

- Merkel's corpuscles are temperature-dependent and subserve the sensory modalities of constant touch or pressure.
- Meissner's corpuscles subserve the sensory modalities of flutter-vibration and moving touch.
- Pacinian corpuscles subserve vibration sense.

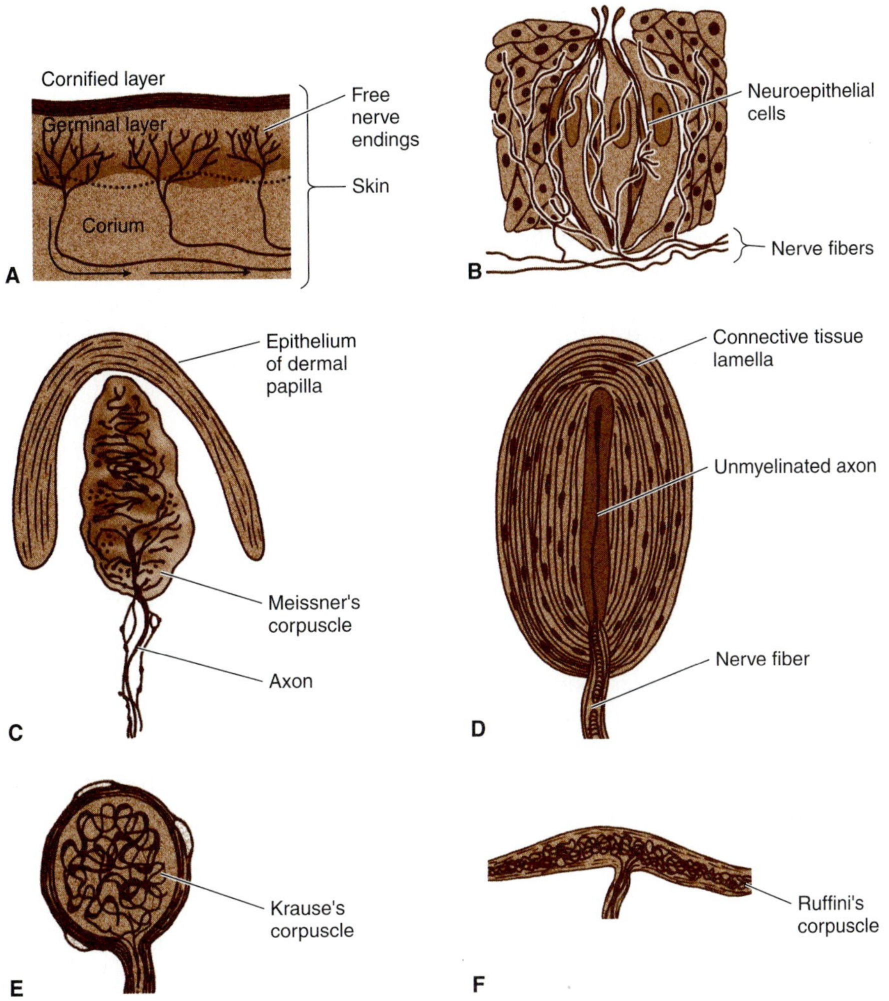

FIGURE 1-12

Schematic diagram of receptor organs. A, Free nerve endings; B, taste bud; C, Meissner's corpuscle; D, Pacinian corpuscle; E, Krause's corpuscle; F, Ruffini's corpuscle.

Vater-Pacini corpuscles. Encapsulated nerve endings with a wide distribution. Rapidly adapting mechanoreceptors. Named after Abraham Vater, a German anatomist, and Filippo Pacini, an Italian anatomist. The corpuscles were first depicted by Lehman in 1741 from a preparation made by Vater, who called them *papillae nervae.* Shekleton (1820–1824) dissected the same nerves and receptors 10 years before they were seen by Pacini. He placed a beautiful specimen in the Museum of the Royal College of Surgeons in Dublin. Pacini then "rediscovered" them in 1830. The name *pacinian corpuscles* was used by Friedrich Henle, a German anatomist, and Rudolph Kolliker, a Swiss anatomist, in 1844. Shekleton's contribution has almost been forgotten.

to 4 mm in length but usually are smaller; they are the only macroscopic receptor organ in the body. The capsule is elliptical in shape and is composed of concentric lamellae of flattened cells (fibroblasts) supported by collagenous tissue that invests the unmyelinated distal segment of a large myelinated (A beta) axon. The interlamellar spaces are filled with fluid. Because of their size, these corpuscles are provided with their own blood supply, which also makes them unique. Histologically, when cut or sectioned, they look like a divided onion, to which they have been likened.

Vater-Pacini corpuscles are mechanoreceptors that are sensitive to vibration. They are maximally responsive at 250 to 300 Hz. These corpuscles are rapidly adapting receptors that respond only transiently to on vibration and off vibration or at the end of a step-wise change in stimulus position. The recovery cycle of this receptor is very short (5 to 6 ms). The rapid adaptation of pacinian corpuscles is a function of the connective tissue capsule that surrounds the central neural elements. The removal of the connective tissue capsule transforms a pacinian corpuscle from a rapidly adapting receptor to a slowly adapting one.

These ubiquitous receptors are distributed profusely in the subcutaneous connective tissue of the hands and feet. They are also found in the external genitalia, nipples, mammary glands, pancreas and other viscera, mesenteries, linings of the pleural and abdominal cavities, walls of blood vessels, periosteum, ligaments, joint capsules, and muscles. Of the estimated 2×10^9 pacinian corpuscles in the human skin, more than one-third are in the digits and more than 1000 can be found in a single finger.

Golgi-Mazzoni corpuscles. End organs distributed in the subcutaneous tissue of the hands, on the surface of tendons, and in the periosteum adjacent to joints. They detect vibration. Described by Camillo Golgi, an Italian anatomist.

Golgi-Mazzoni Corpuscles

Golgi-Mazzoni corpuscles are quickly adapting receptor organs that are lamellated (like the pacinian corpuscles); however, instead of a single receptor terminal, the unmyelinated receptor is arborized with varicosities and terminal expansions. These corpuscles are distributed in the subcutaneous tissue of the hands, on the surface of tendons, in the periosteum adjacent to joints, and elsewhere. Their function is uncertain but probably is related to the detection of vibration with a maximal response under 200 Hz.

Ruffini's corpuscles. Encapsulated nerve endings that are widely distributed but readily found in the dermis of the fingertips and in joint capsules. They convey sensations of pressure and touch. Described by Angelo Ruffini, an Italian anatomist, in 1898.

Ruffini's Corpuscles

Elongated and complex, **Ruffini's corpuscles** (Fig. 1-12) are found in the dermis of the skin, especially the fingertips, but are widely distributed, especially in joint capsules. The receptor endings within the capsule ramify extensively among the supporting connective tissue bundles. These type II slowly adapting receptors have been associated with sensations of pressure and touch as a velocity and position detector. The discharge of Ruffini's corpuscles is temperature-dependent, increasing with skin cooling and decreasing with skin warming. Three types of Ruffini's corpuscles have been identified in joint capsules, based on their position-related discharge. All three maintain constant baseline output, but each type responds differently. One type responds maximally at extreme flexion, another type at extreme extension, and a third midway between flexion and extension of the joint.

End bulbs of Krause. Encapsulated end organs which are widely distributed and are associated with temperature sensation. Named after Wilhelm Johann Friedrich Krause, who described them in 1860.

End Bulbs

The end bulbs resemble the corpuscles of Golgi-Mazzoni. They have a connective tissue capsule enclosing a gelatinous core in which the terminal, unmyelinated endings arborize extensively. The **end bulbs of Krause** (Fig. 1-12) have been associated with sensations of temperature (cold) and are located strategically and distributed widely. The structural complexity of these end bulbs varies remarkably, as does their size. It is likely that they serve a wide variety of different functions; their size and distribution, however, preclude easy analysis. Much confusion has arisen regarding the end bulbs of Krause, since Krause identified and named two morphologically different structures end bulbs.

Neuromuscular Spindles

Neuromuscular spindles are found in skeletal muscle and are highly organized. Muscle spindles are distributed in both flexor and extensor muscles but are more abundant in muscles that control fine movements. Each muscle spindle is less than 1 cm long and contains 2 to 12 specialized striated fibers (so-called intrafusal fibers) in a capsule parallel with the surrounding skeletal muscle fibers [so-called extrafusal (nonencapsulated) muscle fibers]. Histologically, the muscle spindle is composed

KEY CONCEPTS

- Golgi-Mazzoni corpuscles probably subserve the sense of vibration.
- Ruffini's corpuscles subserve velocity and position sense in relation to vibration and touch. Their discharge is temperature-dependent.
- The end bulbs of Krause are related to temperature sensation but probably subserve other sensory functions.

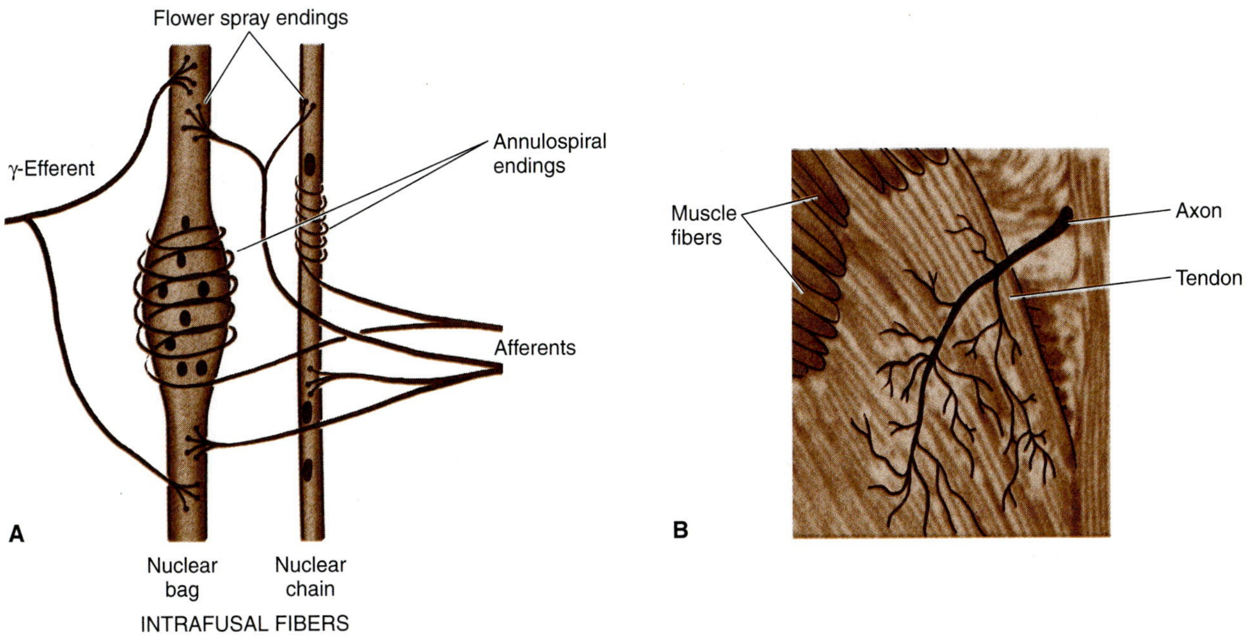

FIGURE 1-13

Schematic diagram of neuromuscular spindle (*A*), and Golgi tendon organ (*B*).

of two types of intrafusal muscle fibers (Fig. 1-13). The nuclear chain fiber is smaller in diameter and shorter in length and contains a single row of centrally located nuclei. The nuclear bag fiber, which is larger and longer, contains a cluster of many nuclei in a baglike dilatation in the central part of the fiber.

Each intrafusal muscle fiber is supplied with both efferent and afferent nerve fibers. The efferent fibers (so-called gamma efferents), which are axons of gamma motor neurons in the anterior horn part of the spinal cord, terminate on the polar ends of both the nuclear chain fibers and the nuclear bag fibers. The afferent nerve fibers originate from two types of receptor endings on the intrafusal fibers: the annulospiral (primary) endings and the flower spray (secondary) endings. The annulospiral endings are reticulated branching endings that are situated around the central portion of both nuclear chain fibers and nuclear bag fibers; they are better developed, however, on the nuclear bag fibers. The so-called flower spray endings are scattered diffusely along the length of the intrafusal fibers but are found especially on each side of the central portion adjacent to the annulospiral endings. Both nuclear chain fibers and nuclear bag fibers contain this type of ending.

The receptor endings of intrafusal muscle fibers respond to the stretching of extrafusal muscle fibers or their tendons. The activity of the spindle ceases with

KEY CONCEPTS

- Intrafusal muscle fibers have two types of receptors: primary (annulospiral) and secondary (flower spray).
- Intrafusal muscle fibers (muscle spindles) respond to stretching of a muscle or its tendons or to stimulation by gamma efferent nerve fibers.
- Brief dynamic stretching of muscle stimulates primary endings, whereas sustained muscle stretching stimulates primary and secondary endings.

the relaxation of tension in the spindle, when the skeletal muscle contracts. The receptor endings also may be stimulated by the stretching of intrafusal muscle fibers secondary to gamma motor nerve activity, which contracts the polar ends of intrafusal muscle fibers, thus stretching the receptor portions of the fibers.

A static stimulus such as that which occurs in sustained muscle stretching stimulates both the annulospiral and the flower spray endings. By contrast, only the annulospiral (primary) endings respond to brief (dynamic) stretching of the muscle or to vibration.

The afferent nerves emanating from the receptor endings project on alpha motor neurons in the spinal cord, which in turn supply the extrafusal fibers. Thus, when a muscle is stretched by tapping its tendon, as is done clinically, the stimulated receptor endings initiate an impulse in the afferent nerves which stimulates the alpha motor neurons and results in a reflex muscle contraction. As soon as the skeletal muscle contracts, the tension in the intrafusal muscle fibers decreases, the receptor response diminishes or ceases, and the muscle relaxes. This is the basis of all monosynaptic stretch reflexes (e.g., knee jerk, biceps jerk). Gamma efferent activity plays a role in sensitizing the receptor endings to a stretch stimulus and helping maintain muscle tone.

Tendon organs of Golgi. Stretch receptors in tendons close to their junction with the muscle fiber. Tension produced in the muscle by stretching is the optimal stimulus for a Golgi tendon organ. Named after Camillo Golgi, an Italian anatomist.

Tendon Organs of Golgi

Tendon organs of Golgi are slowly adapting receptors (Fig. 1-13) located in tendons close to their junction with skeletal muscle fibers and are in series with extrafusal muscle fibers. The organ consists of fascicles of tendon ensheathed by a connective tissue capsule. The capsule encloses the distal end of a large (12 μm) myelinated fiber, which divides repeatedly before it splits into unmyelinated (receptor) segments. These branchlets terminate in ovoid expansions that intermingle with and encircle the fascicles of collagenous tissue that constitute the tendon. Tendon organs respond to tension in skeletal muscle fibers that is developed by stretching the muscle or actively contracting the muscle. The tension thus developed deforms the receptor endings and "sets off" a nerve impulse that is transmitted to the spinal cord. Afferent nerves emanating from Golgi tendon organs project on inhibitory interneurons in the spinal cord. Thus, when a muscle (along with its tendon) is stretched excessively, the muscle relaxes.

REACTION OF NEURONS TO INJURY

The reaction of neurons to injury has been studied extensively in experimental animals, with the findings confirmed in humans; in fact, this has become one of the methods employed in the study of cell group (nuclei) and fiber tracts. Responses can be divided into those which occur proximal to the site of the injury and those which occur distal to it (Fig. 1-14). If death of the nerve cell does not occur, regenerative activity in the form of nerve sprouts emanating from the proximal stump may begin as early as 24 h after an injury.

KEY CONCEPTS

- Golgi tendon organs respond to the tension produced by stretching or active contraction of muscle fibers.
- Neurons react to injury by undergoing characteristic changes that occur proximal (chromatolysis) and distal (wallerian degeneration) to the site of the injury.

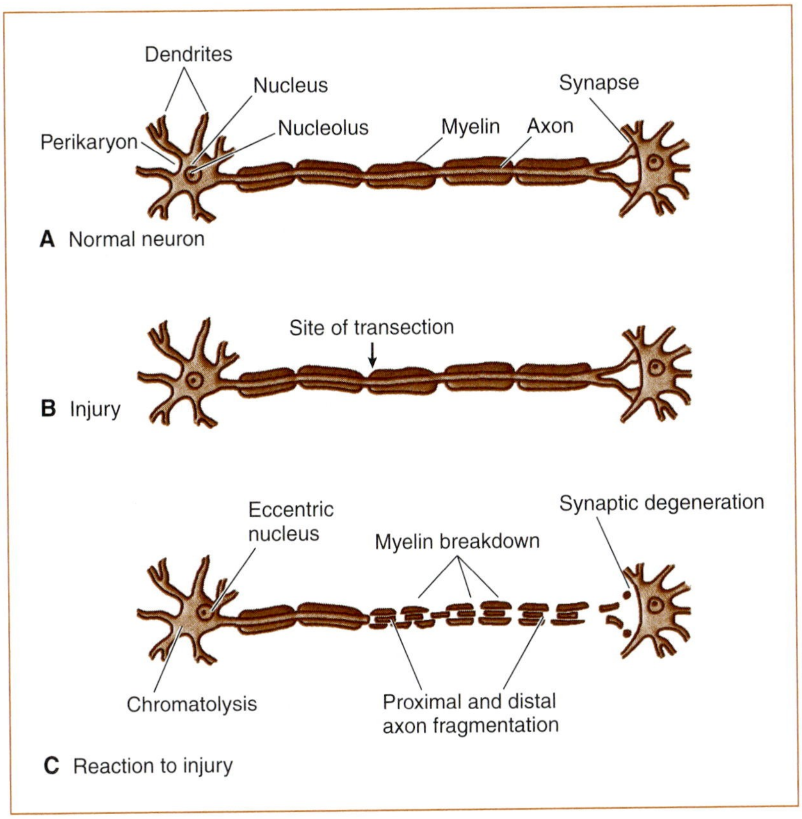

FIGURE 1-14

Schematic diagram of a normal neuron (*A*), site of injury (*B*), and reaction to injury (*C*).

Cell Body and Dendrites

If an axon is severed or crushed, the following reactions can be found in the cell body and dendrites proximal to the site of injury.

1. The entire cell, including the nucleus and nucleolus, swells; the nucleus shifts from its usual central position to a peripheral part of the cell.
2. The Nissl bodies (tigroid substance) undergo **chromatolysis** (i.e., they become dispersed, and the sharp staining pattern disappears). This process is most marked in the central portion of the cell (former perinuclear location) but may extend peripherally to involve Nissl bodies in the dendrites. The process of chromatolysis reflects a change in the metabolic priority from that geared to the production of neurotransmitters needed for synaptic activity to that involving the production of materials needed for axonal repair and growth. The central cell body must synthesize new messenger RNA, lipids, and cytoskeletal proteins. The components of the cytoskeleton most important for axonal regeneration are actin, tubulin, and neurofilament protein. These proteins are carried by slow anterograde axonal transport at a rate of 5 to 6 mm/day, which correlates with the maximal rate of axonal elongation during regeneration. Another group of proteins whose synthesis is increased during regeneration of nerve cells consists of growth-associated proteins (GAPs), which travel by fast axonal transport at a rate of up to 420 mm/day. Although GAPs do not initiate, terminate, or regulate growth, they are essential for regeneration. Neuronotropic factors (NTFs) from the periphery signal to the cell body that an injury has occurred and travel by retrograde axonal transport.

Chromatolysis (Greek *chromatos*, "color"; *lysis*, "dissolution"). Dissolution of the Nissl bodies of a neuron as a result of injury to its axon. The term was introduced by Georges Marinesco, a Romanian neurologist, in 1909.

3. The other organelles, including the Golgi apparatus and mitochondria, proliferate and swell.

The speed at which these changes occur, as well as their degree, depends on several factors, including the location of the injury, the type of injury, and the type of neuron involved. The closer the injury is to the cell body and the more complete the interruption of the axon is, the more severe the reaction is and the poorer are the chances of full recovery. In general, this reaction is seen more often in motor neurons than in sensory neurons.

The reactions of the cell body and dendrites to axonal injury are termed retrograde cell changes. After about 3 weeks, if the cell survives the injury, the cell body and its processes begin to regenerate. Full recovery takes 3 to 6 months. The nucleus returns to its central location and is normal in size and cofiguration. The staining characteristics and structure of the organelles also return to normal. If regeneration fails, the cell atrophies and is replaced by glia.

Axon

After an injury, the axon undergoes both retrograde (proximal) and anterograde (distal) degeneration. Retrograde degeneration usually involves only a short segment of the axon (a few internodes). If the injury to the neuron is reversible, regenerative processes begin with the growth of an axon sprout as soon as new cytoplasm is synthesized and transported from the cell body. The regenerative sprouting of the proximal axon stump requires elongation of the axon. This process is mediated by a growth cone at the tip of the regenerating fiber. Growth cones were first described by Ramon y Cajal, who compared their advance through solid tissue to that of a battering ram. Recent research has revealed that growth cones release a protease that dissolves the matrix, permitting their advance through the tissues. Growth cones have mobile filopodia (extruding from a flattened sheet of lamellipodia), enabling them to move actively and explore the microenvironment of a regenerating axon. Growth cones play an essential role in axon guidance and can respond to contact guidance clues provided by laminin and fibronectin, two major glycoprotein components of the basal laminae of Schwann cells.

Shortly after a nerve injury and before the onset of wallerian degeneration, severe degeneration of the tips of the proximal and distal stumps occurs. This injury is secondary to an influx of sodium and calcium and a massive loss of potassium and protein. The axonal debris and normal tissue scarring may prevent the growth cone of the proximal stump from reaching a healthy distal stump.

Wallerian degeneration. Changes in an axon and its myelin sheath distal to the site of severance of the axon. Named after Augustus Waller, an English physiologist who described the phenomenon between 1850 and 1852.

Distal to the site of the injury, the severed axon and its myelin sheath undergo what is known as secondary, or **wallerian, degeneration,** named in recognition of its description by Augustus Waller in 1852. The axon, deprived of its continuity with the supporting and nutritive materials from the cell body, begins to degenerate within 12 h. The axon degenerates before its Schwann cell sheath does and appears beaded and irregularly swollen within 1 week. The axonal reaction extends distally to involve the synapse. The fragmented portions of the axon are phagocytized by invading macrophages. This process may take considerably longer within the central nervous system.

Along with degeneration of the axon, the myelin sheath begins to fragment and undergo dissolution within the Schwann cell. Macrophages also play an important role in the removal of myelin breakdown products. The degenerative process occurs within the endoneurium and is soon followed by mitotic activity in the Schwann cells, which form a tubelike sleeve within the endoneurium along the entire length of the degenerated axon. Endoneurial tubes persist after the myelin and the axonal debris have been cleared. The proliferating Schwann cells align longitudinally within the endoneurial tube, creating a continuous column of cells named **Büngner's bands.** The growth of axons from the proximal stump begins within 10 h and may traverse the gap between the proximal and distal ends of the axon and enter the Schwann cell tubes (neurolemma). Although many small axonal sprouts may enter a single tube, only one will develop its normal diameter and appropriate sheath; the others will degenerate. This may occur within 2 or 3 weeks, since regenerative growth normally takes place at a rate of 1.5 to 4 mm/day. Failure to establish a pathway for regrowth of the axonal sprouts may result in the formation of a neuroma, which is often a source of pain.

Büngner's bands. Chains of multiplying Schwann cells that facilitate the regeneration of axons after an axonal injury.

It must be pointed out that chance plays a major role in this regenerative activity. If a sensory axon enters a sheath formerly occupied by a motor axon or vice versa, the growing axon will be nonfunctional and the neuron will atrophy. Accurate growth and innervation of the appropriate distal target are thus of critical importance to the success of nerve regeneration. In this context, the target of innervation can exert a guiding "neurotropic" influence on a regenerating axon. Forrsman in 1898 and Ramon y Cajal subsequently showed that the advancing tip of a regenerating axon is chemotropically attracted to its appropriate distal nerve target. Recent experimental studies have confirmed this. In addition, although the process of degeneration is similar in the central and peripheral nervous systems, there is a marked difference in the success of the regenerative process in the two systems. What has been described above applies primarily to regeneration in the peripheral nervous system. Degeneration of a neuron usually is limited to its perikaryon and processes. In certain areas of the nervous system, however, degeneration of a neuron is transmitted to the neuron, with which it makes a connection. This type of degeneration is known as transneuronal degeneration.

Nerve Growth Factors

Successful nerve regeneration requires neuronal growth. Four classes of nerve growth factors are essential for optimal nerve growth: (1) NTFs, or survival factors, (2) neurite-promoting factors (NPFs), which control axonal advance and influence the rate, incidence, and direction of neurite growth, (3) matrix-forming precursors (MFPs), possibly fibrinogen and fibronectin, which contribute fibrin products to the nerve gap and provide a scaffolding for the ingrowth of cells, and (4) metabolic and other factors.

NTFs are macromolecular proteins that promote the survival and growth of neuronal populations. They are present in the target of innervation, where they are taken up by the nerve terminals and transported by retrograde axonal transport back to the cell body. These factors exert a supportive or survival-promoting effect. The best known NTF is nerve growth factor (NGF).

NPFs are substrate-bound glycoproteins that strongly promote the initiation and extension of neurites. Laminin and fibronectin, two components of the basal lamina, have been shown to promote neurite growth. Although NPFs were presumed to exert their neurite-promoting activity by increasing the adhesion of the growth cones to the surface of the basal lamina, recent studies have shown that NPFs promote neurite growth independent of growth cone adhesion.

KEY CONCEPTS

- Growth cones are important in the regeneration of axons distal to the site of an injury.
- Successful nerve regeneration after an injury depends on several nerve growth factors: neuronotropic, neurite-promoting, matrix-forming, and metabolic.

After a nerve injury, a polymerized fibrin matrix is formed from the fibrinogen and fibronectin found in exudates from the cut nerve ends. This matrix is important for the migration of Schwann cells and other cells into the gap between the cut ends.

Metabolic and other factors that promote nerve regeneration include sex hormones, thyroid hormone, adrenal hormones, insulin, and protease inhibitors.

Clinical Correlation

Neurapraxia (Latin *neuralis*, "nerve"; Greek *apraxia*, "absence of action"). Failure of nerve conduction in the absence of structural damage.

Axonotmesis. A lesion of a peripheral nerve that produces discontinuity of axons with preservation of the supporting connective tissue sheaths.

Neurotmesis (Latin *neuralis*, "nerve"; Greek *tmesis*, "cutting"). Partial or complete severance of a nerve with disruption of the axon and myelin sheath and connective tissue elements.

There are at present two classifications of nerve injury that are based on the nature of the lesion in the nerve. The first classification, proposed by Seddon, recognizes three degrees of severity of nerve injury: (1) conduction block (**neurapraxia**), (2) loss of axonal continuity (**axonotmesis**), and (3) loss of nerve trunk continuity (**neurotmesis**). The second classification, proposed by Sunderland, includes five degrees of nerve injury (Table 1-2).

1. The first and least severe degree consists of a temporary physiologic conduction block in which axonal continuity is not interrupted. The conduction across the injured segment of nerve is blocked. Conduction proximal and distal to the block is normal. The three connective tissue sheaths are intact.
2. In the second degree wallerian degeneration is present distal to the nerve lesion. Continuity of the endoneurial sheath is preserved and permits regeneration of the distal segment of the nerve. The peri- and epineurial sheaths are also preserved.
3. The third degree is characterized by the loss of continuity of nerve fibers. The internal fasicular structure is disorganized, the endoneurial sheath becomes discontinuous, and wallerian degeneration is present. Peri- and epineurial sheaths are, however, preserved. Axon regeneration in this type of injury is negligible because of the development of intrafasicular fibrosis and the loss of continuity of the endoneurial sheath.
4. In the fourth degree fasicular nerve structure is destroyed. Endo- and perineurial sheaths are discontinuous. The epineurial sheath is intact. Regenerating axon growth is blocked by fibrous tissue scarring. This type of injury requires excision of the injured nerve segment and nerve repair.
5. The fifth degree represents the complete loss of continuity of the nerve trunk. There is discontinuity of the axon and the endo-, peri-, and epineurial sheaths.

Table 1-2 gives a summary of Sunderland's classification; Fig. 1-15 shows a diagrammatic representation of the different stages of nerve injury.

Neuronal Plasticity

It was thought at one time that the mature central nervous system is incapable of recovering its function after an injury. However, recent studies have demonstrated that the central nervous system may not be so static or rigid. It has been shown that after an injury the neuronal circuitry may reorganize itself by forming new synapses to compensate for those lost to injury. This property of forming new channels of communication after an injury is known as neuronal plasticity.

Neuronal plasticity is most dramatic after partial denervation. In such a situation, the remaining unaffected axons projecting on the partially denervated region de-

KEY CONCEPTS

- Clinically, nerve injury is classified according to the degree of severity into conduction block (neurapraxia), loss of axonal continuity (axonotmesis), and loss of nerve trunk continuity (neurotmesis).
- The ability of the nervous system to form new channels of communication after injury and to adapt to environmental influences constitutes neuronal plasticity.

TABLE 1-2

Nerve Injury

Degree of Severity	Wallerian Degeneration	Endoneurium Continuity	Perineurium Continuity	Epineurium Continuity	Nerve Fiber Continuity	Nerve Trunk Continuity
I	−	+	+	+	+	+
II	+	+	+	+	+	+
III	+	−	+	+	−	+
IV	+	−	−	+	−	+
V	+	−	−	−	−	−

NOTE: +, present; −, absent.

velop axonal sprouts that grow and form new synaptic contacts to replace those lost by denervation.

The ability of the mature central nervous system to form these sprouts and functional synapses varies from one region to another and from one species to another. The factor or factors that promote sprout formation and synaptogenesis in some but not all regions or species are not fully known and are the subject of intensive research. The identification of factors that promote neuronal plasticity in the injured mature central nervous system may have a great impact on the recovery of function in paraplegic patients and stroke victims.

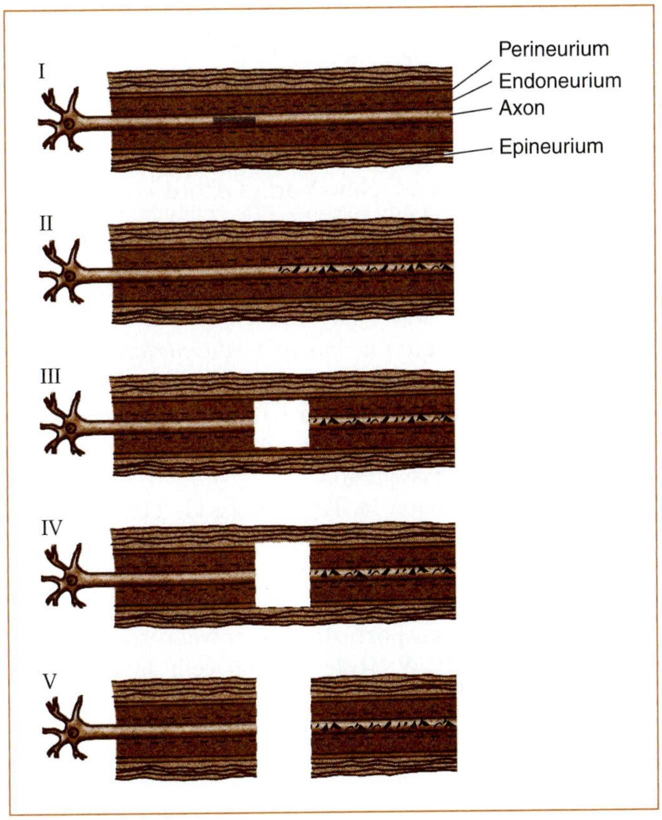

FIGURE 1-15

Schematic diagram of the five types of nerve injury.

This discussion of plasticity has focused on the regenerative ability of the central nervous system after an injury. It must be emphasized, however, that plasticity in its broader sense is an ongoing phenomenon. Although brains are grossly similar anatomically, physiologically, and biochemically, the behavior of humans differs from individual to individual. This difference in behavior reflects the plasticity of the brain in adapting to its environment.

SUGGESTED READINGS

Afifi AK, Bergman RA: *Basic Neuroscience: A Structural and Functional Approach,* 2d ed. Baltimore, Urban & Schwarzenberg, 1986.

Altman J: Microglia emerge from the fog. *Trends Neurosci* 1994; 17:47–49.

Barr ML, Kiernan JA: *The Human Nervous System: An Anatomical Viewpoint,* 6th ed. Philadelphia, Lippincott, 1993.

Bergman RA, et al: *Atlas of Microscopic Anatomy.* Philadelphia, Saunders, 1989.

Bergman RA, et al: *Histology.* Philadelphia, Saunders, 1996.

Edelman G: Cell adhesion molecules in the regulation of animal form and tissue pattern. *Annu Rev Cell Biol* 1986; 2:81–116.

Fawcett D, et al: *A Textbook of Histology*, 12th ed. New York, Chapman & Hall, 1994.

Gluhbegovic N, Williams TH: *The Human Brain: A Photographic Guide.* Philadelphia, Harper & Row, 1980.

Hall ZW: *An Introduction to Molecular Neurobiology.* Sunderland, MA, Sinauer, 1992.

Hillman H, Darman J: *Atlas of the Cellular Structure of the Human Nervous System.* London, Academic Press, 1991.

Hogan MJ, et al: *Histology of the Human Eye.* Philadelphia, Saunders, 1971.

Hudspeth AJ: The hair cells of the inner ear. *Sci Am* 1983; 248:54–64.

Jones E: The nervous tissue. In Weiss L (ed): *Cell and Tissue Biology: A Textbook of Histology*, 6th ed. Baltimore, Urban & Schwarzenberg, 1988:277–352.

Junge D: *Nerve and Muscle Excitation*, 3d ed. Sunderland, MA, Sinauer Associates, 1992.

Kimelberg H, Norenberg M: Astrocytes. *Sci Am* 1989; 260:66–76.

Levi-Montalcini R: The nerve growth factor 35 years later. *Science* 1987; 237:1154–1162.

Levitan I, Kaczmarek L: *The Neuron: Cell and Molecular Biology.* New York, Oxford University Press, 1991.

Lim DJ: Functional structure of the organ of corti: A review. *Hear Res* 1986; 22:117–146.

Matthews GG: *Cellular Physiology of Nerve and Muscle,* 2d ed. Boston, Blackwell, 1991.

Meredith GE, Arbuthnott GW: *Morphological Investigations of Single Neurons in Vitro.* New York, Wiley, 1993.

McDevitt D: *Cell Biology of the Eye.* New York, Academic Press, 1982.

Murphy S: *Astrocytes: Pharmacology and Function.* New York, Academic Press, 1993.

Nicholls JG, Martin AR: *From Neuron to Brain: A Cellular Approach to the Function of the Nervous System,* 3d ed. Sunderland, MA, Sinauer Associates, 1992.

Pappas G, Purpura D: *Structure and Function of Synapses.* New York, Raven Press, 1972.

Peters, A, et al: *The Fine Structure of the Nervous System: The Neurons and Their Supporting Cells,* 3d ed. New York, Oxford University Press, 1990.

Robinson P, et al: Phosphorylation of dynamin I and synaptic vesicle recycling. *Trends Neurosci* 1994; 17:348–353.

Schwartz J: The transport of substances in nerve cells. *Sci Am* 1980; 242:152–171.

Shepherd G: *The Synaptic Organization of the Brain,* 3d ed. New York, Oxford University Press, 1990.

Siegel G, et al: *Basic Neurochemistry.* New York, Raven Press, 1989.

Smith CUM: *Elements of Molecular Neurobiology.* New York, Wiley, 1989.

Steward O: *Principles of Cellular, Molecular and Developmental Neuroscience.* New York, Springer, 1989.

Terzis JK, Smith KL: *The Peripheral Nerve: Structure, Function, and Reconstruction.* New York, Raven Press, 1990.

Thoenen H, Kreutzberg G: The role of fast transport in the nervous system. *Neurosci Res Prog Bull* 1982; 20:1–138.

Vallee RB, Bloom GS: Mechanism of fast and slow transport. *Annu Rev Neurosci* 1991; 14:59–92.

Walz W: Role of glial cells in the regulation of the brain ion microenvironment. *Prog Neurobiol* 1989; 33:309–333.

CHAPTER 2

GROSS TOPOGRAPHY

For didactic purposes, the nervous system is conventionally divided into three major parts: the central nervous system (CNS), peripheral nervous system, and autonomic nervous system. Although this division simplifies the study of a complex system, the three component parts act in concert in the overall control and integration of the motor, sensory, and behavioral activities of the organism. A great deal of effort has been expended to elucidate the structure, connectivity, and function of the nervous system. The methodologic creativity and observational acumen of anatomists, physiologists, psychologists, and physicians have been impressive and rewarding, but their work is far from finished.

The term *central nervous system* refers to the brain and the spinal cord. The term *peripheral nervous system* refers to cranial nerves, the spinal nerves, the ganglia associated with the cranial and spinal nerves, and the peripheral receptor organs. The term *autonomic nervous system* refers to the part of the nervous system involved mainly in the regulation of visceral function; its component parts are located partly within the CNS and partly within the peripheral nervous system.

This chapter is concerned mainly with the gross features of the CNS. Its purposes are to acquaint the student with the terminologic jargon used in the neurologic sciences and provide an orientation to the major components of this system.

KEY CONCEPTS

- The nervous system can be divided into three parts: central, peripheral, and autonomic.
- The central nervous system includes the brain and the spinal cord.
- The peripheral nervous system includes the cranial and peripheral nerves, the ganglia associated with the cranial and spinal nerves, and the peripheral receptor organs.
- The autonomic nervous system includes the parts of the central and peripheral nervous systems that are involved in the regulation of visceral function.

CENTRAL NERVOUS SYSTEM

The CNS usually is considered to have two major divisions: the brain and the spinal cord. The brain is subdivided into the following structures:

1. The two cerebral hemispheres
2. The brain stem, consisting of the diencephalon, mesencephalon (midbrain), pons, and medulla oblongata
3. The cerebellum

The cerebral hemispheres and diencephalon are discussed in this chapter. The gross topography of the rest of the brain stem, the cerebellum, and the spinal cord are presented in other chapters in this book.

BRAIN

The brain is semisolid in consistency and conforms to the shape of its container. It weighs approximately 1400 g in an adult. The male brain is on average slightly heavier than the female brain, although this has no relationship to intelligence. The largest human brain on record weighed 2850 g and came from a mentally defective individual with epilepsy.

The brain is protected from the external environment by three barriers:

1. Skull
2. Meninges
3. Cerebrospinal fluid

The bony skull is the major barrier against physical trauma to the brain.

The meninges are organized into three layers named in order of their proximity to the skull:

1. Dura mater
2. Arachnoid mater
3. Pia mater

The **dura mater** (Latin, "hard mother") is a tough, fibrous connective tissue (Fig. 2-1) arranged in two layers. An outer parietal (periosteal) layer adheres to the skull and forms its periosteum, and an inner meningeal layer is in contact with the arachnoid mater. These two layers of dura are adherent to each other except at the sites of formation of dural venous sinuses such as the superior sagittal (Fig. 2-2).

The meningeal dura mater has three major reflections which separate components of the brain. The falx cerebri (Fig. 2-2) is a vertical reflection between the two

Dura mater (Latin *durus*, "hard"; *mater*, "mother"). The outermost hard meningeal covering of the brain. The term is derived from the Arabic *umm al-dimagh* ("mother of the brain"). Believing that the meninges were the mother of all membranes, the Arabs called the outermost meningeal layer the thick mother and the innermost the thin mother. In 1127 Stephen of Antioch translated these terms into Latin as *dura mater* and *pia mater.* Stephen, a monk, chose *pia* (*pious*) rather than *tenu* to translate the term *thin mother.* The arachnoid membrane (middle meningeal layer) was not known to the Arabs.

KEY CONCEPTS

- The brain is composed of the two cerebral hemispheres, the brain stem, and the cerebellum.
- The brain stem includes the mesencephalon (midbrain), pons, and medulla oblongata.
- The brain of an adult weighs approximately 1400 g.
- The brain is protected from the physical and chemical external environments by the skull, the meninges, and the cerebrospinal fluid.
- There are three layers of meninges: dura mater, arachnoid mater, and pia mater.

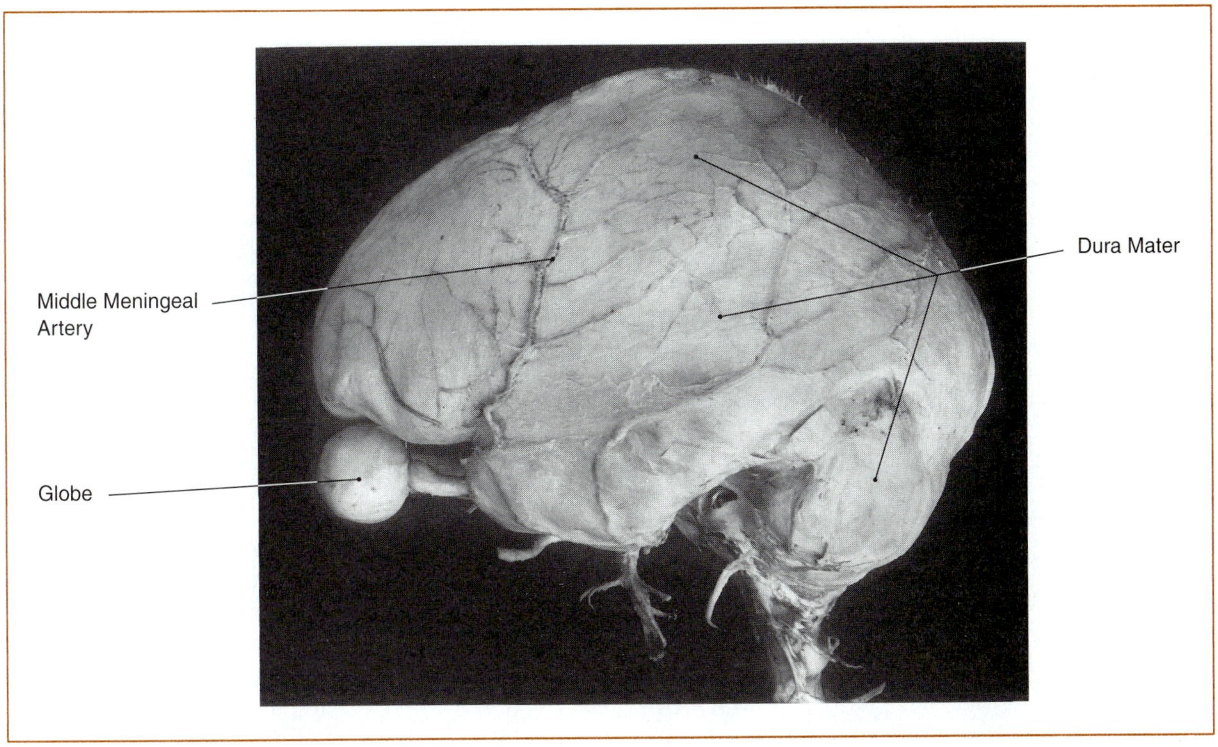

FIGURE 2-1

Lateral view of the brain showing the dura mater meningeal layer and the middle meningeal artery. (*From N. Gluhbegovic and T. H. Williams: The Human Brain: A Photographic Guide. Harper & Row, 1980, courtesy of the authors.*)

cerebral hemispheres. The **tentorium cerebelli** (Fig. 2-2) is a horizontal reflection between the posterior (occipital) parts of the cerebral hemispheres and the cerebellum. The **falx cerebelli** is a vertical reflection which incompletely separates the two cerebellar hemispheres at the inferior surface. The meningeal layer of the dura mater of the brain is continuous with the dura mater that covers the spinal cord.

The **arachnoid mater** (Greek *arachine*, "spider") (Fig. 2-3) is a nonvascular membrane of an external mesothelium that is joined with weblike trabeculae to the underlying pia mater.

The **pia mater** is a thin translucent membrane that is intimately adherent to brain substance. Blood vessels of the brain are located on the pia mater (Fig. 2-3). The arachnoid mater and the pia mater are collectively referred to as the pia-arachnoid membrane because of their close structural and functional relationships.

The meninges are subject to the infection known as meningitis. This is a serious, life-threatening condition that requires immediate medical treatment. The three layers of meninges are separated from each other and from the bony skull by the following spaces.

1. The epidural space is located between the dura mater and the bony skull. Trauma to the skull with rupture of the middle meningeal artery (Fig. 2-1)

KEY CONCEPTS

- Three reflections of the dura mater help separate the parts of the brain: the falx cerebri between the two cerebral hemispheres, the tentorium cerebelli between the occipital lobe and the cerebellum, and the falx cerebelli between the two halves of the cerebellum.
- Cerebral vessels are situated on the pia mater.

Tentorium cerebelli (Latin *tentorium*, "tent" from *tendere*, "to stretch, something stretched out"). A fold of dura mater stretched over the cerebellum like a tent. The term was adopted about the end of the eighteenth century.

Falx cerebelli, cerebri (Latin *falx*, "sickle"). A sickle-shaped structure. The falx cerebelli and cerebri, dural folds separating the two cerebellar and cerebral hemispheres, respectively, are sickle-shaped.

Arachnoid mater (Greek *arachnoeides*, "like a cobweb"). The middle meningeal layer of the brain and spinal cord is so named because of weblike trabeculae that extend from the arachnoid to the underlying pia mater. The arachnoid mater was described by Bichat in 1800.

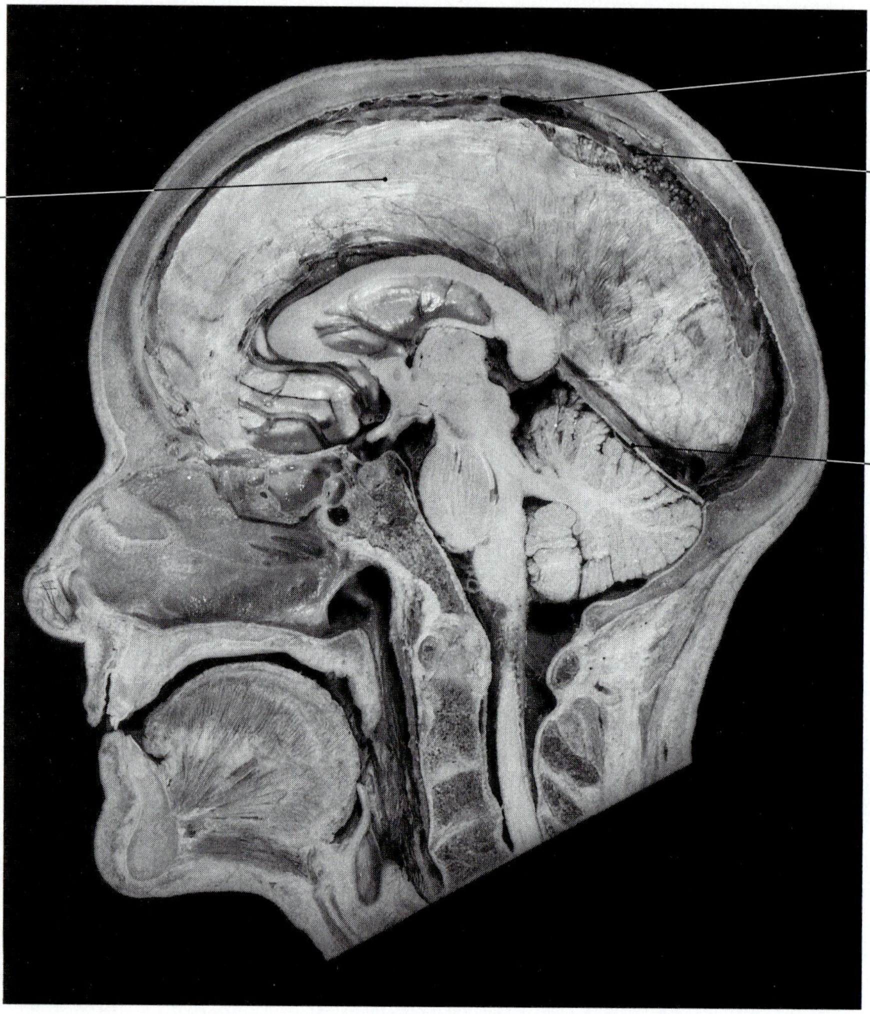

FIGURE 2-2

Midsagittal section of the cranium showing the falx cerebri and tentorium cerebelli. (*From N. Gluhbegovic and T. H. Williams: The Human Brain: A Photographic Guide. Harper & Row, 1980, courtesy of the authors.*)

Pia mater (Latin *pia*, "tender, soft"; *mater*, "mother"). The innermost meningeal layer covering the brain and spinal cord. For further discussion of term, see **dura mater** (p. 38).

leads to epidural hemorrhage, or the accumulation of arterial blood in the epidural space. Because of the pressure produced by a hemorrhage in a closed container such as the skull, an epidural hemorrhage is handled as an acute, life-threatening emergency calling for surgical intervention to evacuate the accumulated arterial blood in the epidural space and control the bleeding.

2. The subdural space lies between the dura mater and the arachnoid mater. Trauma to the skull may rupture the bridging veins, leading to subdural hemor-

KEY CONCEPTS

- The epidural space, a potential space between the skull and the dura mater, is the site of epidural arterial hemorrhage, a life-threatening condition that usually is due to a traumatic rupture of the middle meningeal artery.
- The subdural space, between the dura mater and the arachnoid mater, is the site of subdural venous hemorrhage.

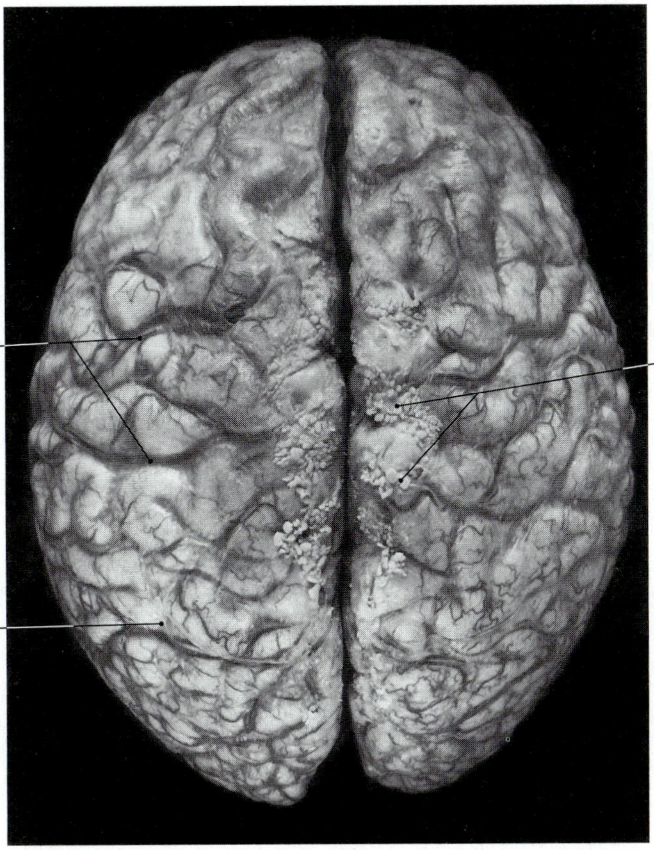
Cerebral Vessels in
Subarachnoid Space
Arachnoid Mater
Arachnoid Mater

FIGURE 2-3

Dorsal view of the brain showing the arachnoid meningeal layer and arachnoid granulations. (*From N. Gluhbegovic and T. H. Williams: The Human Brain: A Photographic Guide. Harper & Row, 1980, courtesy of the authors.*)

rhage, or the accumulation of blood in the subdural space. This condition also calls for surgical intervention to evacuate the accumulated venous blood and control the bleeding.

3. The subarachnoid space is located between the arachnoid mater and the pia mater. This space contains cerebrospinal fluid (CSF) and cerebral blood vessels (Fig. 2-3). Rupture of such vessels leads to subarachnoid hemorrhage, or the accumulation of blood in the subarachnoid space. This condition may result from trauma to the head, congenital abnormalities in vessel structure (aneurysms), or high blood pressure. The subarachnoid space underlying the superior sagittal sinus contains arachnoid granulations (Figs. 2-2 and 2-3), sites of CSF absorption into the superior sagittal sinus.

The third barrier that protects the brain, the CSF, is the subject of Chap. 29.

KEY CONCEPTS

- The subarachnoid space, between the arachnoid mater and the pia mater, contains cerebrospinal fluid. It is also the site of subarachnoid hemorrhage resulting from rupture of cerebral blood vessels on the pia mater.

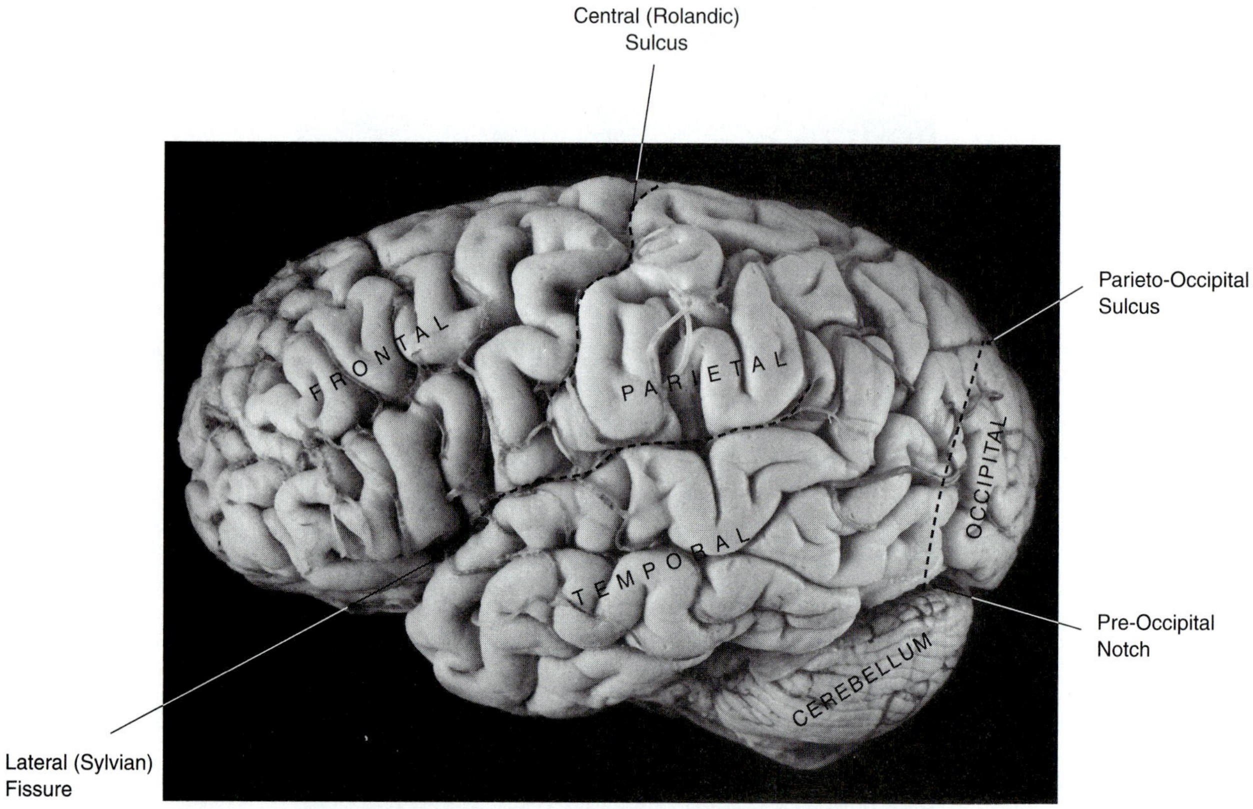

FIGURE 2-4

Lateral view of the brain showing the four lobes (frontal, parietal, temporal, occipital) and the cerebellum. (*From N. Gluhbegovic and T. H. Williams: The Human Brain: A Photographic Guide. Harper & Row, 1980, courtesy of the authors.*)

EXTERNAL TOPOGRAPHY OF THE BRAIN

Sylvian fissure (lateral fissure). A prominent fissure on the lateral surface of the cerebral hemisphere between the frontal and parietal lobes above and the temporal lobe below. Described by Francis de la Boe Sylvius, a French anatomist, in 1641.

Rolandic sulcus (central sulcus). The sulcus that separates the precentral and postcentral gyri of the cerebral hemisphere. Described by Luigi Rolando, an Italian anatomist, in 1825. Named for Rolando by François Leuret in 1839.

For convenience, the topography of the brain will be discussed as it is viewed on the lateral surface, the medial surface, and the ventral surface of the brain.

Lateral Surface

The lateral surface of the brain is marked by two principal landmarks that divide the cerebral hemispheres into lobes (Fig. 2-4). The lateral fissure (**sylvian fissure**) and the central sulcus (**rolandic sulcus**) divide the cerebral hemisphere into the frontal lobe (dorsal to the lateral fissure and rostral to the central sulcus), temporal

KEY CONCEPTS

- On the lateral surface of the cerebral hemisphere three landmarks—the central (rolandic) sulcus, the lateral (sylvian) fissure, and a line connecting the tip of the parieto-occipital sulcus and the preoccipital notch—delineate four lobes: frontal, parietal, temporal, and occipital.

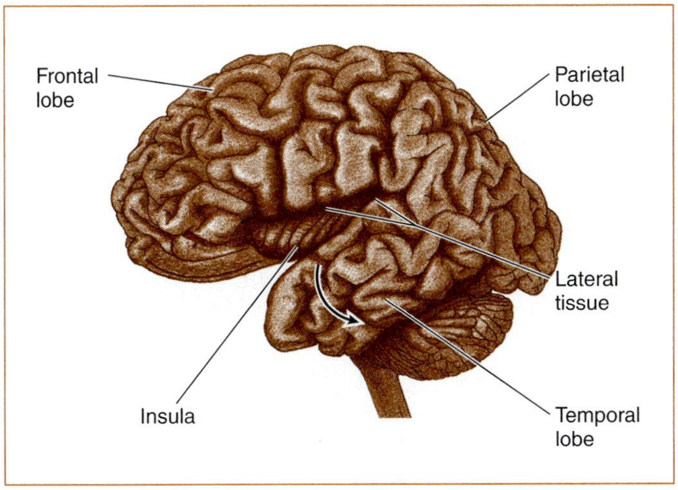

FIGURE 2-5

Schematic diagram of the brain showing the insula in the depth of the lateral fissure.

lobe (ventral to the lateral fissure), and parietal lobe (dorsal to the lateral fissure and caudal to the central sulcus). If a line were drawn from the parieto-occipital sulcus (best seen on the medial aspect of the hemisphere) onto the lateral aspect of the hemisphere down to the preoccipital notch, it would delineate the boundaries of the parietal and temporal lobes rostrally from that of the occipital lobe caudally. The frontal, temporal, parietal, and occipital lobes are named after the skull bones that overlie them. Lying deep within the lateral fissure and seen only when the banks of the fissure are separated is the insula, or **island of Reil** (Fig. 2-5), which is involved primarily with autonomic function.

Island of Reil. The insula of the cerebral cortex. It was noted by Johann Christian Reil, a Danish physiologist, anatomist, and psychiatrist, in 1796 and described by him in 1809.

Frontal Lobe

Rostral to the central sulcus, between it and the precentral sulcus, is the precentral gyrus (primary motor area), which is one of the most important cortical areas involved with movement (Figs. 2-4 and 2-6). Although movement can be elicited by stimulation of a number of cortical areas, movement developed by stimulation of the precentral gyrus is achieved at a relatively low threshold of stimulation. Body parts are disproportionately and somatotopically represented in the primary motor area. The representation of the face is lower than the upper extremity representation, followed in ascending order by the trunk and the lower extremity. The leg and foot are represented on the medial surface of the precentral gyrus. In the face area of the precentral gyrus, the lip representation is disproportionately large compared with its actual size on the face; the same applies to the thumb representation in the hand area. This disproportionate representation of body parts in the primary motor cortex is known as the motor **homunculus**.

Homunculus (Latin, "a little man"). A cortical representation of body parts in the motor and sensory cortices.

Stimulation of specific areas of the precentral gyrus results in the movement of a single muscle or a group of muscles in the contralateral part of the body. Lesions of the precentral gyrus result in contralateral paralysis (loss of movement). This is most marked in muscles used for fine motor performance, such as buttoning a shirt or writing.

Rostral to the precentral sulcus is the premotor area, another important area for movement. Blood flow studies have shown that this area plays a role in initiating new programs for movement and introducing changes in programs that are in progress.

Rostral to the premotor area, the frontal lobe is divided by two sulci—the superior and inferior frontal sulci—into three gyri: the superior, middle, and inferior

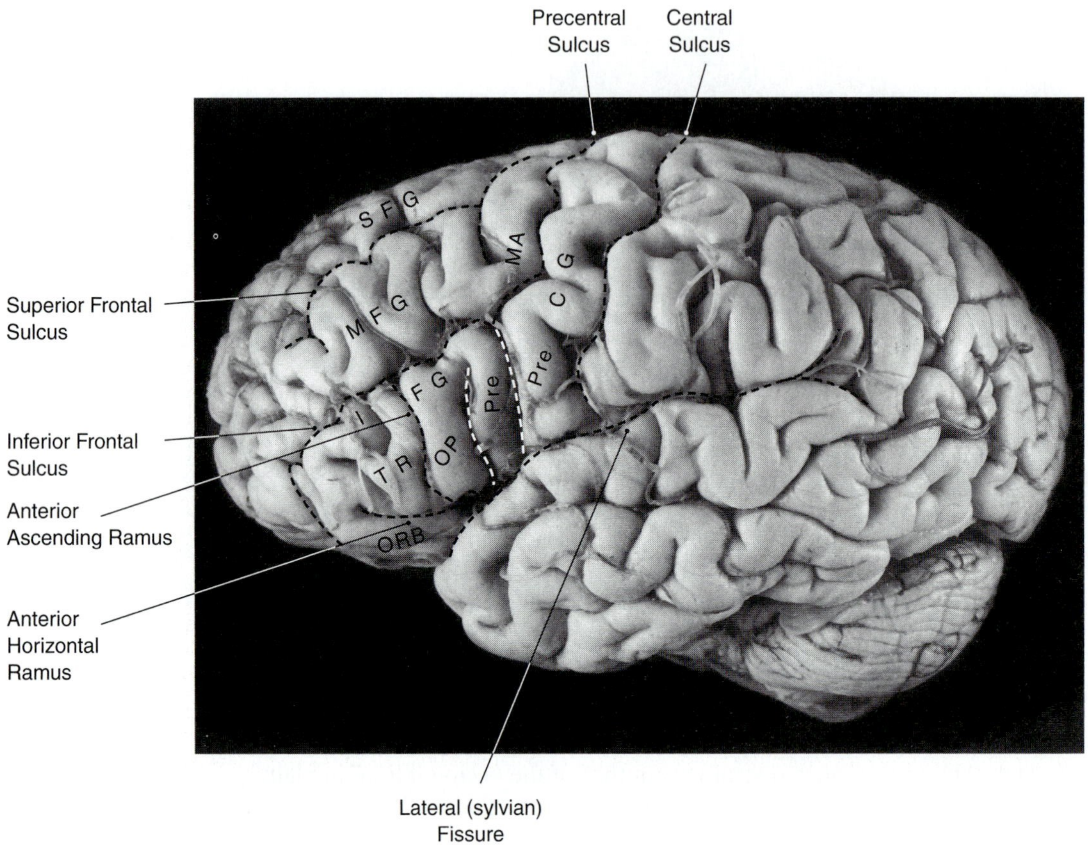

FIGURE 2-6

Lateral view of the brain showing the major sulci and gyri in the frontal lobe. SFG, superior frontal gyrus; MFG, middle frontal gyrus; IFG, inferior frontal gyrus; ORB, orbital gyrus; TR, triangular gyrus; OP, opercular gyrus, Pre CG, precentral gyrus; Pre MA, premotor area. (*From N. Gluhbegovic and T. H. Williams: The Human Brain: A Photographic Guide. Harper & Row, 1980, courtesy of the authors.*)

Brodmann's areas. Fifty-two cortical areas defined on the basis of cytoarchitecture (cellular organization) by Krobinian Brodmann, a German physician, between 1903 and 1908.

Opercular gyrus (Latin *operculum*, "lid" or "cover"). The opercular gyrus of the inferior frontal lobe forms a lid or cover over the lateral (sylvian) fissure.

Broca's area. The motor speech area in the inferior frontal gyrus of the left hemisphere. Named after Pierre-Paul Broca, a French anthropologist, anat-

frontal gyri. The middle frontal gyrus contains **Brodmann's area** 8, which is important for conjugate eye movements. This area is known as the area of frontal eye fields. The inferior frontal gyrus is subdivided by two sulci extending from the lateral (sylvian) fissure: the anterior horizontal and anterior ascending rami. Rostral to the anterior horizontal ramus is the orbital gyrus; between the two rami is the triangular gyrus, and caudal to the anterior ascending ramus is the **opercular gyrus.** The triangular gyrus and the immediately adjacent part of the opercular gyrus constitute **Broca's area,** which in the dominant (left) hemisphere represents the

KEY CONCEPTS

- In the frontal lobe the precentral sulcus separates the precentral gyrus and the premotor area. Two horizontal sulci—superior and inferior frontal—divide the rest of the frontal lobe into superior, middle, and inferior frontal gyri.
- The inferior frontal gyrus is further subdivided by two sulci—anterior horizontal and anterior ascending—into three gyri: orbital, triangular, and opercular. The triangular gyrus and the adjacent part of the opercular gyrus in the left hemisphere constitute Broca's area of speech.

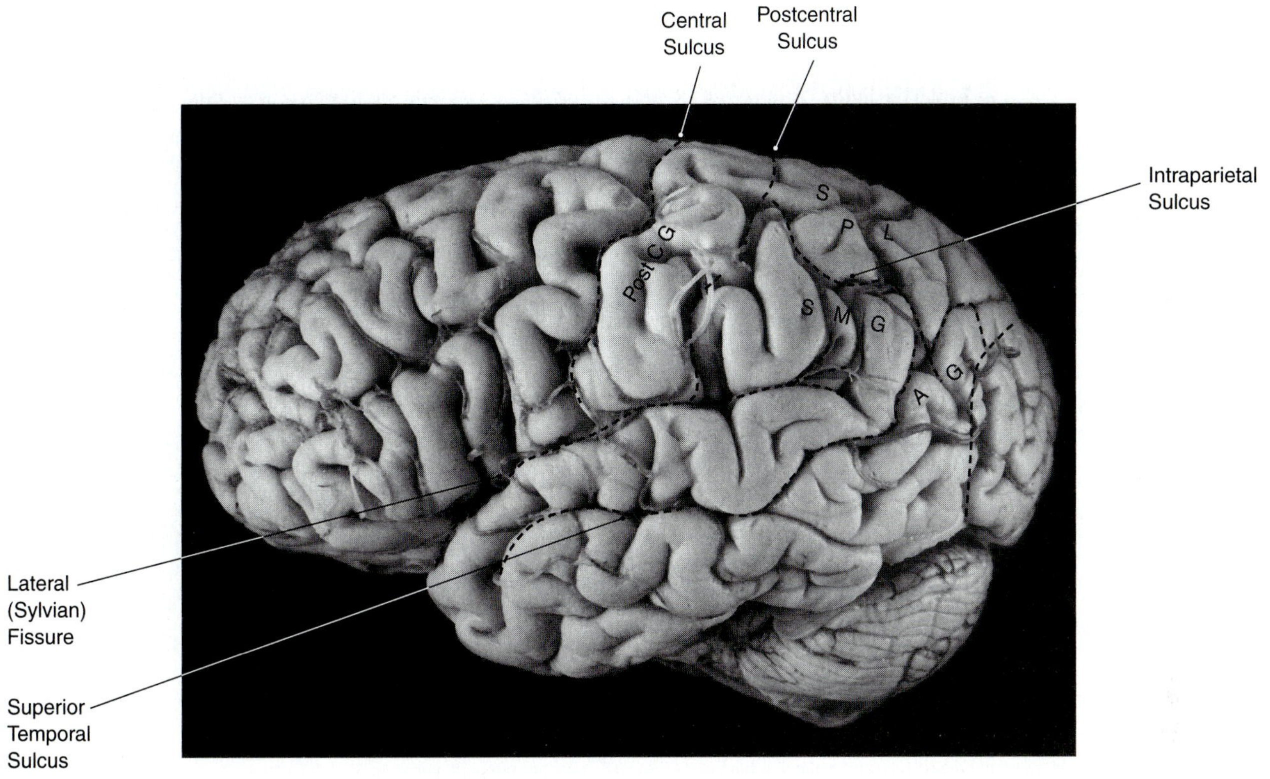

FIGURE 2-7

Lateral view of the brain showing the major sulci and gyri in the parietal lobe. Post CG, postcentral gyrus; SPL, superior parietal lobule; SMG, supramarginal gyrus; AG, angular gyrus. (*From N. Gluhbegovic and T. H. Williams: The Human Brain: A Photographic Guide. Harper & Row, 1980, courtesy of the authors.*)

motor area for speech. Lesions in this area result in an inability to express oneself in spoken language (**aphasia**).

Parietal Lobe

Caudal to the central sulcus, between it and the postcentral sulcus, is the postcentral gyrus, a primary sensory (somesthetic) area involved in general body sensation (Figs. 2-4 and 2-7). Body representation in the primary sensory area is similar to that described above for the primary motor area. The disproportionate and somatotropic representation of body parts in this area is known as the sensory homunculus. Stimulation of this area in humans and other primates elicits sensations of tingling and numbness in the part of the body that corresponds to (and is contralateral to) the area stimulated. A lesion in this area results in the loss of sensation contralateral to the site of the lesion.

Caudal to the postcentral gyrus, the intraparietal sulcus extends horizontally across the parietal lobe, dividing it into superior and inferior parietal lobules. The superior parietal lobule is involved with the behavioral interaction of an individual with the surrounding space. A lesion in this lobule, especially in the right (nondominant) hemisphere, results in neglect of body parts contralateral to the lesion. Such individuals may neglect to shave the face or dress body parts contralateral to the lesion. The inferior parietal lobule contains two important gyri: the supramarginal and angular gyri. The supramarginal gyrus caps the end of the sylvian fissue, whereas

omist, and surgeon who associated lesions of this area with disturbance of speech function (aphasia) in 1861.

Aphasia (Greek *a*, "negative"; *phasis*, "speech"). A defect in language communication, loss of speech. The modern knowledge of the condition dates back to its description by Bouillard in 1825. In 1861 Broca associated this condition with lesions in the inferior frontal gyrus on the left side of the brain and called the condition aphemia. The term *aphasia* was introduced by Armand Trousseau in 1864.

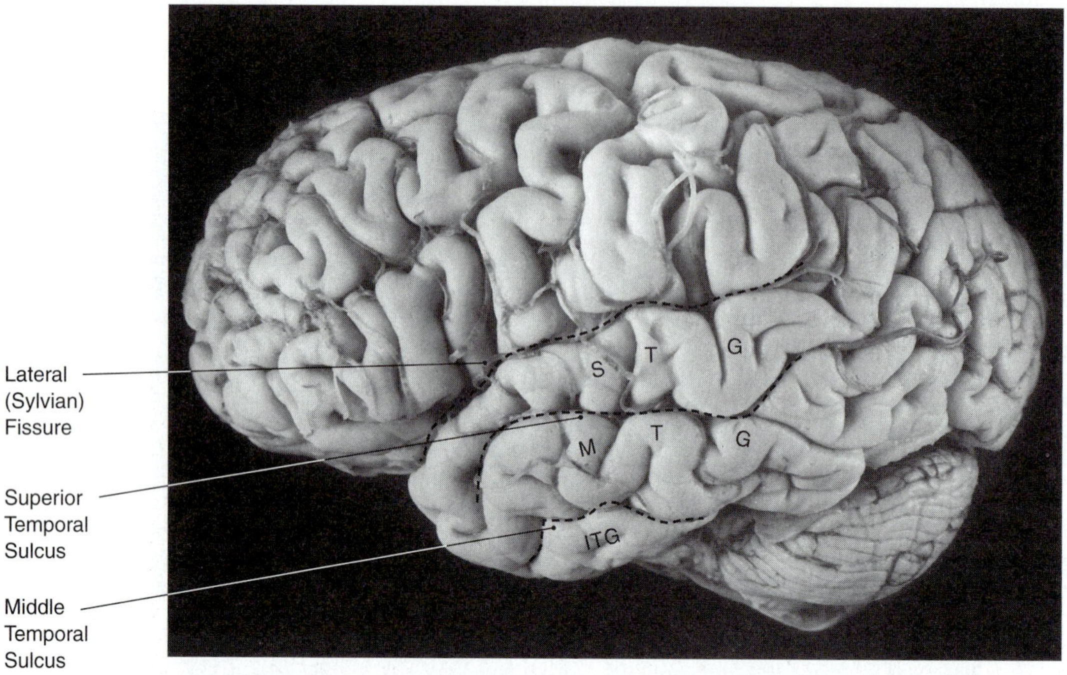

FIGURE 2-8

Lateral view of the brain showing the major sulci and gyri in the temporal lobe. STG, superior temporal gyrus; MTG, middle temporal gyrus; ITG, inferior temporal gyrus. (*From N. Gluhbegovic and T. H. Williams: The Human Brain: A Photographic Guide. Harper & Row, 1980, courtesy of the authors.*)

the angular gyrus caps the end of the superior temporal sulcus. The two gyri are involved in the integration of diverse sensory information for speech and perception. Lesions in these two gyri in the dominant hemisphere result in disturbances in language comprehension and object recognition.

Temporal Lobe

Three gyri constitute the lateral surface of the temporal lobe. The superior, middle, and inferior temporal gyri are separated by the superior and middle sulci (Figs. 2-4 and 2-8). The inferior temporal gyrus extends over the inferior border of the temporal lobe onto the ventral surface of the brain. The superior temporal gyrus contains on its dorsal border (the bank of the lateral fissure) the transverse temporal **gyri of Heschl** (primary auditory area). Caudal to the transverse gyri of Heschl in the superior temporal gyrus is **Wernicke's area,** which is involved in the comprehen-

Heschl's gyri. The transverse temporal gyri, site of the primary auditory cortex. Described by Richard Heschl, an Austrian anatomist, in 1855.

Wernicke's area. The posterior part of the superior temporal gyrus, which is involved with comprehension of spoken language. Lesions in this area are associated with receptive aphasia. Named after Karl Wernicke, a German neuropsychiatrist, who described the area in 1874.

KEY CONCEPTS

- In the parietal lobe the postcentral sulcus delineates the posterior boundary of the postcentral gyrus. A horizontal sulcus, the intraparietal sulcus, divides the rest of the parietal lobe into dorsal and ventral parietal lobules. The ventral parietal lobule contains the supramarginal and angular gyri.
- The temporal lobe is divided by two sulci—the superior and middle temporal sulci—into three gyri: superior, middle, and inferior. The superior temporal gyrus contains Heschl's gyrus and, in the left hemisphere, Wernicke's area of speech.

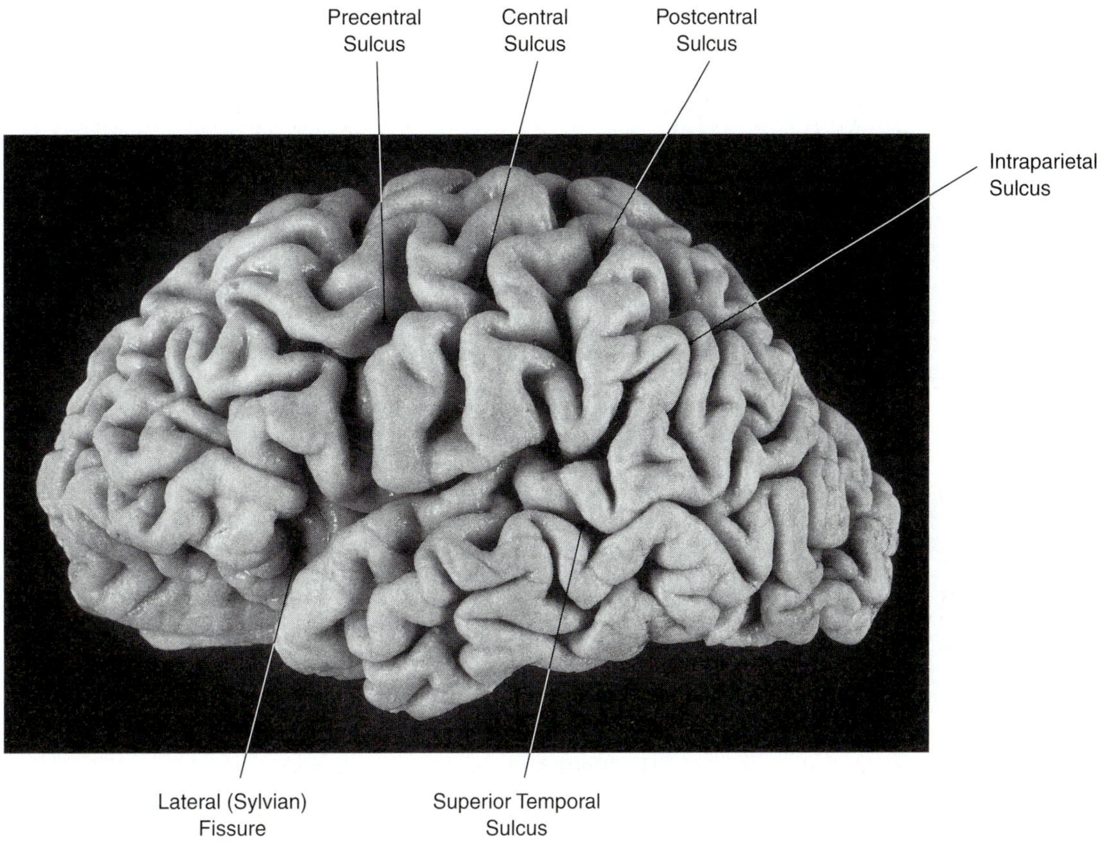
Precentral Sulcus
Central Sulcus
Postcentral Sulcus
Intraparietal Sulcus
Lateral (Sylvian) Fissure
Superior Temporal Sulcus

FIGURE 2-9

Lateral view of the brain in Alzheimer's disease showing prominent sulci and atrophy of gyri. (*Courtesy of G. Van Hoesen.*)

sion of spoken language. The inferior temporal gyrus is involved with the perception of visual form and color.

Occipital Lobe

On the lateral aspect of the brain the occipital lobe (Fig. 2-4) merges with the parietal and temporal lobes, separated from them by an imaginary line drawn between the tip of the parieto-occipital fissure and the preoccipital notch. The occipital pole contains a portion of the primary visual area, which is more extensive on the medial aspect of the occipital lobe. Fissures and sulci of the cerebral hemisphere become much more prominent in degenerative brain disorders such as **Alzheimer's disease** because of atrophy of the gyri (Fig. 2-9).

Medial Surface

The corpus callosum, in a midsagittal section of the brain, stands out prominently as a C-shaped massive bundle of fibers (Fig. 2-10). The corpus callosum generally is subdivided into a head (rostrum) at the rostral extremity, a large body extending across the frontal and parietal lobes, a genu (knee) connecting the rostrum and the body, and a **splenium** at the caudal extremity. It consists of fibers that connect the two cerebral hemispheres. Behavioral studies have shown that the corpus callosum plays an important role in the transfer of information between the two hemispheres. Lesions in the corpus callosum, which disconnect the right hemisphere from the

Alzheimer's disease. A degenerative brain disease (formerly known as senile dementia) characterized by memory loss, cortical atrophy, senile plaques, and neurofibrillary tangles. Described by Alois Alzheimer, a German neuropsychiatrist, in 1907.

Splenium (Greek *splenion*, "bandlike structure," a bandage or compress). The posterior rounded end of the corpus callosum is so named because it is the thick and swollen end of the corpus callosum, resembling a compress. Also named because of its resemblance to the rolled-up leaf of a young fern; *splenium* was used by the Romans as the name of a kind of fern.

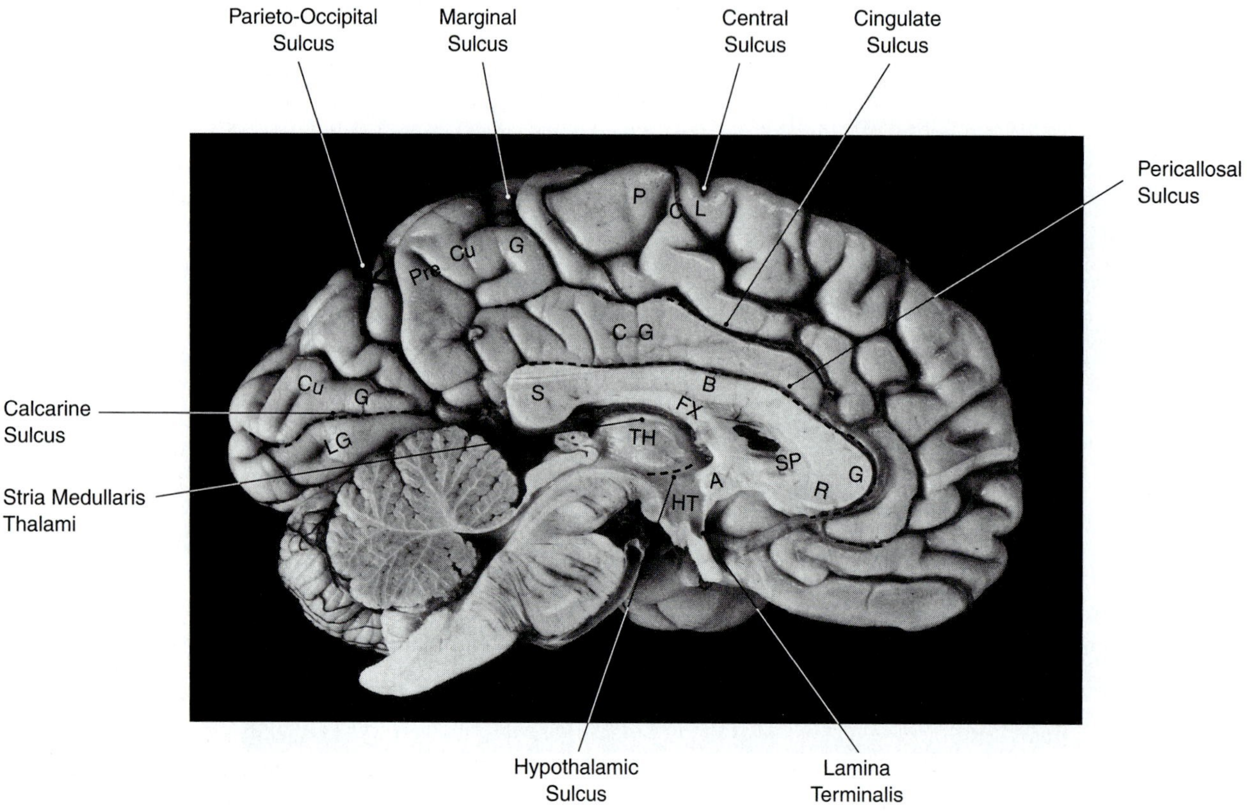

FIGURE 2-10

Midsagittal view of the brain showing major sulci and gyri. PCL, paracentral lobule; Pre Cu G, precuneus gyrus; Cu G, cuneus gyrus; LG, lingual gyrus; CG, cingulate gyrus; S, splenium of corpus callosum; B, body of corpus callosum; G, genu of corpus callosum; R, rostrum of corpus callosum; FX, fornix; TH, Thalamus; HT, hypothalamus; A, anterior commissure; SP, septum pellucidum. (*From N. Gluhbegovic and T. H. Williams: The Human Brain: A Photographic Guide. Harper & Row, 1980, courtesy of the authors.*)

left hemisphere, result in the isolation of both hemispheres so that each will have its own learning processes and memories which are inaccessible to the other.

Dorsal to the corpus callosum, separated from it by the pericallosal sulcus, is the cingulate gyrus, which follows the contours of the corpus callosum and occupies parts of the frontal and parietal lobes. The cingulate gyrus is part of the limbic system, which affects visceral function, emotion, and behavior. The cingulate gyrus is separated from the rest of the frontal and parietal lobes by the cingulate sulcus. Dorsal to the cingulate gyrus, extensions of the pre- and postcentral gyri onto the medial aspect of the brain form the paracentral lobule. The precuneus is the part

KEY CONCEPTS

- The medial surface of the hemisphere shows the corpus callosum, septum pellucidum, fornix, and diencephalon, along with the medial surfaces of the frontal, parietal, occipital, and temporal lobes.
- The paracentral lobule, on the medial surface of the hemisphere, represents medial extensions of the pre- and postcentral gyri.

of the parietal lobe that is caudal to the paracentral lobule, between the marginal and parieto-occipital sulci. The parieto-occipital sulcus is well delineated on this surface of the brain and defines the boundaries between the parietal and occipital lobes. Extending at approximately right angles from the parieto-occipital sulcus in the occipital lobe is the calcarine sulcus, which divides the occipital lobe into a dorsal **cuneus** gyrus and a ventral **lingual gyrus.** The primary visual area is situated on each bank of the calcarine sulcus. Lesions of the primary visual area produce a loss of vision in the contralateral half of the visual field, a condition known as **hemianopia.**

Ventral to the corpus callosum is the **septum pellucidum,** a thin partition which separates the two lateral ventricles. At the inferior border of the septum pellucidum is another C-shaped fiber bundle, the **fornix,** which connects the temporal lobe (hippocampal formation) and the diencephalon. Only a small part of the fornix is seen in midsagittal sections of the brain.

Rostral to the anterior extent of the fornix is a small bundle of fibers, the anterior commissure, which connects the two temporal lobes and olfactory or smell structures in both hemispheres. Recent evidence points to a wider distribution of anterior commissure fibers than was previously believed. The anterior commissure in humans has been shown to be composed of an anterior limb involved with olfaction and a posterior limb containing neocortical fibers that connect visual and auditory areas in the temporal lobes. There is strong support for the theory that the anterior commissure plays a role in the interhemispheric transfer of visual information.

Extending from the ventral border of the anterior commissure to the ventral border of the diencephalon is a thin membrane, the lamina terminalis. This lamina marks the most anterior boundary of the embryologic neural tube.

Behind the rostral extremity of the fornix and extending in an oblique manner caudally is the hypothalamic sulcus. This sulcus divides the diencephalon into a dorsal **thalamus** and a ventral hypothalamus. The midline area between the two thalami and hypothalami is occupied by the slitlike third ventricle. In some brains the two thalami are connected across the midline by the interthalamic adhesion (intermediate mass). The thalamus is the gateway to the cerebral cortex. All sensory inputs except olfaction pass through the thalamus before reaching the cortex. Similarly, motor inputs to the cerebral cortex pass through the thalamus. The hypothalamus is a major central autonomic and endocrine center. It plays a role in activities such as feeding, drinking, sexual behavior, emotional behavior, and growth.

The dorsal border of the thalamus is the stria medullaris thalami, a thin band which extends caudally to merge with the **habenular nuclei.** Above the dorsal and caudal part of the diencephalon lies the pineal gland, which is assumed to have an endocrine function. The stria medullaris thalami, habenular nuclei, and pineal gland constitute the epithalamus.

The continuation of the cingulate gyrus in the temporal lobe (Fig. 2-11) is the parahippocampal gyrus, a component of the **limbic lobe.** The parahippocampal gyrus is continuous with the **uncus** (another component of the limbic lobe) in the tip of the temporal lobe. The collateral sulcus separates the parahippocampal gyrus from the **fusiform** (occipitotemporal) **gyrus.**

KEY CONCEPTS

- On the medial surface of the hemisphere the parieto-occipital sulcus separates the occipital lobe from the parietal and temporal lobes.
- In the occipital lobe the calcarine sulcus separates the lingual and cuneus gyri.
- In the inferomedial surface of the temporal lobe the collateral sulcus separates the parahippocampal gyrus from the occipitotemporal (fusiform) gyrus.

Cuneus (Latin, "wedge"). The cuneus gyrus is a wedge-shaped lobule on the medial surface of the occipital lobe between the parieto-occipital and calcarine sulci.

Lingual gyrus. A gyrus in the occipital lobe on the medial surface of the hemisphere forming the inferior lip of the calcarine sulcus.

Hemianopia (Greek *hemi*, "half"; *an*, "negative"; *ops*, "eye"). Blindness in one-half of the field of vision. The term was introduced by Monoyer. Hirschberg substituted the term *hemianopsia.*

Septum pellucidum (Latin *septum*, "dividing wall, partition"; *pellucidus*, "translucent"). A thin membrane between the corpus callosum and the fornix, separating the anterior horns of the lateral ventricle. Described by Galen.

Fornix (Latin, "arch"). An archlike pathway, below the corpus callosum, connecting mainly the hippocampal formation and the mamillary body. The fornix was noted by Galen and described by Vesalius. It was named by Thomas Willis the *fornix cerebri.*

Thalamus (Greek *thalamos*, "inner chamber," the room occupied in a house by a married couple). A mass of gray matter on each side of the third ventricle. The name was coined by Galen and reaffirmed by Willis in 1664.

Habenular nuclei (Latin *habena*, "a bridle rein or strap"). The habenular nuclei in the caudal diencephalon near the pineal gland constitute part of the epithalamus. The name resulted from the fact that early anatomists considered

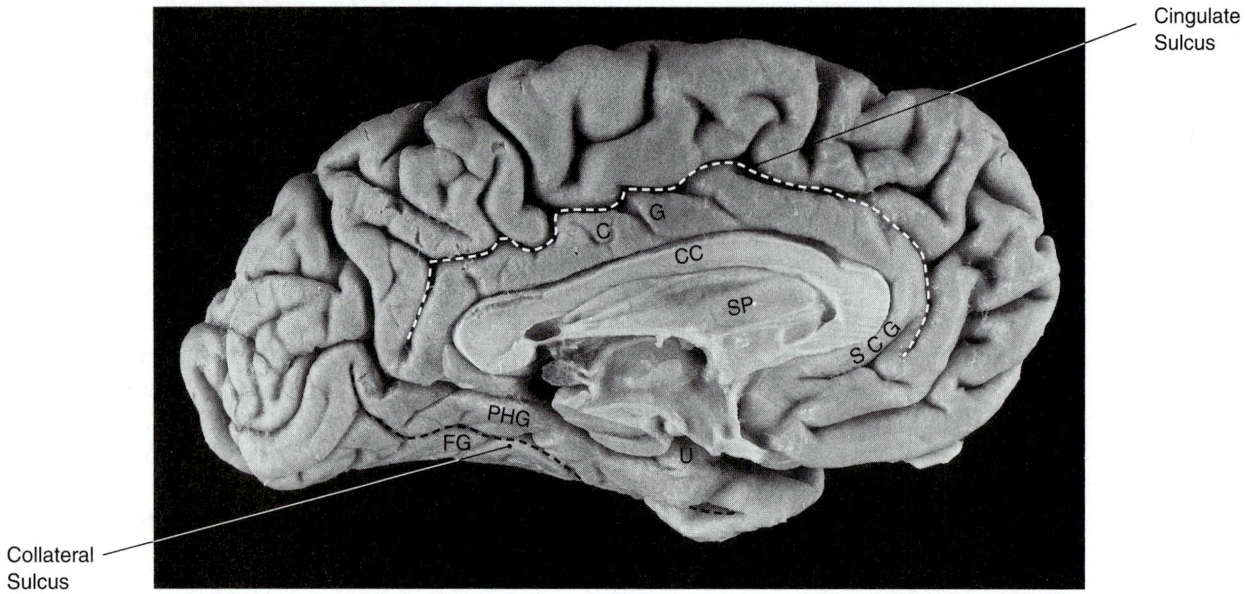

FIGURE 2-11

Midsagittal view of the brain showing components of the limbic lobe. CG, cingulate gyrus; CC, corpus callosum; SP, septum pellucidum; SCG, subcallosal gyrus; PHG, parahippocampal gyrus; U, uncus; FG, fusiform gyrus. (*From N. Gluhbegovic and T. H. Williams: The Human Brain: A Photographic Guide. Harper & Row, 1980, courtesy of the authors.*)

the pineal gland the abode of the soul, likening it to a driver who directed the operations of the mind via the habenula or reins.

Limbic lobe (Latin *limbus*, "border"). The limbic lobe is composed of structures on the medial surface of the cerebral hemisphere bordering the corpus callosum and rostral brain stem.

Uncus (Latin "hook, hook-shaped structure"). The medially curved rostral end of the parahippocampal gyrus resembles a hook, hence the name.

Fusiform gyrus (Latin *fusus*, "spindle"; *forma*, "form"; Greek *gyros*, "circle"). The fusiform gyrus of the temporal lobe has a spindlelike shape, tapering from the middle toward each end. Also called the occipitotemporal gyrus.

Putamen (Latin, "shell", a cutting or paring, that which falls off in pruning or trimming). The outer part of the lentiform nucleus of the basal ganglia.

Extending from the diencephalon caudally are the mesencephalon (midbrain), pons, and medulla oblongata (Fig. 2-12). The cerebellum occupies a position between the occipital lobe, pons, and medulla oblongata (Fig. 2-12).

The medial surface of the brain shows the components of the limbic lobe (Fig. 2-11), including the subcallosal gyrus, cingulate gyrus, parahippocampal gyrus, and uncus. The limbic lobe forms the core of the limbic system, which is discussed in Chap. 21.

Parasagittal sections of the brain show deeper structures that are not seen in midsagittal sections, such as the basal ganglia (caudate nucleus, **putamen, globus pallidus**) and the internal capsule. Lateral extension of the thalamus is also seen in such sections. The caudate nucleus, putamen, and globus pallidus are known collectively as the corpus striatum. They are basal ganglia of the brain and play a role in the regulation of movement. The caudate nucleus and putamen are collectively known as the striatum and are separated by the anterior limb of the internal capsule. The putamen and globus pallidus are collectively known as the lenticular nucleus. Both nuclei are separated from the thalamus by the posterior limb of the internal capsule. The internal capsule carries motor and sensory fibers from the

KEY CONCEPTS

- Components of the limbic lobe, the subcallosal gyrus, the cingulate gyrus, the parahippocampal gyrus, and the uncus are seen to advantage on the medial surface of the cerebral hemisphere.

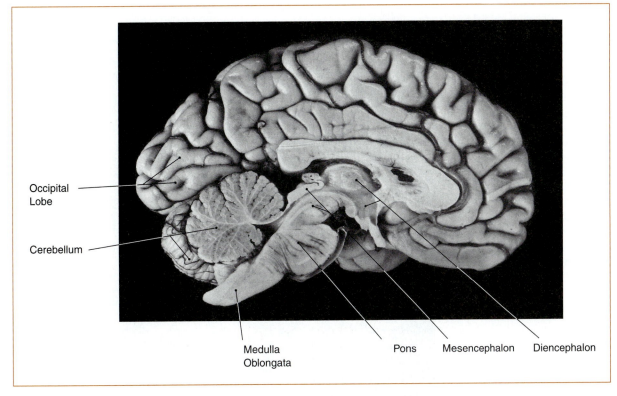

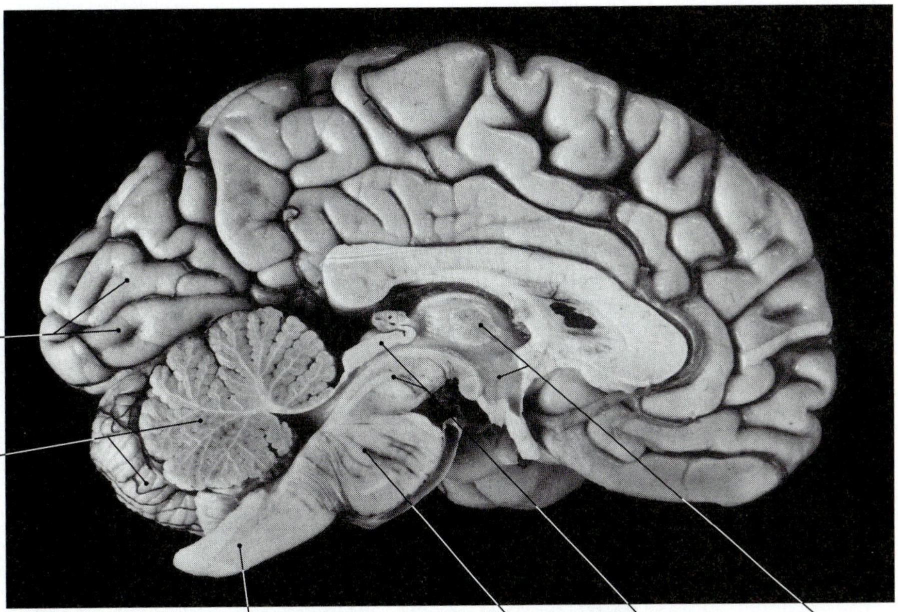
Occipital Lobe
Cerebellum
Medulla Oblongata
Pons
Mesencephalon
Diencephalon

FIGURE 2-12

Midsagittal view of the brain showing components of the brain stem. (*From N. Gluhbegovic and T. H. Williams: The Human Brain: A Photographic Guide. Harper & Row, 1980, courtesy of the authors.*)

cerebral cortex to lower centers and vice versa. Lesions of the internal capsule result in contralateral motor deficits (paralysis) and sensory deficits.

Globus pallidus (Latin *globus*, "sphere" or "ball"; *pallidus*, "pale"). The medial part of the lentiform nucleus of the basal ganglia.

Gyrus rectus (Greek *gyros*, "circle"; Latin *rectus*, "straight"). The gyrus rectus lies along the ventromedial margin of the frontal lobe medial to the olfactory sulcus.

Orbital gyrus. Located on the inferior surface of the frontal lobe lateral to the olfactory sulcus.

Ventral Surface

Portions of the frontal and temporal lobes, the cerebellum, and the brain stem appear on this surface of the brain (Fig. 2-13).

Frontal Lobe

The ventral surface of the frontal lobe shows a longitudinal sulcus—the olfactory sulcus—in which the olfactory tract and bulb are located. Medial to the olfactory sulcus is the **gyrus rectus;** lateral to the olfactory sulcus is the **orbital gyrus.** At the caudal extremity of the olfactory tract is the anterior perforated substance, the site of perforating blood vessels that pass to deeper regions of the brain.

KEY CONCEPTS

- The ventral surface of the brain shows the cerebellum, diencephalon, midbrain, pons, and medulla oblongata.
- The ventral surface of the frontal lobe shows the olfactory tract and bulb between the gyrus rectus medially and the orbital gyrus laterally.

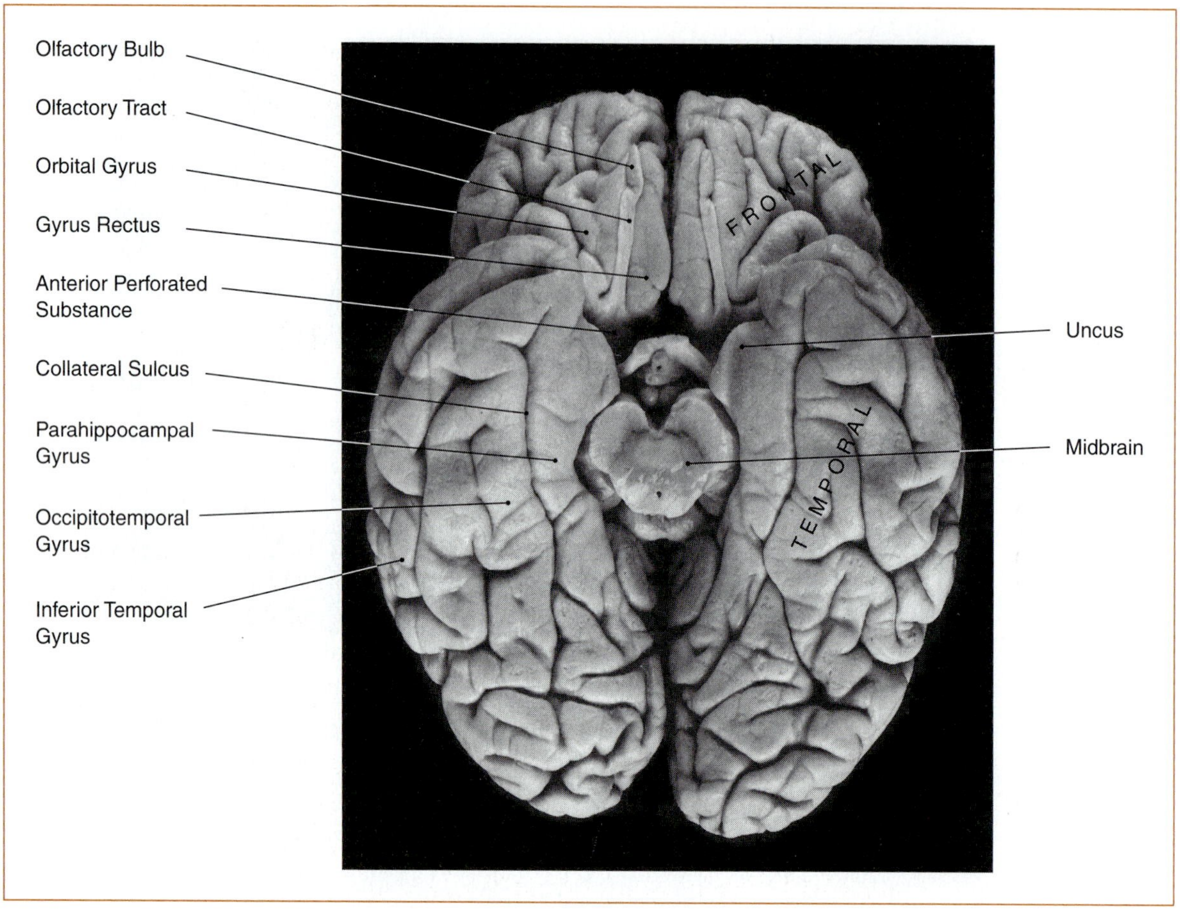

FIGURE 2-13

Ventral view of the brain showing major sulci and gyri. (*From N. Gluhbegovic and T. H. Williams: The Human Brain: A Photographic Guide. Harper & Row, 1980, courtesy of the authors.*)

Tonsil (Latin *tonsilla*, a general term for a small rounded mass). The cerebellar tonsils are rounded masses in the posterior lobe of the cerebellum. Downward extension of the cerebellar tonsils into the foramen magnum leads to compression of the medulla oblongata and is life-threatening.

Flocculus (Latin, "tuft," "small tangle of wool"). A cerebellar lobule that with the nodulus forms the paleocerebellum, which is involved with the maintenance of posture. *Flocculus* was a vulgar Latin word for pubic hair. Its use to name a brain structure illustrates

Temporal Lobe

The ventral surface of the temporal lobe shows the continuation of the inferior temporal gyrus from the lateral surface. Medial to the inferior temporal gyrus is the occipitotemporal (fusiform) gyrus. The collateral sulcus separates the occipitotemporal gyrus from the more medial parahippocampal gyrus and uncus, which constitute parts of the limbic lobe.

Cerebellum and Brain Stem

The ventral surface of the brain also shows the ventral surfaces of the cerebellum, pons, medulla oblongata, and diencephalon as well as the cranial nerves and the circle of Willis (Figs. 2-14 and 2-15).

The ventral surface of the cerebellum (Fig. 2-14) shows the cerebellar hemispheres, including the **tonsils** and **flocculus.** Tonsillar herniation through the foramen magnum under a marked increase in intracranial pressure (from a tumor or intracranial hemorrhage) is a life-threatening condition. The midline cerebellum (**vermis**) is made visible when the medulla oblongata is lifted.

Cranial nerves and related structures that usually are visible on the ventral surface of the brain include the olfactory tract and bulb, the optic chiasm, and the oculomotor, trigeminal, abducens, facial, and cochleovestibular nerves (Fig. 2-15).

The olfactory tract is located in the olfactory sulcus on the ventral surface of the frontal lobe. Tumors in this area may encroach on the olfactory tract and present

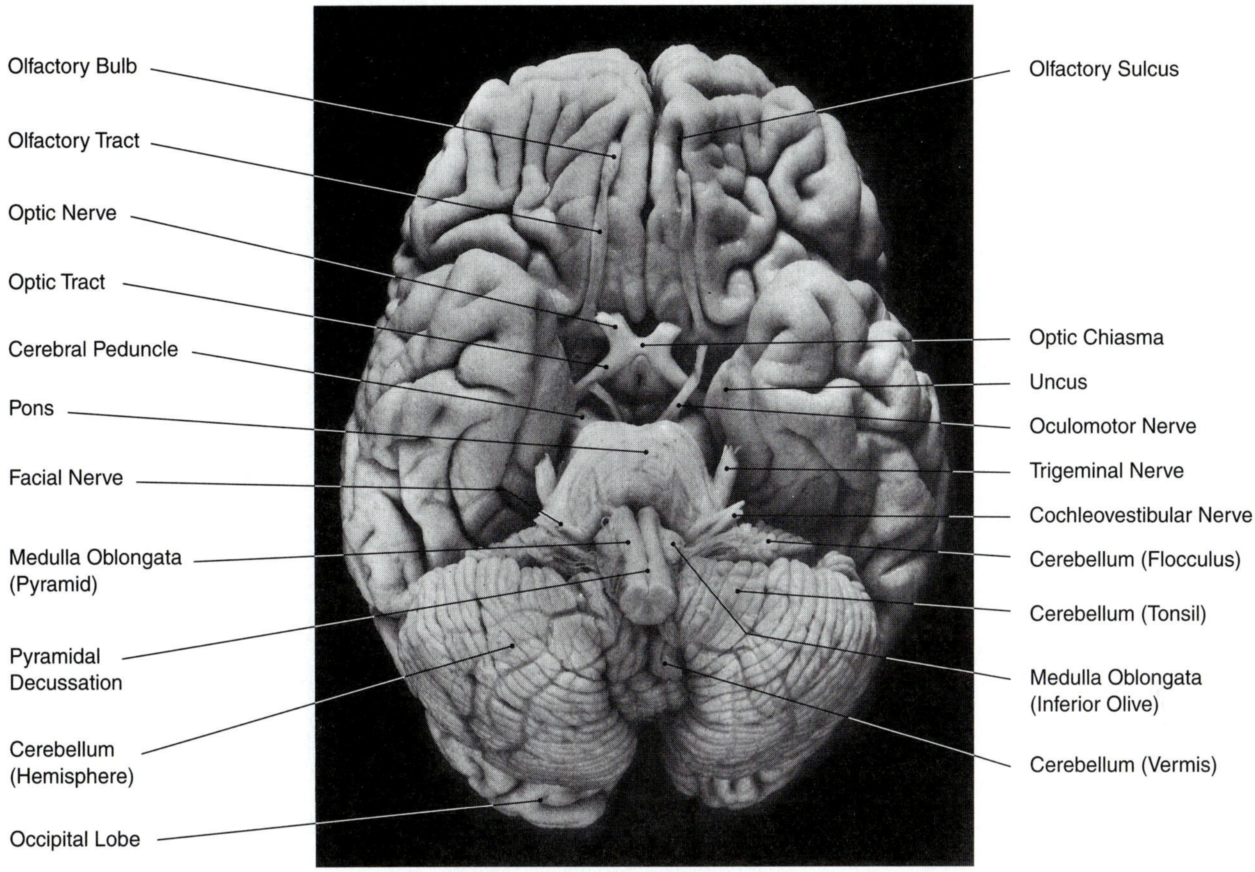

FIGURE 2-14

Ventral view of the brain showing the cranial nerves. (*From N. Gluhbegovic and T. H. Williams: The Human Brain: A Photographic Guide. Harper & Row, 1980, courtesy of the authors.*)

with loss of the sense of smell. The **optic chiasma** is ventral to the diencephalon and rostral to the infundibular stalk. Lesions in this site that encroach on the optic chiasm present with loss of vision in the bitemporal visual fields (bitemporal hemianopia). The **oculomotor nerve** exits on the ventral surface of the brain between the posterior cerebral and superior cerebellar arteries. **Aneurysms** (saccular dilatations) of either of these arteries encroaching on the oculomotor nerve present with oculomotor nerve palsy (drooping of the eyelid, a dilated pupil that is nonresponsive to light stimulation, and deviation of the eye down and out). The **trigeminal nerve** is a robust structure on the ventrolateral surface of the pons. Two components of the nerve are usually visible: a larger (portio major) sensory and a smaller (portio minor) motor component. The **abducens nerve** is visible in a paramedian position in the groove separating the pons from the medulla oblongata. The **facial** and cochleovestibular nerves are visible in the angle between the cerebellum, pons, and medulla oblongata (cerebellopontine angle). Tumors arising in this angle (acoustic neuromas) usually present with hearing loss because of early involvement of the cochleovestibular nerve.

The **trochlear nerve** is slender and often is lost during the process of brain acquisition from the skull. The **glossopharyngeal, vagus, accessory,** and **hypoglossal nerves** are composed of a series of slender filaments aligned along the rostrocaudal surface of the medulla oblongata.

Components of the circle of Willis that usually are visible on the ventral surface

the ancient practice of naming parts of the brain for other parts of the body.

Vermis (Latin "worm"). The vermis of the cerebellum is named for its resemblance to the segmented body of a worm. Galen was the first to liken it to a worm.

Optic chiasma (Greek *optikos*, "of or for sight"; *chiasma*, "a cross," from the letter chi, X). The site of partial decussation (crossing) of the optic nerves. First described by Rufus of Ephesus in the first century A.D. For many years it was thought that the chiasm was responsible for coordinated eye movements.

Oculomotor nerve (Latin *oculus*, "eye"; *motor*, "mover"). The third cranial

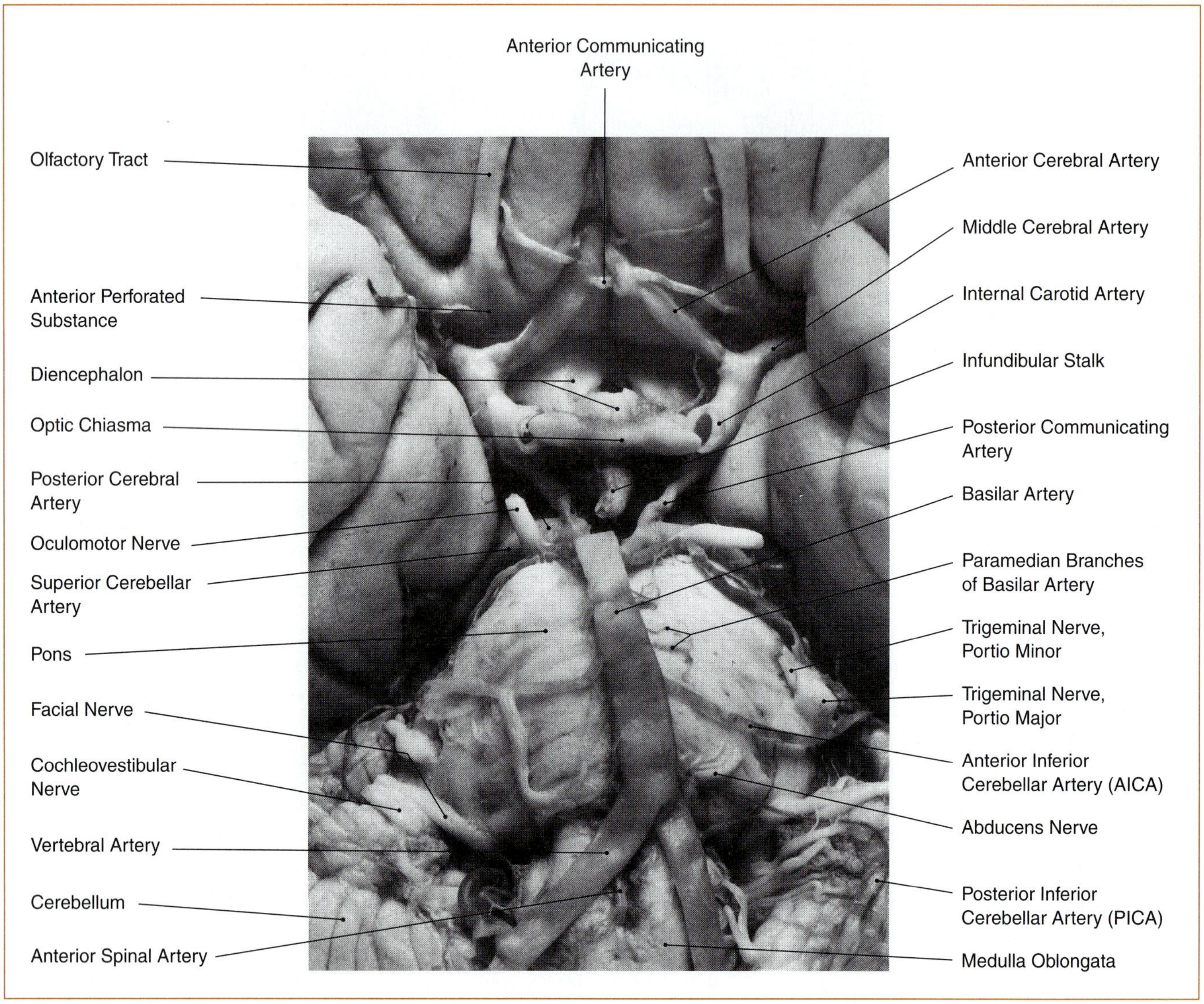

FIGURE 2-15

Ventral view of the brain showing cranial nerves and the circle of Willis.

nerve; affects movements of the eye.

Aneurysm (Greek *aneurysma*, "widening"). A sac formed by dilatation of the wall of an artery, a vein, or the heart as a result of weakening of the wall. The condition was known to Galen.

Trigeminal nerve (Latin *tres*, "three"; *geminus*, "twin"). The fifth cranial nerve was described by Fallopius. So named because the nerve has three divisions: ophthalmic, maxillary, and mandibular.

of the brain include the following arteries (Fig. 2-15): internal carotid, anterior cerebral, anterior communicating, posterior communicating, and posterior cerebral. These arteries form a circle around the diencephalon. The basilar artery occupies a groove (basilar groove) on the ventral surface of the pons. The superior cerebellar, anterior inferior cerebellar, and paramedian arterial branches of the basilar artery usually are visible. The two vertebral arteries are visible on the ventral surface of the medulla oblongata. They give rise to the anterior spinal artery, which supplies the paramedian medulla and spinal cord, and the posterior inferior cerebellar artery

KEY CONCEPTS

- Cranial nerves and related structures commonly seen on the ventral surface of the brain include the olfactory tract and bulb, the optic chiasm, and the oculomotor, trigeminal, abducens, facial, and cochleovestibular nerves.

(PICA), which has a characteristic S configuration and supplies the dorsolateral part of the medulla and the inferior part of the cerebellum.

INTERNAL TOPOGRAPHY OF THE BRAIN

Internal brain topography is presented here in a few selective coronal and axial sections. A more complete set of coronal, axial, and sagittal sections is shown in the Atlas.

Coronal Sections

Four representative rostrocaudal coronal sections are considered. Corresponding illustrations are in the Atlas section of the book.

Section at Level of Anterior Limb of Internal Capsule

At this level the anterior limb of the internal capsule separates the caudate nucleus medially from the putamen laterally. The caudate nucleus shows its characteristic bulge into the lateral ventricle. This bulge is lost in degenerative diseases of the caudate nucleus such as **Huntington's chorea.** The corpus callosum is continuous with the deep white matter of the cerebral hemispheres. The septum pellucidum is ventral to the corpus callosum and forms a partition between the two lateral ventricles.

Section at Level of Anterior Commissure

At this level the anterior commissure courses ventral to the globus pallidus. Dorsal to the corpus callosum is the cingulate gyrus. The caudate nucleus is smaller and retains its characteristic relationship to the lateral ventricle. The putamen is larger and is lateral to the globus pallidus; the two basal ganglia nuclei are separated from the thalamus by the posterior limb of the internal capsule. The fornix is seen in two sites: ventral to the corpus callosum and ventral to the thalamus.

Section at Level of Optic Tract

At this level the optic tracts course in the ventral part of the brain on their way to the lateral geniculate nucleus of the thalamus. Each optic tract carries fibers from the ipsilateral and contralateral retinas. The fornix is dorsal and medial to the optic tracts, separating the hypothalamus into lateral and medial regions. The anterior commissure is seen beneath the putamen. The thalamus is larger and is clearly divided into medial and lateral nuclear groups by the internal medullary lamina. The mamillothalamic tract courses within the thalamus on its way from the **mamillary body** to the anterior nuclear group of the thalamus. The posterior limb of the internal capsule separates the lenticular nucleus (putamen and globus pallidus) from the thalamus. Coursing from the globus pallidus to the thalamus is a bundle of fibers, the ansa lenticularis. Lateral to the putamen is the external capsule, one of the efferent (corticofugal) cortical bundles. Between the external and extreme capsules lies the claustrum.

KEY CONCEPTS

- The circle of Willis usually is visible on the ventral surface of the brain.
- The identification of brain structures in different planes has assumed more importance with the introduction and use of imaging methods in neurologic diagnosis.

Abducens nerve (Latin, "drawing away"). The sixth cranial nerve, which was discovered by Eustachius in 1564, is so named because it supplies the lateral rectus eye muscle, which directs the pupil of the eye to the lateral side away from the midline.

Facial nerve. The seventh cranial nerve. Willis divided the seventh nerve into the portio dura (facial) and the portio mollis (auditory). Soemmering separated the two and numbered them separately.

Trochlear nerve (Latin *trochlearis*, "resembling a pulley"). The fourth cranial nerve supplies the superior oblique eye muscle, whose tendon angles through a ligamentous sling like a pulley. Achillini and Vesalius included this nerve with the third pair of cranial nerves. It was described as a separate root by Fallopius and was named the trochlear nerve by William Molins, an English surgeon, in 1670.

Glossopharyngeal nerve (Greek *glossa*, "tongue"; *pharynx*, "throat"). The ninth cranial nerve. Combined by Galen with the sixth nerve. Fallopius distinguished it as a separate nerve in 1561. Thomas Willis included it as part of the eighth nerve. Soemmering listed it as the ninth cranial nerve.

Vagus (Latin *vagari*, "wanderer"). The tenth cranial nerve is so named because of its long course and wide distribution. This nerve was described by Marinus about A.D. 100. The name *vagus* was coined by Domenico de Marchetti of Padua.

Accessory nerve. The eleventh cranial nerve (accessory nerve of Willis) was described by Thomas Willis in 1664. The name *accessory* was chosen because this nerve receives an additional root from the upper part of the spinal cord (C2–C3 spinal roots).

Hypoglossal nerve (Greek *hypo*, "beneath"; *glossa*, "tongue"). The twelfth cranial nerve was named by Winslow. Willis included it with the ninth cranial nerve. It was considered the twelfth nerve by Soemmering.

Huntington's chorea. A degenerative brain disease caused by abnormal triplet codon repeats at chromosome 4p16.3 inherited in an autosomal dominant pattern. The clinical picture is characterized by abnormal movements (Greek *chorea,* "dancing") and neuropsychological deficits. Named after George Sumner Huntington, an American general practitioner who described the disease in 1872.

Mamillary bodies (Latin, diminutive of *mamma*, "little breast, nipple"). A pair of small round swellings on the ventral surface of the posterior hypothalamus.

Atrium (Greek *atrion*, "court" or "hall"). The atrium was a large area in the center of a Roman house. The term is used in anatomic nomenclature to refer to a chamber that affords entrance to another structure. The atrium of the lateral ventricle affords entrance to the occipital and temporal horns of the lateral ventricle.

Glomus (Latin, "a ball"). The choroid plexus glomus is a ball-like enlargement of the choroid plexus in the atrium (trigone) of the lateral ventricle.

Section at Level of Mamillary Bodies

At this caudal diencephalic level the mamillary bodies occupy the ventral surface of the brain. Emanating from the mamillary bodies are the mamillothalamic tracts on their way to the anterior nucleus of the thalamus. The thalamus at this level is rather large and is separated from the putamen and the globus pallidus by the posterior limb of the internal capsule. Medial to the internal capsule and dorsolateral to the mamillary body is the subthalamic nucleus, a component of the diencephalon that is involved with movement. Lesions of the subthalamic nucleus give rise to a characteristic involuntary movement disorder contralateral to the lesion known as hemiballismus. The caudate nucleus at this level is small. Between the two diencephalons is the cavity of the third ventricle. The insula (island of Reil) is seen deep within the lateral (sylvian) fissure.

Axial Sections

A few representative dorsoventral axial sections are presented.

Section at Level of Corpus Callosum

At this level the corpus callosum interconnects the two halves of the brain and is continuous with the white matter core of both hemispheres. The caudate nucleus is shown bulging into the lateral ventricle. The internal capsule is lateral to the caudate and continuous with the white matter core of the hemispheres.

Section at Level of Thalamus and Basal Ganglia

At this level the frontal, temporal, and occipital lobes are seen. The insula (island of Reil) is buried deep within the sylvian fissure. The frontal (anterior) horn, body, and **atrium** (trigone) of the lateral ventricle are seen. The atrium of the lateral ventricle contains abundant choroid plexus (**glomus**). The septum pellucidum separates the two frontal horns. Ventral to the septum is the fornix. The head of the caudate nucleus is seen bulging into the frontal horn of the lateral ventricle. The tail of the caudate, which is much smaller than the head, is seen more caudally overlying the atrium (trigone). The anterior and posterior limbs of the internal capsule are both seen. The anterior limb separates the caudate and putamen nuclei, whereas the posterior limb separates the thalamus and putamen. The rostral part and the caudal part (splenium) of the corpus callosum are also seen.

Section at Level of Anterior Commissure

At this level the anterior commissure is seen rostral to the putamen, the globus pallidus, and the columns of the fornix. The posterior limb of the internal capsule separates the thalamus from the globus pallidus. Dorsomedial to the thalamus is the stria medullaris thalami. The hippocampus is seen as an involution of the parahippocampal gyrus into the inferior (temporal) horn of the lateral ventricle. The fimbria of the fornix, which contains axons of neurons in the hippocampus, is seen attached to the hippocampus.

Section at Level of Brain Stem

At this level the cerebellum, mesencephalon, mamillary bodies, and optic chiasm are seen. Rootlets of the oculomotor nerve (cranial nerve III) are seen coursing in the mesencephalon. The cerebral peduncles, which are continuations of the internal capsule, are located in the ventral part of the mesencephalon. Dorsal to the cerebral peduncle is the substantia nigra.

The identification of brain structures in sagittal, axial, and coronal sections assumed more importance with the introduction of imaging techniques [magnetic resonance imaging (MRI)] as a diagnostic tool in neurology. In this procedure computerized images of the brain are taken at a predetermined angle to detect the site and nature of lesions in the brain. This is a highly specialized technique that requires a thorough knowledge of the anatomy of the brain in sections. For the purpose of this presentation, only a few representative MRI images will be described.

The first is a midsagittal section of the brain and brain stem that shows the medial surfaces of the frontal, parietal, and occipital lobes; the rostrum, genu, body, and splenium of the corpus callosum; and the lateral and fourth ventricles, thalamus, mesencephalon, pons, medulla, and cerebellum. Also seen in this section are the vertebral, basilar, and anterior cerebral arteries; the internal cerebral vein, basal veins, and great cerebral vein; some of the cerebrospinal fluid cisterns (cisterna magna and medullary, suprasellar, and quadrigeminal cisterns); and the arachnoid granulations.

The second is an axial section through the thalamus that shows the frontal, parietal, and occipital lobes. The third ventricle is in the midline separating the two thalami. Within the thalamus the mamillothalamic tract is seen in cross section. The caudate nucleus forms the lateral wall of the anterior horn of the lateral ventricle. The anterior limb of the internal capsule separates the caudate nucleus and the putamen. The posterior limb of the internal capsule separates the putamen and the thalamus. The genu of the internal capsule lies between the anterior and posterior limbs. The optic radiation is lateral to the atrium (trigone) of the lateral ventricle. The columns of the fornix are above the third ventricle. In the interhemispheric fissure rostrally are pericallosal branches of the anterior cerebral artery. The internal cerebral veins and the straight and superior sagittal sinuses are seen caudally.

The third image is a coronal section through the thalamus and third ventricle. The body of the corpus callosum interconnects the two hemispheres. Dorsal to the corpus callosum are pericallosal branches of the anterior cerebral artery. The third ventricle separates the two thalami. Dorsal to the third ventricle are the internal cerebral veins. The body of the caudate nucleus is in the lateral wall of the body of the lateral ventricle. The insula (island of Reil) is deep within the lateral (sylvian) fissures. Branches of the middle cerebral artery are within the lateral fissure. The inferior (temporal) horns of the lateral ventricle are dorsal to the temporal lobe.

A complete set of MRI images in sagittal, axial, and coronal sections is included in the Atlas.

SUGGESTED READINGS

Gluhbegovic N, Williams TH: *The Human Brain: A Photographic Guide.* Hagerstown, Harper & Row, 1980.

Haines DE: *Neuroanatomy: An Atlas of Structures, Sections, and Systems.* Baltimore, MD, Urban and Schwarzenberg, 1983.

Jouandet ML, Gazzaniga MS: Cortical field of origin of the anterior commissure of the rhesus monkey. *Exp Neurol* 1979; 66:381–397.

Naidich TP, et al: Anatomic relationships along the low-middle convexity: I. Normal specimens and magnetic resonance imaging. *Neurosurgery* 1995; 36:517–532.

Pryse-Phillips W: *Companion to Clinical Neurology.* Boston, Little, Brown, 1995.

Risse GL, et al: The anterior commissure in man: Functional variation in a multisensory system. *Neuropsychologia* 1978; 16:23–31.

Roberts M, Hanaway J: *Atlas of the Human Brain in Sections.* Philadelphia, Lea & Febiger, 1970.

Shipps FC, et al: *Atlas of Brain Anatomy for C.T. Scans*, 2d ed. Springfield, Ill., Charles C Thomas, 1977.

Skinner HA: *The Origin of Medical Terms*, 2d ed. Baltimore, MD, Williams & Wilkins, 1961.

CHAPTER 3

SPINAL CORD

EXTERNAL TOPOGRAPHY

The spinal cord of adult humans extends from the foramen magnum to the level of the first or second lumbar vertebra. Approximately 45 cm long in males and 42 cm in females, it has a cylindrical shape in the upper cervical and thoracic segments and an oval shape in the lower cervical and lumbar segments, which are sites of the brachial and lumbosacral nerve plexuses, respectively. In the early stages of fetal development, the cord occupies the whole length of the vertebral canal; in the term newborn, it extends down to the lower border of the third lumbar vertebra; in late adolescence, the spinal cord attains its adult position, terminating at the level of the intervertebral disk between the L-1 and L-2 vertebrae (Fig. 3-1). The level at which the cord terminates changes with development because the vertebral column grows faster than the spinal cord. The length of the entire adult vertebral column is 70 cm. The spinal cord exhibits two enlargements: cervical (third cervical to second thoracic segments) and lumbar (first lumbar to third sacral segments). These are sites of neurons that innervate the upper and lower extremities, respectively. The **caudal** end of the cord is tapered to form the conus medullaris, from which a pial-glial filament, the filum terminale, extends and attaches to the coccyx to anchor the spinal cord. The spinal cord is also anchored to the dura by two lateral series of **denticulate** ligaments, pial folds that stretch from the surface of the cord to the dural sheath midway between the dorsal and ventral roots. Denticulate

Caudal (Latin "tail"). Pertaining to cauda, toward the tail or posterior end.

Denticulate (Latin *denticulus*, "a small tooth"). The toothlike lateral projections of the pia mater in the spinal cord.

KEY CONCEPTS

- The spinal cord is a cylindrical structure extending in adults from the foramen magnum to the level of the second lumbar vertebra, where it terminates as the conus medullaris.
- The spinal cord has two enlargements, cervical and lumbosacral, corresponding to regions innervating the upper and lower extremities, respectively.

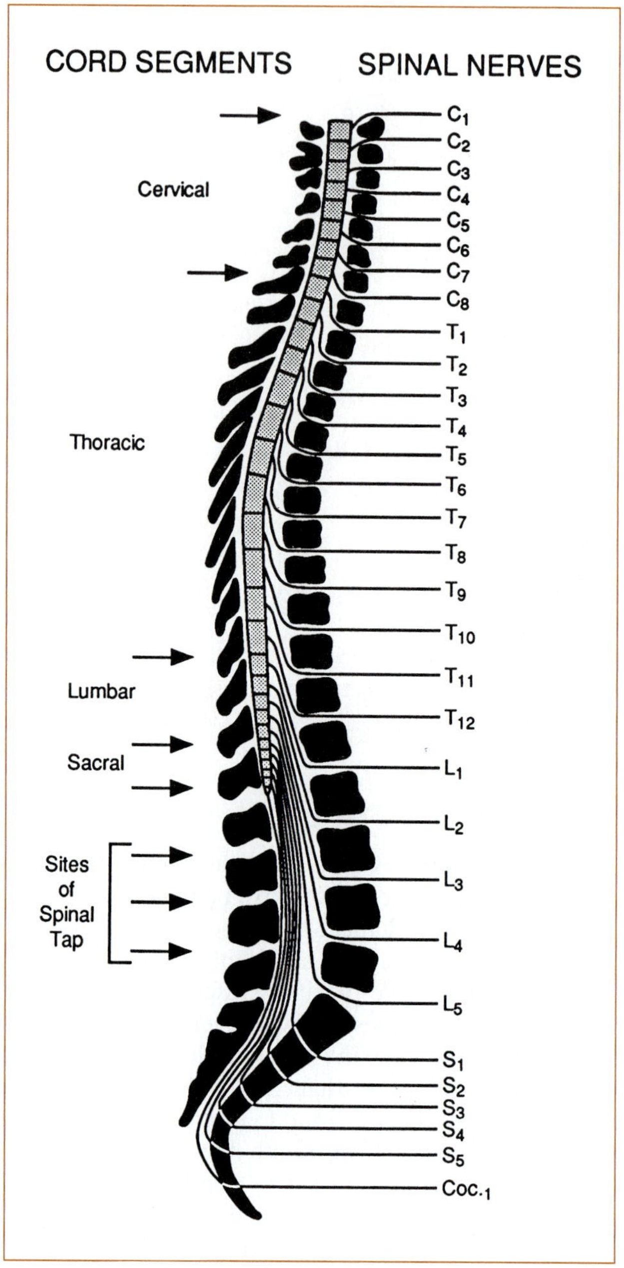

FIGURE 3-1

Schematic diagram showing the relationships of spinal cord segments and spinal nerves to vertebral column levels.

ligaments serve as useful landmarks for the neurosurgeon in identifying the anterolateral segment of the cord when performing operations such as cordotomies for the relief of intractable pain. There are 20 to 21 pairs of denticulate ligaments extending between the first lumbar and first cervical vertebrae.

The human spinal cord comprises 31 segments, each of which, except the first

KEY CONCEPTS

- The spinal cord is anchored to the coccyx by the filum terminale and to the dura mater by the denticulate ligaments.

TABLE 3-1

Relationship of Spinal Cord Segments and Vertebral Spines

Cord Segments	Vertebral Spines
C-1	C-1
C-7	C-6
T-6	T-4
L-1	T-10
S-1	T-12 to L-1

cervical segment, has a pair of **dorsal** and **ventral** roots and a pair of spinal nerves. The first cervical segment has only a ventral root. The dorsal and ventral roots join in the intervertebral foramina to form the spinal nerves. Just proximal to its junction with the ventral root in the intervertebral foramen, each dorsal root has an oval swelling: the dorsal root (spinal) **ganglion** containing pseudounipolar sensory neurons. At the point where the dorsal nerve root enters the spinal cord, glial supporting tissue from the spinal cord extends a short distance into the nerve root to meet the Schwann cell and the collagenous supporting tissue of the peripheral nervous system. The junction zone between the two types of tissues is quite sharp histologically. It is called the *Obersteiner-Redlich space* after two Austrian neurologists, Heinrich Obersteiner and Emil Redlich. The 31 pairs of spinal nerves are divided into 8 cervical nerves, 12 thoracic nerves, 5 lumbar nerves, 5 sacral nerves, and 1 coccygeal nerve (see Fig. 3-1). The fourth and fifth sacral nerves and the coccygeal nerve arise from the conus medullaris. Spinal nerves leave the vertebral canal through the intervertebral foramina. The first cervical nerve emerges above the atlas; the eighth cervical nerve emerges between the seventh cervical (C-7) and the first thoracic (T-1) vertebrae. All other spinal nerves exit beneath the corresponding vertebrae (see Fig. 3-1).

Because of the differential rate of growth of the spinal cord and vertebral column, spinal cord segment levels do not correspond to those of the vertebral column (Table 3-1). Thus, in the cervical region, the tip of the vertebral spine corresponds to the level of the succeeding cord segment; that is, the sixth cervical spine corresponds to the level of the seventh spinal cord segment. In the upper thoracic region, the tip of the spine is two segments above the corresponding cord segment; that is, the fourth thoracic spine corresponds to the sixth cord segment. In the lower

Dorsal (Latin *dorsalis*, from *dorsum*, "back"). Pertaining to or situated near the back of an animal.

Ventral (Latin *ventralis*, "belly"). Pertaining to or toward the belly part of the body, as opposed to dorsal.

Ganglion (Greek "swelling, knot"). A collection of nerve cells outside the central nervous system, as in dorsal root ganglia or autonomic ganglia.

KEY CONCEPTS

- The spinal cord is comprised of 31 segments defined by 31 pairs of spinal nerves. Each spinal nerve is formed by union of a dorsal (sensory) and a ventral (motor) root. The first cervical segment has only a ventral root.
- Because of differential growth rates, spinal cord segments do not correlate with vertebral column segments.
- Whereas upper cervical nerves pass approximately horizontally from their corresponding cord segments to the intervertebral foramina, lower spinal nerves run progressively obliquely downward to reach their corresponding intervertebral foramina.

thoracic and upper lumbar regions, the difference between the vertebral and cord level is three segments; that is, the tenth thoracic spine corresponds to the first lumbar cord segment. Because of this, the root filaments of spinal cord segments have to travel progressively longer distances from cervical to sacral segments to reach the corresponding intervertebral foramina from which the spinal nerves emerge (see Fig. 3-1). The crowding of lumbosacral roots around the filum terminale is known as the **cauda equina.**

Cauda equina (Latin "horse's tail"). Bundle of lumbosacral nerve roots beyoud the tip of the spinal cord that forms a cluster in the spinal canal which resembles the tail of a horse.
Meninges (Greek plural of *meninx*, "membrane"). The membranes covering the spinal cord and brain.
Pia mater (Latin "soft, tender mother"). The thin, delicate innermost meningeal layer.
Arachnoid (Greek *arachne*, "like a cobweb, spider's web"). The middle layer of the meninges between the outer dura and inner pia. Attached to the pia by a spider web-like delicate network of fibers.
Dura mater (Latin "hard mother"). The thick and hard outermost layer of the meninges.

MENINGES

The spinal cord is covered by three meningeal coats; these are the pia, arachnoid, and dura mater. The **pia mater** is composed of an inner membranous layer, the intima pia, and an outer superficial layer, the epipia. The intima pia is intimately adherent to the surface of the spinal cord. The epipia carries blood vessels that supply and drain the spinal cord. It also forms the denticulate ligaments. The **arachnoid** is closely adherent to the dura mater. The space between the dura and arachnoid (subdural space) is a very narrow (potential) space visible with the aid of a microscope in histologic preparations in normal conditions. Bridging veins course across this space. Rupture of these veins results in accumulation of blood and expansion of this space, a condition known as *subdural hematoma.* The space between the arachnoid and pia (subarachnoid space), in contrast, is wider and contains the cerebrospinal fluid. The spinal **dura mater,** unlike the dura within the skull, is firmly attached to bone only at the margin of the foramen magnum. Elsewhere, the spinal dura is separated from the vertebral periosteum by the epidural space. The spinal epidural space contains adipose tissue and a venous plexus and is largest at the level of the second lumbar vertebra. The spinal epidural space is used for injection of local anesthetics to produce paravertebral nerve block known as *epidural anesthesia.* The spinal dura mater ensheaths the dorsal and ventral roots, the dorsal root ganglia, and proximal portions of spinal nerves, and then it becomes continuous with the epineurium of spinal nerves at the level of the intervertebral foramen. The spinal cord terminates at the level of the L-1 and L-2 vertebrae, whereas the dura mater extends down to the level of the S-1 and S-2 vertebrae. Below the site of spinal cord termination (conus medullaris), a sac filled with cerebrospinal fluid and devoid of spinal cord forms in the subarachnoid space. This sac is a favorable site for clinicians to introduce a special spinal needle to obtain cerebrospinal fluid for examination or to inject drugs or dyes into the subarachnoid space for purposes of treatment or diagnosis. This procedure is called *lumbar puncture* or *spinal tap.*

CROSS-SECTIONAL TOPOGRAPHY

In cross section, the spinal cord is composed of a centrally placed butterfly- or H-shaped area of gray matter surrounded by white matter. The two wings of the

KEY CONCEPTS

- The spinal cord is surrounded by three meningeal layers: pia, arachnoid, and dura.
- The epidural space is the site of epidural anesthesia during obstetric delivery.
- The subarachnoid space between the pia and arachnoid contains cerebrospinal fluid. Below the conus medullaris, the subarachnoid space is the most common site for spinal tap to obtain cerebrospinal fluid for examination or to inject drugs for treatment.

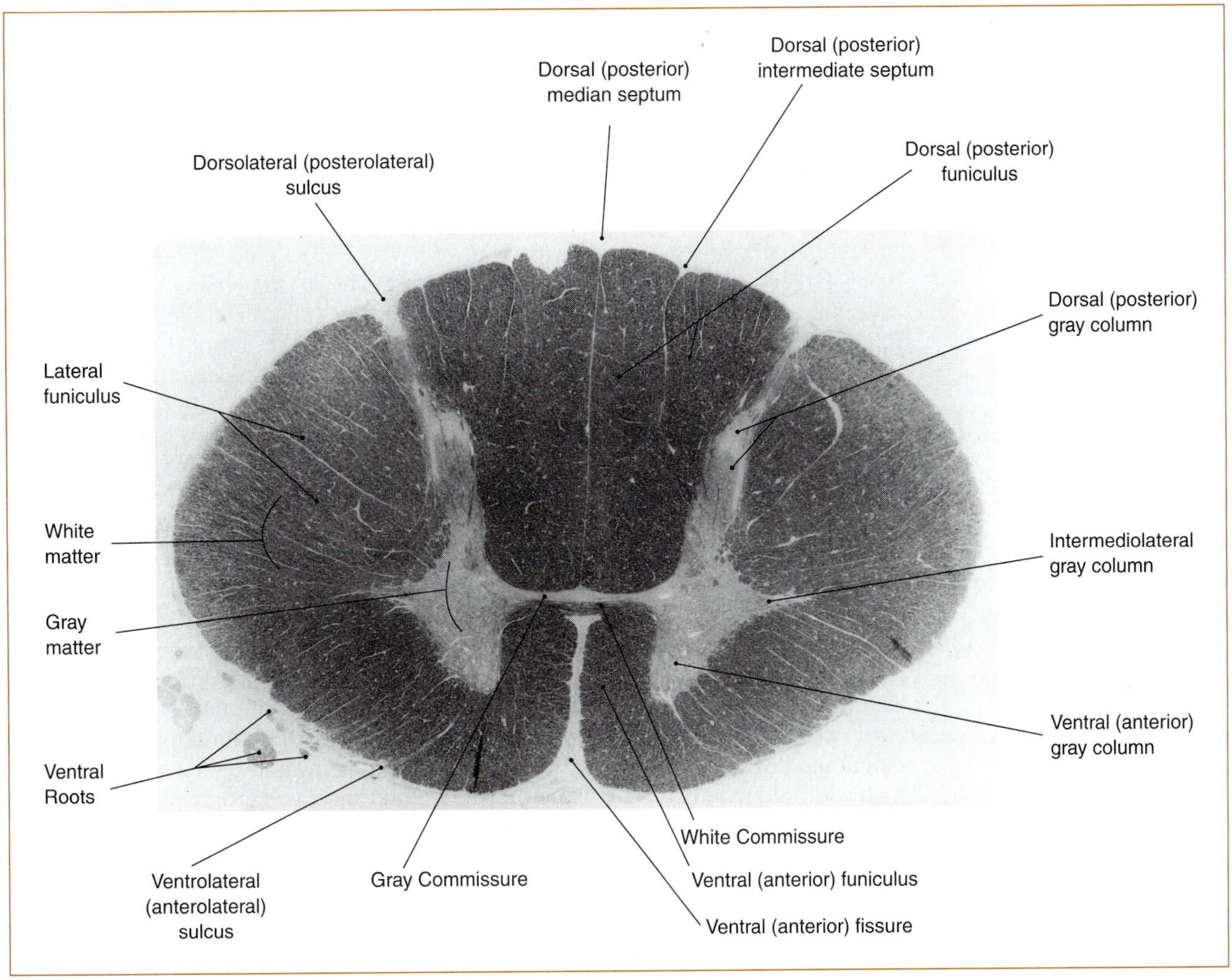

FIGURE 3-2

Photomicrograph of spinal cord showing division into gray and white matter, the sulci and fissures, gray matter columns, and white matter funiculi.

butterfly are connected across the midline by the dorsal and ventral gray **commissures** above and below the central canal, respectively (Fig. 3-2). The gray matter of the cord contains primarily the cell bodies of neurona and glia. The white matter of the cord contains primarily fiber tracts.

The two halves of the spinal cord are separated by the dorsal (posterior) median septum and the ventral (anterior) median fissure (Fig. 3-2). The site of entrance of dorsal root fibers is marked by the dorsolateral (posterolateral) sulcus; similarly, the site of exit of ventral roots is marked by the ventrolateral (anterolateral) **sulcus** (see Fig. 3-2). These landmarks divide the white matter of each half of the cord

Commissure (Latin "joining together"). Axons that connect the two halves of the spinal cord or the two cerebral hemispheres.

Sulcus (Latin "groove"). As in posterolateral and anterolateral sulci of the spinal cord.

KEY CONCEPTS

- The internal structure of the spinal cord consists of central, H-shaped, gray matter and surrounding white matter. The former contains neurons, and the latter contains ascending and descending fiber tracts.

Funiculus (Latin *funis*, "cord"). A bundle of white matter containing one or more fasciculi (tracts).

Ipsilateral (Latin *ipse*, "self"; *latus*, "side"). Pertaining or projecting to the same side.

Fasciculus (Latin "a small bundle"). Small bundle of nerve fibers forming a tract, with common origin and termination.

Gracilis (Latin "slender, thin"). The fasciculus gracilis is so named because it is slender and long.

Cuneatus (Latin "wedge"). The fasciculus cuneatus is so named because of its wedge shape and because it is short.

into a dorsal (posterior) **funiculus,** a lateral funiculus, and a ventral (anterior) funiculus (see Fig. 3-2). Furthermore, in cervical and upper thoracic spinal cord segments, the dorsal (posterior) funiculus is divided into two unequal parts by the dorsal (posterior) intermediate septum (see Fig. 3-2).

The H-shaped gray matter is also divided into a smaller dorsal (posterior) horn or column and a larger ventral (anterior) horn or column. The thoracic and upper lumbar cord segments, in addition, exhibit a wedge-shaped intermediolateral horn or column (Fig. 3-2).

The spinal cord is asymmetric in about 75 percent of humans, with the right side being larger in 75 percent of the asymmetries. The asymmetry is due to more descending corticospinal tract fibers on the larger side. It has been shown that more fibers in the left medullary pyramid cross to reach the right half of the spinal cord and more fibers from the right medullary pyramid remain uncrossed to descend in the right half of the spinal cord. These two occurrences result in a larger complement of corticospinal fibers in the right half of the cord. In essence, then, the right side of the spinal cord receives more fibers from the cortex than the left side. This has no relation to handedness. The amount of uncrossed fibers may be related to the occurrence of the **ipsilateral** hemiplegia (weakness) reported in patients with lesions in the internal capsule. If most fibers do not cross, then the hemiplegia will be mostly ipsilateral.

MICROSCOPIC ANATOMY

The microscopic anatomy of the spinal cord varies in the different regions of the cord. The characteristics of microscopic anatomy in the different regions help define the level of section (Fig. 3-3). As one ascends from low sacral segments to high cervical segments, the volume of white matter increases progressively because the number of nerve fibers, both ascending to higher levels and descending to lower levels, is larger in the high cervical sections and diminishes progressively at more caudal levels. Some tracts are not present at certain levels. The dorsal spinocerebellar tract appears first at the second lumbar segment and is not present below this segment. This is because neurons that give rise to this tract first appear at the level of L-2 and are not present below this level. The cuneate tract (**fasciculus**) appears above the sixth thoracic spinal cord segment and is not present below this level. It follows that the dorsal (posterior) intermediate sulcus, which separates the **gracile** and **cuneate** tracts, is only present above the T-6 segment. Different spinal cord regions also demonstrate distinctive gray matter features. The intermediolateral cell column and the nucleus dorsalis of Clarke extend between the C-8 and L-2 segments and are not seen either below or above these levels. The cervical and lumbar enlargements of the cord are characterized by voluminous ventral horns because of the presence of motor neurons that supply limb musculature at these two levels.

KEY CONCEPTS

- Sulci and fissures divide the white matter of the spinal cord into three funiculi, and each funiculus contains one or more fasciculi (tracts).
- The presence or relative size of some neuronal aggregates and/or fiber tracts in some but not others of spinal cord segments helps identify the rostrocaudal level of a particular spinal cord segment.
- The area of white matter in the spinal cord decreases caudally because of fewer ascending and descending tracts.

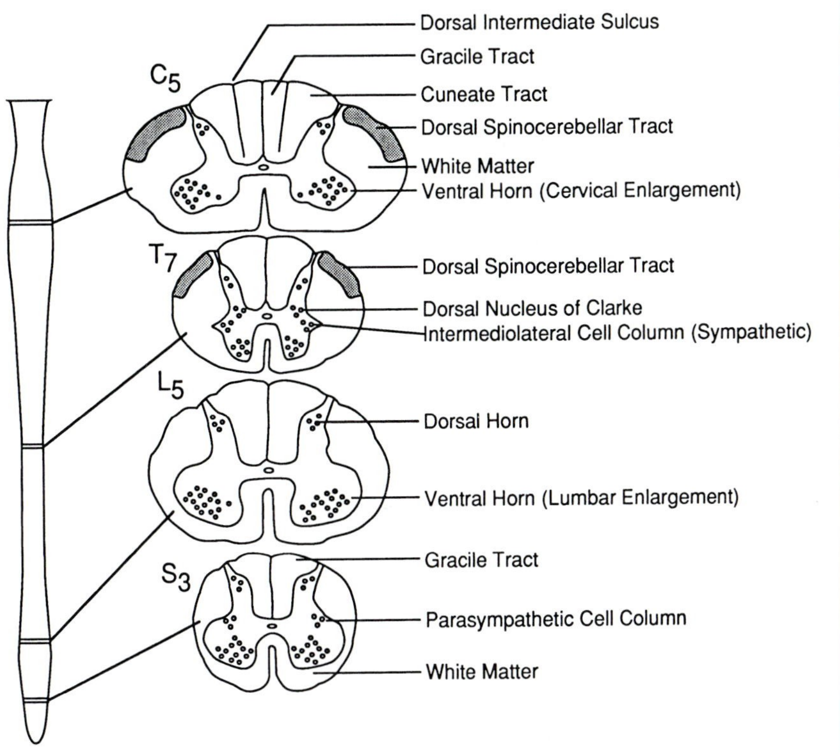

FIGURE 3-3

Schematic diagram showing variations in spinal cord segments at different levels.

Gray Matter

Older Terminology

Prior to 1952, the organization of the gray matter of the spinal cord was presented in the following way.

- *Dorsal Horn* The **dorsal** (posterior) horn or column receives axons of the dorsal root ganglia via the dorsal roots and contains cell clusters concerned with sensory function. These cell clusters are the posteromarginal **nucleus,** the substantia gelatinosa, and the nucleus proprius.
- *Intermediolateral Horn* The intermediolateral horn or column is limited to the thoracic and upper lumbar segments of the cord. It contains cell bodies of the **sympathetic** nervous system, the axons of which form the preganglionic nerve fibers and leave the spinal cord via the ventral root.

Dorsal (Latin *dorsalis*, from *dorsum*, "back"). Pertaining to or situated near the back of an animal.
Nucleus (Latin *nux*, "a nut"). Aggregation of nerve cells concerned with a particular function.
Sympathetic (Greek *sympathein*, "self-responsive"). Sympathetic division of the autonomic nervous system.

KEY CONCEPTS

- The central gray matter is formed of dorsal (sensory), intermediate, and ventral (motor) horns or zones. Each zone is formed of aggregates of neurons called *nuclei.*
- Autonomic sympathetic neurons are located in thoracic and upper lumbar spinal cord segments, whereas autonomic parasympathetic neurons are located in sacral spinal cord segments.

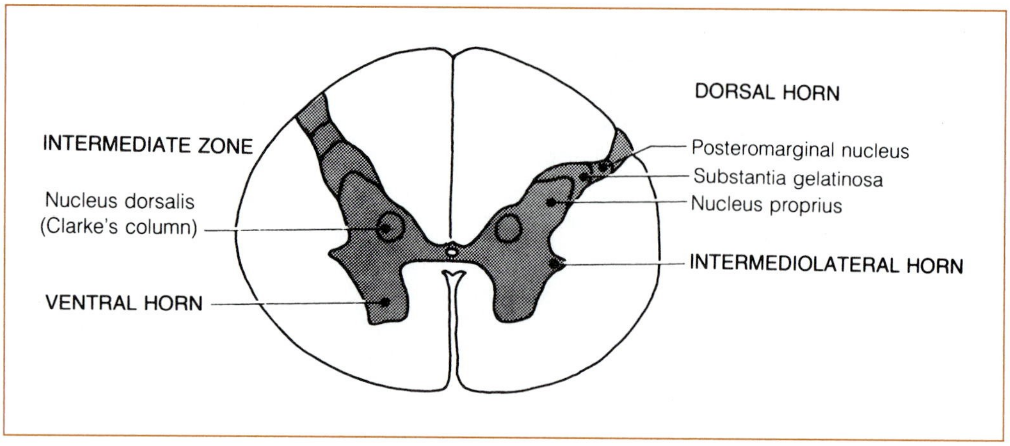

FIGURE 3-4

Cross-sectional diagram of the spinal cord showing the major nuclear groups within the gray columns.

Axon (Greek *axon*, "axis"). The process of the nerve cell that transmits impulses away from the nerve cell.

- *Ventral Horn* The ventral horn or column contains multipolar motor neurons, **axons** of which comprise the major component of the ventral root.
- *Intermediate Zone* This zone contains the nucleus dorsalis of Clarke and a large number of interneurons.

The preceding organizational pattern is illustrated diagrammatically in Fig. 3-4.

Rexed Terminology

In 1952, Rexed investigated the cytoarchitectonics, or cellular organization, of the spinal cord in the cat and found that cell clusters in the cord are arranged with extraordinary regularity into ten zones or **laminae.** His observations subsequently have been confirmed in other species, including humans. Figure 3-5 is a diagrammatic representation of the location of the ten laminae of Rexed. Table 3-2 compares the older terminology with the more recent Rexed terminology.

Lamina (Latin "thin layer"). As in column of nerve cells in Rexed laminae.

Exteroceptive (Latin "to take outside"). To receive from outside. Exteroceptive receptors receive impulses from the outside.

Proprioception (Latin *propius*, "one's own"; *perceptio*, "perception"). The sense of position and movement.

Laminae I to IV are concerned with **exteroceptive** sensations, whereas laminae V and VI are concerned primarily with **proprioceptive** sensations, although they respond to cutaneous stimuli. Lamina VII acts as a relay between midbrain and cerebellum. Lamina VIII modulates motor activity, most probably via gamma neurons. Lamina IX is the main motor area of the spinal cord. It contains large alpha and smaller gamma motor neurons arranged in columns (dorsolateral, ventrolateral, ventromedial, and central). The axons of these neurons supply extrafusal and intrafusal muscle fibers, respectively. From segments S1-2 to S-4, a supplementary column of alpha motor neurons appears in lamina IX. This is the Onuf's (Onufrowicz) nucleus, which lies at the most ventral border of the ventral horn. The nucleus is divided into a dorsomedial cell group innervating the bulbocavernosus and ischiocavernosus muscles and a ventrolateral cell group innervating external anal and urethral sphincters. The dorsomedial portion of Onuf's nucleus contains significantly more neurons in males than in females. Motor neurons in Onuf's nucleus are characteristically spared in motor neuron disease, in marked contrast to motor neurons elsewhere in the spinal cord and brain stem. Alpha motor neurons in lamina IX are somatotopically organized in such a way that neurons supplying flexor muscle groups are located dorsally, whereas neurons supplying extensor

KEY CONCEPTS

- Neuronal aggregates in the spinal cord gray matter are also organized into rostrocaudal laminae (of Rexed).

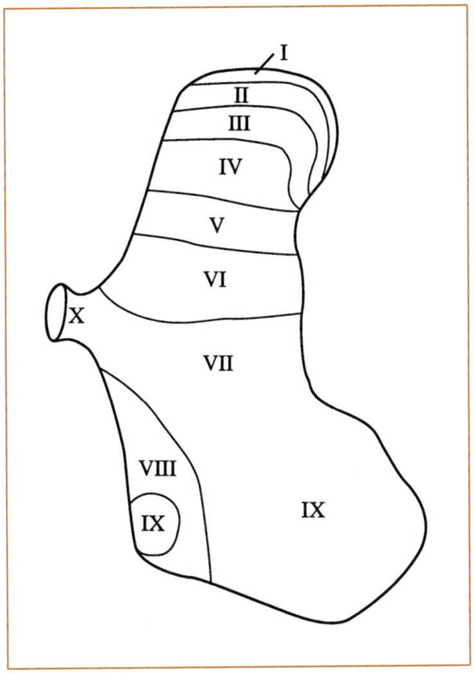

FIGURE 3-5

Schematic diagram of half of the spinal cord showing the location of Rexed laminae.

muscle groups are located ventrally. In addition, neurons supplying trunk musculature are placed medially whereas neurons supplying extremity musculature are placed laterally (Fig. 3-6).

Physiologic studies have demonstrated two types of alpha motor neurons, tonic and phasic. Tonic neurons are characterized by a lower rate of impulse firing and

TABLE 3-2

Cellular Organization of Spinal Cord

Rexed Terminology	Older Terminology
Lamina I	Posteromarginal nucleus
Lamina II	Substantia gelatinosa
Laminae III, IV	Nucleus proprius
Lamina V	Neck of posterior horn
Lamina VI	Base of posterior horn
Lamina VII	Intermediate zone, intermediolateral horn
Lamina VIII	Commissural nucleus
Lamina IX	Ventral horn
Lamina X	Grisea centralis

KEY CONCEPTS

- Alpha motor neurons in the ventral horn are somatotopically organized.

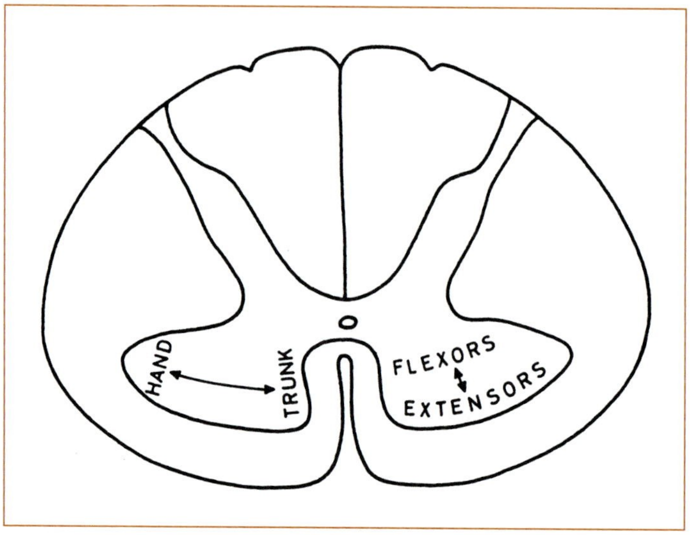

FIGURE 3-6

Schematic diagram of the spinal cord showing somatotopic organization of ventral horn (lamina IX) motor neurons.

slower axonal conduction. No anatomic criteria are available to distinguish tonic from phasic alpha motor neurons.

Physiologic studies also have demonstrated two types of gamma motor neurons, static and dynamic. The static variety is related to the nuclear chain type of intrafusal muscle fiber, which is concerned with the static response of the muscle spindle, whereas the dynamic variety is related to the nuclear bag type of intrafusal muscle fiber, which is concerned with the dynamic response of the spindle. As is the case with alpha motor neurons, no anatomic criteria are available to differentiate static from dynamic gamma motor neurons.

In addition to alpha and gamma motor neurons, lamina IX contains interneurons. One of these interneurons, the Renshaw cell, has received particular attention from neuroscientists. The Renshaw cell is interposed between the recurrent axon collateral of an alpha motor neuron and the dendrite or cell body of the same alpha motor neuron. The axon collateral of the alpha motor neuron excites the Renshaw cell. The axon of the Renshaw cell inhibits (recurrent **inhibition**) the parent alpha motor neuron and other motor neurons. Through this feedback loop, an alpha motor neuron may influence its own activity. Recent studies have shown that Renshaw cell axons project to nearby as well as distant sites, including laminae IX, VIII, and VII. The functional consequences of Renshaw cell inhibition are to curtail the motor output from a particular collection of motor neurons and to highlight the output of motor neurons that are strongly activated. The inhibitory neurotransmitter used by the Renshaw cells is probably glycine.

Inhibition (Latin *inhibere*, "to restrain or check"). Arrest or restraint of process.

Quantitative studies of the dendritic organization of spinal motor neurons have shown that **dendrites** form approximately 80 percent of the receptive area of a neuron. Although dendrites extend up to 1000 μm from the cell body, the proximal third of each dendrite contains most of the **synapses** and thus is the most effective in the reception and subsequent transmission of incoming stimuli. Lamina X surrounds the central canal and contains neuroglia.

Dendrite (Latin *dendron*, "a tree"). The numerous processes of a nerve cell that branch like a tree and that transmit impulses toward the nerve cell.

Synapse (Greek *synapsis*, "contact"). Site of contact between processes of nerve cells (axon to axon, axon to dendrite), between neural process and nerve cell, or between neural process and muscle.

Neurons in the gray matter of the spinal cord are of two types, principal neurons and interneurons. The former have been classified into two general categories on the

KEY CONCEPTS

- Renshaw cells are activated by alpha motor neurons and in turn inhibit the parent alpha motor neurons.

TABLE 3-3

Spinal Cord Ascending Tracts

Tract Name	Origin	Location	Extent	Termination	Function
Gracile	Ipsilateral dorsal root ganglion	Medial in posterior funiculus	Throughout spinal cord	Ipsilateral gracile nucleus in medulla	Conscious proprioception
Cuneate	Ipsilateral dorsal root ganglion	Lateral in posterior funiculus	Above sixth thoracic segment	Ipsilateral cuneate nucleus in medulla	Conscious proprioception
Dorsal spino-cerebellar	Ipsilateral nucleus dorsalis of Clarke	Lateral funiculus	Above second lumbar segment	Ipsilateral cerebellum	Unconscious proprioception
Ventral spino-cerebellar	Contralateral dorsal horn	Lateral funiculus	Throughout spinal cord	Contralateral cerebellum	Unconscious proprioception
Spinocervical thalamic (Morin's)	Ipsilateral dorsal root ganglion	Lateral funiculus	Throughout spinal cord	Ipsilateral lateral cervical nucleus	Conscious proprioception
Lateral spino-thalamic	Contralateral dorsal horn	Lateral funiculus	Throughout spinal cord	Ipsilateral thalamus (ventral posterolateral nucleus)	Pain and thermal sensations
Anterior spinothalamic	Contralateral (largely) dorsal horn	Lateral and anterior funiculi	Throughout spinal cord	Ipsilateral thalamus (ventral posterolateral nucleus)	Light touch

basis of their axonal course. Tract (projection) neurons have axons that contribute to the formation of a tract. Examples of such neurons include the dorsal nucleus of Clarke, which gives rise to the dorsal spinocerebellar tract, and neurons in the dorsal (posterior) horn that give rise to the spinothalamic tract. In contrast, root neurons have axons that contribute to the formation of the ventral root. Examples of such neurons include alpha and gamma motor neurons in the ventral (anterior) horn and the autonomic (sympathetic) neurons in the intermediolateral horn.

White Matter

The white matter of the spinal cord is organized into three funiculi (Fig. 3-2):

1. Posterior (dorsal) funiculus
2. Lateral funiculus
3. Anterior (ventral) funiculus

Each of these funiculi contains one or more tracts or fasciculi (Tables 3-3 and 3-4). A *tract* is composed of nerve fibers sharing a common origin, destination, and

KEY CONCEPTS

- Neurons in gray matter are of two types: principal neurons and interneurons. Principal neurons are classified according to their trajectory into tracts (projection) and root neurons.

TABLE 3-4

Spinal Cord Descending Tracts

Tract Name	Origin	Location	Extent	Termination	Function
Lateral corticospinal	Contralateral cerebral cortex	Lateral funiculus	Throughout spinal cord	Ipsilateral ventral and dorsal horns	Control of skilled movement, modulation of sensory activity
Anterior cortico-pinal (bundle of Türck)	Ipsilateral cerebral cortex (largely)	Anterior funiculus	Variable	Contralateral ventral and dorsal horns	Control of skilled movement, modulation of sensory activity
Of Barns	Ipsilateral cerebral cortex	Lateral funiculus	Throughout spinal cord	Ipsilateral ventral and dorsal horns	Control of skilled movement, modulation of sensory activity
Rubrospinal	Contralateral red nucleus (midbrain)	Lateral funiculus	Throughout spinal cord	Ipsilateral ventral horn	Control of movement
Lateral vestibulo-spinal	Ipsilateral lateral vestibular nucleus	Lateral funiculus	Throughout spinal cord	Ipsilateral ventral horn	Control of muscles that maintain upright posture and balance
Medial vestibulo-spinal	Ipsi- and contralateral medial vestibular nuclei	Anterior funiculus	Cervical spinal cord	Ipsilateral ventral horn	Head position in association with vestibular stimulation
Reticulospinal	Medullary and pontine reticular formation, bilaterally	Lateral and anterior funiculi	Throughout spinal cord	Ipsilateral ventral horn and intermediate zone	Control of movement and posture, modulation of sensory activity
Tectospinal	Contralateral superior colliculus (midbrain)	Anterior funiculus	Cervical spinal cord	Ipsilateral ventral horn	Head position in association with eye movement
Descending autonomic	Ipsilateral hypothalamus	Anterolateral funiculus	Throughout spinal cord	Ipsilateral intermediolateral cell column and sacral preganglionic cell group	Control of smooth muscles and glands
Monoaminergic	Raphe nucleus, locus ceruleus, periaqueductal gray	Lateral and anterior funiculi	Throughout spinal cord	Ipsilateral dorsal horn	Control of pain transmission

function. In general, the name of a tract denotes its origin and destination; for example, the spinocerebellar tract connects the spinal cord and cerebellum and the corticospinal tract connects the cerebral cortex and spinal cord.

Posterior Funiculus

Nerve fibers in this funiculus are concerned with two general modalities related to conscious proprioception. These are **kinesthesia** (sense of position and movement) and discriminative touch (precise localization of touch, including two-point discrimination).

Kinesthesia (Greek *kinesis*, "motion"; *aisthesis*, "sensation"). Sense of perception of movement.

Lesions (Latin *laesia*, laedere, "to hurt or injure"). Morbid changes in tissue due to disease or injury.

Lesions of this funiculus therefore will be manifested clinically as loss or diminution of the following sensations:

1. Vibration sense
2. Position sense
3. Two-point discrimination
4. Touch
5. Weight perception

The presence or absence of these different sensations is tested by the neurologist as follows:

1. Vibration is tested by placing a vibrating tuning fork over a bony prominence.
2. Position sense is tested by moving the tip of the patient's finger or toe dorsally and ventrally and asking the patient (with eyes closed) to identify the position of the part moved.
3. Two-point discrimination is tested by simultaneously pricking or touching the patient in two adjacent areas of skin. Under normal conditions, a person is able to recognize these two simultaneous stimuli as separate stimuli if the distance between them is not less than 5 mm on the fingertips using pins and not less than 10 cm on the shin using fingertips.
4. Touch is tested by placing a cotton ball gently over the skin.
5. Weight perception is tested by asking the patient (with eyes closed) to estimate roughly the weight of an object placed in the hand.

The nerve fibers that contribute to the posterior funiculus have their cell bodies in the dorsal root **ganglia.**

Ganglion (Greek "swelling, knot"). A collection of nerve cells outside the central nervous system, as in dorsal root ganglia or autonomic ganglia.

Receptor (Latin *recipere*, "to receive"). The sensory nerve ending or sensory organ that receives sensory stimuli.

Peripheral **receptors** contributing to this system are (1) cutaneous mechanoreceptors (hair follicle and touch pressure receptors) that convey the sensations of touch, vibration, hair movement, and pressure and (2) proprioceptive receptors (muscle spindle, Golgi tendon organ, and joint receptors). Muscle receptors (muscle spindles and Golgi tendon organs) are the primary receptors conveying position sense. Joint receptors may be concerned with signaling joint movement but not joint position.

Nerve fibers of the posterior funiculus are thickly myelinated and occupy the dorsolateral part of the dorsal root. Those which enter the spinal cord below the sixth thoracic segment are located medially in the posterior funiculus and form the gracile tract. Fibers that enter the spinal cord above the sixth thoracic segment are located more laterally and form the cuneate tract. Thus the nerve fibers in the

KEY CONCEPTS

- Posterior funiculus tracts convey conscious proprioceptive sensory modalities, especially those actively explored by the individual perceived at cortical level.
- The fibers in the posterior funiculus are somatotopically organized into a medial gracile and a lateral cuneate tract. The latter appears in sections above the mid-dorsal level.

posterior funiculus are laminated or layered in such a way that those arising from the sacral region are most medial, whereas those from the cervical region are most lateral (Fig. 3-7). It should be pointed out that the lamination in the posterior funiculus is both segmental (sacral, lumbar, thoracic, cervical) and modality oriented. Physiologic studies have shown that fibers conducting impulses from hair receptors are superficial and are followed by fibers mediating **tactile** and vibratory sensations in successively deeper layers.

Tactile (Latin *tactilis,* "touching"). Pertaining to touch.

The fibers forming the posterior funiculus ascend throughout the spinal cord and synapse on the posterior (dorsal) column nuclei (nucleus gracilis and nucleus cuneatus) in the medulla oblongata. Axons of these nuclei then cross in the midline to form the medial lemniscus, which ascends to the thalamus and from there to the primary sensory (somesthetic) cortex.

Approximately 85 percent of ascending fibers in the posterior funiculus are primary **afferents.** These have cell bodies in the dorsal root ganglia and are activated by stimulation of mechanoreceptors (unimodal afferents). Approximately 15 percent of fibers in the posterior funiculus are nonprimary afferents. These have cell bodies in the dorsal root ganglion, establish synapses in laminae III to V in the posterior (dorsal) horns of the cervical and lumbar enlargements, and are activated by stimulation of both mechanoreceptors and nociceptors (polymodal afferents).

Afferent (Latin *afferre,* "to carry to"). Conveying impulses inward to a part or organ. Toward the spinal cord.

Some of the fibers in the posterior funiculus send collateral branches that terminate (synapse) on neurons in the posterior horn gray matter. Such collaterals give the posterior funiculus a role in modifying sensory activity in the posterior horn. As discussed later, this role is inhibitory to pain impulses.

Lesions in the posterior funiculus decrease the threshold to painful stimuli and augment all forms of sensations conveyed by the spinothalamic pathways. Thus nonpainful stimuli become painful, and painful stimuli are triggered by lower stimulation thresholds.

Stimulation of the posterior funiculus has been used in the treatment of chronic pain. In one large study, 47 percent of treated patients responded initially to this stimulation, but the percentage dropped to 8 percent after 3 years. None of the patients studied had complete relief from pain.

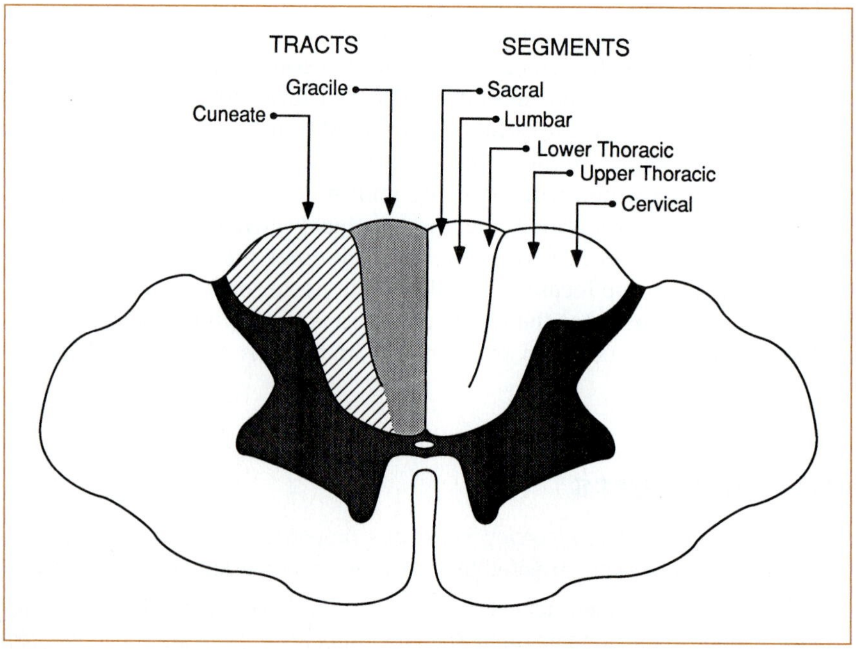

FIGURE 3-7

Schematic diagram of the spinal cord showing spatial arrangement of fibers in the posterior funiculus.

Reports in the literature describe lesions in the posterior funiculus in humans and animals without concomitant deficit in the sesory modalities presumably carried by this system. This is explained by the presence of another system, the spinocervical thalamic, located in the lateral funiculus, which may compensate for some posterior funiculus deficits.

The role of the dorsal (posterior) column (funiculus) system in sensory transmission and appreciation has been studied extensively in both humans and experimental animals (Table 3-5). Sensory stimuli conducted via the posterior column are generally of three types: (1) those which are impressed passively on the organism, (2) those which have temporal or sequential factors added to a spatial cue, and (3) those which cannot be recognized without manipulation and active exploration by the digits. The first type, stimuli that are impressed passively on the organism (e.g., vibrating tuning fork, two-point discrimination, touch with a piece of cotton), are transmitted by the dorsal column. However, much the same information is transmitted by a number of parallel pathways such as the spinocervical thalamic tract. Thus such passive types of sensations remain intact in the absence of the dorsal column. The second type, stimuli, with temporal or sequential factors added to a spatial cue (e.g., determination of the direction of lines that are drawn on the skin), are detected by the dorsal column. The dorsal column has the inherent function of transmission to higher central nervous system centers information concerning the changes in a peripheral stimulus over a period of time. The third type, stimuli that cannot be recognized without manipulation and active exploration by the digits (e.g., detection of shapes and patterns), are appreciated only by the dorsal column.

In addition to its role in sensory transmission, the dorsal column has a role in certain types of motor control. Many movements involving the extremities depend on sensory information that is fed back to the brain from peripheral sensory organs such as muscle spindles, joint receptors, and cutaneous receptors. Many of these feedback inputs travel via the dorsal column. The dorsal column transmits to the motor cortex of the brain (via the thalamus) information necessary to plan, initiate, program, and monitor tasks that involve manipulative movements by the digits. The thalamic nucleus (ventral posterolateral) that receives input from the dorsal column system has been shown to project not only to the primary somesthetic (postcentral gyrus) sensory cortex but also to the primary motor cortex in the precentral gyrus. In addition, the primary sensory cortex projects to the primary motor cortex.

A frequently reported observation in lesions of the posterior column is the discrepancy in loss of vibration and position sense. A possible explanation for this differential loss is that different pathways are used for transmission of the two

TABLE 3-5

Dorsal Column System Function

	Dorsal Column	
Type of Stimulus	Transmits	Essential For
1. Passively impressed (vibration, two-point discrimination, touch)	Yes	No
2. Temporal or sequential (direction of line drawn on skin)	Yes	Yes
3. Actively explored and manipulated (detection of shapes and patterns)	Yes	Yes

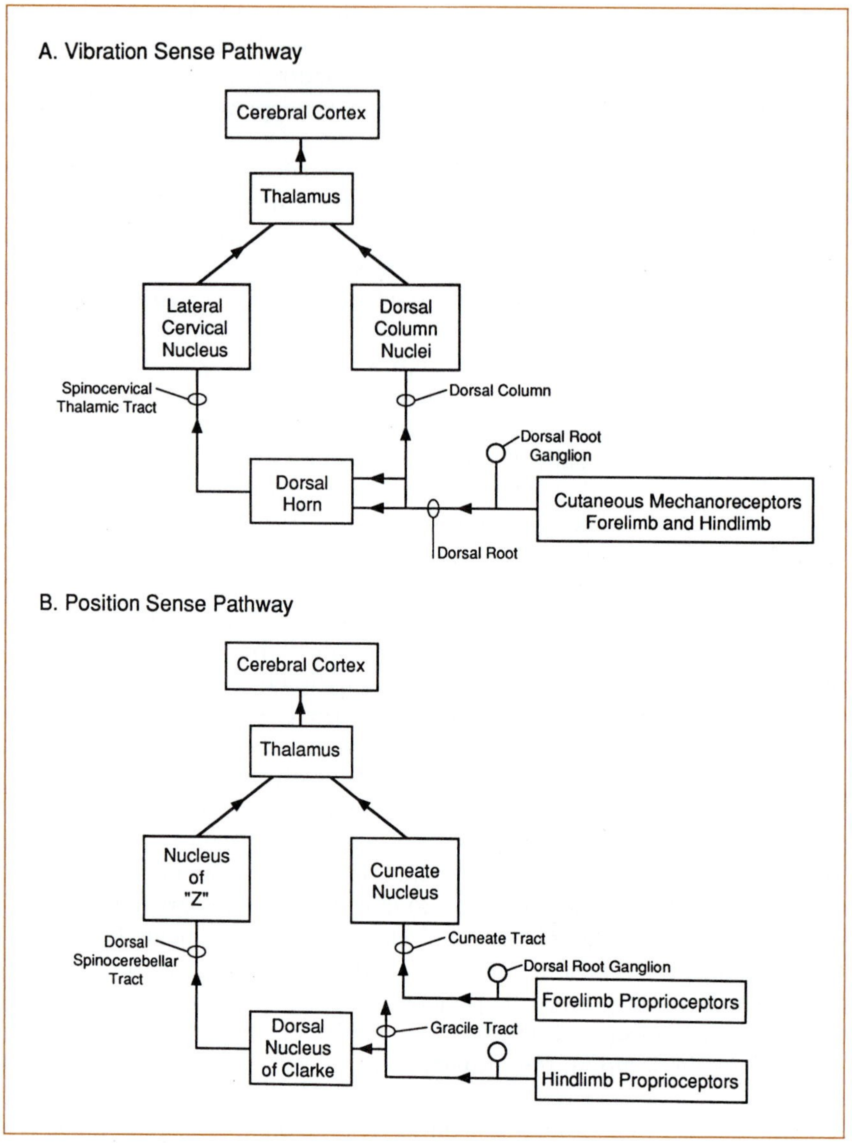

FIGURE 3-8

Schematic diagram showing the different pathways for cutaneous and proprioceptive sensations from fore- and hindlimbs.

modalities. In experimental animals it has been shown that cutaneous mechanoreceptors in forelimbs and hindlimbs (conveying touch, vibration, hair movement, and pressure) transmit their impulses via the dorsal columns (cuneate and gracile tracts, respectively) and the spinocervical thalamic tract (Fig. 3-8). In contrast, proprioceptive sensations [from muscle spindle and Golgi tendon organ (position sense) and joint receptors] from the forelimbs utilize the dorsal column (cuneate tract), while those from the hindlimb travel with the gracile tract to the level of the dorsal nucleus of Clarke. From there they leave the gracile tract, synapse in the nucleus dorsalis of Clarke, and travel with the dorsal spinocerebellar fibers to terminate on the nucleus of Z (of Brodal and Pompeiano), a small collection of cells in the most rostral part of nucleus gracilis in the medulla. From there the fibers join the medial lemniscus to reach the thalamus (see Fig. 3-8).

Lateral and Anterior Funiculi

Whereas the posterior funiculus (see Table 3-3) contains only one ascending tract or fiber system (the posterior column system), the lateral and anterior funiculi

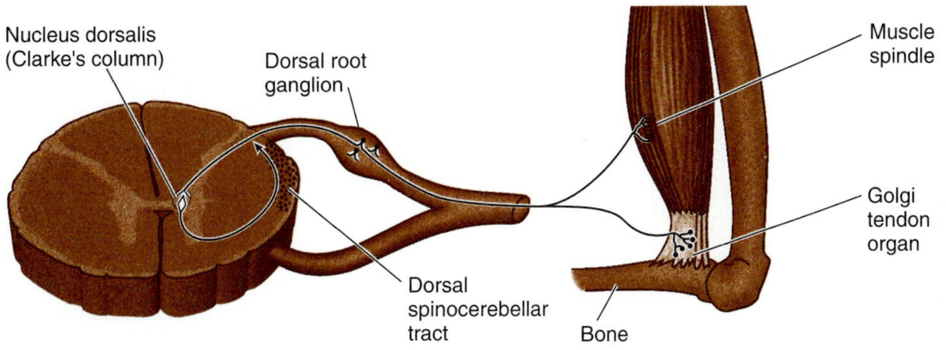

FIGURE 3-9

Schematic diagram of the spinal cord showing the formation of the dorsal spinocerebellar tract.

contain several ascending and descending tracts (see Tables 3-3 and 3-4). Only those tracts with established functional or clinical relevance will be discussed.

Ascending Tracts All the following tracts have their cells of origin in dorsal root ganglia (see Table 3-3).

Dorsal spinocerebellar tract This ascending fiber system conveys to the cerebellum proprioceptive impulses from receptors located in muscles, tendons, and joints. The impulses arising in muscle spindles travel via Ia and II nerve fibers, whereas those arising in Golgi tendon organs travel via Ib nerve fibers. Central processes of neurons in dorsal root ganglia enter the spinal cord via the dorsal root and either ascend or descend in the posterior funiculus for a few segments before reaching the spinal nucleus, or they may reach the nucleus directly. Nerve cells, the axons of which form this tract, are located in the nucleus dorsalis of Clarke (also known as *Clarke's column*) within lamina VII or Rexed (Fig. 3-9). This nucleus is not found throughout the extent of the spinal cord but is limited to the spinal cord segments between the eighth cervical (C-8) and second lumbar (L-2). Because of this, the dorsal spinocerebellar tract is not seen below the second lumbar segment. Nerve fibers belonging to this system and entering below L-2 ascend to the L-2 level, where they synapse with cells located in the nucleus. Similarly, nerve fibers entering above the upper limit of the nucleus ascend in the cuneate tract to reach the accessory cuneate nucleus in the medulla oblongata, which is homologous to the nucleus dorsalis (Fig. 3-10). Fibers in this tract are segmentally laminated in such a way that fibers from lower limbs are placed superficially. The fibers in this tract reach the cerebellum via the inferior cerebellar peduncle (restiform body) and terminate on the rostral and caudal portions of the vermis. The dorsal spinocerebellar tract conveys to the cerebellum information pertaining to muscle contraction, including phase, rate, and strength of contraction.

There is evidence to suggest that some of the fibers forming this tract arise from neurons in laminae V and VI of Rexed, as well as from the nucleus dorsalis of Clarke.

KEY CONCEPTS

- Unconscious proprioception is conveyed by the spinocerebellar tracts in the lateral funiculus.
- The dorsal spinocerebellar tract is seen in spinal cord segments above the second lumbar vertebra.

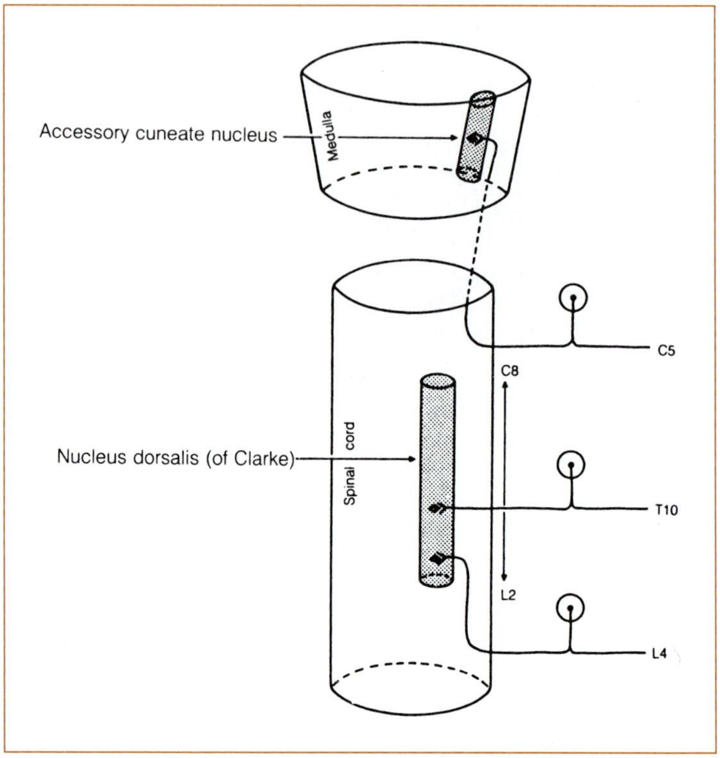

FIGURE 3-10

Schematic diagram of the spinal cord showing the homology of the accessory cuneate nucleus and the nucleus dorsalis of Clarke.

Ventral spinocerebellar tract This fiber system conveys impulses almost exclusively from Golgi tendon organs via Ib afferents. Dorsal root fibers destined for this tract synapse with neurons in laminae V to VII of Rexed. Axons arising from these neurons then cross to form the ventral spinocerebellar tract, which ascends throughout the spinal cord, medulla oblongata, and pons before entering the contralateral cerebellum via the superior cerebellar peduncle (brachium conjunctivum). Thus the fibers of this tract cross twice, once in the spinal cord and again before entering the cerebellum. The majority of fibers in this tract terminate in the vermis and intermediate lobe, mostly homolateral to the limb of origin but also contralateral. The ventral spinocerebellar tract transmits, to the cerebellum, information related to interneuronal activity and the effectiveness of the descending pathways.

In addition to the preceding classic spinocerebellar pathways, there are at least two other indirect pathways from the spinal cord to the cerebellum:

1. The spinoolivocerebellar pathway, with an intermediate station at the inferior olive in the medulla oblongata
2. The spinoreticulocerebellar pathway, with an intermediate synapse in the lateral reticular nucleus of the medulla

The impulses traveling via the indirect spinocerebellar pathways reach the cerebellum after a longer latency than that observed with the more direct spinocerebellar pathways. It is postulated that impulses traveling via the classic direct pathway reach the cerebellum sooner and will condition it for the reception of impulses arriving later via the indirect pathways.

Spinocervical thalamic tract (*Morin's tract*) Nerve fibers destined to form the spinocervical thalamic tract are central processes of dorsal root ganglia. They enter the spinal cord with the thickly myelinated fibers of the medial division of the dorsal root. They travel within the posterior funiculus for several segments before entering the posterior horn gray matter to synapse on neurons there. Axons of neurons in the posterior horn ascend in the lateral funiculus to the upper two or three cervical segments, where they synapse on neurons of the lateral cervical nucleus. Axons of this nucleus cross to the opposite lateral funiculus and ascend to the thalamus (see Fig. 3-8). The lateral cervical nucleus is organized somatotopically (similar to the posterior column nuclei) and similarly receives an input from the cerebral cortex.

The spinocervical thalamic tract accounts for the presence of kinesthesia and discriminative touch after total interruption of the posterior funiculus. Although this tract has not been demonstrated in humans, its presence has been assumed because of the persistence of posterior funiculus sensations after total posterior funiculus lesions. Thus the older concept of the necessity of the posterior funiculus for discriminatory sensation is being challenged. Instead, a newer concept is evolving that attributes to the posterior funiculus a role in the discrimination of those sensations which an animal must explore actively and to the spinocervical thalamic system a role in the discrimination of sensations that are impressed passively on the organism.

Lateral spinothalamic tract This ascending fiber tract is located medial to the dorsal and ventral spinocerebellar tracts (Fig. 3-11) and is concerned with transmission of pain and temperature sensations. Root fibers contributing to this tract (C-fibers and A-delta fibers) have their cell bodies in dorsal root ganglia. They are unmyelinated and thinly myelinated fibers that generally occupy the ventrolateral region of the dorsal root as it enters the spinal cord. C-fibers conduct slowly at 0.5 to 2 m/s. A-delta fibers conduct faster at 5 to 30 m/s. Incoming root fibers establish synapses in laminae I to VI of Rexed. A-delta and C-fibers terminate in laminae I to III; A-delta fibers terminate in addition in deep layer V. Axons of neurons in these laminae in turn establish synapses with neurons in laminae V to VIII. Axons of tract neurons in laminae V to VIII, as well as some axons arising from neurons in lamina I, cross to the opposite lateral funiculus in the anterior white commissure within one to two segments above their entry level to form the lateral spinothalamic tract. Fibers of sacral origin are located most laterally and those of cervical origin more medially in the tract. This segmental lamination is useful clinically in differentiating lesions within the spinal cord from those compressing the spinal cord from outside. In the former, the cervical fibers are affected early, whereas the sacral fibers are affected either late or not at all. This condition, known clinically as *sacral sparing*, is characterized by preservation of pain and temperature sensations in the sacral dermatomes and their loss or diminution in other dermatomes. In addition to this segmental lamination, the lateral spinothalamic tract exhibits modality lamination, in which fibers converying pain sensations are located anteriorly and those conveying thermal sense are located most posteriorly. This segregation of fibers in a modality pattern, however, is incomplete. Once formed, this tract ascends throughout the length of the spinal cord and brain stem to reach the thalamus, where its axons synapse on neurons in the ventral posterolateral nucleus.

KEY CONCEPTS

- Pain and thermal sensations are conveyed by the lateral and anterior spinothalamic tracts.
- Pain-conducting fibers in the lateral spinothalamic tract are somatotopically organized. Sacral-originating fibers are more superficially located in the tract.

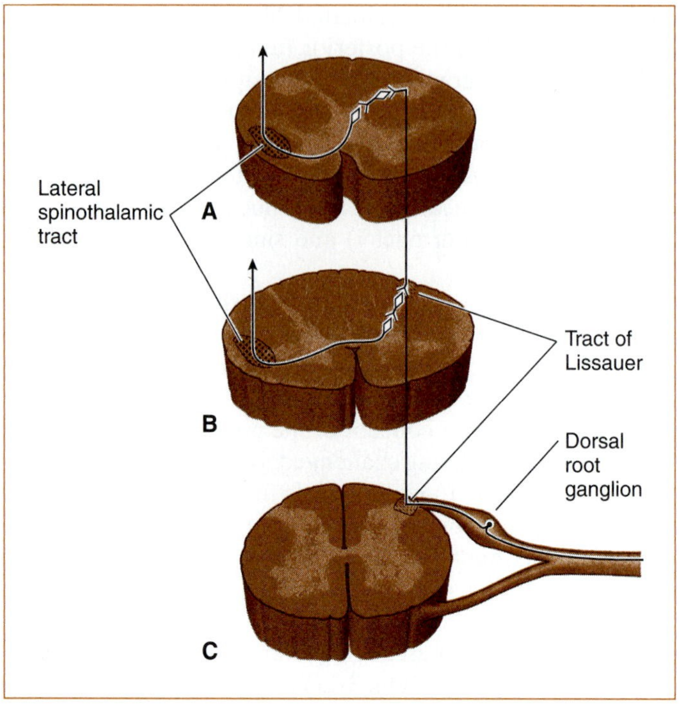

FIGURE 3-11

Schematic diagram showing the formation of the lateral spinothalamic tract.

Lesions of this tract result in loss of pain and thermal sensation in the contralateral half of the body beginning one or two segments below the level of the lesion. In contrast to this pattern of pain and thermal loss, lesions of the dorsal root result in segmental (dermatomal) loss of pain and temperature sensation ipsilateral to the lesion, whereas lesions of the crossing fibers in the anterior white commissure result in bilateral segmental loss of pain and temperature sensation in dermatomes corresponding to the affected spinal segments. This last pattern is often noted in **syringomyelia,** a disease in which the central canal of the spinal cord encroaches on, among other sites, the anterior white commissure.

Syringomyelia (Greek *syrinx*, "a tube"; *myelos*, "marrow"). Tubelike cavitation within the spinal cord.

The lateral spinothalamic tract may be sectioned surgically for the relief of intractable pain. In this procedure, known as *cordotomy*, the surgeon uses the ligamentum denticulatum of the spinal meninges as a landmark and orients the knife anterior to the ligament to reach the tract.

There has been increased interest in pain pathways and pain mechanisms in recent years. These extensive studies have shown that the lateral spinothalamic tract is only one of several pathways carrying pain impulses. Other pathways conveying this modality include a multisynaptic pathway associated with the reticular system and a spinotectal pathway. These studies also have developed the concept of an inhibitory input into the posterior horn from the thickly myelinated fibers of the dorsal root and posterior column. This has led clinicians to stimulate these inhibitory fibers traveling in the posterior column in an attempt to relieve intractable pain.

KEY CONCEPTS

- Sacral sparing of pain sensations in spinal cord lesions denotes an intrinsic lesion.

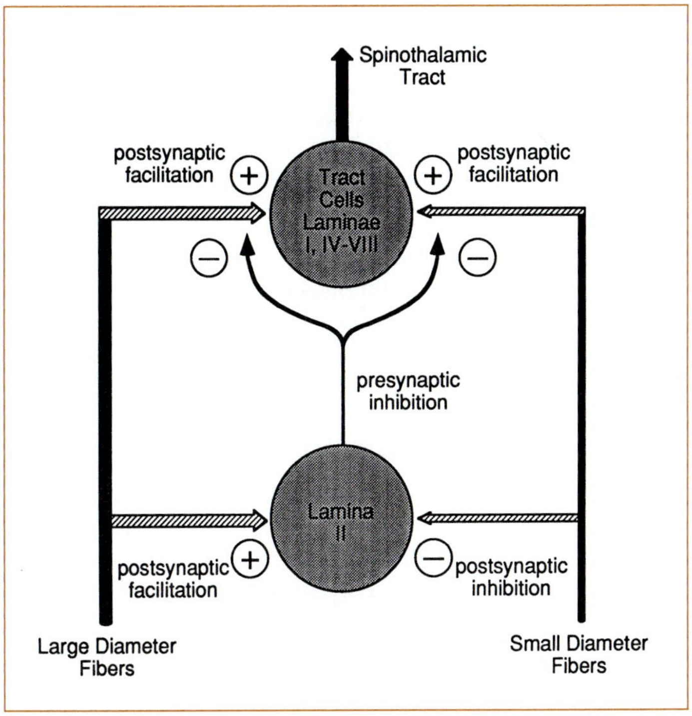

FIGURE 3-12

Schematic diagram of the gate control theory of pain.

Out of these studies on pain mechnaisms has evolved the gate-control theory of pain, proposed by Melzack and Wall (Fig. 3-12). According to this theory, two afferent inputs related to pain enter the spinal cord. One input is via small fibers that are tonic and adapt slowly with a continuous flow of activity, thus keeping the gate open. Impulses along these fibers will activate an excitatory mechanism that increases the effect of arriving impulses. The second input is via large, thickly myelinated fibers that are phasic, adapt rapidly, and fire in response to a stimulus. Both types of fibers project into lamina II of Rexed, which suggests that this lamina is the modular center for pain. The thin fibers inhibit, whereas the thick fibers facilitate, neurons in this lamina. Both types of fibers also project into laminae I and IV to VIII of Rexed, where tract cells are located. Both thin and thick fibers facilitate neurons in these laminae. Furthermore, axons of neurons in lamina II have a presynaptic inhibitory effect on both small and large axons projecting on tract neurons. These different relationships (see Fig. 3-12) can be summarized as follows:

1. Ongoing activity that precedes a stimulus is carried by the tonic, slowly adapting fibers that tend to keep the gate open.
2. A peripheral stimulus will activate both small and large fibers. The discharge of the latter initially will fire the tract cells (T cells) through the direct route

KEY CONCEPTS

- An interplay among thick (fast conducting) and thin (slow conducting) fibers in the transmission of pain impulses is implicated in the gate-control theory of pain transmission.

and then partially close the gate through their action via lamina II (facilitation of presynaptic inhibition).

3. The balance between large- and small-fiber activation will determine the state of the gate. If the stimulus is prolonged, large fibers will adapt, resulting in a relative increase in small-fiber activity that will open the gate further and increase T-cell activity. However, if large-fiber activity is increased by a proper stimulus (vibration), the gate will tend to close, and T-cell activity will diminish.

Since its publication, the gate-control theory has been modified and further clarified. It is now recognized that inhibition occurs by both presynaptic and postsynaptic inputs from the periphery, as well as by descending cortical influences. While it is generally agreed that a gate control for pain exists, its functional role and detailed mechanism need further exploration.

Ongoing research in pain mechanisms has given rise in recent years to much interesting data, some of which are summarized below:

Nociceptive (Latin *noceo*, "to injure"; *capio*, "to take"). Responds to painful injurious stimuli.

1. Two types of pain receptors have been identified: unimodal nociceptors responding to **nociceptive** stimuli and polymodal nociceptors responding to nociceptive, chemical, and mechanical stimuli.
2. Three types of spinothalamic neurons have been identified in the dorsal horn: low-threshold mechanoreceptors in laminae VI to VII, high-threshold, nociceptive-specific nociceptors in lamina I, and wide-dynamic-range neurons in laminae IV and V responding to both mechanoreceptor and nociceptor stimulation. The wide-dynamic-range neurons receive inputs from both low-threshold mechanoreceptors and high-threshold nociceptors and are probably concerned with visceral and referred pain.
3. Only the nociceptor neurons are inhibited by serotonergic fibers from the nucleus raphe magnus of the medulla.
4. Several neurotransmitter substances have been identified in the dorsal horn: norepinephrine and serotonin in the substantia gelantinosa and substance P, somatostatin, and enkephalins in laminae I to III. Substance P has been found to be excitatory, whereas enkephalins are inhibitory.
5. C-fibers entering via the dorsal root terminate on lamina I, lamina II, and lamina III neurons. They excite neurons in all these laminae via axodendritic synapses. Axons of lamina II neurons in turn inhibit neurons of lamina I via axosomatic synapses.
6. A-delta fibers establish excitatory synapses on laminae II and IV neurons. Some terminate on laminae I, III, and V. Since lamina II neurons inhibit lamina I neurons, repetitive stimulation of A-delta fibers can inhibit lamina I neurons significantly. In common practice, this is probably what happens when pain from a cut on the finger is reduced by local pressure (stimulation of A-delta fibers).
7. About 24 percent of sacral and 5 percent of lumbar originating fibers in the lateral spinothalamic tract project to the ipsilateral thalamus.

Anterior spinothalamic tract This tract carries light touch stimuli. Fibers contributing to this tract in the dorsal root establish synapses in laminae VI to VIII. Axons of neurons in these laminae cross in the anterior white commissure over several segments and gather in the lateral and anterior funiculi to form the tract. Somatotopic organization in this tract is similar to that in the lateral spinothalamic tract. The course of this tract in the spinal cord and brain stem is similar to that of the lateral spinothalamic tract. Recent evidence about this tract suggests the following: (1) This tract conveys pain impulses in addition to touch. (2) Some of its fibers ascend ipsilaterally all the way to the midbrain, where they cross in the posterior commissure and project primarily on intralaminar neurons in the thalamus, with some fibers reaching the periaqueductal gray matter in the midbrain. (3) The tract is believed to convey aversive and motivational nondiscriminative pain sensations, in contrast to the lateral spinothalamic tract, which is believed to convey the well-

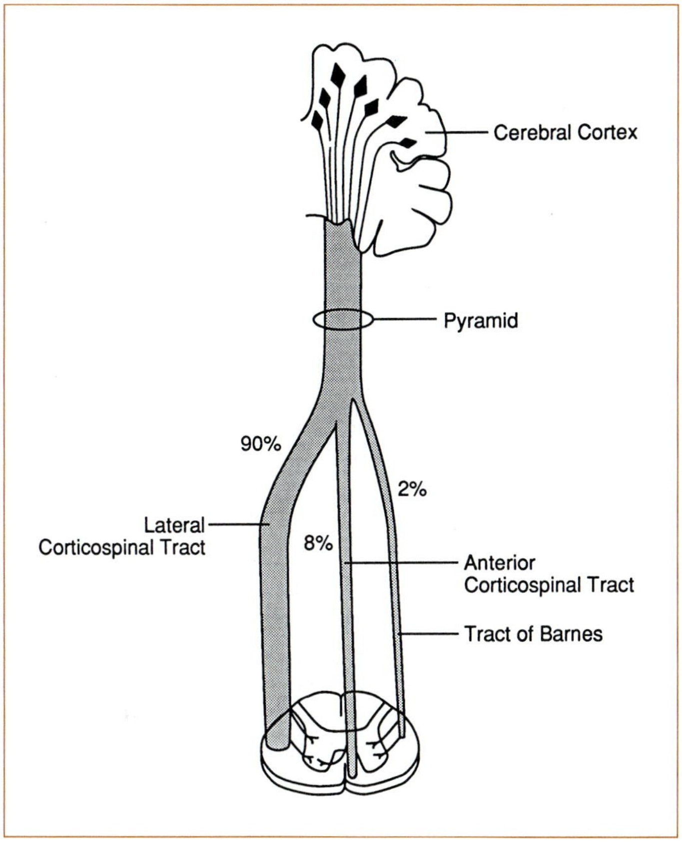

FIGURE 3-13

Schematic diagram showing the three divisions of the corticospinal tract and their patterns of termination in the spinal cord.

localized discriminative pain sensations. The existence of this tract as a separate entity has been questioned. Most authors include this fiber system with the lateral spinothalamic tract. Physiologists tend to refer to the two tracts as the *anterolateral system.*

Other ascending tracts Other ascending tracts of less clinical significance include the spino-olivary, spinotectal, and spinocortical tracts. The functional significance of these multisynaptic pathways is not very well delineated; they may play a role in feedback control mechanisms.

Descending Tracts Whereas all the ascending tracts originate in dorsal root ganglia neurons (see Table 3-3), the descending tracts, in contradistinction, originate from several sites (see Table 3-4). As with the ascending tracts, only the descending tracts of clinical or functional significance will be discussed.

Corticospinal tract The corticospinal tract has the highest level of development in higher primates, especially in humans. The cells of origin of this tract are located in the cerebral cortex. The primary motor cortex (Brodmann's area 4) and the premotor cortex (area 6) contribute 80 percent of the tract. From their site of origin, axons of the corticospinal tract descend throughout the whole length of the neuraxis (brain stem and spinal cord). Approximately one million axons comprise the corticospinal tract on each side. At the caudal end of the medulla oblongata, the majority of corticospinal fibers cross (pyramidal **decussation**) to form the *lateral corticospinal tract*, located in the lateral funiculus of the spinal cord (Fig. 3-13). Fibers in the

Decussation (Latin *decussare*, "to cross like an X"). X-shaped crossing of nerve fiber tracts in the midline, as in pyramidal decussation.

lateral corticospinal tract are organized somatotopically. The cervical fibers are most medial, followed laterally by the thoracic, lumbar, and sacral fibers. The uncrossed fibers remain in the anterior funiculus as the *anterior corticospinal tract* (*bundle of Türck*) (see Fig. 3-13). They, in turn, cross at segmental levels to terminate on **contralateral** motor neurons (see Fig. 3-13). A crossed component of the anterior corticospinal tract has been described, however. It is located in the posterolateral part of the anterior funiculus close to the ventral (anterior) horn. The crossed lateral corticospinal tract extends throughout the spinal cord. The extent of the uncrossed component of the anterior corticospinal tract depends on its size, which is variable. When large, it extends throughout the spinal cord. The crossed component of the anterior corticospinal tract extends to the sixth or seventh cervical segments only. About 2 to 3 percent of the corticospinal fibers remain uncrossed (see Fig. 3-13) in the lateral funiculus (*tract of Barns*) and influence **ipsilateral** motor neurons. The majority of fibers in the corticospinal tract are small in caliber, ranging in diameter from 1 to 4 μm. Only about 3 percent of the fiber population consists of large-caliber fibers (>10 μm in diameter). The large-caliber fibers arise from the giant cells of Betz in the motor cortex. In the spinal cord, corticospinal fibers project on interneurons in laminae IV to VII of Rexed. There is evidence also for a direct projection of a small number of fibers on motor neurons (both alpha and gamma) in lamina IX in the monkey and possibly in humans. The impulses conveyed via the corticospinal tract are facilitatory to flexor motor neurons. Lateral corticospinal tract fibers terminate on motor neurons located in the lateral part of the ventral horn that supply distal limb musculature. Anterior (ventral) corticospinal tract fibers terminate on motor neurons located in the medial part of the ventral horn that supply neck, trunk, and proximal limb musculature (see Fig. 3-13). Stimulation of corticospinal tract fibers results in co-activation of alpha and gamma motor neurons supplying the same muscle and thus simultaneous co-contraction of extrafusal and intrafusal muscles. This co-contraction of the two types of muscles optimizes the sensitivity of the muscle spindle (intrafusal muscle) to changes in muscle length even under conditions of muscle shortening. The termination of the corticospinal tract in laminae IV to VII (which also receive sensory impulses from the periphery) suggests that this tract plays a role in modulation of sensory input to the spinal cord. Evidence for corticospinal tract control of sensory function is provided by terminations of corticospinal tract fibers on primary afferent fibers and sensory relay neurons in the posterior (dorsal) horn of the spinal cord. Corticospinal tract terminals exert presynaptic inhibition on some primary afferents and postsynaptic inhibition or excitation of sensory relay neurons. The presynaptic inhibition of primary afferents determines what type of sensory information is allowed to reach higher levels even before this information is relayed to sensory relay neurons in the dorsal horn or elsewhere. The postsynaptic inhibition or excitation of sensory relay neurons in the dorsal horn modulates activity of those neurons which are involved in the transmission of somesthetic and proprioceptive information to the thalamus and cerebral cortex.

Contralateral (Latin *contra*, "opposite"; *latus*, "side"). Pertaining to or projecting to the opposite side.

Ipsilateral (Latin *ipse*, "self"; *latus*, "side"). Pertaining or projecting to the same side.

The corticospinal tract is essential for skill and precision in movement and the execution of discrete fine finger movements. It cannot by itself, however, initiate these movements. Other corticofugal (cortically originating) fibers are needed. An

KEY CONCEPTS

- The lateral and anterior corticospinal tracts convey motor impulses from wide areas of the cerebral cortex to spinal cord motor and sensory neurons.
- Corticospinal tracts are essential for skilled and precise movements.

intact corticospinal tract is not essential for production of voluntary movement but is necessary for speed and agility during these movements. It also serves to regulate sensory relay processes and thus selects what sensory modality reaches the cerebral cortex.

Lesions of the corticospinal tract result in **paralysis.** If the lesion occurs above the level of the pyramidal decussation, paralysis will be contralateral to the side of the lesion. If the corticospinal tract lesion is below the decussation (i.e., in the spinal cord), the paralysis will be homolateral (ipsilateral) to the side of the lesion. In addition to paralysis, lesions in the corticospinal tract result in a conglomerate of neurologic signs that includes (1) spasticity (resistance to the initial phase of passive movement of a limb or muscle group), (2) hyperactive **myotatic** reflexes (exaggerated response of knee-jerk and other deep tendon reflexes), (3) Babinski sign (abnormal flexor reflex in which stroking the lateral aspect of the sole of the foot results in dorsiflexion of the big toe and fanning out of the other toes), and (4) clonus (an alternating contraction of antagonistic muscles resulting in a series of extension and flexion movements). Collectively, this conglomerate of signs is referred to by clinicians as *upper motor neuron signs.* Usually, there is sparing of muscles of the upper face, mastication, trunk, and respiration, presumably because these muscles are innervated bilaterally from the motor cortex.

Paralysis (Greek *paralusis*, "to disable"). Loss of voluntary movement.

Myotatic (Greek *myo*, "muscle"; *teinein*, "to stretch"). Performed or induced by stretching or extending muscle.

Rubrospinal tract Neurons of origin of the **rubro**spinal tract are located in the posterior two-thirds of the red nucleus in the midbrain. Fibers forming this tract cross in the ventral tegmental decussation of the midbrain and descend throughout the whole length of the neuraxis to reach the lateral funiculus of the spinal cord in close proximity to the corticospinal tract (Fig. 3-14). They terminate in the same laminae as the corticospinal tract and similarly facilitate flexor motor neurons. Because of the similarity in the site of termination of both tracts, and because the red nucleus receives an input from the cortex, the rubrospinal tract has been considered by some as an indirect corticospinal tract. The two tracts constitute the dorsolateral pathway for movement, in which the corticospinal tract initiates movement and the rubrospinal corrects errors in movement.

Rubro (Latin *ruber*, "red"). Rubrospinal tract originates from the red nucleus.

Lateral vestibulospinal tract The neurons of origin of this tract lie in the lateral vestibular nucleus located in the pons. From their site of origin, fibers descend uncrossed and occupy a position in the lateral funiculus of the spinal cord (Fig. 3-15). The fibers in this tract terminate on interneurons in laminae VII and VIII, with some direct terminations on alpha motor neuron dendrites in the same laminae. The impulses conducted in this system facilitate extensor motor neurons that maintain upright posture.

Medial vestibulospinal tract The neurons of origin of the medial vestibulospinal tract are located in the medial vestibular nucleus. From their neurons of origin, fibers join the ipsilateral and contralateral medial longitudinal fasciculi, descend in

KEY CONCEPTS

- Subcortically originating descending tracts in the spinal cord include the vestibulospinal, reticulospinal, and rubrospinal.
- Cortically and subcortically originating tracts facilitate selectively either flexor or extensor motor neurons.
- Subcortically originating tracts contribute to stereotyped movement patterns.

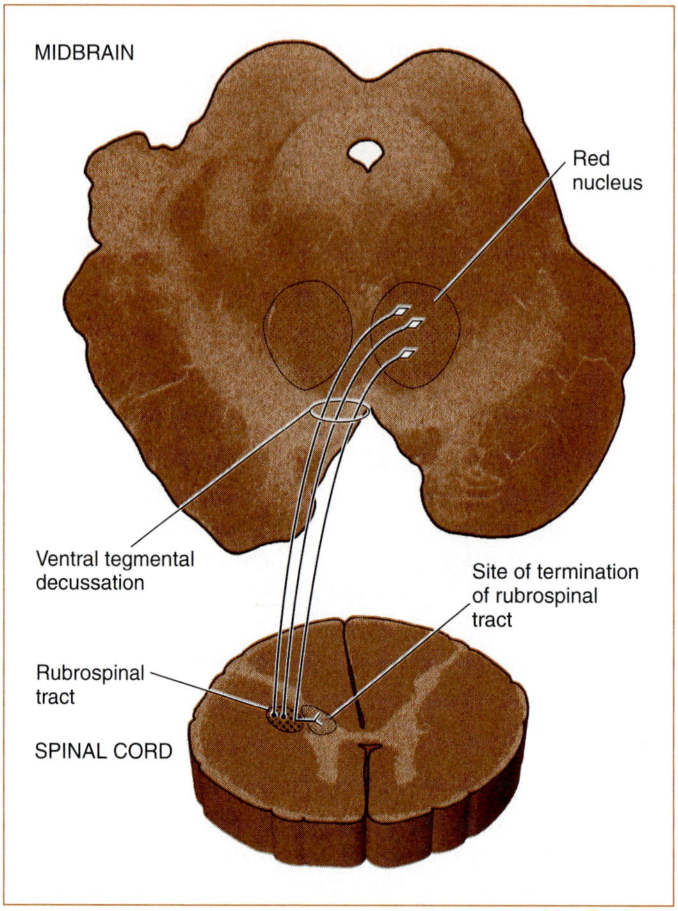
MIDBRAIN
Red nucleus
Ventral tegmental decussation
Site of termination of rubrospinal tract
Rubrospinal tract
SPINAL CORD

FIGURE 3-14

Composite schematic diagram of the origin, course, and termination of the rubrospinal tract.

the anterior funiculus of the cervical cord segments, and terminate on neurons in laminae VII and VIII. They exert a facilitatory effect on flexor motor neurons. The tract plays a role in control of head position.

Reticulospinal tracts The neurons of origin of these tracts are located in the reticular formation of the pons and medulla oblongata. The pontine reticulospinal tract is located in the anterior funiculus of the spinal cord, whereas the medullary reticulospinal tract is located in the lateral funiculus. Both tracts descend predominantly ipsilaterally, but both have, in addition, some crossed components. The pontine reticulospinal tract facilitates extensor motor neurons, whereas the medullary reticulospinal tract facilitates flexor motor neurons.

Earlier studies suggested that reticulospinal fibers arise from large reticular neurons in the medial two-thirds of the medulla and pons. Recent studies show that these fibers originate from many smaller cells. Rostrally originating reticulospinal fibers (pons and rostral medulla) are fast conducting (monosynaptic). Caudally originating reticulospinal fibers (caudal medulla) are slow conducting (multisynaptic). Pontine originating fibers terminate in laminae VII and VIII of Rexed, whereas medullary originating fibers terminate primarily in lamina VII. Some medullary originating fibers interact with motoneuron dendrites in laminae VII and VIII. In addition to influencing motor neurons, reticulospinal fibers modify sensory activity through their interaction with spinothalamic neurons in the dorsal horn.

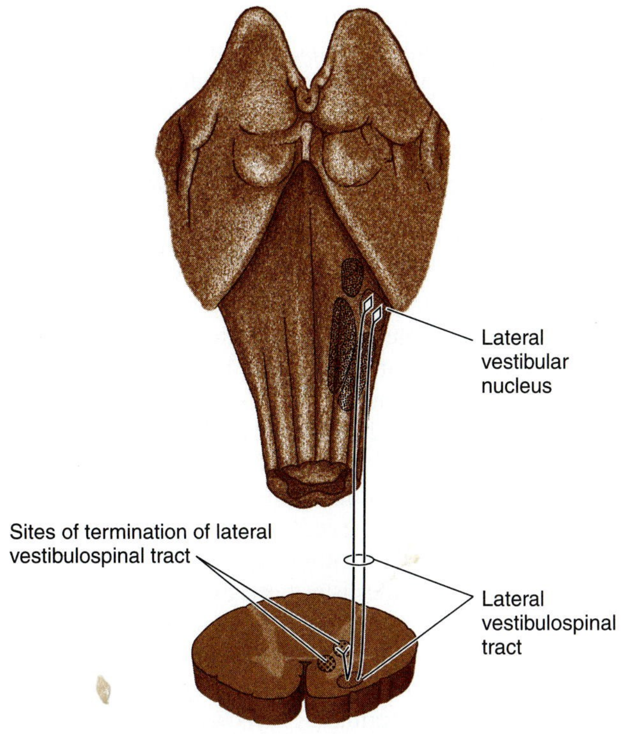
Lateral
vestibular
nucleus
Sites of termination of lateral
vestibulospinal tract
Lateral
vestibulospinal
tract

FIGURE 3-15

Composite schematic diagram of the origin, course, and termination of the lateral vestibulospinal tract.

Tectospinal tract From their neurons of origin in the superior colliculus of the midbrain, fibers of this tract cross in the dorsal tegmental decussation in the midbrain and descend throughout the neuraxis to occupy a position in the anterior funiculus of the cervical spinal cord. Fibers of this tract terminate on neurons in laminae VI, VII, and VIII. The function of this tract is not well understood; it is believed to play a role in the turning of the head in response to light stimulation.

Descending ***autonomic*** *pathway* Fibers belonging to this descending system originate predominantly from the hypothalamus. They are small-caliber fibers that follow a polysynaptic route and are scattered diffusely in the anterolateral funiculus of the spinal cord. They project on neurons in the intermediolateral cell column. Lesions of this system result in autonomic disturbances. If the lesion involves the sympathetic component of this system at or above the T-1 level, a characteristic syndrome known as *Horner's syndrome*, or *Bernard-Horner syndrome*, will result. This syndrome is manifested by (1) miosis (small pupil), (2) pseudoptosis (minimal drooping of the eyelid), (3) anhidrosis (absence of sweating) of the face, and (4) enophthalmos (slight retraction of the eyeball). All these signs occur on the same side as the lesion and are due to interruption of sympathetic innervation to the dilator pupillae, tarsal plate, sweat glands of the face, and retro-orbital fat, respectively.

Autonomic (Greek *autos*, "self"; *nomos*, "law"). Self-governing. The part of the nervous system concerned with visceral (involuntary) processes.

KEY CONCEPTS

- Descending autonomic pathways travel in the anterolateral funiculus.

Descending monoaminergic pathways Serotonergic fibers from the raphe nucleus of the medulla oblongata, noradrenergic fibers from the nucleus locus ceruleus in the rostral pons and caudal midbrain, and enkephalinergic fibers from the periaqueductal gray matter in midbrain descend in the lateral and anterior funiculi. They descend both ipsilateral and contralateral to their site of origin.

Spinal Cord Neurotransmitters and Neuropeptides

The majority of primary sensory neurons in the dorsal horn release glutamate as a rapidly acting excitatory neurotransmitter irrespective of the sensory modality conveyed by the afferent fiber. In addition to glutamate, many small-diameter neurons in the dorsal horn also release neuropeptide transmitters, notably substance P, somatostatin, and vasoactive intestinal peptides. These are believed to mediate slow synaptic transmission. Other neurotransmitters and neuromodulators (peptide neurotransmitters) in the spinal cord include norepinephrine, serotonin, enkephalin, neuropeptide Y, peptide hystidyl isoleucine, and cholecystokinin. Neuropeptides are most abundant in the dorsal horn, followed in decreasing intensity by the intermediate zone and the anterior (ventral) horn. The lumbosacral region has more neuropeptides compared with other regions of the spinal cord. While the exact function of most neuropeptides is not established with absolute certainty, the following observations have been reported: Substance P is the neurotransmitter of primary nociceptive and non-nociceptive afferents in the dorsal horn. The marked reduction of substance P immunoreactivity in lamina II in patients with profound analgesia in the familial dysautonomia (Riley-Day) **syndrome** supports a role for this neuropeptide in pain transmission. Met-enkephalin and somatostatin (SST) in the dorsal horn inhibit release of substance P from primary afferents and inhibit activity in dorsal horn neurons. Vasoactive intestinal peptide (VIP) is the major neurotransmitter in visceral (especially pelvic) afferents and is found abundantly in lumbosacral segments of the cord. Substance P, Met-enkephalin, and cholecystokinin (CCK) in the intermediate zone are terminals from caudal raphe nuclei of the brain stem. Substance P and serotonin from the caudal raphe nuclei participate in the modulation of motor neuron activity in the anterior horn. Norepinephrine from the locus ceruleus has an inhibitory effect on nociceptive activity in the dorsal horn.

Syndrome (Greek *syndromos*, "running together"). A group of symptoms and signs that characterize a disease.

Micturition Pathway and Bladder Control

The urinary bladder receives efferent innervation from three sources: (1) sympathetic supply via the hypogastric nerve, (2) parasympathetic supply via the pelvic nerve, and (3) **somatic** supply via the pudendal nerve. The sympathetic preganglionic neurons are in the intermediolateral cell column in the upper lumbar cord. Preganglionic axons leave the cord via the ventral root and synapse in paravertebral and preaortic sympathetic ganglia. Postganglionic fibers travel in the hypogastric nerve to smooth muscles of bladder wall, internal sphincter, and urethra. Parasympathetic preganglionic neurons are in the intermediolateral-like cell column between the second and fourth sacral segments (S-2 and S-4). Preganglionic axons join the pelvic splanchnic nerves (nervi erigentes) to terminal ganglia and innervate smooth muscles in bladder wall, internal sphincter, and urethra. Somatic neurons are motor

Somatic (Greek *somatikos*, "of the body"). Pertaining to body as distinct from visceral; pertaining to viscera. Includes neurons and neural processes related to skin, muscles, and joints.

KEY CONCEPTS

- Several neuropeptides have been identified in the spinal cord. They are most abundant in the dorsal horn and least abundant in the ventral horn.

neurons in the ventral-ventromedial parta of the anterior (ventral) horn of S-2 to S-4 (nucleus of Onufrowicz). Axons travel with the ventral root, join the pudendal nerve, and innervate the external urethral sphincter.

Afferent impulses from the bladder, urethra, sphincters, and related pelvic muscles enter the cord via the same three nerves. Sympathetic afferents travel via the hypogastric nerve, enter the cord at the upper lumbar level, and may extend rostrally up to the fourth thoracic segment (T-4), but most are in the upper lumbar and low thoracic levels. Parasympathetic afferents travel via the pelvic nerves and enter the cord between S-2 and S-4. Somatic afferents travel via the pudendal nerves and enter the cord at S-2 to S-4 levels.

Descending pathways for micturition travel in the lateral funiculus just ventral to the denticulate ligament and lateral corticospinal tract. They play a role in starting and stopping micturition and in inhibiting the independent reflex activity of the sacral bladder center. The role of the corticospinal tracts in controlling the external sphincter and bladder contractions remains uncertain. In motor neuron disease (amyotrophic lateral sclerosis), patients retain bladder control until very late in the disease despite the degeneration in the corticospinal tract. Furthermore, the nucleus of Onufrowicz is spared in motor neuron disease.

Ascending pathways related to micturition also travel in the lateral funiculus ventral to the denticulate ligament, in the region of the spinothalamic tract. They play a role in the conscious appreciation of the desire to micturate.

FUNCTIONAL OVERVIEW OF THE SPINAL CORD

From the preceding it is evident that the spinal cord is organized into three major functional zones: the dorsal horn, the intermediate zone, and the ventral horn.

1. The dorsal horn receives several varieties of sensory information from receptors in the skin surface (exteroceptive), as well as from deeper-lying receptors in joints, tendons, and muscles (**interoceptive**). Cell characteristics in the dorsal horn vary greatly with respect to the extent of their receptive fields and the degree of specificity of the modality received. Information received from the periphery is not merely relayed in the dorsal horn but is modified by virtue of the various peripheral inputs received, as well as by descending influences from the cerebral cortex and subcortical areas. The sum total of this interaction in the dorsal horn is then mediated to motor neurons in lamina IX, to interneurons, or to ascending tracts.
2. The intermediate zone similarly receives a variety of inputs from the dorsal root and dorsal horn, as well as from cortical and subcortical areas. The information received here is integrated and modified before being projected to other zones.
3. The ventral horn receives inputs from the dorsal root (monosynaptic reflex connections), the dorsal horn, the intermediate zone, and the descending tracts. The descending tracts influence motor neurons either directly or indirectly

Interoceptive. Internal surface field of distribution of receptor organs.

KEY CONCEPTS

- Autonomic innervation of the urinary bladder is related to specific nerve cells in the lower thoracic, upper lumbar, and midsacral region of the spinal cord. Somatic innervation of the urinary bladder originates in the nucleus of Onufrowicz in the ventral horn of midsacral spinal cord segments.
- Sensory neurons in the spinal cord are influenced by dorsal roots and/or descending tracts. They in turn convey signals to segmental spinal motor neurons or, via ascending tracts, to the brain stem or cerebral hemispheres.

through interneurons in the intermediate zone. They selectively facilitate flexor motor neurons (corticospinal, rubrospinal, medial vestibulospinal, and medullary reticulospinal tracts) or extensor motor neurons (lateral vestibulospinal and pontine reticulospinal tracts). The output from the ventral horn is via either alpha motor neurons to influence striated musculature or gamma motor neurons to influence intrafusal muscle fibers.

BLOOD SUPPLY

The spinal cord receives its blood supply from the following arteries.

1. Subclavian via the following branches: vertebral, ascending cervical, inferior thyroid, deep cervical, and superior intercostal
2. Aorta via the following branches: intercostal and lumbar arteries
3. Internal iliac via the following branches: iliolumbar and lateral sacral

Branches of the subclavian artery supply the cervical spinal cord and the upper two thoracic segments; the rest of the thoracic spinal cord is supplied by the intercostal arteries. The lumbosacral cord is supplied by the lumbar, iliolumbar, and lateral sacral arteries. Intercostal arteries supply segmental branches to the spinal cord down to the level of the first lumbar cord segment. The largest of these branches, the great ventral radicular artery, enters the spinal cord between the eighth thoracic and fourth lumbar cord segments. This large artery, also known as the *arteria radicularis magna* or *artery of Adamkiewicz*, usually arises on the left side and may be responsible for most of the arterial blood supply of the lower half of the spinal cord in some people.

The vertebral arteries give rise to anterior and posterior spinal arteries in the cranial cavity. The two anterior spinal arteries unite to form a single anterior spinal artery that descends in the anterior median fissure of the spinal cord. The posterior spinal arteries, smaller than the anterior, remain paired and descend in the posterolateral sulci of the spinal cord. All other arteries send branches that enter the intervertebral foramina, penetrate the dural sheath, and divide into anterior and posterior branches (radicular arteries) that accompany the anterior and posterior nerve roots. These radicular arteries contribute to the three major spinal cord arteries: the anterior spinal and the paired posterior spinal arteries. Since most of the radicular arteries contributing to the anterior spinal artery are small, blood supply is mainly dependent on the four to ten of these that are large, of which one or two are located in the cervical region usually at C-6, one or two in the upper thoracic region, and one to three in the inferior thoracic and lumbosacral region, one of which forms the artery of Adamkiewicz. In contrast, the posterior spinal arteries receive from 10 to 20 well-developed radicular arteries. In the lumbosacral cord, the posterior radicular arteries are vestigial and of no clinical significance. Anastomoses between the anterior and posterior spinal arteries occur caudally around the cauda equina. There are very few anastomoses at each segmental level.

The anterior spinal artery gives off a sulcal branch in the anterior median fissure.

KEY CONCEPTS

- Motor neurons in the spinal cord are influenced by segmental sensory neurons and by descending tracts from cortical and/or subcortical sites. In turn, motor neurons influence extrafusal and intrafusal muscle fibers.
- The blood supply of spinal cord is provided by anterior and posterior spinal arteries derived from vertebal and segmental (radicular) arteries. Some spinal cord segments are particularly susceptible to reduction in blood supply.

This branch turns either right or left to enter the spinal cord; only in the lumbar and sacral cords are there both right and left branches. The sulcal arteries are most numerous in the lumbar region and fewest in the thoracic region. Sulcal arteries supply the anterior and intermediolateral gray horns, the central gray matter, and Clarke's column, that is, all the gray matter except the dorsal horn. They also supply the bulk of the white matter of the anterior and lateral funiculi. Thus the anterior two-thirds of the spinal cord is fed from the anterior spinal artery; the remaining third, including the posterior funiculus and posterior horn, is supplied by the two posterior spinal arteries. The outer rim of the spinal cord is supplied by coronal branches that arise from the anterior spinal artery, pass laterally around the cord, and from imperfect anastomoses with the posterior spinal artery branches.

Certain segments of the spinal cord are more vulnerable than others to a compromise in blood flow. The segments that are particularly vulnerable are T-1 to T-4 and L-1. These are regions of the spinal cord that derive their blood supply from two different sources. At the level of T-1 to T-4, for example, the anterior spinal artery becomes small, and its sulcal branches are not adequate to provide the necessary blood supply. These segments are dependent for their blood supply on the radicular branches of the intercostal arteries. If one or more of the intercostal vessels are compromised, the T-1 to T-4 spinal segments could not be supplied adequately by the small sulcal branches of the anterior spinal artery. As a result, a segment or several segments affected would be damaged.

Venous drainage of the spinal cord corresponds to the arterial supply with the following differences:

1. The venous network is denser on the posterior side of the cord compared with the arterial network, which is more dense anteriorly.
2. There is only one posterior spinal vein.
3. Anastomoses between the anterior and posterior spinal veins are more frequent than between the arteries.
4. The territorial drainage from the anterior two-thirds of the spinal cord by the anterior spinal vein and from the posterior one-third by the posterior spinal vein is generally maintained but not immutable.
5. Venous tributaries within and around the spinal cord are much more numerous than arterial tributaries, so venous obstruction rarely damages the spinal cord. From the perispinal venous network, blood drains into anterior and posterior radicular veins and then into dense longitudinal vertebral plexuses located posteriorly and anteriorly in the epidural space. Blood then reaches the external vertebral venous plexus through the intervertebral and sacral foramina.

SUGGESTED READINGS

Adams RW, et al: The distribution of muscle weakness in upper motoneuron lesions affecting the lower limb. *Brain* 1990; 113:1459–1476.

Angaut-Petit D: The dorsal column system: I. Existence of long ascending post-synaptic fibers in the cat's fasciculus gracilis. *Exp Brain Res* 1975; 22:457–470.

Applebaum AE, et al: Nuclei in which functionally identified spinothalamic tract neurons terminate. *J Comp Neurol* 1974; 188:575–586.

Benarroch EE, et al: Segmental analysis of neuropeptide concentrations in normal human spinal cord. *Neurology* 1990; 40:137–144.

Bishop B: Pain: Its physiology and rationale for management. Part I: Neuroanatomical substrate of pain. *Phys Ther* 1980; 60:13–20.

Boivie J: An anatomical reinvestigation of the termination of the spinothalamic tract in the monkey. *J Comp Neurol* 1979; 186:343–370.

Brodal A, Pompeiano O: The vestibular nuclei in the cat. *J Anat* (*Lond*) 1957; 91:438–454.

Broucker TD, et al: Diffuse noxious inhibitory controls in man: Involvement of the spinoreticular tract. *Brain* 1990; 113:1223–1234.

Craig AD, Burton H: The lateral cervical nucleus in

the cat: Anatomic organization of cervicothalamic neurons. *J Comp Neurol* 1979; 185:329–346.

Davidoff RA: The dorsal columns. *Neurology* 1989; 39:1377–1385.

Davidoff RA: The pyramidal tract. *Neurology* 1990; 40:332–339.

Guttmann L: Clinical symptomatology of spinal cord lesions. In Vinken PJ, Bruyn GW (eds): *Handbook of Clinical Neurology,* vol 2. Amsterdam, North-Holland, 1978:178.

Hall JG: Supraspinal inhibition of spinal neurons responding to nociceptive stimulation. *Neurosci Lett* 1979; 14:165–169.

Hughes JT: Vascular disorders. In *Pathology of the Spinal Cord*, vol 6: *Major Problems in Pathology.* Philadelphia, Saunders, 1978:61.

Jankowski E, Lindström S: Morphological identification of Renshaw cells. *Acta Physiol Scand* 1971; 81:428–430.

Kerr FWL, Fukushima T: New observations on the nociceptive pathways in the central nervous system. In Bonica JJ (ed): *Pain: Research Publication: Association for Research in Nervous and Mental Diseases*, vol 58. New York, Raven Press, 1980:47.

Landgren S, Silfvenius H: Nucleus Z, the medullary relay in the projection path to the cerebral cortex of group I muscle afferents from the cat's hind limb. *J Physiol* (*Lond*) 1971; 218:551–571.

Matsushita M, et al: Anatomical organization of the spinocerebellar system in the cat as studied by retrograde transport of horseradish peroxidase. *J Comp Neurol* 1979; 184:81–106.

Moberg E: The role of cutaneous afferents in position sense, kinesthesia, and motor function of the hand. *Brain* 1983; 106:1–19.

Nathan PW, et al: Sensory effects in man of lesions of the posterior columns and of some other afferent pathways. *Brain* 1986; 109:1003–1041.

Nathan PW, et al: The corticospinal tract in man: Course and location of fibers at different segmental levels. *Brain* 1990; 113:303–324.

Priestley JV: Neuroanatomy of the spinal cord: Current research and future prospects. *Paraplegia* 1987; 25:198–204.

Rustioni A, et al: Dorsal column nuclei and ascending spinal afferents in macaque. *Brain* 1979; 102:95–125.

Scheibel ME, Scheibel AB: Inhibition and the Renshaw cell: A structural critique. *Brain Behav Evol* 1971; 4:53–93.

Schmahmann JD, et al: The mysterious relocation of the bundle of Türck. *Brain* 1992; 115:1911–1924.

Schoenen J: The dendritic organization of the human spinal cord: The dorsal horn. *Neuroscience* 1982; 7:2057–2087.

Schoenen J: Dendritic organization of the human spinal cord: The motoneurons. *J Comp Neurol* 1982; 211:226–247.

Smith MC, Deacon P: Topographical anatomy of the posterior columns of the spinal cord in man: The long ascending fibers. *Brain* 1984; 107:671–698.

Triggs WJ, Beric A: Sensory abnormalities and dysoethesias in the anterior spinal artery syndrome. *Brain* 1992; 115:189–198.

Van Keulen LCM: Axon trajectories of Renshaw cells in the lumbar spinal cord of the cat as reconstructed after intracellular staining with horseradish peroxidase. *Brain Res* 1979; 167:157–162.

Wall PD: The role of substantia gelatinosa as a gate control: In Bonica JJ (ed): *Pain: Research Publication: Association for Research in Nervous and Mental Diseases,* vol 58. New York, Raven Press, 1980:205.

Willis D: The case for the Renshaw cell. *Brain Behav Evol* 1971; 4:5–52.

Willis WD, et al: Spinothalamic tract neurons in the substantia gelatinosa. *Science* 1978; 202:986–988.

Willis WD: Studies of the spinothalamic tract. *Tex Rep Biol Med* 1979; 38:1–45.

Willis WD, et al: The cells of origin of the primate spinothalamic tract. *J Comp Neurol* 1979; 188:543–574.

Young RF: Evaluation of dorsal column stimulation in the treatment of chronic pain. *Neurosurgery* 1978; 3:373–379.

CHAPTER 4

CLINICAL CORRELATES OF SPINAL CORD ANATOMY

CLINICALLY IMPORTANT SPINAL CORD STRUCTURES

The following structures (Fig. 4-1) are useful in clinical localization of spinal cord disorders:

1. Descending tracts (motor function): Lateral corticospinal (pyramidal) tract

KEY CONCEPTS

- Lesions of each of the clinically relevant ascending and descending tracts and spinal motor neurons give rise to well-defined and characteristic neurologic signs.

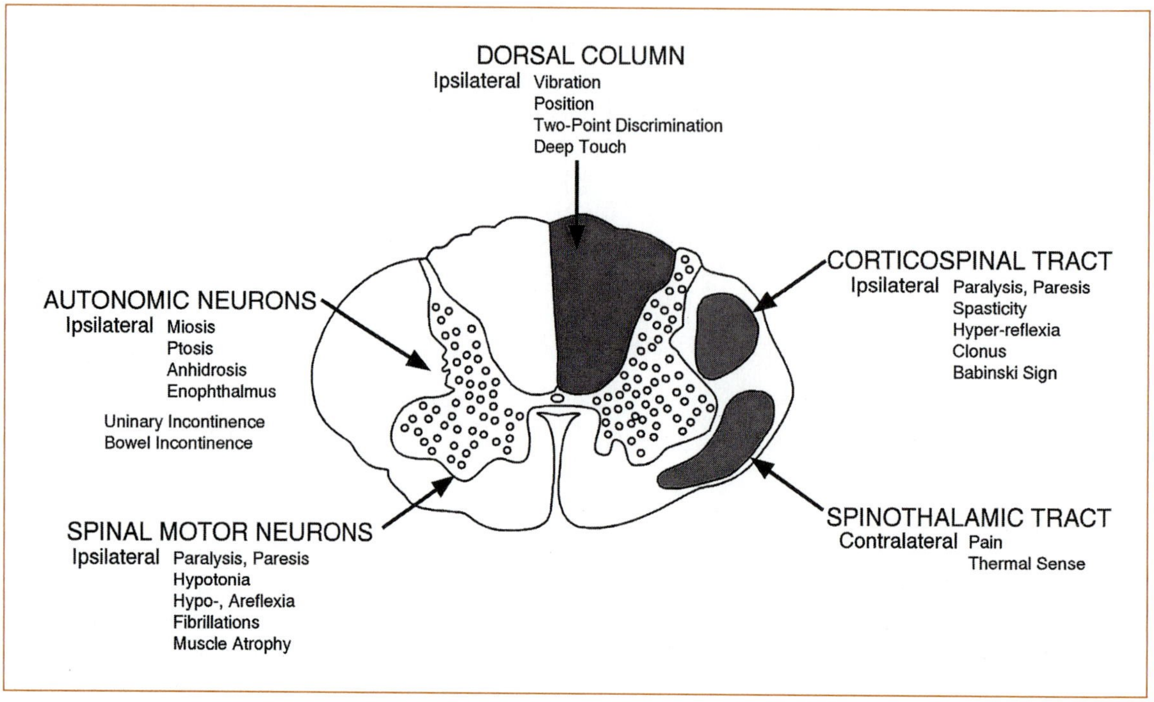

FIGURE 4-1

Schematic diagram of clinically important spinal cord structures and effects of lesions in each.

Kinesthesia (Greek *kinesis,* "motion"; *aisthesis,* "sensation"). Sense of perception of movement.

2. Ascending tracts (sensory function)
   a. Dorsal (posterior) column (**kinesthesia** and discriminative touch)
   b. Lateral spinothalamic tract (pain and temperature)
3. Neuronal populations
   a. Anterior horn cells (somatic motor function)
   b. Intermediolateral cell column (autonomic sympathetic function)
   c. Sacral autonomic neurons (autonomic parasympathetic function)

MOTOR SIGNS OF SPINAL CORD DISORDERS (see Fig. 4-1)

Clonus (Greek *klonos,* "turmoil"). Repetitive involuntary contractions of agonist and antagonist muscles in response to stretch. A sign of upper motor neuron disease.

Babinski Sign. An upper motor neuron sign consisting of dorsiflexion of the big toe and fanning out of the rest of the toes in response to stimulation of the sole of the foot. Described in detail by Josef-Francois-Felix Babinski, French neurologist, in 1896.

It is customary to classify motor signs of spinal cord disease into upper and lower motor neuron signs:

1. Upper motor neuron signs (lesion of corticospinal tract)
   a. Loss (paralysis) or diminution (paresis) of voluntary movement
   b. Increase in muscle tone (spasticity)
   c. Hyperreflexia [exaggerated deep tendon (myotatic) reflexes]
   d. **Clonus** (repetitive involuntary alternating contractions of agonist and antagonist muscle groups in response to sudden maintained stretching force)
   e. Abnormal superficial plantar reflex (**Babinski sign**). The Babinski sign, described by the French neurologist Josef-François-Feleix as "the phenomenon of the toes," consists of dorsiflexion of the hallux and fanning of the toes in response to painful stimulation of the sole of the foot.

   All these signs occur ipsilateral and below the level of the spinal cord lesion.
2. Lower motor neuron signs (lesion of anterior horn cells)
   a. Loss (paralysis) or diminution (paresis) of voluntary movement
   b. Decrease in muscle tone (hypotonia)
   c. Hyporeflexia (decrease) or areflexia (absence) of deep tendon (myotatic) reflexes

   d. **Fibrillations** and/or **fasciculations** (spontaneous activity of muscle fibers at rest)
   e. Muscle atrophy

   All these signs occur ipsilateral and in muscles (myotomes) supplied by the affected motor neurons.

3. Autonomic neuron signs
   a. Intermediolateral (sympathetic) cell column (T-1 to L-2): Lesions in the intermediolateral cell column are associated with the following conglomerate of signs collectively known as the **Horner's syndrome**: miosis (small pupil), pseudoptosis (minimal drooping of eyelids), anhidrosis (absence of sweating over the face), and enophthalmus (slight retraction of eyeball)

   All these signs occur ipsilateral to the lesion in the spinal cord. Johann Friedrich Horner, a Swiss ophthalmologist, is credited with the first complete description of this syndrome in humans, although Claude Bernard described the same ocular changes in animals 7 years earlier. (The syndrome is also known as the *Bernard-Horner syndrome.*)

   b. Sacral autonomic (parasympathetic) neurons (S-2 to S-4): Lesions in the sacral autonomic area are associated with urinary incontinence and bowel incontinence.

Fibrillations. Spontaneous contraction of a single muscle fiber not visible by the naked eye but recorded by electromyography. A sign of denervation.

Fasciculations. Local, spontaneous, contraction of a group of muscle fibers, usually visible under the skin due to denervation. The term was introduced by Derek Denny Brown, English neurologist.

Horner's Syndrome. Drooping of the eyelid (ptosis), constriction of the pupil (miosis), retraction of the eyeball (enophthalmus), and loss of sweating on the face (anhidrosis) comprise a syndrome described by Johann Friedrich Horner, Swiss ophthalmologist, in 1869. The syndrome is due to interruption of descending sympathetic fibers. The syndrome was described in animals by Francois du Petit in 1727. Claude Bernard in France in 1862, and E. S. Hare in England in 1838 gave precise accounts of the syndrome before Horner.

SENSORY SIGNS OF SPINAL CORD DISORDERS

Dorsal (Posterior) Column Signs (Figs. 4-1 and 4-2)

Lesions in the dorsal column are usually associated with diminution or loss of

1. Vibration sense
2. Position sense
3. Two-point discrimination
4. Deep touch

All these signs occur ipsilateral to the affected posterior column in dermatomes at and below the level of the spinal cord lesion.

Lateral Spinothalamic Tract Signs (Figs. 4-1 and 4-3)

Lesions affecting the lateral spinothalamic tract are associated with diminution or loss of

1. Pain sensations
2. Temperature sensations

Deficits in pain and temperature sensations occur contralateral to the affected tract in dermatomes beginning one or two segments below the level of the spinal cord lesions.

Sacral Sparing

Because of the pattern of lamination of nerve fibers in the spinothalamic tract (sacral fibers lateral, cervical fibers medial), extrinsic cord lesions (such as a tumor

KEY CONCEPTS

- A conglomerate of neurologic signs characterizes each of the upper and lower motor neuron syndromes.

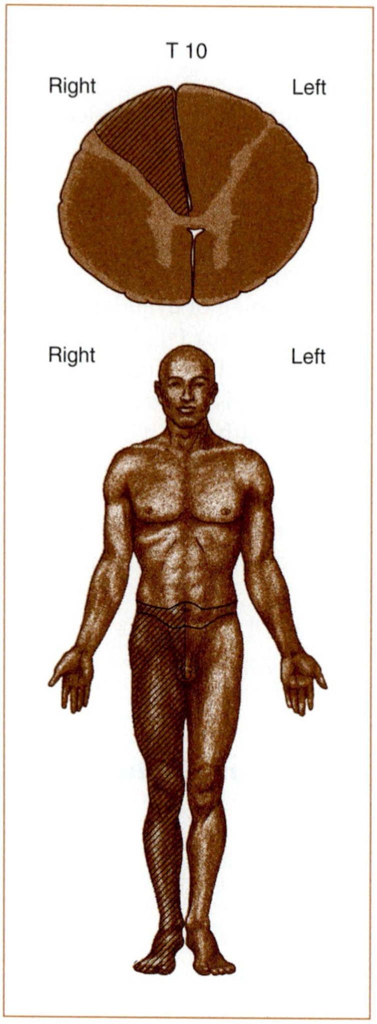

FIGURE 4-2

Schematic diagram showing the pattern of sensory deficit resulting from a lesion in the posterior column.

in the meninges that compresses the spinal cord from the outside) will affect sacral fibers early, whereas intrinsic spinal cord lesions (such as a tumor arising within the spinal cord) will affect cervical fibers early and sacral fibers late or not at all (sacral sparing).

Dorsal Root Signs (Fig. 4-4)

Lesions affecting one or more dorsal roots are associated with diminution or loss of all sensory modalities ipsilateral and in dermatomes supplied by the involved dorsal root(s).

KEY CONCEPTS

- Lesions in the dorsal root, anterior white commissure, or spinothalamic tract give rise to distinct and different patterns of pain and thermal sensation deficits.
- Sacral sparing helps differentiate intrinsic from extrinsic cord lesions.

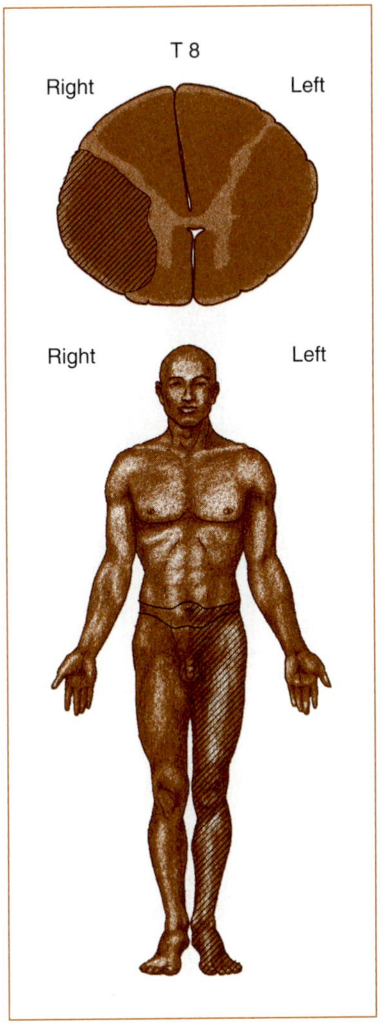

FIGURE 4-3

Schematic diagram showing the pattern of sensory deficit resulting from a lesion in the lateral funiculus involving the lateral spinothalamic tract.

Anterior White Commissure Signs (Fig. 4-5)

Lesions in the anterior white commissure are associated with bilateral diminution or loss of pain and temperature (sensory modalities that cross in the anterior white commissure) sensations in dermatomes supplied by the involved spinal cord segments. Although fibers carrying light touch also travel in the anterior white commissure, no deficit in light touch occurs because this sensory modality is also represented in the posterior column.

SPINAL CORD SYNDROMES

The following clinicopathologic syndromes are encountered in clinical practice.

KEY CONCEPTS

- Signs and symptoms of the different spinal cord syndromes reflect the involvement of neural structures affected in each of the syndromes.

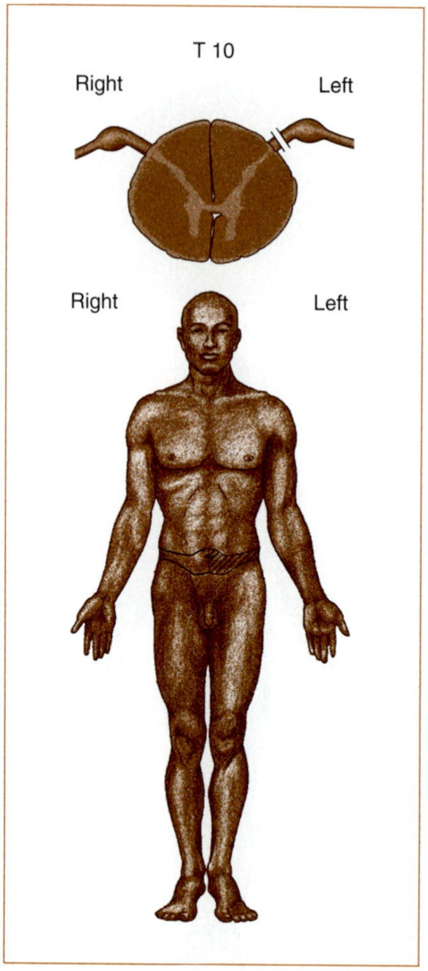
T 10
Right
Left
Right
Left

FIGURE 4-4

Schematic diagram showing the distribution of sensory deficit resulting from a lesion in the dorsal root.

Segmental Lower Motor Neuron Syndrome (Fig. 4-6)

Lesions of spinal motor neurons in the anterior horn are associated with a lower motor neuron syndrome (paralysis, hypotonia, areflexia, muscle atrophy, fasciculations) ipsilateral to the cord lesion and in muscles supplied by the affected spinal cord segments. This syndrome is commonly seen in the disease poliomyelitis.

Hemisection (Brown-Séquard Syndrome) (Fig. 4-7)

Brown-Séquard Syndrome. A spinal cord syndrome characterized by ipsilateral loss of pyramidal and posterior column signs and contralateral spinothalamic signs, due to cord hemisection. Described by Charles Edouard Brown-Séquard, Eurasian and Irish American neurologist, in 1850.

This syndrome is named after the neurologist Charles Edouard Brown-Séquard, who first described the syndrome. The following signs will be detected in hemisection of the spinal cord. The nuclear groups or tracts giving rise to these signs are indicated.

1. *Ipsilateral signs.* Signs ipsilateral to the spinal cord lesion are
   a. Corticospinal tract signs. The following upper motor neuron signs occur below the level of the hemisection:
      (1) Muscle paralysis
      (2) Spasticity
      (3) Hyperactive myotatic reflexes
      (4) Babinski sign
      (5) Clonus

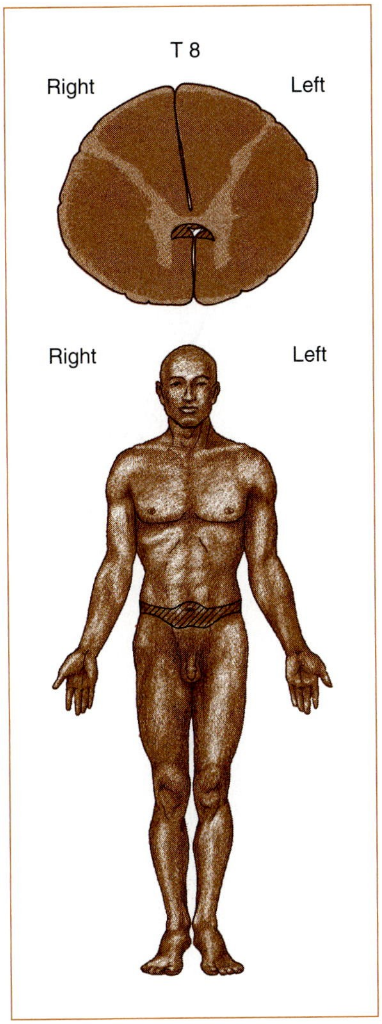
T 8
Right
Left
Right
Left

FIGURE 4-5

Schematic diagram showing the distribution of sensory deficit resulting from a lesion in the anterior white commissure.

b. Posterior column signs. These include loss of the following sensations at and below the level of the hemisection:
   (1) Vibration
   (2) Position
   (3) Two-point discrimination
   (4) Deep touch

c. Ventral horn signs. The following lower motor neuron signs are found in muscles (myotomes) supplied by the affected spinal cord segment(s):
   (1) Muscle paralysis
   (2) Muscle atrophy
   (3) Loss of myotatic reflexes
   (4) Fibrillations and fasciculations
   (5) Hypotonia

KEY CONCEPTS

- Spinal cord hemisection generates characteristic ipsi- and contralateral signs.

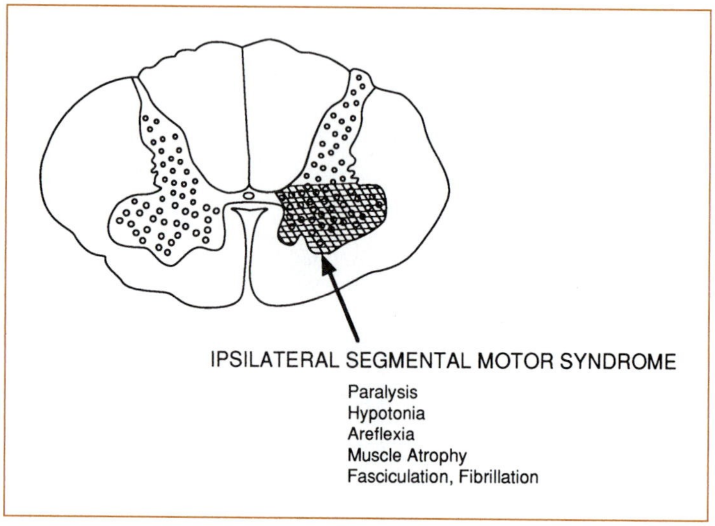

FIGURE 4-6

Schematic diagram showing the site of the lesion in segmental lower motor neuron syndrome and associated neurologic signs.

2. *Contralateral signs.* Signs contralateral to the spinal cord lesion are lateral spinothalamic tract signs. Loss of pain and thermal sense in the contralateral half of the body beginning one or two segments below the level of hemisection.
3. *Bilateral signs.* Segmental loss of pain and thermal sense one or two segments below the level of the hemisection due to interruption of spinothalamic fibers crossing in the anterior white commissure.

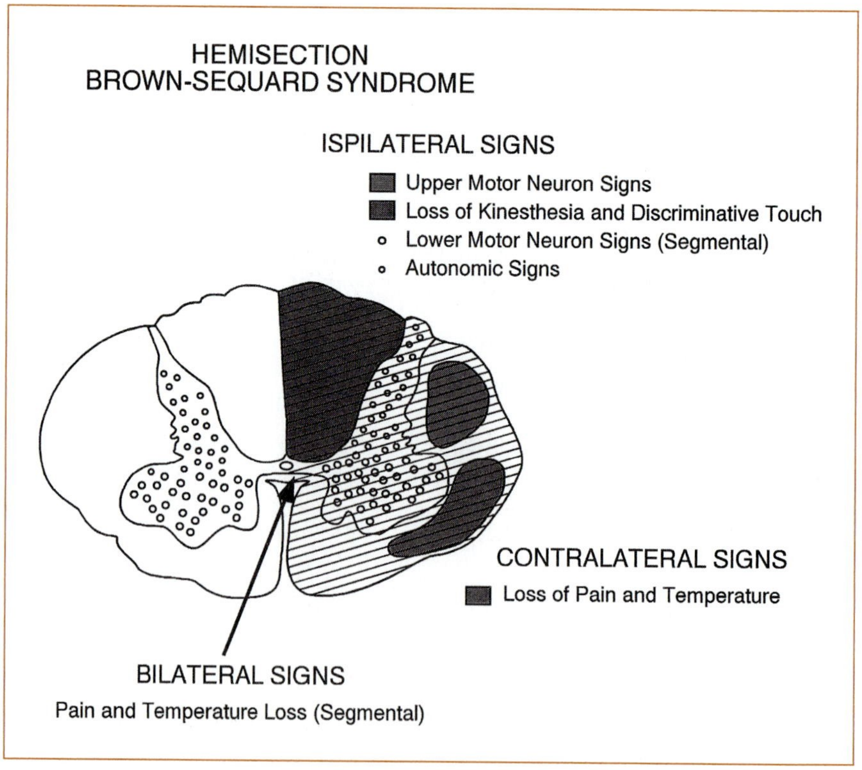

FIGURE 4-7

Schematic diagram showing the site of the lesion in spinal cord hemisection and associated neurologic signs.

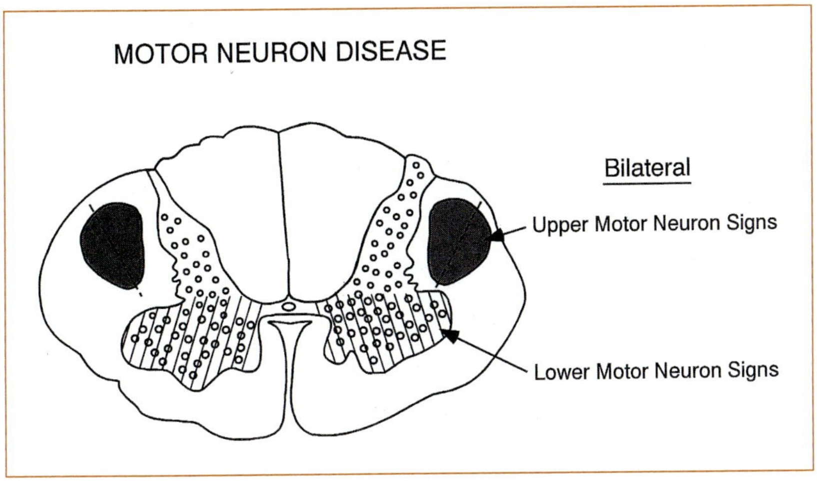

FIGURE 4-8

Schematic diagram showing the spinal cord structures involved in motor neuron disease and associated neurologic signs.

Anterior Horn and Lateral Corticospinal Tract Syndrome (Motor Neuron Disease) (Fig. 4-8)

This syndrome is known clinically as *motor neuron disease* or **amyotrophic lateral sclerosis.** This disorder is also known as *Lou Gehrig's disease.* It is a degenerative disease affecting the anterior horn and the lateral corticospinal tract bilaterally. It is thus manifested by a combination of lower and upper motor neuron signs, including paralysis, muscular atrophy, fasciculation and fibrillation, exaggerated myotatic reflexes, and a Babinski sign. This is a progressive condition that involves the spinal cord as well as motor nuclei of cranial nerves in the brain stem.

Lesions around Central Canal (Syringomyelia) (Fig. 4-9)

Lesions in or around the central canal will encroach initially on the fibers conveying pain and temperature in the anterior white commissure. The effect of such encroachment will be segmental and bilateral loss of temperature and pain sensations in the corresponding dermatomes. Such a lesion is characteristic of the clinical condition known as **syringomyelia.** This type of lesion usually affects the cervical spinal segments but may effect other segments of the spinal cord as well. In some patients, the lesion (**syrinx**) may extend to the brain stem (**syringobulbia**). In most instances, the original lesion may progress to involve, in addition to the anterior white commissure, the anterior, lateral, and/or posterior columns of the spinal cord, with symptoms and signs corresponding to the affected structures.

KEY CONCEPTS

- Upper and lower motor neuron signs coexist in motor neuron disease syndrome.
- Spinal cord lesions around the central canal characteristically present early with bilateral segmental pain and thermal sensory loss.

Amyotrophic Lateral Sclerosis. Progressive degenerative central nervous system disorder characterized by muscle weakness and wasting combined with pyramidal tract signs. The pathology primarily affects spinal and cranial nerve motor neurons and the corticospinal (pyramidal) tract. The condition is also known as motor neuron disease, Charcot syndrome, progressive muscular atrophy, Aran-Duchenne disease, and Lou Gehrig's disease.

Syringomyelia (Greek *syrinx,* "pipe, tube"; *myelos,* "marrow"). Cavitation within the spinal cord of developmental or acquired etiology. Clinical signs were described by Sir William Withey Gull, English physician, in 1862. The term was introduced by Hans Chiari, Austrian pathologist in 1888.

Syrinx (Greek *syrinx,* "pipe, tube"). Fluid filled space cavitation of the spinal cord or brain stem of developmental or acquired etiology.

Syringobulbia (Greek *syrinx,* "pipe, tube"; *bolbos,* "bulb"). Extension of syringomyelic cavity from the spinal cord to the brain stem.

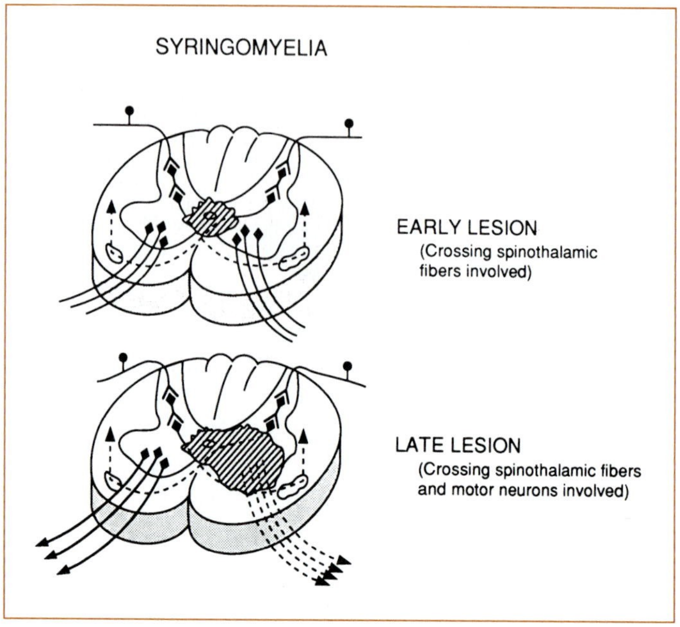

FIGURE 4-9

Schematic diagram showing the site of the lesion in syringomyelia and associated neurologic signs.

Combined System Degeneration Syndrome (Fig. 4-10)

Friedreich's Ataxia. Progressive hereditary degenerative central nervous system disorder characterized by combination of posterior column, lateral corticospinal, and spinocerebellar tracts signs. Described by Nikolaus Friedreich, Germany pathologist in 1863.

In this syndrome, there is bilateral but selective degeneration of some of the posterior and lateral column tracts with loss of kinesthesia and discriminative touch, as well as upper motor neuron signs. It is seen in patients with pernicious anemia. In a hereditary form of this syndrome, known as **Friedreich's ataxia** (after the German pathologist Nikolaus Friedreich, who described the condition), the spinocerebellar tracts are also involved bilaterally in the degenerative process.

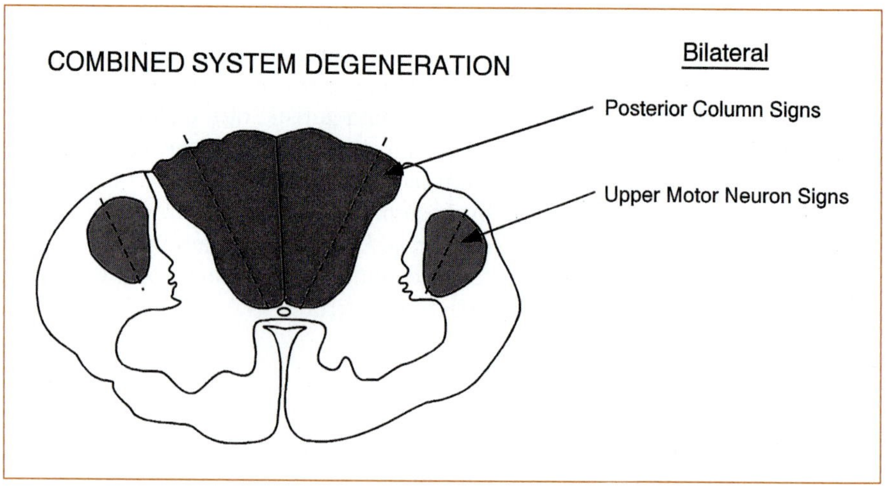

FIGURE 4-10

Schematic diagram showing the affected spinal cord tracts in combined system degeneration and associated neurologic signs.

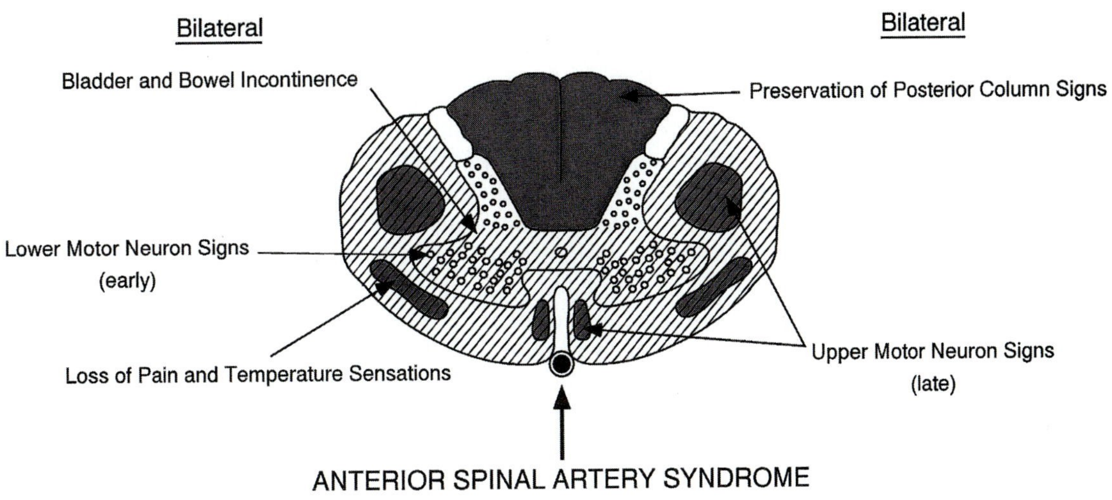

FIGURE 4-11

Schematic diagram showing the extent of the spinal cord lesion in the anterior spinal artery syndrome and associated neurologic signs.

Anterior Spinal Artery Syndrome (Fig. 4-11)

This syndrome is due to occlusion of the anterior spinal artery that supplies the anterior two-thirds of the spinal cord. The syndrome is characterized by abrupt onset of symptoms and signs. Flaccid (lower motor neuron) paralysis (spinal shock) occurs within minutes or hours below the level of the lesion and is associated with impaired bowel and bladder functions. Dissociated sensory loss characterized by loss of pain and temperature sensations (lateral spinothalamic tract lesion) and preservation of kinesthesia and discriminative touch sensations (sparing of posterior column) occurs below the level of the spinal cord lesion. With time, upper motor neuron signs predominate (withdrawal of supraspinal inhibition). Some patients develop painful dysesthesia about 6 to 8 months after onset of neurologic symptoms. This is attributed either to sparing of spinoreticulothalamic tract or to alteration of central nervous system interpretation of sensory input as a result of the imbalance produced by an intact posterior column and impaired lateral spinothalamic sensory input.

Transection

The following signs will be detected in transection of the spinal cord, as occurs in transverse myelitis due to a demyelinating lesion as in multiple sclerosis or to trauma.

KEY CONCEPTS

- The anterior part of the spinal cord is characteristically preferentially involved in ischemic lesions.

Spinal Shock

Complete transection of the spinal cord results in disturbances of motor, sensory, and autonomic functions. The manifestations of such a lesion in the immediate and early stages (2 to 3 weeks) differ from those in later stages.

1. *Motor manifestations.* In the immediate and early stages following transection, there is flaccid and bilateral paralysis of all muscles (myotomes) innervated by segments of the spinal cord affected by the transection, as well as those myotomes below the level of the transection. The flaccid paralysis of muscles below the level of the lesion, however, will change into the spastic (upper motor neuron) variety in later stages. Flaccid paralysis of muscles innervated by the affected spinal cord segments is attributed to injury of motor neurons in the anterior horn or their ventral roots. The early flaccid paralysis below the level of the lesion is attributed to the sudden withdrawal of a predominantly facilitating or excitatory influence from supraspinal centers. The spastic type of paralysis that follows later is attributed to release of segmental reflexes below the level of the lesion from supraspinal inhibitory influences. This spastic paralysis results in the development of flexor spasms that eventually change into extensor spasms. During the stage of flexor spasm, the patient's paralyzed limbs are kept in almost permanent hip and knee flexion (**paraplegia**-in-flexion). In the extension spasm stage, the limbs are kept extended at the knee and ankle (paraplegia-in-extension). Experience with war victims has shown that paraplegia-in-flexion occurs in complete [whole segment(s)] cord transection, whereas paraplegia-in-extension occurs in incomplete (partial) cord lesion.
2. *Sensory manifestations.* All sensations are lost bilaterally at and below the level of the transection. In addition, there is a hyperpathic zone at the border of the lesion and for one or two dermatomes above it. In this **hyperpathic** zone, the patient complains of pain of a burning character.
3. *Bladder function.* In the immediate and early stages following transection, all volitional or reflex functions of the urinary bladder are lost, resulting in urinary retention. This may last from 8 days to 8 weeks. Subsequently, a state of automatic bladder emptying develops. In this state, once a sufficient degree of bladder distension occurs, sensory receptors in the bladder wall evoke reflex contraction of the detrusor muscle, thus emptying the bladder.
4. *Bowel function.* Similar to bladder function, the immediate and early effect of cord transection is paralysis of bowel function and fecal retention. This is changed in later stages to intermittent automatic reflex defecation.
5. *Sexual function.* Erection and ejaculatory functions are lost in males in the immediate and early stages. Later on, reflex erection and ejaculation appear as a component of the automatic activity of the isolated cord and are evoked by extrinsic and intrinsic stimuli. In the female, there may be temporary cessation of menstruation and irregularities in the menstrual cycle.

Paraplegia (Greek *para,* "beside"; *plege,* "stroke"). Paralysis of the legs.

Hyperpathic (Greek *hyper,* "above or excessive"; *pathia,* "pain"). Abnormally exaggerated subjective response to painful stimuli.

Conus Medullaris Syndrome

Lesions of the conus (usually tumors) are characterized by early sphincter dysfunction, urinary incontinence, loss of voluntary emptying of the bladder, increased residual urine volume, and absent sensation of the urge to urinate occur. In addition, constipation and impairments in erection and ejaculation occur. Symmetric loss of sacral sensations (**saddle anesthesia**) along the distribution of S-2 to S-4 dermatomes

Saddle Anesthesia. Sensory deficit in the anal, perianal, and genital regions, buttocks and posterior upper thighs due to a lesion in the second to the fourth sacral segments of the spinal cord or their roots.

KEY CONCEPTS

- Neurologic signs and symptoms following spinal cord transection vary with the extent of the transection and with the time lapse after the transection.

is found. Pain is unusual, but dull aching pain may occur over the region of the tumor. Usually there is no motor deficit until S-1 and L-5 roots are involved. Loss of ankle jerk may then be the early sign.

Cauda Equina Syndrome

Lesions of the cauda equina give rise to symptoms and signs related to the affected nerve roots. In general, there is early occurrence of radicular pain in dermatomes supplied by the affected roots. Lower motor neuron-type paresis or paralysis occurs in muscles supplied by the affected nerves. In high cauda equina lesions, for example, affecting the L-2 to L-4 nerves, on the right side, the patient will have ipsilateral wasting and weakness of quadriceps and adductor thigh muscles and absent knee jerk. Sensory loss will be evident in L-2 to L-4 dermatomes. If the tumor compresses the spinal cord, upper motor neuron-type signs will be present. For example, in L-2 to L-4 tumor, there will be ipsilateral Babinski sign, ankle clonus, and weakness of dorsiflexion of foot. Sphincter disturbances are usually late occurrences in cauda equina lesions.

Autonomic Syndromes

Respiratory Dysfunction

Three patterns of respiratory insufficiency may occur in spinal cord lesions. The first is reduction in respiratory vital capacity due to weakness of the diaphragm and intercostal muscles as a result of interruption of the descending motor pathways. The second is reduction in CO_2 responsivity without reduction in vital capacity and without overt weakness of the diaphragm or chest wall muscles. The basis of this phenomenon is presumed to be interruption of ascending ventrolateral quadrant nerve fibers, which augment the response of the respiratory center to CO_2. The third is a combination of the preceding two syndromes, namely, reduced vital capacity from muscle weakness as well as reduced responsivity to CO_2. This deficit may indicate interruption of both ascending and descending pathways.

Autonomic Respiratory Dysfunction Syndrome

Interruption of the ventrolateral white matter of the cervical region causes a distinct autonomic respiratory dysfunction syndrome. The full syndrome consists of (1) respiratory arrest or sleep apnea (core sign) and variable onset of one or more of the following: (2) hypotension, (3) hyponatremia, (4) **inappropriate antidiuretic hormone secretion,** (5) **hypohidrosis,** and (6) urinary retention. The syndrome may appear suddenly or within hours following cordotomy. It may last days to weeks.

Inappropriate Antidiuretic Hormone Secretion. Excessive section of antidiuretic hormone (ADH) by the posterior pituitary gland leading to excessive urine output, and hyponatremia associated with serum hypoosmolarity and urine hyperosmolarity.

Autonomic Dysfunction Syndrome

This is an episodic autonomic dysreflexia syndrome seen in the chronic stages after cord section rostral to T-5. In this syndrome, a specific stimulus (usually distension of bladder or rectum) sets off excessive sweating (especially rostral to the level of the lesion), cutaneous flushing, hypertension, pounding headache, and reflex bradycardia.

Hypohidrosis (Greek *hypo,* "below"; *hidros,* "sweat"). Decreased sweating, as seen in the face in those with Horner's syndrome.

KEY CONCEPTS

- A number of autonomic signs and symptoms are associated with rostral lesions of the spinal cord.

SUGGESTED READINGS

Biller J, Brazis PW: The localization of lesions affecting the spinal cord. In Brazis PW, et al (eds): *Localization in Clinical Neurology*. Boston, Little, Brown, 1985:63.

Guttman L: Clinical symptomology of spinal cord lesions. In Vinken RJ, Bruyn GW (eds): *Handbook of Clinical Neurology*, vol 2. Amsterdam, North-Holland, 1978:178.

Nathan PW, et al: Sensory effects in man of lesions of the posterior columns and of some other afferent pathways. *Brain* 1986; 109:1003–1041.

Triggs WJ, Beric A: Sensory abnormalities and dysaesthesias in the anterior spinal artery syndrome. *Brain* 1991; 115:189–198.

CHAPTER 5

MEDULLA OBLONGATA

GROSS TOPOGRAPHY

Ventral (Anterior) Surface

The anterior median fissure of the spinal cord continues on the ventral (anterior) surface of the medulla (Fig. 5-1). On each side of this fissure are the medullary pyramids. These pyramids carry descending corticospinal fibers from the cerebral cortex to the lateral and anterior corticospinal tracts in the spinal cord and carry corticobulbar fibers to cranial nerve nuclei in the brain stem. In the lower part of the medulla, the corticospinal fibers in the pyramid partly cross to the opposite side to form the lateral corticospinal tract. This decussation, or crossing, forms the basis for the motor control of one cerebral hemisphere over the contralateral half

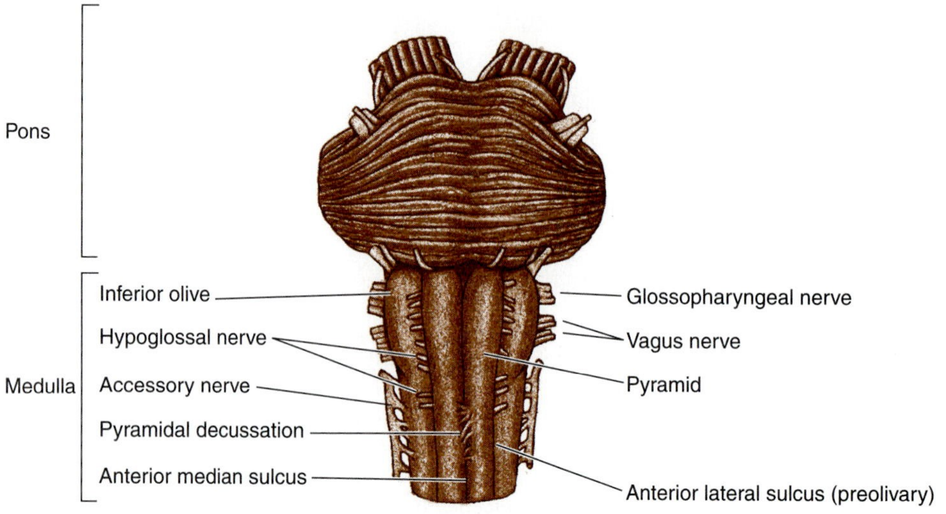
Pons
Medulla
Inferior olive
Hypoglossal nerve
Accessory nerve
Pyramidal decussation
Anterior median sulcus
Glossopharyngeal nerve
Vagus nerve
Pyramid
Anterior lateral sulcus (preolivary)

FIGURE 5-1

Schematic diagram showing the major structures seen on the ventral surface of the medulla oblongata.

of the body and is known as the motor or pyramidal decussation. The pyramids are bounded laterally by the anterolateral (ventrolateral) sulcus, a continuation of the same structure in the spinal cord. Lateral to this sulcus, approximately in the middle of the medulla, are the inferior olives. Lateral to each olive is the posterolateral (dorsolateral) sulcus. Rootlets of the hypoglossal nerve (cranial nerve XII) exit between the pyramids and olives in the anterolateral sulcus. Rootlets of the accessory (cranial nerve XI), vagus (cranial nerve X), and glossopharyngeal (cranial nerve IX) cranial nerves exit lateral to the olives.

Dorsal (Posterior) Surface

The posterior (dorsal) median sulcus and the posterolateral (dorsolateral) sulcus of the spinal cord continue on the dorsal surface of the medulla (Fig. 5-2). Between these two surface landmarks are the rostral prolongations of the gracile and cuneate tracts and their nuclei. On the dorsal surface of the medulla, the gracile and cuneate nuclei form protuberances known as the clava and cuneate tubercles, respectively. Lateral to the cuneate tubercle, between it and the posterolateral sulcus, is the tuberculum **cinereum,** which represents the surface marking of the spinal nucleus of the trigeminal nerve (cranial nerve V).

Cinereum (Latin *cinerius*, "ashen-hued," for the gray matter of the brain). The term *tuberculum cinereum* refers to the spinal trigeminal nucleus, which is part of the gray matter of the medulla oblongata.

KEY CONCEPTS

- The ventral surface of the medulla oblongata shows the pyramids, the pyramidal decussation, and the inferior olive.
- Hypoglossal nerve rootlets exit the medulla oblongata between the pyramid and the inferior olive. Rootlets of the accessory, vagus, and glossopharyngeal nerves exit the medulla lateral to the inferior olive.
- The dorsal surface of the medulla forms the caudal half of the floor of the fourth ventricle.

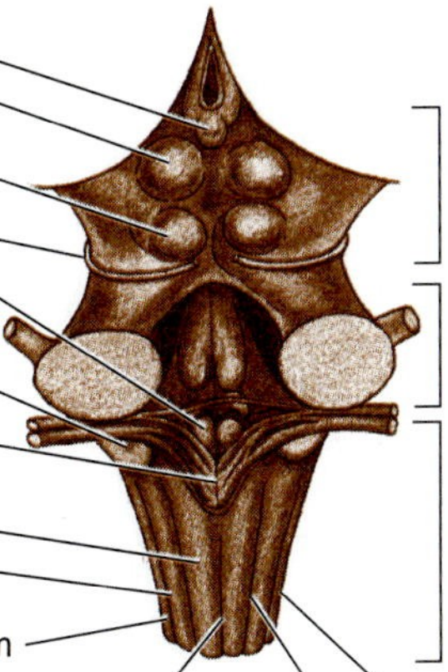

FIGURE 5-2

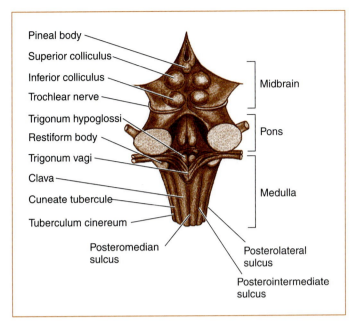

Schematic diagram showing the major structures seen on the dorsal surface of the brain stem.

Fourth Ventricle

Floor

The caudal part of the floor of the fourth ventricle is formed by the dorsal surface of the medulla oblongata (Fig. 5-3). The rostral part of the floor is formed by the pons. The medullary and pontine parts of the floor form a diamond-shaped structure. The medullary part of the floor has the following surface landmarks.

Posterior Median Fissure This fissure is a continuation of the posterior median sulcus of the spinal cord.

Hypoglossal Trigone This **trigone** is a protuberance of the nucleus of the hypoglossal nerve (cranial nerve XII) into the floor of the fourth ventricle.

Trigone (Latin, "triangular area"). The hypoglossal and vagal trigones are so named because of their triangular shape.

Vagal Trigone Lateral to the hypoglossal trigone is a protuberance of the dorsal motor nucleus of the vagus nerve (cranial nerve X) into the floor of the fourth ventricle.

The pontine part of the floor contains the facial colliculus, which represents the surface markings of the subependymal bundle of the facial nerve (cranial nerve VII), making a loop around the nucleus of the abducens nerve (cranial nerve VI).

KEY CONCEPTS

- The dorsal surface of the medulla shows the clava (gracile nucleus), the cuneate tubercle (cuneate nucleus), and the hypoglossal and vagal trigones (surface markings of the hypoglossal nucleus and dorsal motor nucleus of the vagus, respectively).
- The tuberculum cinereum on the dorsal surface of the medulla represents the surface marking of the spinal nucleus of the trigeminal nerve.

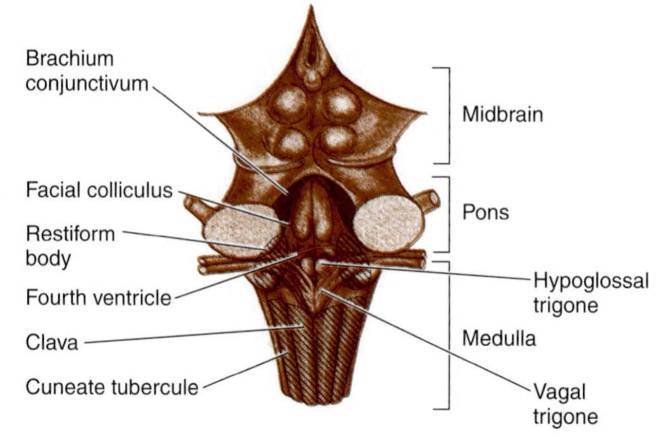

FIGURE 5-3

Schematic diagram showing the major structures seen in the floor of the fourth ventricle.

Between the rostral (pontine) and caudal (medullary) parts of the floor of the fourth ventricle is an intermediate zone containing the stria medullaris, a fiber bundle which courses laterally. This is the surface landmark of the arcuatocerebellar bundle of fibers running from the arcuate nucleus of the medulla oblongata to the cerebellum.

Roof

Three structures form the roof of the fourth ventricle: the anterior medullary **velum,** the cerebellum, and the **tela choroidea** (Fig. 5-4). The tela choroidea is formed by the neural ependyma [the original posterior (inferior) medullary velum] covered by a mesodermal pia mater.

From the tela choroidea in the posterior part of the roof of the fourth ventricle, the choroid plexus projects as two vertical and two lateral ridges, forming a T-shaped structure with a double vertical stem.

Lateral Boundaries

The lateral boundaries of the fourth ventricle (see Fig. 5-3) are formed from rostral to caudal by the following structures.

Brachium Conjunctivum This structure connects the cerebellum and the midbrain.

Restiform Body This structure connects the medulla oblongata and the cerebellum.

KEY CONCEPTS

- The roof of the fourth ventricle is formed by the superior and inferior medullary vela and the cerebellum. The inferior medullary velum contains choroid plexus.
- The lateral boundaries of the fourth ventricle are formed by the brachium conjunctivum, the restiform body, and the rostral extensions of the clava and cuneate tubercles.

Velum (Latin, "curtain or veil"). A term used for various thin membranes or veils in the brain, such as the superior medullary velum and inferior medullary velum, that constitute the roof of the fourth ventricle.

Tela choroidea (Latin *tela*, "a web"; *chorion*, "membrane"; *eidos*, "form"). A membrane of pia and ependyma that includes the choroid plexus. Found in the lateral ventricles, the roof of the third ventricle, and the posterior roof of the fourth ventricle.

Brachium (Latin, Greek *brachion*, "arm"). Any structure resembling an arm.

Brachium conjunctivum (Latin, Greek *brachion*, "arm"; *conjunctiva*, "connecting"). An armlike bundle of fibers that connect the cerebellum and midbrain.

Restiform body (Latin *restis*, "rope"; *forma*, "form"). The restiform body (inferior cerebellar peduncle) is shaped like a rope. This body was described by Humphrey Ridley, an English anatomist, in 1695.

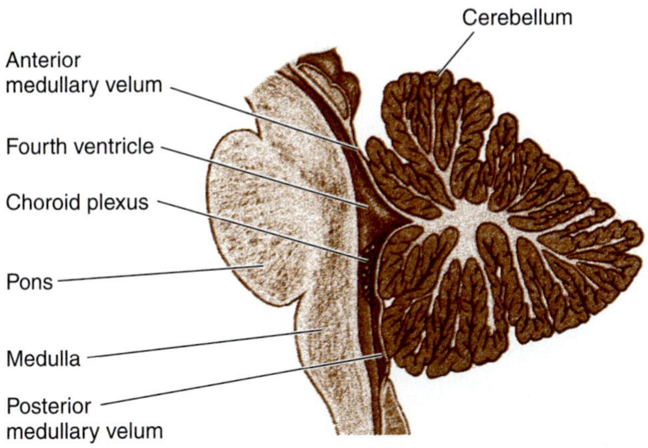
Cerebellum
Anterior medullary velum
Fourth ventricle
Choroid plexus
Pons
Medulla
Posterior medullary velum

FIGURE 5-4

Schematic diagram showing structures that form the roof and floor of the fourth ventricle.

Clava and Cuneate Tubercles These are the surface markings of the gracile and cuneate nuclei, respectively.

The lateral angles of the fourth ventricle are the lateral recesses.

INTERNAL STRUCTURE

The internal structure of the medulla is best understood when examined at three caudorostral representative levels: the level of motor (pyramidal) decussation, the level of sensory (lemniscal) decussation, and the level of the inferior olive.

Level of Motor (Pyramidal) Decussation

The two main distinguishing features of this level (Fig. 5-5) are the pyramidal decussation and the dorsal column nuclei.

Pyramidal Decussation

Although the concept of the control of one side of the body by the contralateral hemisphere (law of cruciate conduction) has existed since the time of Hippocrates, the actual crossing of the pyramids was not observed until 1709; it was described in the following year. This description was ignored, however, until **Gall** and **Spurzheim** called attention to it in 1810. Many anatomists denied the existence of the pyramidal decussation until 1835, when **Cruveilhier** traced the pyramidal bundles to the opposite side.

The pyramids contain two types of descending cortical fibers: corticospinal and corticobulbar. The corticospinal fibers are somatotopically organized. The fibers of the lower extremities are more lateral than are those of the upper extremities. As they descend in the medulla oblongata, corticobulbar fibers leave the pyramid to project on the nuclei of cranial nerves. Near the caudal border of the medulla, roughly 75 to 90 percent of the corticospinal fibers in the pyramid decussate to the

KEY CONCEPTS

- At the pyramidal decussation, 75 to 90 percent of corticospinal fibers decussate to form the lateral corticospinal tract.

Clava (Latin, "stick"). The surface marking of the nucleus gracilis on the dorsal surface of the medulla oblongata.

Cuneate (Latin, "wedge"). The cuneate fasciculus and cuneate tubercle are so called because of their wedgelike shape.

Motor decussation. The crossing of most of the pyramidal fibers in the caudal medulla oblongata to form the lateral corticospinal tract. Also called the pyramidal decussation.

Pyramidal decussation. Crossing of pyramidal fibers in the caudal medulla to form the lateral corticospinal tract. Also called motor decussation.

Gall, F. J. (1758–1828). A Viennese physician and neuroanatomist who founded the discipline of phrenology and cerebral localization.

Spurzheim, Johann Caspar (1776–1832). A french physician. A student of and collaborator with F. J. Gall in the discipline of phrenology and cerebral localization. With Gall, he called attention in 1810 to the crossing of the pyramids, which had been described in 1709.

Cruveilhier, Jean (1791–1874). A French surgeon and pathologist who traced the crossing of the pyramids at the pyramidal decussation.

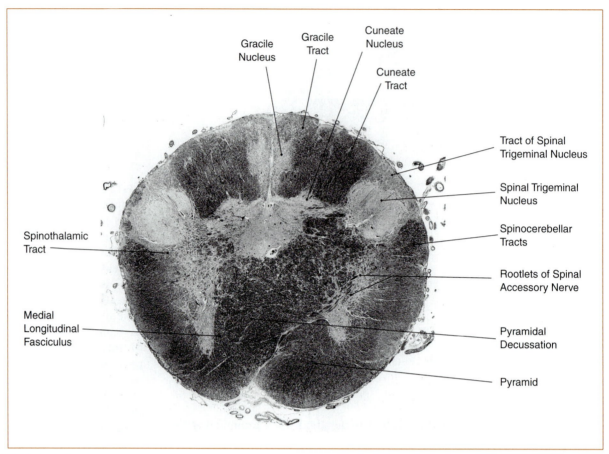

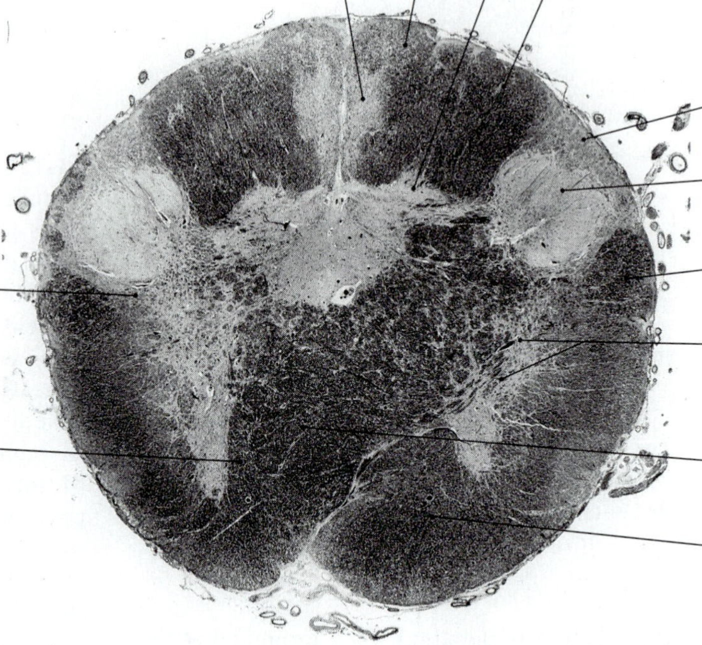
Gracile Nucleus
Gracile Tract
Cuneate Nucleus
Cuneate Tract
Tract of Spinal Trigeminal Nucleus
Spinal Trigeminal Nucleus
Spinocerebellar Tracts
Rootlets of Spinal Accessory Nerve
Pyramidal Decussation
Pyramid
Spinothalamic Tract
Medial Longitudinal Fasciculus

FIGURE 5-5

Photograph of caudal medulla oblongata at the level of the motor (pyramidal) decussation showing major structures seen at this level.

opposite side to form the lateral corticospinal tract. The rest of the corticospinal fibers descend homolaterally to form the anterior corticospinal tract. It has been observed that the left pyramid decussates first in 73 percent of humans; this, however, bears no relationship to the handedness of an individual. The corticospinal fibers that convey impulses to the neck and upper extremity musculature cross first. These fibers are separate from and rostral to those conveying impulses to the lower extremities; they are also more superficially located and are identified in the lower medulla in close proximity to the odontoid process of the second cervical vertebra. Because of this anatomic location, fractures of the odontoid process or mass lesions in that location result in paralysis of the muscles of the upper extremities but may spare the muscles of the lower extremities. By contrast, paralysis of an ipsilateral arm and a contralateral leg (**hemiplegia cruciata**) can result from a lesion in the lower medulla that injures the crossed fibers to the arm as well as the uncrossed fibers to the leg.

Cruciate hemiplegia (alternate brachial diplegia). Paralysis of one arm and the contralateral leg caused by a lesion within the pyramidal decussation at a point below the decussation of fibers destined for the arm and above the decussation of fibers destined for the leg.

Gracile (Latin, "slender, thin"). The fasciculus gracilis and nucleus gracilis are so named because they are slender and long.

The pyramidal decussation constitutes the anatomic basis for the voluntary motor control of one-half of the body by the opposite cerebral hemisphere. As the pyramidal fibers decussate, the fibers of the medial longitudinal fasciculus are displaced laterally.

Dorsal Column Nuclei

In the dorsal (posterior) column two nuclei appear: the nucleus **gracilis** in the tractus gracilis and the nucleus cuneatus in the tractus cuneatus. They are collectively referred to as the dorsal column nuclei. The gracile nucleus appears and disappears

TABLE 5-1

Dorsal Column Nuclei

	Core Region	Reticular Zone
Location	Middle and caudal	Rostral and deeper
Neuron Type	Relay	Interneurons and relay
Input	Posterior column (long ascending primary fibers)	Posterior column (second-order post-synaptic fibers, and dorsolateral fasciculus)
Output	Ventral posterolateral nucleus of thalamus	Diffusely to thalamus, brain stem nuclei, cerebellum
Primary receptors	Cutaneous (distal extremities)	Cutaneous (distal and proximal extremities and axial)
Other receptors	Joint and muscle proprioceptors (minority)	Muscle and joint
Receptive fields	Small	Large
Other	Selective response to activation of a particular cutaneous receptor excited by specific stimuli	Input from cortical areas and reticular formation

caudal to the cuneate nucleus. Caudally, both the nuclei and the tracts capping them are seen; rostrally, only the nuclei are seen. The surface projections of these two nuclei into the dorsal (posterior) surface of the medulla form the clava and cuneate tubercles.

The dorsal column nuclei are organized for the spatial origin of afferent fibers. Afferent fibers from C1 to T7 project to the nucleus cuneatus, whereas fibers below T7 project to the nucleus gracilis. It has been shown in animal experiments that overlapping terminations are more extensive and irregular in the gracile nucleus than in the cuneate nucleus, with less autonomous terminal representation of individual dorsal roots.

The dorsal column nuclei are not homogeneous cell masses. They contain several different types of nerve cells, and on the basis of the distribution of these cells and their afferent and efferent connections, the dorsal column nuclei are divided into two distinct areas (Table 5-1): a core region and a reticular zone. The core region

KEY CONCEPTS

- The dorsal column nuclei (gracile and cuneate) contain two distinct areas: a core region and a surrounding reticular zone.

includes the middle and caudal parts of each dorsal column nucleus. The reticular zone surrounds the core region and consists of the rostral and deeper portions of the dorsal column nuclei.

Activity in the dorsal column nuclei is controlled by peripheral afferent inputs and is modulated by input from the cerebral cortex and other suprasegmental sites (reticular formation, caudate nucleus, cerebellum). In general, descending afferents are restricted in their distribution to the reticular zone.

Peripheral afferent inputs from cutaneous mechanoreceptors that are activated by mechanical stimulation (touch, pressure, vibration, hair movement) in both forelimbs and hindlimbs are transmitted to the core region of the dorsal column nuclei by primary afferents in the dorsal column. From the dorsal column nuclei, this information reaches the thalamus [ventral posterolateral (VPL) nucleus] via the medial lemniscus. This primary pathway accounts for roughly 20 percent of the fibers in the dorsal column. Collateral branches from these primary afferents in the dorsal column synapse on second-order sensory neurons in the posterior horn of the spinal cord. The second-order (sensory) neurons then travel in the spinocervical thalamic tract, synapse on neurons in the lateral cervical nucleus, and from there join the medial lemniscus to reach the VPL nucleus of the thalamus. The existence of two pathways by which information from peripheral mechanoreceptors reaches the thalamus (dorsal column and spinocervical thalamic tract) explains the preservation of sensations related to these mechanoreceptors (touch, pressure, vibration) after a dorsal column lesion.

Proprioceptive pathways from joint (Golgi tendon organ) and muscle (spindle) receptors convey joint movement and position sense, respectively, and are more complicated than the cutaneous mechanoreceptor pathways. Afferents from upper extremity proprioceptors travel in the dorsal column (cuneate tract) and synapse on relay cells in the cuneate nucleus and from there travel via the medial lemniscus to the thalamus. Afferents from lower extremity proprioceptors, in contrast, reach the thalamus via two pathways. Those from some joint receptors (rapidly adapting) travel through the dorsal column (gracile tract) to the dorsal column nuclei (gracile nucleus) and from there project to the thalamus via the medial lemniscus. Afferents from muscle spindles and slowly adapting joint receptors leave the gracile tract and synapse on cells of the dorsal (Clarke's) nucleus in the spinal cord. Second-order neurons then travel via the dorsolateral fasciculus to nucleus of Z, a small collection of cells situated in the medulla in the most rostral part of the nucleus gracilis. Fibers from this nucleus cross the midline to join the medial lemniscus to reach the thalamus. The differential channeling of cutaneous and proprioceptive information presumably is responsible for the differential loss of vibration and position senses in some patients with spinal cord lesions.

Descending afferents to the dorsal column nuclei arise mainly from the primary somatosensory cortex with contributions from the secondary somatosensory cortex

KEY CONCEPTS

- Dorsal column nuclei receive input from the dorsal column (gracile and cuneate tracts) as well as from the cerebral cortex and other suprasegmental sites.
- Afferent input from cutaneous mechanoreceptors in both forelimbs and hindlimbs are transmitted to the thalamus via the dorsal column system and the spinocervical thalamic system.
- Afferent input from joint and muscle receptors in the forelimbs reaches the thalamus via the dorsal column system, whereas receptors in the hindlimb travel via the dorsal column system or the dorsolateral fasciculus and the nucleus of Z.

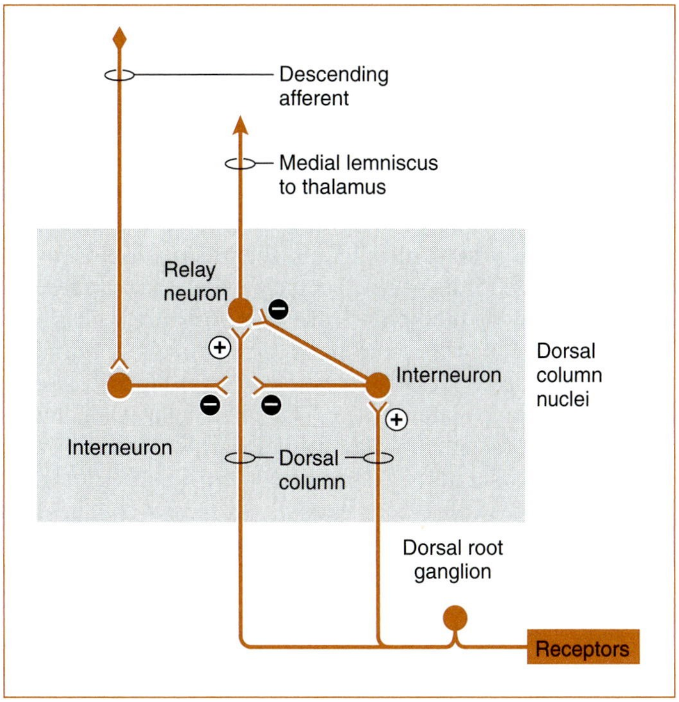

FIGURE 5-6

Schematic diagram depicting the major input and output of the posterior column nuclei, as well as their internal circuitry.

and the primary motor and premotor cortices. This input is somatotopically organized so that forelimb cortical areas project on the cuneate nucleus and hindlimb cortical areas project on the gracile nucleus. Cortical inputs to the dorsal column nuclei travel via the internal capsule and reach the nuclei via the pyramid. They project on interneurons in the reticular zone. Activation of descending cortical input generally inhibits, via interneurons, the excitation of relay neurons.

Neurons in the dorsal column nuclei are influenced by facilitatory as well as inhibitory inputs (Fig. 5-6). Inhibition is mediated by reticular zone interneurons and is both presynaptic and postsynaptic. Presynaptic inhibition is mediated by interneurons that form axoaxonic synapses on the terminals of dorsal column afferents. These terminals in turn form excitatory synapses on relay neurons. Postsynaptic inhibition, in contrast, is mediated by interneurons that form axodendritic and axosomatic synapses on relay neurons. Interneurons in the reticular zone are excited by primary as well as postsynaptic fibers in the dorsal column. In turn, interneurons modulate the transmission of impulses from dorsal column afferents to relay neurons.

The main efferent projection of the dorsal column nuclei is the medial lemniscus, which terminates in the thalamus. Other projections, which have been confirmed recently, include those to the inferior olive, tectum, spinal cord, and cerebellum. The cerebellar fibers originate mainly from the cuneate nucleus with minor contributions

KEY CONCEPTS

- The output of the dorsal column nuclei projects to the thalamus via the medial lemniscus.

from the gracile nucleus. The function of these extrathalamic connections is not well understood.

Trigeminal nerve (Latin *tres*, "three"; *geminus*, "twin"). The fifth cranial nerve was described by Fallopius. So named because the nerve has three divisions: ophthalmic, maxillary, and mandibular.

Onion-skin (peel) pattern. A pattern of sensory loss in the face which is complete centrally around the nose and mouth but shades off peripherally and occurs with a rostral spinal trigeminal nucleus and tract lesion. This pattern was described by Dejerine in 1914. The onion-skin segmental distribution reflects the rostral-caudal somatotopic arrangement of the cutaneous distribution of the spinal trigeminal nucleus, with the perioral area being rostral and the lateral face being caudal in the nucleus.

Tractotomy. A surgical operation that involves severing a specific nerve fiber tract in the central nervous system, usually to relieve pain.

Dejerine, Joseph-Jules (1849–1917). A French neurologist who increased knowledge about cerebral localization, clinical neurology, and the alexias.

Locus ceruleus (Latin, "place, dark blue"). A pigmented noradrenergic nucleus in the rostral pons that is dark blue in sections.

Spinal Trigeminal Nucleus

Another feature seen at the level of the motor decussation is the spinal nucleus of the trigeminal nerve. This nuclear mass occupies a dorsolateral position in the medulla and is capped by the descending (spinal) tract of the **trigeminal nerve.** The spinal trigeminal nucleus extends throughout the medulla oblongata and descends caudally to the level of C3 in the cervical spinal cord. It is continuous caudally with the substantia gelatinosa of the spinal cord and rostrally with the main sensory nucleus of the trigeminal nerve in the pons. The spinal tract and nucleus of the trigeminal nerve are concerned with exteroceptive sensations (pain, temperature, and light touch) from the ipsilateral face. The spinal nucleus is divided into three parts along its rostrocaudal extent. The caudal part, the caudal nucleus, extends from the obex of the medulla oblongata rostrally to the substantia gelatinosa of the spinal cord, with which it is continuous caudally. It mediates pain and temperature sensations from the ipsilateral side of the face. Rostral to the obex is the nucleus interpolaris, which is distinct cytologically from the nucleus caudalis; it mediates dental pain. Rostral to the interpolar nucleus and just caudal to the main sensory nucleus of the trigeminal is the nucleus oralis, which mediates tactile sensations from the oral mucosa.

Fibers of the spinal tract of the trigeminal nerve that originate from the mandibular region of the face project down to the third and fourth cervical segments. Those from the perioral region of the face project to lower medullary levels. Those originating between the mandible and the perioral region terminate in the upper cervical region. Evidence in support of this "**onion-skin**" distribution pattern is found in patients in whom the spinal tract of the trigeminal nerve is cut (**tractotomies**) to relieve pain. Thus, tractotomies that spare the lower medulla spare pain and temperature sensations around the mouth. In contrast to the onion-skin pattern of distribution of exteroceptive sensations on the face described by **Dejerine** in 1914, some recent observations suggest that all fibers carrying pain impulses from the face, not only those from the mandible, reach lower cervical levels. Pain neurons in the spinal trigeminal nucleus, like their counterparts in the spinal cord, have been classified physiologically into high-threshold (HT), low-threshold (LT), and wide-dynamic-range (WDR) neurons. Specific thermoreceptive neurons have been localized on the outer rim of the nucleus. In addition to the major input from exteroreceptors in the face, the spinal trigeminal nucleus has been shown to receive an input from the nucleus **locus ceruleus** in the pons and to send fibers back to the locus ceruleus. The input from the locus ceruleus is inhibitory. It should be pointed out that the spinal tract of the trigeminal conveys, in addition to exteroceptive sensations from the face, general somatic fibers belonging to the facial (cranial nerve, VII), glossopharyngeal (cranial nerve IX), and vagus (cranial nerve X) nerves.

KEY CONCEPTS

- The spinal trigeminal nucleus is concerned with exteroceptive sensations (pain, temperature, light touch) from the ipsilateral face.
- The spinal trigeminal nucleus has three subnuclei: caudalis, interpolaris, and oralis.
- Afferent fibers from the face are somatotopically organized in the spinal trigeminal nucleus.

Other Tracts

The following ascending tracts are also seen at the level of the motor decussation. The spinothalamic tracts traverse the medulla in close proximity to the spinal nucleus and tract of the trigeminal nerve (Fig. 5-5). Lesions of the medulla in this location therefore produce sensory loss of pain and temperature sensation on the face ipsilateral to the medullary lesion (spinal tract and nucleus of the trigeminal nerve) as well as loss of the same sensations on the body contralateral to the medullary lesion (spinothalamic tract). Although the lateral and anterior spinothalamic tracts retain their spinal cord positions in the caudal medulla, the position of the anterior spinothalamic tract in the rostral medulla has not been definitively delineated in humans, and its fibers probably run along with the lateral spinothalamic tract.

The spinal cord positions of the dorsal and ventral spinocerebellar tracts remain unchanged in the medulla (Fig. 5-5).

Other ascending and descending tracts encountered in the spinal cord traverse the medulla on their way to higher or lower levels.

Level of Sensory (Lemniscal) Decussation

Medial Lemniscus

The distinguishing feature of the level of sensory decussation (Fig. 5-7) is the crossing of second-order neurons of the dorsal column system. Axons of relay neurons in the dorsal column nuclei course ventromedially (internal arcuate fibers) and cross to the opposite side (sensory decussation) above the pyramids to form the medial lemniscus. In the decussation, fibers derived from the gracile nucleus come to lie ventral to those derived from the cuneate nucleus. The medial lemniscus thus carries the same modalities of sensation carried by the dorsal column. Lesions in the medial lemniscus result in a loss of kinesthesia and discriminative touch contralateral to the side of the lesion in the medulla. The sensory decussation provides part of the anatomic basis for the sensory representation of one-half of the body in the contralateral hemisphere. The other part is provided by the crossing of the spinothalamic system in the spinal cord.

Lemniscal decussation. Crossing of axons of the posterior column nuclei in the medulla oblongata to form the medial lemniscus. Also known as sensory decussation.

Sensory decussation. Crossing of axons of the posterior column nuclei (gracilis and cuneatus) in the medulla oblongata to form the medial lemniscus. Also known as the lemniscal decussation.

Medial Longitudinal Fasciculus

The medial longitudinal fasciculus (MLF), which is displaced dorsolaterally by the pyramidal decussation, is pushed farther upward by the sensory decussation so that it comes to lie dorsal to the medial lemniscus (Fig. 5-7). It retains this position throughout the extent of the medulla oblongata. Descending fibers in this bundle are derived from various brain stem nuclei. Vestibular fibers in the bundle are derived from the medial and inferior vestibular nuclei. The pontine reticular forma-

KEY CONCEPTS

- The proximity of the spinal trigeminal nucleus to the spinothalamic tract in the medulla is responsible for the crossed sensory deficit (ipsilateral face and contralateral body) described in patients with medullary lesions.
- In the medial lemniscus fibers from the lower extremities are ventral to those from the upper extremities.
- The medial lemniscus conveys dorsal column sensations (kinesthesia and discriminative touch) to the thalamus.

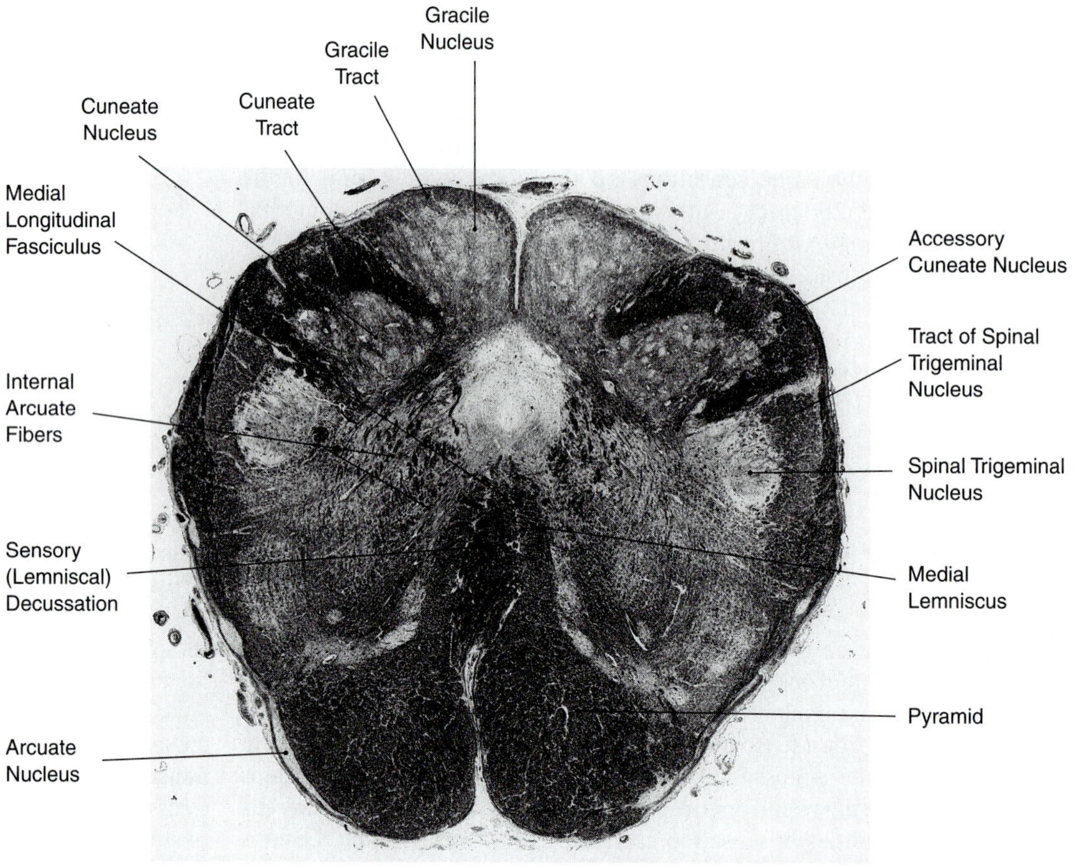

FIGURE 5-7

Photograph of medulla oblongata at the level of sensory (lemniscal) decussation showing major structures seen at this level.

tion contributes the largest number of descending fibers. Smaller groups of fibers arise from Cajal's interstitial nucleus in the rostral midbrain.

Accessory Cuneate Nucleus

A group of large neurons situated dorsolateral to the cuneate nucleus is known as the accessory (lateral or external) cuneate nucleus. Although this nucleus shares its name with the cuneate nucleus, it does not belong functionally to the dorsal column system; it is part of the dorsal spinocerebellar system. Fibers of the dorsal spinocerebellar system entering the spinal cord above the level of C8 [upper extent of the dorsal (Clarke's) nucleus] ascend with the posterior column fibers and terminate on neurons of the accessory cuneate nucleus. Second-order neurons from the accessory cuneate nucleus course dorsolaterally as dorsal external arcuate fibers

KEY CONCEPTS

- The medial longitudinal fasciculus contains descending reticular (main component) and vestibular fibers.
- The accessory (lateral) cuneate nucleus is homologous to the nucleus dorsalis (Clarke's nucleus) in the spinal cord and thus is part of the spinocerebellar system of unconscious proprioception.

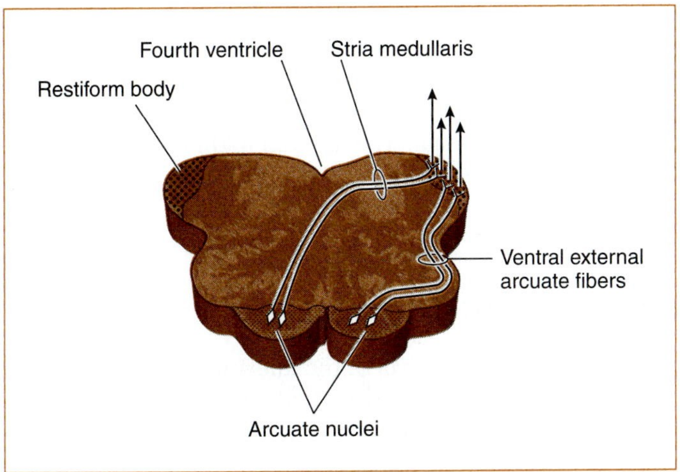

FIGURE 5-8

Schematic diagram illustrating the course of arcuatocerebellar fibers within the medulla oblongata.

and reach the cerebellum (cuneocerebellar fibers) via the restiform body. Like the spinocerebellar system, the cuneocerebellar tract is concerned with unconscious proprioception. Recently, neurons in the accessory cuneate nucleus have been shown to receive fibers from the glossopharyngeal (cranial nerve IX) and vagus (cranial nerve X) nerves as well as from the vasopressor and cardioacceleratory areas of the posterior hypothalamus. Stimulation of the accessory cuneate nucleus has been shown to produce bradycardia and hypotension. This response has been shown to be due to vagal stimulation. It has been suggested that hypertension triggers the accessory cuneate nucleus, via cardiovascular reflexes, to produce bradycardia and hypotension.

Arcuate Nuclei

A group of neurons on the anterior (ventral) aspect of the pyramid is known as the arcuate nucleus. The arcuate nuclei increase in size significantly in rostral levels of the medulla and become continuous with the pontine nuclei in the pons. The afferent and efferent connections of the arcuate nuclei are identical to those of the pontine nuclei. Their major input is from the contralateral cerebral cortex; their major output is to the homolateral and contralateral cerebellum via the restiform body. The arcuatocerebellar fibers reach the restiform body via two routes (Fig. 5-8). One route courses along the outer surface of the medulla (ventral external arcuate fibers); the other route courses along the midline of the medulla and turns laterally in the floor of the fourth ventricle, forming the stria medullaris of the floor of the fourth ventricle.

Arcuate nucleus (Latin *arcuatus*, "bow-shaped"). The arcuate nucleus in the medulla oblongata is an archlike structure lateral and inferior to the pyramid.

Area Postrema

In the floor of the caudal fourth ventricle, just rostral to the obex, is the area postrema, which is formed of astroblast-like cells, arterioles, sinusoids, and some

Area postrema. One of the circumventricular organs devoid of a blood-brain barrier. Located in the floor of the fourth ventricle.

KEY CONCEPTS

- The arcuate nuclei are homologous to the pontine nuclei and similarly serve as a relay between the cerebral cortex and the cerebellum.
- The area postrema in the caudal fourth ventricle belongs to the group of circumventricular organs devoid of blood-brain barrier.

apolar or unipolar neurons. It is one of several central nervous system areas that lack a blood-brain barrier. Collectively referred to as the circumventricular organs, they include, in addition to the area postrema, the subfornical organ, subcommissural organ, pineal gland, median eminence, neurohypophysis, and organum vasulosum. All except the area postrema are unpaired midline structures that are related to the diencephalon. Stimulation of the area postrema in experimental animals induces vomiting, suggesting the presence of a chemosensitive emetic center in this area.

Level of Inferior Olive

The distinguishing feature of the level of the inferior olive (Fig. 5-9) of the medulla is the appearance of the inferior olivary nuclei, which are convoluted laminae of gray matter dorsal to the pyramids. They project from the ventrolateral surface of the medulla as olive-shaped structures (Fig. 5-1). The inferior olivary nuclear complex consists of three nuclear groups:

1. Principal olive (the largest of the complex)
2. Dorsal accessory olive
3. Medial accessory olive

The olivary complex in humans is estimated to contain 0.5 million neurons. The complex is surrounded by a mass of fibers known as the amiculum olivae.

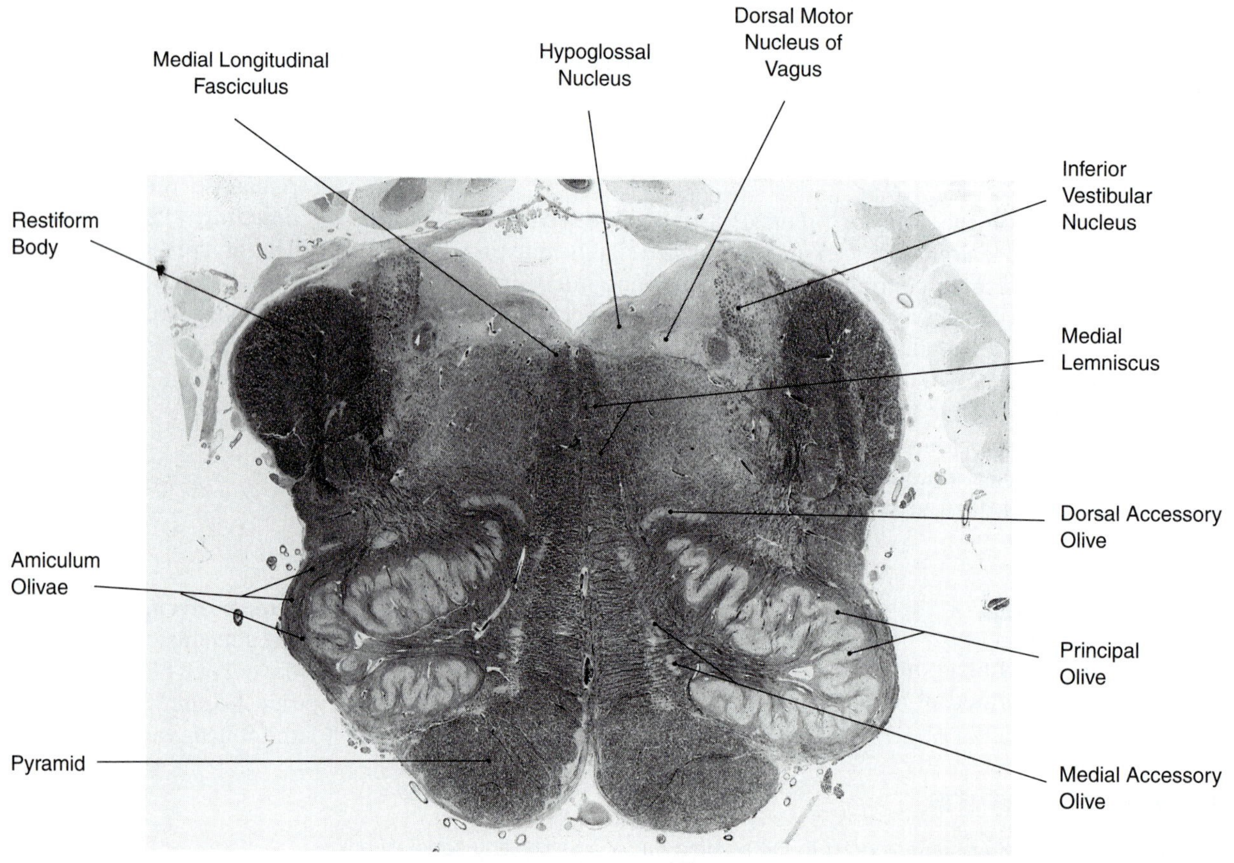

FIGURE 5-9

Photograph of medulla oblongata at the inferior olive level showing major structures seen at this level.

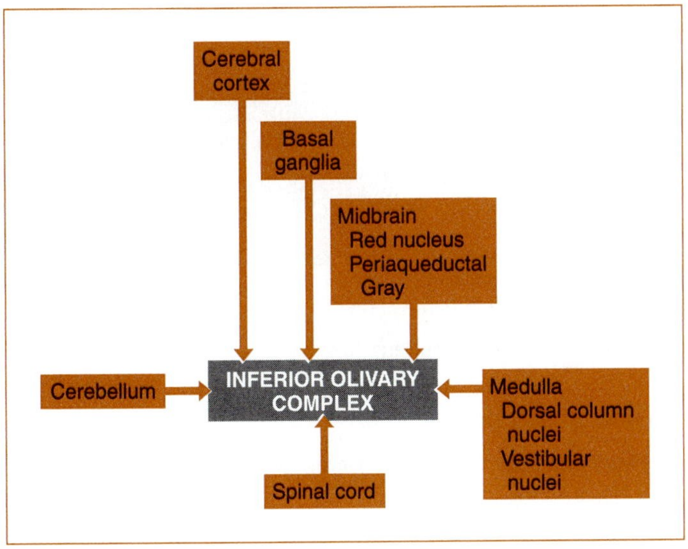

FIGURE 5-10

Schematic diagram showing major sources of input to the inferior olive.

The inferior olives receive fibers from the following sources (Fig. 5-10):

1. Cerebral cortex via the corticospinal tract to both principal olives.
2. Basal ganglia to both principal olives via the central tegmental tract.
3. Mesencephalon from the periaqueductal gray matter of the midbrain and the red nucleus to the homolateral principal olive via the central tegmental tract.
4. In the medulla oblongata, the dorsal column nuclei project to the contralateral accessory olive. The inferior and medial vestibular nuclei project to both inferior olives. The two inferior olives are interconnected.
5. In the cerebellum, the deep cerebellar nuclei (dentate and interposed nuclei) project to the principal and accessory inferior olives via the superior cerebellar peduncle.
6. From the spinal cord, to the accessory olives of both sides via the spino-olivary tract.

The major output of the inferior olivary complex is to the cerebellum (olivocerebellar tract). Olivocerebellar fibers arise from both olivary complexes but come primarily from the contralateral complex. They pass through the hilum of the olive, traverse the medial lemniscus, and course through the opposite olive to enter the restiform body on their way to the cerebellum. Olivocerebellar fibers constitute the major component of the restiform body and are localized in the ventromedial part. Olivocerebellar fibers originating from the accessory olives and the medial parts of the principal olives project onto the vermis of the cerebellum, whereas fibers originating from the rest of the principal olive project to the cerebellar hemispheres. The deep cerebellar nuclei also receive fibers from the olivocerebellar tract.

KEY CONCEPTS

- Olivocerebellar fibers reach the cerebellum via the restiform body and are somatotopically organized.

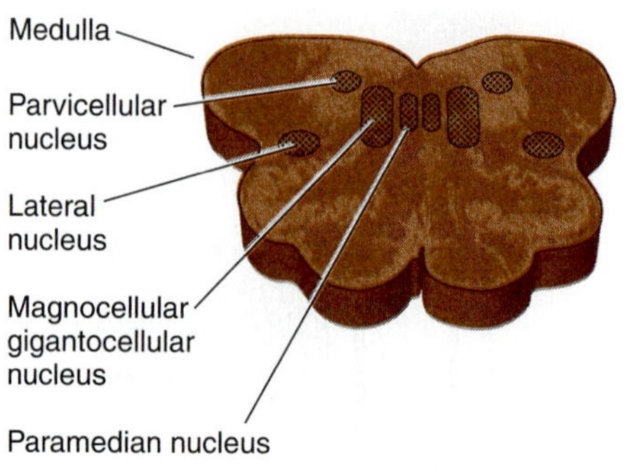

FIGURE 5-11

Schematic diagram showing the major subdivisions of the reticular nuclear complex in the medulla oblongata.

Thus, the inferior olivary complex is a relay station between the cortex, subcortical structures, the spinal cord, and the cerebellum.

The ascending and descending fiber tracts, as well as the nuclear complexes encountered in more caudal levels of the medulla, are present at this level. The cranial nerve nuclei of the medulla are discussed in "Cranial Nerve Nuclei of the Medulla," below.

MEDULLARY RETICULAR FORMATION

The medullary reticular formation is characterized by a great number of neurons of various sizes and shapes intermingled with a complex network of fibers. It spans the area between the pyramids (ventrally) and the floor of the fourth ventricle (dorsally). It is phylogenetically old and in lower forms constitutes the major part of the central nervous system. Caudally, the reticular formation appears at about the level of the pyramidal decussation. Rostrally, it is continuous with the reticular formation of the pons. Physiologically, the reticular formation is a polysynaptic system that is rich in collateral fibers for the dispersion of impulses.

Cellular Organization

Although the reticular formation was previously considered an unorganized network of neurons and fibers, more recent studies have suggested that it is organized into well-defined subdivisions with known afferent and efferent connections. In general, the medullary reticular formation is organized into three subgroups (Fig. 5-11):

1. Paramedian (**raphe**) nuclear group (caudal nucleus of the raphe)
2. Central group (gigantocellular and ventral reticular nuclei)
3. Lateral group (lateral reticular nucleus and **parvicellular nucleus**)

Raphe nucleus (Greek *raphe*, "a seam or suture"). This word was used by Homer in the *Odyssey* in connection with the sewing of harnesses for horses. The term is used in anatomy to refer to a seamlike formation that suggests that adjacent structures have been sewn together. The midline reticular nuclei are called the raphe nuclei.

Parvicellular nucleus (Latin *parvus*, "small"; *cellula*, "cell"). So named because it is composed of small cells.

KEY CONCEPTS

- The inferior olivary complex serves as a relay between cortical and subcortical areas and the cerebellum.
- The medullary reticular formation is organized into three subgroups: paramedian (raphe), central, and lateral.

The caudal nucleus of the raphe is a small-celled, slender structure that is continuous from the medulla to the lower pons. It produces the neurotransmitter serotonin and sends inhibitory projections to spinothalamic neurons in the dorsal horn of the spinal cord. The analgesic effects of electric stimulation of the midbrain periaqueductal gray matter appear to be mediated through connections with raphe nuclei in the lower brain stem.

The gigantocellular nucleus lies in the rostral medulla and is characterized by large neurons. The ventral reticular nucleus contains small neurons and is caudal to the gigantocellular nucleus.

The lateral reticular nucleus is found dorsal to the inferior olive. The medullary vomiting center is believed to be within, or close to, the lateral reticular nucleus. The parvicellular nucleus contains both large and small neurons and is located lateral to the gigantocellular nucleus.

Afferent Connections

The paramedian nuclear group receives fibers from the following structures:

1. Cerebral cortex (homolateral and contralateral)
2. Homolateral cerebellum

The central nuclear group (gigantocellular nucleus) receives fibers from the following structures:

1. Homolateral and contralateral cerebral cortex
2. Lateral nuclear group (parvicellular nucleus)
3. Spinal cord (spinoreticular tract).

The lateral nuclear group receives fibers from the following structures:

1. Contralateral red nucleus (lateral reticular nucleus)
2. Spinothalamic tract (lateral reticular nucleus)
3. Spinoreticular tract (lateral reticular nucleus)
4. Second-order neurons of some (trigeminal, auditory, and vestibular) sensory systems (parvicellular nucleus)

As a rule, the medullary reticular formation receives no fibers from the medial lemniscus.

Figure 5-12 is a composite diagram of the afferent connections of the medullary reticular formation. In summary, the afferent connections of the medullary reticular formation come from the following structures:

1. Cerebral cortex
2. Red nucleus
3. Cerebellum
4. Spinal cord
5. Second-order neurons of some sensory systems

KEY CONCEPTS

- The raphe reticular nucleus contains serotonin and mediates the analgesic effect of stimulation of the midbrain periaqueductal gray matter.
- The medullary vomiting center is within or close to the lateral reticular nucleus.

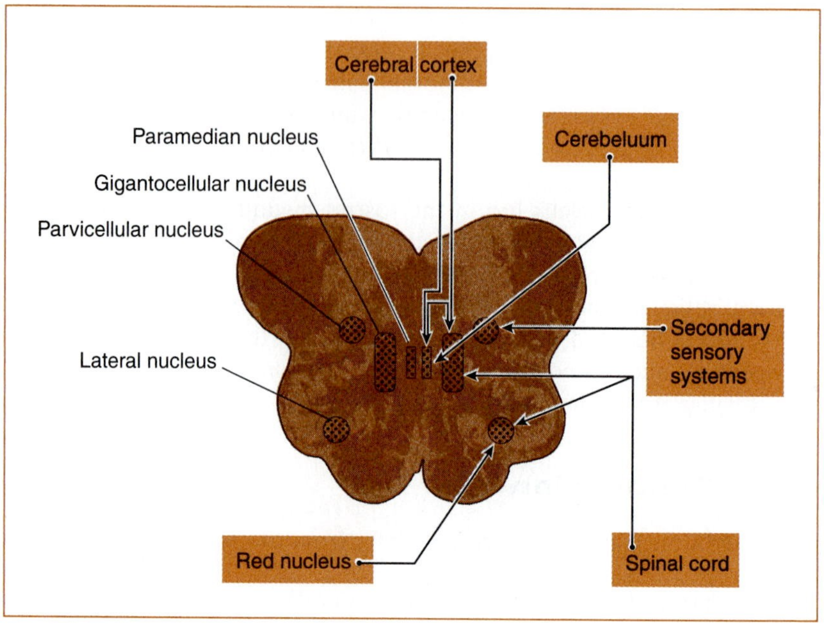

FIGURE 5-12

Composite schematic diagram of the afferent connections of the medullary reticular formation.

Efferent Connections

The major efferent flow from the paramedian nuclear group is to the cerebellum (vermis) via the restiform body. The cerebellum receives fibers from the homolateral and contralateral paramedian groups. The caudal nucleus of the raphe (raphe magnus) has been shown to project to the dorsal horn of the spinal cord. The transmitter in this projection is serotonin, which inhibits neurons in the spinothalamic tract.

The central nuclear group has two major outputs. These outputs are mostly to the homolateral thalamus (intralaminar nuclei and reticular nucleus) via the central tegmental tract but also to the spinal cord (the medullary reticulospinal tract). The medullary reticulospinal tract has been shown to originate from both the ventral reticular and the gigantocellular nuclei and to be topographically organized. Fibers originating from the dorsal parts of these nuclei project to the cervical spinal cord and supply upper limb neurons; fibers originating from the ventral parts project to the lower thoracic and lumbar spinal cord and supply lower limb neurons.

The lateral nuclear group projects to both cerebellar hemispheres, but mostly to the homolateral one (lateral reticular nucleus), as well as to the central nuclear group (parvicellular nucleus).

Figure 5-13 is a composite diagram of the efferent connections of the medullary reticular formation. In summary, the efferent connections of the medullary reticular formation are to the following structures:

1. Thalamus (a part of the reticular activating system which is important in the arousal response)

KEY CONCEPTS

- The central reticular nucleus is the major, but not the only, source of the medullary reticulospinal tract and the ascending reticulothalamic tract.

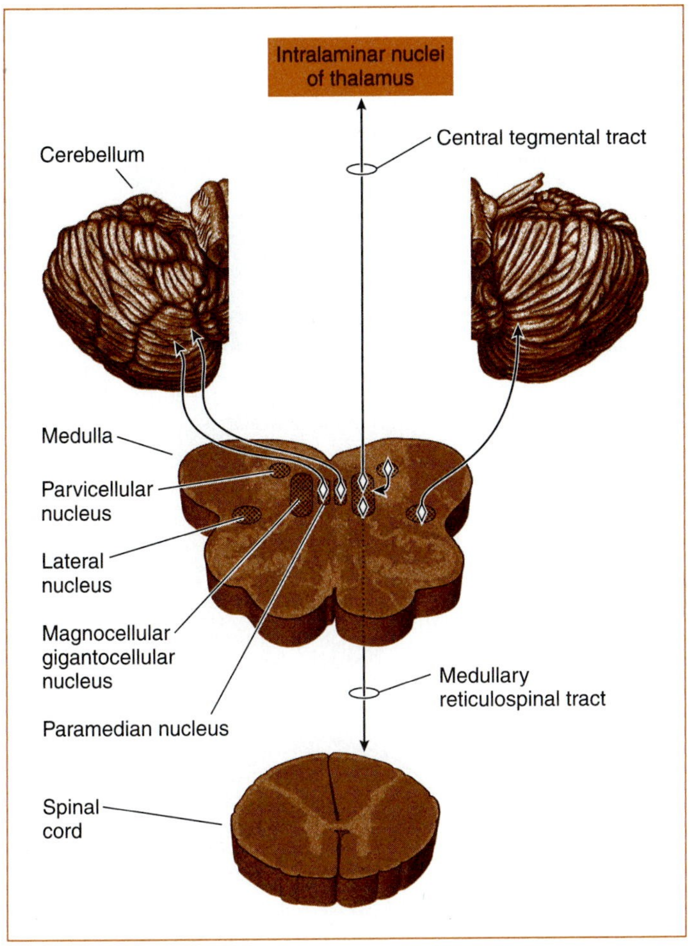

FIGURE 5-13

Composite schematic diagram of the efferent connections of the medullary reticular formation.

2. Spinal cord
3. Cerebellum

Various studies suggest that the reticular formation is concerned with (1) somatic motor functions, (2) visceral motor functions, and (3) consciousness, sleep, and attention. Stimulation of the medullary reticular formation facilitates flexor spinal motor neurons and inhibits extensor motor neurons. It also results in visceral changes such as an increase in blood pressure and an increase or decrease in heart rate (depending on the area stimulated). The connection between the central group of reticular neurons and the thalamus belongs to the reticular activating system, which is concerned with sleep, wakefulness, and attention.

KEY CONCEPTS

- The medullary reticular formation serves as a relay between the cerebral cortex, subcortical sites, and the spinal cord, and the cerebellum.
- The medullary reticular formation is concerned with somatic and visceral motor functions as well as with consciousness, attention, and sleep.

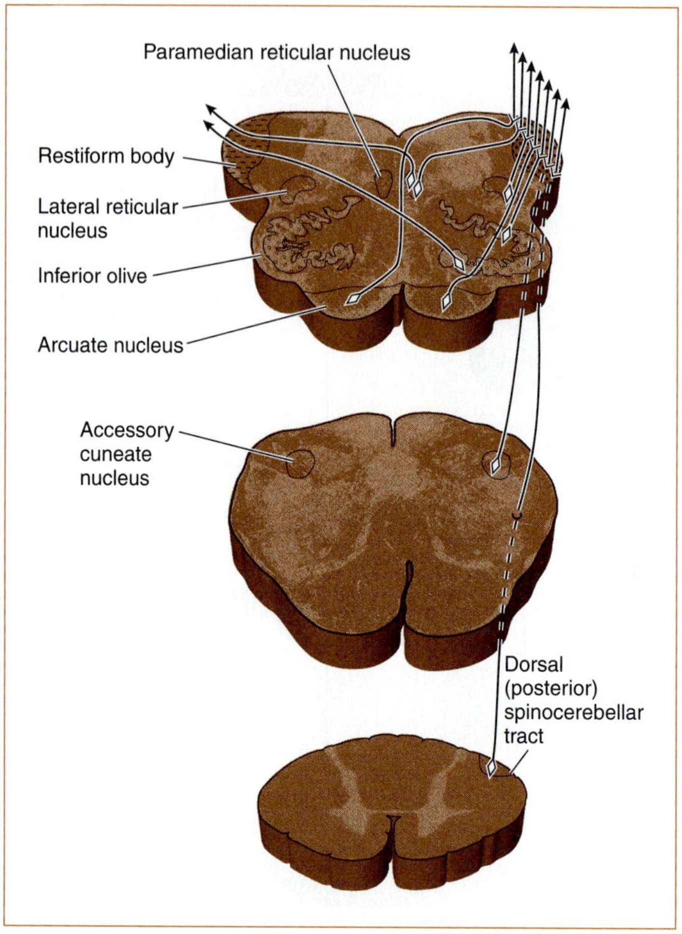
Paramedian reticular nucleus
Restiform body
Lateral reticular nucleus
Inferior olive
Arcuate nucleus
Accessory cuneate nucleus
Dorsal (posterior) spinocerebellar tract

FIGURE 5-14

Composite schematic diagram of the components of the inferior cerebellar peduncle (restiform body).

INFERIOR CEREBELLAR PEDUNCLE (RESTIFORM BODY)

The brain stem and cerebellum are connected by three peduncles:

1. The inferior cerebellar peduncle (Figs. 5-3 and 5-14) between the medulla and the cerebellum
2. The middle cerebellar peduncle (**brachium pontis**) between the pons and the cerebellum
3. The superior cerebellar peduncle (brachium conjunctivum) between the cerebellum and the midbrain

Brachium pontis. An armlike bundle of fibers that link the pons and the cerebellum.

The inferior cerebellar peduncle (restiform body) is located on the dorsolateral border of the medulla oblongata. It appears rostral to the clava and cuneate tubercles and forms a distinct bundle at about the midolivary level. The fiber tracts contained within the inferior cerebellar peduncle include the following afferent and efferent

KEY CONCEPTS

- The inferior cerebellar peduncle (restiform body) links the spinal cord and medulla with the cerebellum.

(medullary and spinal originating or destined) tracts:

1. Olivocerebellar tract (the largest component of this peduncle) connecting the inferior olive and cerebellum
2. Dorsal spinocerebellar tract from the nucleus dorsalis (Clarke's nucleus) to the cerebellum
3. Reticulocerebellar tract connecting the reticular formation with the cerebellum
4. Cuneocerebellar tract from the accessory cuneate nucleus to the cerebellum (homologous to the dorsal spinocerebellar tract)
5. Arcuatocerebellar tract from the arcuate nucleus to the cerebellum
6. Cerebello-olivary tract from the cerebellum to the inferior olive
7. Trigeminocerebellar tract from the spinal nucleus of the trigeminal nerve (medulla) and the principal nucleus of the trigeminal nerve (pons) to the cerebellum
8. Fibers from the perihypoglossal nuclei to the cerebellum

A small inner (medial) part of the restiform body is known as the juxtarestiform body. It contains the following fiber tracts:

1. Cerebelloreticular tract from the cerebellum to the reticular formation
2. Cerebellovestibular tract from the cerebellum to the vestibular nuclei
3. Vestibulocerebellar secondary vestibular fibers form the vestibular nuclei to the cerebellum
4. Direct vestibular nerve fibers to the cerebellum (with no synapse in the vestibular nuclei)
5. Cerebellospinal tract (from the cerebellum to motor neurons of the cervical spinal cord)

Lesions in the inferior cerebellar peduncle result in the following symptoms and signs:

1. **Ataxia** (lack of coordination of movement) with a tendency to fall toward the side of the lesion
2. **Nystagmus** (involuntary rapid eye movement)
3. Muscular hypotonia

Ataxia (Greek *a*, "negative"; *taxis*, "order"). Without order, disorganized. Incoordination of movement frequently seen in cerebellar disease. The term was used by Hippocrates and Galen for disordered action of any type, such as irregularity of pulse.

Nystagmus (Greek *nystagmos*, "drowsiness, nodding"). Nodding or closing of the eyes in a sleepy person. Today the term refers to involuntary rhythmic oscillation of the eyes.

Hypoglossal nerve (Greek *hypo*, "beneath"; *glossa*, "tongue"). The twelfth cranial nerve was so named by Winslow. Willis included it with the ninth cranial nerve. It was named the twelfth nerve by Soemmering.

CRANIAL NERVE NUCLEI OF THE MEDULLA

The following cranial nerves have their nuclei in the medulla oblongata: (1) hypoglossal (cranial nerve XII), (2) accessory (cranial nerve XI), (3) vagus (cranial nerve X), (4) glossopharyngeal (cranial nerve IX), and (5) vestibulocochlear (cranial nerve VIII).

Hypoglossal Nerve (Cranial Nerve XII)

The hypoglossal nerve contains primarily somatic motor nerve fibers that innervate the intrinsic and extrinsic muscles of the tongue. It also contains afferent proprioceptive fibers from the muscle spindles of tongue muscles.

KEY CONCEPTS

- The juxtarestiform body is the medial part of the restiform body. It contains fibers linking the cerebellum with the vestibular and reticular nuclei.
- Four cranial nerve nuclei are situated in the medulla oblongata: hypoglossal, accessory, glossopharyngeal, and vagus.

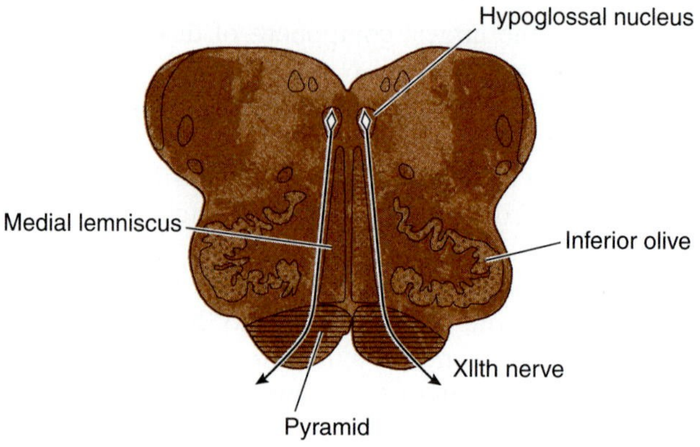

FIGURE 5-15

Schematic diagram of the origin and intramedullary course of filaments of the hypoglossal nerve.

The nucleus of the hypoglossal nerve extends throughout the medulla oblongata except for its most rostral and caudal levels. It is divided into cell groups that correspond to the tongue muscles they supply. The surface markings of the nucleus in the floor of the fourth ventricle are known as trigonum hypoglossi. The nucleus receives both crossed and uncrossed corticoreticulobulbar fibers. The root fibers of the nerve course in the medulla oblongata lateral to the medial lemniscus and emerge on the ventral surface of the medulla between the pyramid and the inferior olive (Fig. 5-15).

A number of nuclear masses in close proximity to the hypoglossal nerve (cranial nerve XII) nucleus are believed to be reticular neurons; they do not contribute fibers to the hypoglossal nerve. They are known as perihypoglossal or satellite nuclei (nucleus intercalatus, nucleus prepositus, and Roller's nucleus). They receive input from the (1) cerebral cortex, (2) vestibular nuclei, (3) accessory oculomotor nuclei, and (4) paramedian pontine reticular formation.

The output of these nuclei terminates in (1) cranial nerve nuclei involved in extraocular movement (oculomotor, trochlear, abducens), (2) the cerebellum, and (3) the thalamus.

The perihypoglossal nuclei and their connections are part of a complex circuitry related to eye movements.

Immediately posterior to the hypoglossal nucleus, in the periventricular area, is a small bundle of descending fibers, visceral in function, known as the dorsal longitudinal fasciculus of Schütz.

Lesions in the hypoglossal nerve or nucleus result in lower motor neuron paralysis of the tongue musculature homolateral to the lesion (Fig. 5-16*A*), which is manifested by the following symptoms:

1. Decrease or loss of movement of the homolateral half of the tongue
2. Atrophy of muscles in the homolateral half of the tongue

KEY CONCEPTS

- The hypoglossal nucleus is subdivided into subnuclei that represent the muscles supplied by the hypoglossal nerve.
- Lesions of the hypoglossal nucleus or nerve result in ipsilateral tongue atrophy, fasciculations, and weakness. The protruded tongue deviates towards the weak atrophic side.

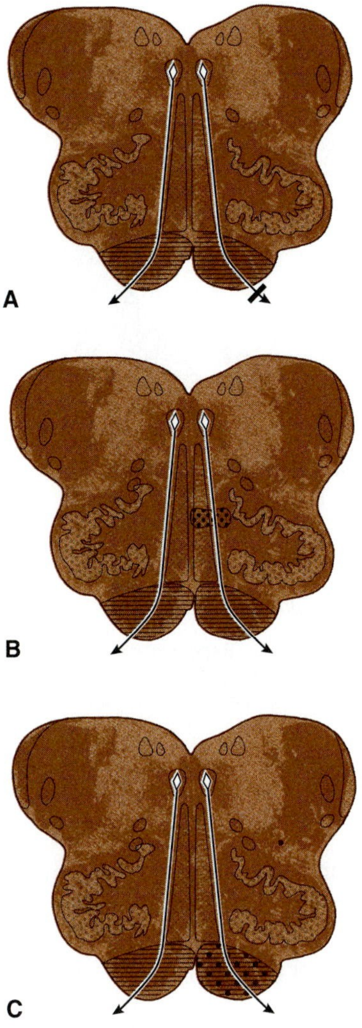

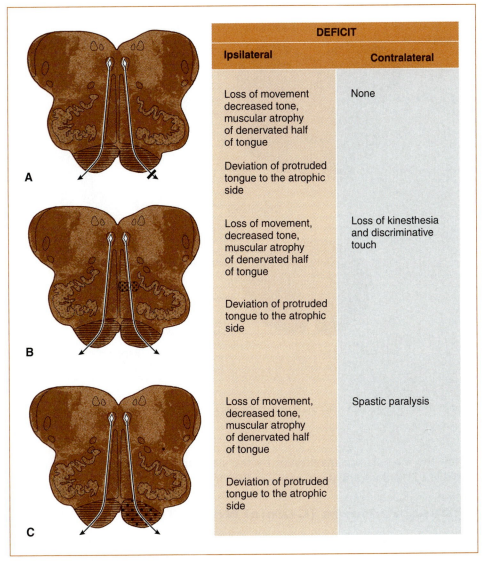

DEFICIT	
Ipsilateral	**Contralateral**
Loss of movement decreased tone, muscular atrophy of denervated half of tongue Deviation of protruded tongue to the atrophic side	None
Loss of movement, decreased tone, muscular atrophy of denervated half of tongue Deviation of protruded tongue to the atrophic side	Loss of kinesthesia and discriminative touch
Loss of movement, decreased tone, muscular atrophy of denervated half of tongue Deviation of protruded tongue to the atrophic side	Spastic paralysis

FIGURE 5-16

Schematic diagram illustrating lesions of the hypoglossal nerve in its extra- and intramedullary course, and the resulting clinical deficits of each.

3. **Fasciculations** of muscles in the homolateral half of the tongue
4. Deviation of the protruding tongue to the atrophic side (by action of the normal genioglossus muscle)

Lesions involving the rootlets of the hypoglossal nerve and the adjacent medial lemniscus within the medulla result in the signs of hypoglossal nerve lesion detailed above and contralateral loss of kinesthesia and discriminative touch (Fig. 5-16*B*).

Lesions involving the rootlets of the hypoglossal nerve and the adjacent pyramid

Fasciculation. Spontaneous contraction of muscle fibers visible through the skin as a result of denervation of a number of muscle fibers innervated by a single motor nerve fiber (motor unit).

KEY CONCEPTS

- Vascular occlusion of the anterior spinal artery in the medulla produces crossed motor and/or sensory syndromes characterized by ipsilateral tongue paralysis and contralateral loss of kinesthesia and discriminative touch (medial lemniscus) and/or the contralateral upper motor neuron syndrome (pyramid).

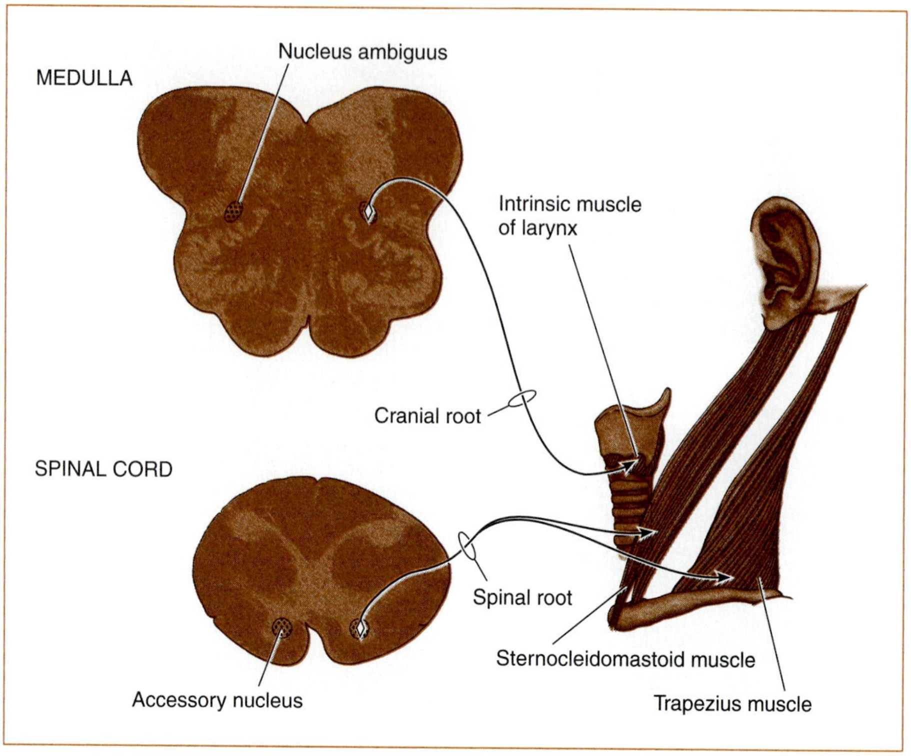

FIGURE 5-17

Schematic diagram illustrating the neurons of origin of the accessory nerve, and muscles supplied by the nerve.

within the medulla are manifested by the signs and symptoms of a hypoglossal nerve lesion and contralateral upper motor neuron paralysis (Fig. 5-16*C*).

Accessory nerve. The eleventh cranial nerve (accessory nerve of Willis) was described by Thomas Willis in 1664. The name *accessory* was used because this nerve receives an additional root from the upper part of the spinal cord.

Accessory Nerve (Cranial Nerve XI)

The accessory nerve (Fig. 5-17) has two roots: spinal and cranial. The spinal root arises from the accessory nucleus, a collection of motor neurons in the anterior horn of the upper five or six cervical spinal segments and the caudal part of the medulla. From their cells of origin, the rootlets course dorsolaterally and exit from the lateral part of the spinal cord between the dorsal and ventral roots. The spinal root of the accessory nerve enters the cranial cavity through the foramen magnum and leaves it through the jugular foramen. The spinal root contains somatic motor fibers that supply the sternocleidomastoid and trapezius (upper part) muscles.

The cranial root arises from the caudal pole of the nucleus ambiguus in the medulla oblongata. This root emerges from the lateral surface of the medulla, joins rootlets of the vagus nerve (forming its recurrent laryngeal branch), and supplies the intrinsic muscles of the larynx. Thus, the cranial root of the accessory nerve is in essence part of the vagus nerve.

KEY CONCEPTS

- The accessory nerve has two components: the spinal, which supplies the sternocleidomastoid and the upper part of the trapezius muscles, and the cranial, which forms the recurrent laryngeal nerve of the vagus and supplies the intrinsic muscles of the larynx.

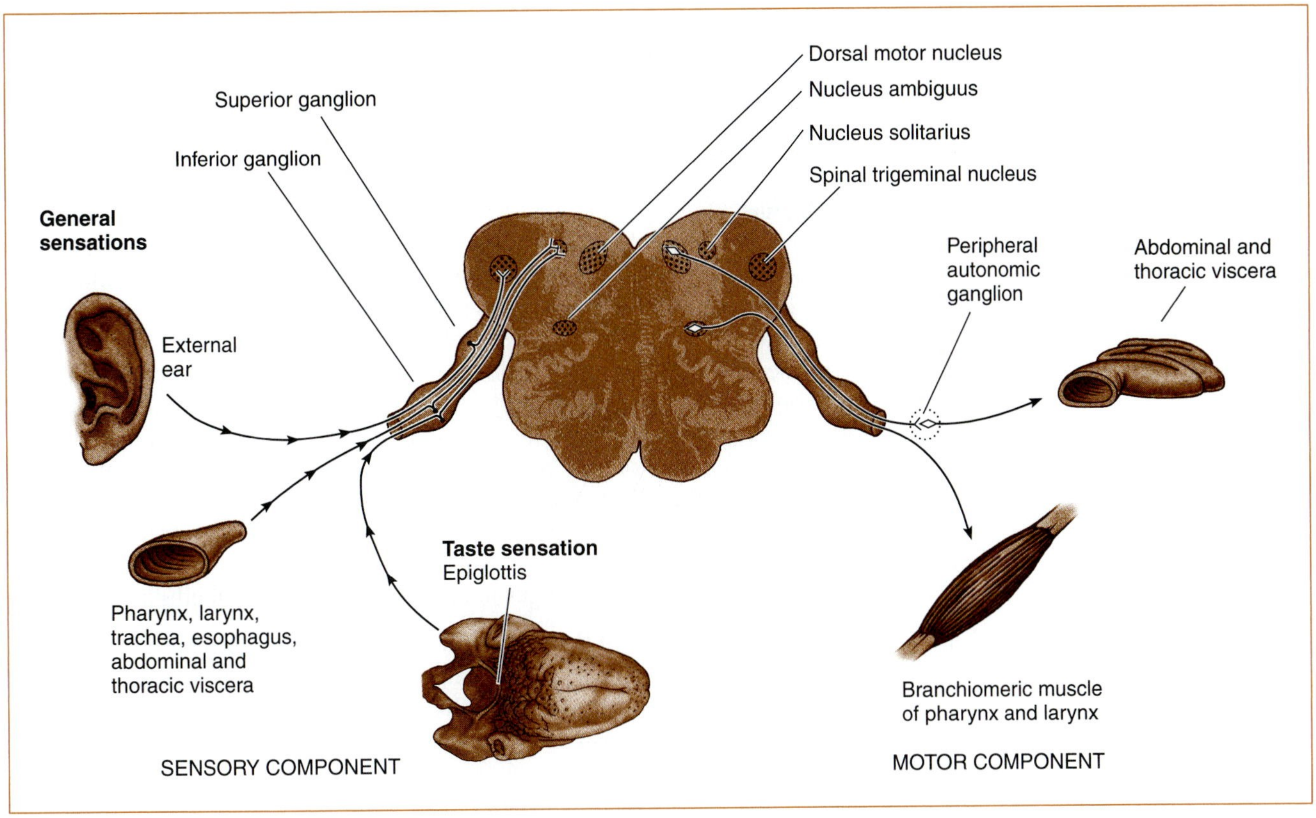
Dorsal motor nucleus
Nucleus ambiguus
Nucleus solitarius
Spinal trigeminal nucleus
Superior ganglion
Inferior ganglion
General sensations
External ear
Peripheral autonomic ganglion
Abdominal and thoracic viscera
Pharynx, larynx, trachea, esophagus, abdominal and thoracic viscera
Taste sensation
Epiglottis
Branchiomeric muscle of pharynx and larynx
SENSORY COMPONENT
MOTOR COMPONENT

FIGURE 5-18

Schematic diagram of the components of the vagus nerve and the areas they supply.

The recurrent laryngeal nerve is also known as Galen's nerve after Galen of Pergamon (A.D. 130–200), who took pride in his discovery that the recurrent laryngeal nerves control the voice. Some scholars argue that the function of the recurrent laryngeal nerve was described centuries before Galen.

The following are manifestations of unilateral lesions of the accessory nerve:

1. Downward and outward rotation of the scapula ipsilateral to the lesion
2. Moderate sagging of the ipsilateral shoulder
3. Weakness on turning the head to the side opposite the lesion
4. No observable abnormality of head position in repose

The first two signs are due to impaired function of the trapezius muscle, and the third is due to impaired function of the sternocleidomastoid muscle.

Vagus Nerve (Cranial Nerve X)

The vagus nerve (Fig. 5-18), a mixed nerve containing both afferent and efferent fibers, is associated with four nuclei in the medulla oblongata. The efferent components of the nerve are related to two medullary nuclei.

Vagus (Latin *vagari*, "wanderer"). The tenth cranial nerve is so named because of its long course and wide distribution. The nerve was described by Marinus in about A.D. 100. The name *vagus* was coined by Domenico de Marchetti of Padua.

Dorsal Motor Nucleus of the Vagus

The dorsal motor nucleus of the vagus is a column of cells dorsolateral or lateral to the hypoglossal nucleus and extending both rostrally and caudally a little beyond the hypoglossal nucleus. Axons of neurons in this column course ventrolaterally in the medulla and emerge from the lateral surface of the medulla between the inferior olive and the inferior cerebellar peduncle. Axons arising from this nucleus are preganglionic parasympathetic fibers that convey general visceral efferent impulses to the viscera in the thorax and abdomen. Postganglionic fibers arise from terminal ganglia situated within or on the innervated viscera in the thorax and abdomen. The dorsal motor nucleus of the vagus receives fibers from the vestibular nuclei; thus, excessive vestibular stimulation (e.g., motion sickness) results in nausea, vomiting, and a change in heart rate.

Nucleus ambiguus (Latin, "changeable or doubtful"). The boundaries of the nucleus ambiguus are indistinct.

Nucleus Ambiguus

The nucleus ambiguus is also known as the ventral motor nucleus of the vagus. It is a column of cells situated about halfway between the inferior olive and the nucleus of the spinal tract of the trigeminal nerve. Axons of neurons in this nucleus course dorsomedially and then turn ventrolaterally to emerge from the lateral surface of the medulla between the inferior olive and the inferior cerebellar peduncle. These axons convey special visceral efferent impulses to the branchiomeric muscles of the pharynx and larynx (pharyngeal constrictors, cricothyroid, intrinsic muscles of the larynx, levator veli palatini, palatoglossus, palatopharyngeus, and uvula). In addition to the vagus nerve, the nucleus ambiguus contributes efferent fibers to the glossopharyngeal (cranial nerve IX) and accessory (cranial nerve XI) nerves.

The afferent components of the vagus nerve are related to two medullary nuclei:

1. Nucleus of the spinal tract of the trigeminal nerve. This nucleus receives general somatic afferent fibers from the external ear. The neurons of origin of these fibers are in the superior ganglion of the vagus nerve. The general somatic afferent component of the vagus nerve is small, and its ganglion contains relatively few neurons.
2. Nucleus solitarius. This nucleus receives two types of visceral afferent fibers.
   a. General visceral afferent fibers. These fibers convey general visceral sensations from the pharynx, larynx, trachea, and esophagus as well as the thoracic and abdominal viscera.
   b. Special visceral afferent fibers. These fibers convey taste sensations from the region of the epiglottis.

The neurons of origin of both types of afferent fibers reside in the inferior ganglion of the vagus. The central processes of neurons in this ganglion enter the lateral surface of the medulla oblongata, course dorsomedially, and form the tractus solitarius, which projects on cells of the nucleus solitarius. Neurons in the latter nucleus are organized so that those receiving general visceral afferent fibers are located in the caudal and medial part of the nucleus, whereas those receiving special visceral afferent fibers (taste) are located in the rostral and lateral part. Caudally, the two solitary nuclei merge to form the commissural nucleus of the vagus nerve. In addition to the vagus nerve, the nucleus solitarius receives general visceral afferent fibers from the glossopharyngeal nerve (cranial nerve IX) and special visceral (taste) afferent fibers from the glossopharyneal (cranial nerve IX) and facial (cranial nerve VII) nerves.

Bilateral lesions of the vagus nerve are fatal as a result of complete laryngeal paralysis and asphyxia.

KEY CONCEPTS

- The vagus nerve has two motor nuclei (the dorsal motor nucleus and the nucleus ambiguus) and two sensory nuclei (the nucleus solitarius and the spinal trigeminal nucleus).
- The nucleus ambiguus contributes fibers to three cranial nerves: accessory, vagus, and glossopharyngeal.

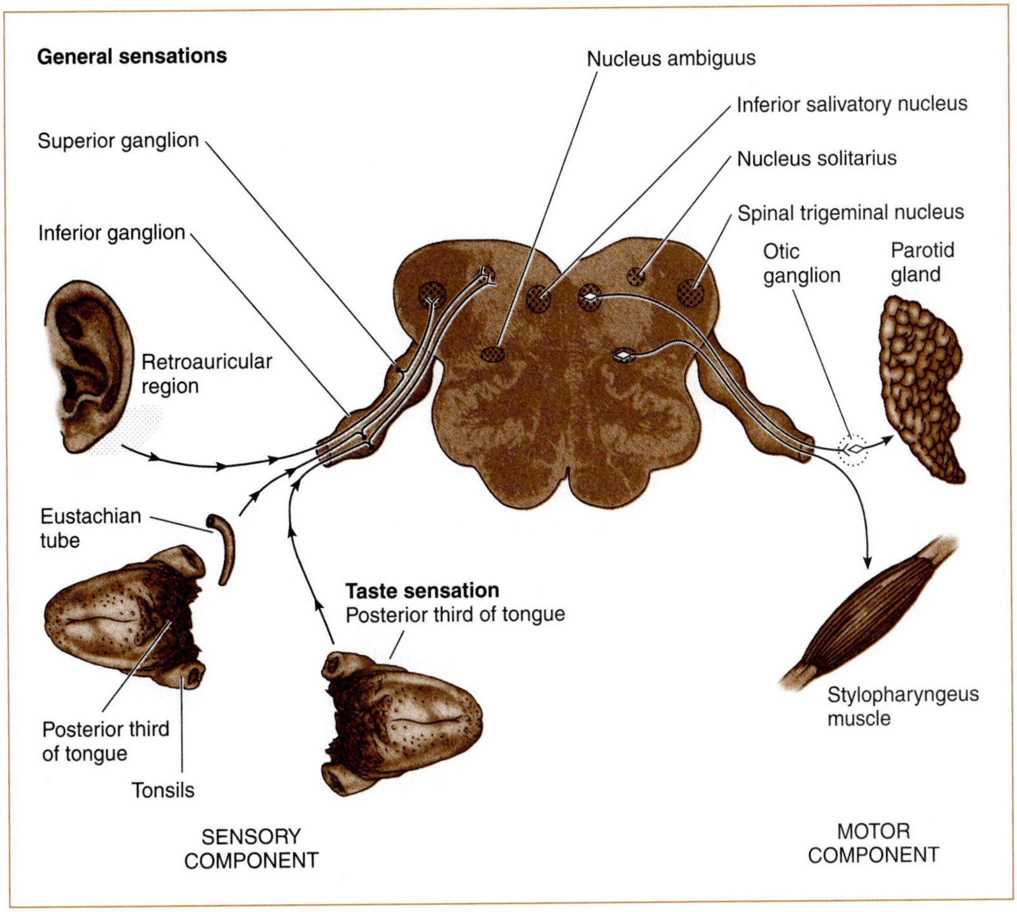

FIGURE 5-19

Schematic diagram of the components of the glossopharyngeal nerve and the structures they supply.

Unilateral vagal lesions result in ipsilateral paralysis of the soft palate, pharynx, and larynx. This is manifested by hoarseness of the voice, **dysphagia** (difficulty swallowing), and **dyspnea** (difficulty breathing).

Glossopharyngeal Nerve (Cranial Nerve IX)

The glossopharyngeal nerve (Fig. 5-19), which is also a mixed nerve (containing both afferent and efferent components), is associated with four nuclei in the medulla. The efferent components of the glossopharyngeal nerve are related to two nuclei.

Nucleus Ambiguus

Axons that travel with the glossopharyngeal nerve arise from neurons in the rostral part of the nucleus ambiguus and supply special visceral efferent fibers to the stylopharyngeus muscle. This efferent component of the glossopharyngeal nerve is small.

Inferior Salivatory Nucleus

The inferior salivatory nucleus is a group of neurons that are difficult to distinguish from reticular neurons in the dorsal aspect of the medulla. The axons of neurons in this nucleus leave the medulla from its lateral surface. They are preganglionic general visceral efferent fibers that convey secretomotor impulses to the parotid

Dysphagia (Greek *dys*, "difficult"; *phagien*, "to eat"). Difficulty swallowing.

Dyspnea (Greek *dyspnoia*, "difficulty breathing"). Difficulty breathing.

Glossopharyngeal (Greek *glossa*, "tongue"; *pharynx*, "throat"). The ninth cranial nerve. Included by Galen with the sixth nerve. Fallopius distinguished it as a separate nerve in 1561. Thomas Willis included it as part of the eighth nerve. Soemmering listed it as the ninth cranial nerve.

gland. They travel via the lesser petrosal nerve to the otic ganglion, from which postganglionic fibers supply the parotid gland.

The afferent components of the glossopharyngeal nerve are related to the same two nuclei associated with the vagus nerve:

1. Nucleus of the spinal tract of the trigeminal nerve. This nucleus receives general somatic afferent fibers from the retroauricular region. Neurons of origin of these fibers are located in the superior ganglion within the jugular foramen.
2. Nucleus solitarius. This nucleus receives two types of visceral afferent fibers.
   a. General visceral afferent fibers. These fibers convey tactile, pain, and thermal sensations from the mucous membranes of the posterior third of the tongue, the tonsils, and the eustachian tube.
   b. Special visceral afferent fibers. These fibers convey taste sensations from the posterior third of the tongue.

Neurons of origin of the visceral afferent fibers are located in the inferior ganglion. Within the medulla, they form the tractus solitarius and project on the nucleus solitarius in a manner similar to that described above for the vagus nerve.

The glossopharyngeal nerve also contains a special afferent branch, the carotid sinus nerve. This branch innervates the carotid body and carotid sinus, which are chemoreceptor and baroreceptor centers. Elevation of carotid arterial pressure stimulates the carotid sinus nerve, which upon reaching the medulla sends collaterals to the dorsal motor nucleus of the vagus. General visceral efferent components of the vagus nerve then reach ganglion cells in the wall of the heart to slow the heart rate and reduce blood pressure. This glossopharyngeal-vagal reflex is especially sensitive in elderly people. Therefore, extreme care should be taken in manipulating the carotid sinus region in the neck of an elderly person.

Unilateral lesions of the glossopharyngeal nerve are manifested by the following signs:

1. Loss of the pharyngeal (gag) reflex homolateral to the nerve lesion. This reflex is elicited by stimulation of the posterior pharyngeal wall, the tonsillar area, or the base of the tongue. Normally, tongue retraction is associated with elevation and constriction of the pharyngeal musculature.
2. Loss of the carotid sinus reflex homolateral to the nerve lesion.
3. Loss of taste in the homolateral posterior third of the tongue.
4. Deviation of the uvula to the unaffected side.

Vestibulocochlear Nerve (Cranial Nerve VIII)

The vestibular component of the vestibulocochlear nerve is discussed in Chap. 7. The two vestibular nuclei that appear at rostral levels of the medulla are the inferior vestibular nucleus and the medial vestibular nucleus.

The inferior vestibular nucleus is located medial to the restiform body and is characterized in histologic preparations by the presence of dark-staining bundles

KEY CONCEPTS

- The glossopharyngeal nerve has two motor nuclei (the nucleus ambiguus and the inferior salivatory nucleus) and two sensory nuclei (the nucleus solitarius and the spinal trigeminal nucleus).
- Two vestibular nuclei are seen in the dorsolateral medulla: inferior vestibular and medial vestibular.

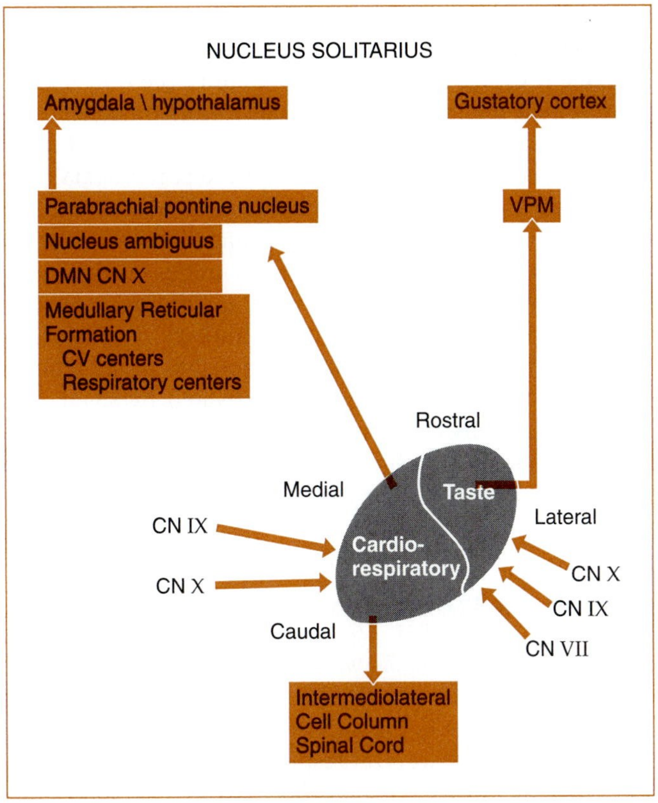

FIGURE 5-20

Schematic diagram showing major inputs and outputs of the nucleus solitarius.

of fibers coursing through it. The medial vestibular nucleus, which is located medial to the inferior nucleus, is poorly stained in myelin preparations because of the relatively few fibers it contains.

Nucleus Solitarius

The nucleus solitarius is divided into two zones (Fig. 5-20). The caudal and medial zone is concerned with general visceral sensation and primarily cardio-respiratory function. The rostral and lateral zone is concerned with special visceral (taste) function. Caudally, the two solitary nuclei merge to form the commissural nucleus of the vagus nerve.

The **gustatory** (taste) zone receives taste sensations via three cranial nerves: The facial nerve (cranial nerve VII) conveys taste sensations from the anterior two-thirds of the tongue, the glossopharyngeal nerve (cranial nerve IX) conveys taste sensations from the posterior third of the tongue, and the vagus nerve (cranial nerve X) conveys taste sensations from the epiglottis. The output of the gustatory zone is to the posterior thalamus (ventral posterior medial nucleus), which in turn projects to the primary gustatory cortex.

Gustatory (Latin *gustatorius*, "pertaining to the sense of taste").

KEY CONCEPTS

- The nucleus solitarius is divided into two subnuclei: the caudal and medial general visceral subnucleus and the rostral and lateral special visceral (taste) subnucleus.

The zone concerned with general visceral sensations receives input via two cranial nerves: the glossopharyngeal (cranial nerve IX) and the vagus (cranial nerve X). Neurons in this zone project to the nucleus ambiguus, the dorsal motor nucleus of the vagus, centers within the medullary reticular formation concerned with cardiovascular and respiratory function, the intermediolateral cell column in the spinal cord, and the parabrachial pontine nucleus. From the parabrachial pontine nucleus, visceral sensory information is relayed to the amygdala and hypothalamus. Lesions in the nucleus or tractus solitarius and their connections with the area postrema have been associated in humans and experimental animals with a change in feeding behavior characterized by early satiety and poor appetite. The nucleus solitarius is coextensive with the physiologically defined medullary respiratory center, which includes the nucleus ambiguus and surrounding portions of the reticular formation. Cells of the medullary respiratory center are activated by vagal impulses and by changes in their chemical environment (CO_2 accumulation). The caudal zone of the nucleus solitarius, along with the dorsal motor nucleus of the vagus and the medial reticular formation, has been implicated in the genesis of neurogenic pulmonary edema.

The Medulla and Respiratory Function

Experimental studies have identified two medullary regions related to respiratory function. The dorsal respiratory group in the nucleus solitarius contains primary inspiratory neurons that project to the nucleus ambiguus and to spinal cord neurons that supply the diaphragm. The ventral respiratory group in the nucleus ambiguus and nucleus retroambiguus contains inspiratory and expiratory neurons. The inspiratory neurons are driven by the nucleus solitarius. Neurons in the ventral respiratory group project to spinal cord neurons that supply the intercostal and abdominal muscles.

There is a paucity of information about centers of respiration in the brain stem in humans. Structures implicated in apnea in humans include the nucleus solitarius, the nucleus ambiguus, the nucleus retroambiguus, the dorsal motor nucleus of the vagus, the region of the medial lemniscus, the region of the spinothalamic tract, and the medullary reticular formation, all bilaterally.

Discrete unilateral lesions in the nucleus ambiguus and the adjacent reticular formation in humans have been reported to result in failure of automatic respiratory function (sleep apnea, **Ondine's curse**). Lesions that also involve the nucleus solitarius result in failure of both automatic and voluntary respiration.

Ondine's curse. A syndrome characterized by the cessation of breathing in sleep because of failure of the medullary automatic respiratory center. Named after the story of Ondine, a water nymph who punished her unfaithful husband by depriving him of the ability to breathe while asleep.

Neurogenic Pulmonary Edema

The classic anatomic substrate for the generation of neurogenic pulmonary edema in experimental models is an "edemagenic center" in the preoptic hypothalamus. This observation was based on the development of pulmonary edema in rats after preoptic hypothalamic lesions. Subsequent studies demonstrated that these hypo-

KEY CONCEPTS

- The nucleus solitarius receives input from three cranial nerves: facial, glossopharyngeal, and vagus.
- Two regions in the medulla are concerned with respiratory function: dorsal in the nucleus solitarius and ventral in the nuclei ambiguus and retroambiguus.

thalamic lesions are associated with systemic hypertension followed by cardiac failure and pulmonary edema.

Clinical reports of neurogenic pulmonary edema from focal lesions support a caudal brain stem site for the induction of pulmonary edema. These cases include focal puncture wounds of the medulla, posterior fossa stroke, localized brain stem hemorrhage, bulbar poliomyelitis, and multiple sclerosis. Recent high-resolution brain imaging studies have suggested an anatomic substrate for neurogenic pulmonary edema in the caudal brain stem that includes the nucleus solitarius, the dorsal motor nucleus of the vagus, and the medial medullary reticular formation. Both indirect evidence and direct evidence support the nucleus solitarius as the effector site inducing neurogenic pulmonary edema. The caudal portion of the nucleus solitarius appears phylogenetically only in air-breathing animals and contains the neuronal pools involved in the regulation of ventilation. The nucleus is also the site of termination of afferent fibers from the lung (via cranial nerves IX and X) and from chemoreceptors and baroreceptors of the carotid sinus. Efferent fibers from the ventral lateral zone of the nucleus solitarius terminate in the thoracic region of the spinal cord. The caudal zone of the nucleus plays well-defined roles in the regulation of other peripheral cardiovascular functions, particularly systemic vascular pressure.

The Medulla and Sneezing

The sneezing reflex is triggered by a variety of stimuli, the most common of which is stimulation of the nasal mucosa (trigeminal nerve sensory endings) by mechanical or chemical stimuli. Other stimuli include exposure to bright or blue light (solar sneeze) and male orgasm. The latter two stimuli elicit sneezing via pathways that converge on the sneezing center. The sneezing center is in the medulla oblongata at the ventromedial margin of the descending tract and nucleus (spinal nucleus) of the trigeminal nerve and includes the adjacent reticular formation and nucleus solitarius. The sneezing reflex has two phases: nasal and respiratory.

The afferent limb of the nasal phase consists of the ethmoidal and olfactory nerves, which project to the sneezing center in the medulla oblongata. The efferent limb consists of preganglionic fibers to the greater petrosal nerve and the sphenopalatine ganglion, which innervate glands and blood vessels in the nose, resulting in nasal secretion and edema, further stimulation of the nasal mucosa, and more impulses to the sneezing center.

The respiratory phase of the sneezing reflex commences when a critical number of inspiratory and expiratory neurons are recruited by the sneezing center. Recruitment of these neurons increases activity in the vagus, phrenic, and intercostal nerves to the appropriate musculature. Manifestations of this phase consist of the following sequence of events: eye closure, deep inspiration, pharyngeal closure, forceful expiration, dilation of the glottis, explosive air release through the mouth and nose, and expulsion of mucus and irritants.

Sneezing disorders consist of those of excessive sneezing (more common) and the inability to sneeze (less common). Inability to sneeze has been reported in psychiatric disorders and in medullary neoplasms affecting the sneezing center.

KEY CONCEPTS

- Lesions in the medulla oblongata in or near the nucleus solitarius have been linked to the development of neurogenic pulmonary edema.
- A sneezing center is believed to exist in the medulla oblongata near the spinal trigeminal nucleus and tract.

The Medulla and Swallowing

The process of swallowing involves three functionally distinct phases: oral, pharyngolaryngeal, and esophageal. In the oral phase, food is broken into sufficiently small pieces for transport through the pharynx and esophagus and the food is propelled into the pharynx after mastication. The pharyngolaryngeal phase propels the bolus to the esophagus while coordinating the protection of the respiratory tract by means of inhibition of respiration, closure of the palatopharyngeal isthmus, and constriction of the larynx. The esophageal phase involves both striated and smooth esophageal muscles and propels the food to the stomach. The pharyngolaryngeal and esophageal phases are controlled by neurons in the medullary reticular formation.

Stimulation studies suggest that two regions in the medulla are involved in swallowing: a dorsal area around and including the nucleus solitarius and a ventral area around the nucleus ambiguus. Lesion studies demonstrate loss of swallowing in patients with lesions within the rostral tractus solitarius or nucleus solitarius. The swallowing centers in the medulla are influenced by peripheral stimuli from sensory receptors and by descending suprasegmental input. The peripheral fields from which swallowing can be evoked include the posterior tongue and the oropharyngeal region. The most important afferent impulses are carried in the glossopharyngeal and vagus nerves. Descending pathways that modify swallowing arise from the prefrontal cortex, the limbic system, the hypothalamus, the midbrain, and the pons. Descending pathways are important in the process of learning to integrate orofacial movements in the oral phase but are not essential in the coordination of the pharyngeal and esophageal phases. Swallowing continues in humans and experimental animals with lesions in the descending pathways.

Neuroanatomy of Vomiting

Clinical and experimental studies have shown the existence of a vomiting center in the dorsolateral medullary reticular formation (parvicellular nucleus) with a chemoreceptor trigger zone for vomiting in the area postrema, an area devoid of a blood-brain barrier, in the floor of the caudal fourth ventricle. In experimental animals, stimulation of the vomiting center in the lateral reticular formation (in the vicinity of the fasciculus solitarius) results in projectile vomiting. Centrally acting emetic drugs (apomorphine) do not act directly on the reticular medullary vomiting center. Instead, they stimulate the chemoreceptor zone in the area postrema, which secondarily stimulates the vomiting center. Ablation of the area postrema thus abolishes the emetic response to intravenous apomorphine. Several afferent and efferent connections to the vomiting center have been demonstrated or speculated about (Fig. 5-21). The major afferents arise from the area postrema and the nucleus solitarius. Other afferents include inputs from the cerebellum, vestibular system, salivary nucleus, sensory nuclei of the trigeminal nerve, respiratory and vasomotor centers, vagus nerve, and sympathetic **splanchnic nerves.** The

Splanchnic nerves (Greek *splanchnikos*, "pertaining to the viscera"). The sympathetic nerves to the abdominal viscera. Originally investigated by Scarpa. The term appeared in English in 1694.

KEY CONCEPTS

- Two regions in the medulla oblongata are linked to swallowing: a dorsal region in and near the nucleus solitarius and a ventral region around the nucleus ambiguus.
- A vomiting center has been identified in the dorsolateral medullary reticular formation, and a chemoreceptor trigger zone for vomiting has been identified in the area postrema.

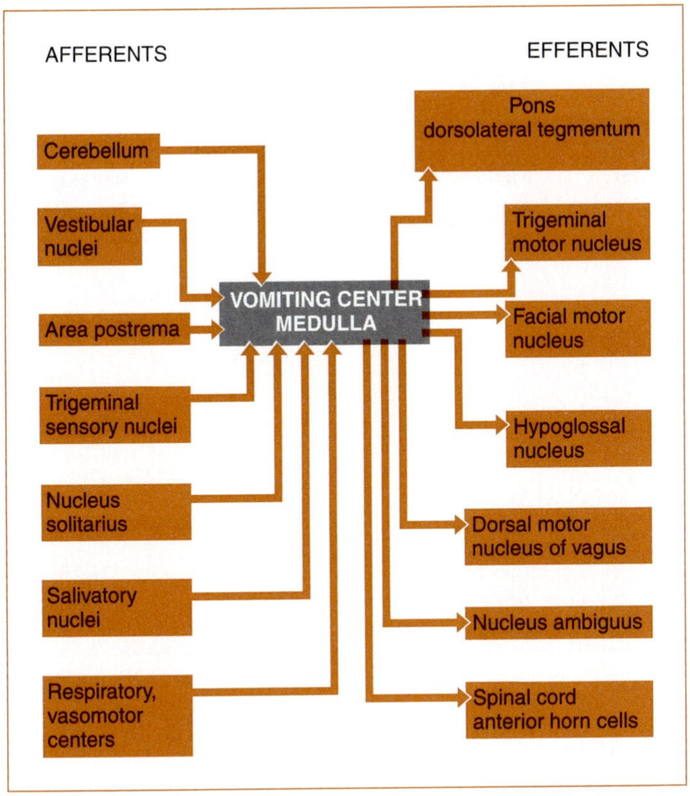

FIGURE 5-21

Schematic diagram showing major sources of input and targeted output of the medullary vomiting center.

area postrema mediates the effects of drugs and toxins on the vomiting center. The nucleus solitarius acts as an intermediary for the inputs from taste receptors (via cranial nerves VII, IX, and X) and for autonomic input from the large intestine via the vagus (parasympathetic) and splanchnic nerves (sympathetic). The vagal and splanchnic inputs also may reach the vomiting center directly. The input from the vestibular system explains the vomiting of motion sickness.

Major efferent pathways are to the motor nuclei of the cranial nerves that control jaw, mouth, and tongue movements (trigeminal, facial, and hypoglossal nerves) and to nuclei that control the respiratory and abdominal muscles that are of prime importance in the expulsive phase of vomiting (dorsal motor nucleus of the vagus, nucleus ambiguus, and anterior horn of the spinal cord, which supply the respiratory and abdominal muscles). Ascending fibers from the medullary vomiting center and the area postrema have been traced to the dorsolateral pontine tegmentum, where they terminate on or ventral to the parabrachial nuclei.

Lesions in the dorsolateral pontine tegmentum have been associated with vomiting. Descending projections from the dorsolateral pontine tegmentum reach the facial and hypoglossal motor nuclei, the nucleus ambiguus, and motor neurons of the spinal cord.

Neurotransmitters and Neuropeptides

The following neurotransmitters and neuropeptides have been identified in the medulla oblongata: acetylcholine, norepinephrine, serotonin, enkephalin, substance P, somatostatin, cholecystokinin, and neuropeptide Y (Table 5-2).

TABLE 5-2

Medulla Oblongata: Neurotransmitters and Neuropeptides

	Hypoglossal Nucleus	Dorsal Motor Nucleus of Vagus	Nucleus Ambiguus	Nucleus Solitarius	Spinal Trigeminal Nucleus	Reticular Formation	Raphe Nucleus
Acetylcholine	+	+	+				
Norepinephrine						+	
Serotonin							+
Enkephalin				+	+	+	+
Substance P				+	+		+
Somatostatin				+			
Cholecystokinin				+			
Neuropeptide Y				+			

BLOOD SUPPLY OF THE MEDULLA

The medulla oblongata receives its blood supply from the following arteries:

1. Vertebral
2. Anterior spinal
3. Posterior spinal
4. Posterior inferior cerebellar (PICA)

The medulla is divided into the following four vascular territories: paramedian, olivary, lateral, and dorsal (Fig. 5-22).

The paramedian territory receives its blood supply from the vertebral and/or anterior spinal arteries. It includes the pyramid, the medial lemniscus, the medial longitudinal fasciculus, and the hypoglossal nucleus and nerve. The olivary territory receives an inconstant blood supply from the vertebral artery. It includes most of the inferior olivary complex. The lateral territory receives a constant blood supply from the vertebral artery and a dorsally variable supply from the posterior inferior cerebellar artery. It includes the dorsal motor nucleus of the vagus, the nucleus solitarius and tract, vestibular nuclei, the nucleus ambiguus, the spinal trigeminal nucleus and tract, the lateral spinothalamic tract, the restiform body, and the inferior olivary complex. The dorsal territory is supplied rostally by the posterior inferior cerebellar artery and caudally by the posterior spinal artery. This includes the vestibular nuclei, the dorsal column nuclei and tracts, and part of the restiform body.

KEY CONCEPTS

- The blood supply to the medulla oblongata comes from the following arteries: vertebral, anterior spinal, posterior spinal, and posterior inferior cerebellar (PICA).
- The medulla oblongata is divided into four vascular territories: paramedian, olivary, lateral, and dorsal.

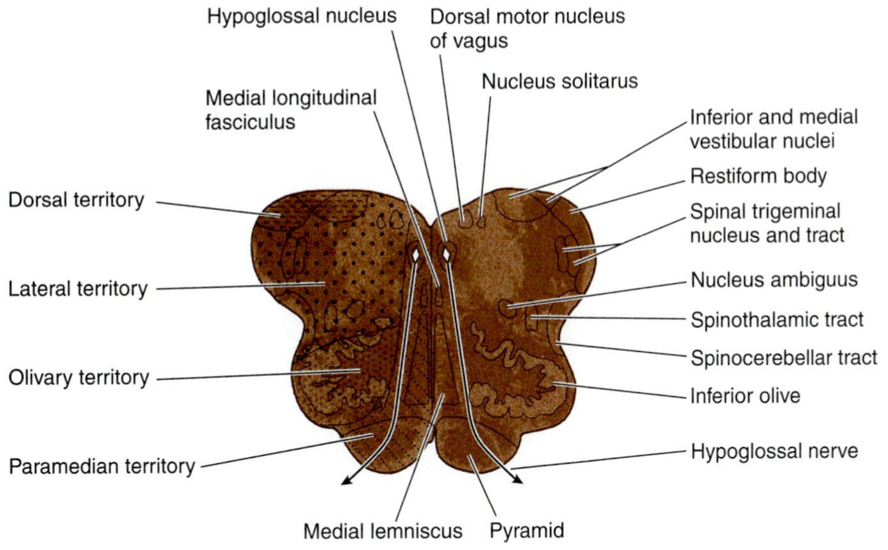

FIGURE 5-22

Schematic diagram of vascular territories of the medulla oblongata.

SUGGESTED READINGS

Amarenco P, et al: Infarction in the territory of the medial branch of the posterior inferior cerebellar artery. *J Neurol Neurosurg Psychiatry* 1990; 53:731–735.

Baker P, Bernat JL: The neuroanatomy of vomiting in man: Association of projectile vomiting with a solitary metastasis in the lateral tegmentum of the pons and the middle cerebellar peduncle. *J Neurol Neurosurg Psychiatry* 1985; 48:1165–1168.

Beckstead RM, et al: The nucleus of the solitary tract in the monkey: Projections to the thalamus and brain stem nuclei. *J Comp Neurol* 1980; 190:259–282.

Bogousslavsky J, et al: Respiratory failure and unilateral caudal brainstem infarction. *Ann Neurol* 1990; 28:668–673.

Ciriello J, Calaresu FR: Vagal bradycardia elicited by stimulation of the external cuneate nucleus in the cat. *Am J Physiol* 1978; 235:R286–293.

Glendinning DS, Vierck CJ: Lack of proprioceptive deficit after dorsal column lesions in monkeys. *Neurology* 1993; 43:363–366.

Iwata M, Hirano A: Localization of olivo-cerebellar fibers in inferior cerebellar peduncle in man. *J. Neurol Sci* 1978; 38:327–335.

Kalil K: Projections of the cerebellar and dorsal column nuclei upon the inferior olive in the Rhesus monkey: An autoradiographic study. *J Comp Neurol* 1979; 188:43–62.

Kawamura K, Hashikawa T: Olivocerebellar projections in the cat studied by means of anterograde axonal transport of labeled amino acids as tracers. *Neuroscience* 1979; 4:1615–1633.

Kotchabhakdi N, et al: Afferent projections to the thalamus from the perihypoglossal nuclei. *Brain Res* 1980; 187:457–461.

Martin RA, et al: Inability to sneeze as a manifestation of medullary neoplasm. *Neurology* 1991; 41:1675–1676.

Masdeu JC, Ross ER: Medullary satiety. *Neurology* 1988; 38:1643–1645.

Miller AJ: Neurophysiological basis of swallowing. *Dysphagia* 1986; 1:91–100.

Poulos DA, et al: Localization of specific thermoreceptors in spinal trigeminal nucleus of the cat. *Brain Res* 1979; 165:144–148.

Saint-Cyr JA, Courville J: Projection from the vestibular nuclei to the inferior olive in the cat: An autoradiographic and horseradish peroxidase study. *Brain Res* 1979; 165:189–200.

Simon RP, et al: Medullary lesions inducing pulmonary edema: A magnetic resonance imaging study. *Ann Neurol* 1991; 30:727–730.

Somana R, Walberg F: A re-examination of the cerebellar projections from the gracile, main and external cuneate nuclei in the cat. *Brain Res* 1980; 186:33–42.

Uemura M, et al: Topographical arrangement of hypoglossal motoneurons: An HRP study in the cat. *Neurosci Lett* 1979; 13:99–104.

Waespe W, Wichmann W: Oculomotor disturbances during visual vestibular interactions in Wallenberg's lateral medullary syndrome. *Brain* 1990; 113:821–846.

Weisberg JA, Rustioni A: Differential projections of cortical sensorimotor areas upon the dorsal column nuclei of cats. *J Comp Neurol* 1979; 184:401–422.

Zemlan FP, Pfaff DW: Topographical organization in medullary reticulospinal systems as demonstrated by the horseradish peroxidase technique. *Brain Res* 1979; 174:161–166.

CHAPTER 6

MEDULLA OBLONGATA: CLINICAL CORRELATES

Vascular lesions in the medulla oblongata are best suited to anatomicoclinical correlation. In the past, these syndromes were designated by the artery of supply (e.g., anterior spinal artery syndrome, posterior inferior cerebellar artery syndrome, vertebral artery syndrome). Because of variations in the source of blood supply, however, these syndromes are currently designated by the anatomic region affected by the lesion. Two such syndromes are particularly illustrative: the medial medullary syndrome and the lateral medullary syndrome.

MEDIAL MEDULLARY SYNDROME (DEJERINE'S ANTERIOR BULBAR SYNDROME)

The medial medullary syndrome (Fig. 6-1) is caused by occlusion of the anterior spinal artery or the paramedian branches of the vertebral artery. The affected area

Dejerine, Joseph-Jules (1849–1917). A French neurologist who described, among other syndromes, the medial medullary syndrome.

KEY CONCEPTS

- Vascular lesions of the medulla oblongata are designated by the anatomic region affected rather than by the arterial supply.
- Vascular syndromes that are illustrative of occlusive vascular disease in the medulla oblongata include the medial medullary syndrome, the lateral medullary syndrome, combined medial and lateral syndromes, and the dorsal medullary syndrome.

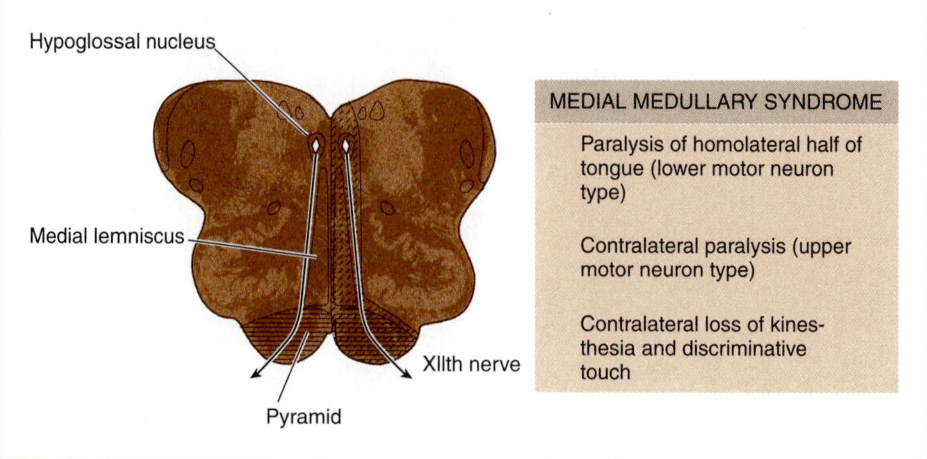

FIGURE 6-1

Schematic diagram of medullary structures involved in the medial medullary syndrome, and the resulting clinical manifestations.

usually includes the following structures:

1. Medial lemniscus
2. Pyramid
3. Rootlets of the hypoglossal nerve or its nucleus within the medulla

The neurologic signs resulting from the involvement of these areas are as follows:

1. Contralateral loss of kinesthesia and discriminative touch resulting from involvement of the medial lemniscus
2. Contralateral paralysis of the upper motor neuron type (weakness, hyperactive reflexes, **Babinski's sign, clonus,** and spasticity) with sparing of the face caused by involvement of the pyramid
3. Lower motor neuron paralysis of the homolateral half of the tongue (weakness, atrophy, and **fibrillation**) and deviation of the protruded tongue to the atrophic side caused by involvement of the hypoglossal nucleus or nerve

The medial medullary syndrome may occur bilaterally, resulting in bilateral upper motor neuron weakness or paralysis (with facial sparing), bilateral paralysis of the tongue of the lower motor neuron type, and bilateral loss of kinesthesia and discriminative touch.

LATERAL MEDULLARY SYNDROME

The lateral medullary syndrome (Fig. 6-2) is caused by occlusion of the vertebral artery or, less frequently, the medial branch of the posterior inferior cerebellar artery when this artery supplies the lateral medulla. It is also known as the posterior

KEY CONCEPTS

- The anatomic structures that are affected in the medial medullary syndrome include the medial lemniscus, the pyramid, and the hypoglossal nerve rootlets or nucleus.
- The clinical signs of the medial medullary syndrome include contralateral weakness of the upper motor neuron type, contralateral loss of kinesthesia and discriminative touch, and ipsilateral tongue weakness of the lower motor neuron type.

Babinski's sign. An upper motor neuron lesion sign characterized by dorsiflexion of the big toe and fanning out of the rest of the toes upon painful stimulation or stroking of the sole. The sign was described "as the phenomenon of the toes" by Josef-François-Felix Babinski (1857–1932), a French neurologist, in 1896. The phenomenon had previously been noted by Hall and Remak. Babinski investigated the phenomenon in depth in papers published between 1896 and 1903.

Clonus (Greek *klonos*, "turmoil"). Alternate muscular contraction of agonist and antagonist muscle groups in rapid succession in response to sudden stretching of the muscle tendon. Usually seen in an upper motor neuron lesion caused by the loss of suprasegmental inhibition of the local spinal reflex arc. The term was originally used by Greek physicians for the convulsing movements of epileptics.

Fibrillation. Local involuntary contraction of muscle that is invisible under the skin and is recorded by electromyography after the placement of a recording needle in the muscle. A sign of denervation.

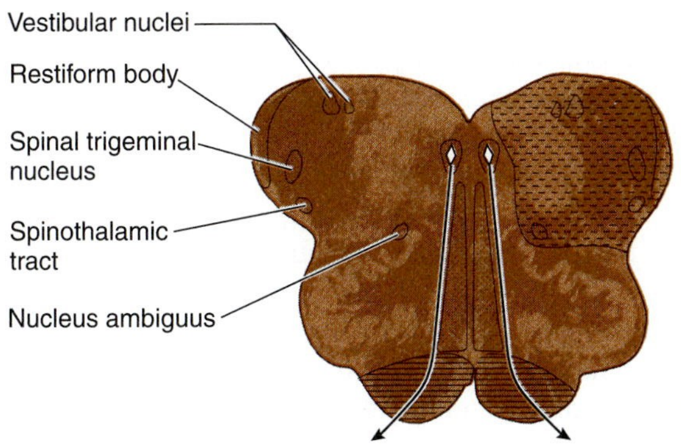

LATERAL MEDULLARY SYNDROME

- Loss of pain and temperature sensations over the ipsila-eral face and contralateral half of the body
- Ataxia (loss of coordination)
- Vertigo (hallucination of movement)
- Loss of gag reflex, difficulty in swallowing, and difficulty in articulation
- Ipsilateral Horner's syndrome
- Vomiting

FIGURE 6-2

Schematic diagram of medullary structures involved in the lateral medullary syndrome, and the resulting clinical manifestations.

inferior cerebellar artery (PICA) syndrome or **Wallenberg's syndrome.** The affected area usually includes the following structures:

1. Spinal nucleus of the trigeminal nerve and its tract
2. Adjacent spinothalamic tract
3. **Nucleus ambiguus** or its axons
4. Base of the inferior cerebellar peduncle
5. Vestibular nuclei
6. Descending sympathetic fibers from the hypothalamus

The neurologic signs and symptoms resulting from the involvement of these areas include the following:

1. Loss of pain and temperature sensations from the ipsilateral face as a result of involvement of the spinal nucleus of the trigeminal nerve and its tract.
2. Loss of pain and temperature sensation over the contralateral half of the body because of involvement of the spinothalamic tract.
3. Loss of the gag reflex, difficulty swallowing (dysphagia), hoarseness, and difficulty in articulation (dysarthria) caused by paralysis of muscles supplied by the nucleus ambiguus ipsilateral to the medullary lesion.
4. Ipsilateral loss of coordination (ataxia) resulting from involvement of the base of the inferior cerebellar peduncle.

Wallenberg's (lateral medullary) syndrome. Also known as the lateral bulbar syndrome and the posterior inferior cerebellar artery syndrome. A syndrome consisting of vertigo, vomiting, hiccups, dysarthria, dysphagia, hoarseness, ataxia, Horner's syndrome, and crossed sensory loss. The syndrome was described in detail by Adolph Wallenberg, a German neurologist, in 1895. An earlier account of the syndrome was provided by the Swiss physician Gaspard Vieusseux in 1810.

Nucleus ambiguus (Latin, "changeable, doubtful"). So called because its boundaries are indistinct.

KEY CONCEPTS

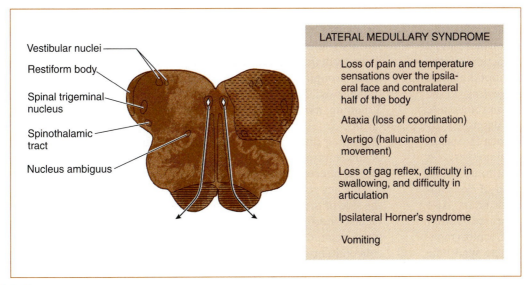

- The anatomic structures affected in the lateral medullary syndrome include the spinal trigeminal nucleus and tract, the spinothalamic tract, the nucleus ambiguus, the vestibular nuclei, the inferior cerebellar peduncle, and the descending sympathetic fibers.
- The clinical signs of the lateral medullary syndrome include loss of pain and temperature sense in the ipsilateral face and the contralateral half of the body, ipsilateral loss of the gag reflex, hoarseness, dysphagia, dysarthria, ataxia, vertigo, ipsilateral Horner's syndrome, nystagmus, and ocular lateropulsion.

5. Hallucination of turning (vertigo) resulting from involvement of the vestibular nuclei.
6. **Horner's syndrome** caused by involvement of the descending sympathetic fibers from the hypothalamus. This syndrome consists of a small pupil (miosis), slight drooping of the upper eyelid (ptosis), and warm dry skin of the face (**anhidrosis**), all ipsilateral to the lesion.
7. Vomiting, **nystagmus,** and nausea resulting from involvement of the vestibular nuclei.
8. **Hiccuping** that is of uncertain cause but usually is attributed to involvement of the respiratory center in the reticular formation of the medulla.
9. Ocular **lateropulsion** occurs almost universally in this syndrome. It consists of a tendency toward saccadic eye movement overshoot or hypermetria toward the side of the lesion and a tendency toward hypometria away from the lesion. Ocular lateropulsion is believed to result from involvement of olivocerebellar fibers related to ocular movement traveling in the lateral medulla or to a concomitant cerebellar lesion.
10. Difficulty pursuing contralateral moving targets as a result of involvement of the vestibular pathways in nuclei of extraocular movement

Although credit for the description of the lateral medullary syndrome in 1895 is often given to Adolph Wallenberg, as evidenced by the term *Wallenberg's syndrome*, the Swiss physician Gaspard Vieusseux provided an account in 1810, reporting in detail his own stroke to the Medical and Surgical Society of London.

Clinical manifestations of the lateral medullary syndrome may vary depending on the caudal-rostral level of the lesion. Dysphagia, hoarseness, and ipsilateral facial paresis are more common in patients with lesions in the rostral medulla. Gait ataxia, vertigo, and nystagmus are more common in patients with caudal medullary lesions. The ipsilateral facial paresis reported in rostral medullary lesions is attributed to involvement of aberrant corticobulbar fibers in the medulla or extension of the medullary lesion to the pons.

Besides Wallenberg's syndrome, occlusion of the medial branch of PICA can present with a pseudolabyrinthine syndrome characterized by cerebellar and vestibular signs (vertigo, **dysmetria,** ataxia, and axial lateropulsion) that overshadow the medullary signs. Occlusion of the medial branch of the posterior inferior cerebellar artery also may result in a silent infarct that is detected only at autopsy. There are no clinical reports of occlusion of the lateral branch of the posterior inferior cerebellar artery. Silent infarcts have been reported as a chance autopsy finding.

BABINSKI-NAGEOTTE SYNDROME

The Babinski-Nageotte syndrome, also known as medullary tegmental paralysis, is a combined lateral and medial medullary syndrome. The lesion is at the pontomedullary junction. Manifestations include ipsilateral Horner's syndrome (autonomic sympathetic fibers); ipsilateral weakness of the soft palate, pharynx, larynx (nucleus ambiguus), and tongue (hypoglossal nucleus); loss of taste in the posterior third of the tongue (nucleus solitarius); cerebellar ataxia (restiform body) and nystagmus

KEY CONCEPTS

- The signs of the lateral medullary syndrome vary, depending on the rostrocaudal level of the lesion.
- The clinical signs of combined lateral and medial medullary syndromes constitute the Babinski-Nageotte syndrome.

Horner's syndrome. Drooping of the eyelid (ptosis), constriction of the pupil (miosis), retraction of the eyeball (enophthalmos), and loss of sweating on the face (anhidrosis) constitute a syndrome described by Johann Friedrich Horner, a Swiss ophthalmologist, in 1869. The syndrome is due to interruption of descending sympathetic fibers. Also known as Bernard-Horner syndrome and oculosympathetic palsy. The syndrome was described in animals by François du Petit in 1727. Claude Bernard in France in 1862 and E. S. Hare in Great Britain in 1838 gave precise accounts of the syndrome before Horner.

Anhidrosis (Greek *an*, "negative"; *hidros*, "sweat"). Absence or deficiency of sweating.

Nystagmus (Greek *nystagmos*, "drowsiness, nodding"). Nodding or closing of the eye in a sleepy person. The modern use of the term refers to involuntary rhythmic oscillation of the eyes.

Hiccup. An involuntary spasmodic contraction of the diaphragm that causes a beginning of inspiration, which is suddenly checked by closure of the glottis, causing a characteristic sound. Also called singultus.

Lateropulsion (Latin *latero*, "side"; *pellere*, "to drive"). An involuntary tendency to go to one side. A characteristic sign of a cerebellar or lateral medullary lesion.

Dysmetria (Greek *dys*, "difficult"; *metron*, "measure"). Improper measuring of distance, disturbed control of range of move-

(vestibular nuclei); and contralateral **hemiparesis** (pyramid) and **hemianesthesia** (medial lemniscus).

DORSAL MEDULLARY SYNDROME

The dorsal medullary syndrome is caused by occlusion of the medial branch of the posterior inferior cerebellar artery. Affected structures include the vestibular nuclei and the restiform body (inferior cerebellar peduncle). The associated neurologic signs include the following:

1. Ipsilateral limb or gait ataxia resulting from involvement of the restiform body
2. Vertigo, vomiting, and ipsilateral gaze-evoked nystagmus resulting from involvement of the vestibular nuclei

PSEUDOBULBAR PALSY

Pseudobulbar palsy is a clinical syndrome caused by the interruption of the corticobulbar fibers to motor nuclei of the cranial nerves. Most cranial nerve nuclei in the brain stem receive bilateral inputs from the cerebral cortex arising primarily from the precentral cortex. The majority of these fibers reach cranial nerve nuclei via the reticular formation (corticoreticulobulbar system). Some cranial nerve nuclei, however, receive corticobulbar fibers directly. These nuclei include the sensory and motor trigeminal nuclei, the nucleus solitarius, the facial motor nucleus, the spinal accessory (supraspinal) nucleus, and the hypoglossal nucleus.

Bilateral interruption of the indirect corticoreticulobulbar or direct corticobulbar fibers in the brain stem results in the syndrome of pseudobulbar palsy. The neurologic manifestations of this syndrome include the following:

1. Weakness (upper motor neuron variety) of muscles supplied by the corresponding cranial nerve nuclei
2. Inappropriate outbursts of laughter and crying

KEY CONCEPTS

- The anatomic structures involved in the dorsal medullary syndrome include the vestibular nuclei and the restiform body.
- The clinical signs of the dorsal medullary syndrome include ipsilateral ataxia, nystagmus, vomiting, and vertigo.
- Bilateral interruption of the corticobulbar or corticoreticulobulbar fibers results in the pseudobulbar syndrome.

ment. A sign of cerebellar disease.

Nageotte, Jean (1866–1948). A French neurologist who with Babinski described the combined lateral and medial medullary syndrome (medullary tegmental paralysis).

Hemiparesis (Greek *hemi*, "half"; *paresis*, "relaxation"). Weakness of one side of the body.

Hemianesthesia (Greek *hemi*, "half"; *an*, "negative"; *aisthesis*, "sensation"). Loss of feeling or sensation in half the body.

SUGGESTED READINGS

Amarenco P, et al: Infarction in the territory of the medial branch of the posterior inferior cerebellar artery. *J Neurol Neurosurg Psychiatry* 1990; 53:731–735.

Brazius PW: The localization of lesions affecting the brainstem. In Brazis PW, et al (eds): *Localization in Clinical Neurology.* Boston, Little, Brown, 1985:225–238.

Milandre L, et al: Bilateral infarction of the medullary pyramids. *Neurology* 1990; 40:556.

Norrving B, Cronquist S: Lateral medullary infarction: Prognosis in an unselected series. *Neurology* 1991; 41:244–248.

Pryse-Phillips W: *Companion to Clinical Neurology.* Boston, Little, Brown, 1995.

Romano J, Merritt HH: The singular affection of

Gaspard Vieusseux: An early description of the lateral medullary syndrome. *Bull Hist Med* 1941; 9:72–79.

Sacco RL, et al: Wallenberg's lateral medullary syndrome: Clinical-magnetic resonance imaging correlations. *Arch Neurol* 1993; 50:609–614.

Troost BT: Signs and symptoms of stroke syndromes of the brain stem. In Hofferberth, B, et al (eds): *Vascular Brain Stem Diseases.* Basel, Karger, 1990:112–124.

Vuilleumier P, et al: Infarction of the lower brainstem: Clinical, aetiological and MRI-topographical correlations. *Brain* 1995; 118:1013–1025.

Waepse W, Wichmann W: Oculomotor disturbances during visual vestibular interactions in Wallenberg's lateral medullary syndrome. *Brain* 1990; 113:821–846.

CHAPTER 7

PONS

GROSS TOPOGRAPHY

The **pons** is the part of the brain stem that lies between the medulla oblongata caudally and the midbrain rostrally. The cerebral peduncles and the superior pontine sulcus mark its rostral boundary, the middle cerebellar peduncles (**brachium pontis**) mark its lateral boundary, and the inferior pontine sulcus marks its caudal boundary. The dorsal surface of the pons is covered by the cerebellum.

Ventral Surface

The ventral surface (Fig. 7-1) of the pons forms a bulge known as the pontine protuberance. In the middle of this protuberance is the pontine sulcus, which contains the basilar artery. Several cranial nerves leave the ventral surface of the pons. The abducens nerve (cranial nerve VI) emerges from the boundary between the pons and the medulla oblongata. In the angle between the caudal pons, the rostral medulla, and the cerebellum (the **cerebellopontine angle**), the facial (cranial nerve VII) and cochleovestibular (cranial nerve VIII) nerves appear. From the lateral and rostral parts of the pons emerge the two components of the trigeminal nerve (cranial nerve V): the larger sensory portion (portio major) and the smaller motor portion (portio minor). The crowding of the facial and cochleovestibular nerves in the cerebellopontine angle explains the early involvement of these two nerves in tumors (**acoustic neuromas**) that arise in this angle.

Pons (Latin, "bridge"). A bridge between the medulla oblongata, midbrain, and cerebellum. Described by Eustachius and Varolius. The illustrations of Eustachius were superior to those of Varolius but were not published until 1714, whereas those of Varolius were published in 1573; hence the name *pons varolii.*

Brachium pontis (Latin, Greek, *brachion*, "arm"; *pontis*, "bridge"). An armlike bundle of fibers that connect the pons and cerebellum.

Cerebellopontine angle. The angle between the medulla oblongata, pons, and cerebellum. Contains the seventh (facial) and eighth (cochleovestibular) cranial nerves.

KEY CONCEPTS

- The ventral surface of the pons shows the basilar artery in the pontine sulcus and four cranial nerves: the abducens at the medullary pontine junction, the facial and cochleovestibular in the cerebellopontine angle, and the trigeminal at the midpontine level.

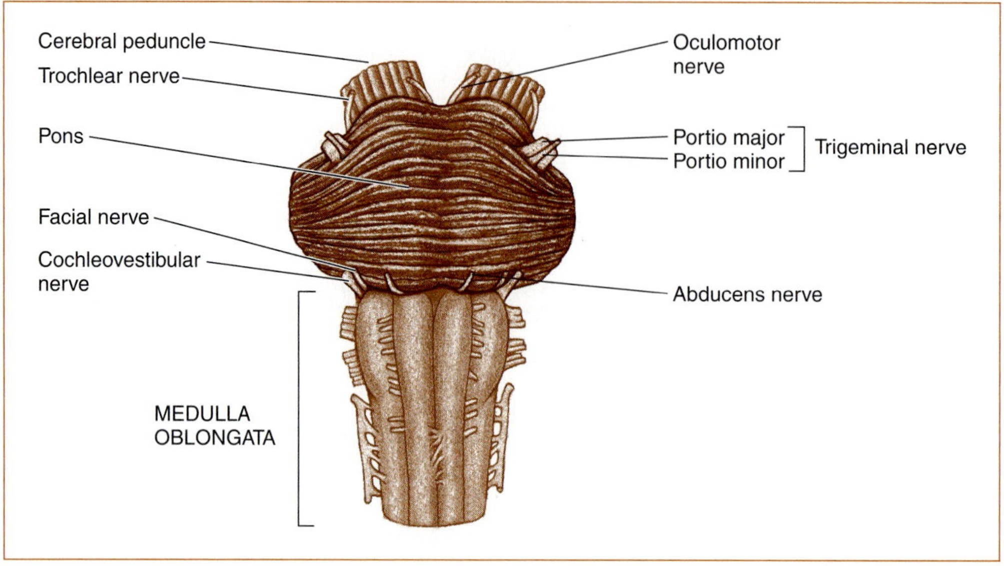

FIGURE 7-1

Schematic diagram of the ventral surface of the brain stem showing the major structures on the ventral surface of the pons.

Acoustic neuroma. A tumor of the eighth cranial nerve characterized by deafness and vertigo. May involve adjacent structures in the brain stem. Described by Harvey Cushing, an American neurosurgeon, in 1917.

Facial colliculus (Latin *colliculus*, "small elevation"). An elevation in the floor of the fourth ventricle overlying the genu of the facial nerve and the abducens nucleus.

Dorsal Surface

The dorsal surface (see Fig. 5-3) of the pons forms the rostral portion of the floor of the fourth ventricle. This part of the floor features the **facial colliculi,** one on each side of the midline sulcus (median sulcus). These colliculi represent the surface landmarks of the genu of the facial nerve and the underlying nucleus of the abducens nerve.

MICROSCOPIC STRUCTURE

Coronal sections of the pons reveal a basic organizational pattern made of two parts: a ventral basis pontis and a dorsal tegmentum.

Basis Pontis (Ventral)

The basis pontis (Fig. 7-2) corresponds to the pontine protuberance described in "Gross Topography," above. It contains the pontine nuclei and multidirectional nerve fiber bundles.

The multidirectional nerve fiber bundles in the basis pontis belong to three fiber systems.

KEY CONCEPTS

- The dorsal surface of the pons forms the rostral floor of the fourth ventricle, in which the facial colliculi are seen.
- Coronal sections of the pons reveal two components: a ventral and phylogenetically newer basis pontis and a dorsal and phylogenetically older tegmentum.
- The basis pontis contains pontine nuclei and the following nerve fiber bundles: corticospinal, corticobulbar, and corticopontocerebellar (the largest).

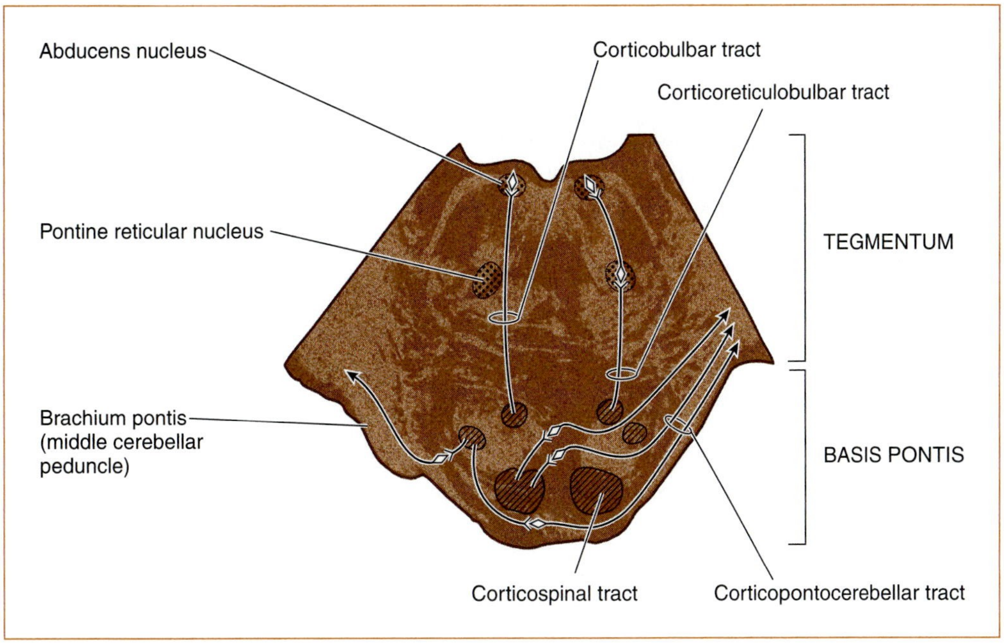

FIGURE 7-2

Schematic diagram of the pons showing its major divisions into tegmentum and basis pontis, and types of fiber bundles traversing the basis pontis.

1. Corticospinal fibers from the cerebral cortex to the spinal cord pass through the basis pontis and continue caudally as the pyramids of the medulla oblongata.
2. Corticobulbar fibers from the cerebral cortex to the cranial nerve nuclei of the brain stem. Some of these fibers project directly on the nuclei of cranial nerves (corticobulbar); the majority, however, synapse on an intermediate reticular nucleus before reaching the cranial nerve nucleus (corticoreticulobulbar). Corticobulbar and corticoreticulobulbar fibers usually arise from both cerebral hemispheres.
3. Corticopontocerebellar fibers constitute the largest group of fibers in the basis pontis. This fiber system originates from wide areas of the cerebral cortex, projects on ipsilateral pontine nuclei, and crosses the midline on its way to the cerebellum via the middle cerebellar peduncle. It is estimated that in humans this fiber system contains approximately 19 million fibers on each side. The number of pontine neurons in humans is estimated to be approximately 23 million in each half of the pons. Thus, the ratio of corticopontine fibers to pontine neurons is approximately 1:1. Although the corticopontine projection is believed to arise from wide areas of the cerebral cortex, it arises principally from the prerolandic and postrolandic sensorimotor cortices with minor to moderate contributions from the parietal and temporal association cortices, the premotor and prefrontal association cortices, and the cingulate gyrus. The fact that cortical input to the pontine nuclei arises chiefly from primary cortical areas suggests that the corticopontocerebellar fiber system is concerned with the rapid correction of movements. The functional significane of the cingulopontine fiber connection is not known, but it may represent the anatomic substrate for the effect of emotion on motor function. The input from the association cortices suggests a role for this fiber system in behavioral and cognitive processes.

A cortical region usually projects to more than one cell column of the pontine nuclei, and some pontine columns receive projections from more than one cortical region. Like the cortico-olivocerebellar system, the corticopontocerebellar system is somatotopically organized. Thus, the prerolandic cortex (primary motor cortex) projects to medial pontine nuclei, the postrolandic cortex (primary somatosensory cortex) to lateral pontine nuclei, the arm area of the sensorimotor cortex to dorsal pontine nuclei, and the leg area to ventral pontine nuclei. The projection from the cingulate gyrus also has been shown to be somatotopically organized, with the anterior cingulate cortex projecting to the medial pontine nuclei and the posterior cingulate cortex projecting to the lateral pontine nuclei.

The pontocerebellar projection is primarily crossed; however, it has been estimated that 30 percent of the pontine projection to the cerebellar vermis and 10 percent of the projection to the cerebellar hemisphere are ipsilateral. The density of projection to the cerebellar hemispheres is three times that to the vermis. Like the corticopontine projection, the pontocerebellar projection is somatotopically organized, with the caudal half of the pons projecting to the anterior lobe of the cerebellum and the rostral half projecting to the posterior lobe.

The basilar portion of the pons is the phylogenetically newer part and is present only in animals with well-developed cerebellar hemispheres.

Tegmentum (Latin, a "covering"). The dorsal parts of the pons and midbrain.

Tegmentum (Dorsal)

The tegmentum is the phylogenetically older part of the pons and is composed largely of the reticular formation. Lesions that destroy more than 25 percent of the tegmentum may result in loss of consciousness. In the basal part of the tegmentum, the medial lemniscus (which maintains a vertical orientation on each side of the midline in the medulla) becomes flattened in a mediolateral direction (Fig. 7-3). Fibers originating from the cuneate nucleus are located medially; gracile fibers are laterally placed. Lateral to the medial lemniscus lies the trigeminal tract, which conveys sensations of pain, temperature, touch, and proprioception from the contralateral face. The spinothalamic tract is lateral to the trigeminal tract and carries pain and temperature sensations from the contralateral half of the body. Thus, in the basal part of the tegmentum lies the specific sensory lemniscal system, which includes the medial lemniscus, trigeminal lemniscus, and spinothalamic tract.

Intermingled with the ascending fibers of the lemniscal system are transversely oriented fibers of the trapezoid body. These fibers arise from the cochlear nuclei, course through the tegmentum, and gather in the lateral portion of the pons to form the lateral lemniscus. This fiber system will be discussed below in connection with the cochlear division of the cochleovestibular nerve (cranial nerve VIII).

Dorsal to the medial lemniscus is the central tegmental tract, which originates in the basal ganglia and midbrain and projects on the inferior olive; it shifts position in the tegmentum of the pons and lies dorsal to the lateral part of the medial lemniscus in the caudal pons (Fig. 7-3).

The medial longitudinal fasciculus and the tectospinal tract retain the same dorsal and paramedian positions they occupied in the medulla just beneath the floor of the fourth ventricle (Fig. 7-3).

KEY CONCEPTS

- The tegmentum contains the following nerve fiber bundles: medial lemniscus, trigeminal lemniscus, spinothalamic, trapezoid body, central tegmental tract, medial longitudinal fasciculus, tectospinal, and descending sympathetic fibers.
- The tegmentum contains the cranial nerve nuclei (cochleovestibular, facial, abducens, and trigeminal), the nucleus locus ceruleus, and the pontine reticular formation.

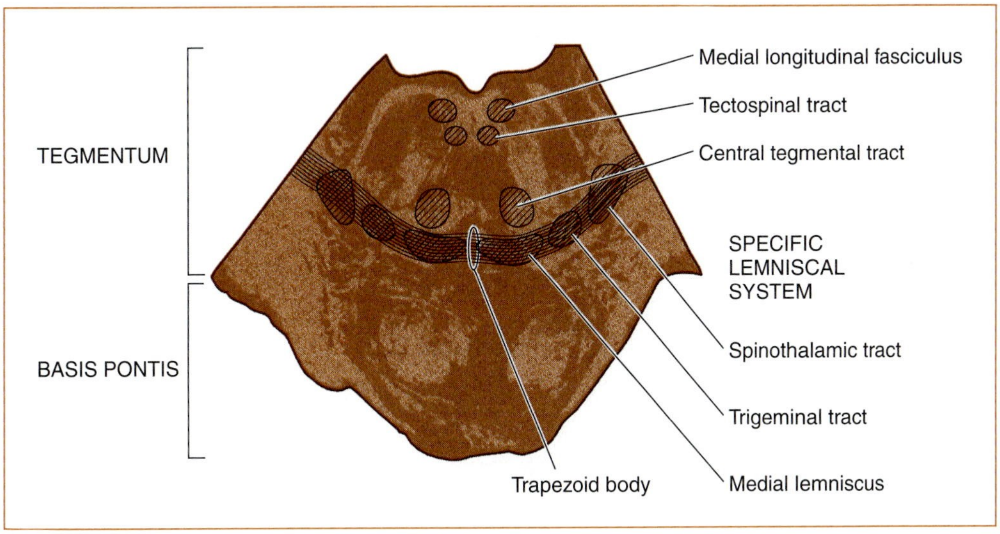

FIGURE 7-3

Schematic diagram of the pons showing the major tracts traversing the tegmentum.

Other tracts coursing through the tegmentum of the pons include the rubrospinal tract medial to the spinal trigeminal nucleus and the ventral spinocerebellar tract medial to the restiform body. The ventral spinocerebellar tract enters the superior cerebellar peduncle to reach the cerebellum. The tegmentum of the pons also contains descending sympathetic fibers from the hypothalamus; these fibers are located in the lateral part of the tegmentum. Interruption of these fibers produces **Horner's syndrome** (Chap. 5). Corticobulbar fibers and corticoreticulobulbar fibers on their way from the basis pontis to cranial nerve nuclei also pass through the tegmentum (Fig. 7-2).

In the rostral pons, lying dorsally in the tegmentum, is the nucleus **locus ceruleus** (group A-6 of primates). It contains on each side an average of 16,000 to 18,000 melanin-containing neurons which are involved in **Parkinson's disease, Alzheimer's disease,** and **Down syndrome.** It is the major source of the widespread noradrenergic innervation to most central nervous system regions. This nucleus is subdivided into four subnuclei: central (largest), anterior (rostral end), the nucleus subceruleus (caudal and ventral), and a small posterior and dorsal nucleus. The nucleus spans a rostral-caudal distance of 11 to 14 mm. Rostrally, the nucleus begins at the level of the inferior colliculus (midbrain), where it is situated ventral and lateral to the cerebral aqueduct (aqueduct of Sylvius) in the periaqueductal gray matter of the midbrain. Caudally, at the junction of the cerebral aqueduct and the fourth ventricle, the nucleus is displaced laterally. The number of cells in the nucleus increases from rostral to caudal. Two projection bundles emanate from the nucleus: a dorsal ascending bundle to the hypothalamus, hippocampus, neocortex, and cerebellum and a descending bundle to the spinal cord. Cell loss in the nucleus is generalized in Parkinson's disease, whereas it is limited to the rostral portion of the nucleus (which projects mainly to the cerebral cortex) in Alzheimer's disease and Down syndrome.

Horner's syndrome. Drooping of the eyelids (ptosis), constriction of the pupil (miosis), retraction of the eyeball (enophthalmos), and loss of sweating on the face (anhidrosis) constitute a syndrome described by Johann Friedrich Horner, a Swiss ophthalmologist, in 1869. The syndrome is due to interruption of descending sympathetic fibers. Also known as Bernard-Horner syndrome and oculosympathetic palsy. Described in animals by François du Petit in 1727. Claude Bernard in France in 1862 and ES. Hare in Great Britain in 1838 gave precise accounts of the syndrome before Horner did.

Locus ceruleus (Latin, "place, dark blue"). A pigmented noradrenergic nucleus in the rostral pons that is dark blue in sections.

KEY CONCEPTS

- The nucleus locus ceruleus is the source of noradrenergic innervation to most regions of the central nervous system.

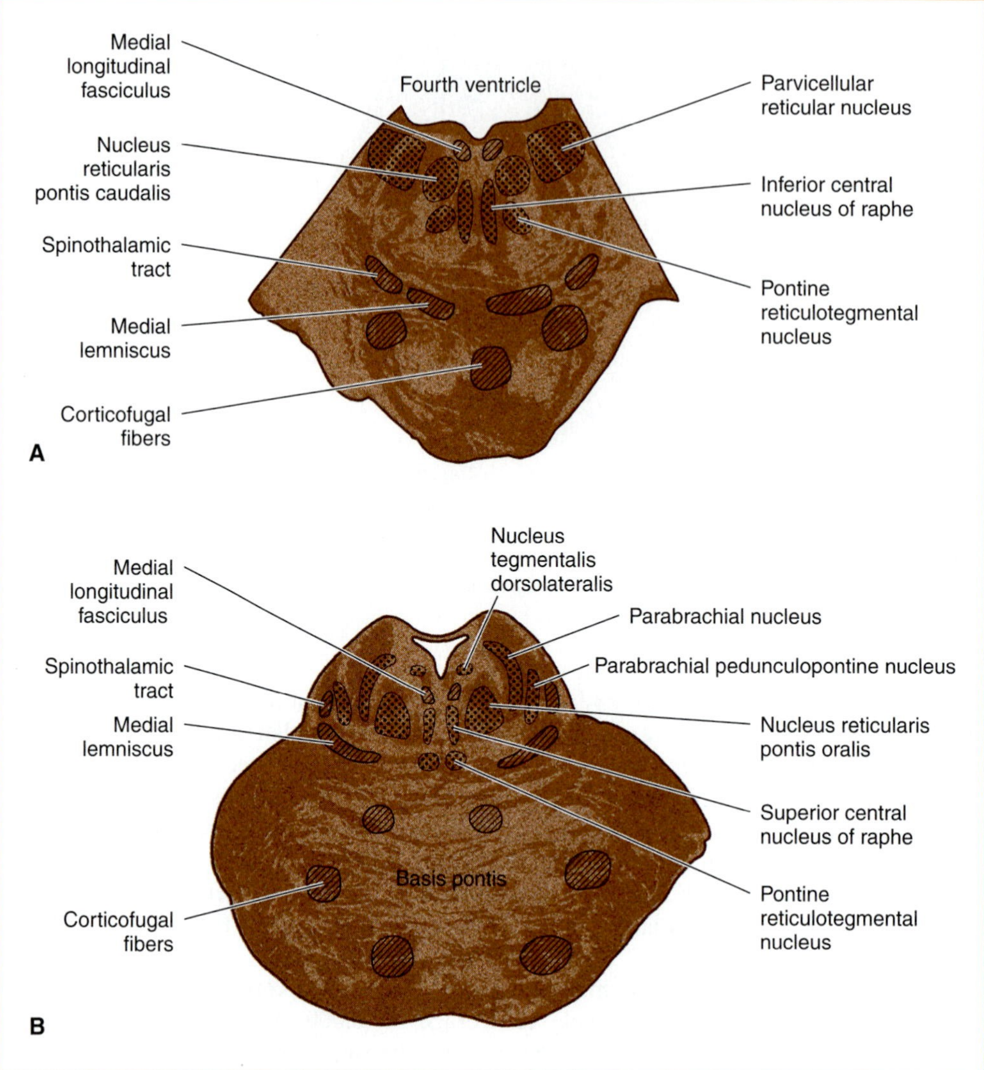

FIGURE 7-4

Schematic diagram of the pons showing reticular nuclei in the caudal (*A*), and rostral (*B*) levels of the pons.

Parkinson's disease. A degenerative disease of the brain characterized by postural tremor and rigidity from loss of dopaminergic neurons in the substantia nigra. Described by James Parkinson, an English physician, in 1817 under the name of *shaking palsy*.

Alzheimer's disease. A degenerative disease of the brain formerly known as senile dementia. Characterized by memory loss, cortical atrophy, senile plaques, and neurofibrillary tangles. Described by Alois Alzheimer, a Germany neuropsychiatrist, in 1907.

PONTINE RETICULAR FORMATION

The pontine reticular formation constitutes the major part of the tegmental portion of the pons and is a rostral continuation of the medullary reticular formation. As in the medulla, the pontine reticular nuclei are located medially and laterally (Fig. 7-4).

The bulk of the pontine reticular nuclei is composed of two medially located nuclei: the nucleus reticularis pontis caudalis and the nucleus reticularis pontis oralis. The pontis caudalis is a continuation of the gigantocellular reticular nucleus

KEY CONCEPTS

- The two major reticular nuclei are the medially located nuclei reticularis pontis caudalis and oralis, both of which contribute to the pontine reticulospinal tract and the ascending reticular activating system.

of the medulla oblongata. It extends from the caudal pons to the level of the motor nucleus of the trigeminal nerve at midpontine levels, where it becomes the nucleus reticularis pontis oralis. The oralis nucleus does not have large cells and extends from the midpons to the caudal midbrain.

From the nuclei reticularis pontis caudalis and oralis arise the pontine reticulospinal tract and the ascending reticular activating fiber system. Reticulospinal fibers travel with the medial longitudinal fasciculus and influence ipsilateral spinal motor neurons. The ascending reticular activating fiber system (reticulothalamic fibers) travels in the central tegmental tract to the intralaminar nuclei of the thalamus. The nucleus reticularis pontis caudalis has been associated with paradoxical sleep. Bilateral lesions in this nucleus result in the complete elimination of paradoxical sleep.

Paramedian reticular nuclei (also known as **raphe nuclei**) occupy a position on each side of the central raphe. In the caudal pons they include the inferior central nucleus, which is a continuation of the nucleus raphe magnus of the medulla oblongata, and in the rostral pons they include the superior central Bekhterew's nucleus (median nucleus of the raphe), which is best developed at the level of the isthmus.

In the ventral tegmentum, on each side of the midline, is the reticulotegmental nucleus, which represents displaced pontine nuclei. The lateral pontine reticular nuclei include caudally the parvicellular reticular nucleus (lateral to the nucleus reticularis pontis caudalis), an association nucleus that relates ascending and descending fiber systems to the medial group of reticular nuclei; rostrally, in the dorsolateral part of the pontine tegmentum, is the nucleus tegmentalis dorsolateralis, which is the pontine micturition center. Stimulation of this nucleus results in bladder contraction and micturition. Fiber connections have been shown between this nucleus and the intermediolateral autonomic (parasympathetic) cell column in the sacral spinal cord.

At the level of the **isthmus,** in the dorsolateral pons, between the lateral edge of the **brachium conjunctivum** (superior cerebellar peduncle) and the lateral lemniscus, is the parabrachial nucleus, a synaptic station for gustatory (taste) pathways. In humans the parabrachial nucleus has been shown to have neuromelanin-containing catecholamine neurons. The pigmented neurons in the nucleus are rather small (compared with neuromelanin-containing neurons in the locus ceruleus or the substantia nigra), and their granules have a very delicate appearance; this may explain why pigmented neurons in this nucleus have been overlooked in reports on the distribution of catecholamine neurons in the human brain. In humans the parabrachial nucleus is subdivided into lateral and medial segments. Pigmented neurons are more abundant in the lateral segment. Pigmented neurons in the parabrachial nucleus undergo a significant reduction in number in patients with Parkinson's disease. The parabrachial nucleus has fiber connections with the hypothalamus, amygdala, stria terminalis, and brain stem nuclei, including the nucleus of the solitary tract and the dorsal raphe nucleus. It is believed that the parabrachial nucleus plays an important role in autonomic regulation, and its involvement in parkinsonism may explain the autonomic disturbances that occur in that disease.

Between the spinal lemniscus, brachium conjunctivum, and medial lemniscus is the parabrachial pedunculopontine nucleus. It is composed of a ventral subnucleus dissipatus (group A-8 of primates) and a subnucleus compactus, a cholinergic nucleus which projects to the intralaminar thalamic nuclei, substantia nigra (pars compacta), subthalamic nucleus, and cerebral cortex.

Down syndrome. A genetic syndrome caused by trisomy of chromosome 21 or translocation of chromosomal material. Characterized by unique facial features, mental retardation, skeletal abnormalities, congenital cardiac lesions, and a single transverse palmar crease. Described by James Langdon Haydon Down, an English physician, in 1866.

Raphe nucleus (Greek *raphe*, "a seam or suture"). The word *raphe* was used by Homer in the *Odyssey* in connection with the sewing of harnesses for horses. The term is used in anatomy to refer to a seamlike formation that suggests that adjacent structures have been sewn together. The midline reticular nuclei are called the raphe nuclei.

Isthmus (Greek *isthmos*, "a narrow connection between two large bodies or spaces"). The narrowest portion of the hindbrain. It is situated between the pons and the midbrain.

Brachium conjunctivum (Latin, Greek *brachion*, "arm"; *conjunctiva*, "connecting"). An armlike bundle of fibers that connect the cerebellum and midbrain.

KEY CONCEPTS

- Other reticular nuclei include the paramedian (raphe nucleus), lateral parvicellular, nucleus tegmentalis dorsolateralis (pontine micturition center), and parabrachial.

Paradoxical sleep. Rapid eye movement sleep. So named because electroencephalography shows a wakefulness pattern when the person is asleep.

Spiral ganglion. The sensory ganglion of the cochlear nerve. Contains bipolar cells.

Modiolus (Latin, "nave, hub"). The central pillar (axis) of the cochlea. Described and named by Eustachius in 1563. Its structure suggests the hub of the wheel with radiating spokes (lamina spiralis) attached to it.

Organ of Corti. The cochlear receptor organ in the inner ear. Described by Marchese Alfonso Corti, an Italian histologist, in 1851.

Restiform body (Latin *restis*, "rope"; *forma*, "form"). A body (inferior cerebellar peduncle) shaped like a rope. Described by Humphrey Ridley, an English anatomist, in 1695.

Cochlea (Latin, "snail shell"). So named because it has a spiral form resembling a snail shell.

Trapezoid body (Latin *trapezoides*, "table-shaped"). The ventral acoustic stria in the tegmentum of the pons constitutes the trapezoid body.

Both serotonin- and norepinephrine-containing neurons in the reticular formation play a role in sleep. Inhibition of serotonin synthesis or destruction of serotonin-containing neurons in the raphe system leads to insomnia. Serotonin may be involved in the neural mechanism related to slow wave sleep. In addition, serotonin may have an effect on cells of the locus ceruleus that trigger paradoxical sleep. Bilateral lesions of locus ceruleus in animals cause selective suppression of **paradoxical sleep** for about 2 weeks, after which it returns to normal.

CRANIAL NERVE NUCLEI

Cochleovestibular Nerve (Cranial Nerve VIII)

The cochleovestibular nerve has two divisions: cochlear and vestibular. The two divisions travel together from the peripheral end organs in the inner ear to the pons, where they separate; each then establishes its own distinct connections.

Cochlear Division

The cochlear division (Fig. 7-5) of the cochleovestibular nerve is the larger of the two divisions. Nerve fibers in the cochlear nerve are central processes of bipolar neurons in the **spiral ganglion** located in the **modiolus** of the inner ear. The peripheral processes of these bipolar neurons are linked to the hair cells of the auditory end organ in the **organ of Corti.** As fibers of the cochlear nerve reach the caudal part of the pons, they enter its lateral surface caudal and lateral to the vestibular division and project on the dorsal and ventral cochlear nuclei. The dorsal cochlear nucleus, which is situated on the dorsolateral surface of the **restiform body,** receives fibers originating in the basal turns of the **cochlea** (mediating high-frequency sound). The ventral cochlear nucleus, which is situated on the ventrolateral aspect of the restiform body, receives fibers from apical turns of the cochlea (mediating low-frequency sound). The total number of neurons in the cochlear nuclei far exceeds the total number of cochlear nerve fibers, and so each fiber is believed to project on several neurons.

The human dorsal cochlear nucleus is not laminated as is the case in other mammals. The ventral cochlear nucleus includes a rostral area of spherical cells, a central area of multipolar and globular cells, a caudal area of octopus cells, and a laterodorsal cap of small neurons.

Second-order neurons from the cochlear nuclei course through the tegmentum of the pons to form the three acoustic striae: dorsal, ventral, and intermediate. The dorsal acoustic stria is formed by axons of neurons in the dorsal cochlear nucleus, the ventral acoustic stria (**trapezoid body**) is formed by axons from the inferior cochlear nucleus, and the intermediate acoustic stria originates in the inferior and superior cochlear nuclei.

KEY CONCEPTS

- The cochleovestibular nerve is made up of two divisions: cochlear and vestibular.
- Cells of origin of the cochlear nerve are bipolar neurons in the spiral ganglion.
- The cochlear receptor organ is the organ of Corti in the inner ear.
- Cochlear nerve fibers terminate selectively on neurons in the dorsal or ventral cochlear nuclei.
- Second-order cochlear fibers within the acoustic striae establish synapses in one or more of the following brain stem nuclei to form the lateral lemniscus: superior olivary nuclear complex and the nucleus of the trapezoid body.

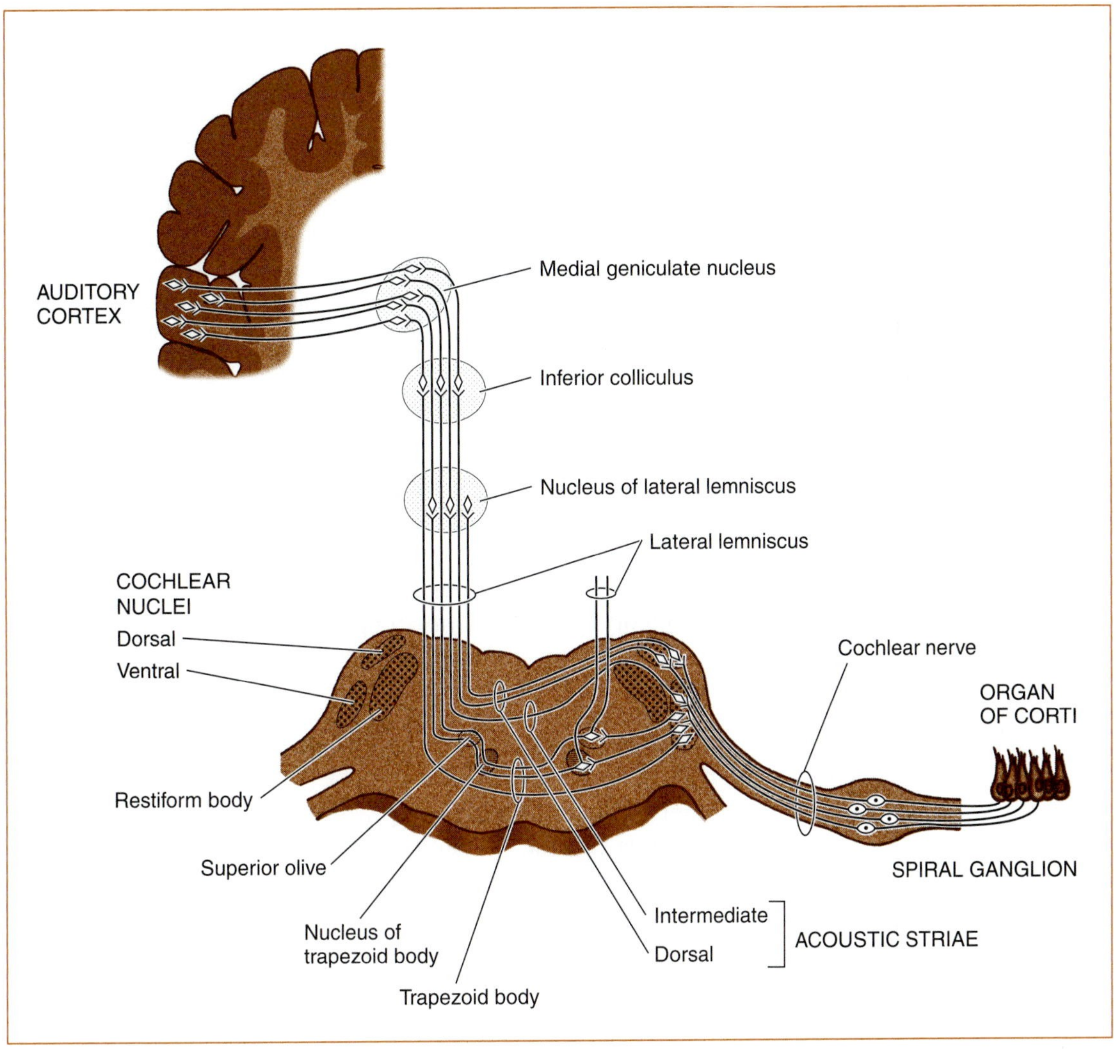

FIGURE 7-5

Schematic diagram of the auditory pathways.

The ventral acoustic stria (the trapezoid body) is the largest of the three striae. Fibers in this stria project on neurons in the superior olivary complex and the nucleus of the trapezoid body. The superior olivary nuclear complex is embedded in the trapezoid body. It includes the lateral and medial superior olivary nuclei. The olivary nuclei are elongated cell masses of which the medial superior olivary nucleus is much better developed in humans, whereas the lateral superior olivary nucleus and the nucleus of the trapezoid body are poorly developed. The nucleus of the trapezoid body consists of small cells situated at the caudal half of the superior olivary nucleus. The two superior olivary nuclei and the nucleus of the trapezoid body are surrounded by a zone of cells of varying sizes and shapes known collectively as the periolivary nuclei. It was originally believed that the periolivary nuclei are exclusively involved in descending auditory pathways, but it has been established that these cells are involved in descending as well as ascending auditory projections. Third-order neurons from the superior olivary complex, the nucleus of the trapezoid body, and the periolivary nuclei contribute mainly to the contralateral **lateral lemniscus,** with some projection to the homolateral lateral lemniscus. The lateral lemniscus also receives fibers from the dorsal and intermediate acoustic striae. Fibers in the lateral lemniscus project on the nucleus of the lateral lemniscus. The nucleus of

Lateral lemniscus (Latin from Greek *lemniskos,* "ribbon"). A fiber bundle carrying second-order and third-order auditory fibers in the brain stem.

the lateral lemniscus is an elongated strand of cells embedded within the lateral lemniscus at the isthmus level. Two subnuclei are recognized: dorsal and ventral. Subsequent stations in the auditory system include synapses in the inferior colliculus and the medial geniculate body.

The inferior colliculus is the most important relay station in the ascending and descending auditory projections. It consists of a large compact central nucleus and a more diffuse laterally situated zone. The majority of ascending auditory fibers to the inferior colliculus terminate in the central nucleus. The lateral zone of the inferior colliculus receives afferents from the central nucleus as well as from the nucleus of the lateral lemniscus. Only a limited number of fibers belonging to the ascending auditory projection bypass the inferior colliculus to reach the medial geniculate body directly. These fibers usually arise from the cochlear nuclei and the nucleus of the lateral lemniscus. The two inferior colliculi are connected to each other by the commissure of the inferior colliculus and to the medial geniculate nucleus by the brachium of the inferior colliculus (inferior quadrigeminal brachium).

Heschl's gyri (Greek *gyros*, "circle"). The transverse gyri in the temporal lobe are the sites of the primary auditory cortex. Named after Richard Heschl, an Austrian anatomist who described them in 1855.

The final station is the primary auditory cortex (transverse **Heschl's gyri**) in the temporal lobe. The auditory projection (auditory radiation) from the medial geniculate body to the primary auditory cortex traverses the sublenticular portion of the internal capsule. From the level of the inferior colliculus onward to the primary auditory cortex, the auditory projection is subdivided into "core" and "belt" projections. The core projection terminates in the primary auditory cortex; the belt projection terminates in cortical areas surrounding the primary auditory cortex. The core and belt projections also have distinct zones of origin within the inferior colliculus, where the central nucleus is related to the core projection, whereas the lateral zone is related to the belt projection. Tonotopic localization exists throughout the auditory system.

In addition to this "classic" auditory pathway, evidence suggests the existence of another multisynaptic auditory pathway through the reticular formation. The evidence for a reticular pathway is based on several experimental observations.

1. Reticular thalamic neurons project to the medial geniculate nucleus.
2. The nucleus of the lateral lemniscus and the inferior colliculus are connected with the mesencephalic reticular formation.
3. Auditory-responding cells have been identified in the mesencephalic reticular formation and the pretectum.
4. An increase in 2-deoxy-D-glucose metabolism throughout the auditory pathways has been obtained by means of electric stimulation of the mesencephalic reticular formation.

KEY CONCEPTS

- The lateral lemniscus establishes synapses in the nucleus of the lateral lemniscus and the inferior colliculus.
- Auditory impulses are transmitted from the inferior colliculus to the medial geniculate body via the brachium of the inferior colliculus.
- Auditory impulses travel from the medial geniculate body via the thalamic radiation to the primary auditory cortex in the temporal lobe (transverse Heschl's gyri).
- Lesions in or proximal to the cochlear nuclei result in complete unilateral hearing loss.
- Unilateral lesions in the auditory pathway distal to the cochlear nuclei (within the neuraxis) result in a partial bilateral auditory deficit that is more marked in the ear contralateral to the lesion.

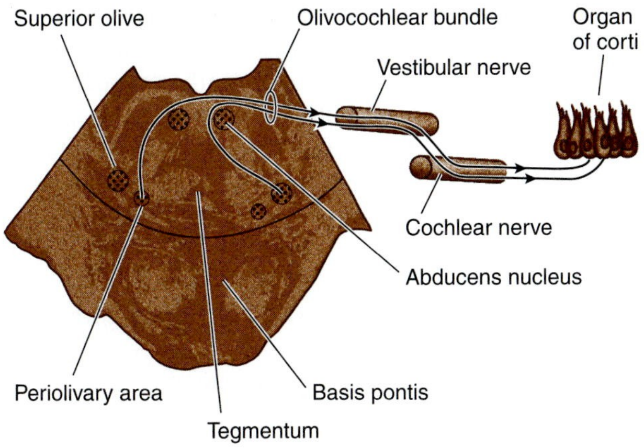

FIGURE 7-6

Schematic diagram showing the origins and course of the olivocochlear bundle.

Several fiber bundles of the auditory system decussate at various levels.

1. In the pontine tegmentum, the superior, middle, and inferior acoustic striae decussate and link the right and left cochlear nuclear complexes.
2. The olivocochlear bundle (**bundle of Rasmussen**), which will be discussed below, also decussates in the pontine tegmentum.
3. The nuclei of the lateral lemniscus are connected via **Probst's commissure,** which passes through the brachium conjunctivum and the most rostral part of the pontine tegmentum. Probst's commissure also carries fibers from the nuclei of the lateral lemniscus to the contralateral inferior colliculus.
4. At the midbrain level, the two inferior colliculi communicate via the commissure of the inferior colliculus. This commissure also carries fibers passing from the inferior colliculus to the medial geniculate body.

Efferent bundle of Rasmussen The olivocochlear efferent bundle in the pons extends from the periolivary nuclei to the hair cells of the organ of Corti. Suppresses the receptivity of the cochlear end organ. Described by Theodor Rasmussen, a Canadian neurosurgeon, in 1946.

Probst's commissure. A bundle of fibers connecting the nuclei of the lateral lemniscus with each other and with the inferior colliculus.

The auditory system is characterized by the presence of several inhibitory feedback mechanisms that consist of descending pathways linking the different cortical and subcortical auditory nuclei. Thus, a system of descending fibers links the primary auditory cortex, the medial geniculate body, the inferior colliculus, the nucleus of the lateral lemniscus, the superior olivary nuclear complex, and the cochlear nuclei. However, the most important feedback mechanism is served by the olivocochlear bundle, which is also known as the efferent bundle of Rasmussen (Fig. 7-6). This bundle of fibers arises from cholinergic neurons of the periolivary nuclei and projects on hair cells in the organ of Corti. It has both crossed and uncrossed components which differentially innervate the two types of hair cells.

The crossed bundle originates from large cells in the ventromedial part of the periolivary area, courses dorsally in the pontine tegmentum, bypasses the nucleus of the abducens nerve, and crosses to the contralateral side to terminate by large

KEY CONCEPTS

- Reciprocal feedback circuits exist throughout the extent of the auditory pathways.
- The most effective feedback circuit in the auditory system is the olivocochlear efferent bundle (bundle of Rasmussen) between the superior olivary complex and the organ of Corti.

synaptic terminals abutting the basal parts of the outer hair cells. The uncrossed component is smaller and originates from small neurons in the vicinity of the lateral superior olivary nucleus. It terminates by en passant synapases on primary afferent cochlear fibers just beneath the inner hair cells. Both components initially join the vestibular division of the cochleovestibular nerve (cranial nerve VIII) but at the vestibulocochlear anastomosis leave it and travel with the cochlear division as far as the hair cells of the organ of Corti. Stimulation of the olivocochlear bundle suppresses the receptivity of the organ of Corti, and thus activity in the auditory nerve.

The hair cells of the organ of Corti transduce mechanical energy into nerve impulses and exhibit a graded generator potential. Spike potentials appear in the cochlear nerve.

Cochlear nerve fibers respond to both displacement and velocity of the basilar membrane of the organ of Corti. Displacement of the basilar membrane toward the scala vestibuli produces inhibition, whereas displacement toward the scala tympani produces excitation. A single fiber in the cochlear nerve may respond to both displacement and velocity.

Reflex movements of the eyes and neck toward a sound source are mediated via two reflex pathways. The first runs from the inferior colliculus to the superior colliculus and from there via tectobulbar and tectospinal pathways to the nuclei of eye muscles and the cervical musculature. The other pathway runs from the superior olive to the abducens nerve (cranial nerve VI) nucleus and then via the medial longitudinal fasciculus to the nuclei of cranial nerves of extraocular muscles.

Other reflex pathways include those between cochlear nuclei and the ascending reticular activating system, which give rise to the auditory-evoked startle response, and those between the ventral cochlear nuclei and the motor nuclei of the trigeminal and facial nerves. The latter pathways constitute reflex arcs that link the organ of Corti with the tensor tympani and stapedius muscles. Thus, in response to sounds of high intensity, these muscles reflexly contract and dampen the vibration of the ear ossicles.

Vestibular Division

Vestibular nerve fibers are central processes of bipolar cells in **Scarpa's ganglion.** Peripheral processes of these bipolar cells are distributed to the vestibular end organ in the three semicircular canals, the **utricle,** and **saccule.** The semicircular canals are concerned with angular acceleration (detecting a simultaneous increase in velocity and direction when one is rotating or turning); the utricle and saccule are concerned with linear acceleration (detecting a change in velocity without a change in direction, the gravitational effect). The superior portion of Scarpa's ganglion receives fibers from the utricle and saccule. The inferior portion of the ganglion receives fibers from the posterior semicircular canal and the saccule (Fig. 7-7). The vestibular nerve accompanies the cochlear nerve from the internal auditory

Scarpa's ganglion (Greek *ganglion*, "knot"). A structure containing bipolar cells that give rise to the vestibular nerve. Located in the internal auditory meatus. Described by Antonius Scarpa, an Italian surgeon and anatomist, in 1779.

Saccule (Latin *sacculus*, "little bag or sac"). One of the vestibular end organs in the inner ear. Detects linear displacement of the body.

Utricle (Latin *utriculus*, "small sac"). A sensory vestibular end organ that detects linear displacement of the body.

KEY CONCEPTS

- Reflex eye and neck movements to sound are carried out via two pathways: from the inferior colliculus to the superior colliculus and then via the tectobulbar and tectospinal tracts to the nuclei of eye and neck muscles and from the superior olive to the abducens nucleus and then via the medial longitudinal fasciculus to the nuclei of extraocular movements.
- The vestibular receptor organs are in the semicircular canals, utricle, and saccule.
- Cells of origin of the vestibular nerve are bipolar neurons in the Scarpa's ganglion.

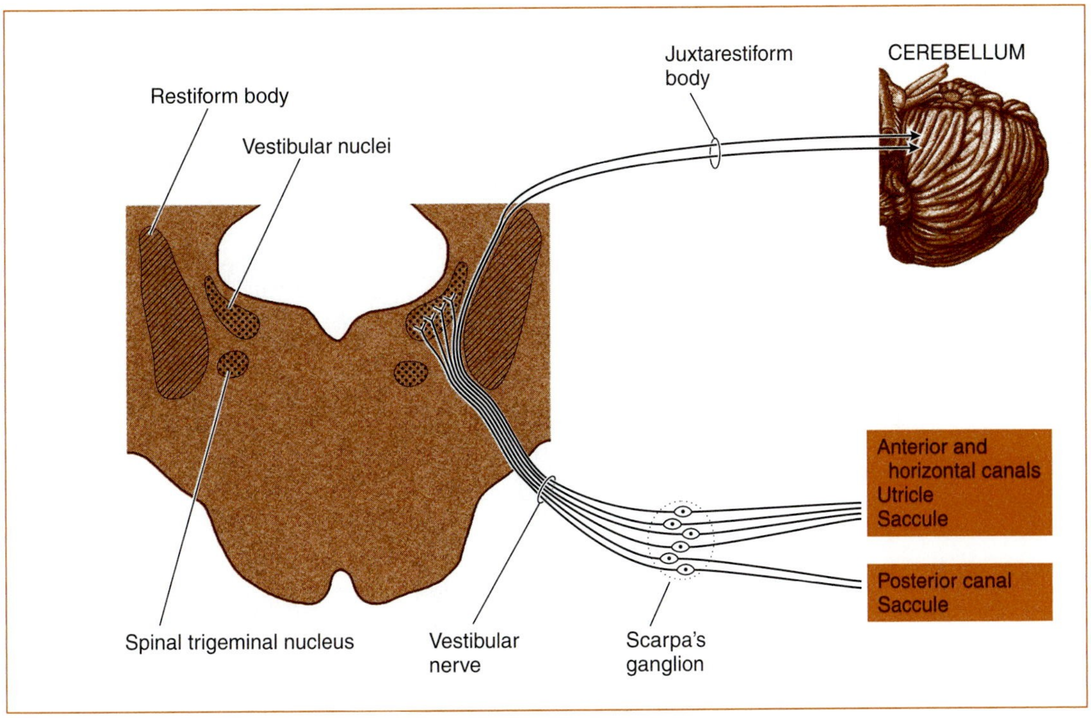

FIGURE 7-7

Schematic diagram showing the origin and termination of the vestibular nerve.

meatus to the pons, where it enters the lateral surface at the pontomedullary junction medial to the cochlear nerve.

Within the pons, vestibular nerve fibers course in the tegmentum between the restiform body and the spinal trigeminal complex. The major portion of these fibers projects on the four vestibular nuclei; a smaller portion goes directly to the cerebellum via the juxtarestiform body. In the cerebellum, these fibers terminate as mossy fibers on neurons in the flocculonodular lobe and the uvula. There are four vestibular nuclei: medial, inferior, lateral, and superior. The medial nucleus [principal nucleus (**Schwalbe's nucleus**)] appears in the medulla oblongata at the rostral end of the inferior olive and extends to the caudal part of the pons. The inferior nucleus (spinal nucleus) lies between the medial nucleus and the restiform body. The inferior nucleus, which is characterized in histologic sections by myelinated fibers that traverse it from the vestibular nerve, extends from the rostral extremity of the gracile nucleus to the pontomedullary junction. The lateral nucleus (**Deiters' nucleus**), which is characterized in histologic sections by the presence of large multipolar neurons, extends from the pontomedullary junction to the level of the abducens nerve (cranial nerve VI) nucleus. The superior nucleus (**Bekhterew's nucleus**) is smaller than the other nuclei and lies dorsal and medial to the medial and lateral nuclei. The number of neurons in the vestibular nuclei far exceeds the number of vestibular nerve fibers. Vestibular nerve fibers project only to limited regions within each vestibular nucleus. In addition to input from the vestibular

Schwalbe's nucleus. The medial vestibular nucleus. Described by Gustav Schwalbe (1844–1916), a German anatomist.

Deiters' nucleus. The lateral vestibular nucleus. Described by Otto Friedrich Karl Deiters, a German anatomist, in 1865.

Bekhterew's nucleus. The superior nucleus of the vestibular nerve. Described by Vladimir Bekhterew, a Russian neurologist, in 1908.

KEY CONCEPTS

- Vestibular nerve fibers terminate selectively on four vestibular nuclei: medial (Schwalbe's principal), inferior (spinal), lateral (Deiters'), and superior (Bekhterew's). Some fibers project directly to the cerebellum.

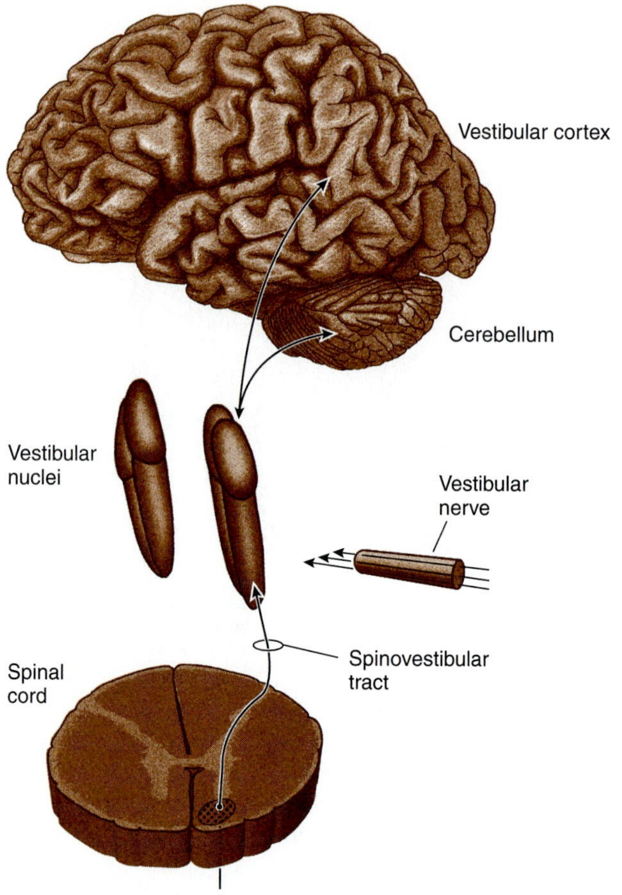

FIGURE 7-8

Schematic diagram showing the major inputs to the vestibular nuclei.

nerve, the vestibular nuclei receive fibers from (1) the spinal cord, (2) the cerebellum, and (3) the vestibular cortex (Fig. 7-8). The output from the vestibular nuclei is to (1) the spinal cord, (2) the cerebellum, (3) the thalamus, (4) the nuclei of the extraocular muscles, (5) the vestibular cortex, and (6) the vestibular end organ.

The vestibular projection to the spinal cord (Fig. 7-9) is through the lateral vestibulospinal tract (from the lateral vestibular nucleus) and the medial vestibulospinal tract (from the medial vestibular nucleus) via the descending component of the medial longitudinal fasciculus. The lateral vestibulospinal tract facilitates extensor motor neurons, whereas the medial tract facilitates flexor motor neurons. The medial vestibulospinal tract sends fibers to the dorsal motor nucleus of the vagus;

KEY CONCEPTS

- The output of vestibular nuclei is to the following areas: spinal cord, cerebellum, thalamus, nuclei of extraocular movement, vestibular cortex, and vestibular end organ.
- The medial and lateral vestibulospinal tracts link the medial and lateral vestibular nuclei, respectively, with the spinal cord.

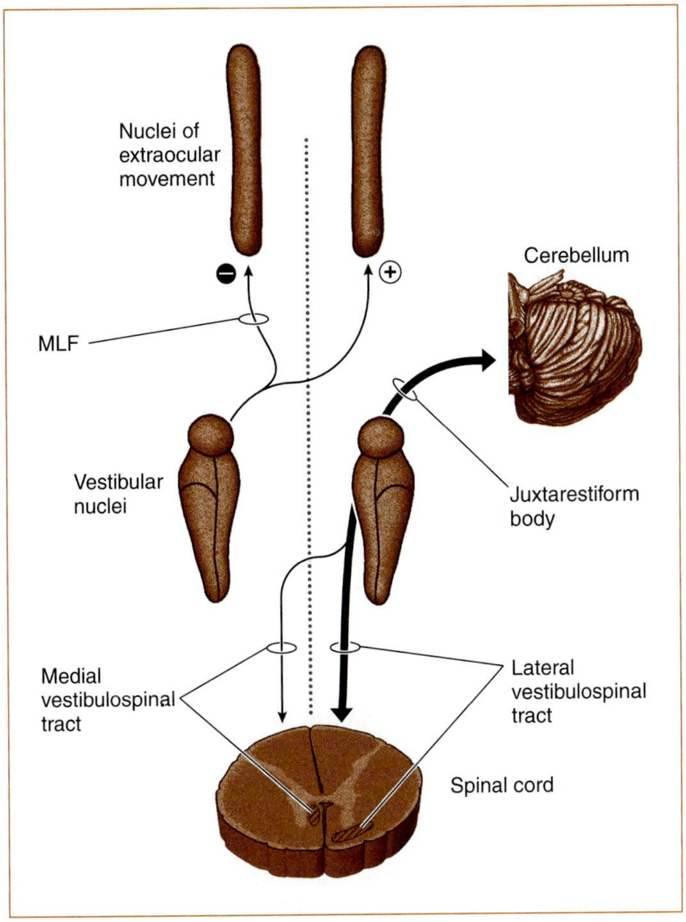

FIGURE 7-9

Schematic diagram showing the efferent connections of the vestibular nuclei.

this explains the nausea, sweating, and vomiting that occur after stimulation of the vestibular end organ.

Projections from the vestibular nuclei to the cerebellum (Fig. 7-9) travel via the **juxtarestiform body** along with the primary vestibulocerebellar fibers. These projections arise from the superior, inferior, and medial vestibular nuclei and terminate mainly ipsilaterally (but also bilaterally) on neurons in the flocculonodular lobe, the uvula, and the nucleus fastigii. Cerebellovestibular connections are much more abundant than are vestibulocerebellar connections.

Juxtarestiform body (Latin *juxta*, "near, close by"; *restis*, "rope"; *forma*, "shape"). A bundle of nerve fibers in close proximity to the restiform body (inferior cerebellar peduncle). Carries vestibular and reticular fibers from and to the cerebellum.

Vestibulothalamic projections arise from the medial, lateral, and superior vestibular nuclei and project bilaterally on several thalamic nuclei (ventral posterolateral, centrolateral, lateral geniculate, and posterior group). They reach their destinations via several pathways (lateral lemniscus, brachium conjunctivum, reticular formation), with a few traveling via the medial longitudinal fasciculus.

KEY CONCEPTS

- Vestibulocerebellar fibers travel via the juxtarestiform body.
- Vestibulothalamic fibers travel via several pathways to reach the vestibular cortex.

Vestibular projections to the nuclei of extraocular muscles travel via the ascending component of the medial longitudinal fasciculus. They arise from all four vestibular nuclei and project on nuclei of the oculomotor (cranial nerve III), trochlear (cranial nerve IV), and abducens (cranial nerve VI) nerves. The crossed component of this system exerts an excitatory effect, whereas the uncrossed component exerts an inhibitory effect, on nuclei of extraocular movement.

A projection from the vestibular nuclei to the primary vestibular cortex in the temporal lobe probably reaches the vestibular cortex via relays in the thalamus.

A projection to the vestibular end organ has been described. Axons travel with the vestibular nerve and terminate in a bilateral fashion on hair cells in cristae of the semicircular canal and the maculae of the utricle and saccule. In contrast to the olivocochlear bundle, which exerts an inhibitory effect on the cochlear end organ, this bundle is excitatory to the vestibular end organ.

The vestibular output to the nuclei of extraocular muscles plays an important role in the control of **conjugate eye movements** (Fig. 7-9). This control is mediated via two pathways: the ascending component of the medial longitudinal fasciculus and the reticular formation. Reflex conjugate deviation of the eyes in a specific direction, which is known as nystagmus, has two components: a slow component away from the stimulated vestibular system and a fast component toward the stimulated side. In clinical medicine, the term **nystagmus** refers to the fast component. Although the mechanism of the slow component is fairly well understood in terms of neuronal connections, the same cannot be said of the fast component, which is believed to represent a corrective attempt to return the eyes to a neutral position. Stimulation of the right horizontal semicircular canal (turning to the right in a **Bárány chair** or pouring warm water in the right ear) or the right medial, lateral, or inferior vestibular nucleus results in a reflex conjugate horizontal deviation of the eyes (horizontal nystagmus) with a slow component to the left and a fast component to the right. Bilateral stimulation of the anterior semicircular canal results in upward movement of the eyes, while stimulation of the posterior canal produces downward movement. Sectioning of the medial longitudinal fasciculus rostral to the abducens nuclei abolishes these primary oculomotor responses. Nystagmus, however, can still result from labyrinthine stimulation, confirming that pathways essential for nystagmus probably pass via the reticular formation. Stimulation of the superior vestibular nucleus produces vertical nystagmus.

Lesions of the medial longitudinal fasciculus (MLF) rostral to the abducens nucleus interfere with normal conjugate eye movements. In this condition, which is known as **internuclear ophthalmoplegia** or the MLF syndrome, there is paralysis of adduction ipsilateral to the MLF lesion and horizontal monocular nystagmus of the abducting eye (Fig. 7-10). This condition is known to occur in multiple sclerosis and vascular disorders of the pons. Experimental evidence has shown that this type of lesion interrupts MLF fibers destined for the part of the oculomotor nuclear complex which innervates the medial rectus; this explains the loss of adduction.

Conjugate eye movement (Latin *conjugatus*, "yoked together"). The lateral deviation of the two eyes in parallel.

Nystagmus (Greek *nystagmos*, "drowsiness, nodding"). Nodding or closing of the eyes in a sleepy person. The terms now refers to involuntary rhythmic oscillation of the eyes.

Bárány chair test. A test of labyrinthine function in which the subject, wearing opaque lenses, is rotated while seated on a chair with the head tilted 30 degrees forward to bring the horizontal semicircular canal into the true horizontal plane. Rotation normally elicits horizontal nystagmus opposite to the direction of rotation.

Internuclear ophthalmoplegia (MLF syndrome). A condition characterized by paralysis of ocular adduction ipsilateral to the medial longitudinal fasciculus lesion and monocular nystagmus in the contralateral abducting eye.

KEY CONCEPTS

- Vestibular fibers to the nuclei of extraocular muscles (cranial nerves III, IV, and VI) travel via the medial longitudinal fasciculus and the reticular formation.
- Vestibular projections to the nuclei of extraocular movement play important roles in controlling conjugate eye movements.
- Lesions in the medial longitudinal fasciculus rostral to the abducens nucleus result in internuclear ophthalmoplegia (the MLF syndrome), or paralysis of adduction (ipsilateral to the lesion), and monocular nystagmus of the abducting eye (contralateral to the lesion).

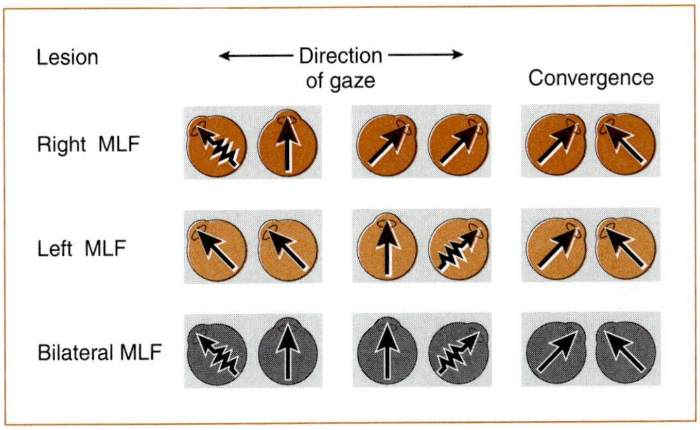

FIGURE 7-10

Schematic diagram showing the effects of lesions in the medial longitudinal fasciculus (MLF) on conjugate eye movements. Zigzag arrows indicate nystagmus.

There is no satisfactory explanation for the monocular horizontal nystagmus of the abducting eye. Two theories have been proposed to explain this phenomenon. The first suggests that nystagmus is due to the utilization of convergence mechanisms to adduct the ipsilateral eye. This induces adduction of the contralateral eye, which then jerks back to the position of fixation. The second theory suggests that the medial longitudinal fasciculus carries facilitatory fibers to the ipsilateral medial rectus neurons and inhibitory fibers to the contralateral medial rectus neurons. In lesions of the medial longitudinal fasciculus, failure of inhibition of adduction in the contralateral eye thus causes an abducting (corrective) nystagmus in that eye.

Facial Nerve (Cranial Nerve VII)

The facial nerve (Fig. 7-11) is a mixed nerve with both sensory and motor components.

Facial nerve. The seventh cranial nerve. Willis divided the seventh nerve into a portio dura (facial) and a portio mollis (auditory). Soemmering separated the two and numbered them separately.

Sensory Components

The facial nerve carries two types of sensory afferents: exteroceptive fibers from the external ear and taste fibers from the anterior two-thirds of the tongue.

The exteroceptive fibers from the external ear are peripheral processes of neurons in the geniculate ganglion. Central processes project on neurons in the spinal trigeminal nucleus [similar to fibers from the same area carried by the glossopharyngeal (cranial nerve IX) and vagus (cranial nerve X) nerves].

The taste fibers have their neurons of origin in the geniculate ganglion. Peripheral processes of these neurons reach the taste buds in the anterior two-thirds of the tongue; central processes enter the brain stem with the nervus intermedius and project on neurons in the gustatory part of the nucleus solitarius, along with fibers carried by the glossopharyngeal (from the posterior third of the tongue) and vagus (from the epiglottic region) nerves. The sensory and gustatory fibers, along with the visceral motor component, form a separate lateral root of the facial nerve, the **nervus intermedius** (Wrisberg's nerve).

Nervus intermedius (Wrisberg's nerve). Lateral root of the facial nerve containing visceral motor and sensory components. Named by Heinrich August Wrisberg, a German anatomist.

KEY CONCEPTS

- The facial nerve is composed of sensory and motor components.
- The sensory facial nuclei are the spinal trigeminal nucleus (exteroceptive sensation) and the nucleus solitarius (taste).

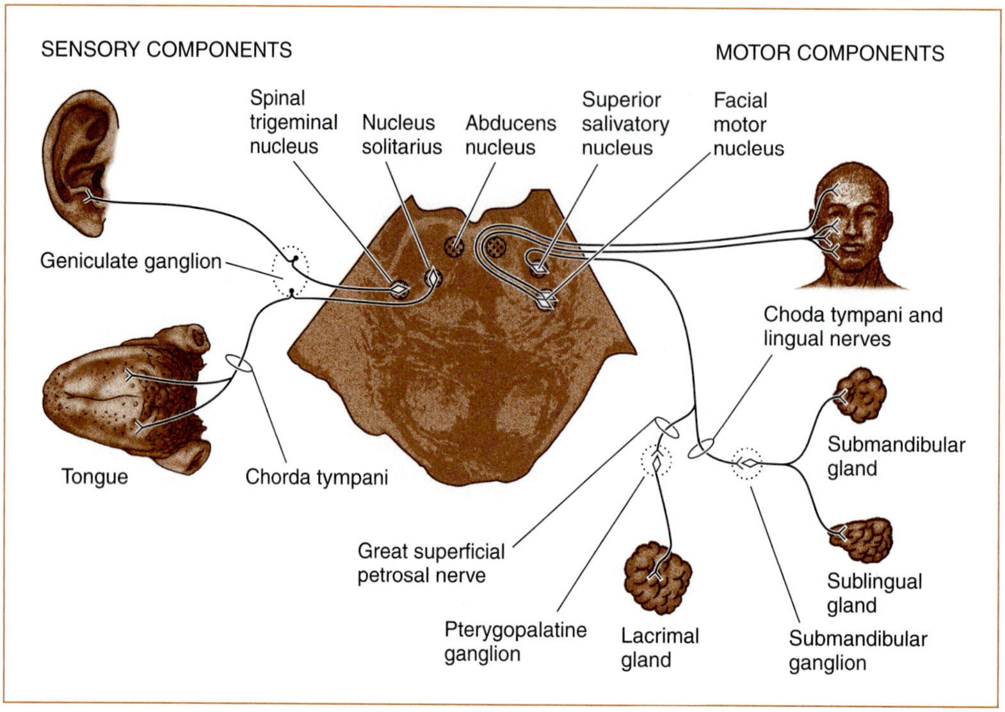
SENSORY COMPONENTS
MOTOR COMPONENTS
Spinal trigeminal nucleus
Nucleus solitarius
Abducens nucleus
Superior salivatory nucleus
Facial motor nucleus
Geniculate ganglion
Choda tympani and lingual nerves
Tongue
Chorda tympani
Submandibular gland
Great superficial petrosal nerve
Sublingual gland
Pterygopalatine ganglion
Lacrimal gland
Submandibular ganglion

FIGURE 7-11

Schematic diagram showing the nuclei of origin, course, and areas of supply of the facial (CN VII) nerve.

Motor Components

The facial nerve carries two types of motor fibers: somatic and secretomotor.

Somatic Motor Fibers Somatic motor fibers supply the muscles of facial expression and the stapedius, the stylohyoid, and the posterior belly of the digastric. These fibers arise from the facial motor nucleus in the pontine tegmentum. From their neurons of origin, fibers course dorsomedially and then rostrally in the tegmentum and form a compact bundle near the abducens (cranial nerve VI) nucleus in the floor of the fourth ventricle (the facial colliculus). They bend (genu) laterally over the abducens nucleus and turn ventrolaterally to emerge at the lateral border of the pons. This peculiar course of the somatic motor component of the facial nerve fibers in the tegmentum results from the migration of facial motor neurons from a dorsal position in the floor of the fourth ventricle caudally and ventrally, pulling its axons with it. The migration of the facial motor nucleus is explained by neurobiotaxis, in which neurons tend to migrate toward major sources of stimuli. In the case of the facial motor nucleus, this migration brings it closer to the trigeminal spinal nucleus and its tract. Visceral motor and sensory components of the facial nerve do not make a loop around the abducens nucleus. Instead, they form a separate lateral root of the facial nerve, the nervus intermedius.

The motor nucleus of the facial nerve is organized into longitudinally oriented motor columns (subnuclei) concerned with specific facial muscles: the medial, dorsal,

KEY CONCEPTS

- The motor facial nuclei are the facial motor nucleus (somatic motor) and the superior salivatory nucleus (visceral motor).

intermediate, and lateral subnuclei. Motor neurons that supply upper facial muscles are located in the dorsal part of the nucleus, those innervating lower facial muscles are primarily located in the lateral part of the nucleus, and those supplying the platysma and the posterior auricular muscles are in the medial part of the nucleus.

The facial motor nucleus receives fibers from the following sources:

Cerebral cortex These fibers travel as direct corticobulbar or indirect corticoreticulobulbar fibers. The cortical input to the facial nucleus is bilateral to the part of the nucleus that supplies the upper facial muscles and only contralateral to the part that innervates the perioral musculature. In lesions affecting one hemisphere, only the lower facial muscles contralateral to the lesion are affected (Fig. 7-12). This is referred to as central facial paresis, in contradistinction to peripheral facial paralysis or paresis (resulting from lesions of the facial motor nucleus or the facial nerve), in which all the muscles of facial expression ipsilateral to the lesion are affected. Two types of central facial paresis (**palsy**) have been described: voluntary and involuntary (mimetic). Voluntary central facial palsy results from lesions involving the contralateral corticobulbar or corticoreticulobulbar fibers. Mimetic or emotional innervation of the muscles of facial expression is involuntary and of uncertain origin. It allows contraction of the lower facial muscles in response to genuine emotional stimuli. Certain neural lesions can produce mimetic central facial paralysis without voluntary central facial paralysis. More extensive lesions produce combined voluntary and mimetic central facial paralysis.

Central facial palsy. Weakness of the lower facial muscles contralateral to a lesion in the cerebral cortex or corticobulbar fibers.

Recent experimental evidence provides an alternative explanation for the sparing of the upper facial musculature in patients with central (hemispheral) lesions. Sparse

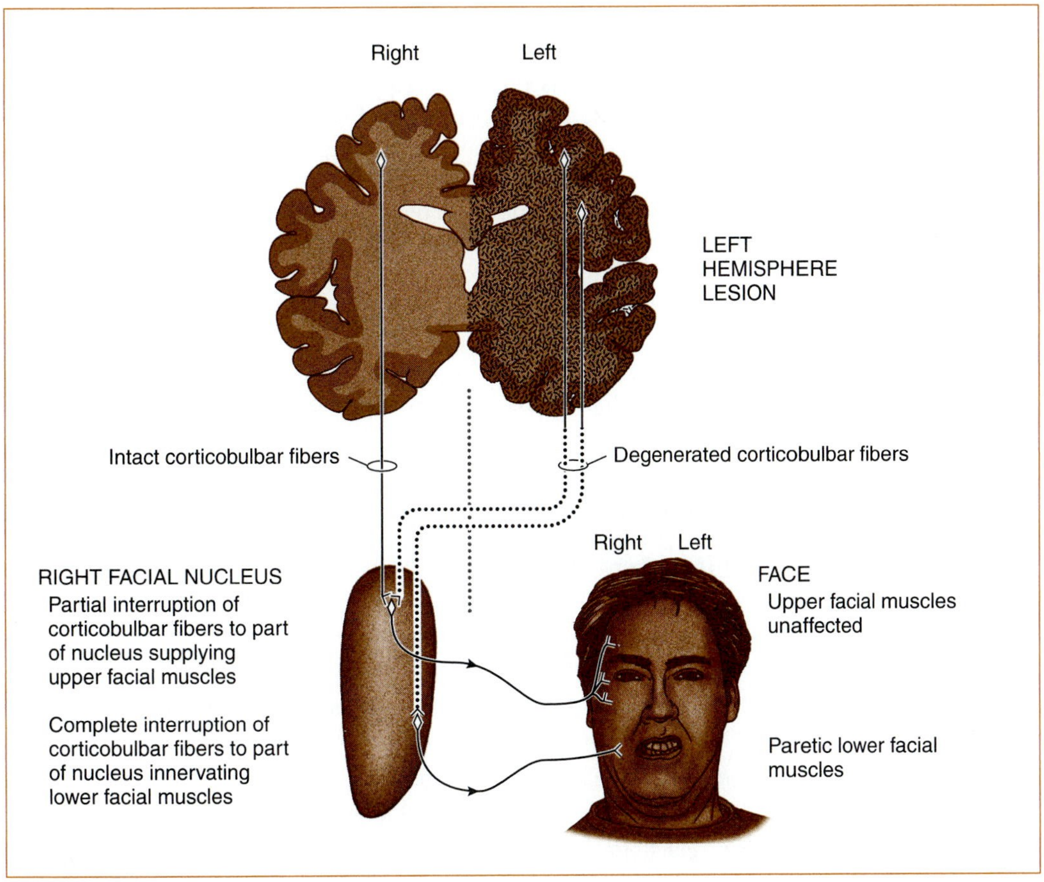

FIGURE 7-12

Schematic diagram illustrating the concept of central facial paresis.

data from human studies coupled with the results of experimental studies in a variety of mammals, including monkeys, have shown that (1) the bilateral cortical input to facial motor neurons that innervate upper facial muscles is sparse, (2) motor neurons of the facial nucleus that innervate the lower facial muscles receive significant and bilateral cortical input which is threefold heavier on the contralateral side, and (3) cortical innervation of the ipsilateral lower facial motor subnucleus is considerably heavier than that of the ipsilateral upper facial motor subnucleus. On the basis of these findings, it has been proposed that the deficit of facial muscles seen after unilateral hemispheral lesions reflects the extent to which direct cortical innervation of facial motor neuron is lost. Thus, motor neurons innervating the upper face would be little affected because they do not receive much direct cortical input. Also, lower facial motor neurons contralateral to the lesion would suffer loss of function because they are most dependent on direct contralateral cortical innervation and because the remaining ipsilateral cortical projection apparently is insufficient to drive them. The small loss of cortical input to lower facial motor neurons ipsilateral to the lesion is compensated by the remaining, much more intense, input from the intact hemisphere. Alternately, it is possible that the lower facial muscles ipsilateral to the lesion display some mild weakness but that this is obscured by the much more profound contralateral weakness.

Basal ganglia This input to the facial motor nucleus explains the movement of paretic facial muscles in response to emotional stimulation. Patients with central facial paralysis who are unable to move the lower facial muscles voluntarily may be able to do so reflexly in response to emotional stimulation.

Superior olive This input is part of a reflex involving the facial and auditory nerves. It explains the grimacing of facial muscles that occurs in response to a loud noise.

Trigeminal system This input is also reflex in nature, linking the trigeminal and facial nerves. It underlies the blinking of the eyelids in response to corneal stimulation.

Superior colliculus This input via tectobulbar fibers is reflex in nature and provides for closure of the eyelids in response to intense light or a rapidly approaching object.

Secretomotor (Visceral Motor) Fibers These fibers arise from the superior salivatory nucleus in the tegmentum of the pons. They are preganglionic fibers that leave the brain stem with the nevus intermedius (Wrisberg's nerve) and synapse in collateral ganglia. Fibers destined for the lacrimal gland travel in the greater

KEY CONCEPTS

- The facial motor nucleus receives fibers from the following sources: cerebral cortex, basal ganglia, superior olive, and secondary trigeminal pathways.
- Cortical input to the facial motor nucleus is bilateral to the upper face motor neurons and only contralateral to the lower face motor neurons.
- Unilateral interruption of cortical input to the facial motor nucleus results in paralysis of the contralateral lower facial muscles.
- The input to the motor facial nucleus from the basal ganglia allows movement of the paralyzed lower facial muscles in response to emotional stimuli.
- The input from the superior olive and secondary trigeminal pathways to the motor facial nucleus allows reflex grimacing to sound stimuli and blinking to corneal stimulation, respectively.

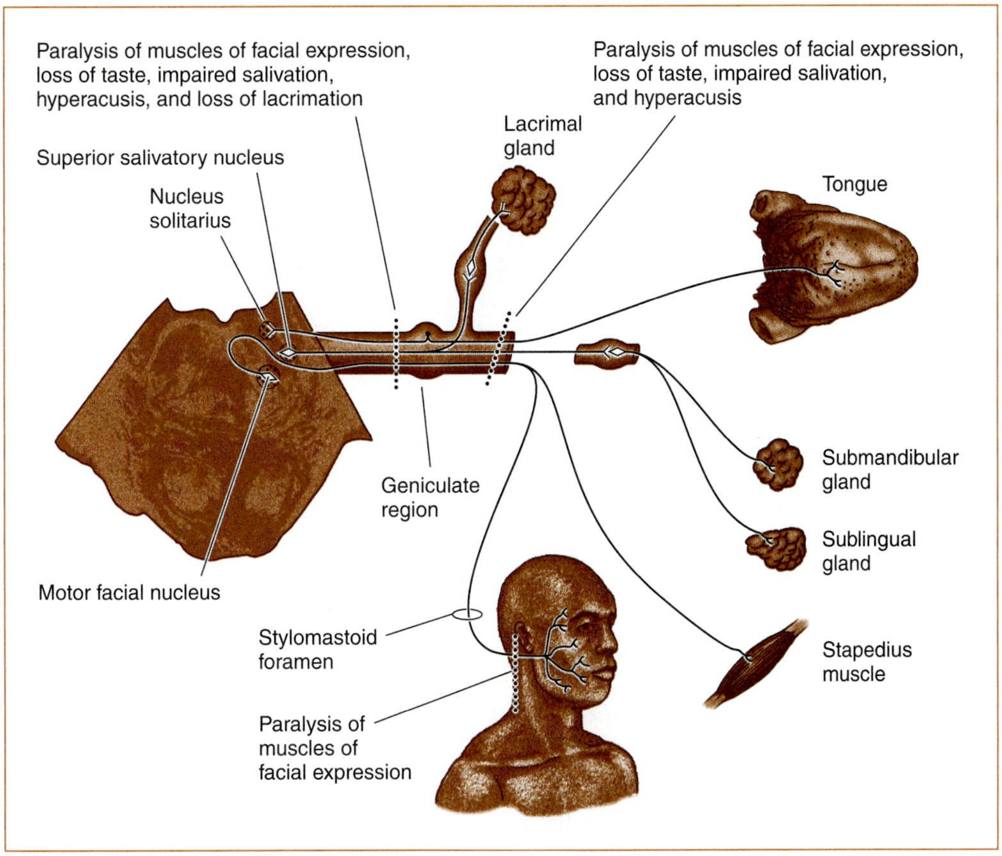

FIGURE 7-13

Schematic diagram showing lesions in the facial nerve at different sites and the resulting clinical manifestations of each.

superficial petrosal nerve and synapse in the pterygopalatine ganglion, from which postganglionic parasympathetic fibers reach the lacrimal gland. Fibers destined for the submandibular and sublingual glands join the chorda tympani and the lingual nerves and synapse in the submandibular ganglion, from which postganglionic parasympathetic fibers arise. Because fibers for the lacrimal, submandibular, and sublingual glands leave the brain stem together, lesions of the facial nerve proximal to the geniculate ganglion may result in abberant growth of regenerating fibers so that fibers destined to innervate the lacrimal glands reach the submandibular and sublingual salivary glands. This aberrant growth is responsible for the phenomenon of "**crocodile tears,**" in which the presence of food in the mouth is followed by lacrimation rather than salivation.

Facial Nerve Lesions

Signs of facial nerve paralysis (**Bell's palsy**) vary with the location of the lesion (Fig. 7-13). Bell's palsy is named after Sir Charles Bell (1774–1842), a British anatomist, physiologist, surgeon, and neurologist who was also a pioneer in the study of facial expression.

Proximal to Geniculate Ganglion Lesions of the facial nerve proximal to the geniculate ganglion result in the following signs:

1. Paralysis of all the muscles of facial expression
2. Loss of taste in the anterior two-thirds of the ipsilateral half of the tongue
3. Impaired salivary secretion
4. Impaired lacrimation

Crocodile tears (Bogorad syndrome). Shedding of tears while eating as a result of aberrant innervation of facial nerve fibers so that fibers destined to innervate the lacrimal glands reach the submandibular and sublingual glands. Named after F. A. Bogorad, a Russian physiologist who suggested the name and the physiologic mechanism in 1928. The phenomenon had been described by Hermann Oppenheim, a German neurologist, in 1913.

Bell's palsy. Facial paralysis ipsilateral to a facial nerve lesion. Described by Sir Charles Bell, a Scottish anatomist and surgeon, in 1821.

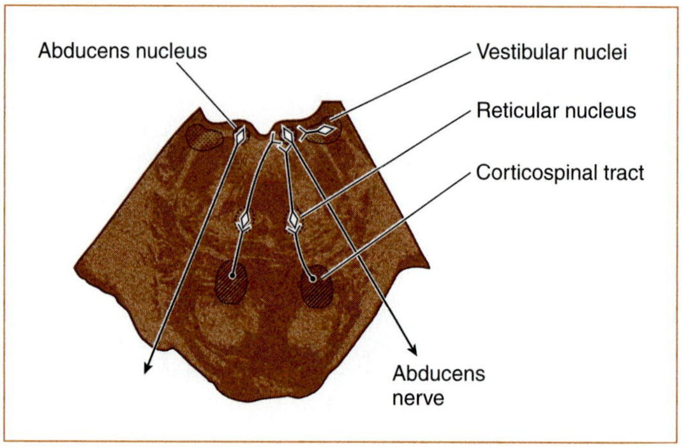

FIGURE 7-14

Schematic diagram showing sources of modulating inputs into the abducens (CN VI) nucleus and intrapontine course of the abducens nerve.

Hyperacusis (Greek *hyper*, "above"; *akousis*, "hearing"). Abnormal sensitivity to loud sounds. Commonly seen in persons with facial nerve lesions and subsequent paralysis of the stapedius muscle.

5. **Hyperacusis** (hypersensitivity to sound as a result of paralysis of the stapedius muscle)
6. Crocodile tears in some patients with aberrant growth of regenerating fibers

Distal of Geniculate Ganglion Lesions of the facial nerve distal to the geniculate ganglion but proximal to the chorda tympani result in the following ipsilateral signs:

1. Paralysis of all the muscles of facial expression
2. Loss of taste in the anterior two-thirds of the tongue
3. Impaired salivary secretion
4. Hyperacusis

Lacrimation is not affected by this type of lesion, since the fibers destined for the lacrimal gland leave the nerve proximal to the level of the lesion.

Stylomastoid Foramen Lesions of the facial nerve at the stylomastoid foramen (where the motor fibers destined for the muscles of facial expression leave the cranium) result only in paralysis of the muscles of facial expression that are ipsilateral to the lesion.

Abducens nerve (Latin, "drawing away"). The sixth cranial nerve, discovered by Eustachius in 1564, is so named because it supplies the lateral rectus muscle, whose function is to direct the eye to the lateral side away from the midline.

Abducens Nerve (Cranial Nerve VI)

The abducens nerve (Fig. 7-14) is a purely motor nerve that innervates the lateral rectus muscle. The abducens nucleus is located in a paramedian site in the tegmentum of the pons, in the floor of the fourth ventricle. It extends from the rostral limit of the lateral vestibular nucleus to the rostral portion of the descending vestibular nucleus. The abducens nucleus has two populations of neurons: large (motoneurons) and small (interneurons). Two types of interneurons (fusiform and circular) have been reported in the abducens nucleus on the basis of shape and differences in organelle content. While differences in shape may indicate different functions, this is not supported by the available physiologic data.

KEY CONCEPTS

- Characteristic conglomerate clinical signs occur in lesions of the facial nerve at or distal to the stylomastoid foramen, distal to the geniculate ganglion, and proximal to the geniculate ganglion.

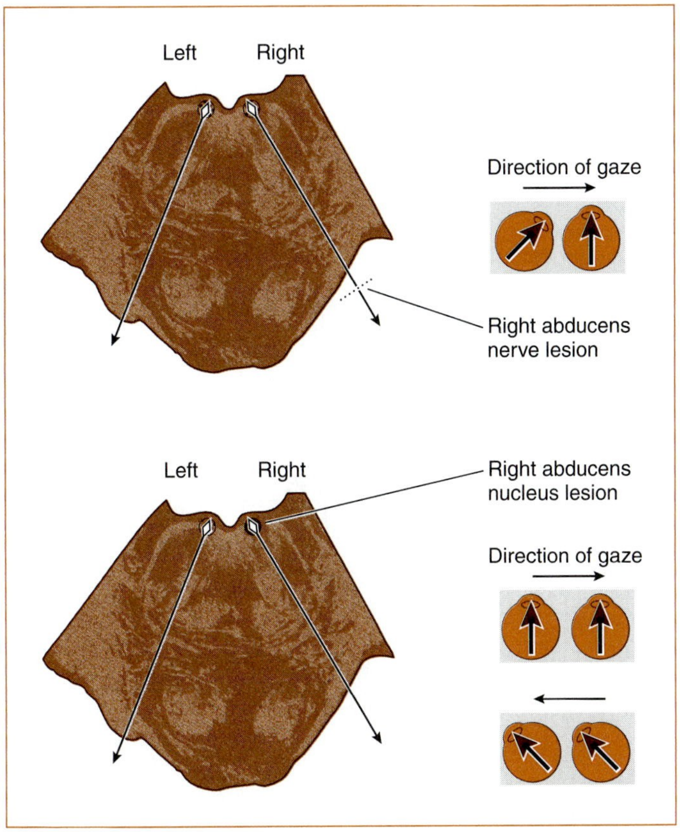

FIGURE 7-15

Schematic diagram showing the clinical manifestations resulting from lesions in the abducens nucleus and nerve.

Axons of the large neurons (motoneurons) form the abducens nerve and supply the lateral rectus muscles. Axons of the small neurons (interneurons) join the contralateral medial longitudinal fasciculus and terminate on neurons in the oculomotor nucleus that supply the medial rectus muscle (medial rectus subnucleus). Axons of the abducens nerve course through the tegmentum and basis pontis and exit on the ventral surface of the pons in the groove between the pons and the medulla oblongata (Fig. 7-14). The abducens nucleus (Fig. 7-14) receives fibers from (1) the cerebral cortex (corticoreticulobulbar fibers), (2) the medial vestibular nucleus via the medial longitudinal fasciculus, (3) the paramedian pontine reticular formation (PPRF), and (4) the **nucleus prepositus** hypoglossi. The corticobulbar input is bilateral, the inputs from the PPRF and the nucleus prepositus are uncrossed, and the input from the medial vestibular nucleus is predominantly uncrossed. Direct afferent fibers from Scarpa's ganglion to the abducens nucleus have been described.

Lesions of the abducens nerve result in paralysis of the ipsilateral lateral rectus muscle and **diplopia** (double vision) on attempted horizontal gaze toward the side of the paralyzed muscle (Fig. 7-15*A*); the two images are horizontal, and the distance between them increases as the eyes move in the direction of action of the paralyzed

Nucleus prepositus. One of the perihypoglossal reticular nuclei in the medulla oblongata. Related to ocular movement.

Diplopia (Greek *diplos*, "double"; *ops*, "eye") The perception of two images of a single object. Double vision resulting from extraocular muscle weakness.

KEY CONCEPTS

- The abducens nucleus contains two types of neurons: principal, which provide a nerve supply to the ipsilateral lateral rectus muscle, and interneurons, which send axons to the contralateral medial rectus subnucleus within the oculomotor nucleus.

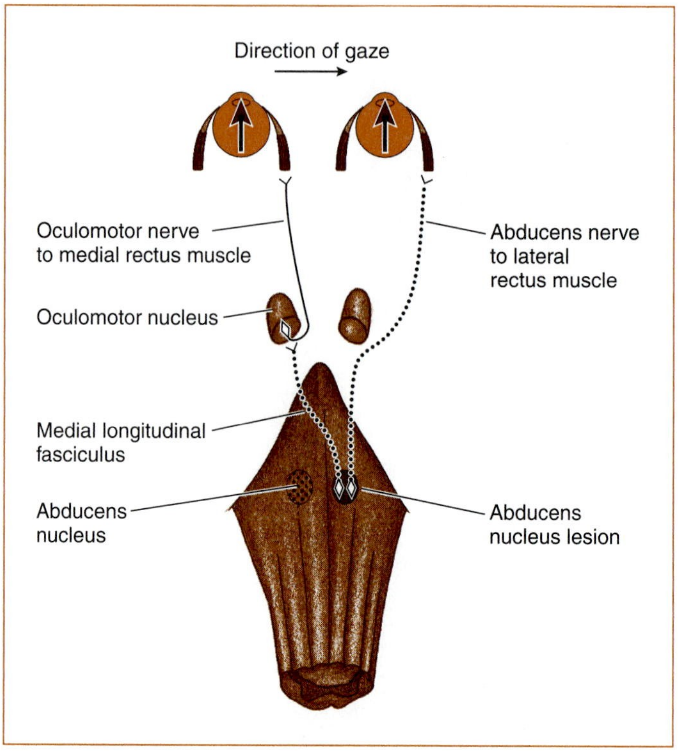

FIGURE 7-16

Schematic diagram illustrating the basis of lateral gaze paralysis in abducens nucleus lesions.

muscle. The abducens nerve has a long intracranial course and therefore is commonly affected in intracranial diseases of varying etiologies and sites. In contrast to lesions of the abducens nerve, lesions of the abducens nucleus do not result in paralysis of abduction but instead in paralysis of horizontal gaze ipsilateral to the lesion; this is manifested by the failure of both eyes to move on attempted ipsilateral horizontal gaze (Fig. 7-15*B*).

Paralysis of lateral gaze after abducens nucleus lesions is explained by involvement of the large neurons which supply the ipsilateral lateral rectus muscle and the small neurons (interneurons) which supply the contralateral medial rectus neurons (medial rectus subnucleus) within the oculomotor nucleus (Fig. 7-16). The notion that pontine reticular neurons are responsible for paralysis of adduction no longer appears tenable. Tritiated amino acids injected into the paramedian pontine reticular formation do not reveal terminations in the oculomotor nucleus but instead in the abducens nucleus and the interstitial nucleus of the medial longitudinal fasciculus, which is believed to be involved in vertical (downward) gaze. The pontine center for lateral gaze and the abducens nucleus probably constitute a single entity. The PPRF (pontine center for lateral gaze) is a physiologically defined neuronal pool that is rostral to the abducens nucleus. It is composed of caudal and rostral

KEY CONCEPTS

- Lesions of the abducens nerve outside the neuraxis result in ipsilateral lateral rectus paralysis.
- Lesions of the abducens nucleus result in paralysis of ipsilateral lateral gaze.

parts. The caudal part is connected to the ipsilateral abducens nucleus. Stimulation of the caudal part results in conjugate horizontal deviation of the eyes. The rostral part is connected to the rostral interstitial nucleus of the MLF (RiMLF), which in turn projects to the ipsilateral oculomotor nucleus by pathways other than the MLF. Stimulation of the rostral PPRF results in vertical gaze. Lesions in the caudal PPRF abolish conjugate lateral gaze, whereas lesions in the rostral PPRF abolish vertical gaze. Extensive lesions in PPRF result in paralysis of both horizontal and vertical gaze.

Abducens nerve rootlets along their course within the pons may be involved in a variety of intraaxial vascular lesions.

1. Lesions in the basis pontis involving the corticospinal fibers and the rootlets of the abducens nerve result in **alternating hemiplegia** manifested by ipsilateral lateral rectus paralysis (and diplopia) as well as an upper motor neuron paralysis of the contralateral half of the body (Fig. 7-17*A*).
2. Lesions in the pontine tegmentum involving the abducens rootlets and the medial lemniscus result in ipsilateral lateral rectus paralysis (and diplopia) and contralateral loss of kinesthesia and discriminative touch (Fig. 7-17*B*).
3. More dorsal lesions involving the abducens nucleus, the medial longitudinal fasciculus, and the curving rootlets of the facial nerve produce paralysis of horizontal gaze and peripheral-type facial paralysis, both ipsilateral to the lesion (Fig. 7-17*C*).

Alternating hemiplegia. Paresis of the cranial nerves ipsilateral to a brain stem lesion and of the trunk and limbs contralateral to the lesion.

Trigeminal Nerve (Cranial Nerve V)

The trigeminal nerve has two roots: a smaller (portio minor) efferent root and a larger (portio major) afferent root. The motor root is composed of as many as 14 separately originating rootlets that are joined about 1 cm from the pons. At the pons, the first division of the trigeminal sensory root (V1) usually is located in a dorsomedial position adjacent to the motor root and the third division (V3) is in a caudolateral position. V3, however, may vary from being directly lateral to directly caudal to V1. Aberrant sensory roots exist in about 50 percent of individuals and may explain the persistence of facial pain (**trigeminal neuralgia**) after surgical sectioning of the sensory root. Aberrant sensory rootlets enter the sensory root within 1 cm of the pons and contribute mainly to V1. Some rootlets between the motor and sensory roots may join either root farther away from the pons. Anastomosis between the motor and sensory roots has been described and may explain the failure of sensory root sectioning to relieve facial pain.

Trigeminal nerve (Latin *tres*, "three"; *geminus*, "twin"). The fifth cranial nerve was described by Fallopius. So named because it has three divisions: ophthalmic, maxillary, and mandibular.

Trigeminal neuralgia (tic douloureux, Fothergill's syndrome). Paroxysmal attacks of severe facial pain in the trigeminal sensory distribution. Described by John Fothergill, an English physician, in 1773.

Efferent Root

The efferent root of the trigeminal nerve arises from the motor nucleus of the trigeminal nerve in the tegmentum of the pons. The efferent root supplies the muscles of mastication and the tensor tympani, the tensor palati, the myelohyoid, and the anterior belly of the digastric. The motor nucleus receives fibers from the

KEY CONCEPTS

- Lesions of the abducens nerve within the pons result in crossed sensory or motor syndromes.
- The trigeminal nerve has two components: smaller motor (portio minor) and larger sensory (portio major).
- The motor nucleus of the trigeminal nerve supplies the muscles of mastication, the tensor tympani, the tensor palati, the mylohyoideus, and the anterior belly of the digastric.

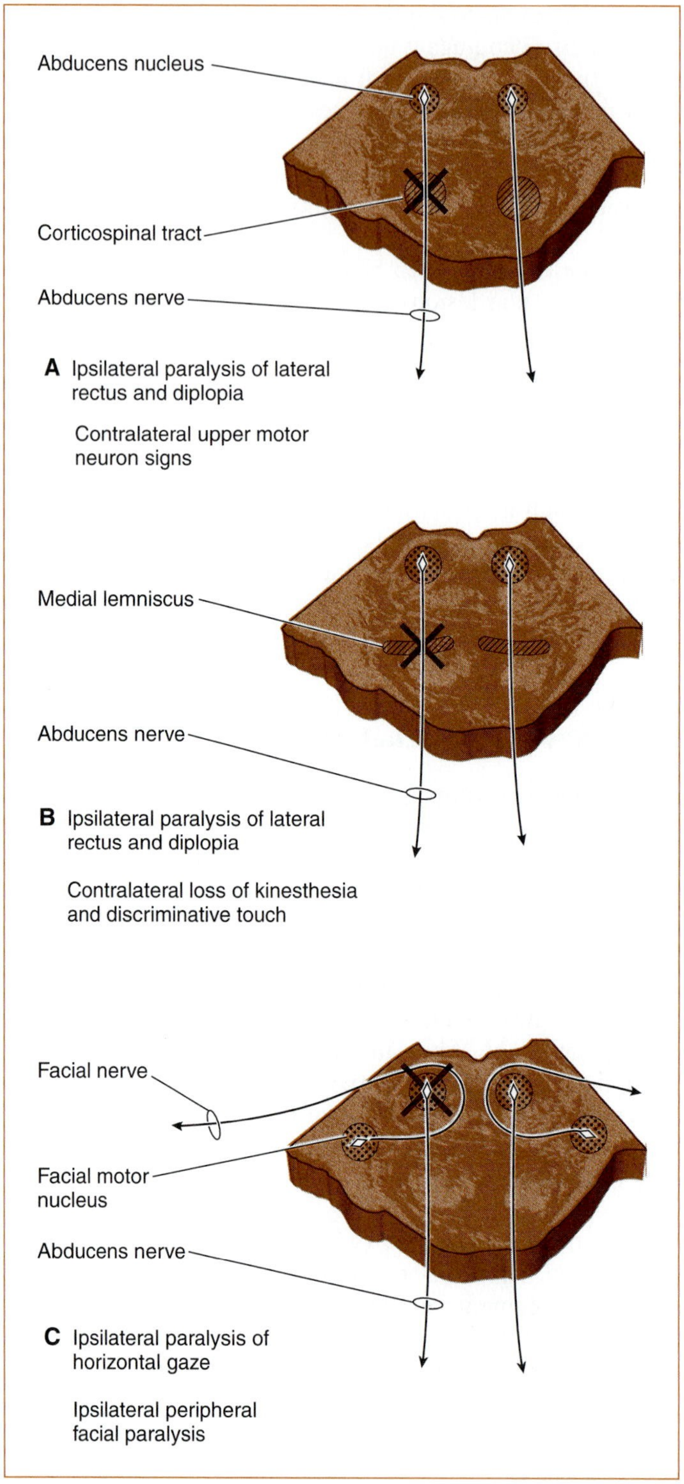
Abducens nucleus
Corticospinal tract
Abducens nerve
A Ipsilateral paralysis of lateral rectus and diplopia
Contralateral upper motor neuron signs
Medial lemniscus
Abducens nerve
B Ipsilateral paralysis of lateral rectus and diplopia
Contralateral loss of kinesthesia and discriminative touch
Facial nerve
Facial motor nucleus
Abducens nerve
C Ipsilateral paralysis of horizontal gaze
Ipsilateral peripheral facial paralysis

FIGURE 7-17

Schematic diagram of lesions of the abducens (CN VI) nerve and nucleus and the resulting clinical manifestations.

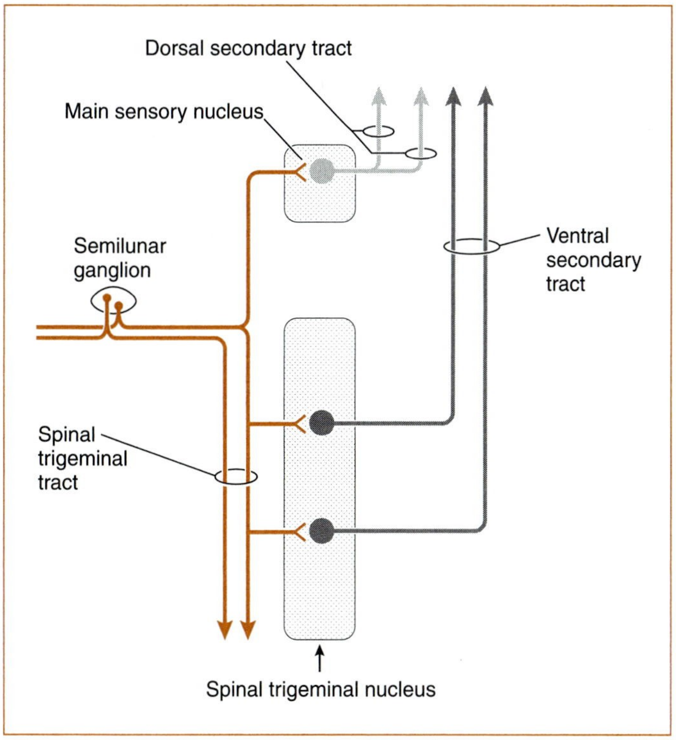

FIGURE 7-18

Schematic diagram showing the cells of origin and course of the sensory root of the trigeminal (CN V) nerve.

cerebral cortex (corticobulbar) and the sensory nuclei of the trigeminal nerve. The cortical projections to trigeminal motoneurons are bilateral and symmetric via direct corticobulbar and indirect corticoreticulobulbar fibers. Lesions affecting the motor nucleus or efferent root result in paralysis of the lower motor neuron type of the muscles supplied by this root.

Afferent Root

The afferent root (Fig. 7-18) of the trigeminal nerve contains two types of afferent fibers.

Proprioceptive Fibers Proprioceptive fibers from deep structures of the face travel via the efferent and afferent roots. They are peripheral processes of unipolar neurons in the mesencephalic nucleus of the trigeminal nerve located at the rostral pontine and caudal mesencephalic levels. This nucleus is unique in that it is homologous to the dorsal root ganglion yet is centrally placed. Proprioceptive fibers to the mesencephalic nucleus convey pressure and kinesthesia from the teeth, periodontium, hard palate, and joint capsules as well as impulses from stretch receptors in the muscles of mastication. The output from the mesencephalic nucleus is destined for the cerebellum, the thalamus, the motor nuclei of the brain stem, and the reticular formation. The mesencephalic nucleus is concerned with mechanisms that control the force of the bite.

Exteroceptive Fibers Exteroceptive fibers are general somatic sensory fibers that convey pain, temperature, and touch sensations from the face and the anterior aspect of the head. The neurons of origin of these fibers are situated in the **semilunar (Grasserian) ganglion.** The peripheral processes of neurons in the ganglion are

Semilunar ganglion (Latin *semi*, "half"; *luna*, "moon"). Resembling a crescent or half moon. The semilunar (gasserian) ganglion of the trigeminal nerve lies on the medial end of the petrous bone.

Gasserian ganglion. The sensory trigeminal (semilunar) ganglion was named after Johann Gasser, an Austrian anatomist, by one of his students in 1765. Gasser had described the ganglion in his thesis.

distributed in the three divisions of the trigeminal nerve: ophthalmic, maxillary, and mandibular. The central processes of these unipolar neurons enter the lateral aspect of the pons and distribute themselves as follows.

Some of these fibers descend in the pons and medulla and run down to the level of the second or third cervical spinal segment as the descending (spinal) tract of the trigeminal nerve. They convey pain and temperature sensations. Throughout their caudal course these fibers project on neurons in the adjacent nucleus of the descending tract of the trigeminal nerve (spinal trigeminal nucleus). The spinal trigeminal nucleus is divided into three parts on the basis of its cytoarchitecture: (1) an oral part which extends from the entry zone of the trigeminal nerve in the pons to the level of the rostral third of the inferior olivary nucleus in the medulla oblongata and receives tactile sensibility from oral mucosa, (2) an interpolar part which extends from the caudal extent of the oral part to just rostral to the pyramidal decussation in the medulla oblongata and receives dental pain, and (3) a caudal part which extends from the pyramidal decussation down to the second or third cervical spinal segments and receives pain and temperature senations from the face.

Axons of neurons in the spinal trigeminal nucleus cross the midline and form the ventral secondary ascending trigeminal tract, which courses rostrally to terminate in the thalamus. During their rostral course these second-order fibers send collateral branches to several motor nuclei of the brain stem [hypoglossal (cranial nerve XII), vagus (cranial nerve X), glossopharyngeal (cranial nerve IX), facial (cranial nerve VII), and trigeminal (cranial nerve V)] to establish reflexes. Trigeminal fibers establish three kinds of synapses with facial nerve nuclei: (1) disynaptic with the ipsilateral facial nerve nucleus, (2) polysynaptic with the ipsilateral facial nucleus, (3) indirect and polysynaptic with the contralateral facial nerve nucleus. The spinal tract of the trigeminal nerve is concerned mainly with the transmission of pain and temperature sensations. It sometimes is cut surgically at a low level (trigeminal tractotomy) to relieve intractable pain. These operations may relieve pain but leave touch sensation intact. The spinal tract of the trigeminal nerve also carries somatic afferent fibers traveling with other cranial nerves [facial (cranial nerve VII), glossopharyngeal (cranial nerve IX), and vagus (cranial nerve X)], as was outlined previously.

Other incoming fibers of the trigeminal nerve bifurcate on entry into the pons into ascending and descending branches. These fibers convey touch sensation. The descending branches join the spinal tract of the trigeminal nerve and follow the course that was outlined above. The shorter ascending branches project on the main sensory nucleus of the trigeminal nerve. From the main sensory nucleus, second-order fibers ascend ipsilaterally and contralaterally as the dorsal ascending trigeminal tract to the thalamus. Some crossed fibers also travel in the ventral ascending trigeminal tract. Once they are formed, both secondary trigeminal tracts (dorsal and ventral) lie lateral to the medial lemniscus between it and the spinothalamic tract. Since fibers that convey touch sensation bifurcate on entry to the pons and terminate on both the spinal and the main sensory trigeminal nuclei, touch sensations are not abolished when the spinal trigeminal tract is cut (trigeminal tractotomy). A schematic summary of the afferent and efferent trigeminal roots

KEY CONCEPTS

- The sensory nuclei of the trigeminal nerve are the spinal (pain, temperature, touch), principal (main) sensory (touch), and mesencephalic (proprioception).
- Dorsal and ventral trigeminothalamic tracts link the main sensory and spinal trigeminal nuclei, respectively, with the thalamus.

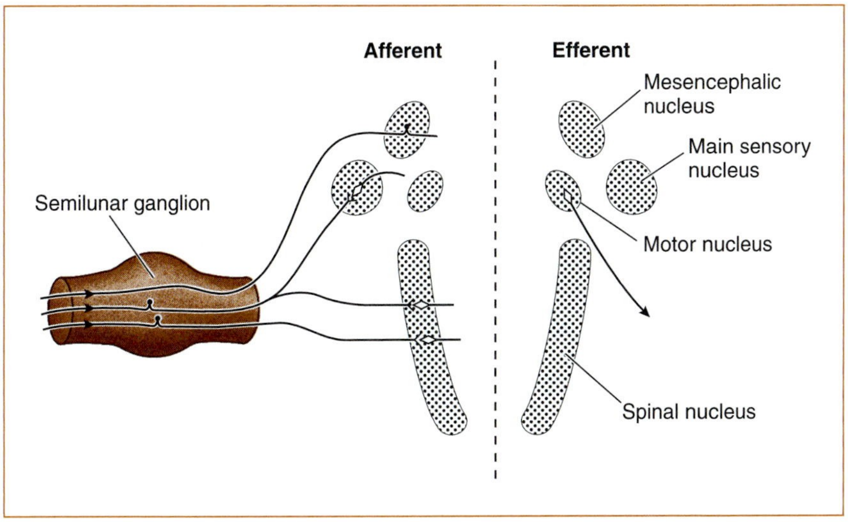
Afferent
Efferent
Mesencephalic nucleus
Main sensory nucleus
Semilunar ganglion
Motor nucleus
Spinal nucleus

FIGURE 7-19

Composite schematic diagram of the afferent and efferent roots of the trigeminal (CN V) nerve and their nuclei.

and their nuclei is shown in Figure 7-19. Recent studies of trigeminothalamic fibers have revealed that the bulk of these fibers arise from the main sensory nucleus and the interpolaris segment of the spinal nucleus. The majority of these fibers terminate in the contralateral thalamus [ventral posterior medial (VPM) nucleus] with few terminations ipsilaterally. Other efferents of the trigeminal nuclei include projections to the ipsilateral cerebellum via the inferior cerebellar peduncle (from the spinal and main sensory nuclei), the spinal cord dorsal horn (bilaterally) from the spinal nucleus, and the cerebellum (from the mesencephalic nucleus).

Trigeminal neuralgia (tic douloureux) is a disabling painful sensation in the distribution of the branches of the trigeminal nerve. The pain is paroxysmal, stabbing, or like lightning in nature and usually is triggered by eating, talking, or brushing the teeth. Several methods of treatment, including drugs, alcohol injection of the nerve, electrocoagulation of the ganglion, and surgical interruption of the nerve or spinal tract in the medulla oblongata (**trigeminal tractotomy**), have been tried with varying degrees of success.

Trigeminal Reflexes

Collaterals from the secondary ascending trigeminal tracts establish synapses with the following cranial nerve nuclei to establish reflex responses:

1. The motor nucleus of the trigeminal to elicit the **jaw reflex**
2. The facial motor nuclei on both sides, resulting in a bilateral blink reflex, the **corneal reflex** (direct and consensual), in response to unilateral corneal stimulation
3. The nucleus ambiguus, the respiratory center of the reticular formation, and the spinal cord (phrenic nerve nuclei and anterior horn cells to intercostal muscles), resulting in the **sneezing reflex** in response to stimulation of the nasal mucous membrane
4. The dorsal motor nucleus of the vagus as part of the **vomiting reflex**
5. The inferior salivatory nucleus for the **salivatory reflex**
6. The hypoglossal nucleus for reflex movements of the tongue in response to tongue stimulation

Trigeminal tractotomy. Cutting of the spinal trigeminal tract in the brain stem to relieve severe intractable facial pain.

Jaw reflex. Contraction of the masseter and the temporalis muscle in response to a tap just below the lower lip. The afferent limb of the reflex is via the trigeminal nerve; the efferent limb is via the facial nerve. The reflex is evident in upper motor neuron lesions.

Corneal reflex. Blinking in response to corneal stimulation. The afferent limb of the reflex is via the trigeminal nerve, and the efferent limb is via the facial nerve.

Sneezing (nasal) reflex. Sneezing in response to a nasal tickle. The afferent limb of the reflex is via the trigeminal nerve; the efferent limbs are via the vagus, phrenic, and intercostal nerves.

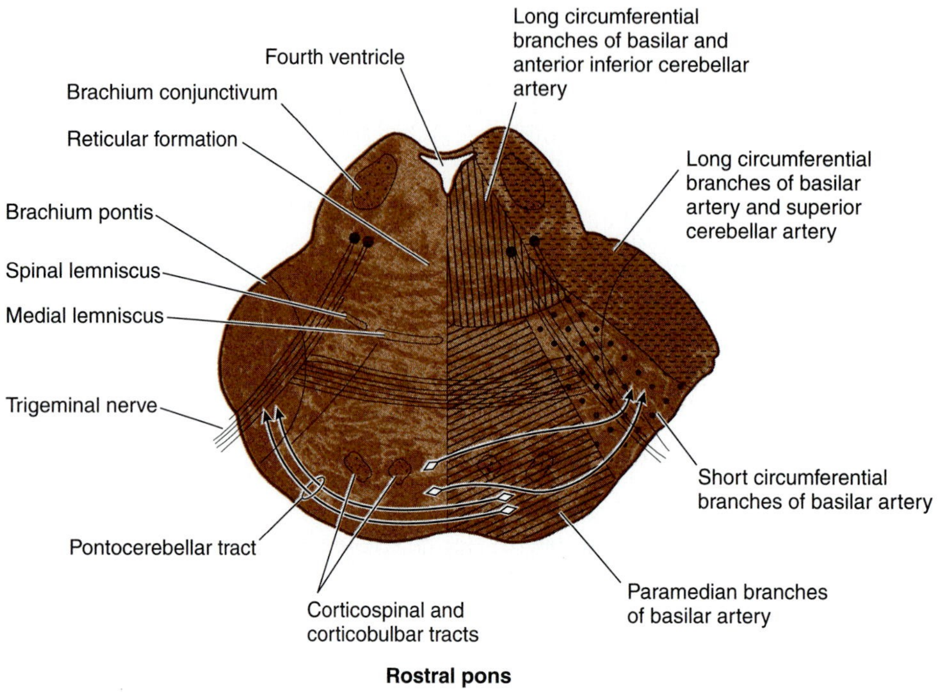
Long circumferential branches of basilar and anterior inferior cerebellar artery
Fourth ventricle
Brachium conjunctivum
Reticular formation
Long circumferential branches of basilar artery and superior cerebellar artery
Brachium pontis
Spinal lemniscus
Medial lemniscus
Trigeminal nerve
Short circumferential branches of basilar artery
Pontocerebellar tract
Paramedian branches of basilar artery
Corticospinal and corticobulbar tracts
Rostral pons

FIGURE 7-20

Schematic diagram of vascular territories in the rostral pons.

Vomiting reflex. Vomiting in response to stimulation of the pharyngeal wall. The afferent limb of the reflex is via the trigeminal nerve; the efferent limb is via the vagus nerve.

Salivatory reflex. Salivation in response to trigeminal stimulation. The afferent limb of the reflex is via the trigeminal nerve; the efferent limb is via the glossopharyngeal nerve.

Tearing reflex. Production of tears in response to corneal stimulation. The afferent limb of the reflex is via the trigeminal nerve; the efferent limb is via the facial nerve.

7. The superior salivatory nucleus, resulting in tears in response to corneal irritation, the **tearing reflex**

Blood Supply

The blood supply of the pons (Figs. 7-20 and 7-21) is derived from the basilar artery. Three groups of vessels provide blood to specific regions of the pons: the paramedian and the short and long circumferential.

The paramedian vessels (four to six in number) arise from the basilar artery and enter the pons ventrally, supplying the medial basis pontis and the tegmentum. Pontine nuclei, corticospinal tract bundles within the basis pontis, and the medial lemniscus are among the structures supplied by these vessels.

Short circumferential arteries arise from the basilar artery, enter the brachium pontis, and supply the ventrolateral region of the basis pontis.

KEY CONCEPTS

- Trigeminothalamic fibers establish reflex connections via collaterals to the following cranial motor nuclei: hypoglossal, vagus, glossopharyngeal, facial, and trigeminal.
- Blood supply to the pons is provided by the basilar artery via three branches: paramedian, short circumferential, and long circumferential.
- Paramedian arteries supply the medial basis pontis and tegmentum.

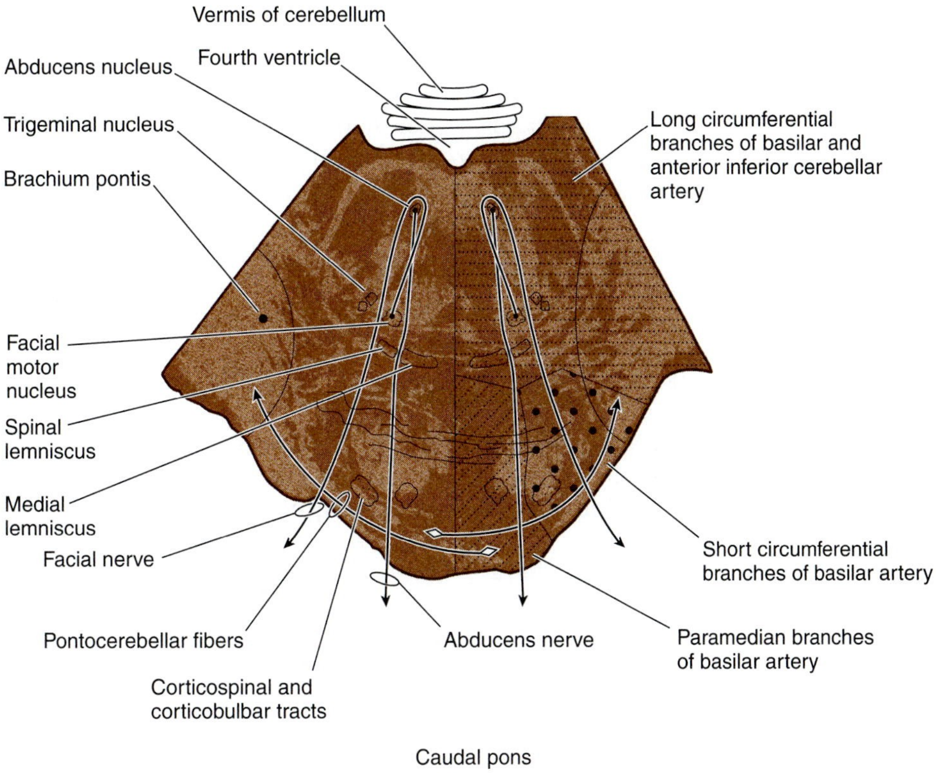

FIGURE 7-21

Schematic diagram of vascular territories in the caudal pons.

Long circumferential arteries include the anterior inferior cerebellar artery (AICA), the internal auditory artery, and the superior cerebellar artery. The AICA supplies the lateral tegmentum of the lower two-thirds of the pons as well as the ventrolateral cerebellum. The internal auditory artery, which may arise from the AICA or the basilar aratery, supplies the auditory, vestibular, and facial cranial nerves. The superior cerebellar artery supplies the dorsolateral pons, brachium pontis, brachium conjunctivum, and dorsal reticular formation. Occasionally the ventrolateral pontine tegmentum is also supplied by this vessel.

KEY CONCEPTS

- Short circumferential arteries supply the ventrolateral region of the pons.
- Long circumferential arteries include the anterior inferior cerebellar artery (AICA), the internal auditory artery, and the superior cerebellar artery.
- The anterior inferior cerebellar artery supplies the lateral tegmentum of the lower two-thirds of the pons and the ventrolateral cerebellum.
- The internal auditory artery supplies the cochleovestibular and facial cranial nerves.
- The superior cerebellar artery supplies the dorsolateral pons.

SUGGESTED READINGS

Ash PR, Keltner JL: Neuro-ophthalmic signs in pontine lesions. *Medicine (Baltimore)* 1979; 58:304–320.

Brodal P: The pontocerebellar projection in the Rhesus monkey: An experimental study with retrograde axonal transport of horseradish peroxidase. *Neuroscience* 1979; 4:193–208.

Burton H, Craig AD: Distribution of trigeminothalamic projection cells in cat and monkey. *Brain Res* 1979; 161:515–521.

Carpenter MB, Batton RR: Abducens internuclear neurons and their role in conjugate horizontal gaze. *J Comp Neurol* 1980; 189:191–209.

Fisher CM: Ataxic hemiparesis: A pathologic study. *Arch Neurol* 1978; 35:126–128.

Gacek RR: Location of abducens afferent neurons in the cat. *Exp Neurol* 1979; 64:342–353.

Gudmundsson K, et al: Detailed anatomy of the intracranial portion of the trigeminal nerve. *J Neurosurg* 1971; 35:592–600.

Haymaker W: *The Founders of Neurology.* Springfield, IL, Charles C Thomas, 1953.

Hu JW, Sessle BJ: Trigeminal nociceptive and non-nociceptive neurons: Brain stem intranuclear projections and modulation by orofacial, periaqueductal gray and nucleus raphe magnus stimuli. *Brain Res* 1979; 170:547–552.

Jenny AB, Saper CB: Organization of the facial nucleus and corticofacial projection in the monkey: A reconsideration of the upper motor neuron facial palsy. *Neurology* 1987; 37:930–939.

Jones BE: Elimination of paradoxical sleep by lesions of the pontine gigantocellular tegmental field in the cat. *Neurosci Lett* 1979; 13:285–293.

Korte GE, Mugnaini E: The cerebellar projection of the vestibular nerve in the cat. *J Comp Neurol* 1979; 184:265–278.

Kotchabhakdi N, et al: The vestibulothalamic projections in the cat studied by retrograde axonal transport of horseradish peroxidase. *Exp Brain Res* 1980; 40:405–418.

Kushida CA, et al: Cortical asymmetry of REM sleep EEG following unilateral pontine hemorrhage. *Neurology* 1991; 41:598–601.

Lang W, et al: Vestibular projections to the monkey thalamus: An autoradiographic study. *Brain Res* 1979; 177:3–17.

Loewy AD, et al: Descending projection from the pontine micturition center. *Brain Res* 1979; 172:533–538.

Nakao S, Sasaki S: Excitatory input from interneurons in the abducens nucleus to medial rectus motoneurons mediating conjugate horizontal nystagmus in the cat. *Exp Brain Res* 1980; 39:23–32.

Nieuwenhuys R: Anatomy of the auditory pathways, with emphasis on the brain stem. *Adv Otorhinolaryngol* 1984; 34:25–38.

Pryse-Phillips W: *Companion to Clinical Neurology.* Boston, Little, Brown, 1995.

Stiller, J, et al: Brainstem lesion with pure motor hemiparesis: Computed tomographic demonstration. *Arch Neurol* 1982; 39:660–661.

Venna N, Sabin TD: Universal dissociated anesthesia, due to bilateral brain-stem infarcts. *Arch Neurol* 1985; 42:918–922.

Vilensky JA, Van Hoesen GW: Corticopontine projections from the cingulate cortex in the Rhesus monkey. *Brain Res* 1981; 205:391–395.

Wiesendanger R, et al: An anatomical investigation of the corticopontine projection in the primate (Macaca fascicularis and Saimiri sciureus): II. The projection from frontal and parietal association areas. *Neuroscience* 1979; 4:747–765.

CHAPTER 8

PONS: CLINICAL CORRELATES

Vascular lesions of the pons are best suited to anatomicoclinical correlations. The following syndromes are particularly illustrative.

BASAL PONTINE SYNDROMES

Basal pontine syndromes are caused by lesions in the basal part of the pons, affecting the rootlets of cranial nerves and corticospinal tract bundles in the basis pontis.

KEY CONCEPTS

- Vascular lesions in the pons may involve structures in the basis pontis (basal pontine syndromes), the tegmentum (tegmental pontine syndromes), or both.

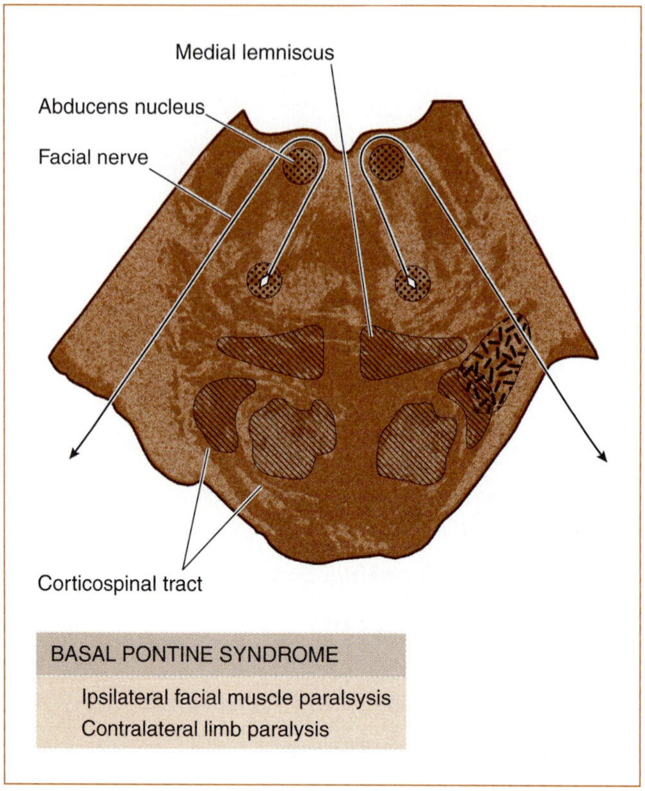
Medial lemniscus
Abducens nucleus
Facial nerve
Corticospinal tract
BASAL PONTINE SYNDROME
Ipsilateral facial muscle paralsysis
Contralateral limb paralysis

FIGURE 8-1

Schematic diagram of the structures involved in the caudal pontine syndrome (Millard-Gubler) and the resulting clinical manifestations.

Caudal Basal Pontine Syndrome (Millard-Gubler Syndrome)

Millard-Gubler syndrome (caudal basal pontine syndrome). A vascular syndrome of the caudal basis pontis characterized by ipsilateral facial nerve palsy and contralateral hemiplegia. The syndrome may include abducens nerve palsy. Described by Auguste Millard and Adolphe-Marie Gubler, French physicians, in 1856.

The manifestations of the caudal basal pontine syndrome include ipsilateral facial paralysis of the peripheral type and contralateral hemiplegia of the upper motor neuron type (Fig. 8-1). Frequently, the lesion may extend medially and rostrally to include the rootlets of the sixth nerve (Fig. 8-2). In this situation, the patient also manifests signs of ipsilateral sixth nerve paralysis.

Rostral Basal Pontine Syndrome

If the basal pontine lesion occurs more rostrally, at the level of the trigeminal nerve (Fig. 8-3), the manifestations include ipsilateral trigeminal signs (sensory and motor) and a contralateral hemiplegia of the upper motor neuron variety.

KEY CONCEPTS

- Manifestations of the Millard-Gubler syndrome consist of ipsilateral facial nerve palsy and contralateral hemiplegia. In some patients the abducens nerve may be involved ipsilateral to the lesion.
- Manifestations of the rostral basal pontine syndrome consist of ipsilateral trigeminal nerve palsy (motor and sensory) and contralateral hemiplegia.

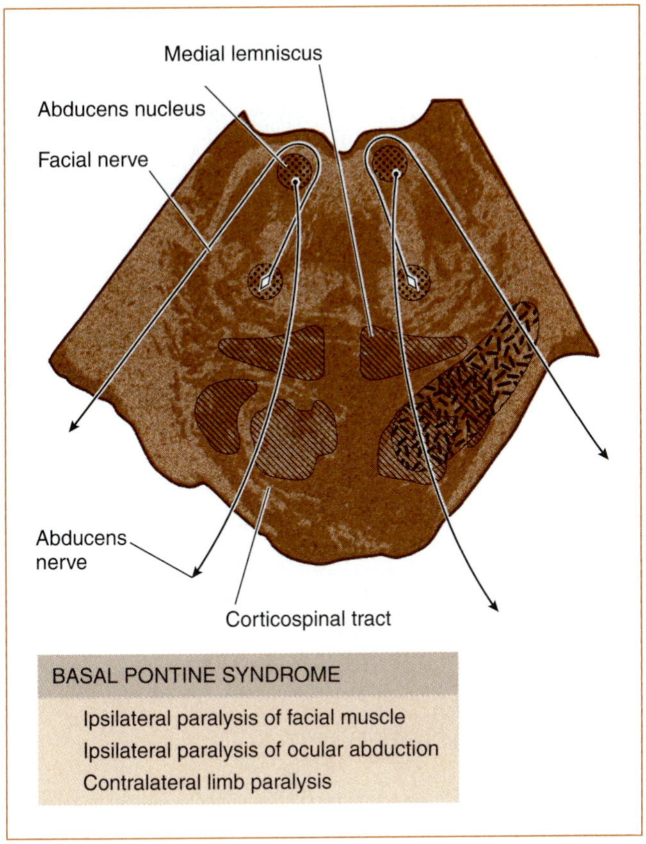
Medial lemniscus
Abducens nucleus
Facial nerve
Abducens nerve
Corticospinal tract
BASAL PONTINE SYNDROME
Ipsilateral paralysis of facial muscle
Ipsilateral paralysis of ocular abduction
Contralateral limb paralysis

FIGURE 8-2

Schematic diagram of the structures involved in medial and rostral extensions of the caudal basal pontine syndrome and the resulting clinical manifestations.

Pure Motor and Ataxic Hemiparesis

Discrete lesions in the basis pontis have been reported to result in pure motor hemiparesis or ataxic hemiparesis. Pure motor hemiparesis is secondary to involvement of corticospinal tract fascicles within the basis pontis. Atactic hemiparesis is due to involvement of corticospinal tract fascicles along with pontocerebellar fascicles in the basis pontis.

Dysarthria–Clumsy Hand Syndrome

Vascular lesions of the basis pontis at the junction of the upper third and lower two-thirds of the pons have been associated with the dysarthria–clumsy hand syn-

Dysarthria (Greek *dys*, "difficult"; *arthroun*, "to utter distinctly"). Imperfect articulation of speech caused by a disturbance of muscular control.

KEY CONCEPTS

- Pure motor hemiparesis and ataxic hemiparesis in discrete lesions in the basis pontis are due to involvement of corticospinal and pontocerebellar fibers, respectively.
- Lesions in the basis pontis at the junction of the rostral third with the caudal two-thirds of the pons are manifested by dysarthria, dysphagia, hand paresis, and clumsiness.

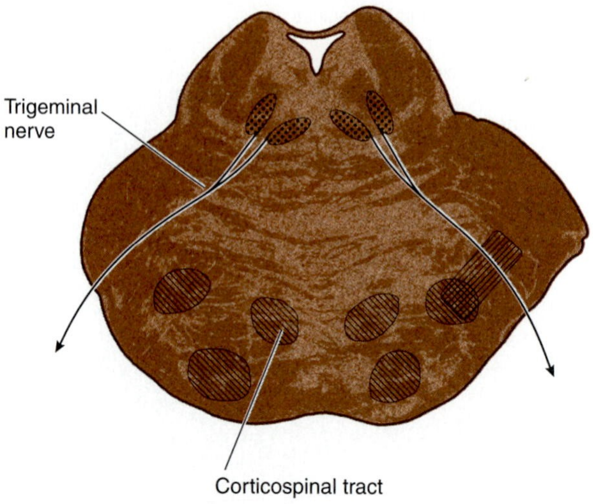

Basal pontine syndrome

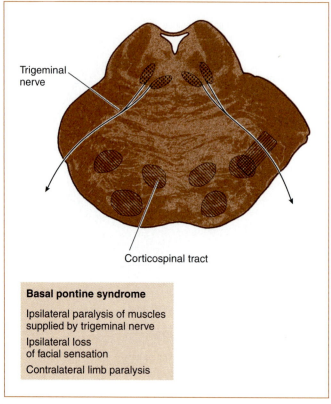

Ipsilateral paralysis of muscles supplied by trigeminal nerve

Ipsilateral loss of facial sensation

Contralateral limb paralysis

FIGURE 8-3

Schematic diagram showing structures involved in the rostral basal pontine syndrome and the resulting clinical manifestations.

drome. This syndrome is characterized by central (supranuclear) facial weakness, severe dysarthria and **dysphagia,** hand paresis, and clumsiness.

Dysphagia (Greek *dys*, "difficult"; *phagien*, "to eat"). Difficulty swallowing.

The Locked-in Syndrome

The locked-in syndrome is a severely disabling basal pontine syndrome which is due to an infarct in the ventral half of the pons. In this syndrome there is paralysis of all motor activity as a result of involvement of corticospinal tracts in the basis pontis and aphonia (loss of voice) caused by the involvement of corticobulbar fibers coursing in the basis pontis. Vertical gaze and blinking are spared and are the only means by which such patients communicate. Such patients have been described as "corpses with living eyes."

Crying and Laughter

Discrete unilateral or bilateral vascular lesions in the basis pontis have been associated with pathologic crying and, rarely, laughter. These episodes consist of a sudden

KEY CONCEPTS

- Lesions in the basis pontis may be manifested by generalized paralysis, loss of voice (aphonia), and maintenance of vertical gaze and blinking, by which such patients communicate (the locked-in syndrome).

onset of involuntary crying (rarely laughter) lasting about 15 to 30 s. Such emotional "incontinence" may herald a brain stem stroke, be part of it, or follow the onset of a stroke by a few days. The anatomic basis for pontine lesion–associated emotional incontinence has not been established. Most cases of pathologic crying or laughter are associated with bilateral frontal or parietal lesions with pseudobulbar palsy. Some investigators have postulated that lesions in the basis pontis interrupt an inhibitory corticobulbar pathway to the pontine tegmental center for laughing and crying, essentially releasing that center from cortical inhibition.

TEGMENTAL PONTINE SYNDROMES

Tegmental pontine syndromes are caused by lesions in the tegmentum of the pons that affect cranial nerve nuclei or rootlets and long tracts in the tegmentum.

The Medial Tegmental Syndrome

Structures affected in the medial tegmental syndrome include the nucleus and rootlets of the abducens nerve (cranial nerve VI), the genu of the facial nerve, and the medial lemniscus (Fig. 8-4). The manifestations of the lesion therefore include ipsilateral sixth nerve paralysis and a lateral gaze paralysis, ipsilateral facial paralysis of the peripheral variety, and contralateral loss of kinesthesia and discriminative touch.

The One and a Half Syndrome

The one and a half syndrome is characterized by ipsilateral lateral gaze paralysis resulting from involvement of the abducens nucleus and **internuclear ophthalmoplegia** (paralysis of adduction of the eye ipsilateral to the lesion and nystagmus of the abducting eye) as a result of involvement of the medial longitudinal fasciculus. The vascular lesion is discrete in the dorsal paramedian tegmentum.

Internuclear ophthalmoplegia (MLF syndrome). A condition characterized by paralysis of ocular adduction ipsilateral to a medial longitudinal fasciculus (MLF) lesion and monocular nystagmus in the contralateral abducting eye.

Dorsolateral Tegmental Pontine Syndrome

Vascular lesions in the dorsolateral pontine tegmentum that affect structures supplied by the anterior inferior cerebellar artery (AICA) on one side coupled with a vascular lesion in the dorsolateral medulla that affects structures supplied by the posterior inferior cerebellar artery (PICA) on the other side have been reported to produce dissociated sensory loss (loss of pain and temperature sense with preservation of vibration and position sense) enveloping the entire body, accompanied

KEY CONCEPTS

- Crying and laughter may be manifestations of vascular lesions in the basis pontis.
- The medial tegmental syndrome is manifested by ipsilateral abducens and facial nerve palsies and contralateral loss of kinesthesia and discriminative touch.
- The one and a half syndrome is manifested by ipsilateral horizontal gaze paralysis and internuclear ophthalmoplegia.
- The dorsolateral pontine tegmental syndrome is manifested by dissociated sensory loss (loss of pain and temperature sense with preservation of kinesthesia and discriminative touch) over the ipsilateral face and contralateral trunk and extremities.

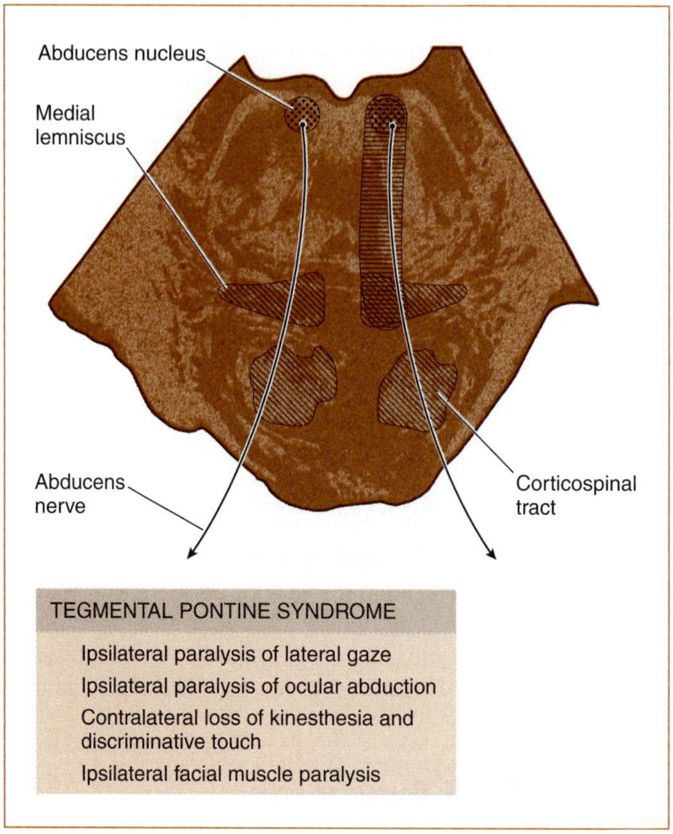

FIGURE 8-4

Schematic diagram showing structures involved in the tegmental pontine syndrome and the resulting clinical manifestations.

by truncal and limb ataxia without weakness. The dissociated sensory loss is due to simultaneous and bilateral involvement of the spinothalamic tracts and the trigeminal system with sparing of the lemniscal system. The **ataxia** is due to involvement of cerebellar-destined fibers coursing in the tegmentum or, alternatively, the cerebellum itself.

Ataxia (Greek *an*, "negative"; *taxis*, "order"). Without order, disorganized. Incoordination of movement seen in cerebellar disease. The term was used by Hippocrates and Galen for disordered action of any type, such as irregularity of pulse.

Foville's syndrome (Raymond-Foville syndrome). A syndrome of alternating hemiplegia caused by vascular lesions in the tegmentum of the caudal pons. Characterized by ipsilateral facial nerve palsy and conjugate gaze paralysis and contralateral hemiparesis. Described by Achille-Louis-François Foville in 1858.

Caudal Tegmental Pontine Syndrome (Foville's Syndrome, Raymond-Foville Syndrome)

Other tegmental pontine vascular syndromes include Foville's syndrome, which is characterized by an ipsilateral peripheral type of facial nerve palsy and conjugate gaze palsy and contralateral hemiparesis. The lesion usually is in the caudal pons and involves the corticospinal tract (contralateral hemiparesis), the paramedian pontine reticular formation (PPRF), and/or the abducens nucleus (conjugate gaze palsy) as well as the nucleus or fascicles of the facial nerve (facial muscle weakness).

KEY CONCEPTS

- Foville's syndrome is manifested by ipsilateral facial nerve palsy, ipsilateral conjugate gaze paralysis, and contralateral hemiparesis.

Rostral Tegmental Pontine Syndrome (Raymond-Cestan-Chenais Syndrome)

In the Raymond-Cestan-Chenais syndrome the lesion is in the rostral pons and involves the medial lemniscus, medial longitudinal fasciculus, spinothalamic tract, corticospinal tract, and cerebellar fibers. The manifestations are internuclear ophthalmoplegia (medial longitudinal fasciculus), ipsilateral ataxia (cerebellar fibers), and contralateral mild hemiparesis (corticospinal tract) and hemisensory loss (medial lemniscus and spinothalamic tract).

Extreme Lateral Tegmental Pontine Syndrome (Marie-Foix Syndrome)

In the Marie-Foix syndrome there is ipsilateral cerebellar ataxia and contralateral hemiparesis with or without hemisensory loss. The lesion in the rostral extreme lateral pons involves the brachium pontis (ataxia), the spinothalamic tract (hemisensory loss), and the corticospinal tract (hemiparesis). The full clinical picture of the Marie-Foix syndrome has rarely been reported and includes ipsilateral cranial nerve palsies, Horner's syndrome, hemiataxia, palatal myoclonus, and contralateral spinothalamic sensory loss.

Ocular Bobbing and Dipping

A variety of oscillatory eye movement abnormalities have been described in patients with pontine vascular lesions. These abnormalities have been referred to as ocular bobbing, inverse ocular bobbing, ocular dipping, and inverse ocular dipping on the basis of the predominant oscillatory abnormality.

REM Sleep

The pons is also necessary and sufficient to generate rapid eye movement (REM) sleep. In humans, bilateral pontine damage may prevent REM sleep.

Central Neurogenic Hyperventilation

Reports in humans suggest that medial tegmental pontine lesions, possibly affecting the PPRF bilaterally, are associated with the syndrome of central neurogenic hyperventilation. This syndrome is characterized by sustained **tachypnea** that persists despite an elevated arterial P_{O_2} and pH and a low arterial P_{CO_2}. It has been hypothesized that a pontine lesion of this type disinhibits inhibitory pontine influences on medullary respiratory neurons.

KEY CONCEPTS

- The Raymond-Cestan-Chenais syndrome is manifested by ipsilateral internuclear ophthalmoplegia, and ataxia and contralateral hemiparesis and hemisensory loss.
- The Marie-Foix syndrome is manifested by ipsilateral ataxia and contralateral hemiparesis with or without hemisensory loss.
- Ocular bobbing and ocular dipping are oscillatory eye movement abnormalities that occur in patients with pontine vascular lesions.
- Disturbances in rapid eye movement (REM) sleep, central neurogenic hyperventilation, and loss of voluntary and/or automatic respiration are associated with pontine lesions.

Raymond-Cestan-Chenais syndrome. A vascular syndrome of the rostral tegmentum of the pons characterized by internuclear ophthalmoplegia, ipsilateral ataxia, and contralateral mild hemiparesis and hemisensory loss. Described by Fulgence Raymond, Etienne Jacques-Marie-Raymond Cestan, and L. G. Chenais, French physicians, in 1903.

Marie-Foix syndrome. A vascular pontine syndrome characterized by ipsilateral cerebellar ataxia and contralateral hemiparesis with or without hemisensory loss. Described by Pierre Marie, a French neurologist, and his student Charles Foix in 1913.

Ocular bobbing. Saccadic repetitive fast movement of the eyes downward with a slow return to the primary position. Seen in patients with severe pontine dysfunction, who are usually unresponsive. Described by C. M. Fisher in 1964.

Ocular dipping (inverse ocular bobbing). Spontaneous eye movement in comatose patients with slow downward movement and a fast return to the primary position. The reverse of ocular bobbing. Seen in patients with disorders of the pons, basal ganglia, or cerebral cortex.

Tachypnea (Greek *tachys*, "swift"; *pnoia*, "breath"). Excessive rapidity of respiration.

The Pons and Respiration

Ondine's curse. A syndrome characterized by cessation of breathing in sleep because of failure of the medullary automatic center. Named after the story of Ondine, a water nymph who punished her unfaithful husband by depriving him of the ability to breathe while asleep.

Respiration is of two types: voluntary and automatic. Selective loss of voluntary respiration occurs in patients with lesions of the basis pontis. Selective loss of voluntary or automatic respiration also has been described as part of the locked-in syndrome.

Automatic respiratory pathways are presumed to be initiated in limbic cortex and involve diencephalic structures, the reticular system of the brain stem, the lateral or dorsal pons, the medullary nuclei mediating automatic respirations, and respiratory neurons of the spinal cord. Selective loss of automatic respiration occurs in patients with **Ondine's curse,** lesions of the medulla oblongata, or bilateral high cervical cord lesions.

SUGGESTED READINGS

Asfora WT, et al: Is the syndrome of pathological laughing and crying a manifestation of pseudobulbar palsy? *J Neurol Neurosurg Psychiatry* 1989; 52:523–525.

Ash PR, Keltner JL: Neuro-ophthalmic signs in pontine lesions. *Medicine (Baltimore)* 1979; 58:304–320.

Bassetti C, et al: Isolated infarcts of the pons. *Neurology* 1996; 46:165–175.

Brazis PW: The localization of lesions affecting the brainstem. In Brazis PW, et al (eds): *Localization in Clinical Neurology.* Boston, Little, Brown, 1985: 225–238.

Carter JE, Rauch RA: One-and-a-half syndrome, type II. *Arch Neurol* 1994; 51:87–89.

Deleu D, et al: Dissociated ipsilateral horizontal gaze palsy in one-and-a-half syndrome: A clinicopathologic study. *Neurology* 1988; 38:1278–1280.

Fisher CM: Ocular bobbing. *Arch Neurol* 1964; 11: 543–546.

Fisher CM: Some neuro-ophthalmologic observations. *J Neurol Neurosurg Psychiatry* 1967; 30:383–392.

Fisher CM: Ataxic hemiparesis: A pathologic study. *Arch Neurol* 1978; 35:126–128.

Goebel HH, et al: Lesions of the pontine tegmentum and conjugate gaze paralysis. *Arch Neurol* 1971; 24:431–440.

Jaeckle KA, et al: Central neurogenic hyperventilation: Pharmacologic intervention with morphine sulfate and correlative analysis of respiratory, sleep, and ocular motor dysfunction. *Neurology* 1990; 40:1715–1720.

Kushida CA, et al: Cortical asymmetry of REM sleep EEG following unilateral pontine hemorrhage. *Neurology* 1991; 41:598–601.

Matlis, A, et al: Radiologic-clinical correlation, Millard-Gubler syndrome. *AJNR* 1994; 15:179–181.

Munschauer FE, et al: Selective paralysis of voluntary but not limbically influenced automatic respiration. *Arch Neurol* 1991; 48:1190–1192.

Pryse-Phillips W: *Companion to Clinical Neurology.* Boston, Little, Brown, 1995.

Rothstein TL, Alvord EC: Posterior internuclear ophthalmoplegia: A clinicopathologic study. *Arch Neurol* 1971; 24:191–202.

Silverman IE, et al: The crossed paralyses. The original brain-stem syndromes of Millard-Gubler, Foville, Weber, and Raymond Cestan. *Arch Neurol* 1995; 52:635–638.

Stiller J, et al: Brainstem lesions with pure motor hemiparesis. Computed tomographic demonstration. *Arch Neurol* 1982; 39:660–661.

Tatemichi TK, et al. Pathological crying: A pontine pseudobulbar syndrome. *Ann Neurol* 1987; 22:133.

Troost BT: Signs and symptoms of stroke syndromes of the brain stem. In Hofferberth B, et al (eds): *Vascular Brain Stem Diseases.* Basel, Karger, 1990:112.

Venna N, Sabin TD: Universal dissociated anesthesia due to bilateral brain-stem infarcts. *Arch Neurol* 1985; 42:918–922.

Wall, M, Wray SH: The one-and-a-half syndrome: A unilateral disorder of the pontine tegmentum: A study of 20 cases and review of the literature. *Neurology* 1983; 33:971–980.

Yarnell PR: Pathological crying localization. *Ann Neurol* 1987; 22:133–134.

CHAPTER 9

MESENCEPHALON (MIDBRAIN)

GROSS TOPOGRAPHY

Ventral View

The inferior surface of the mesencephalon (midbrain) is marked by the divergence of two massive bundles of fibers—the cerebral peduncles—which carry corticofugal fibers to lower levels (Fig. 9-1). Caudally, the cerebral peduncles pass into the basis pontis; rostrally, they continue into the internal capsule. Between the cerebral peduncles lies the interpeduncular fossa, from which exit the **oculomotor nerve** (cranial nerve III). The trochlear nerve (cranial nerve IV) emerges from the dorsal aspect of the mesencephalon, curves around, and appears at the lateral borders of the cerebral peduncles. The optic tract passes under the cerebral peduncles before the peduncles disappear into the substance of the cerebral hemispheres.

Oculomotor nerve (Latin *oculus*, "eye"; *motor*, "mover"). The third cranial nerve affects movements of the eye.

Corpora quadrigemina (Latin *corpus*, "body"; *quadrigeminus*, "fourfold"). Four bodies in the dorsal aspect of the midbrain, consisting of two inferior colliculi and two superior colliculi.

Dorsal View

The dorsal surface of the mesencephalon features four elevations (**corpora quadrigemina**) (see Fig. 5-2). The rostral and larger two are the superior colliculi; the

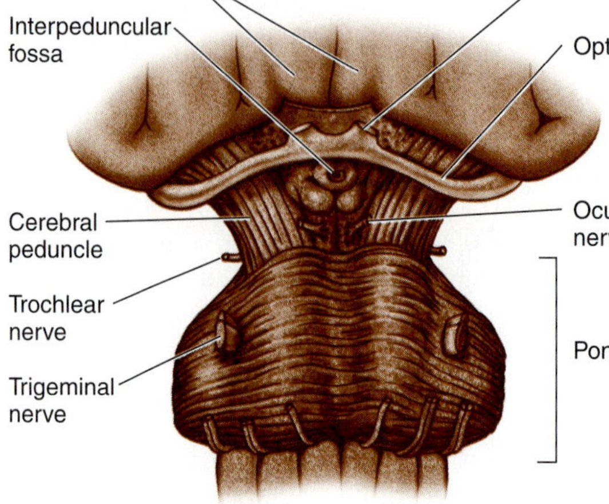

FIGURE 9-1

Schematic diagram of the ventral surface of the midbrain and pons showing major midbrain structures encountered on this surface.

Trochlear nerve (Latin *trochlearis*, "resembling a pulley"). The fourth cranial nerve supplies the superior oblique eye muscle, whose tendon angles through a ligamentous sling like a pulley. Achillini and Vesalius included this nerve with the third pair of nerves. It was described as a separate root by Fallopius and was named the trochlear nerve by William Molins, an English surgeon, in 1670.

Tectum ("rooflike structure"). A structure that forms the roof of the midbrain.

Tegmentum (Latin *tegmenta*, "covering"). A structure that covers the cerebral peduncles.

caudal and smaller two are the inferior colliculi. The **trochlear nerves** emerge just caudal to the inferior colliculi.

MICROSCOPIC STRUCTURE

General Organization

Three subdivisions are generally recognized in sections of the mesencephalon (Fig. 9-2).

1. The **tectum** is a mixture of gray and white matter that is dorsal to the central gray matter. It includes the superior and inferior colliculi (quadrigeminal plates). The term *quadrigeminal plate* was coined by Vesalius to refer to the tectum. Anatomists of that time wanted to name the superior and inferior colliculi after the Latin equivalents for the testes and buttocks. The overlying pineal gland, which looked like a pinecone to the Greeks, was mistaken for a penis. This was too explicit for Vesalius, who renamed the tectum the quadrigeminal plate.
2. The **tegmentum,** the main portion of the mesencephalon, lies inferior to the central gray matter and contains ascending and descending tracts, reticular nuclei, and well-delineated nuclear masses.

KEY CONCEPTS

- In cross sections the mesencephalon is divided into three regions: the tectum, the tegmentum, and the basal portion.
- The tectum consists of the quadrigeminal plates: two inferior and two superior colliculi.
- The tegmentum contains ascending and descending tracts, reticular nuclei, and well-delineated nuclear masses (cranial nerve nuclei and red nucleus).

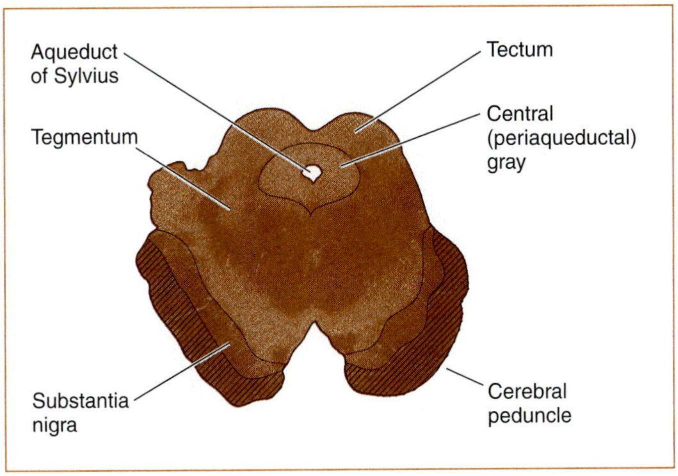

FIGURE 9-2

Cross-sectional diagram of the midbrain showing its major subdivisions.

3. The basal portion includes the cerebral peduncles, a massive bundle of corticofugal fibers on the ventral aspect of the mesencephalon, and the substantia nigra, a pigmented nuclear mass that lies between the dorsal surface of the cerebral peduncle and the tegmentum.

The components of these subdivisions are discussed below under two characteristic levels of the mesencephalon: the inferior colliculus and the superior colliculus. The inferior colliculus level is characterized in histologic sections by the decussation of the superior cerebellar peduncle and by the fourth nerve (trochlear) nucleus. The superior colliculus level is characterized by the red nucleus, the third nerve (oculomotor) nucleus, and the posterior commissure.

Inferior Colliculus Level

Colliculus (Latin, a "small elevation"). The inferior and superior colliculi are small elevations in the dorsal surface of the midbrain.

Tectum

The nucleus of the inferior colliculus occupies the tectum at the level of the inferior colliculus. This nucleus is an oval mass of small and medium-size neurons organized into three parts: (1) main laminated mass of neurons, called the central nucleus, (2) a thin dorsal cellular layer, the pericentral nucleus, and (3) a group of neurons that surround the central nucleus laterally and ventrally, the external nucleus. The central nucleus is the major relay nucleus in the auditory pathway. High-frequency sounds are represented in the ventral part, and low-frequency sounds in the dorsal part of the nucleus (similar to that in the cochlea). The pericentral nucleus receives only contralateral monaural input and serves to direct auditory attention. The external nucleus is related primarily to acousticomotor reflexes. The inferior colliculus has the following afferent and efferent connections.

KEY CONCEPTS

- The basal portion contains the substantia nigra and the cerebral peduncle.
- The inferior colliculus is a major subcortical auditory relay center.

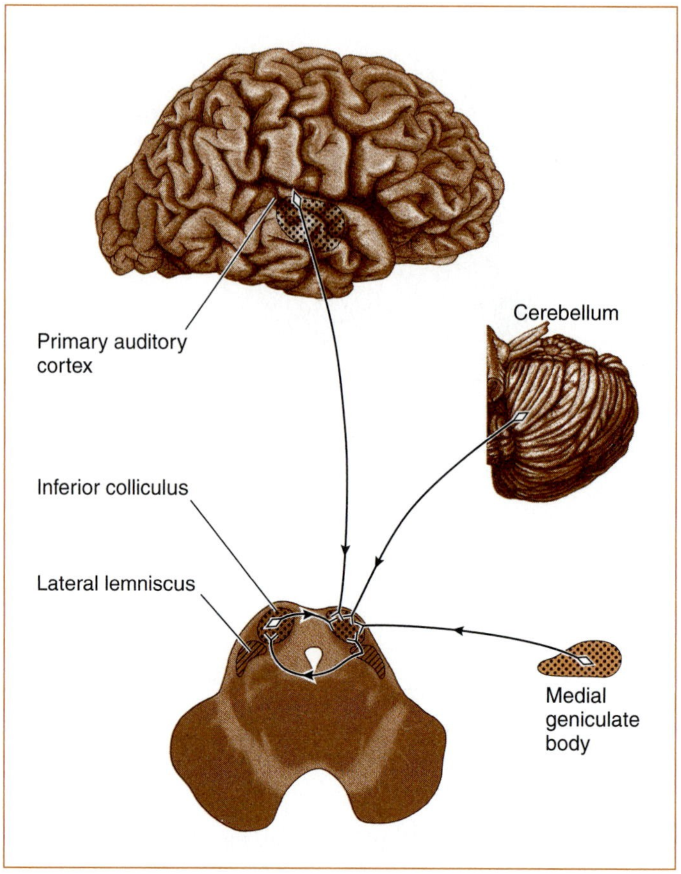

FIGURE 9-3

Schematic diagram showing the major afferent connections of the inferior colliculus.

Afferent Connections (Fig. 9-3) Fibers come from the following sources.

1. *Lateral lemniscus.* These fibers terminate on the ipsi- and contralateral inferior colliculi. Some lateral lemniscus fibers bypass the inferior colliculus to reach the medial geniculate body.
2. *Contralateral inferior colliculus.*
3. *Ipsilateral medial geniculate body.* This connection serves as a feedback mechanism in the auditory pathway.
4. *Cerebral cortex (primary auditory cortex).*
5. *Cerebellar cortex via the anterior medullary velum.*

Efferent Connections The inferior colliculus projects to the following areas (Fig. 9-4).

1. *Medial geniculate body via the brachium of the inferior colliculus.* This pathway is concerned with audition.
2. *Contralateral inferior colliculus.*

KEY CONCEPTS

- The inferior colliculus receives inputs from the lateral lemniscus, medial geniculate body, primary auditory cortex, and cerebellar cortex.

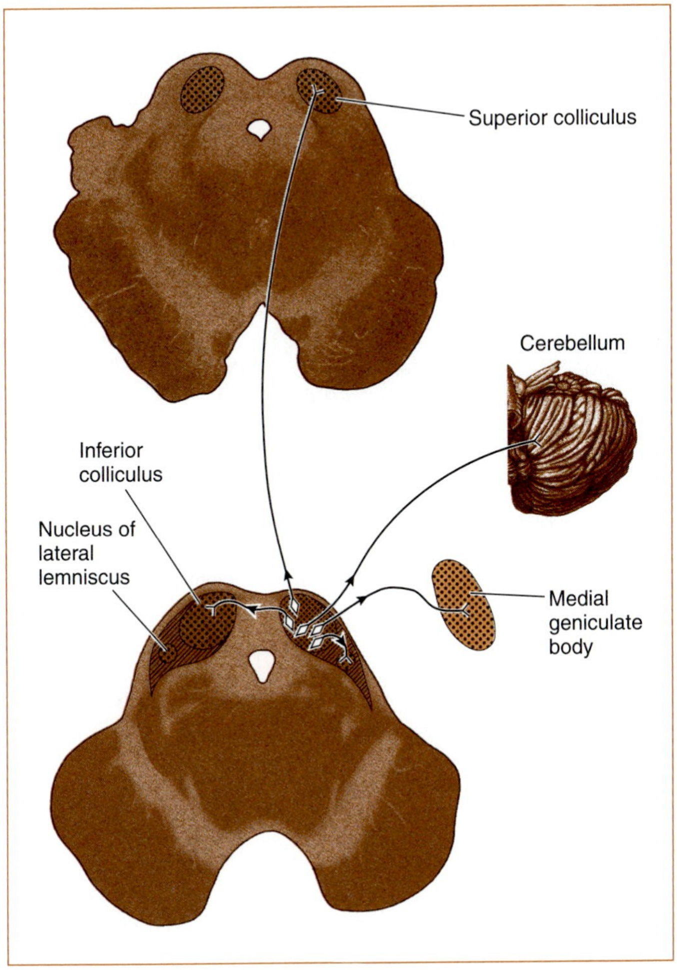

FIGURE 9-4

Schematic diagram showing the major efferent connections of the inferior colliculus.

3. *Superior colliculus.* This pathway establishes reflexes for turning the neck and eyes in response to sound.
4. *Nucleus of the lateral lemniscus and other relay nuclei of the auditory system for feedback.*
5. *Cerebellum.* The inferior colliculus is a major center for the transmission of auditory impulses to the cerebellum via the anterior medullary velum. The inferior colliculus thus is a relay nucleus in the auditory pathway to the cerebral cortex and cerebellum. In addition, the inferior colliculus plays a role in the localization of the source of sound.

Tegmentum

At the level of the inferior colliculus, the tegmentum of the mesencephalon contains fibers of passage (ascending and descending tracts) and nuclear groups.

KEY CONCEPTS

- The output of the inferior colliculus is to the medial geniculate body, nucleus of the lateral lemniscus, superior colliculus, and cerebellum.
- The two inferior colliculi are interconnected.

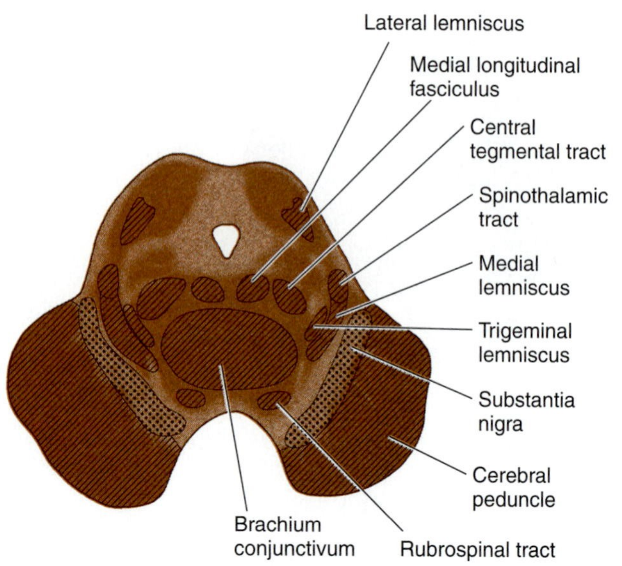

FIGURE 9-5

Schematic diagram of the midbrain at the inferior colliculus level, showing the major ascending and descending tracts.

Fibers of Passage The following fiber tracts pass through the mesencephalon (Fig. 9-5).

Brachium conjunctivum (Latin, Greek *brachion*, "arm"; *conjunctiva*, "connecting"). An armlike bundle of fibers that connects the cerebellum and midbrain.

Brachium conjunctivum (*superior cerebellar peduncle*) The **brachium conjunctivum** is a massive bundle of fibers arising in the deep cerebellar nuclei. These fibers decussate in the tegmentum of the midbrain at this level. A few proceed rostrally to terminate on the red nucleus; the others form the capsule of the red nucleus and continue rostrally to terminate on the ventrolateral nucleus of the thalamus.

Medial lemniscus The medial lemniscus lies lateral to the decussating brachium conjunctivum and above the substantia nigra. This fiber system, which conveys kinesthesia and discriminative touch from more caudal levels, continues its course toward the thalamus.

Trigeminal lemniscus The trigeminal lemniscus is composed of the ventral secondary trigeminal tracts and travels in close proximity to the medial lemniscus on its way to the thalamus.

Spinothalamic tract The spinothalamic tract conveys pain and temperature sensations from the contralateral half of the body and lies lateral to the medial lemniscus. Mingled with the spinothalamic fibers are the spinotectal fibers on their way to the tectum.

Lateral lemniscus The lateral lemniscus conveys auditory fibers and occupies a position lateral and dorsal to the spinothalamic tract.

Medial longitudinal fasciculus The medial longitudinal fasciculus maintains its position dorsally in the tegmentum in a paramedian position.

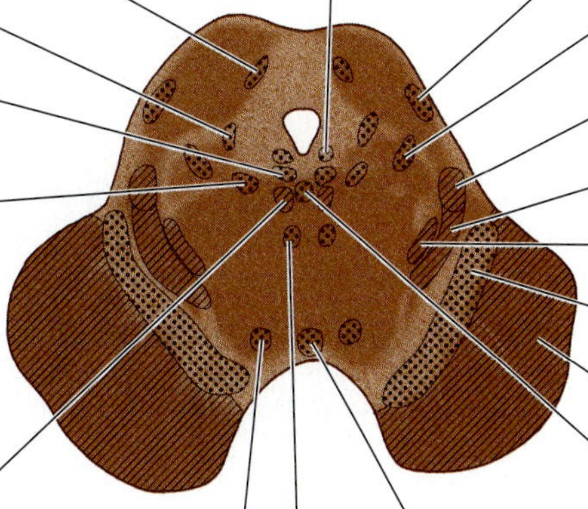

FIGURE 9-6

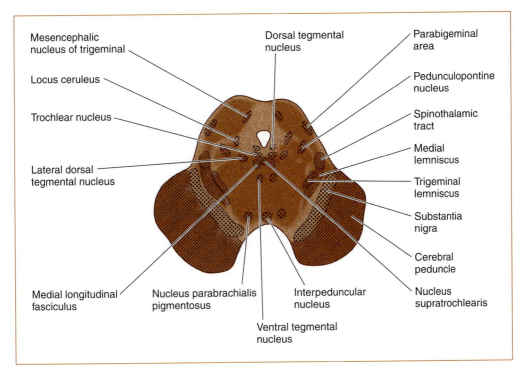

Schematic diagram of the midbrain at the inferior colliculus level showing major nuclear groups seen at this level.

Central tegmental tract The central tegmental tract conveys fibers from the basal ganglia and midbrain to the inferior olive and occupies a dorsal position in the tegmentum, ventrolateral to the medial longitudinal fasciculus.

Rubrospinal tract The rubrospinal tract conveys fibers from the red nucleus to the spinal cord and is located dorsal to the medial lemniscus.

Nuclear Groups

The following nuclei are seen at the level of the inferior colliculus (Fig. 9-6).

Mesencephalic Nucleus The mesencephalic nucleus of the trigeminal nerve is homologous in structure to the dorsal root ganglion but is uniquely placed within the central nervous system. It contains unipolar neurons with axons (the mesencephalic root of the trigeminal nerve) which convey proprioceptive impulses from the muscles of mastication and the periodontal membranes. As these fibers approach the nucleus, they gather in a bundle close to the nucleus: the mesencephalic tract.

KEY CONCEPTS

- At the level of the inferior colliculus the tegmentum contains the decussating fibers of the brachium conjunctivum, medial lemniscus, trigeminal lemniscus, spinothalamic tract, lateral lemniscus, medial longitudinal fasciculus, central tegmental tract, and rubrospinal tract.

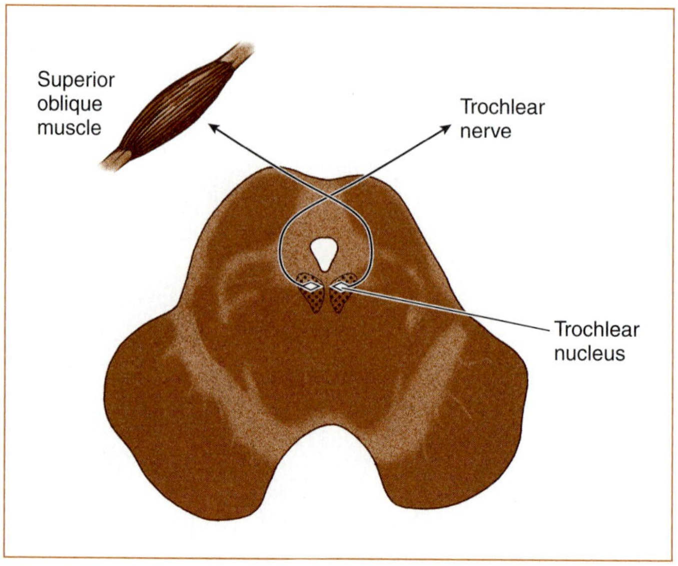

FIGURE 9-7

Schematic diagram of the midbrain showing origin, intraaxial course of the trochlear nerve, and the extraocular muscle supplied by the nerve.

Intorsion (Latin *in*, "toward"; *torsio*, "twisting"). Inward rotation of eye.
Diplopia (Greek *diploos*, "double"; *ops*, "eye"). Double vision.

Nucleus of the Trochlear Nerve (Cranial Nerve IV) The nucleus of the trochlear nerve lies in the V-shaped ventral part of the central gray matter. Axons of this nerve arch around the central gray matter, cross in the anterior medullary velum, and emerge from the dorsal aspect of the mesencephalon (Fig. 9-7). These axons supply the superior oblique eye muscle. The trochlear nerve is thus unique in two respects: It is the only cranial nerve that crosses before emerging from the brain stem, and it is the only cranial nerve that emerges on the dorsal aspect of the brain stem. Because of decussation, lesions of the trochlear nucleus result in paralysis of the contralateral superior oblique muscle, whereas lesions of this nerve after it emerges from the brain stem result in paralysis of the ipsilateral superior oblique muscle. The superior oblique muscle has three actions: primary of **intorsion,** secondary of depression, and tertiary of abduction. It thus acts by intorsion of the abducted eye and depression of the adducted eye. Patients with trochlear nerve lesions complain of vertical **diplopia** (double vision that is especially marked in looking contralaterally downward while descending stairs and usually is corrected by head tilt (toward the normal nerve) to compensate for the action of the paralyzed muscle. Tilting the head toward the paretic nerve increases double vision. The trochlear nucleus receives contralateral and probably some ipsilateral corticobulbar fibers and vestibular fibers from the medial longitudinal fasciculus, that are concerned with coordination of eye movements. Vestibular fibers to the trochlear nucleus

KEY CONCEPTS

- Nuclear groups in the tegmentum at the level of the inferior colliculus include the mesencephalic nucleus of the trigeminal, trochlear nucleus, interpeduncular nucleus, nucleus parabrachialis pigmentosus, dorsal tegmental nucleus, ventral tegmental nucleus, lateral dorsal tegmental nucleus, pedunculopontine nucleus, dorsal raphe nucleus, and locus ceruleus.
- Axons of trochlear neurons form the trochlear nerve, the smallest cranial nerve and the only one that decussates before exiting the neuraxis from the dorsal surface of the midbrain.

originate from the superior and medial vestibular nuclei. The fibers from the superior vestibular nucleus are ipsilateral and inhibitory; those from the medial vestibular nucleus are contralateral and excitatory.

Interpeduncular Nucleus The interpeduncular nucleus, which is indistinct in humans, is a poorly understood nuclear group in the base of the tegmentum between the cerebral peduncles. It receives fibers mainly from the **habenular** nuclei (in the diencephalon) through the habenulointerpeduncular tract and sends fibers to the dorsal tegmental nucleus through the pedunculotegmental tract.

Habenula (Latin *habena*, "small strap or bridle rein"). The habenular nuclei in the caudal diencephalon near the pineal gland form part of the epithalamus. Early anatomists considered the pineal gland the abode of the soul; it was likened to a driver who directs the operations of the mind via the habenula, or reins.

Nucleus Parabrachialis Pigmentosus The nucleus parabrachialis pigmentosus, which lies between the substantia nigra and the interpeduncular nucleus, is a ventral extension of the ventral tegmental area of Tsai.

Dorsal Tegmental Nucleus The dorsal tegmental nucleus lies dorsal to the medial longitudinal fasciculus (MLF) in the central gray matter in close proximity to the dorsal raphe nucleus. It is made up of conspicuously small cells. It receives fibers from the interpeduncular nucleus and projects on autonomic nuclei of the brain stem and the reticular formation.

Ventral Tegmental Nucleus The ventral tegmental nucleus lies ventral to the MLF in the midbrain tegmentum. Cells in this nucleus are rostral continuations of the superior central nucleus of the pons. This nucleus receives fibers from the mamillary bodies in the hypothalamus. The dorsal and ventral tegmental nuclei are part of a circuit concerned with emotion and behavior.

Pedunculopontine (Nucleus Tegmenti Pedunculopontis) and Lateral Dorsal Tegmental Nuclei These two cholinergic nuclei lie within the tegmentum of the caudal mesencephalon (inferior colliculus level) and rostral pons dorsolateral to and overlapping the lateral margin of the rostral superior cerebellar peduncle, between that peduncle and the lateral lemniscus. Neurons of the pedunculopontine nucleus are affected in patients with progressive supranuclear palsy, a degenerative central nervous system disease. The pedunculopontine nucleus receives inputs from the cerebral cortex, the medial pallidal segment, and the pars reticulata of the substantia nigra. It projects to the thalamus and the pars compacta of the substantia nigra. This nucleus lies in a region from which walking movements can be elicited on stimulation (locomotor center).

Nucleus Supratrochlearis (Dorsal Raphe Nucleus) The nucleus supratrochlearis lies in the ventral part of the periaqueductal (central) gray matter between the two trochlear nuclei. It is equivalent in humans to the B-7 cell group in primates. It sends serotonergic fibers to the substantia nigra, neostriatum (caudate and putamen), and neocortex.

Parabigeminal Area The parabigeminal area is an oval collection of cholinergic neurons ventrolateral to the nucleus of the inferior colliculus and lateral to the lateral lemniscus. It receives fibers from superficial layers of the superior colliculus and projects bilaterally back into superficial layers of the superior colliculus. Cells in this area play a role, along with the superior colliculus, in processing visual information. They respond to visual stimuli and are activated by both moving and stationary visual stimuli.

Nucleus Pigmentosus (Locus Ceruleus) The nucleus pigmentosus is seen in the rostral pons and caudal mesencephalon. It contains 30,000 to 35,000 neurons and corresponds to the A-6 cell group of primates. At the level of the inferior colliculus it is situated at the edge of the central gray matter, between the mesencephalic

Locus ceruleus (Latin, "place, dark blue"). The pigmented noradrenergic nucleus in the rostral pons is dark blue in sections.

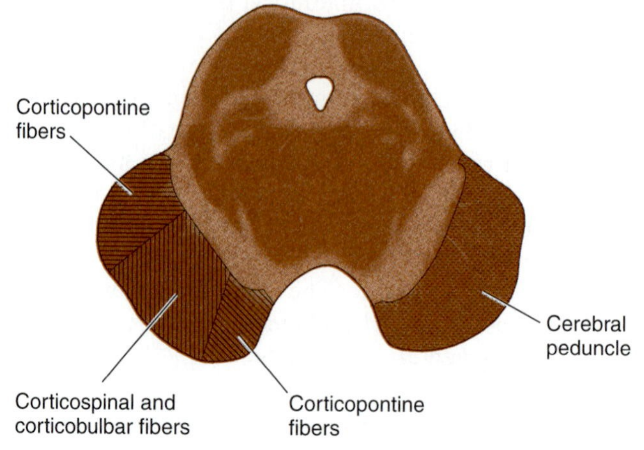

FIGURE 9-8

Schematic diagram of the midbrain showing the major subdivisions of the cerebral peduncle.

nucleus of the trigeminal and the dorsal tegmental nucleus. It is made up of four subnuclei: central (largest); anterior (rostral end); ventral (caudal and ventral), also known as the nucleus subceruleus; and posterior dorsal (small). Its pigmented cells contain melanin granules which are lost in patients with Parkinson's disease. The neurons of the locus ceruleus provide noradrenergic innervation to most central nervous system regions. Axons of the neurons in the locus ceruleus are elaborately branched and ramify practically throughout the brain. These axons reach their destinations via three major ascending tracts: the central tegmental tract, the dorsal longitudinal fasciculus, and the medial forebrain bundle. Through these tracts, the locus ceruleus innervates the thalamus, hypothalamus, and basal telencephalon. In addition, the locus ceruleus projects to the cerebellum (via the brachium conjunctivum), to the spinal cord and to sensory nuclei of the brain stem. This nucleus is believed to play a role in the regulation of respiration as well as in the rapid eye movement (REM) stage of sleep.

Basal Portion

At the level of the inferior colliculus, the basal portion of the mesencephalon includes the cerebral peduncles and the substantia nigra.

Cerebral Peduncle The cerebral peduncle (Fig. 9-8) is a massive fiber bundle that occupies the most ventral part of the mesencephalon. It is continuous with the internal capsule rostrally and merges caudally into the basis pontis. This massive fiber bundle carries corticofungal fibers from the cerebral cortex to several subcorti-

KEY CONCEPTS

- Nuclear groups in the tegmentum at the level of the inferior colliculus include the mesencephalic nucleus of the trigeminal, trochlear nucleus, interpeduncular nucleus, nucleus parabrachialis pigmentosus, dorsal tegmental nucleus, ventral tegmental nucleus, lateral dorsal tegmental nucleus, pedunculopontine nucleus, dorsal raphe nucleus, and locus ceruleus.

cal centers. The middle three-fifths of the cerebral peduncle is occupied by the corticospinal tract, which is continuous caudally with the pyramids. Fibers destined to the arm are medially located, those to the leg are laterally placed, and trunk fibers lie in between. The corticopontine fibers occupy the areas of the cerebral peduncle on each side of the corticospinal tract. The medially located corticopontine fibers constitute the frontopontine projection; the laterally located fibers constitute the parieto-occipito-temporo-pontine projections. Corticopontine fibers originate in wide areas of the cerebral cortex, synapse on pontine nuclei, and enter the contralateral cerebellar hemisphere via the middle cerebellar peduncle (brachium pontis). The corticobulbar fibers destined for cranial nerve nuclei occupy a dorsomedial position among the corticospinal fibers. According to some studies, the cerebral peduncle in humans has two groups of corticobulbar tracts. Those in the medial portion of the peduncle descend to the pontine neurons responsible for gaze; those in the lateral portion descend to the motor nuclei of cranial nerves V, VII, and XII and the nucleus ambiguus.

Substantia Nigra The substantia nigra is a pigmented mass of neurons sandwiched between the cerebral peduncles and the tegmentum. It is composed of two zones: a dorsal zona compacta containing melanin pigment and a ventral zona reticulata containing iron compounds. It has been observed that the dendrites of neurons in the zona compacta arborize in the zona reticulata. The pars lateralis represents the oldest part of this nucleus. The neuronal population of the substantia nigra consists of pigmented and nonpigmented neurons. Pigmented neurons outnumber nonpigmented neurons two to one. The neurotransmitter in pigmented neurons is dopamine. Nonpigmented neurons are either cholinergic or GABAergic. There is a characteristic pattern of neuronal loss in the substantia nigra in different disease states (Table 9-1). Both pigmented and nonpigmented neurons are lost in patients with Huntington's chorea. Only pigmented (dopaminergic) neurons, especially those in the center of the substantia nigra, are lost in idiopathic **Parkinson's disease.** In the postencephalitic type of Parkinson's disease, pigmented (dopaminergic) neurons are lost uniformly. In the Parkinson's disease–dementia complex, there is a uniform loss of both pigmented and nonpigmented neurons. Finally, in multiple system atrophy, pigmented neurons are lost in medial and lateral nigral zones. Nigral neurons (variable number) show abnormal (reduced) immunostaining for complex I of the mitochondrial electron transport system in patients with Parkinson's disease. This reduction is believed to be related to the pathogenesis of the disease. The neural connectivity of the substantia nigra suggests an important role in the regulation of motor activity. Lesions of the substantia nigra are almost always seen in Parkinson's disease, which is characterized by tremor, rigidity, and slowness of motor activity. The known afferent and efferent connections of the substantia nigra are outlined below.

Parkinson's disease. A chronic progressive degenerative disease characterized by tremor, rigidity, and akinesia. It was initially described in 1817 by the English physician James Parkinson under the rubric *shaking palsy.*

KEY CONCEPTS

- In the cerebral peduncle, corticospinal fibers occupy the middle three-fifths, flanked on each side by corticopontine fibers.
- Corticobulbar fibers in the cerebral peduncle lie in a dorsomedial position among corticospinal fibers.
- The substantia nigra is divided into a pars compacta, a pars reticulata, and a pars lateralis.
- Pigmented neurons in the pars compacta of the substantia nigra are lost in Parkinson's disease patients.

TABLE 9-1

Substantia Nigra: Pattern of Cell Loss in Disease

Type of Cell	Huntington's Disease	Idiopathic Parkinson's Disease	Postencephalitic Parkinson's Disease	Parkinson's Dementia Complex	Multiple System Atrophy
Pigmented neurons	x	x	x	x	x
Nonpigmented neurons	x			x	
Distribution					
Uniform loss			x	x	
Central loss		x			
Medial					x
Lateral					x

Afferent connections (Fig. 9-9)

Neostriatum The neostriatal input to the substantia nigra is the largest and projects primarily to the pars reticulata with a smaller input to the pars compacta. It arises from the associative region of the neostriatum primarily from the caudate nucleus. The neurotransmitter is gamma-aminobutyric acid (GABA). The matrix region is the source of input to the pars reticulata, whereas the striosomal region projects to the pars compacta and the adjacent ventral tegmental area. The striatonigral fibers are topographically organized so that the head of the caudate nucleus projects to the rostral third of the substantia nigra while the putamen projects to all the other parts of the nigra.

Cerebral cortex The corticonigral projection is not as massive as was previously believed. Most of these fibers are fibers of passage, and relatively few of them terminate on nigral neurons.

Globus pallidus The input to the substantia nigra from the globus pallidus arises from the external (lateral) segment. It is composed of GABAergic fibers that terminate mainly on the pars reticulata neurons of the substantia nigra, with some in the pars compacta of the substantia nigra.

Subthalamic nucleus The subthalamic nucleus projects in a patchy manner to pars reticulata of the substantia nigra. The transmitter here is glutamine.

Tegmentonigral tracts The tegmentonigral tracts arise from the midbrain raphe nuclei, which have serotonin and cholecystokinin, and from the pedunculopontine nucleus, which is cholinergic.

Efferent connections (Fig. 9-9)

Nigrostriate fibers Nigrostriate fibers from the pars compacta of the substantia nigra project to the neostriatum (caudate and putamen) and are dopaminergic. The nigrostriate projection is somatotopically organized so that neurons in the lateral part of the pars compacta of the substantia nigra project to the putamen, whereas the caudate nucleus receives its nigral input mainly from the medial part.

KEY CONCEPTS

- The substantia nigra receives inputs from the neostriatum, cerebral cortex, globus pallidus, subthalamic nucleus, and midbrain reticular formation.

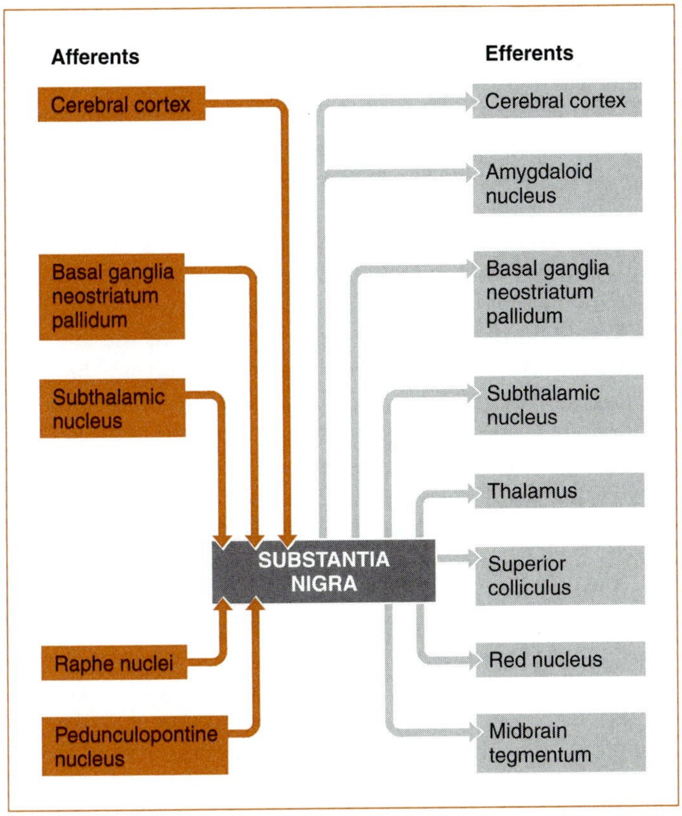

FIGURE 9-9

Schematic diagram showing the major afferent and efferent connections of the substantia nigra.

The nigrostriate projections terminate on the associative sensorimotor and limbic striatum. The sites of origin of the projections to the caudate and putamen are segregated in the pars compacta. Cells in the pars compacta of the substantia nigra project to the caudate nucleus or the putamen but not to both. Dopaminergic nigral projections to the neostriatum terminate on distal dendrites of medium spiny (projection) neurons. They facilitate neostriatal neurons that project to the pars reticulata of the substantia nigra and the internal (medial) segment of the globus pallidus and inhibit neostriatal neurons that project to the external (lateral) segment of the globus pallidus.

Nigrocortical tract The nigrocortical fibers originate in the medial zona compacta and the adjacent ventral tegmental area, course through the medial forebrain bundle, and terminate in the limbic cortex. The involvement of this pathway in parkinsonism may explain the **akinesia** seen in that disease. Another projection from the substantia nigra and the ventral tegmental area terminates in the neocortex. The function of this projection is not known but may be related to cognition.

Akinesia (Greek *a*, "negative"; *kinesis*, "motion"). Poverty or absence of movement.

Nigropallidal tract Nigropallidal projections are more abundant in the associative pallidal territory compared with the sensorimotor territory.

Nigrorubral tract A projection to the red nucleus from the substantia nigra has been described in experimental animals.

Nigrosubthalamic tract The connections between the substantia nigra and subthalamic nucleus are reciprocal.

Nigrothalamic tract The nigrothalamic GABAergic tract runs from the pars reticulata to the ventral anterior, ventral lateral, and dorsomedial nuclei of the thalamus.

Nigrotegmental tract and nigrocollicular tract The nigrotegmental and nigrocollicular tracts originate from separate regions of the pars reticularis of the substantia nigra. They are both GABAergic. The nigrotegmental tract links the substantia nigra with the reticular formation and with the spinal cord via the reticulospinal projection. The nigrocollicular tract links the substantia nigra with the superior colliculus and secondarily with the control of ocular movement as well as with the spinal cord (tectospinal tract). Through its connections with the basal ganglia and the superior colliculus and reticular formation, the substantia nigra acts as a link through which the basal ganglia exert an effect on spinal and ocular movements.

Nigroamygdaloid tract The nigromygdaloid tract originates from dopaminergic neurons in the zona compacta and the pars lateralis of the substantia nigra and projects on the lateral and central amygdaloid nuclei.

The nigral origin of many of these efferent fiber systems requires further exploration. The GABAergic outputs from the pars reticulata of the substantia nigra to the thalamus, superior colliculus, and reticular formation are believed to play a role in suppressing the progression of epileptic discharge. A marked increase in metabolic activity in the substantia nigra has been reported to occur during epileptic discharge. Nigrothalamic, nigrotectal, and nigrotegmental pathways originate from separate regions in the pars reticulata.

Mesencephalic dopaminergic cell groups Besides the pars compacta of the substantia nigra, two other cell groups in the mesencephalic tegmentum are dopaminergic: the ventral tegmental area of Tsai in close proximity to the medial substantia nigra and the retrorubral cell group (substantia nigra, pars dorsalis) in close proximity to the red nucleus. The pars compacta of the substantia nigra in humans corresponds to area A-9 of primates, the ventral tegmental area corresponds to area A-10, and the retrorubral nucleus corresponds to area A-8. The dopaminergic neurons of the ventral tegmental area of Tasi project to the ventral striatum (nucleus accumbens, olfactory tubercle), the limbic forebrain, and the prefrontal cortex and usually are spared in Parkinson's disease. The retrorubral cell group projects selectively on the matrix zones of the neostriatum (caudate and putamen). This cell group is moderately affected in Parkinson's disease. The pars compacta of the substantia nigra, by contrast, projects to both matrix and striosome zones of the neostriatum (caudate and putamen) and is severely affected in Parkinson's disease.

Recent studies in primates and humans have identified three subdivisions of the mesencephalic dopaminergic system on the basis of their projection sites. One subdivision is related to the striatum (mesostriatal subdivision) and terminates on the caudate nucleus, putamen, globus pallidus, and nucleus accumbens. The second subdivision is related to the allocortex (mesoallocortical subdivision) and terminates on the amygdala, olfactory tubercle, septal area, and piriform cortex. The third subdivision is related to the neocortex (mesoneocortical) and terminates in all neocortical areas (frontal, temporal, parietal, and occipital cortices). Recently, a dopaminergic projection to the cerebellar cortex from the ventral tegmental area of Tsai was described, possibly as part of the hypothalamo-tegmental-cerebellar hypothalamic loop.

The term *mesostriatal* is used to describe the first subdivision in preference to the term *nigrostriatal system*, since evidence suggests that both the ventral tegmental

KEY CONCEPTS

- The output of the substantia nigra is to the neostriatum, limbic cortex, globus pallidus, red nucleus, subthalamic nucleus, thalamus, superior colliculus, midbrain reticular formation, and amygdala.
- Mesencephalic dopaminergic cell groups include the substantia nigra, the ventral tegmental area of Tsai, and the retrorubral cell group.
- On the basis of its projection sites, the mesencephalic dopaminergic system is subdivided into mesostriatal, mesoallocortical, and mesoneocortical subdivisions.

TABLE 9-2

Disorders of the Mesencephalic Dopaminergic System

Subdivision	Hypoactivity	Hyperactivity
Mesostriatal	Parkinson's disease	Huntington's chorea
Mesoallocortical	Cognitive impairment (Parkinson's disease)	Psychotic disorders
Mesoneocortical	?Cognitive impairment (Parkinson's disease) Photosensitive epilepsy (visual cortex)	Undetermined

area and the substantia nigra contribute to this projection. A reduction in dopaminergic neurotransmission in this system is associated with parkinsonism. Hyperactivity of this system has been implicated in **Huntington's chorea.** Hyperactivity in the mesoallocortical subdivision is believed to play a role in the symptomatology of psychotic disorders, whereas a reduction in function may contribute to the cognitive abnormalities found in patients with Parkinson's disease.

Very little is known about the functional role of the mesoneocortical system. Some researchers have suggested a role in human cognition. A decrease in dopamine in this system may explain cognitive impairments in patients with Parkinson's disease. A decrease in dopamine in the visual cortex has been implicated in photosensitive epilepsy (Table 9-2).

Two types of response mode have been demonstrated in mesencephalic dopamine neurons: (1) a phasic mode response to reward and reward-predicting stimuli that have to be processed by the subject with high priority and (2) a tonic mode response involved in maintaining states of behavioral alertness. Thus, the dopamine system is involved in both the setting and the maintenance of levels of alertness through the phasic and tonic mode responses.

Huntington's chorea (Greek *choreia*, "dance"). A progressive neurodegenerative disorder inherited as an autosomal dominant trait. The disease was imported to America from Suffolk in the United Kingdom by the emigrant wife of an Englishman in 1630. Her father was choreic, and the groom's father disapproved of the match because of the bride's father's illness. The disorder is named after George Sumner Huntington, a general practitioner who described it in 1872. Characterized by the ceaseless occurrence of a wide variety of rapid, complex, jerky movements performed involuntarily and resembling a dance.

Superior Colliculus Level

Tectum

The nucleus of the superior colliculus occupies the tectum at the level of the superior colliculus. The superior colliculus is a laminated mass of gray matter that plays a role in visual reflexes and control of eye movement. The laminated appearance results from alternating strata of white and gray matter. Superficial layers of the superior colliculus contain cells aligned in an orderly fashion with well-defined visual receptive fields and apparently represent a map of visual space. In contrast, the deep layers contain cells whose activity is related to the goal points of saccadic eye movements. It thus appears that a sensory map of the visual space in the

KEY CONCEPTS

- The mesencephalic dopaminergic system is involved in the setting and maintenance of levels of alertness.
- The superior colliculus plays a role in visual reflexes and control of eye movements.

superficial layers is transformed in the deeper layers into a motor map on which a vector from an initial eye position to a goal eye position is represented. The vector is then translated into command signals for saccade generators such as the paramedian pontine reticular formation (PPRF).

Afferent connections to the superior colliculus (Fig. 9-10) come from the following sources.

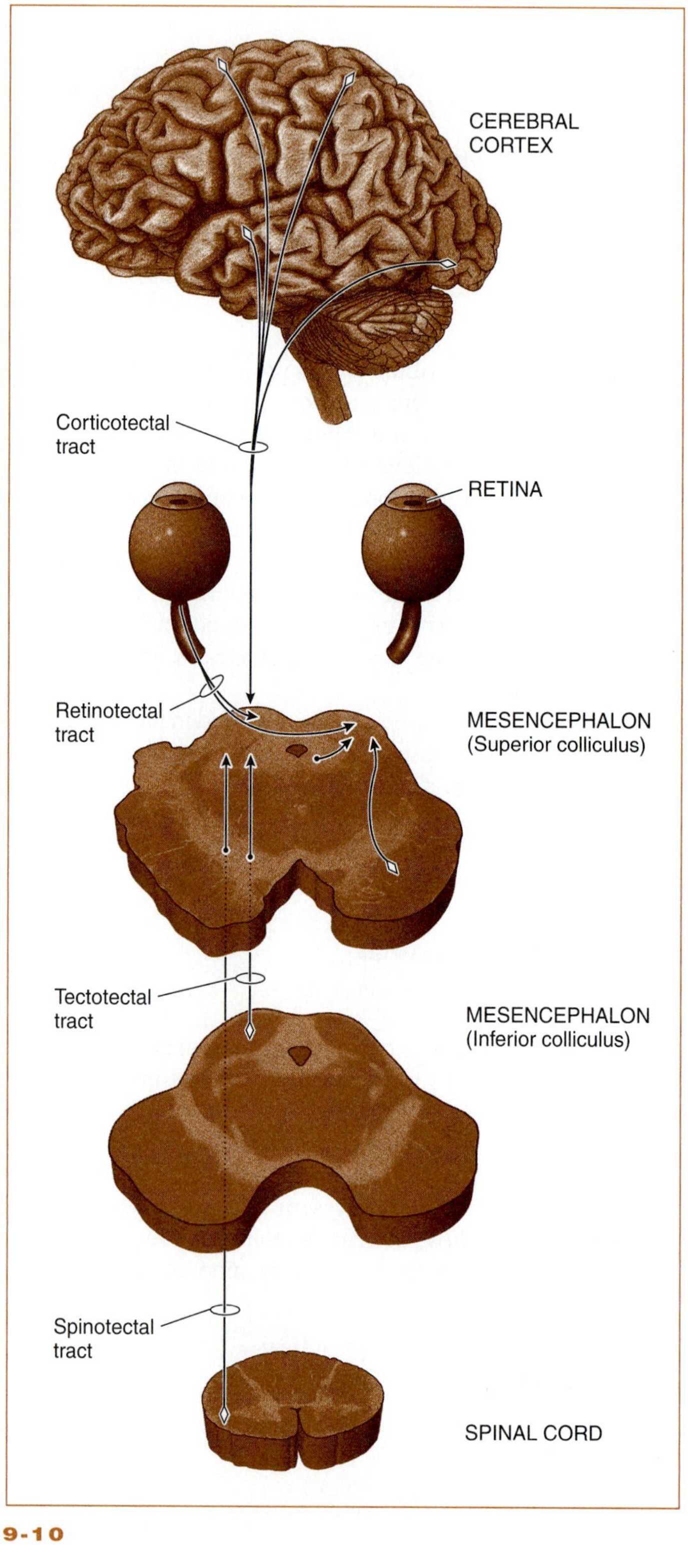
CEREBRAL
CORTEX
Corticotectal
tract
RETINA
Retinotectal
tract
MESENCEPHALON
(Superior colliculus)
Tectotectal
tract
MESENCEPHALON
(Inferior colliculus)
Spinotectal
tract
SPINAL CORD

FIGURE 9-10

Schematic diagram showing the major afferent connections of the superior colliculus.

Cerebral Cortex Corticocollicular fibers arise from all over the cerebral cortex, but most abundantly from the occipital (visual) cortex. Fibers originating from the frontal lobe are concerned with conjugate eye movements and reach the superior colliculus by a transtegmental route. Occipitotectal fibers are concerned with reflex scanning eye movements in pursuit of a passing object and reach the colliculus via the brachium of the superior colliculus. Corticotectal fibers are ipsilateral. Occipitotectal and frontotectal fibers terminate in the superficial and middle layers of the superior colliculus. Temporotectal fibers (from the auditory cortex), in contrast, project into deep collicular layers.

Retina Retinal fibers project on the same layer of the superior colliculus as do those of the cerebral cortex. In contrast to cortical fibers, fibers from the retina are bilateral, with a preponderance of contralateral input. Retinal fibers reach the superior colliculus by way of the brachium of the superior colliculus; they leave the optic tract proximal to the lateral geniculate body. Retinotectal fibers arise from homonymous portions of the retina of each eye, but crossed fibers are the most numerous. The contralateral homonymous halves of the visual field are thus represented in each superior colliculus. The retinotectal fibers are retinotopically organized so that upper retinal quadrants of the contralateral visual fields are in the medial parts of the superior colliculus and lower retinal quadrants are in the lateral parts of the colliculus. Peripheral visual fields are represented in the caudal superior colliculus, and central visual fields are rostrally placed in the colliculus.

Spinal Cord Spinotectal fibers ascend in the anterolateral part of the cord (with the spinothalamic tract) to reach the superior colliculus. They belong to a multisynaptic system that conveys pain sensation.

Inferior Colliculus The input from the inferior colliculus and a number of other auditory relay nuclei is part of a reflex arc which turns the neck and eyes toward the source of a sound.

Other inputs to the superior colliculus have been reported to arise from the midbrain tegmentum, central (periaqueductal) gray matter, substantia nigra (pars reticulata), and spinal trigeminal nucleus.

Efferent connections (Fig. 9-11) leave the superior colliculus via the following tracts.

Tectospinal Tract From their neurons of origin in the superior colliculus, fibers of the tectospinal tract system cross in the dorsal tegmental decussation in the midbrain tegmentum and descend as part of or in close proximity to the medial longitudinal fasciculus to reach the cervical spinal cord and terminate on Rexed's laminae VII and VIII. They are concerned with reflex neck movement in response to visual stimuli.

Tectopontocerebellar Tract The tectopontocerebellar tract descends to the ipsilateral pontine nuclei, which also receive fibers from visual and auditory cortex. This tract is believed to convey visual impulses from the superior colliculus to the cerebellum via the pontine nuclei.

Tectoreticular Tract The tectoreticular tract projects profusely and bilaterally on reticular nuclei in the midbrain as well as on the accessory oculomotor nuclei.

KEY CONCEPTS

- The superior colliculus receives inputs from the cerebral cortex, retina, spinal cord, and inferior colliculus.

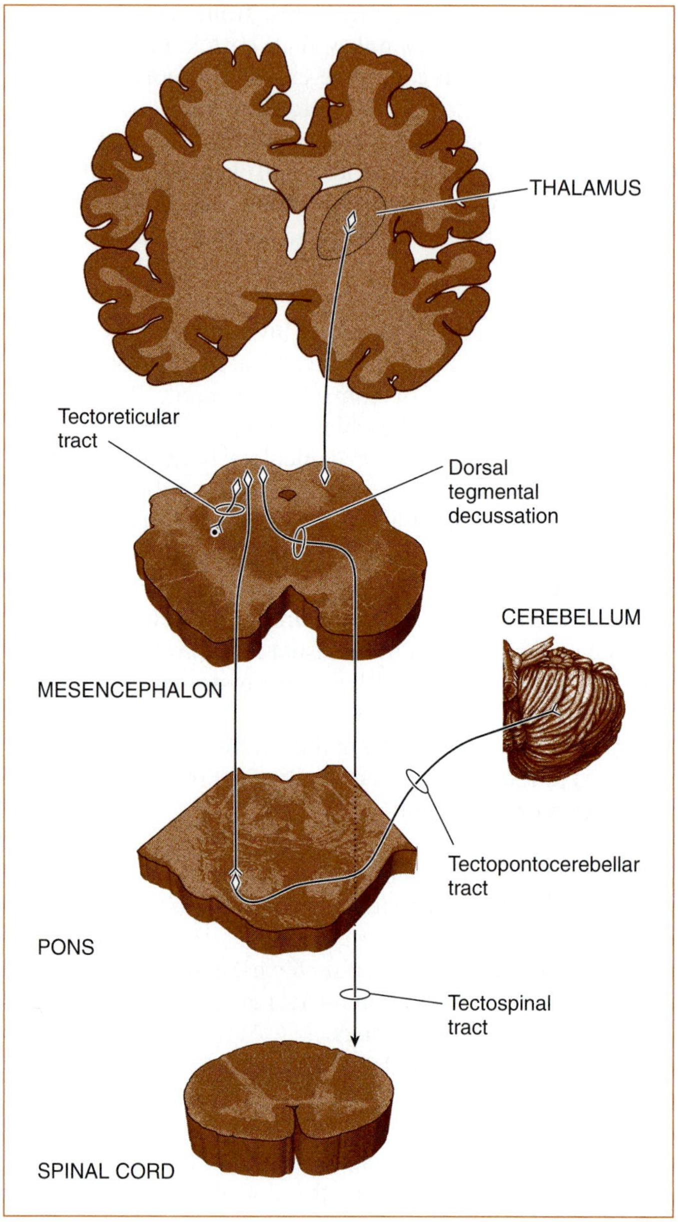

FIGURE 9-11

Schematic diagram showing the major efferent connections of the superior colliculus.

Tectothalamic Tract The tectothalamic tract projects to the lateral posterior nucleus of the thalamus, the lateral geniculate, and the pulvinar. The pulvinar receives extensive projections from superficial layers of the superior colliculus and relays them to extrastriate cortical areas 18 and 19. Input to the lateral geniculate nucleus arises from superficial layers of the superior colliculus and is relayed to the striate cortex.

As with the afferent connections of the superior colliculus, the efferent connec-

KEY CONCEPTS

- The output of the superior colliculus is to the spinal cord, pontine nuclei, reticular formation of the midbrain, and thalamus.

tions originate from different laminae of the superior colliculus. In general, the ascending tectothalamic projections originate from superficial laminae, whereas the descending tectospinal, tectopontine, and tectoreticular projections originate in deeper laminae.

Unilateral lesions of the superior colliculus in animals have been associated with the following functional deficits: relative neglect of visual stimuli in the contralateral visual field, heightened responses to stimuli in the ipsilateral visual field, and deficits in perception involving spatial discrimination and the tracking of moving objects.

Stimulation of the superior colliculus results in contralateral conjugate deviation of the eyes. Since there are no demonstrable direct connections of the superior colliculus to the nuclei of extraocular movement, this effect may be mediated via connections to the rostral interstitial nucleus of the medial longitudinal fasciculus (RiMLF) and the PPRF.

Most collicular neurons respond only to moving stimuli, and most also show directional selectivity.

Pretectal Area Rostral to the superior colliculus at the mesencephalic-diencephalic junction is the pretectal area (pretectal nucleus). This area is an important station in the reflex pathway for the pupillary light reflex. It receives fibers from the retinas and projects fibers bilaterally to both oculomotor nuclei. Several nuclei in the pretectal region have been identified, including the nucleus of the optic tract, along the dorsolateral border of the pretectum at its junction with the pulvinar, and the pretectal olivary nucleus, which is seen best at the level of the caudal posterior commissure.

Experiments in which the pretectal area and/or the posterior commissure were ablated suggest strongly that these structures are essential for vertical gaze. This may explain the paralysis of vertical gaze in patients with pineal tumors, which compress these structures. In humans, a group of signs and symptoms resulting from a lesion in the pretectal area are referred to as the pretectal syndrome. Synonyms include the sylvian aqueduct syndrome, the dorsal midbrain syndrome, **Koerber-Salus-Elschnig syndrome,** the pineal syndrome, and **Parinaud's syndrome.** The conglomerate signs and symptoms that constitute this syndrome include vertical gaze palsies, pupillary abnormalities (**anisocoria,** light-near dissociation), conversion retraction nystagmus, lid retraction (**Collier's sign**), impaired convergence, skewed eye deviation in the neutral position, papilledema, and lid flutter. This syndrome has been reported in a variety of clinical states, including brain tumors (pineal, thalamic, midbrain, third ventricle), hydrocephalus, stroke, infection, trauma, and tentorial herniation.

Tegmentum

At the level of the superior colliculus, the tegmentum contains fibers of passage and nuclear groups.

Fibers of Passage The fibers of passage include all the fiber tracts encountered at the level of the inferior colliculus except the lateral lemniscus, which terminates

KEY CONCEPTS

- The pretectal area is located at the mesencephalic-diencephalic junction.
- The pretectal area is involved in the pupillary light reflex and vertical gaze.
- The tegmentum at the level of the superior colliculus includes all fiber tracts encountered at the level of the inferior colliculus except the lateral lemniscus, which terminates in the inferior colliculus.

Koerber-Salus-Elschnig syndrome. A syndrome of vertical gaze palsy, anisocoria, light-near dissociation, conversion retraction nystagmus, lid retraction, impaired convergence, skewed eye deviation, papilledema, and lid flutter associated most commonly with pineal tumors or disorders of the pretectal region. Also known as Parinaud's syndrome, the pretectal syndrome, the sylvian aqueduct syndrome, and the syndrome of the posterior commissure.

Parinaud's syndrome. Paralysis of upward gaze associated with pretectal lesions. Described by Henri Parinaud, a French neuro-ophthalmologist, in 1883.

Anisocoria (Greek *anisos,* "unequal, uneven"; *kore,* "pupil"). Inequality in the diameters of the pupils.

Collier's sign. Bilateral lid retraction seen in the pretectal syndrome.

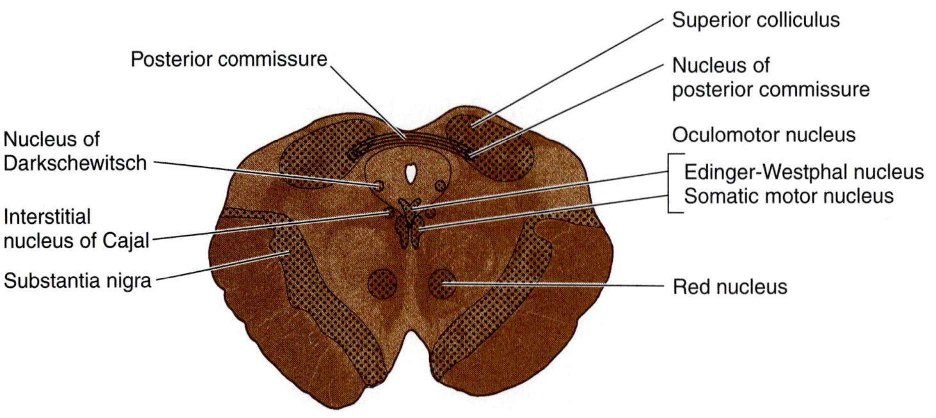

FIGURE 9-12

Schematic diagram of the midbrain at the superior colliculus level, showing its major nuclear groups.

on inferior colliculus neurons and is not seen at superior colliculus levels. The brachium conjunctivum fibers, which decussate at inferior colliculus levels, terminate in the red nucleus at this level or form the capsule of the red nucleus on their way to the thalamus. The other tracts discussed under "Inferior Colliculus Level" above maintain approximately the same positions at this level.

Nuclear Groups The nuclear groups include the red nucleus, the oculomotor nucleus, and accessory oculomotor nuclei (Fig. 9-12).

Red nucleus The red nucleus, so named because in fresh preparations its rich vascularity gives it a pinkish hue, is a prominent feature of the tegmentum at this level. It is composed of a rostral, phylogenetically recent small cell part (**parvicellular**) and a caudal, phylogenetically older large cell part (magnicellular). The rostral part is well developed in humans. The nucleus is traversed by the following fiber systems: (1) the superior cerebellar peduncle (brachium conjunctivum), (2) the oculomotor nerve (cranial nerve III) rootlets, and (3) the habenulointerpeduncular tract. Of the three systems, only the brachium conjunctivum projects on this nucleus; the other two are related to the red nucleus only by proximity. The red nucleus has the following afferent and efferent connections.

Afferent connections that are most documented come from two sources (Fig. 9-13).

Deep cerebellar nuclei The cerebellorubral fibers arise from the **dentate, globose,** and **emboliform nuclei** of the cerebellum. They travel via the brachium conjunctivum, decussate in the tegmentum of the inferior colliculus, and project

Parvicellular nucleus (Latin *parvus*, "small"; *cellula*, "cell"). The parvicellular nucleus is composed of small cells.

Dentate nucleus (Latin *dentatus*, "toothlike"). A nucleus in the cerebellum that is serrated like a tooth.

Globose (Latin *globus*, "a ball, sphere-shaped"). The globose nucleus in the cerebellum is spherical in shape.

Emboliform (Greek *embolos*, "plug"). The emboliform nucleus in the cerebellum "plugs" the dentate nucleus.

KEY CONCEPTS

- Nuclear groups encountered in the tegmentum at the level of the superior colliculus include the red nucleus, oculomotor, and accessory oculomotor nuclei.
- The red nucleus is traversed by the brachium conjunctivum, oculomotor nerve rootlets, and habenulointerpeduncular tract.
- Input to the red nucleus comes mainly from the deep cerebellar nuclei and the cerebral cortex.

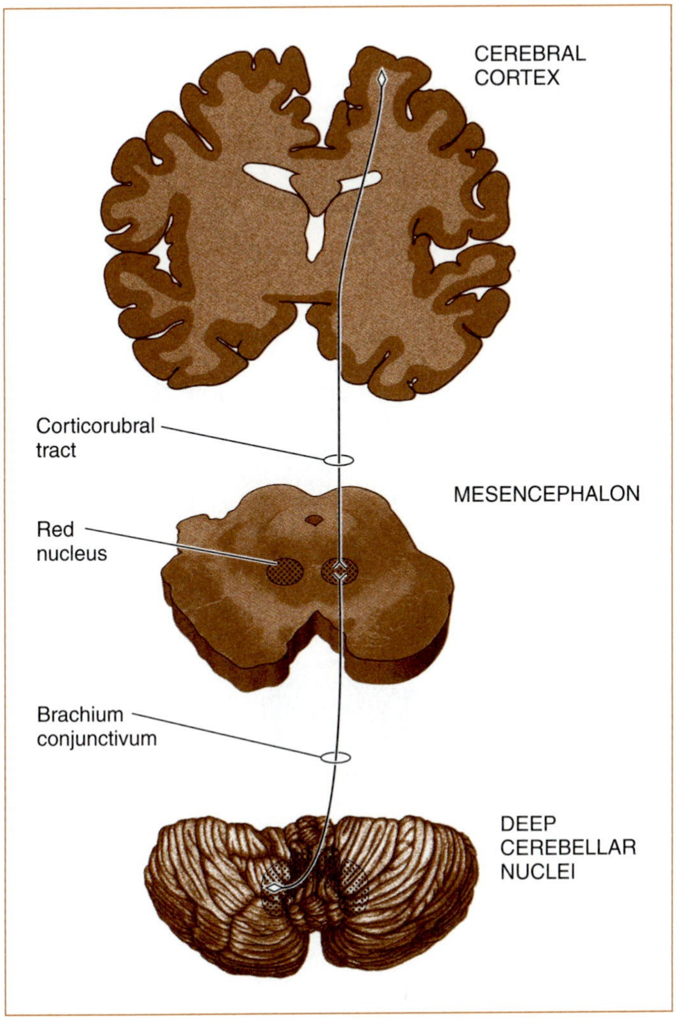

FIGURE 9-13

Schematic diagram showing the major afferent connections of the red nucleus.

partly to the contralateral red nucleus. Fibers from the dentate nucleus terminate on the rostral (parvicellular) part of the red nucleus, while fibers from the globose and emboliform nuclei project on the caudal part (magnicellular) of the nucleus, which projects to the spinal cord. Interruption of the cerebellorubral fiber system results in a volitional type of tremor that is manifested when the extremity is in motion (e.g., attempting to reach for an object). Electron microscopic studies have shown that the cerebellorubral input establishes mainly axosomatic synapses in the red nucleus. The triangular area bounded by the red nucleus, the inferior olive (in the medulla oblongata), and the dentate nucleus of the cerebellum is known as Mollaret's triangle. Lesions that interrupt connectivity among these three structures result in spontaneous rhythmic movement of the palate (palatal myoclonus).

Cerebral cortex Corticorubral fibers arise mainly from the motor and premotor cortices and project mainly to the ipsilateral red nucleus. This projection is somatotopically organized. Projections from the medial part of area 6 (supplementary motor area MII) are crossed and end in the magnicellular region of the nucleus. Projections from the precentral (motor) cortex are ipsilateral to the magnicellular part of the nucleus and correspond to the somatotopic origin of the rubrospinal

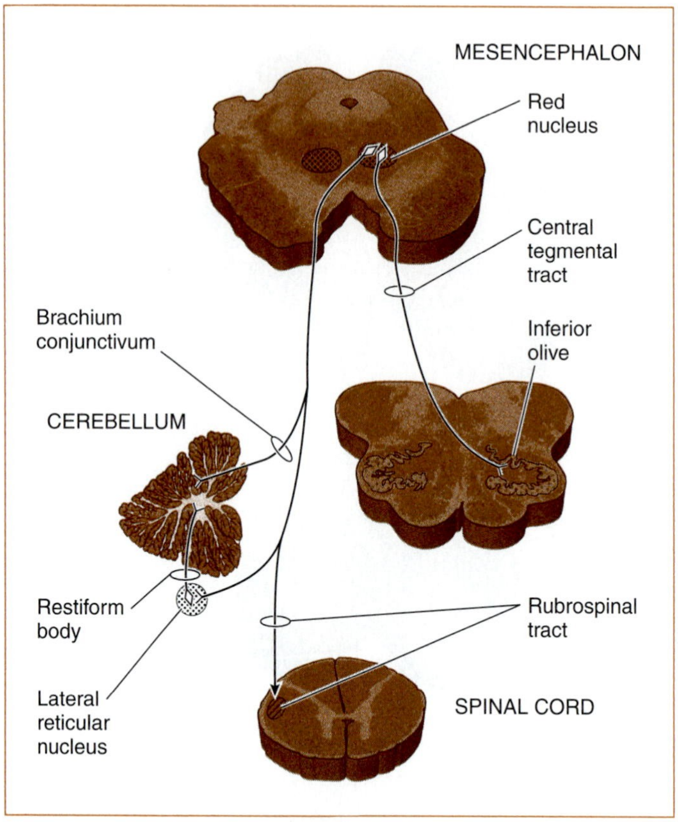

FIGURE 9-14

Schematic diagram showing the major efferent connections of the red nucleus.

fibers. The corticorubral and rubrospinal tracts are considered an indirect corticospinal fiber system. The corticorubral input to the red nucleus establishes primarily axodendritic synapses. Deafferentation experiments have shown that after cerebellar ablation the cerebral input to the red nucleus establishes axosomatic synapses to replace the deafferented cerebellar input.

The two afferent connections mentioned above are the best established. Other possible afferent tracts include tectorubral from the superior colliculus and the pallidorubral from the globus pallidus.

Efferent connections project to the following areas (Fig. 9-14).

Spinal cord Rubrospinal fibers arise from the caudal part (magnicellular) of the nucleus, cross in the ventral tegmental decussation, and descend to the spinal cord. They project on the same spinal cord laminae as does the corticospinal tract. Like the corticospinal tract, the rubrospinal tract facilitates flexor motor neurons and inhibits extensor motor neurons. Because of their common termination and the fact that the red nucleus receives cortical input, the rubrospinal tract has been considered an indirect corticospinal tract. In most mammals, the red nucleus sends its major output to the spinal cord and clearly subserves a motor function. The projection to the spinal cord has diminished with evolution, and in humans the red nucleus sends its major output to the inferior olive. In turn, the inferior olive is connected to the cerebellum.

Cerebellum In most mammals the rubrocerebellar fibers are collaterals from the rubrospinal tract. In the upper pons some rubrospinal fibers leave the descending tract and accompany the superior cerebellar peduncle to the cerebellum. In the cerebellum these fibers terminate on cells of the interposed nuclei (emboliform and globose).

Reticular formation Rubroreticular fibers are also offshoots from the rubrospinal tract. They separate from the descending tract in the medulla oblongata and terminate in the ipsilateral lateral reticular nucleus. The lateral reticular nucleus, which is described in Chap. 5, in turn projects to the cerebellum. Thus, a feedback circuit is established between the cerebellum, the red nucleus, the lateral reticular nucleus, and back to the cerebellum.

Inferior olive The rubro-olivary tract is a fiber system which arises in the rostral small cell part (parvicellular) of the nucleus and projects to the ipsilateral inferior olive via the central tegmental tract. The inferior olive in turn projects to the cerebellum, thus establishing another feedback circuit between the cerebellum, the red nucleus, the inferior olive, and back to the cerebellum. The rubro-olivary tract in humans is more important than is the rubrospinal tract.

Other projections Recently described efferent projections include fibers to Darkschewitsch's nucleus, the Edinger-Westphal nucleus, the mesencephalic reticular formation, the tectum, the pretectum, principal sensory and spinal trigeminal nuclei, and the facial motor nucleus.

Thus, the red nucleus is a synaptic station in neural systems concerned with movement, linking the cerebral cortex, cerebellum, and spinal cord.

Lesions of the red nucleus result in contralateral tremor.

Oculomotor nucleus The oculomotor nucleus lies dorsal to the MLF at the level of the superior colliculus. It is composed of a lateral somatic motor cell column and a medial visceral cell column. It is approximately 10 mm in length. This nucleus receives fibers from the following sources.

Cerebral cortex Corticoreticulobulbar fibers are bilateral but come mainly from the contralateral hemisphere.

Mesencephalon Mesencephalic projections to the oculomotor nucleus originate from Cajal's interstitial nucleus, the RiMLF, and the pretectal olivary nucleus. Fibers from Cajal's interstitial nucleus course in the posterior commissure and project mainly on the contralateral oculomotor nucleus. Interruption of these fibers results in paralysis of upward gaze. The RiMLF is just rostral to Cajal's interstitial nucleus. The projection from the RiMLF to the oculomotor nucleus is mainly ipsilateral. Lesions of the RiMLF lead to paralysis of downard gaze. Physiologic studies have shown that neurons in Cajal's interstitial nucleus and the RiMLF are active just before vertical eye movements. Cajal's interstitial nucleus and the RiMLF project fibers to the somatic motor cell column of the oculomotor nucleus, whereas the pretectal area projects mainly to the Edinger-Westphal nucleus of the visceral cell column. The pretectal area receives fibers from both retinas and projects to both oculomotor nuclei. This connection plays a role in the pupillary light reflex.

KEY CONCEPTS

- The output of the red nucleus is mainly to the spinal cord, cerebellum, reticular formation, and inferior olive.
- In humans, the major descending output of the red nucleus is to the inferior olive.
- Lesions of the red nucleus result in contralateral tremor.
- The oculomotor nucleus contains somatic motor neurons [that supply the levator palpebrae muscle and all the muscles of extraocular movement except the lateral rectus (supplied by abducens nerve) and the superior oblique (supplied by trochlear nerve)] and autonomic neurons of the Edinger-Westphal nucleus (which supplies the constrictor pupillae muscle), and Perlia's nucleus (which probably is concerned with accommodation).

Pons and medulla Pontine and medullary projections to the oculomotor nucleus arise from the vestibular nuclei, the nucleus prepositus, and the abducens nucleus. The vestibular projections originate in the superior and medial vestibular nuclei. Projections from the medial vestibular nuclei via the MLF are bilateral, while those from the superior vestibular nucleus, via the MLF, are ipsilateral. Other fibers from the superior vestibular nucleus that are not contained in the MLF cross in the caudal midbrain and project to the superior rectus and the inferior oblique subnuclei of the oculomotor complex. The projection from the abducens nucleus arises from interneurons, is crossed, and reaches the oculomotor nucleus via the MLF along with vestibular fibers. The connection between the abducens and oculomotor nuclei provides the anatomic substrate for the coordination between the lateral rectus and medial rectus muscles in conjugate horizontal gaze. The nucleus prepositus projects ipsilaterally to the oculomotor complex and may be involved in vertical eye movement.

Cerebellum Cerebello-oculomotor fibers to the somatic motor cell column arise from the contralateral dentate nucleus and are concerned with the regulation of eye movements. In addition, the cerebellum exerts an influence on autonomic neurons of the oculomotor nucleus. Short-latency (direct) as well as long-latency (indirect) responses have been elicited in the Edinger-Westphal nucleus after stimulation of the interposed and **fastigial cerebellar nuclei.** This connection is believed to course in the brachium conjunctivum and plays a role in pupillary constriction and accommodation. The short-latency connection is facilitatory, whereas the long-latency connection is inhibitory.

Nucleus fastigii (Latin *fastigium*, "pointed, roof"). The roof nucleus. Located in the pointed roof of the fourth ventricle.

The somatic motor cell column is organized into subgroups for each of the eye muscles supplied by the oculomotor nerve. From the most rostral extension of the oculomotor nucleus to its middle third are the Edinger-Westphal nuclei and the inferior rectus subnuclei. Inferior rectus subnuclei extend rostrally like a peninsula and are the only subnuclei seen in the most rostral part of the nucleus. A discrete lesion of the oculomotor nucleus at its most rostral level may result in an isolated inferior rectus paresis with or without pupillary abnormalities.

The inferior oblique subnuclei are the most laterally placed subnuclei in the middle and caudal thirds of the nuclear complex. Superior rectus subnuclei are medially located in the middle and caudal thirds of the nucleus and are the only subnuclei in the third nuclear complex that supply contralateral eye muscles (superior rectus muscle). All other subnuclei supply corresponding ipsilateral eye muscles. The superior rectus subnucleus is adjacent to and caudal to the inferior rectus subnucleus. A lesion slightly caudal to a lesion that produces an isolated inferior rectus palsy can affect the inferior and superior rectus subnuclei, producing an ipsilateral inferior rectus and contralateral superior rectus paresis. The medial rectus subnuclei are located primarily in the ventral oculomotor nuclear complex in close

KEY CONCEPTS

- Inputs to the oculomotor nucleus are from the cerebral cortex, accessory oculomotor nuclei, vestibular nuclei, abducens nucleus, nucleus prepositus (parahypoglossal nuclei), and dentate nucleus.
- Somatic motor neurons of the oculomotor nucleus are organized into subnuclei that correspond to the eye muscles supplied by the oculomotor nerve. All these subnuclei supply ipsilateral muscles except the superior rectus subnucleus, which supplies the contralateral superior rectus muscle, and the levator palpebrae subnucleus, which supplies both levator palpebrae muscles.

proximity to the MLF. The levator palpebrae subnucleus is a single central nucleus in the caudal third of the nucleus. Axons from the neurons of this single nucleus divide into right and left bundles to supply the two levator palpebrae muscles. Discrete lesions in individual subnuclei of the oculomotor nuclear complex have been reported (using magnetic resonance imaging) with isolated unilateral inferior rectus paresis, bilateral inferior rectus paresis and unilateral superior rectus weakness, and isolated unilateral inferior rectus and contralateral superior rectus weakness.

Axons of neurons in the somatic motor column course through the tegmentum of the midbrain, pass near or through the red nucleus, and emerge from the interpeduncular fossa medial to the cerebral peduncle. In their course in the midbrain tegmentum, oculomotor nerve fascicles are organized so that fascicles to the inferior oblique are most laterally placed, followed from lateral to medial by superior rectus, medial rectus, inferior rectus, and pupillary fascicles. The levator palpebrae fascicles lie dorsally close to those of the medial rectus. Discrete lesions involving one or more of these fascicles may result in partial oculomotor nerve paresis.

The oculomotor nerve leaves the brain stem between the superior cerebellar artery and the posterior cerebral artery. Once it leaves the brain stem, this nerve courses anteriorly in the subarachnoid space until it pierces the dura covering the roof of the cavernous sinus. In the anterior part of the cavernous sinus, the oculomotor nerve divides into superior and inferior divisions. The superior division innervates the levator palpebrae superioris and superior rectus muscles. The inferior division innervates the inferior rectus, medial rectus, and inferior oblique muscles and the iris sphincter. The inferior oblique muscle lowers the eye when one is looking medially, and the superior and inferior rectus muscles elevate and lower the eye, respectively, when one is looking laterally. The medial rectus **adducts** the eye. The levator palpebrae elevates the lid.

The visceral cell column includes the **Edinger-Westphal nucleus** and **Perlia's nucleus.** The Edinger-Westphal nucleus is concerned with the light reflex. Perlia's nucleus is probably concerned with accommodation but has not been identified in humans.

The axons of neurons in the visceral cell column accompany those of the somatic motor column as far as the orbit. In the orbit they part company, and the visceral axons project to the ciliary ganglion. Postganglionic fibers from the ciliary ganglion innervate the sphincter pupillae and ciliaris muscles. Lesions in this component of the oculomotor nerve result in a dilated pupil that is unresponsive to light or accommodation.

Lesions of the oculomotor nerve outside the brain stem (Fig. 9-15*A*) result in (1) paralysis of the muscles supplied by the nerve, manifested by drooping of the ipsilateral eyelid (**ptosis**) and deviation of the ipsilateral eye downward and outward by the action of the intact lateral rectus and superior oblique muscles (supplied by the abducens and trochlear nerves, respectively), (2) double vision (diplopia), and (3) paralysis of the sphincter pupillae and ciliaris muscles, manifested by an ipsilateral dilated pupil that is unresponsive to light and accommodation.

KEY CONCEPTS

- Discrete lesions in the oculomotor nucleus or in the rootlets within the midbrain may result in selective paralysis of individual extraocular muscles.
- Lesions of the oculomotor nerve outside the neuraxis result in ptosis, deviation of the eye down and out, and a dilated pupil that is nonresponsive to light stimulation, all ipsilateral to the nerve lesion (oculomotor nerve palsy).

Adduction (Latin *adducere*, "to draw toward"). The process of drawing toward the median plane.

Edinger-Westphal nucleus. The parasympathetic component of the oculomotor nuclear complex. Described by Ludwig Edinger, a German anatomist and neurologist, in 1885 and by Carl Friedreich Otto Westphal, a German psychiatrist, neurologist, and anatomist, 2 years later.

Perlia's nucleus. A component of the autonomic oculomotor nuclear complex related to ocular conversion. Described by Richard Perlia, a German ophthalmologist, in 1899.

Ptosis (Greek *ptosis*, "fall"). Drooping of the upper lid from oculomotor nerve palsy (levator palpebrae muscle paralysis) or sympathetic nerve palsy (tarsal plate paralysis) as in Horner's syndrome.

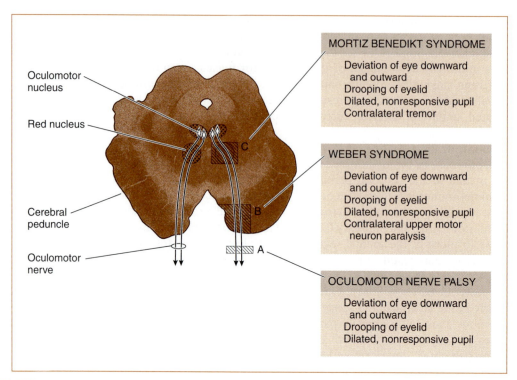

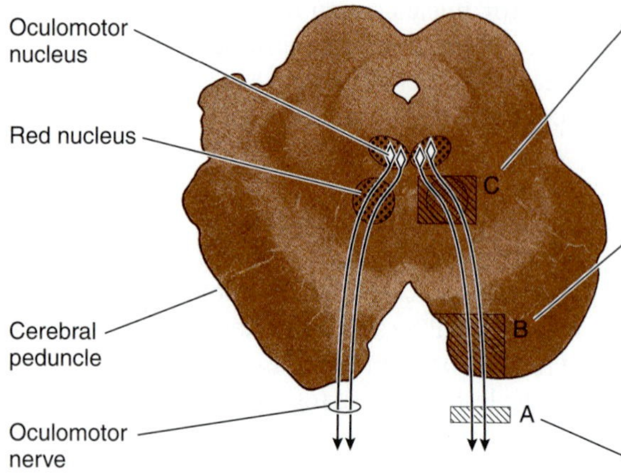
Oculomotor nucleus
Red nucleus
Cerebral peduncle
Oculomotor nerve
C
B
A
MORTIZ BENEDIKT SYNDROME
Deviation of eye downward and outward
Drooping of eyelid
Dilated, nonresponsive pupil
Contralateral tremor
WEBER SYNDROME
Deviation of eye downward and outward
Drooping of eyelid
Dilated, nonresponsive pupil
Contralateral upper motor neuron paralysis
OCULOMOTOR NERVE PALSY
Deviation of eye downward and outward
Drooping of eyelid
Dilated, nonresponsive pupil

FIGURE 9-15

Schematic diagram showing lesions of the oculomotor nerve in its intra- and extraaxial course and their respective clinical manifestations.

Lesions at the interpeduncular fossa (Fig. 9-15*B*) involving the cerebral peduncle and the rootlets of the oculomotor nerve result in (1) deviation of the ipsilateral eye downward and outward, with drooping of the eyelid, (2) diplopia, (3) ipsilateral loss of light and accommodation reflexes, (4) dilatation of the ipsilateral pupil, and (5) contralateral upper motor neuron paralysis.

Lesions in the mesencephalon involving the red nucleus and the rootlets of the oculomotor nerve (Fig. 9-15*C*) are manifested by (1) deviation of the ipsilateral eye downward and outward, with drooping of the eyelid, (2) diplopia, (3) ipsilateral loss of light and accommodation reflexes, (4) dilatation of the ipsilateral pupil, and (5) contralateral tremor.

The relationship of the oculomotor nerve to the posterior cerebral and superior cerebellar arteries makes this nerve vulnerable to aneurysms in those vessels. Rupture of these aneurysms is usually manifested by the sudden onset of headache and signs of oculomotor nerve lesion.

It is worth noting that the parasympathetic fibers concerned with the pupillary light reflex travel on the superficial aspect of the oculomotor nerve in its cisternal portion and thus are the most susceptible to extrinsic compression by extraneural masses such as posterior communicating artery aneurysms. Conversely, in the major-

KEY CONCEPTS

- Lesions of the oculomotor nerve within the midbrain result in oculomotor nerve palsy and either contralateral tremor (if the red nucleus is concomitantly involved) or contralateral upper motor neuron paralysis (if the cerebral peduncle is involved).
- Autonomic fibers of the oculomotor nerve travel in the superficial part of the nerve and usually are spared in ischemic lesions of the nerve, as in patients with diabetes.

ity of cases of vascular ischemic disease of the nerve, such as diabetes mellitus, which affect centrally located fibers, the pupillary fibers are spared. The blood supply of the oculomotor nerve dips deep into the nerve, and thus interruption of the blood supply adversely affects deeper fibers and spares the more superficial ones concerned with the pupillary light reflex. The pupillary fibers are also of the small unmyelinated type and are relatively resistant to ischemia.

The sparing of parasympathetic pupillary fibers in ischemic disease and their dysfunction in compressive disease are not, however, absolute. In 3 to 5 percent of aneurysms the pupil may be spared. Pupil-sparing oculomotor nerve palsy is not, however, unique to nerve involvement outside the brain stem (in the subarachnoid space or cavernous sinus). These palsies also have been reported with intraaxial (within the midbrain) lesions. Many, however, are associated with other neurologic signs (e.g., tremor), suggesting the involvement of adjacent structures such as the red nucleus. Few cases of pupil-sparing oculomotor nerve palsy from intraaxial lesions have been reported without another associated neurologic sign. Such cases are explained by isolated involvement of the appropriate nerve fascicles by the ischemic process.

Accessory oculomotor nuclei The accessory oculomotor nuclei include the following nuclei (see Fig. 9-2).

CAJAL'S INTERSTITIAL NUCLEUS Cajal's nucleus is composed of a mass of small cells in the rostral midbrain lateral to the MLF. Cajal's interstitial nucleus has extensive connections with rostral and caudal structures. It receives inputs from the ipsilateral frontal cortex (frontal eye fields), the contralateral deep cerebellar nuclei, and the pretectum. It also receives, via the MLF, an excitatory input from the contralateral labyrinth as well as an inhibitory input from the ipsilateral labyrinth after relays in the superior vestibular nucleus. Cajal's interstitial nucleus projects to the contralateral oculomotor nucleus, both trochlear nuclei, the ipsilateral medial vestibular nucleus, the inferior olive, the nucleus prepositus hypoglossi, the spinal cord, and Cajal's contralateral interstitial nucleus. This nucleus is concerned with slow rotatory and vertical eye movements and smooth pursuit eye patterns.

ROSTRAL INTERSTITIAL NUCLEUS OF THE MEDIAL LONGITUDINAL FASCICULUS The RiMLF (also known as the nucleus of the prerubral field) is composed of a mass of small cells just rostral to Cajal's interstitial nucleus and the third nerve nuclear complex at the junction of the rostral midbrain and the caudal diencephalon. Input to this nucleus comes from the superior vestibular nucleus via the MLF and from the PPRF via the reticular formation. Axons of neurons in this nucleus project to the inferior rectus subnucleus of the oculomotor nuclear complex and are concerned with downgaze.

DARKSCHEWITSCH'S NUCLEUS **Darkschewitsch's nucleus** lies dorsal and lateral to the somatic motor cell column of the oculomotor nerve. It projects to the nuclei of the posterior commissure but does not project to the oculomotor nuclear complex.

Darkschewitsch's nucleus. One of the accessory oculomotor nuclei. Named after Liverij Osipovich Darkschewitsch, a Russian anatomist.

NUCLEUS OF THE POSTERIOR COMMISSURE This nucleus is located within the posterior commissure. It has connections with pretectal and posterior thalamic nuclei. Lesions involving nuclei of the posterior commissure and crossing fibers from Cajal's interstitial nuclei of Cajal produce bilateral eyelid retraction and impairment of vertical eye movement.

KEY CONCEPTS

- Accessory oculomotor nuclei include Cajal's interstitial nucleus, rostral interstitial nucleus of the medial longitudinal fasciculus (RiMLF), Darkschewitsch's nucleus, and nucleus of the posterior commissure.

The accessory oculomotor nuclei are directly or indirectly connected with the oculomotor complex. Cajal's interstitial nucleus also sends fibers to the spinal cord via the MLF.

Aqueduct of Sylvius (cerebral aqueduct) (Latin *aqua*, "water"; *ductus*, "canal"). The narrow passage in the midbrain linking the third and fourth ventricles. Described by Jacques Dubois (Sylvius) in 1555.

Dorsal longitudinal fasciculus (Fasciculus of Schütz). A periventricular ascending and descending fiber system that connects the hypothalamus with the periaqueductal gray matter and with autonomic nuclei in the pons and medulla oblongata.

Central (Periaqueductal) Gray

The central gray region of the mesencephalon surrounds the **aqueduct of Sylvius** and contains scattered neurons, several nuclei, and some fine myelinated and unmyelinated fibers. The oculomotor, accessory oculomotor, and trochlear nuclei, as well as the mesencephalic nucleus of the trigeminal nerve, lie at the edge of this region. The **dorsal longitudinal fasciculus (Fasciculus of Schütz)** courses in the central gray matter. It arises in part from the hypothalamus and contains autonomic fibers. Its projections are not well delineated but probably include cranial nerve nuclei. Recent interest in the central gray has been focused on its role in pain. The neuropeptide enkephalin has been identified in the central gray matter. Stimulation of certain sites within the central gray matter release enkephalins which act on serotonergic neurons in the medulla oblongata, which in turn project on primary afferent axons (concerned with pain conduction) in the dorsal horn of the spinal cord to produce analgesia. Stimulus-produced analgesia has been achieved by stimulation of ventrolateral regions of the central gray matter. In contrast, stimulation of the rostral and lateral central gray matter facilitates pain sensations.

In addition to its role in central analgesic mechanisms, the central (periaqueductal) gray region has been implicated in vocalization, control of reproductive behavior, modulation of medullary respiratory centers, aggressive behavior, and vertical gaze. Afferents to this region arise from the hypothalamus, the amygdala, the brain stem reticular formation, the locus ceruleus, and the spinal cord. Immunoreactivity to a variety of neuropeptides has been demonstrated in periaqueductal neurons; these neuropeptides include enkephalin, substance P, cholecystokinin, neurotensin, serotonin, dynorphin, and somatostatin.

LIGHT REFLEX

Stimulation of the retina by light sets off a reflex with the following afferent and efferent pathways (Fig. 9-16).

Afferent Pathway

From the retina the impulse travels via the optic nerve and optic tract to the pretectal area. After synapsing on neurons of the pretectal area, the impulse travels via the posterior commissure to both Edinger-Westphal nuclei in the oculomotor complex.

Efferent Pathway

From the Edinger-Westphal nucleus, parasympathetic preganglionic fibers travel with the somatic motor component of the oculomotor nerve as far as the orbit. In the orbit, the parasympathetic fibers project on neurons in the ciliary ganglion.

KEY CONCEPTS

- The periaqueductal (central) gray region is concerned with modulation of pain, vocalization, control of reproductive behavior, modulation of medullary respiratory centers, aggressive behavior, and vertical gaze.
- The light reflex is conveyed by the optic nerve (afferent) and the oculomotor nerve (efferent) with synapses in the pretectal area and the Edinger-Westphal nucleus.

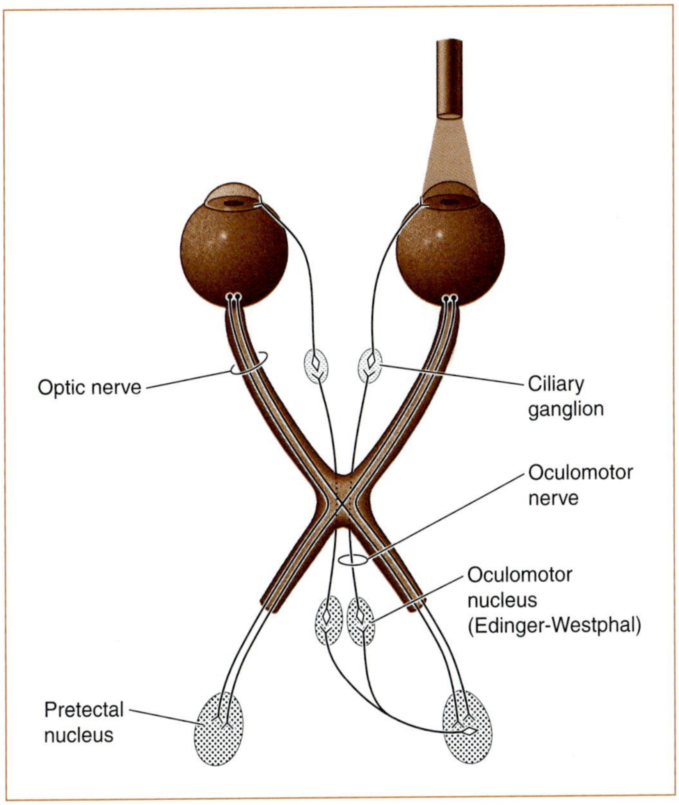

FIGURE 9-16

Schematic diagram showing the afferent and efferent pathways of the pupillary light reflex.

Postganglionic fibers arise from the ciliary ganglion (short ciliary nerves) and innervate the sphincter pupillae and ciliaris muscles.

Thus, when light is thrown on one retina, both pupils respond by constricting. The response of the ipsilateral pupil is the direct light reflex, whereas that of the contralateral pupil is the consensual light reflex. A consensual light reflex is possible because of the projection of the pretectal area to both oculomotor nuclei.

Lesions of the optic nerve (Fig. 9-17) abolish both direct and consensual light reflexes in response to light stimulation of the ipsilateral retina. Lesions of the oculomotor nerve (Fig. 9-18) abolish the direct light reflex but not the consensual light reflex in response to light stimulation of the ipsilateral retina.

The **Marcus Gunn** phenomenon is a paradoxical dilatation of both pupils that occurs when light is shown in the symptomatic eye (optic nerve lesion) after having

Marcus Gunn pupil. Paradoxical dilatation of both pupils when light is shone in a symptomatic eye with an optic nerve lesion after having been shone in the normal eye (swinging flashlight test). When light is shone in the normal eye, both pupils constrict. When light is then swung to the symptomatic eye, less light reaches the oculomotor nucleus because of the optic nerve lesion. The oculomotor nucleus senses the less intense light and shuts off the parasympathetic response, resulting in paradoxical pupillary dilatation. In 1902 Robert Marcus Gunn (1850–1909), a Scottish ophthalmologist, observed the reaction of both eyes to stimulation of one of them, while Levatin described the swinging flashlight test and observed the paradoxical dilatation of the pupil of the affected eye when the light was swung to it from the normal eye.

KEY CONCEPTS

- Constriction of the pupil ipsilateral to light stimulation constitutes the direct light reflex; constriction of the pupil contralateral to light stimulation constitutes the consensual light reflex.
- Lesions of the optic nerve (afferent limb of the reflex) abolish both the direct and the consensual light reflexes, while lesions of the oculomotor nerve (efferent limb of the reflex) abolish the direct light reflex.
- The Marcus Gunn reflex or phenomenon consists of paradoxical dilation of both pupils when light is shone in an eye with an optic nerve lesion after having been shone in the normal eye.

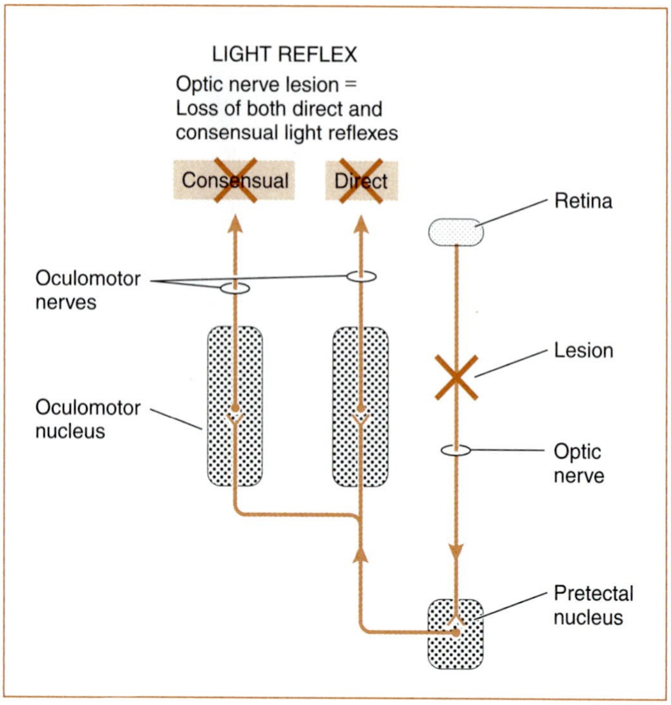

FIGURE 9-17

Schematic diagram showing the effects of optic nerve lesions on the direct and consensual pupillary light reflexes.

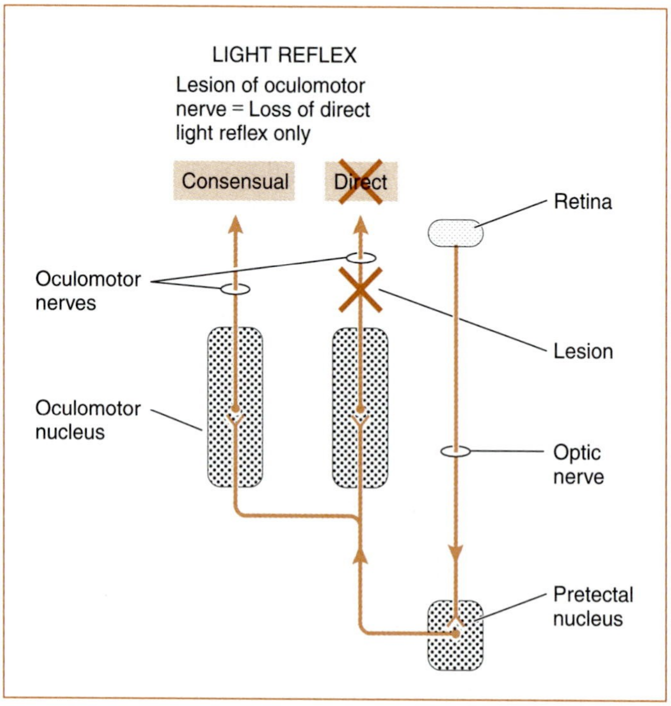

FIGURE 9-18

Schematic diagram showing the effects of oculomotor nerve lesions on the direct and consensual pupillary light reflexes.

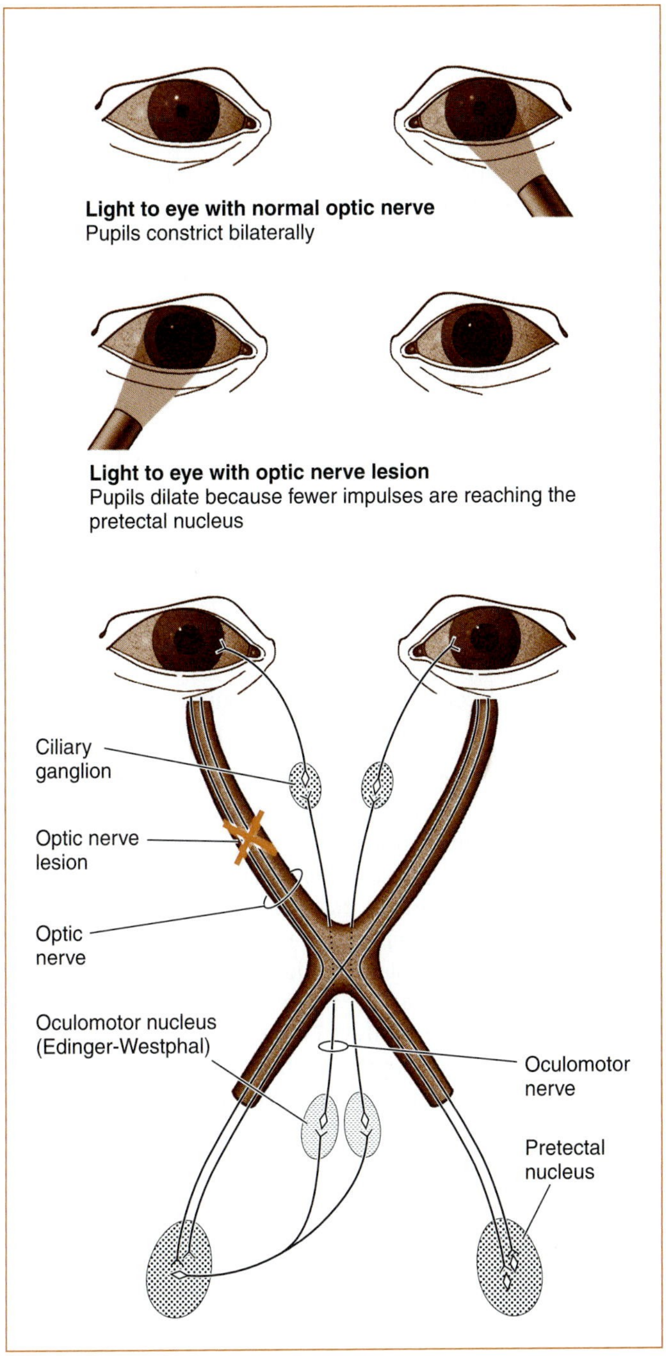
Light to eye with normal optic nerve
Pupils constrict bilaterally
Light to eye with optic nerve lesion
Pupils dilate because fewer impulses are reaching the pretectal nucleus
Ciliary ganglion
Optic nerve lesion
Optic nerve
Oculomotor nucleus (Edinger-Westphal)
Oculomotor nerve
Pretectal nucleus

FIGURE 9-19

Schematic diagram showing response to light stimulation of the Marcus Gunn pupil.

been shown in the normal eye. When light is shone in the normal eye, both pupils constrict (direct and consensual light reflexes). When light is then swung to the symptomatic eye, less light reaches the oculomotor nucleus because of the optic nerve lesion (optic neuropathy). The oculomotor nucleus senses the less intense light and shuts off the parasympathetic response, resulting in paradoxical pupillary dilatation (Fig. 9-19).

Adie's pupil, or tonic pupil, is characterized by a sluggish, prolonged pupillary contraction in reaction to light. When it is constricted, the pupil takes a long time to dilate. The affected pupil is larger than the normal pupil, but in darkness it may

Adie's Pupil (tonic pupil, Holmes-Adie syndrome). A condition in which the pupil exhibits sluggish prolonged constriction to light and, when it is constricted, takes a long time to dilate. The phenomenon results from pathology in the ciliary ganglion. Described by James Ware in 1812, by Piltz in 1899, and by others before William Joh Adie, an Australian neurologist, described it in 1931.

be smaller, since the normal pupil is free to dilate widely. Adie's pupil results from pathology in the ciliary ganglion within the orbit. Normally, 90 percent of parasympathetic nerves in the ciliary ganglion innervate the ciliary body and the remaining 10 percent innervate the iris sphincter. When the ciliary ganglion is damaged, the pupil becomes dilated and unresponsive to light or accommodation. During recovery reinnervation takes place in a random fashion. As a result, 90 percent of the parasympathetic fibers that previously innervated the pupil now innervate the ciliary body. When light is shone in the eye, 90 percent of the parasympathetic instruction to constrict the pupil is dissipated in the ciliary body, leaving only 10 percent for pupillary constriction.

ACCOMMODATION-CONVERGENCE REFLEX

The accommodation-convergence reflex involves the following processes:

1. The assumption of a convex shape by the lens is secondary to contraction of the ciliary muscle, which causes relaxation of the suspensory ligament. This is a process of accommodation of the lens, which thickens to keep the image in sharp focus.
2. Contraction of both medial recti muscles for convergence brings the eyes into alignment.
3. Pupillary constriction occurs as an aid in regulating the depth of focus for sharper images.

The accommodation-convergence reflex occurs when the eyes converge voluntarily to look at a nearby object or make a reflex response to an approaching object.

The pathway of the accommodation-convergence reflex has not been well delineated. It is believed, however, that afferent impulses from the retina reach the occipital cortex and that the efferent pathway from the occipital cortex reaches the oculomotor complex after synapsing in the pretectal nucleus and/or superior colliculus. In the oculomotor complex, Perlia's nucleus has been assumed to play a role in convergence. The pathway for the accommodation-convergence reflex is thus different from that of the light reflex. This is supported clinically by a condition known as the **Argyll Robertson pupil,** in which the light reflex is lost while the accommodation-convergence reflex persists. The site of the lesion in this condition has not been established with certainty, but its etiology is known to be syphilis of the nervous system.

Argyll-Robertson pupil. A pupil that reacts to accommodation but not to light. Described by Argyll Robertson, a Scottish ophthalmologist, in 1869. Syphilis is the classical etiology, but diabetes and lesions in the midbrain can cause this phenomenon.

MESENCEPHALIC RETICULAR FORMATION

The mesencephalic reticular formation is a continuation of the pontine reticular nuclei and merges rostrally with the zona incerta. The mesencephalic reticular

KEY CONCEPTS

- Adie's (tonic) pupil is characterized by a sluggish prolonged contraction in reaction to light and by prolonged dilatation when constricted because of pathology in the ciliary ganglion.
- The pathway for the accommodation convergence reaction is not well delineated but is different from that of the light reflex.
- In an Argyll Robertson pupil, light reflex is lost while accommodation convergence is preserved.

formation is less extensive than that of the pons. It receives fibers from most of the ascending fiber pathways (except the medial lemniscus) and from the limbic lobe. Although the mesencephalic reticular formation does not send direct reticulospinal fibers, it influences spinal activity indirectly through the reticular nuclei of the pons and medulla. The major output from the mesencephalic reticular formation ascends to the diencephalon and cerebral cortex and is involved in behavior mechanisms as well as sleep mechanisms. Unilateral lesions in this formation in monkeys result in profound neglect of tactile, auditory, and visual sensations in the contralateral half of the body. This neglect is believed to be due to interruption of the corticolimbic reticular alerting system, which includes the mesencephalic reticular formation.

The following reticular nuclei are situated in the mesencephalon: the nucleus cuneiformis, the nucleus subcuneiformis, the nucleus tegmenti pedunculopontis, and the interpeduncular nucleus. The cuneiform and subcuneiform nuclei lie ventral to the tectum and dorsal to the pedunculopontine nucleus. The central tegmental tract is medial to these nuclei. Pedunculopontine and interpeduncular nuclei are discussed under "Inferior Colliculus: Nuclear Groups," earlier in this chapter.

VERTICAL GAZE

Whereas control of lateral gaze is a function of the pons, the rostral midbrain at the mesencephalic-diencephalic junction is critical in the mediation of vertical gaze.

At this level, a lesion may give rise to several disorders of eye movements, including (1) conjugate vertical gaze palsy syndromes, including upward gaze palsy, downward gaze palsy, and combined upward and downward gaze palsy, and (2) dysconjugate vertical disturbances such as supranuclear monocular elevation palsy and the vertical **one and a half syndrome.** Some researchers have claimed that a vertical gaze palsy must be related to bilateral lesions, but a single unilateral lesion near the midline may interrupt fibers involved in vertical gaze before and after they decussate, resulting in a functionally bilateral lesion.

One and a half syndrome. A neuro-ophthalmic syndrome characterized by horizontal conjugate gaze palsy and internuclear ophthalmoplegia resulting from a lesion in the dorsal tegmentum of the pons that affects the nucleus of the abducens nerve (ipsilateral horizontal gaze palsy) and the medial longitudinal fasciculus (failure of adduction of the ipsilateral eye on contralateral horizontal gaze).

The critical areas involved in vertical gaze are the RiMLF and the posterior commissure. The RiMLF in the monkey contains burst and tonic cells that are involved in vertical gaze. The RiMLF lies just above the dorsal and medial part of the oral pole of the red nucleus, close to the midline. In monkeys, the areas involved in downgaze are dorsal and medial to the oral pole of the red nucleus, corresponding to the medial part of the RiMLF. In humans, the existence of this nucleus has been demonstrated, but its divisions are still a matter of debate. It has been suggested that the pathways for upward and downward gaze emanating from the RiMLF are separate. Those involved in downgaze are directed medially toward both (predominantly ipsilateral) oculomotor and trochlear nuclei with an unknown level of decussation. The tracts involved in upgaze are more lateral with a decussation in the posterior commissure before reaching the oculomotor complex. The longer course of the upgaze tracts may explain the higher frequency of upgaze palsies compared with downgaze palsies. It also may explain why a unilateral lesion that destroys the fibers reaching the posterior commissure may result in a lesion of the axons originating in both RiMLFs and may induce an upward gaze palsy.

KEY CONCEPTS

- The midbrain reticular formation is involved in modulation of spinal motor activity, behavior mechanisms, and sleep.
- The rostral midbrain is critical in the mediation of vertical gaze. Important structures for vertical gaze include the rostral interstitial nucleus of the medial longitudinal fasciculus and the posterior commissure.

TABLE 9-3

Vertical Gaze Palsy: Clinicopathologic Correlates

Direction of Gaze	Site of Lesion: Unilateral	Site of Lesion: Bilateral
Upward	Interstitial nucleus of MLF *or* connection of nucleus with posterior commissure "Functional bilateral interruption of afferent and efferent fibers of posterior commissure"	Tectum, pretectum, and fibers of posterior commisure *or* posterior commissure
Downward	Not reported	Interstitial nucleus of MLF *or* periaqueductal gray *or* interstitial nucleus of Cajal
Combined upward and downward	Interstitial nucleus of MLF *or* its efferents and periaqueductal gray *or* posterior commissure	Interstitial nucleus of MLF and posterior commissure *or* periaqueducal gray fiber tracts

Clinicopathologic correlation of cases of upward gaze palsy (Table 9-3) has shown that in unilateral cases the lesions were in either the RiMLF or the connections of the nucleus with the posterior commissure. The functional consequence of this anatomic unilateral lesion is bilateral interruption of the afferent or efferent fibers of the posterior commissure. In bilateral upgaze palsy, the lesions involve the tectum and pretectum, the fibers of the posterior commissure, or the posterior commissure itself.

Clinicopathologic correlations of cases with downgaze palsy (Table 9-3) have shown that the lesions are bilateral, involving the RiMLF or the periaqueductal

KEY CONCEPTS

- Paralysis of upward gaze is produced by unilateral or bilateral lesions in the rostral midbrain.
- Bilateral lesions in the rostral midbrain are required to produce paralysis of downgaze.

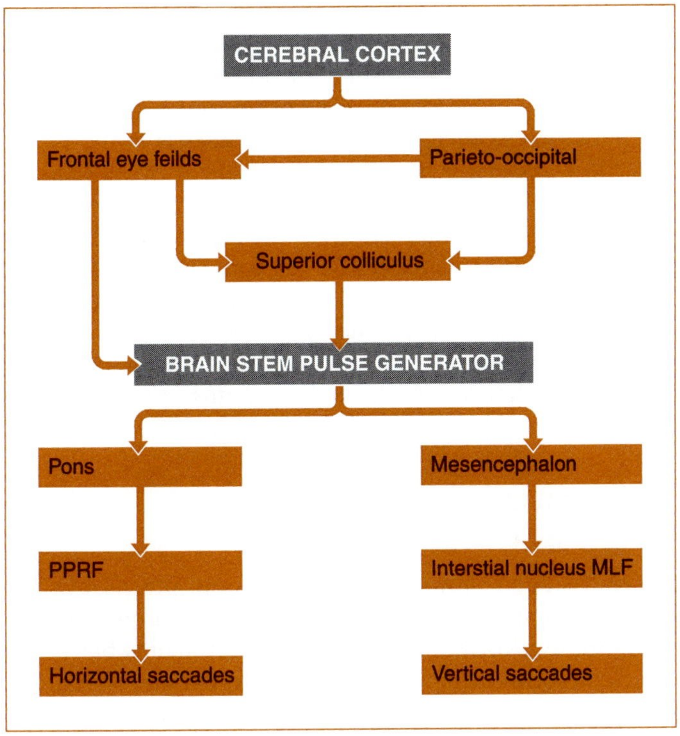

FIGURE 9-20

Schematic diagram showing cortical and subcortical control of saccadic eye movements.

gray or Cajal's interstitial nucleus on both sides. Unilateral lesions have not been associated with downgaze palsies.

In combined upgaze and downgaze palsies (Table 9-3) the lesion may be unilateral or bilateral. In the bilateral cases the RiMLF and posterior commissure or tracts of the periaqueductal gray matter are interrupted on both sides. In unilateral cases a lesion of the RiMLF or its efferent fibers and the periaqueductal area or a lesion of the posterior commissure has been described. These lesions interrupt fibers related to upward gaze. The concomitant occurrence of downgaze palsy has not been explained.

Reflex eye movements in response to head turning (oculocephalic response) are mediated by vestibular originating fibers destined for the oculomotor and trochlear nuclear complexes with a relay in Cajal's nucleus. These fibers do not traverse the posterior commissure. Lesions of Cajal's nucleus are thus associated with abolition of the oculocephalic response. Lesions of Cajal's nucleus also have been associated with downgaze palsy.

CONTROL OF SACCADIC EYE MOVEMENT

Commands for saccadic eye movements are initiated from the cerebral cortex (Fig. 9-20). The frontal eye field (area 8 in the frontal lobe), the angular gyrus (area 39),

KEY CONCEPTS

- Oculocephalic reflex eye movements are mediated by vestibular fibers destined for the oculomotor and trochlear nuclei after relays in Cajal's nucleus. These fibers do not travel in the posterior commissure.

Saccades (French, "jerking"). Abrupt, rapid movements or jerks of the eyes when one is changing points of fixation.

and the adjacent area 19 of the parieto-occipital cortices project to the superior colliculus. The cortical areas of ocular motility are interconnected. The superior colliculus in turn projects to the brain stem pulse generators in the pons and midbrain. The pulse generators also receive cortical input directly from the frontal eye fields. The pulse generator for horizontal **saccades** is in the PPRF. The pulse generator for vertical saccades is in the mesencephalic RiMLF. Thus, there are two pathways concerned with saccadic movements: (1) an anterior pathway from the frontal eye fields directly and indirectly (via the superior colliculus) to the brain stem centers for saccadic movements (PPRF for horizontal saccades and the mesencephalic RiMLF for vertical saccades) and (2) a posterior pathway from the parieto-occipital cortex to the superior colliculus and then to the brain stem centers for saccadic movements. The anterior pathway generates intentional saccades; the posterior pathway generates reflexive saccades. Each pathway can compensate partially for the other.

SMOOTH PURSUIT EYE MOVEMENTS

Each hemisphere has been shown to mediate smooth pursuit eye movements to the ipsilateral side. The cortical areas involved in smooth pursuit are not as well delineated as are those involved in saccadic eye movements but probably include the posterior parietal cortex or the temporo-occipito-parietal region. The pathogenesis of the pursuit deficits and pathways involved in smooth pursuit eye movements are not completely understood. Specific lesions in the temporo-occipito-parietal cortex that are associated with smooth pursuit deficits in humans correspond to Brodmann areas 19, 37, and 39. Lesions in the frontal eye field also have been associated with deficits in smooth pursuit.

The corticofugal pathway for smooth pursuit movements remains controversial. Two pathways have been described. The first courses from the temporo-occipito-parietal cortex through the posterior limb of the internal capsule to the dorsolateral pontine nucleus. The second courses from the frontal eye field to the dorsolateral pontine nucleus and the nucleus reticularis tegmenti pontis. Pursuit pathways in the brain stem and cerebellum are less well defined, although the dorsolateral pontine nucleus and the cerebellar flocculus are important in the monkey. Cerebral hemisphere lesions impair ocular pursuit ipsilaterally or bilaterally, whereas posterior fossa lesions impair ocular pursuit contralaterally or ipsilaterally. This variability probably reflects the involvement of a presumed pursuit pathway that crosses from the pontine nuclei to the cerebellum and then consists of a unilateral projection from the cerebellum to the vestibular nuclei.

BLOOD SUPPLY

Compared with the vascular supply of the pons, the midbrain vasculature is complex (Fig. 9-21). The mesencephalon (midbrain) receives its blood supply from the basilar artery via paramedian as well as superior cerebellar and posterior cerebral branches.

KEY CONCEPTS

- Saccadic eye movements are controlled by cortical inputs to the brain stem pulse generators either directly or indirectly via the superior colliculus. Brain stem pulse generators for horizontal saccades are in the pons paramedian pontine reticular formation, and for vertical saccades they are in the midbrain (RiMLF).
- Smooth-pursuit eye movements are controlled by input from cortical areas 8, 19, 37, and 39 to the dorsolateral pontine nucleus and the nucleus reticularis tegmenti pontis and cerebellum.

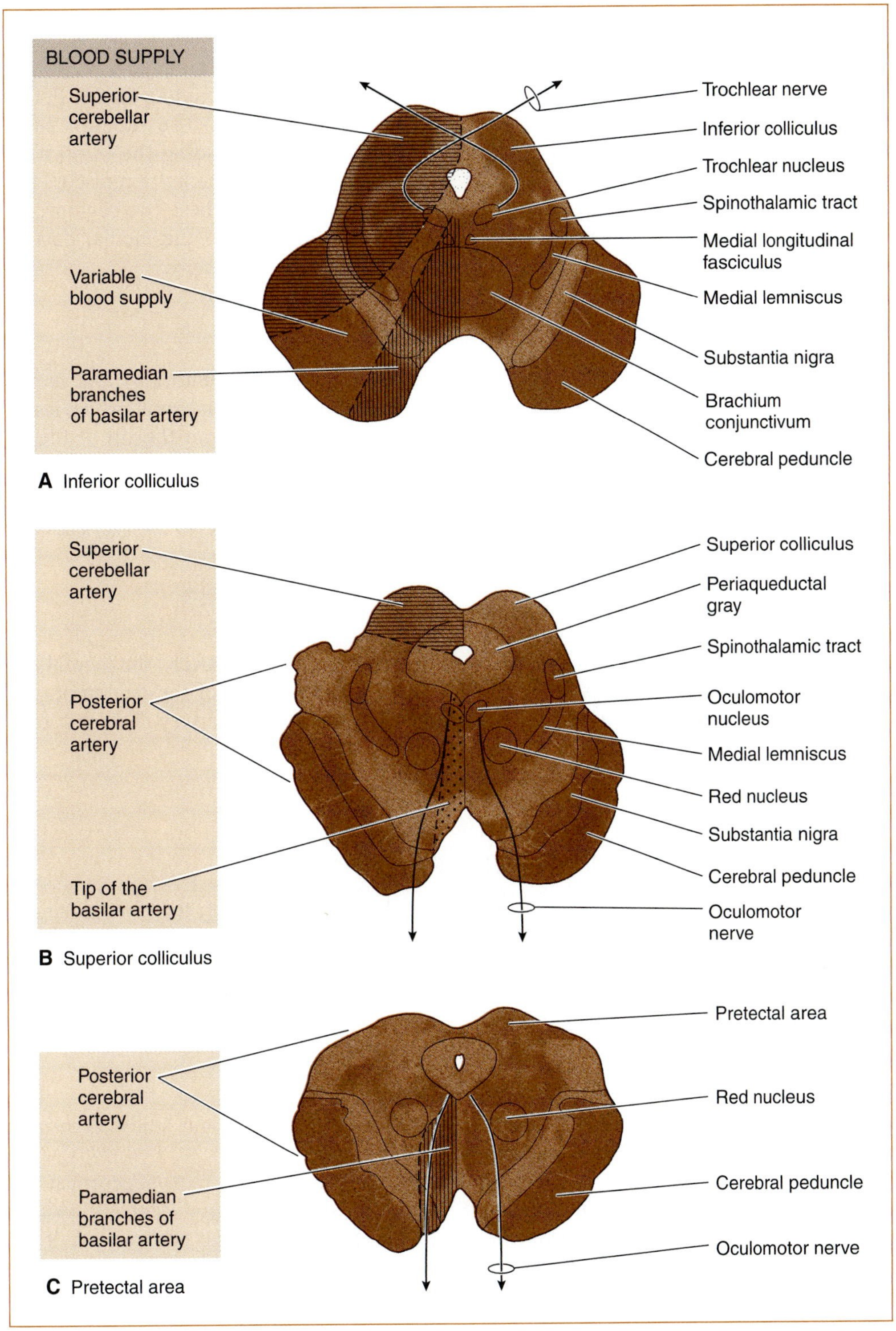
BLOOD SUPPLY
Superior cerebellar artery
Variable blood supply
Paramedian branches of basilar artery
Trochlear nerve
Inferior colliculus
Trochlear nucleus
Spinothalamic tract
Medial longitudinal fasciculus
Medial lemniscus
Substantia nigra
Brachium conjunctivum
Cerebral peduncle
A Inferior colliculus
Superior cerebellar artery
Posterior cerebral artery
Tip of the basilar artery
Superior colliculus
Periaqueductal gray
Spinothalamic tract
Oculomotor nucleus
Medial lemniscus
Red nucleus
Substantia nigra
Cerebral peduncle
Oculomotor nerve
B Superior colliculus
Posterior cerebral artery
Paramedian branches of basilar artery
Pretectal area
Red nucleus
Cerebral peduncle
Oculomotor nerve
C Pretectal area

FIGURE 9-21

Schematic diagram showing vascular territories of the midbrain at three caudorostral levels.

Inferior Colliculus Level

At the level of the inferior colliculus (lower midbrain), the paramedian branches supply the medial region of the mesencephalon, including the MLF, the paramedian reticular nuclei, and the brachium conjunctivum. The superior cerebellar artery supplies the lateral region of the midbrain, including the inferior colliculus, the rootlets of the trochlear nerve, the spinal and medial lemniscus, and the lateral part of the cerebral peduncle. A wedge between these two regions, which includes the trochlear nucleus, the cerebral peduncle, and the medial part of the medial lemniscus, has a variable and inconstant blood supply.

Superior Colliculus Level

At the level of the superior colliculus (middle midbrain), the mesencephalon is divided into three zones of blood supply. The medial zone, which includes the third cranial nerve nuclear complex, receives blood from the tip of the basilar artery. The tectum (dorsal zone) is supplied by the superior cerebellar artery. The rest of the midbrain is supplied by the posterior cerebral artery. This zone includes the spinal and medial lemnisci, the substantia nigra, the cerebral peduncle, the red nucleus, and the third cranial nerve rootlets.

Pretectal Level

At the level of the upper midbrain (the pretectal level), the medial zone, including the medial part of the red nucleus, and rootlets of the oculomotor nerve receive blood from paramedian branches of the basilar artery. The rest of the midbrain receives blood from the posterior cerebral artery.

KEY CONCEPTS

- The midbrain receives the bulk of its blood supply from the basilar artery via the paramedian, superior cerebellar, and posterior cerebral branches.

SUGGESTED READINGS

Afifi AK, Kaelber WW: Efferent connections of the substantia nigra: An experimental study in cats. *Exp Neurol* 1965; 11:474–482.

Anderson ME, Yoshida M: Axonal branching patterns and location of nigrothalamic and nigrocollicular neurons in the cat. *J Neurophysiol* 1980; 43:883–895.

Bogousslavsky J, et al: Pure midbrain infarction: Clinical syndromes, MRI, and etiologic patterns. *Neurology* 1994; 44:2032–2040.

Breen LA, et al: Pupil-sparing oculomotor nerve palsy due to midbrain infarction. *Arch Neurol* 1991; 48:105–106.

Castro O, et al: Isolated inferior oblique paresis from brain-stem infarction: Perspective on oculomotor fascicular organization in the ventral midbrain tegmentum. *Arch Neurol* 1990; 47:235–237.

Dehaene I, Lammens M: Paralysis of saccades and pursuit: Clinicopathologic study. *Neurology* 1991; 41: 414–415.

DeKeyser J, et al: The mesoneocortical dopamine neuron system. *Neurology* 1990; 40:1660–1662.

Deleu D, et al: Vertical one-and-a-half syndrome: Supranuclear downgaze paralysis with monocular elevation palsy. *Arch Neurol* 1989; 46:1361–1363.

Doraiswamy PM, et al: Morphometric changes of the human midbrain with normal aging: MR and stereologic findings. *AJNR* 1992; 13:383–386.

Fallon JH, Moore RY: Catecholamine innervation of the basal forebrain: IV. Topography of the dopamine projection to the basal forebrain and neostriatum. *J Comp Neurol* 1978; 180:545–580.

Felice KJ, et al: "Rubral" gait ataxia. *Neurology* 1990; 40:1004–1005.

Fog M, Hein-Sørenson O: Mesencephalic syndromes.

In Vinken PJ, Bruyn GW (eds): *Handbook of Clinical Neurology*. Amsterdam, North-Holland, 1969, vol 2, pp 272–285.

Gale K: Role of the substantia nigra in GABA-mediated anticonvulsant actions. *Adv Neurol* 1986; 44:343–364.

Galetta SL, et al: Pretectal eyelid retraction and lag. *Ann Neurol* 1993; 33:554–557.

Gebhart GF, Toleikis JR: An evaluation of stimulation-produced analgesia in the cat. *Exp Neurol* 1980; 62:570–579.

Gonzalez-Vegas JA: Nigro-reticular pathway in the rat: An intracellular study. *Brain Res* 1981; 207:170–173.

Halmagyi GM, et al: Tonic contraversive ocular tilt reaction due to unilateral meso-diencephalic lesion. *Neurology* 1990; 40:1503–1509.

Hartmann-von Monakow K, et al: Projections of precentral and premotor cortex to the red nucleus and other midbrain areas in *Macaca fascicularis*. *Exp Brain Res* 1979; 34:91–105.

Hattori N, et al: Immunohistochemical studies on complexes I, II, III, and IV of mitochondria in Parkinson's disease. *Ann Neurol* 1991; 30:563–571.

Hommel M, Bogousslavsky J: The spectrum of vertical gaze palsy following unilateral brain stem stroke. *Neurology* 1991; 41:1229–1234.

Hopf HC, Gutman L: Diabetic 3rd nerve palsy: Evidence for a mesencephalic lesion. *Neurology* 1990; 40:1041–1045.

Juncos JL, et al: Mesencephalic cholinergic nuclei in progressive supranuclear palsy. *Neurology* 1991; 41:25–30.

Kaelber WW, Afifi AK: Nigroamygdaloid fiber connections in the cat. *Am J Anat* 1977; 148:129–135.

Kaplan PW, Lesser RP: Vertical and horizontal epileptic gaze deviation and nystagmus. *Neurology* 1989; 39:1391–1393.

Keane JR: Isolated brain-stem third nerve palsy. *Arch Neurol* 1988; 45:813–814.

Keane JR: The pretectal syndrome: 206 patients. *Neurology* 1990; 40:684–690.

Liu GT, et al: Unilateral oculomotor palsy and bilateral ptosis from paramedian midbrain infarction. *Arch Neurol* 1991; 48:983–986.

Liu GT, et al: Midbrain syndromes of Benedikt, Claude, and Nothnagel: Setting the record straight. *Neurology* 1992; 42:1820–1822.

Marshall RS, et al: Dissociated vertical nystagmus and internuclear ophthalmoplegia from a midbrain infarction. *Arch Neurol* 1991; 48:1034–1305.

Mehler MF: The neuro-ophthalmologic spectrum of the rostral basilar artery syndrome. *Arch Neurol* 1988; 45:966–971.

Meibach RC, Katzman R: Origin, course and termination of dopaminergic substantia nigra neurons projecting to the amygdaloid complex in the cat. *Neuroscience* 1981; 6:2159–2171.

Moore RY: Catecholamine neuron systems in the brain. *Ann Neurol* 1982; 12:321–327.

Oyanagi K, et al: Quantitative investigation of the substantia nigra in Huntington's disease. *Ann Neurol* 1989; 26:13–19.

Pierrot-Deseilligny CH, et al: Parinaud's syndrome. Electro-oculographic and anatomical analysis of six vascular cases with deductions about vertical gaze organization in the premotor structures. *Brain* 1982; 105:667–696.

Pryce-Phillips W: *Companion to Clinical Neurology*. Boston, Little, Brown, 1995.

Pusateri TJ, et al: Isolated inferior rectus muscle palsy from a solitary metastasis to the oculomotor nucleus. *Arch Ophthalmol* 1987; 105:675–677.

Ranalli PJ, et al: Palsy of upward and downward saccadic, pursuit, and vestibular movements with a unilateral midbrain lesion: Pathophysiologic correlations. *Neurology* 1988; 38:114–122.

Remy P, et al: Peduncular "rubral" tremor and dopaminergic denervation: A PET study. *Neurology* 1995; 45:472–477.

Skinner HL: *The Origin of Medical Terms*. Baltimore, Williams & Wilkins, 1961.

Smith JL: The "nuclear third" question. *J Clin Neuro Ophthalmol* 1982; 2:61–63.

Steiger HJ, Buttner-Ennever JA: Oculomotor nucleus afferents in the monkey demonstrated with horseradish peroxidase. *Brain Res* 1979; 160:1–15.

Thurston SE, Saul RF: Superior oblique myokymia: Quantitative descriptive of the eye movement. *Neurology* 1991; 41:1679–1681.

Trojanowski JQ, Wray SH: Vertical gaze ophthalmoplegia: Selective paralysis of downgaze. *Neurology* 1980; 30:605–610.

Usunoff KG, et al: Electron microscopic evidence for the existence of a corticonigral tract in the cat. *J Hirnforsch* 1982; 23:17–23.

Vanooteghem P, et al: Combined trochlear nerve palsy and internuclear ophthalmoplegia. *Arch Neurol* 1992; 49:108–109.

Walberg F, Nordby T: A re-examination of the rubro-olivary tract in the cat, using horseradish peroxidase as a retrograde and an anterograde neuronal tracer. *Neuroscience* 1981; 6:2379–2391.

Warren W, et al: Atypical oculomotor paresis. *J Clin Neuro Ophthalmol* 1982; 2:13–18.

Weber JT, et al: The precise origin of the tectospinal pathway in three common laboratory animals: A study using the horseradish peroxidase method. *Neurosci Lett* 1979; 11:121–127.

CHAPTER 10

MESEN-CEPHALON (Midbrain): CLINICAL CORRELATES

MESENCEPHALIC VASCULAR SYNDROMES

Midbrain infarcts have not been studied extensively. There have been only a few reports of single cases, well described clinically and by magnetic resonance imaging (MRI), of isolated midbrain infarcts. (Table 10-1).

The most commonly affected region is the middle midbrain, and the most frequently involved territory is the paramedian territory, followed by the posterior cerebral artery territory and the territory intermediate between the two. Involvement of the territory of the superior cerebellar artery is rare.

Patients with middle midbrain infarcts have a localizing clinical picture that is linked to involvement of the third nerve or its nucleus. Paramedian infarcts are associated with the nuclear syndrome of the oculomotor nerve, whereas more lateral

KEY CONCEPTS

- Midbrain infarcts occur most frequently at the middle midbrain level in the paramedian territory.

TABLE 10-1

Midbrain Vascular Syndromes

Syndrome	Ipsilateral	Contralateral	Lesion Site
Weber's	Oculomotor palsy	Hemiparesis	CN III, CP
Benedikt	Oculomotor palsy	Tremor ± hemianesthesia	CN III, RN ± ML, ST
Claude's	Oculomotor palsy	Tremor and ataxia	CN III, RN, BC
Nothnagel's	Oculomotor palsy and ataxia	Oculomotor palsy ± ataxia	CN III, BC
Parinaud's	Upward gaze paralysis Pupillary abnormalities Large pupil Light-near dissociation Convergence retraction nystagmus on upgaze Lid retraction (Collier's sign)		Pretectal region
Walleyed	Internuclear ophthalmoplegia (MLF syndrome)	Internuclear ophthalmoplegia (MLF syndrome)	MLF, bilateral
Vertical one and a half	Downgaze palsy Monocular elevation palsy	Downgaze palsy	Efferents of RiMLF, CBF
Locked-in	Mute quadriplegia		Ventral mesencephalon
Peduncular hallucinosis	Hallucinations, somnolence		Tegmentum, CP

NOTE: CN III, third cranial nerve; CP, cerebral peduncle; RN, red nucleus; BC, brachium conjunctivum; ML, medial lemniscus; ST, spinothalamic tract; MLF, medial longitudinal fasciculus; RiMLF, rostral interstitial nucleus of the medial longitudinal fasciculus; CBF, corticobulbar fibers.

infarcts are associated with fascicular involvement of the third nerve in isolation or with contralateral hemiparesis (syndrome of Weber) or hemiataxia (Claude's syndrome).

Patients with rostral or caudal midbrain infarcts have a less localizing neurologic picture except for vertical gaze impairment in those with dorsal rostral midbrain infarcts. Ipsilateral trochlear nerve palsy, **Horner's syndrome,** and contralateral

Horner's syndrome. Drooping of the eyelid (ptosis), constriction of the pupil (miosis), retraction of the eyeball (enophthalmos), and loss of sweating on the face (anhidrosis) constitute a syndrome described by Johann Friedrich Horner, a Swiss ophthalmologist, in 1869. The syndrome is caused by interruption of descending sympathetic fibers. Also known as Bernard-Horner syndrome and oculosympathetic palsy. The syndrome was de-

KEY CONCEPTS

- Midbrain infarcts are characterized by oculomotor nerve signs ipsilateral to the lesion and a contralateral red nucleus lesion sign (hemiataxia) or cerebral peduncle lesion sign (hemiparesis).
- Dorsal midbrain infarcts are associated with vertical gaze abnormalities and trochlear nerve signs.

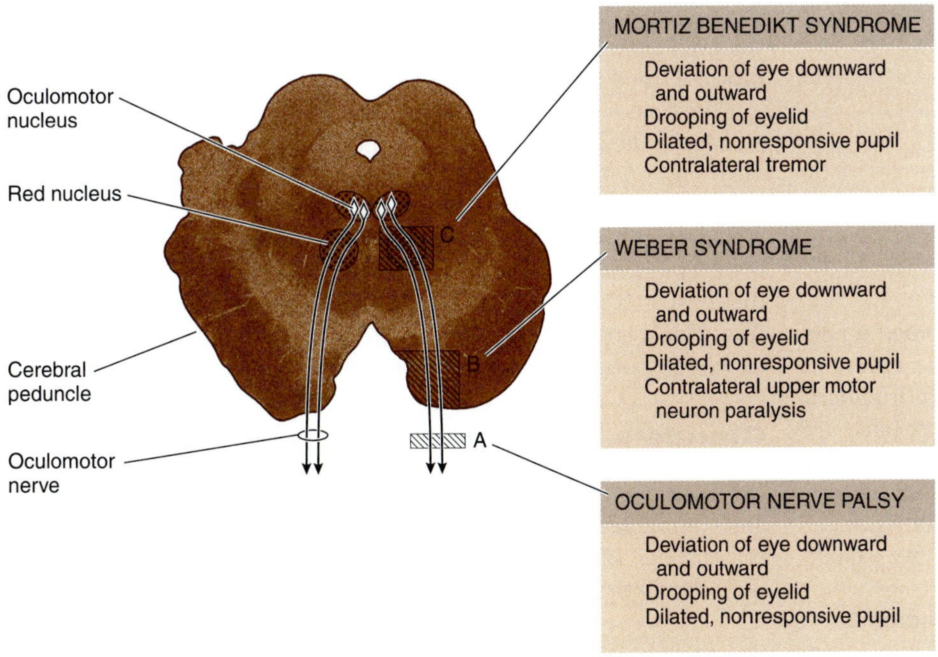
MORTIZ BENEDIKT SYNDROME
Deviation of eye downward and outward
Drooping of eyelid
Dilated, nonresponsive pupil
Contralateral tremor
Oculomotor nucleus
Red nucleus
Cerebral peduncle
Oculomotor nerve
C
B
A
WEBER SYNDROME
Deviation of eye downward and outward
Drooping of eyelid
Dilated, nonresponsive pupil
Contralateral upper motor neuron paralysis
OCULOMOTOR NERVE PALSY
Deviation of eye downward and outward
Drooping of eyelid
Dilated, nonresponsive pupil

FIGURE 10-1

Schematic diagram showing lesions of the oculomotor nerve in its intra- and extraaxial course and their respective clinical manifestations.

ataxia point to the territory of the superior cerebellar artery. Hand-foot-mouth hyperesthesia is due to involvement of the medial lemniscus and the ventral ascending tract of the trigeminal nerve.

Syndrome of Weber

In the syndrome of Weber the patient presents with signs of ipsilateral oculomotor nerve paralysis and contralateral upper motor neuron paralysis that includes the lower face. The vascular lesion, usually an infarct, affects rootlets of the oculomotor nerve and the underlying cerebral peduncle (Fig. 10-1). This syndrome was described by Gubler 4 years before Weber reported his case. The syndrome is therefore referred to by some researchers as the Gubler-Weber syndrome.

Syndrome of Benedikt

In the syndrome of Benedikt the patient presents with signs of ipsilateral oculomotor nerve paralysis and contralateral tremor. The vascular lesion affects rootlets of the oculomotor nerve within the tegmentum of the mesencephalon and the underlying

KEY CONCEPTS

- The syndrome of Weber consists of oculomotor nerve paralysis ipsilateral to the midbrain lesion and contralateral hemiplegia.
- The syndrome of Benedikt consists of oculomotor nerve paralysis ipsilateral to the midbrain lesion and contralateral tremor. Contralateral hemianesthesia may occur.

scribed in animals by François du Petit in 1727. Claude Bernard in France in 1862 and E. S. Hare in Great Britain in 1838 gave precise accounts of the syndrome before Horner did.

Syndrome of Weber. A midbrain vascular syndrome characterized by ipsilateral oculomotor nerve palsy and contralateral hemiplegia. Named after Sir Herman David Weber, a German-English physician who described the syndrome in 1863.

Syndrome of Benedikt. A midbrain vascular syndrome characterized by ipsilateral oculomotor nerve palsy and contralateral tremor with or without hemianesthesia. Described in a 4-year-old patient by Moritz Benedikt, an Austrian physician, in 1889.

red nucleus (see Fig. 10-1). Contralateral hemianesthesia has been described by some researchers and is attributed to involvement of the medial lemniscus and spinothalamic tract. This syndrome was first described by a Viennese physician, Moritz Benedikt, in 1889.

The tremor in this syndrome has been called rubral tremor on the basis of damage to the red nucleus or the superior cerebellar peduncle. The tremor is usually of low frequency and may have resting, postural, and kinetic components. The kinetic component may be explained by the involvement of the superior cerebellar peduncle and/or the red nucleus. The resting and postural components are due to the involvement of dopaminergic nigrostriatal fibers that arise from the pars compacta of the substantia nigra and run ventral to the red nucleus and through field H of Forel (prerubral) on their way to the hypothalamus and striatum. This component of the tremor responds well to treatment with levodopa.

Claude's syndrome. A midbrain vascular syndrome characterized by ipsilateral oculomotor nerve palsy and contralateral tremor and ataxia. Described by a French psychiatrist and neurologist, Henri Claude, in 1912.

Nothnagel's syndrome. A midbrain vascular syndrome characterized by ipsilateral or bilateral oculomotor nerve palsy and ataxia. Described by Carl Wilhelm Hermann Nothnagel, an Austrian internist, neurologist, and pathologist, in 1879.

Parinaud's syndrome. Paralysis of upward gaze associated with pretectal lesions. Described by Henri Parinaud, a French neuro-ophthalmologist, in 1883.

Koerber-Salus-Elschnig syndrome. A syndrome of vertical gaze palsy, anisocoria (unequal pupil sizes), light-near dissociation, conversion retraction nystagmus, lid retraction, impaired convergence, skewed eye deviation, papilledema, and lid flutter associated most commonly with pineal tumors or disorders of the pretectal region. Also known as Parinaud's syndrome, the sylvian aqueduct syndrome, and the syndrome of the posterior commissure.

Collier's sign. Bilateral lid retraction seen in the pretectal syndrome.

Claude's Syndrome

In Claude's syndrome the patient presents with ipsilateral oculomotor nerve palsy and contralateral tremor and ataxia. The lesion involves the oculomotor nerve, the red nucleus, and the brachium conjunctivum. This syndrome was first described by the French psychiatrist and neurologist Henry Claude in 1912.

Nothnagel's Syndrome

Nothnagel's syndrome has been variably described by different authors. In 1879, Nothnagel, an Austrian physician, described a patient with bilateral asymmetric oculomotor palsies of varying degree and gait ataxia. Subsequently, the syndrome was variously described in patients with oculomotor nerve palsy and ipsilateral or contralateral ataxia and patients with oculomotor nerve palsy and vertical gaze palsy. The lesion in the original report involved the superior and inferior colliculi. Subsequent reports described pathology in the oculomotor nerve fascicles and the brachium conjunctivum.

Parinaud's Syndrome

Parinaud's syndrome is also known as the sylvian aqueduct syndrome, the dorsal midbrain syndrome, **Koerber-Salus-Elschnig syndrome,** the pineal syndrome, and the syndrome of the posterior commissure. The lesion is in the pretectal region. Patients with this syndrome present with upward gaze paralysis, pupillary abnormalities (large pupil, light-near dissociation), lid retraction (**Collier's sign**), and convergence retraction nystagmus on upward gaze. This syndrome was described in 1883 by Parinaud, who vaguely speculated about the lesion site. Definitive localization of the lesion in the pretectal area resulted from experimental and human observations made between 1969 and 1974 by Bender, who coined the term *pretectal syndrome.*

KEY CONCEPTS

- Claude's syndrome consists of oculomotor nerve paralysis ipsilateral to the midbrain lesion and contralateral ataxia and tremor.
- Nothnagel's syndrome is variably described as consisting of bilateral oculomotor nerve paralysis, ipsi or contralateral gait ataxia, and vertical gaze palsy.
- Parinaud's syndrome consists of upgaze palsy, pupillary abnormalities, lid retraction, and convergence retraction nystagmus on upward gaze.

Walleyed Syndrome

The walleyed syndrome is also known as the walleyed bilateral internuclear ophthalmoplegia (WEBINO) syndrome. The lesion is bilateral and involves the rostral medial longitudinal fasciculus. This syndrome is characterized by exotropic gaze and the absence of ocular adduction.

Walleyed syndrome. A midbrain vascular syndrome characterized by lateral deviation of both eyes and bilateral absence of ocular adduction.

Vertical One and a Half Syndrome

The vertical one and a half syndrome is characterized by bilateral impairment of downgaze (the one) and monocular paralysis of elevation (the half). The lesion usually consists of bilateral infarcts in the mesencephalic-diencephalic region that involve efferent tracts of the rostral interstitial nucleus of the medial longitudinal fasciculus [MLF (RiMLF)] bilaterally and premotor fibers to the contralateral superior rectus subnucleus and the ipsilateral inferior oblique subnucleus before or after decussation in the posterior commissures. A variant of this syndrome consists of bilateral impairment of upgaze (the one) with monocular downgaze palsy (the half).

Vertical one and a half syndrome. A midbrain vascular syndrome characterized by bilateral downgaze palsy combined with monocular elevation palsy. A variant consists of bilateral upgaze palsy and monocular downgaze palsy.

Locked-in Syndrome

The locked-in syndrome is also known as the bilateral pyramidal system syndrome. It is characterized by mute quadriplegia, preservation of consciousness, and communication by ocular movements and blinking. In most patients the lesion is bilateral in the ventral half of the pons; in some patients the lesion may be bilateral in the ventral mesencephalon or both internal capsules. The term *locked-in syndrome* was proposed by Plum and Posner in 1987. This syndrome is also known as pseudocoma, the deefferented state, the ventral pontine or brain stem syndrome, and the Monte Cristo syndrome in reference to Alexander Dumas's novel *The Count of Monte Cristo,* in which the elderly Noirtier communicated only by eye blinks.

Locked-in syndrome. A brain stem syndrome characterized by mute quadriplegia, preservation of consciousness, and communication by ocular movements and blinking. This term was proposed by Plum and Posner in 1987.

Top of the Basilar Syndrome

In the top of the basilar syndrome the lesion is not limited to the mesencephalon but also involves other structures (the thalamus and portions of the temporal and occipital cortices). The conglomerate signs and symptoms of this syndrome include (1) visual defects such as hemianopia, cortical blindness (loss of vision with intact pupillary light reflexes), and **Balint's syndrome (optic ataxia)** caused by involvement of the occipital, parietal, and temporal cortices, (2) abnormalities of eye movements, including vertical gaze abnormalities, lid retraction (Collier's sign), and convergence disorder, (3) pupillary abnormalities, including light-near dissociation and a small reactive or large fixed pupil, (4) behavioral disturbances (somnolence, memory

Balint's syndrome. Also known as Balint-Holmes syndrome, ocular apraxia, and optic ataxia. A rare syndrome resulting from bilateral parieto-occipital disease and characterized by an inability to direct the eyes to a certain point in the visual field despite intact eye movements. Discovered by Rudolph Balint, a Hungarian neurologist, in 1909.

Optic ataxia. A rare syndrome resulting from bilateral parieto-occipital disease and characterized by inability to direct the eyes to a certain point in the visual field despite intact eye movements. Also known as Balint's syndrome, Balint-Holmes syndrome, and ocular apraxia.

KEY CONCEPTS

- The walleyed syndrome consists of exotropic gaze and an absence of ocular adduction. This syndrome is also known as the walleyed bilateral internuclear ophthalmoplegia (WEBIO) syndrome.
- The vertical one and a half syndrome consists of bilateral impairment of downgaze and monocular paralysis of eye elevation. A variant syndrome consists of bilateral impairment of upgaze and monocular downgaze paralysis.
- The locked-in syndrome consists of mute quadriplegia, preservations of consciousness, and communication by ocular movement and blinking.

defects, agitation, hallucination), and (5) motor and sensory deficits. The usual etiology of this syndrome is occlusion of the rostral basilar artery.

Peduncular hallucinosis. A syndrome of vividly colored hallucinations in somnolent patients in association with lesions in the midbrain, thalamus, and occipitotemporal cortex. The condition was first described by Jean Jacques Lhermitte, a French neurologist, in 1922, and the name was suggested by Ludo Van Bogaert, a Belgian neurologist, in 1924.

Peduncular Hallucinosis Syndrome

The peduncular hallucinosis syndrome is characterized by hallucinations, often formed nonstereotypically, colored, and vivid, that usually occur in somnolent patients with presumed tegmental and cerebral peduncle lesions. The symptoms probably arise from thalamic or occipitotemporal lesions rather than from the midbrain. This condition was first described by Jean Jacques Lhermitte, a French neurologist, in 1922. The name was suggested by Ludo Van Bogaert, a Belgian neurologist, in 1924.

DISTURBANCES OF CONSCIOUSNESS

Akinetic mutism. A clinical condition characterized by a state of apparent wakefulness in which the patient maintains a sleep-wake cycle but is unable to communicate in any way. Also known as the persistent vegetative state and Cairns syndrome. The pathology is in the brain stem reticular formation. Described by Sir Hugh William Bell Cairns, an Australian neurosurgeon, in 1941.

Various levels of unconsciousness occur in patients with lesions of the mesencephalic reticular formation. Evidence from experimental work points to a tonic role of the mesencephalic reticular formation in cortical excitability and the maintenance of awareness. Bilateral limited lesions of the mesencephalic reticuar formation have been associated with **akinetic mutism** (Cairns syndrome), a clinical condition characterized by absolute mutism and complete immobility except for the eyes, which are kept open and move in all directions. The patient appears awake and maintains a sleep-wake cycle, but no communication with the patient through either painful or auditory stimuli can be established. The condition was first reported by an Australian neurologist, Sir Hugh Cairns, in 1941. This condition may result from injury to the mesencephalic reticular formation caused by transtentorial brain herniation with edema, hemorrhage, or occlusion of branches of the basilar artery.

DECEREBRATE RIGIDITY

Decerebrate rigidity in humans results from lesions of the brain stem caudal to the red nucleus and rostral to the vestibular nuclei. The body is forced backward with the head bent extremely dorsally. The shoulders are internally rotated, the elbows are extended, and the distal parts of the upper limbs are hyperpronated with finger extension at the metacarpophalangeal joints and flexion at the interphalangeal joints. The hips and knees are extended; the feet and toes are plantar flexed. This syndrome is associated with severe head trauma and compression of the brain stem by herniation.

KEY CONCEPTS

- The top of the basilar syndrome consists of a variety of visual defects, abnormalities of eye movements, pupillary abnormalities, and behavioral disturbances.
- The peduncular hallucinosis syndrome consists of hallucinations and somnolence.
- Akinetic mutism characterized by complete immobility except in the eyes occurs with lesions in the midbrain reticular formation.
- Decerebrate rigidity is associated with midbrain lesions caudal to the red nucleus, between it and the vestibular nuclei.

SUGGESTED READINGS

Bogousslavsky J, et al: Pure midbrain infarction: Clinical syndromes, MRI, and etiologic patterns. *Neurology* 1994; 44:2032–2040.

Breen LA, et al: Pupil-sparing oculomotor nerve palsy due to midbrain infarction. *Arch Neurol* 1991; 48:105–106.

Deleu D, et al: Vertical one-and-a-half syndrome: Supranuclear downgaze paralysis with monocular elevation palsy. *Arch Neurol* 1989; 46:1361–1363.

Felice KJ, et al: "Rubral" gait ataxia. *Neurology* 1990; 40:1004–1005.

Keane JR: The pretectal syndrome: 206 patients. *Neurology* 1990; 40:684–690.

Liu GT, et al: Midbrain syndromes of Benedikt, Claude, and Nothnagel: Setting the record straight. *Neurology* 1992; 42:1820–1822.

Mehler MF: The neuro-ophthalmologic spectrum of the rostral basilar artery syndrome. *Arch Neurol* 1988; 45:966–971.

Pryse-Phillips W: *Companion to Clinical Neurology.* Boston, Little, Brown, 1995.

Ranalli PJ, et al: Palsy of upward and downward saccadic, pursuit, and vestibular movements with a unilateral midbrain lesion: Pathophysiologic correlation. *Neurology* 1988; 38:114–122.

CHAPTER 11

DIENCEPHALON

GROSS TOPOGRAPHY (Figs. 11-1 and 11-2)

The **diencephalon,** or "in-between brain," is completely surrounded by the cerebral hemispheres except at its ventral surface. It is limited posteriorly by the posterior commissure and anteriorly by the lamina terminals and the foramen of Monro. The posterior limb of the internal capsule limits the diencephalon laterally. Medially, the diencephalon forms the lateral wall of the third ventricle. The dorsal surface forms the floor of the lateral ventricle and is marked medially by a band of nerve fibers, the stria medullaris thalami. The ventral surface contains hypothalamic structures. A groove extending between the foramen of Monro and the aqueduct of Sylvius (the hypothalamic sulcus) divides the diencephalon into a dorsal portion, the **thalamus,** and a ventral portion, the **hypothalamus.** The two thalami are connected across the midline in about 70 percent of humans through the interthalamic adhesion (**massa intermedia**). The diencephalon develops from the caudal vesicle of the embryologic prosencephalon.

Diencephalon (Greek *dia*, "between"; *enkephalos*, "brain"). The part of the central nervous system between the two hemispheres. It includes the epithalamus, thalamus (including the metathalamus), subthalamus, and hypothalamus. The diencephalon is the posterior of the two brain vesicles formed from the prosencephalon of the developing embryo.

DIVISIONS OF DIENCEPHALON

The diencephalon is divided into four major subdivisions. These are (1) the epithalamus, (2) the thalamus and metathalamus, (3) the subthalamus, and (4) the hypothalamus. The first three subdivisions will be discussed in this chapter. The fourth subdivision, the hypothalamus, will be discussed in Chap. 19.

Thalamus (Greek *thalamos*, "inner chamber"). Also meant "a bridal couch," so the pulvinar nucleus is its cushion or pillow. Part of the diencephalon on each side of the third ventricle and above the hypothalamic sulcus. Galen made up the word *thalamus*, and Willis was the first to use the term in its modern sense.

KEY CONCEPTS

- The two thalami are connected by the mass intermedia (interthalamic adhesion) in 70 percent of humans.
- The diencephalon develops from the prosencephalon of the embryologic brain.
- The term *diencephalon* includes the following structures: epithalamus, thalamus (including the metathalamus), hypothalamus, and subthalamus.

Hypothalamus (Greek *hypo*, "under, below"; *thalamos*, "inner chamber"). The region of the diencephalon below the thalamus.

Massa intermedia. Bridge of gray matter that connects the thalami of the two sides across the third ventricle; also called *interthalamic adhesion.*

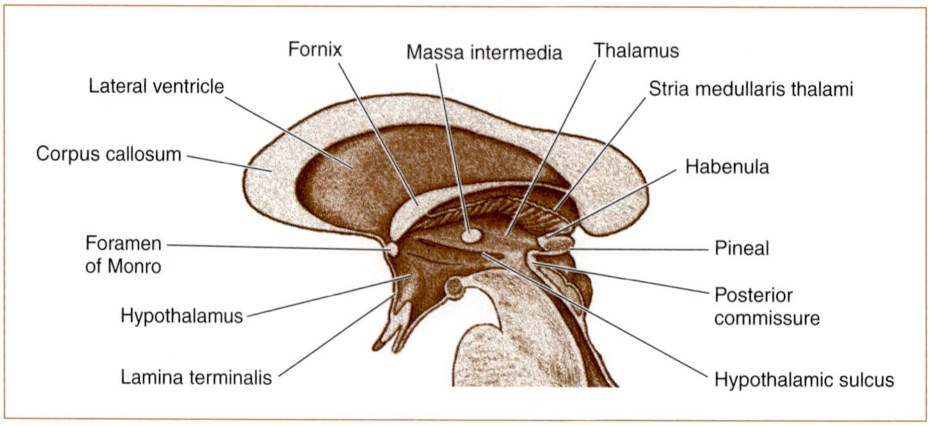

FIGURE 11-1

Schematic diagram showing the subdivisions of the diencephalon as seen in a midsagittal view.

Epithalamus

Epithalamus (Greek *epi*, "upon"; *thalamos*, "inner chamber"). Part of the diencephalon dorsal to the thalamus. It includes the stria medullaris thalami, habenular nucleus, and pineal gland.

The **epithalamus** occupies a position dorsal to the thalamus and includes the following structures (Fig. 11-1).

Stria Medullaris Thalami

This band of nerve fibers courses dorsomedial to the thalamus and connects the septal (medial olfactory) area, located underneath the rostral end of the corpus callosum in the frontal lobe, with the habenular nuclei.

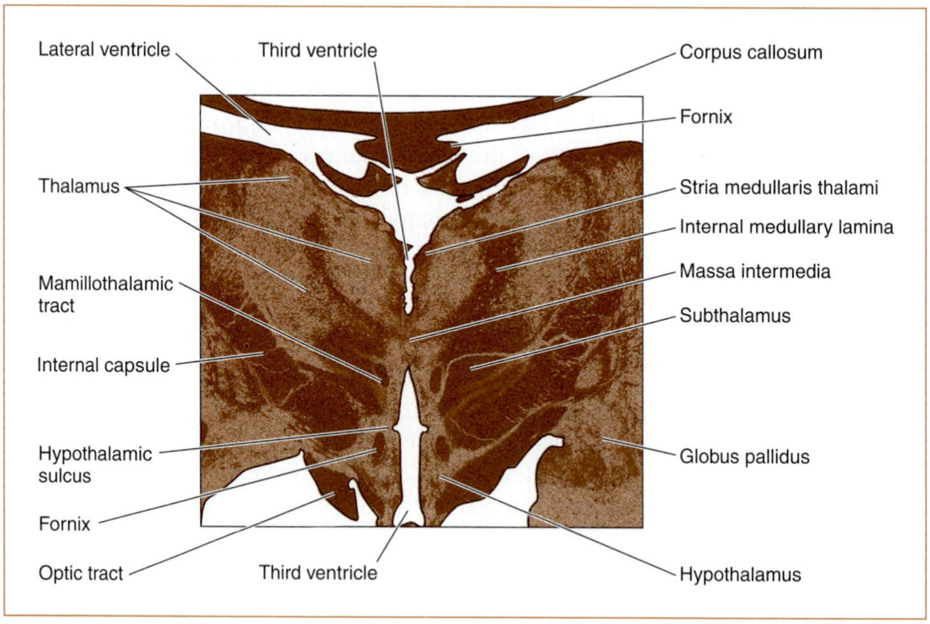

FIGURE 11-2

Schematic diagram showing the subdivisions of the diencephalon as seen in a composite coronal view.

KEY CONCEPTS

- The term *epithalamus* includes the stria medullaris thalami, habenular nuclei, and the pineal gland.

Habenular Nuclei

These nuclei are located in the caudal diencephalon; one is on each side, dorsomedial to the thalamus. They receive the stria medullaris and project via the habenulointerpeduncular tract (fasciculus retroflexus of Meynert) to the interpeduncular nucleus of the midbrain. The two habenular nuclei are connected by the habenular commissure. The habenular nuclei, part of a neural network that includes the limbic and olfactory systems, are concerned with mechanisms of emotion and behavior.

Habenula (Latin diminutive of *habena*, "a small strap or rein"). The habenular nuclei are part of the epithalamus.

Pineal Gland

This endocrine gland is located just rostral to the superior colliculi in the roof of the third ventricle. The functions of the pineal gland are not well understood. It may have roles in gonadal function and circadian rhythm. It secretes the biogenic amines serotonin, norepinephrine, and melatonin and contains several hypothalamic peptides including thyrotropin-releasing hormone (TRH), leutinizing hormone–releasing hormone (LHRH), and somatostatin (SRIF). It synthesizes melatonin from serotonin in a rhythmic fashion that fluctuates with the daily cycle of light. The pineal gland usually calcifies after the age of 16 years. This fact is used in the detection of midline shifts in skull x-rays. In normal skull x-rays, pineal calcifications are seen in the midline. Shifts of pineal calcification away from the midline suggest the presence of space-occupying lesions displacing the pineal. Such a lesion could be blood in the subdural or epidural space, a hematoma within the brain, or a brain tumor. Pineal gland tumors (pinealomas) depress gonadal function and delay the onset of puberty. In contrast, lesions that destroy the pineal gland may be associated with precocious onset of puberty, suggesting that the pineal gland exerts an inhibitory influence on gonadal function. Tumors in the region of the pineal gland usually interfere with vertical gaze. This loss of vertical gaze, known as *Parinaud's syndrome,* results from pressure of the pineal lesion on the pretectal area and/or the posterior commissure.

Pineal gland (Latin *pinea*, "a pine cone"). A small midline organ shaped like a pine cone.

Thalamus and Metathalamus

The term *thalamus* derives from a Greek word that means "inner chamber." Use of the terms *optic thalamus* and *chamber of vision* relates to the tracing, in the secondary century A.D., of optic nerve fibers to the thalamus by **Galen.** The prefix *optic* was dropped when it was discovered that sensory modalities other than vision are also processed in the thalamus.

Galen, Claudius (A.D. 130–200). Hellinistic physician who practiced mainly in Rome and Pergamon. He was the leading medical authority of the Christian world for 1400 years. The great cerebral vein is named after him.

The thalamus is the largest component of the diencephalon and is subdivided into the following major nuclear groups (Fig. 11-3) on the basis of their rostrocaudal and mediolateral location within the thalamus:

1. Anterior
2. Medial
3. Lateral
4. Intralaminar and reticular
5. Midline
6. Posterior

The thalamus is traversed by a band of myelinated fibers, the internal medullary lamina, which runs along the rostrocaudal extent of the thalamus. The internal

KEY CONCEPTS

- Based on their rostrocaudal and mediolateral location, thalamic nuclei are divided into the following groups: anterior, medial, lateral, intralaminar and reticular, midline, and posterior.

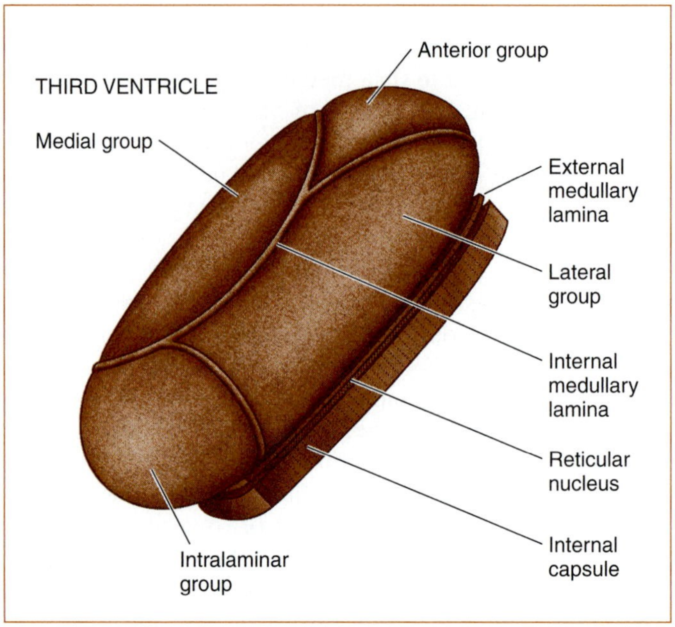

FIGURE 11-3

Schematic diagram showing the major nuclear groups of the thalamus.

medullary lamina separates the medial from the lateral group of nuclei. Rostrally and caudally, the internal medullary lamina splits to enclose the anterior and intralaminar nuclear groups, respectively. The internal medullary lamina contains intrathalamic fibers connecting the different nuclei of the thalamus with each other. Another medullated band, the external medullary lamina, forms the lateral boundary of the thalamus medial to the internal capsul. Between the external medullary lamina and the internal capsule is the reticular nucleus of the thalamus. The external medullary lamina contains nerve fibers leaving or entering the thalamus on their way to or from the adjacent capsule.

Anterior Nuclear Group

The anterior tubercle of the thalamus (dorsal surface of the most rostral part of the thalamus) is formed by the anterior nuclear group. In humans, the anterior nuclear group of thalamic nuclei consists of two nuclei: *principal anterior* and *anterodorsal.* The principal anterior nucleus of humans corresponds to the anteromedial and anteroventral nuclei of other species. The anterior group of thalamic nuclei has reciprocal connections (Fig. 11-4) with the hypothalamus (**mamillary bodies**) and the cerebral cortex (cingulate gyrus). The anterior group also receives significant input from the hippocampal formation of the cerebral cortex (subiculum and presubiculum) via the fornix.

Mamillary bodies (Latin diminutive of *mamma*, "breast, nipple"). A pair of small round swellings on the ventral surface of the hypothalamus mimicking the mammas.

The reciprocal fibers between the anterior thalamic nuclear group and the mamillary bodies travel via the mamillothalamic tract (tract of Vicq d'Azyr). The projections from the mamillary bodies to the anterior group of thalamic nuclei is topo-

KEY CONCEPTS

- The anterior group of thalamic nuclei have reciprocal connections with the mamillary bodies and cingulate gyrus. They belong to the modality-specific and limbic group of thalamic nuclei.

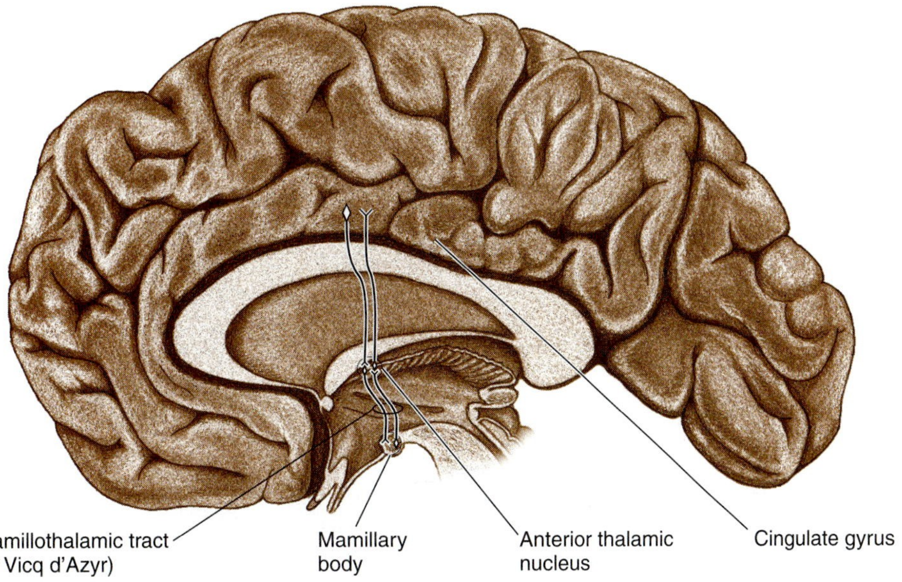

FIGURE 11-4

Schematic diagram showing the reciprocal connections among the anterior nucleus of the thalamus, mamillary body, and cingulate gyrus.

graphically organized such that the medial mamillary nucleus projects to the ipsilateral principal anterior nucleus, whereas the lateral mamillary nucleus projects to both anterodorsal nuclei. The reciprocal connections between the anterior nuclear group and the cingulate gyrus accompany the anterior limb of the internal capsule. The projection from the anterior thalamic group to the cingulate gyrus is topographically organized such that the medial part of the principal anterior nucleus projects to rostral parts of the cingulate gyrus, whereas the lateral part of the principal nucleus and the anterodorsal nucleus project to caudal parts of the cingulate gyrus. The anterior nuclear group of the thalamus is part of the limbic system, which is concerned with emotional behavior and memory mechanisms.

Medial Nuclear Group

Of the medial nuclear group, the *dorsomedial nucleus* is the most highly developed in humans. In histologic sections stained for cells, three divisions of the dorsomedial nucleus are recognized: a dorsomedial magnocellular division located rostrally, a dorsolateral parvicellular division located caudally, and a paralaminar division adjacent to the internal medullary lamina. The dorsomedial nucleus develops in parallel with and is reciprocally connected with the prefrontal cortex (areas 9, 10, 11, and 12) and the frontal eye fields (area 8) (Fig. 11-5). It also receives inputs from the temporal neocortex, amygdaloid nucleus, substantia nigra pars reticulata, and adjacent thalamic nuclei, particularly the lateral and intralaminar groups. The

KEY CONCEPTS

- The medial group of thalamic nuclei have reciprocal relationship with the prefrontal cortex. They belong to the multimodal associative group of thalamic nuclei and play a role in affective behavior, memory, and the integration of somatic visceral activities.

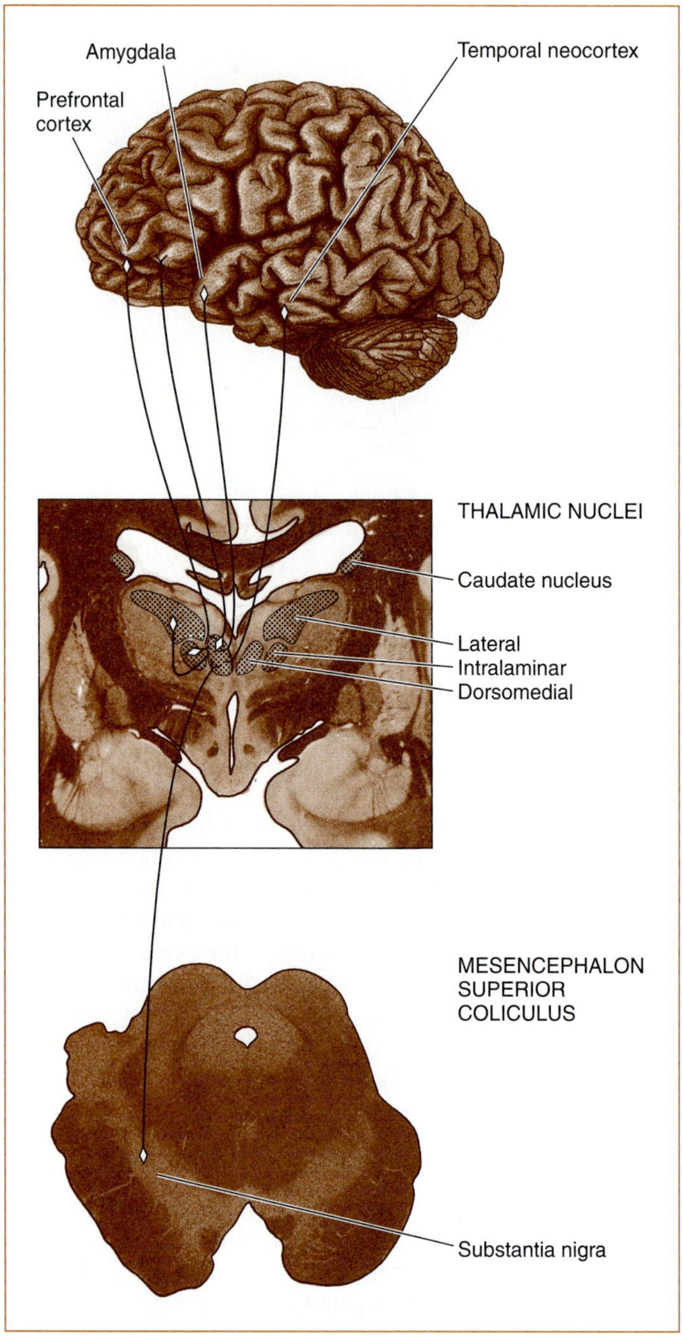
Amygdala
Temporal neocortex
Prefrontal cortex
THALAMIC NUCLEI
Caudate nucleus
Lateral
Intralaminar
Dorsomedial
MESENCEPHALON
SUPERIOR
COLICULUS
Substantia nigra

FIGURE 11-5

Schematic diagram showing the major afferent and efferent connections of the dorsomedial nucleus of the thalamus.

dorsomedial nucleus belongs to a neural system concerned with affective behavior, memory, and the integration of somatic and visceral activities. The reciprocal connections between the prefrontal cortex and the dorsomedial nucleus can be interrupted surgically to relieve severe anxiety states and other psychiatric disorders. This operation, known as *prefrontal lobotomy* (ablation of prefrontal cortex) or *prefrontal leukotomy* (severance of the prefrontal-dorsomedial nucleus pathway), is rarely practiced nowadays, having been replaced largely by medical treatment that achieves the same result without undesirable side effects.

Lateral Nuclear Group

The lateral nuclear group of the thalamus is subdivided into two groups, dorsal and ventral.

Dorsal Subgroup This subgroup includes, from rostral to caudal, the lateral dorsal, lateral posterior, and pulvinar nuclei. The *lateral dorsal nucleus*, although anatomically part of the dorsal tier of the lateral group of thalamic nuclei, is functionally part of the anterior group of thalamic nuclei, with which it collectively forms the *limbic thalamus.* Similar to the anterior group of thalamic nuclei, the lateral dorsal nucleus receives inputs from the hippocampus (via the fornix) and an uncertain input from the mamillary bodies and projects to the cingulate gyrus. In histologic sections stained for myelin, the lateral dorsal nucleus is characterized by a distinct capsule of myelinated fibers surrounding it.

The borderline between the *lateral posterior nucleus* and the **pulvinar** *nucleus* is vague, and the term *pulvinar–lateral posterior complex* has been used to refer to this nuclear complex.

Pulvinar (Latin, *pulvinar*, "a cushioned reclining seat"). The pulvinar nucleus is located in the posterior pole of the thalamus overhanging the superior colliculus and geniculate bodies.

The pulvinar–lateral posterior complex has reciprocal connections caudally with the lateral geniculate body and rostrally with the association areas of the parietal, temporal, and occipital cortices (Fig. 11-6). It also receives inputs from the pretectal area and superior colliculus. The pulvinar is thus a relay station between subcortical visual centers and their respective association cortices in the temporal, parietal, and occipital lobes. There is evidence that the pulvinar nucleus plays a role in speech mechanisms. Stimulation of the pulvinar nucleus of the dominant hemisphere has produced anomia (nominal aphasia). The pulvinar nucleus also has been shown to play a role in pain mechanisms. Lesions in the pulvinar nucleus have been effective in the treatment of intractable pain. Experimental studies have demonstrated connections between the pulvinar nucleus and several cortical and subcortical areas concerned with pain mechanisms.

The pulvinar–lateral posterior complex and the dorsomedial nucleus are known collectively as *multimodal association thalamic nuclei.* They all have the following in common:

1. They do not receive a direct input from the long ascending tracts.
2. Their input is mainly from other thalamic nuclei.
3. They project mainly to the association areas of the cortex.

Ventral Subgroup This subgroup includes the ventral anterior, ventral lateral, and ventral posterior nuclei. The neural connectivity and functions of this subgroup are

KEY CONCEPTS

- The lateral group of thalamic nuclei are divided into dorsal and ventral tiers (subgroups).
- The lateral dorsal nucleus belongs to the modality-specific and limbic nuclei of the thalamus. It is functionally part of the anterior group.
- The dorsal tier of the lateral group of thalamic nuclei includes the lateral dorsal, lateral posterior, and pulvinar nuclei.
- The pulvinar and lateral posterior nuclei form a single nuclear complex based on their anatomic connections and functions.
- The pulvinar–lateral posterior complex links subcortical visual areas with the association cortical visual areas. The pulvinar–lateral posterior complex belongs to the multimodal associative group of thalamic nuclei.
- The ventral tier of the lateral group of thalamic nuclei includes the ventral anterior, ventral lateral, and ventral posterior nuclei.

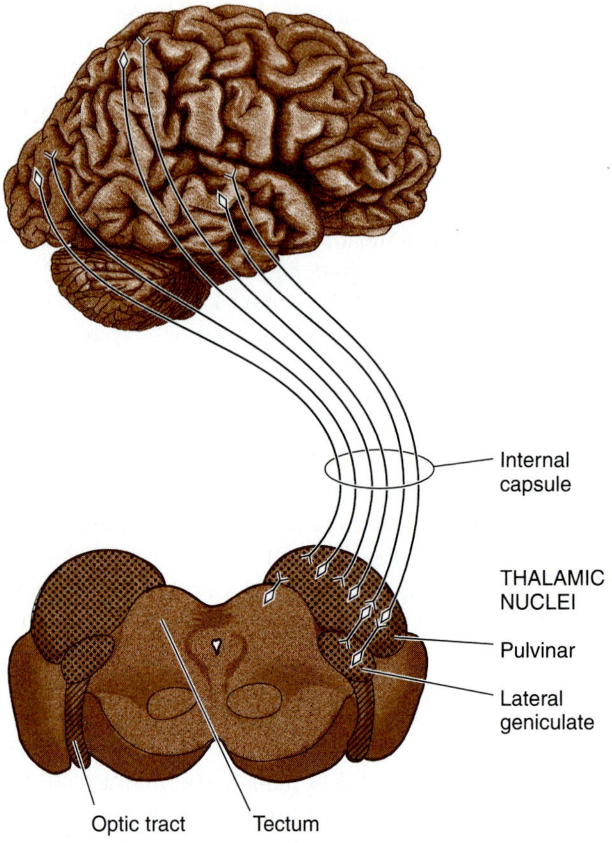
Internal
capsule
THALAMIC
NUCLEI
Pulvinar
Lateral
geniculate
Optic tract
Tectum

FIGURE 11-6

Schematic diagram showing the major afferent and efferent connections of the pulvinar.

much better understood than those of the dorsal subgroup. In contast to the dorsal subgroup, which belongs to the multimodal association thalamic nuclei, the ventral subgroup belongs to the modality-specific thalamic nuclei. These nuclei share the following characteristics:

1. They receive a direct input from the long ascending tracts.
2. They have reciprocal relationships with specific cortical areas.
3. They degenerate on ablation of the specific cortical area to which they project.

Ventral anterior nucleus This is the most rostrally placed of the ventral subgroup. It receives fibers from several sources (Fig. 11-7).

Global pallidus. A major input to this nucleus is from the globus pallidus. Fibers from the globus pallidus form the ansa and lenticular fasciculi and reach the nucleus via the thalamic fasciculus.

Substantia nigra, pars reticulata

Intralaminar thalamic nuclei

Premotor and prefrontal cortices (areas 6 and 8)

KEY CONCEPTS

- The ventral anterior nucleus links the basal ganglia and the cerebral cortex. It belongs to the modality-specific and motor groups of thalamic nuclei.

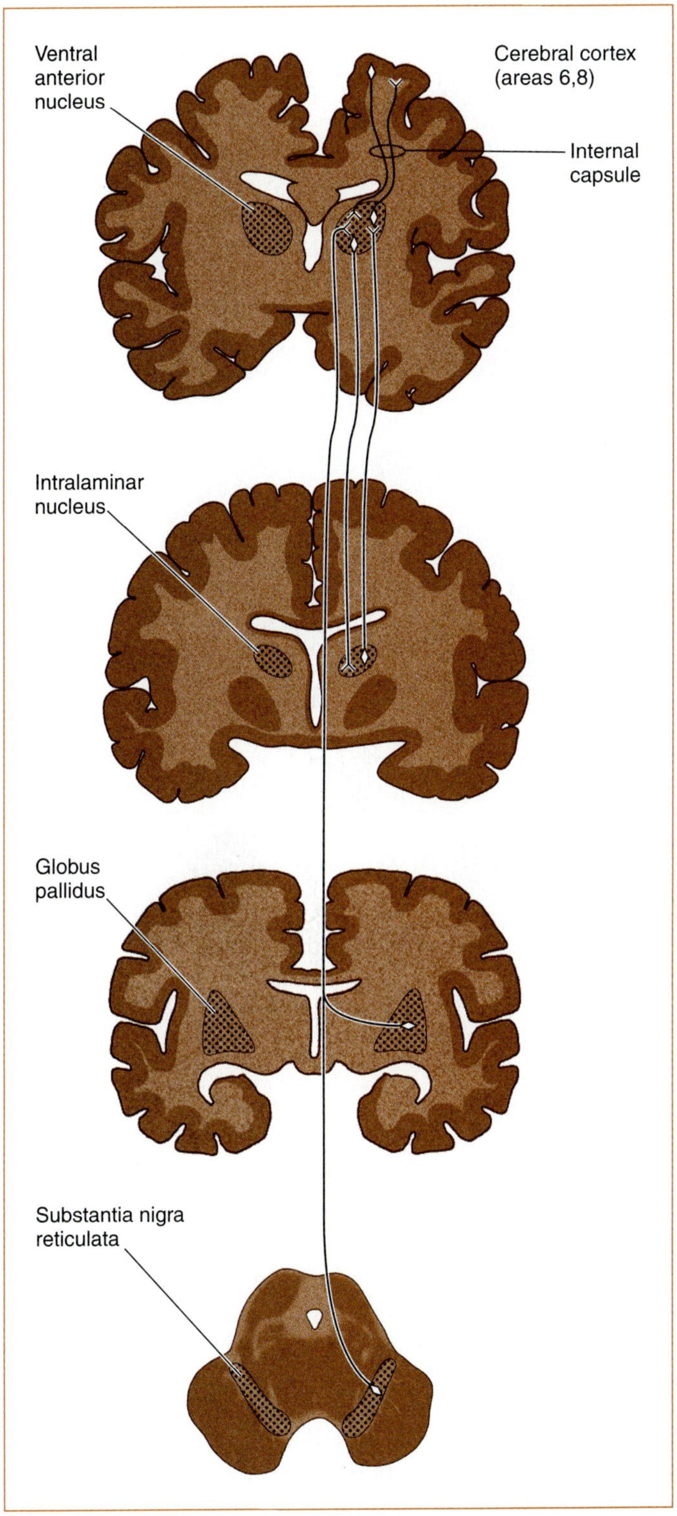
Ventral
anterior
nucleus
Cerebral cortex
(areas 6,8)
Internal
capsule
Intralaminar
nucleus
Globus
pallidus
Substantia nigra
reticulata

FIGURE 11-7

Schematic diagram showing the major connections of the ventral anterior nucleus of the thalamus.

The inputs from globus pallidus and substantia nigra are GABAergic inhibitory. The inputs from the cerebral cortex are excitatory.

The major output of the ventral anterior nucleus goes to the premotor cortices and to wide areas of the prefrontal cortex, including the frontal eye fields. It also

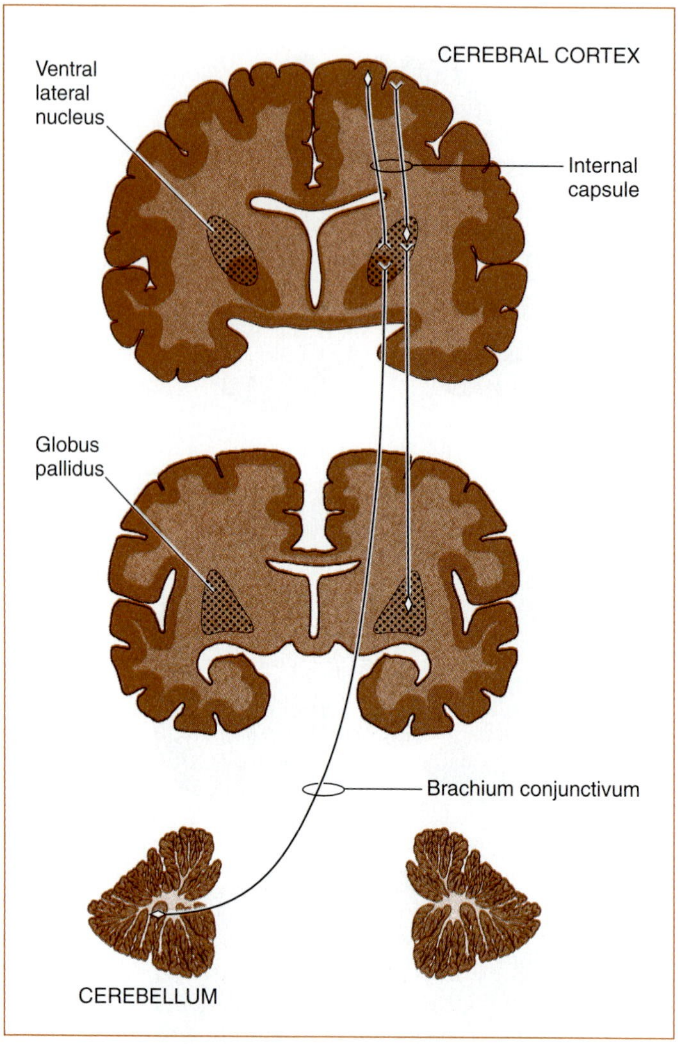
Ventral lateral nucleus
CEREBRAL CORTEX
Internal capsule
Globus pallidus
Brachium conjunctivum
CEREBELLUM

FIGURE 11-8

Schematic diagram showing the major afferent and efferent connections of the nucleus ventralis lateralis of the thalamus.

has reciprocal connections with the intralaminar nuclei. A cortical projection to the motor cortex has been described.

Thus the ventral anterior nucleus is a major relay station in the motor pathways from the basal ganglia to the cerebral cortex. As such, it is involved in the regulation of movement. The medial (magnocellular) part of the ventral anterior nucleus is concerned with control of voluntary eye, head, and neck movements. The lateral (parvicellular) part of the nucleus is concerned with control of body and limb movements. Lesions in this nucleus and adjacent areas of the thalamus have been placed surgically (thalamotomy) to relieve disorders of movement, especially parkinsonism.

Ventral lateral nucleus This nucleus is located caudal to the ventral anterior nucleus and, similar to the latter, plays a major role in motor integration. The ventral anterior and ventral lateral nuclei together comprise the motor thalamus. The afferent fibers to the ventral lateral nucleus come from the following sources (Fig. 11-8).

Deep cerebellar nuclei. The dentatothalamic system constitutes the major input to the ventral lateral nucleus. As detailed in Chap. 15, this fiber system originates

TABLE 11-1

Motor Thalamus Cell Population

Cell Type	Activation: Active Movement	Activation: Somatosensory Stimulation
Voluntary cells[a]	+	−
Sensory cells	−	+
Combined cells[b]	+	+
No-response cell	−	−

[a]Cells involved in parkinsonian tremor.
[b]Site of tremor-relieving lesion.

in the deep cerebellar nuclei (mainly dentate), leaves the cerebellum via the superior cerebellar peduncle, and decussates in the mesencephalon. Some fibers synapse in the red nucleus, while others bypass it to reach the thalamus.

Globus pallidus. Although the pallidothalamic fiber system projects primarily on ventral anterior neurons, some fibers reach the ventral lateral nucleus.

Primary motor cortex. There is a reciprocal relationship between the primary motor cortex (area 4) and the ventral lateral nucleus.

The efferent fibers of the ventral lateral nucleus go primarily to the primary motor cortex in the precentral gyrus. Other cortical targets include nonprimary somatosensory areas in the parietal cortex (areas 5 and 7) and the premotor and supplementary motor cortices. The parietal cortical targets play a role in decoding sensory stimuli that provide spatial information for targeted movements.

Thus the ventral lateral nucleus, like the ventral anterior nucleus, is a major relay station in the motor system linking the cerebellum, the basal ganglia, and the cerebral cortex. Deep cerebellar nuclei have been shown to project exclusively to ventral lateral thalamic nuclei, whereas the projection from the globus pallidus targets mainly the ventral anterior nucleus. Physiologic studies have shown that the cerebellar and pallidonigral projection zones in the thalamus are separate; very few cells have been identified that respond to both cerebellar and pallidonigral stimulation.

As in the case of the ventral anterior nucleus, lesions in the ventral lateral nucleus have been produced surgically to relieve disorders of movement manifested by tremor. Physiologic recordings during surgical procedures (thalamotomy) for relief of parkinsonian tremor have identified four types of neurons in the ventral thalamic nuclear group (Table 11-1): (1) cells with activity related to somatosensory stimulation (sensory cells), (2) cells with activity related to active movement (voluntary cells), (3) cells with activity related to both somatosensory stimulation and active movement (combined cells), and (4) cells with activity related to neither somatosensory stimulation nor active movement (no-response cells). Combined voluntary and no-response cells are located in the region of the thalamus, where a lesion will stop tremor, and anterior to the region, where sensory cells were found. These findings

KEY CONCEPTS

- The ventral lateral nucleus links the cerebellum with the cerebral cortex. It belongs to the modality-specific and motor groups of thalamic nuclei.

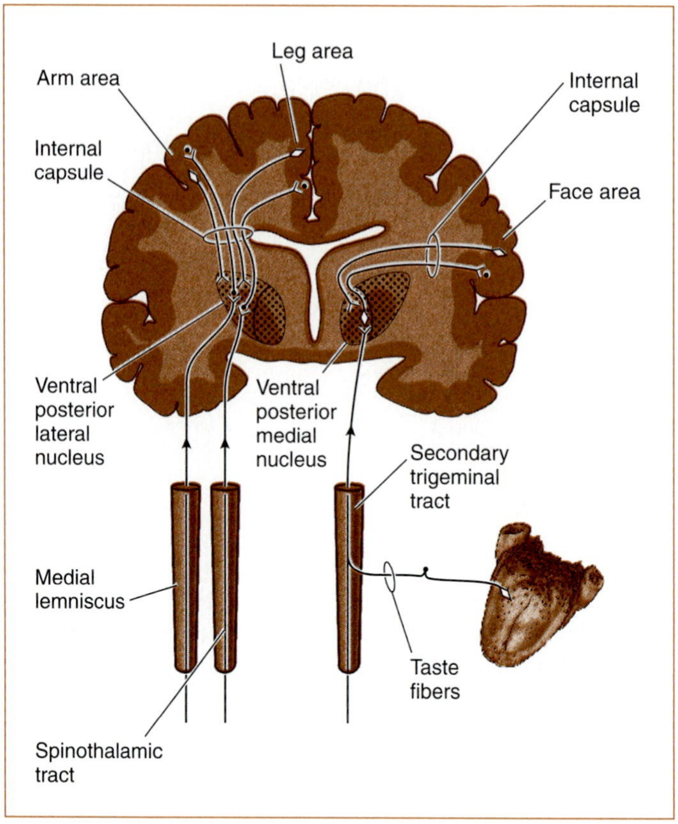

FIGURE 11-9

Schematic diagram showing the major afferent and efferent connections of the ventral posterior lateral and ventral posterior medial nuclei of the thalamus.

suggest that thalamic cells unresponsive to somatosensory stimulation (voluntary and no-response cells) and those responsive to somatosensory stimulation (combined cells) are involved in the mechanism of parkinsonian tremore. Activity in sensory cells lags behind tremor, while activity of combined cells leads the tremor.

Ventral posterior nucleus This nucleus is located in the caudal part of the thalamus. It receives the long ascending tracts conveying sensory modalities (including taste) from the contralateral half of the body and face. These tracts (Fig. 11-9) include the medial lemniscus, trigeminal lemniscus (secondary trigeminal tracts), and spinothalamic tract.

Vestibular information is relayed to the cortex via the ventral posterior as well as the intralaminar and posterior group of thalamic nuclei.

The ventral posterior nucleus is made up of two parts: the *ventral posterior medial (VPM) nucleus*, which receives the trigeminal lemniscus and taste fibers, and the *ventral posterior lateral (VPL) nucleus*, which receives the medial lemniscus and spinothalamic tracts. Both nuclei also receive input from the primary somatosensory cortex.

KEY CONCEPTS

- The ventral posterior nucleus belongs to the modality-specific and sensory groups of thalamic nuclei. It is subdivided into ventral posterior lateral and ventral posterior medial nuclei.

The output from both nuclei is to the primary somatosensory cortex (SI) in the postcentral gyrus (areas 1, 2, and 3). The projection to the cortex is somatotopically organized in such a way that fibers from the ventral posterior medial nucleus project to the face area, while different parts of the ventral posterior lateral nucleus project to corresponding areas of body representation in the cortex. A cortical projection from the part of the ventral posterior medial nucleus that receives taste fibers to the parietal operculum (area 43) has been demonstrated.

A group of cells located ventrally between the ventral posterior lateral and ventral posterior medial nuclei comprises the *ventral posterior inferior* (*VPI*) *nucleus.* Cells in this nucleus provide the major thalamic projection to somatosensory area II (SII).

The ventral posterior lateral and ventral posterior medial nuclei are collectively referred to as the *ventrobasal complex.*

Intralaminar, Midline, and Reticular Nuclei

The intralaminar nuclei, as their name suggests, are enclosed within the internal medullary lamina in the caudal thalamus. The reticular nuclei occupy a position between the external medullary lamina and the internal capsule (Fig. 11-3).

The intralaminar nuclei include several nuclei, of which the most important functionally, in humans, are the *centromedian* and *parafascicular nuclei.* Others, more rostrally located, include the *paracentral, centrolateral,* and *centromedial nuclei.* The intralaminar nuclei have the following afferent and efferent connections.

Afferent Connections (Fig. 11-10) Fibers projecting on the intralaminar nuclei come from the following sources.

Reticular formation of the brain stem This constitutes the major input to the intralaminar nuclei.

Cerebellum The dentatorubrothalamic system projects on the ventral lateral nucleus of the thalamus. Collaterals of this system project on the intralaminar nuclei.

Spinothalamic and Trigeminal Lemniscus Afferent fibers from the ascending pain pathways project largely on the ventral posterior nucleus but also on the intralaminar nuclei.

Globus pallidus Pallidothalamic fibers project mainly on the ventral anterior nucleus. Collaterals of this projection reach the intralaminar nuclei.

Cerebral cortex Cortical fibers arise primarily from the motor and premotor areas. Fibers originating in the motor cortex (area 4) terminate on neurons in the centromedian, paracentral, and centrolateral nuclei. Those originating from the premotor cortex (area 6) terminate on the parafascicular and centrolateral nuclei. In contrast to other thalamic nuclei, the connections between the intralaminar nuclei and cerebral cortex are not reciprocal.

KEY CONCEPTS

- The ventral posterior lateral nucleus links the somatosensory (medial lemniscus and spinothalamic) neural system from the contralateral half of the body with the somatosensory cortex.
- The ventral posterior medial nucleus links the somatosensory neural system from the contralateral face (trigeminothalamic) and taste system with the somatosensory cortex.

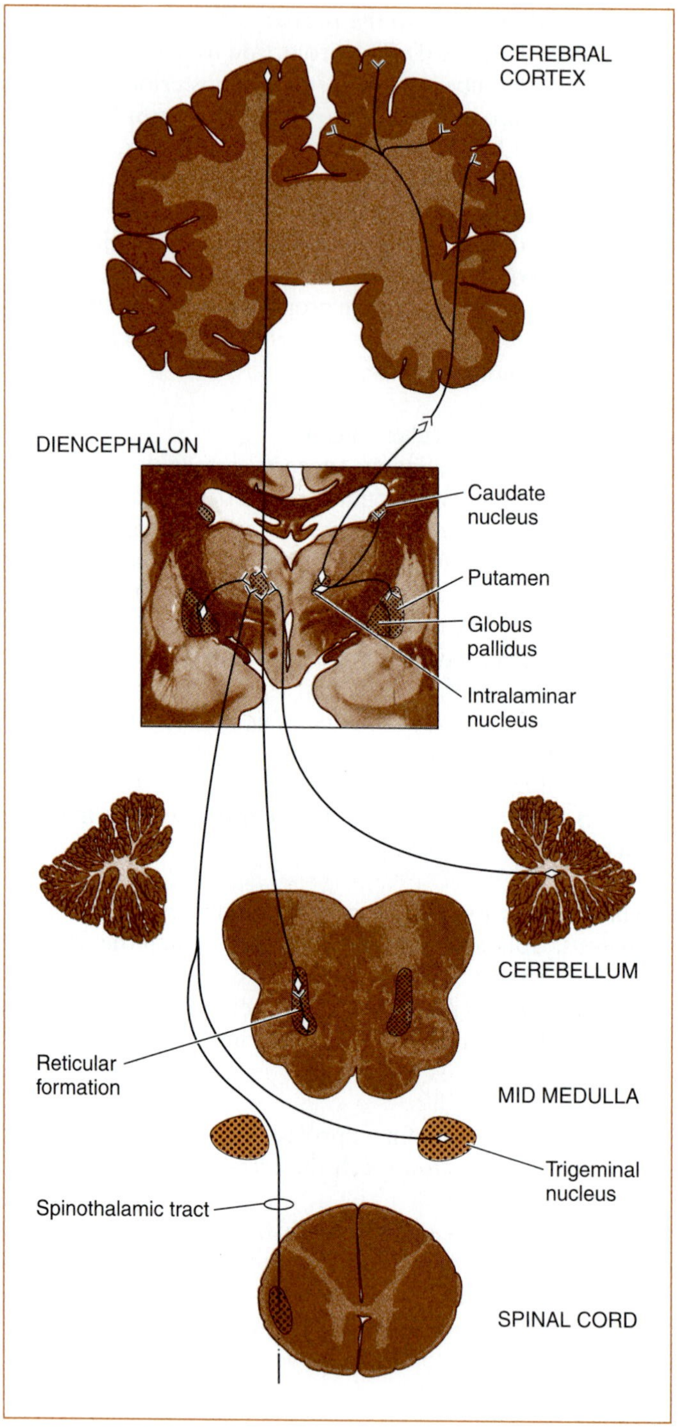
CEREBRAL CORTEX
DIENCEPHALON
Caudate nucleus
Putamen
Globus pallidus
Intralaminar nucleus
CEREBELLUM
Reticular formation
MID MEDULLA
Trigeminal nucleus
Spinothalamic tract
SPINAL CORD

FIGURE 11-10

Schematic diagram showing the major afferent and efferent connections of the intralaminar nuclei of the thalamus.

Other Connections Retrograde transport studies of horseradish peroxidase recently have identified afferent connections to the intralaminar nuclei from the vestibular nuclei, periaqueductal gray matter, superior colliculus, pretectum, and the locus ceruleus.

Efferent Connections The intralaminar nuclei project to the following structures.

Other thalamic nuclei The intralaminar nuclei influence cortical activity through other thalamic nuclei. There are no direct cortical connections for the intralaminar nuclei. One exception has been demonstrated recently, with both the horseradish peroxidase technique and autoradiography showing a direct projection from one of the intralaminar nuclei (centrolateral) to the primary visual cortex (area 17) in the cat. The significance of this finding is twofold. First, it shows that intralaminar nuclei, contrary to previous concepts, do project directly to cortical areas. Second, it explains the reported response of area 17 neurons to nonvisual stimuli (e.g., pinprick or sound); such responses would be mediated through the intralaminar nuclei.

The striatum (caudate and putamen) The striatal projection is topographically organized such that the centromedian nucleus projects to the putamen and the parafascicular nucleus to the caudate nucleus.

Midline Nuclei Consist of numerous cell groups, poorly developed in humans, located in the medial border of the thalamus along the banks of the third ventricle. They include the paraventral, central, and reunien nuclei. Their input includes projections from the hypothalamus, brain stem nuclei, amygdala, and parahippocampal gyrus. Their output is to the limbic cortex and ventral striatum. They have a role in emotion, memory, and autonomic function.

The intralaminar and midline nuclei comprise the *nonspecific thalamic nuclear group.*

Reticular Nuclei The *reticular nucleus* is a continuation of the reticular formation of the brain stem into the diencephalon. It receives inputs from the cerebral cortex and other thalamic nuclei. The former are collaterals of corticothalamic projections, and the latter are collaterals of thalamocortical projections. The reticular nucleus projects to other thalamic nuclei. The inhibitory neurotransmitter in this projection is GABA. The reticular nucleus is unique among thalamic nuclei in that its axons do not leave the thalamus. Based on its connections, the reticular nucleus plays a role in integrating and gating activities of thalamic nuclei.

Thus the intralaminar nuclei and reticular nucleus collectively receive fibers from several sources, motor and sensory, and project diffusely to the cerebral cortex (through other thalamic nuclei). Their multisource inputs and diffuse cortical projections enable them to play a role in the cortical arousal response. The intralaminar nuclei, by virtue of their basal ganglia connections, are also involved in motor control mechanisms, and by virtue of the input from ascending pain-mediating pathways, they are also involved in the awareness of painful sensory experience. The awareness of sensory experience in the intralaminar nuclei is poorly localized and has an emotional quality, in contrast to cortical awareness, which is well localized.

Metathalamus (Greek *meta*, "after"; *thalamos*, "inner chamber"). The metathalamus includes the lateral and medial geniculate bodies.

Geniculate (Latin *geniculare*, "to bend the knee"). Abrubtly bent, as in lateral and medial geniculate nuclei of the thalamus.

Metathalamus

The term **metathalamus** refers to two thalamic nuclei, the medial **geniculate** and lateral geniculate.

KEY CONCEPTS

- The intralaminar, reticular, and midline nuclei belong to the nonspecific system of thalamic nuclei. They are concerned with arousal, motor control, and the awareness of sensory experiences.
- The term *metathalamus* refers to the lateral and medial geniculate nuclei.

Medial Geniculate Nucleus This is a relay thalamic nucleus in the auditory system. It receives fibers from the lateral lemniscus directly or, more frequently, after a synapse in the inferior colliculus. These auditory fibers reach the medial geniculate body via the brachium of the inferior colliculus (inferior quadrigeminal brachium). The medial geniculate nucleus also receives feedback fibers from the primary auditory cortex in the temporal lobe. The efferent outflow from the medial geniculate nucleus forms the auditory radiation of the internal capsule (sublenticular part) to the primary auditory cortex in the temporal lobe (areas 41 and 42).

Lateral Geniculate Nucleus This is a relay thalamic nucleus in the visual system. It receives fibers from the optic tract conveying impulses from both retinae. The lateral geniculate nucleus is laminated, and the inflow from each retina projects on different laminae (ipsilateral retina to laminae II, III, and V; contralateral retina to laminae I, IV, and VI). Feedback fibers also reach the nucleus from the primary visual cortex (area 17) in the occipital lobes. The efferent outflow from the lateral geniculate nucleus forms the optic radiation of the internal capsule (retrolenticular part) to the primary visual cortex in the occipital lobe. Some of the efferent outflow projects to the pulvinar nucleus and to the secondary visual cortex (areas 18 and 19).

Posterior Thalamic Nuclear Group

This group embraces the caudal pole of the ventral posterior group of thalamic nuclei medial to the pulvinar nucleus and extends caudally to merge with the medial geniculate body and the gray matter medial to it. It receives inputs from all somatic ascending tracts (medial lemniscus and spinothalamic), as well as from the auditory pathways and possibly the visual pathways. Neurons in this part of the thalamus are multimodal and respond to a variety of stimuli. The outflow from the posterior group projects to the association cortices in the parietal, temporal, and occipital lobes. The posterior nuclear group is thus a convergence center for varied sensory modalities. It lacks the modal and spatial specificity of the classic ascending sensory systems but allows for interaction among the divergent sensory systems that project on it. Unlike the specific sensory thalamic nuclei, the posterior group does not receive reciprocal feedback connections from the cerebral cortex.

Nomenclature

There are several nomenclature systems for thalamic nuclei based on shared features of fiber connectivity and function. Two such nomenclature systems are used commonly. The first nomenclature system groups thalamic nuclei into three general categories: (1) modality-specific, (2) multimodal associative, and (3) nonspecific and reticular. The *modality-specific group* of nuclei shares the following features in common: (1) they receive direct inputs from long ascending tracts concerned with somatosensory, visual, and auditory information (ventral posterior lateral and

KEY CONCEPTS

- The medial geniculate nucleus is a relay station in the auditory pathway. It belongs to the modality-specific and sensory groups of thalamic nuclei.
- The lateral geniculate nucleus is a relay station in the visual pathway. It belongs to the modality-specific and sensory groups of nuclei.
- The posterior thalamic nucleus belongs to the multimodal associative group of thalamic nuclei. It is a convergence center for multimodal sensory modalities.
- Based on their neural connectivity, thalamic nuclei are grouped into the following categories: modality-specific, multimodal associative, nonspecific, and reticular.

medial, lateral geniculate, medial geniculate) or else process information derived from the basal ganglia (ventral anterior, ventral lateral), the cerebellum (ventral lateral), or the **limbic system** (anterior, lateral dorsal); (2) they have reciprocal connections with well-defined cortical areas (primary somatosensory, auditory, and visual areas, premotor and primary motor areas, cingulate gyrus); and (3) they undergo degeneration on ablation of the specific cortical area to which they project. The *multimodal associative group*, in contrast, receives no direct inputs from long ascending tracts and projects to association cortical areas in the frontal, parietal, and temporal lobes. These nuclei include the dorsomedial nucleus and the pulvinar–lateral posterior nuclear complex.

Limbic system (Latin "a border"). The limbic system exerts an important influence on the endocrine and autonomic systems. Its function also appears to affect motivational and mood states.

The *nonspecific and reticular group* of nuclei is characterized by diffuse and widespread indirect cortical projections and by inputs from the brain stem reticular formation. These nuclei include the intralaminal, midline, and reticular nuclei.

Low-frequency stimulation of the modality-specific thalamic nuclei result in a characteristic cortical response known as the *augmenting response.* This response consists of a primary excitatory postsynaptic potential (EPSP) followed by augmentation of the amplitude and latency of the primary EPSP recorded from the specific cortical area to which the modality-specific nucleus projects.

Stimulation of the nonspecific nuclear group, on the other hand, gives rise to the characteristic recruiting response in the cortex. This is a bilateral generalized cortical response (in contrast to the localized augmenting response) characterized by a predominantly surface-negative EPSP that increases in amplitude and, with continued stimulation, will wax and wane.

The other nomenclature system groups thalamic nuclei into the following categories: (1) motor, (2) sensory, (3) limbic, (4) associative, and (5) nonspecific and reticular. The *motor group* receives motor inputs from the basal ganglia (ventral anterior, ventral lateral) or the cerebellum (ventral lateral) and projects to the premotor and primary motor cortices. The *sensory group* receives inputs from ascending somatosensory (ventral posterior lateral and medial), auditory (medial geniculate), and visual (lateral geniculate) systems. The *limbic group* is related to limbic structures (mamillary bodies, hippocampus, cingulate gyrus). The *associative*

KEY CONCEPTS

- The modality-specific group of thalamic nuclei shares the following: (1) receive direct inputs from long ascending sensory tracts (somatosensory, visual, auditory) or process information from basal ganglia, cerebellum, or the limbic system; (2) have reciprocal connections with well-defined cortical areas; and (3) undergo degeneration upon ablation of the specific cortical area to which they project. Stimulation of the modality-specific group of nuclei elicits a cortical augmenting response.
- The multimodal associative group of thalamic nuclei receives no direct inputs from long ascending tracts and projects to association cortical areas.
- The nonspecific and reticular groups of thalamic nuclei receive inputs from the brain stem and reticular nuclei and have indirect and diffuse cortical projections. Stimulation of the nonspecific nuclear group elicits the cortical recruiting response.
- Based on their function, thalamic nuclei are grouped into the following categories: motor, sensory, and limbic.
- The motor group of thalamic nuclei links the basal ganglia and cerebellum with the premotor and motor cortices.
- The sensory group of thalamic nuclei links the subcortical somatosensory, visual, and auditory systems with their respective cortical areas.
- The limbic group of thalamic nuclei is related to limbic structures.

TABLE 11-2

Thalamus Nuclear Groups

	Modality Specific	Multimodal Associative	Nonspecific and Reticular
Motor			
Ventral anterior	X		
Ventral lateral	X		
Sensory			
Ventral posterior	X		
Lateral geniculate	X		
Medial geniculate	X		
Limbic			
Anterior	X		
Lateral dorsal	X		
Associative			
Dorsomedial		X	
Pulvinar		X	
Posterior		X	
Reticular/nonspecific			
Reticular			X
Intralaminar			X
Midline nuclei			X

and *nonspecific and reticular groups* correspond to the same groupings in the other nomenclature system. Table 11-2 combines the two nomenclature systems.

Neurotransmitters and Neuropeptides The following neurotransmitters have been identified in the thalamus: (1) gamma-aminobutyric acid (GABA) is the inhibitory neurotransmitter in terminals from the globus pallidus, in local circuit neurons, and in projection neurons of the reticular nucleus and lateral geniculate nucleus, and (2) glutamate and aspartate are the excitatory neurotransmitters in corticothalamic and cerebellar terminals and in thalamocortical projection neurons. Several neuropeptides have been identified in terminals of long ascending tracts. They include substance P, somatostatin, neuropeptide Y, enkephalin, and cholecystokinin.

KEY CONCEPTS

- Within the thalamus, gamma-aminobutyric acid (GABA) is the inhibitory neurotransmitter in terminals from the globus pallidus, reticular nucleus, and local circuit neurons. Glutamate and aspartate are the excitatory neurotransmitters in corticothalamic, cerebellothalamic, and thalamocortical terminals.

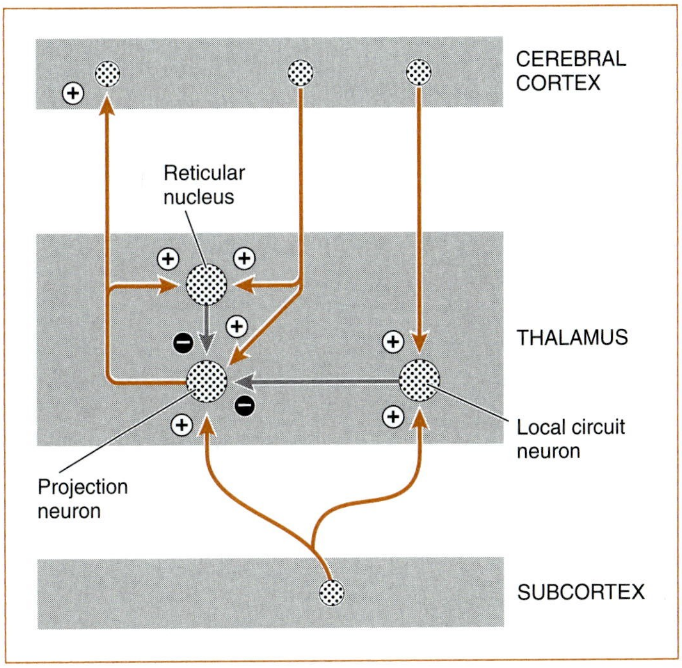

FIGURE 11-11

Schematic diagram showing neuronal circuitry within the thalamus.

Neuronal Circuitry

Thalamic nuclei contain two types of neurons. The predominant type is the principal (projection) neuron, whose axon projects on extrathalamic targets. The other neuron is the local-circuit interneuron. Inputs to thalamic nuclei from subcortical and cortical sites facilitate both the projection and local-circuit neurons, the neurotransmitter being glutamate or aspartate. An exception to this is the subcortical input from the basal ganglia, which is inhibitory GABAergic. The local-circuit neuron, in turn, inhibits the projection neuron. The neurotransmitter is GABA. Thus afferent inputs to the thalamus influence projection (thalamocortical) neurons via two pathways: a direct excitatory pathway and an indirect (via the local-circuit neuron) inhibitory pathway (Fig. 11-11). The local-circuit neuron thus modulates activity of the projection neuron. Projection neurons send their axons to the extrathalamic targets (cerebral cortex, striatum). Neurons in the reticular nucleus act like local-circuit neurons. They are facilitated by collaterals of corticothalamic and thalamocortical projections, and they, in turn, inhibit projection neurons by GABAergic transmission (Fig. 11-11).

Internal Capsule (Fig. 11-12)

The internal capsule is a broad, compact band of nerve fibers that are continuous rostrally with the corona radiata and caudally with the cerebral peduncles. It contains

KEY CONCEPTS

- Thalamic nuclei contain two types of neurons: principal (projection) and local circuit (interneuron).
- Principal neurons are facilitated by cortical and subcortical projection. The exception is the projection from the basal ganglia, which is inhibitory.
- Principal neurons are inhibited by projections from the local circuit neurons, the reticular nucleus, and the globus pallidus.

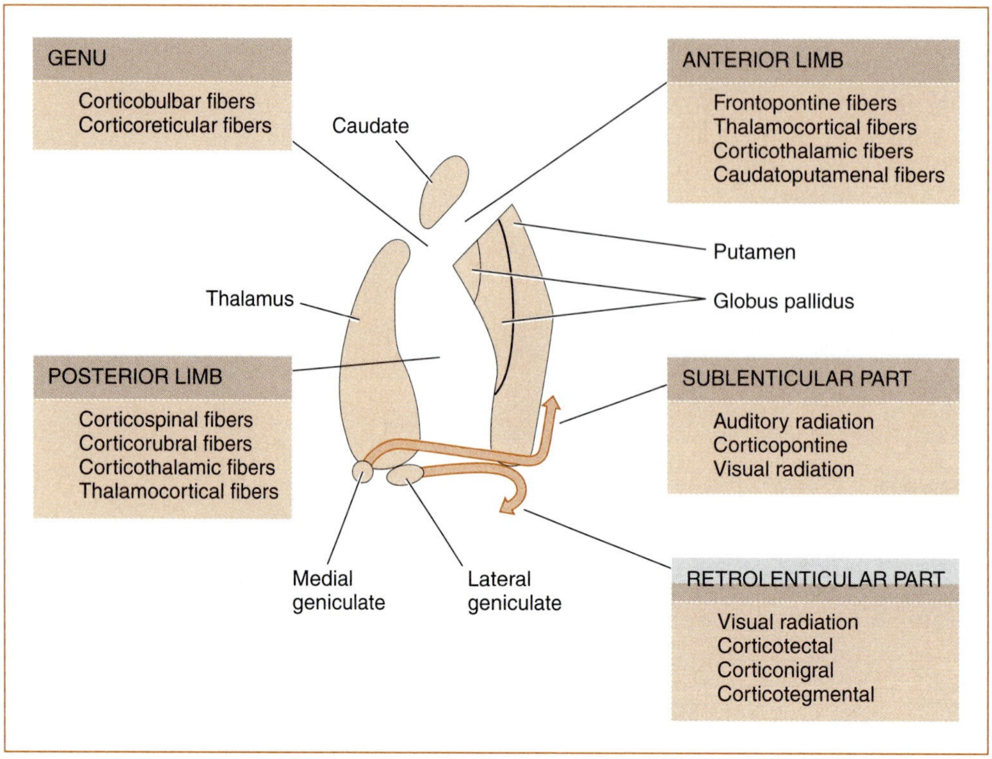
GENU
Corticobulbar fibers
Corticoreticular fibers
Caudate
ANTERIOR LIMB
Frontopontine fibers
Thalamocortical fibers
Corticothalamic fibers
Caudatoputamenal fibers
Putamen
Thalamus
Globus pallidus
POSTERIOR LIMB
Corticospinal fibers
Corticorubral fibers
Corticothalamic fibers
Thalamocortical fibers
SUBLENTICULAR PART
Auditory radiation
Corticopontine
Visual radiation
Medial geniculate
Lateral geniculate
RETROLENTICULAR PART
Visual radiation
Corticotectal
Corticonigral
Corticotegmental

FIGURE 11-12

Schematic diagram showing component parts of the internal capsule and the fiber bundles within each component.

Genu (Latin "knee"). A kneelike structure. The genu of the corpus callosum.

afferent and efferent nerve fibers passing to and from the brain stem to the cerebral cortex. In axial sections of the cerebral hemispheres, the internal capsule is bent with a lateral concavity to fit the wedge-shaped lentiform nucleus. It is divided into an anterior limb, **genu,** posterior limb, retrolenticular part, and sublenticular part.

The anterior limb is sandwiched between the head of the caudate nucleus medially and the lentiform nucleus (putamen and globus pallidus) laterally. It contains frontopontine, thalamocortical, and corticothalamic bundles; the latter two bundles reciprocally connect the dorsomedial and anterior thalamic nuclei with the prefrontal cortex and cingulate gyrus, respectively. Some investigators add the caudatoputamenal interconnections to components of the anterior limb.

The genu of the internal capsule contains corticobulbar fibers that terminate on motor nuclei of the brain stem. Evidence obtained from stimulation of the internal capsule during stereotaxic surgery and from vascular lesions of the internal capsule suggest, however, that corticobulbar fibers are located in the posterior third of the posterior limb rather than in the genu.

The posterior limb is bounded medially by the thalamus and laterally by the lentiform nucleus. It contains corticospinal and corticorubral fibers, as well as fibers that reciprocally connect the lateral group of thalamic nuclei (ventral lateral and ventral posterior) with the cerebral cortex. The corticospinal bundle is somatotopically organized in such a way that the fibers to the upper extremity are located more anteriorly, followed by fibers to the trunk and the lower extremity. Recent data suggest that the corticospinal fiber bundle is largely confined to the caudal

KEY CONCEPTS

- The internal capsule contains afferent and efferent fibers connecting the cerebral cortex and subcortical structures.

half of the posterior limb. The thalamocortical projections from the ventral lateral nucleus to the precentral gyrus (area 4) and from the ventral posterior nucleus to the postcentral gyrus (areas 1, 2, and 3) are segregated in the internal capsule. Small focal capsular lesions may selectively involve one of the two sites of these thalamocortical projections.

The retrolenticular part of the internal capsule contains corticotectal, corticonigral, and corticotegmental fibers, as well as part of the visual radiation. The sublenticular part of the internal capsule contains corticopontine fibers, the auditory radiation, and part of the visual radiation.

Because of the crowding of corticothalamic and thalamocortical fibers in the internal capsule, lesions in the capsule produce more widespread clinical signs than similar lesions elsewhere in the neuraxis. Vascular lesions in the posterior limb of the internal capsule are associated with contralateral hemiplegia and hemisensory loss. Lesions in the most posterior region will, in addition, be associated with contralateral visual loss (hemianopsia) and hearing deficit (hemi**hypacusis**). Lesions involving the genu of the internal capsule will be associated with cranial nerve signs.

Hypacusis (Greek *hypo*, "under, below"; *akousis*, "hearing"). Decreased hearing.

Blood Supply

Blood supply of the thalamus is derived from four parent vessels: basilar root of the posterior cerebral, posterior cerebral, posterior communicating, and internal carotid. The basilar root of the posterior cerebral artery, via paramedian branches, supplies the medial thalamic territory. The posterior cerebral artery, via its geniculothalamic branch, supplies the posterolateral thalamic territory. The posterior communicating artery, via the tuberothalamic branch, supplies the anterolateral thalamic territory. The internal carotid artery, via its anterior choroidal branch, supplies the lateral thalamic territory. Because different authors use different terminology to refer to the same vessel, accounts of blood supply of the thalamus may be confusing. Table 11-3 is a summary of blood supply of the thalamus and clinical manifestations of thalamic infarcts.

Functions

The function of the thalamus is to integrate sensory and motor activities. In addition, it has roles to play in arousal and consciousness, as well as in affective behavior and memory. In a sense, it is the gateway to the cortex.

The thalamus plays a central role in sensory integration. All somatic and special senses, except olfaction, pass through the thalamus before reaching the cerebral cortex. Sensory activity within the thalamus is channeled in one of three routes.

The first route is through the modality-specific sensory relay nuclei (medial geniculate, lateral geniculate, and ventral posterior). Sensations relayed in the modality-specific sensory relay nuclei have direct access to the respective sensory cortical areas. They are strictly organized with regard to topographic and modal specificities and are discriminative and well localized.

KEY CONCEPTS

- The internal capsule is divided into anterior limb, genu, posterior limb, and sublenticular and retrolenticular parts.
- Vascular lesions in the posterior limb of the internal capsule are associated with contralateral hemiplegia and hemisensory loss. Lesions that involve the visual and auditory radiations are in addition associated with contralateral visual loss and hearing deficit. Lesions that involve the genu are associated with cranial nerve signs.
- The thalamus receives its blood supply from four parent vessels: basilar, posterior cerebral, posterior communicating, and internal carotid.

TABLE 11-3

Blood Supply of Thalamus

Thalamic Territory	Blood Supply	Synonyms	Parent BV	Structures Supplied		Clinical Manifestations of Thalamic Infarcts
Posterolateral	Geniculothalamic	Posterolateral Thalamogeniculate	Posterior cerebral (PCA)	VPL, VPM, MG, pulvinar, CM, ±DM, PL, ret, Pf, LG (primary sensory nuclei)	*Complete:* (Dejerine-Roussy syndrome)	(Concomitant PCA infarction) **Pansensory loss (clinical hallmark)** (Pure hemisensory loss) Dysthesia Hemiparesis Visual field defect Choreiform movements Hemispatial neglect (with associated PCA infarct)
					Partial:	↓ Pain and touch in part of body (face, arm, leg) Occasional dysarthria Visual field defect No hemiparesis Visual perceptual defect (with associated PCA infarct)
Anterolateral	Tuberothalamic	Polar Anterior internal optic Premamillary pedicle	Posterior communicating	VA, VL, DM, AV		Facial paresis for emotional movement Hemiparesis Visual field defect (PCA infarct) Sensory loss rarely **Severe neuropsychologic inpairment** (L) Speech, intellect, language, memory (R) Visuospatial

Medial	Paramedian	Posteromedial Deep interpeduncular profunda Posterior internal optica Thalamoperforating	Basilar root of posterior cerebral	CM, Pf, DM (bilateral or unilateral), CP ±VL, AV, VPL, VPM	**Drowsiness** Vertical gaze paresis Memory, attention, intellect defects Hemiparesis occasionally No sensory deficit
Lateral	Anterior choroidal	—	Internal carotid	IC (posterior limb), GP, amygdala, optic tract, lateral thalamus (LG, VPL, pul, ret), medial temporal lobe	**Hemiparesis** Sensory loss for pain and touch **Dysarthria** Visual field defect, occasionally Neuropsychologic defect (L) Memory, (R) visuospatial Pure motor hemiparesis
Posterior	Posterior choroidal	—	Posterior cerebral	LG, pul, DL ±DM, AV, ±hippocampus, ±rostral midbrain	Homonymous quadrantaposia Hemisensory dysfunction (hemihypesthesia) Neuropsychological disturbances (memory, transcortical aphasia) +Hemiparesis ±Choreoathetosis

NOTE: AV, anterior ventral; CM, centromedian; CP, cerebral peduncle; DM, dorsomedial; GP, globus pallidus; IC, internal capsule; LG, lateral geniculate; MG, medial geniculate; PCA, posterior cerebral artery; PL, posterior lateral; Pf, parafascicular; Pul, pulvinar; Ret, reticular; VA, ventral anterior; VL, ventral lateral; VPL, ventral posterior lateral; VPM, ventral posterior medial; L, left; R, right.

The second route is through the nonspecific nuclei. With its many sources of input and diffuse projections to the cortex, this route serves the low extreme of the modality-specificity gradient.

The third route is through the posterior nuclear group. This route receives from multiple sensory sources and projects to the association cortical areas. It plays an intermediate role between the modality-specific and nonspecific routes described above.

Some sensory modalities are perceived at the thalamic level and are not affected by ablation of the sensory cortex. Following sensory cortical lesions, all sensory modalities are lost, but soon pain, thermal sense, and crude touch return. The sense of pain that returns is the aching, burning type of pain that is carried by C-fibers. It is this type of pain that is believed to terminate in the thalamus, whereas the pricking, well-localized pain carried by the A-fibers terminates in the sensory cortex and is lost with its ablation. In patients with intractable pain, placement of a surgical lesion in the ventral posterior and/or intralaminar nuclei (centromedian) may provide relief. Vascular lesions of the thalamus result in a characteristic clinical syndrome known as the *thalamic syndrome.* Following an initial period of loss of all sensations contralateral to the thalamic lesion, pain, thermal sense, and some crude touch return. However, the threshold of stimulation that elicits these sensations is elevated, and the sensations are exaggerated and unpleasant when perceived. The syndrome is usually associated with a marked affective response attributed to the intact dorsomedial nucleus, usually unaffected by the vascular lesion.

The role of the thalamus in motor control is evident from the input it receives from the cerebellum, basal ganglia, and motor areas of the cortex. A tremorogenic center has been postulated for the ventral lateral nucleus. Lesions have been placed in the ventral lateral nucleus to relieve abnormal movement resulting from cerebellar and basal ganglia disorders.

The thalamus, as part of the ascending reticular activating system, has a central role in the conscious state and attention. The role of the thalamus as essential for arousal and wakefulness has been challenged recently, in part by the recognition that the cerebral cortex can be activated directly by cholinergic, serotonergic, noradrenergic, and histaminergic arousal systems that originate in brain stem, basal forebrain, or hypothalamus and do not pass through the thalamus.

The connections of the medial thalamus with the prefrontal cortex reflect its role in affective behavior. Ablation of the prefrontal cortex or its connections with the dorsomedial nucleus causes changes in personality characterized by lack of drive, flat affect, and indifference to pain.

The connections of the anterior thalamic nuclei with the hypothalamus and cingulate gyrus enable them to play a role in memory, visceral function, and emotional behavior. Other thalamic nuclei have been implicated singly or in combination in memory mechanisms. They include the dorsomedial nucleus and the midline nuclei. Two distinct types of memory impairment (amnesia) have been associated with diencephalic lesions: (1) severe amnesia associated with damage to the mamillary bodies, midline thalamic nuclei, mamillothalamic tract, and/or dorsomedial thalamic nucleus, characterized by encoding defects that never approximate normal performance, and (2) milder memory deficit associated with lesions in the intralaminar and medial thalamic nuclei, characterized by severe distractibility.

KEY CONCEPTS

- The thalamus is the gateway to the cortex. It plays roles in arousal and consciousness, affective behavior, and memory. It also integrates sensory and motor activities.
- Vascular lesions in the thalamus are associated with a characteristic pain syndrome, the thalamic syndrome.

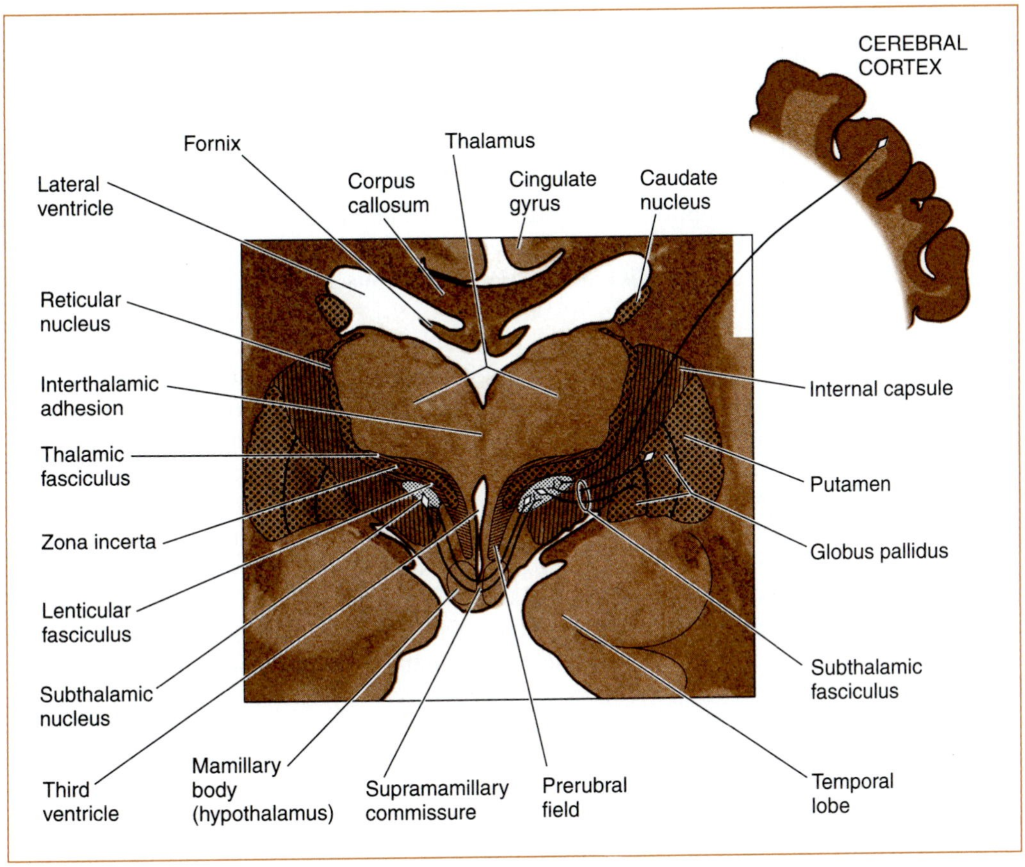

FIGURE 11-13

Schematic diagram of the subthalamic region showing its component parts, and the major afferent and efferent connections of the subthalamic nucleus.

Subthalamus

The subthalamus is a mass of gray and white substance in the caudal diencephalon. it is bordered medially by the hypothalamus, laterally by the internal capsule, dorsally by the thalamus, and ventrally by the internal capsule. The subthalamus consists of three main structures; these are the subthalamic nucleus, the fields of Forel, and the zona incerta.

Subthalamus (Latin *sub*, "under"; Greek *thalamos*, "inner chamber"). Region of the diencephalon beneath the thalamus.

Subthalamic Nucleus (Fig. 11-13)
The subthalamic nucleus (of **Luys**) is a biconvex gray mass that replaces the substantia nigra in caudal diencephalic levels. The subthalamic nucleus receives a massive GABAergic (inhibitory) input from the external segment of globus pallidus and a glutamatergic (excitatory) input from the cerebral cortex (areas 4 and 6). The input from the globus pallidus travels in the subthalamic fasciculus, whereas the input from the cerebral cortex travels in the internal capsule. Other inputs include those from the thalamus (primarily from the intralaminar nuclei) and the brain stem reticular formation. The two subthalamic nuclei communicate via the supramamillary commissure. Recent studies have shown that projections to the subthalamic

Luys, Jules Bernard (1828–1895). French clinical neurologist who described the subthalamic nucleus (nucleus of Luys).

KEY CONCEPTS

- The subthalamus includes the subthalamic nucleus, the fields of Forel, and the zone incerta.

nucleus are arranged in distinct sensorimotor, associative, and limbic territories similar to those reported for other basal ganglionic nuclei. The output from the subthalamic nucleus is to both segments of the globus pallidus and to the substantia nigra pars reticulata. The neurotransmitter in both these projections is glutamate (excitatory). It has been shown that the projections to the external and internal segments of the globus pallidus arise from different subthalamic neurons.

Interruption of the subthalamopallidal pathways or the subthalamic nucleus is responsible for the involuntary violent hyperkinesia of the contralateral upper and lower extremities known as **hemiballismus**. Facial and neck muscles may be involved.

Hemiballismus (Greek *hemi*, "half"; *ballismos*, "jumping about"). Violent flinging involuntary movements of one side of the body due to a lesion in the contralateral subthalamic nucleus.

Fields of Forel (Fig. 11-13)

This term refers to fiber bundles containing pallidal and cerebellar efferents to the thalamus. Efferent pallidal fibers that course across the internal capsule gather dorsal to the subthalamic nucleus to form the lenticular fasciculus or H_2 field of Forel. Dentatorubrothalamic fibers gather in the caudal diencephalon in a bundle known as the *prerubral field* or *H field of Forel*, which also contains pallidothalamic fibers. Both the prerubral field fibers and the lenticular fasciculus contribute to the thalamic fasciculus or H_1 field of Forel, which enters the ventral lateral and ventral anterior nuclei of the thalamus. The fields of Forel are named after **August Forel,** the Swiss psychiatrist, neurologist, and anatomist who is best remembered for his anatomic studies on the basal ganglia and subthalamic region. The H is from the German word *Haube,* meaning "a cap" or "hood."

Forel, August Henri (1848–1931). Swiss neuropsychiatrist who described the fiber bundles of the subthalamus (H fields of Forel).

Zona Incerta

The **zona incerta** (Fig. 11-13) is the rostral continuation of the mesencephalic reticular formation that extends laterally into the reticular nucleus of the thalamus. It is sandwiched between the lenticular fasciculus and the thalamic fasciculus. The neural connectivity of the zona incerta is not well delineated. It receives fibers from the precentral cortex (area 4). Lesions have been placed in the zona incerta to relieve abnormal movement. The zona incerta also has been implicated in drinking behavior.

"Zona incerta (Latin *zona*, "zone, belt"; *incerta*, "in between"). A rostral extension of the brain stem reticular formation into the subthalamus. Inserted between the lenticular and thalamic fasciculi.

KEY CONCEPTS

- Lesions of the subthalamic nucleus or of the subthalamopallidal pathways are associated with contralateral hemiballismus.
- The H-fields of Forel contain pallidal and cerebellar efferents to the thalamus.
- The zona incerta is a continuation of the brain stem reticular formation. It has been implicated in drinking behavior.

SUGGESTED READINGS

Bertrand G: Stimulation during stereotactic operation for dyskinesia. *J Neurosurg* 1996; 24:419–423.

Blum PS, et al: Thalamic components of the ascending vestibular system. *Exp Neurol* 1979; 64:587–603.

Carpenter MB, et al: Interconnections and organization of pallidal and subthalamic nucleus neurons in the monkey. *J Comp Neurol* 1981; 197:579–603.

Carpenter MB, et al: Connections of the subthalamic nucleus in the monkey. *Brain Res* 1981; 224:1–29.

Cramon DY, et al: A contribution to the anatomical basis of thalamic amnesia. *Brain* 1985; 108:993–1008.

Donnan GA, et al: A prospective study of lacunar infarction using computerized tomography. *Neurology* 1982; 32:49–56.

Englander RN, et al: Location of human pyramidal tract in the internal capsule: Anatomic evidence. *Neurology* 1975; 25:823–826.

Goldman PS: Contralateral projections to the dorsal

thalamus from frontal association cortex in the rhesus monkey. *Brain Res* 1979; 166:166–171.

Graff-Radford NR, et al: Nonhaemorrhagic thalamic infarction: Clinical, neuropsychological and electrophysiological findings in four anatomical groups defined by computerized tomography. *Brain* 1985; 108:485–516.

Groothuis DR, et al: The human thalamocortical sensory path in the internal capsule: Evidence from a small capsular hemorrhage causing a pure sensory stroke. *Ann Neurol* 1977; 2:328–331.

Hanaway J, et al: Localization of the pyramidal tract in the internal capsule. *Neurology* 1981; 31:365–366.

Hartman-von Monakow R, et al: Projections of the precentral motor cortex and other cortical areas of the frontal lobe to the subthalamic nucleus in the monkey. *Exp Brain Res* 1978; 33:395–403.

Hendry SHC, et al: Thalamic relay nuclei for cerebellar and certain related fiber systems in the cat. *J Comp Neurol* 1979; 185:679–714.

Hirai T, Jones EG: A new parcellation of the human thalamus on the basis of histochemical staining. *Brain Res Rev* 1989; 14:1–34.

Hirayama K, et al: The representation of the pyramidal tract in the internal capsule and basis pedunculi: A study based on three cases of amyotrophic lateral sclerosis. *Neurology* 1962; 12:337–342.

Ilinsky IA, Kultas-Ilinsky K: An autoradiographic study of topographical relationships between pallidal and cerebellar projections to the cat thalamus. *Exp Brain Res* 1984; 54:95–106.

Ilinsky IA, et al: quantitative evaluation of crossed and uncrossed projections from basal ganglia and cerebellum to the cat thalamus. *Neuroscience* 1987; 21:207–227.

Kultas-Ilinsky K, et al: A description of the GABAergic neurons and axon terminals in the motor nuclei of the cat thalamus. *J Neurosci* 1985; 5:1346–1369.

Lenz FA, et al: Single unit analysis of the human ventral thalamic nuclear group: Tremor-related activity in functionally identified cells. *Brain* 1994; 117:531–543.

Madarasz M, et al: A combined horseradish peroxidase and Golgi study on the afferent connections of the ventrobasal complex of the thalamus in the cat. *Cell Tissue Res* 1979; 199:529–538.

McGuiness CM, Krauthamer GM: The afferent projections to the centrum medianum of the cat as demonstrated by retrograde transport of horseradish peroxidase. *Brain Res* 1980; 184:255–269.

Mennemeir M, et al: Contributions of the left intraluminar and medial thalamic nuclei to memory: Comparisons and report of a case. *Arch Neurol* 1992; 49:1050–1058.

Miller JW, Benevento LA: Demonstration of a direct projection from the intralaminar central lateral nucleus to the primary visual cortex. *Neurosci Lett* 1979; 14:229–234.

Nauta HJW, Cole M: Efferent projections of the subthalamic nucleus: An autoradiographic study in monkey and cat. *J Comp Neurol* 1978; 180:1–16.

Nomura S, et al: Topographical arrangement of thalamic neurons projecting to the orbital gyrus in the cat. *Exp Neurol* 1980; 67:601–610.

Royce GJ: Cells of origin of subcortical afferents to the caudate nucleus: A horseradish peroxidase study in the cat. *Brain Res* 1978; 153:465–475.

Sandson TA, et al: Frontal lobe dysfunction following infarction of the left-sided medial thalamus. *Arch Neurol* 1991; 48:1300–1303.

Schell GR, Strick PL: The origin of thalamic inputs to the arcuate premotor and supplementary motor areas. *J Neurosci* 1984; 4:539–560.

Smith Y, et al: Efferent projections of the subthalamic nucleus in the squirrel monkey as studied by the PHA-L anterograde tracing method. *J Comp Neurol* 1990; 294:306–323.

Tekian A, Afifi AK: Efferent connections of the pulvinar nucleus in the cat. *J Anat* 1981; 132:249–265.

C H A P T E R 12

DIENCEPHALON: CLINICAL CORRELATES

CLINICAL CORRELATES OF THALAMIC ANATOMY

A multiplicity of neurologic signs and symptoms has been reported in disorders of the **thalamus**. These reflect (1) the anatomic and functional heterogeneity of the thalamus, (2) simultaneous involvement of several nuclei even by discrete vascular **lesions** due to the fact that arterial vascular territories in the thalamus cross nuclear boundaries, and (3) simultaneous involvement of neighboring areas such as the midbrain in paramedian thalamic vascular lesions, the internal capsule in lateral thalamic vascular lesions, and the subthalamus in posterior thalamic vascular lesions.

The conglomerate of signs and symptoms associated with thalamic lesions includes the following: sensory disturbances, thalamic pain, hemiparesis, dyskinesias, disturbances of consciousness, memory disturbances, affective disturbances, and disorders of language.

Correlation of signs and symptoms with affected thalamic territory is best with vascular lesions (infarcts) of the thalamus (Table 12-1). Clinicoanatomic correlation

Thalamus (Greek *thalamos*, "inner chamber", especially "bridal chamber"). The name was given by Galen to "chambers" at the base of the brain that were thought to supply animal spirits to the optic nerves.

Lesion (Lesion *laesum*, "hurt or wounded"). The term is applied to an abnormality that may destroy tissue, as in infarction, hemorrhage, or tumor, or stimulate tissue, as in epilepsy.

KEY CONCEPTS

- Variability in the clinical picture of thalamic lesions is accounted for by the anatomic and functional heterogeneity of the thalamus, overlap of vascular territories, and involvement of extrathalamic structures.

TABLE 12-1

Blood Supply of Thalamus

Thalamic Territory	Blood Supply	Synonyms	Parent BV	Structures Supplied		Clinical Manifestations of Thalamic Infarcts
Posterolateral	Geniculothalamic	Posterolateral Thalamogeniculate	Posterior cerebral (PCA)	VPL, VPM, MG, pulvinar, CM, ±DM, PL, ret, Pf, LG (primary sensory nuclei)	*Complete:* (Dejerine-Roussy syndrome)	(Concommitant PCA infarction) **Pansensory loss (clinical hallmark)** (Pure hemisensory loss) Dysthesia Hemiparesis Visual field defect Choreiform movements Hemispatial neglect (with associated PCA infarct)
					Partial:	↓ Pain and touch in part of body (face, arm, leg) Occasional dysarthria Visual field defect No hemiparesis Visual perceptual defect (with associated PCA infarct)
Anterolateral	Tuberothalamic	Polar Anterior internal optic Premamillary pedicle	Posterior communicating	VA, VL, DM, AV		Facial paresis for emotional movements Hemiparesis Visual field defect (PCA infarct) Sensory loss rarely **Severe neuropsychological inpairment** (L) Speech, intellect, language, memory (R) Visuospatial

Medial	Paramedian	Posteromedial Deep interpeduncular profunda Posterior internal optic Thalamoperforating	Basilar root of posterior cerebral	CM, Pf, DM (bilateral or unilateral), CP ±VL, AV, VPL, VPM	**Drowsiness** Vertical gaze paresis Memory, attention, intellect defects Hemiparesis occasionally No sensory deficit
Lateral	Anterior choroidal	—	Internal carotid	IC (posterior limb), GP, amygdala, optic tract, lateral thalamus, (LG, VPL, pul, ret) medial temporal lobe	**Hemiparesis** Sensory loss for pain and touch **Dysarthria** Visual field defect, occasionally Neuropsychological defect, (L) memory, (R) visuospatial Pure motor hemiparesis
Posterior	Posterior choroidal	—	Posterior cerebral	LG, pul, DL, ±DM, AV, ±hippocampus ±rostral midbrain	Homonymous quadrantaposia Hemisensory dysfunction (hemihypesthesia) Neuropsychological disturbances (memory, transcortical aphasia) ±Hemiparesis ±Choreoathetosis

NOTE: AV, anterior ventral; CM, centromedian; CP, cerebral peduncle; DM, dorsomedial; GP, globus pallidus; IC, internal capsule; LG, lateral geniculate; MG, medial geniculate; PCA, posterior cerebral artery; PL, posterior lateral; Pf, parafascicular; Pul, pulvinar; Ret, reticular; VA, ventral anterior; VL, ventral lateral; VPL, ventral posterior lateral; VPM, ventral posterior medial; L, left; R, right.

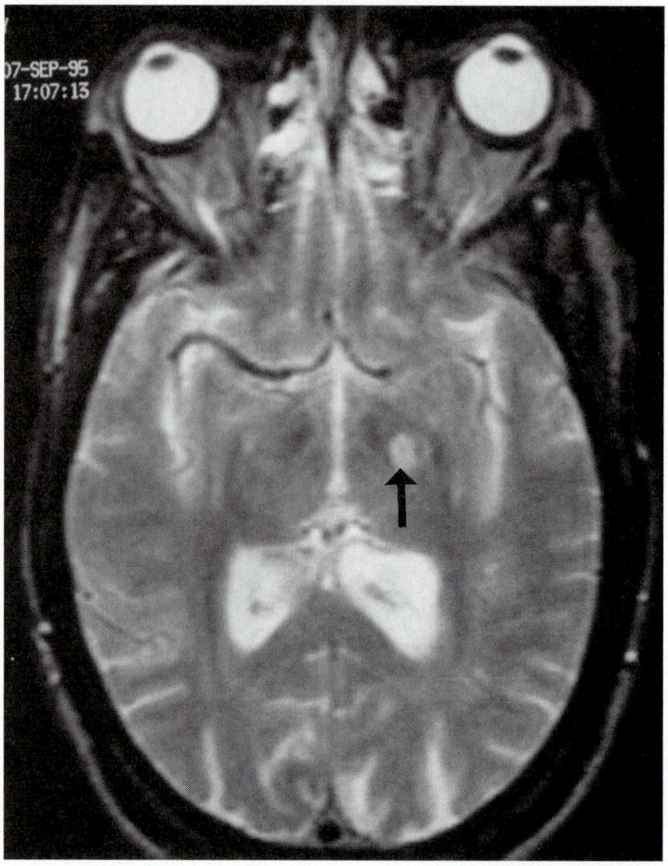

FIGURE 12-1

T2-weighted axial magnetic resonance image (MRI) showing an infarct (*arrow*) in the posterolateral thalamic territory.

in patients with occlusion of thalamic arteries has been greatly facilitated by neuroimaging methods (computed tomography and magnetic resonance imaging). The different vascular territories of the thalamus and associated neurologic signs and symptoms are outlined below.

THALAMIC INFARCTS

Posterolateral Thalamic Territory

(Fig. 12-1)

Infarction (Latin *infarcire*, "to stuff into"). Vascular occlusion leading to death of tissue.

Infarcts in this thalamic territory are due to occlusion of the geniculothalamic (thalamogeniculate, posterolateral) artery, a branch of the posterior cerebral artery. Thalamic structures involved by the infarct are the primary sensory thalamic nuclei, which include the ventral posterior lateral, ventral posterior medial, medial genicu-

KEY CONCEPTS

- Thalamic lesions are associated with one or more of the following: sensory deficits, thalamic pain, motor deficits, and disturbances in consciousness, memory, behavior, and language.

late, pulvinar, and centromedian nuclei. Other nuclei that are inconsistently involved include the dorsomedial, posterior lateral, **reticular,** parafascicular, and lateral geniculate nuclei. The clinical hallmark of posterolateral thalamic territory infarcts is a pansensory loss **contralateral** to the lesion, **paresthesia,** and thalamic pain. In addition, one or more of the following may occur: transient hemiparesis, homonymous **hemianopsia,** hemi**ataxia,** tremor, choreiform movements, and spatial neglect, all contralateral to the lesion in the thalamus. An athetoid posture of the contralateral hand (thalamic hand) may appear 2 or more weeks following lesions in this territory. The hand is flexed and pronated at the wrist and metacarpophalangeal joints and extended at the interphalangeal joints. The fingers may be abducted. The thumb is either abducted or pushed against the palm. The conglomerate of signs and symptoms associated with posterolateral thalamic territory infarcts comprises the *thalamic syndrome of Dejerine and Roussy.* In this **syndrome,** severe, persistent, paroxysmal, and often intolerable pain (thalamic pain) resistant to analgesic medications occurs at the time of injury or following a period of transient hemiparesis, hemiataxia, choreiform movements, and hemisensory loss. Cutaneous stimuli trigger paroxysmal exacerbations of the pain that outlast the stimulus. Because the perception of "epicritic" pain (from a pinprick) is reduced on the painful areas, this symptom is known as *anesthesia dolorosa,* or *painful anesthesia.* The syndrome is named after Joseph-Jules Dejerine, a French neurologist, and his assistant, Gustave Roussy, a Swiss-French neuropathologist. The etiology of the thalamic pain syndrome is not clear but may be the result of alterations in frequencies and patterns of inputs to the thalamus, qualities of injured neurons, or changes in quality of output to the cortex.

Reticular (Latin *reticularis,* "resembling a net"). Reticular formation of the brain stem is a network of neurons and nerve fibers.

Contralateral (Latin *contra,* "opposite"; *lateris,* "of a side"). Of the other side of the body.

Paresthesia (Greek *para,* "beside, near, beyond"; *aisthesis,* "perception"). Distorted sensation, tingling, "pins and needles."

Hemianopsia (Greek *hemi,* "half"; *an,* "negative"; *opsis,* "vision"). Defect of half the field of vision.

Ataxia (Greek *a,* "without"; *taxis,* "order"). Loss of muscle coordination with irregularity of movement.

Syndrome (Greek *syndromos,* "a running together, combining"). A group of co-occuring symptoms and signs that characterize a disease.

Anterolateral Thalamic Territory

Infarcts in the anterolateral territory of the thalamus are usually secondary to occlusion of the tuberothalamic branch of the posterior communicating artery. Synonyms for this branch include the *polar, anterior internal optic,* and *premamillary pedicle.* Thalamic nuclei involved in the infarct include the ventral anterior, ventral lateral, dorsomedial, and anterior. The clinical manifestations include contralateral hemiparesis, visual field defects, facial paresis with emotional stimulation, and rarely, hemisensory loss. Severe, usually transient neuropsychological impairments predominate in lesions in this thalamic territory. **Abulia,** lack of spontaneity and initiative, and reduced quantity of speech are the predominant findings. Other impairments consist of defects in intellect, language, and memory in left-sided lesions and visuospatial deficits in right-sided lesions.

Abulia (Greek *a,* "without"; *boulé,* "will"). A state in which the patient manifests lack of initiative and spontaneity with preserved consciousness.

Medial Thalamic Territory (Fig. 12-2)

Infarcts in the medial territory of the thalamus are associated with occlusion of the paramedian branches of the basilar root of the posterior cerebral artery. These branches include the posteromedial, deep interpeduncular profunda, posterior internal optic, and thalamoperforating. The thalamic nuclei involved include the intralaminar (centromedian, parafascicular) and dorsomedial, either unilaterally or bilat-

KEY CONCEPTS

- Posterolateral (thalamogeniculate) thalamic territory lesions are characterized by pansensory loss associated with thalamic pain, the Dejerine-Roussy syndrome.
- Anterolateral (tuberothalamic) thalamic territory lesions are characterized by neuropsychological impairment.

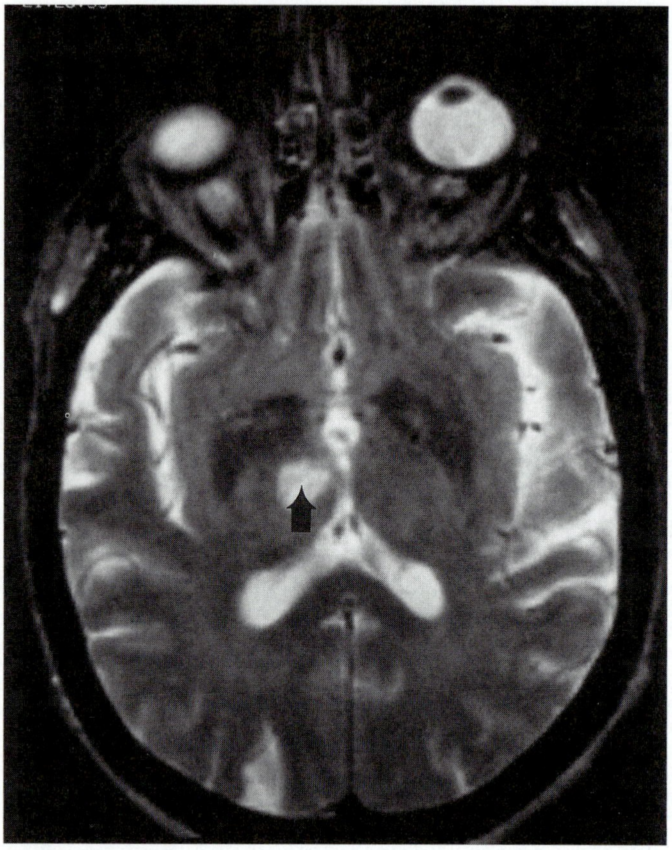

FIGURE 12-2

T2-weighted axial magnetic resonance image (MRI) showing an infarct (*arrow*) in the medial thalamic territory.

erally. The paramedian territory of the midbrain is often involved by the lesion. The following nuclei are inconsistently involved: the ventral lateral, anterior, and ventral posterior. The hallmark of the clinical picture is drowsiness. In addition, there are abnormalities in recent memory, attention, intellect, vertical gaze, and occasionally, mild hemiparesis or hemiataxia. No sensory deficits are as a rule associated with lesions in this territory. Utilization behavior (instrumentally correct but highly exaggerated response to environmental cues and objects) that is characteristic of frontal lobe damage has been reported in medial thalamic territory infarcts.

Two syndromes also have been reported in medial thalamic territory infarcts: akinetic mutism and the Kleine-Levin syndrome. In akinetic mutism (persistent

KEY CONCEPTS

- Medial (paramedian) thalamic territory lesions are characterized by alteration in state of consciousness. Akinetic mutism and the Kleine-Levin syndrome occur with lesions in this thalamic territory.

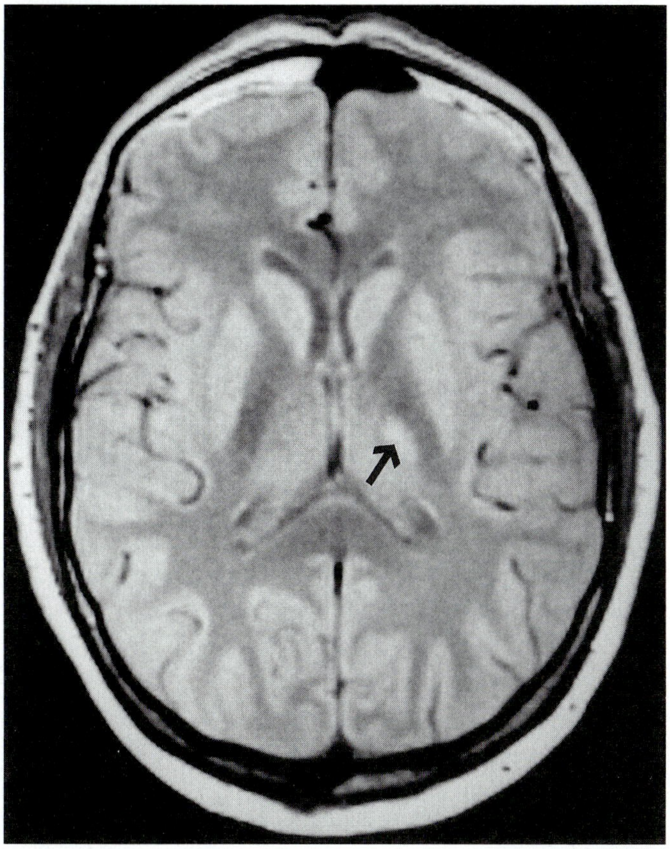

FIGURE 12-3

Proton density magnetic resonance image (MRI) showing an infarct (*arrow*) in the lateral thalamic territory.

vegetative state), patients appear awake and maintain a sleep-wake cycle but are unable to communicate in any way. In addition to thalamic infarcts, akinetic mutism has been reported to occur with lesions in the basal ganglia, anterior cingulate gyrus, and pons. The Kleine-Levin syndrome (hypersomnia-bulimia syndrome) is characterized by recurrent periods (lasting 1 to 2 weeks every 3 to 6 months) in adolescent males of excessive somnolence, hyperphagia (compulsive eating), hypersexual behavior (sexual disinhibition), and impaired recent memory. A confusional state, hallucinosis, irritability, or a schizophreniform state may occur around the time of the attacks. The syndrome was first reported by Antimoff in 1898 but more fully by Kleine in 1925 in German and by Levin 4 years later in English.

Lateral Thalamic Territory (Fig. 12-3)

Infarcts in the lateral territory of the thalamus are associated with occlusion of the anterior choroidal branch of the internal carotid artery. Structures involved in the lesion include the posterior limb of the internal capsule, lateral thalamic nuclei (lateral geniculate, ventral posterior lateral, pulvinar, reticular), and medial temporal lobe. The clinical hallmarks of the infarct are contralateral hemiparesis and **dysarthria.** Lesions in the lateral thalamic territory may manifest with only pure motor hemiparesis. Other clinical manifestations include hemisensory loss of pain

Dysarthria (Greek *dys*, "difficult"; *arthroun*, "to articulate"). Difficulty in speaking.

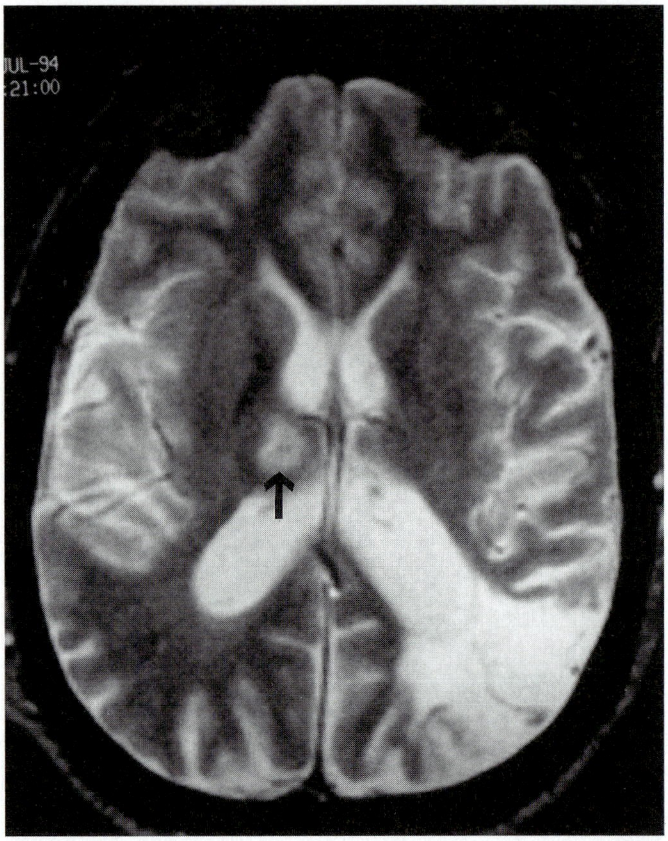

FIGURE 12-4

T2-weighted magnetic resonance image (MRI) showing an infarct (*arrow*) in the posterior thalamic territory.

and touch, occasional visual field defects, and neuropsychological defects. The latter consist of memory defects in left-sided lesions and visuospatial defects in right-sided lesions.

Posterior Thalamic Territory (Fig. 12-4)

Infarcts in the posterior thalamic territory are associated with occlusion of the posterior choroidal branch of the posterior cerebral artery. Thalamic nuclei involved include the lateral geniculate, pulvinar, and dorsolateral nuclei. The following structures are inconsistently involved in the lesion: dorsomedial and anterior thalamic nuclei, hippocampus, and rostral midbrain. Clinical manifestations include contralateral homonymous quadrantanopsia and hemihypesthesia, as well as neuropsycho-

KEY CONCEPTS

- Lateral (anterior choroidal) thalamic territory lesions are characterized by hemiparesis and dysarthria.

TABLE 12-2

Thalamic Pain Syndromes Subtypes

Type	Central Pain	Vibration, Touch, Joint	Pain, Temperature	Somatosensory Evoked Potentials (SSEPs)
I (analgetic)	Absent	Lost	Lost	Absent
II	Present	Lost	Present	Absent
III	Present	Present	Present	Reduced
IV (pure algetic)	Present	Present	Present	Normal

logical deficits, including memory defects and transcortical **aphasia.** Inconsistent signs include contralateral hemiparesis and choreoathetosis.

Aphasia (Greek *a*, "without"; *phasis*, "speech"). Defect in communication by language.

Thalamic Pain Syndromes

Four types of pain syndromes have been described in association with thalamic lesions (Table 12-2). The four types are differentiated from each other on the basis of the presence or absence in each of central (thalamic) pain, **proprioceptive** sensations (vibration, touch, joint), **exteroceptive** sensations (pain and temperature), and abnormalities in somatosensory evoked potentials.

In type I (analgetic type), central pain is absent, both proprioceptive and exteroceptive sensations are lost, and no somatosensory evoked potentials are elicitable. In type II, both central pain and exteroceptive sensations are present, whereas proprioceptive sensations are lost and somatosensory evoked potentials are absent. In type III, central pain as well as proprioceptive and exteroceptive sensations are present, whereas somatosensory evoked potentials are reduced in amplitude. In type IV (pure algetic), central pain is present, proprioceptive and exteroceptive sensations are unimpaired, and somatosensory evoked potentials are normal.

Proprioceptor (Latin *proprius*, "one's own"; *receptor*, "receiver"). Sensory endings in muscles, tendons, and joints that provide information about movement and position of body parts.

Exteroceptor (Latin *exterus*, "external"; *receptor*, "receiver"). Sensory receptor that serves to acquaint the individual with the external environment. Includes pain and temperature receptors.

Memory Deficits

Discrete lesions of the thalamus can cause severe and lasting memory deficits. Although it remains uncertain which thalamic structures are critical for memory, evidence from human and animal research suggests that one or more of the following structures are important: anterior nuclei, midline and intralaminar nuclei, dorso-

KEY CONCEPTS

- Posterior (posterior choroidal) thalamic territory lesions are characterized by hemisensory dysfunction and visual field defects.
- Four types of thalamic pain syndromes have been described based on the presence or absence of each of thalamic pain, proprioceptive and exteroceptive sensations, and abnormalities in somatosensory evoked potentials.

Diencephalon (Greek *dia*, "between"; *enkephalos*, "brain"). The part of the brain between the telencephalon and midbrain. It includes the epithalamus, thalamus, subthalamus, and hypothalamus.

Mamillary bodies (Latin diminutive of *mamma*, "little breast, nipple"). A pair of small round swellings on the ventral surface of the hypothalamus.

medial nucleus, mamillothalamic tract, and amygdalofugal tract. There are three distinct behavioral and anatomic types of memory impairment associated with **diencephalic** lesions: (1) Severe encoding defects are associated with lesions in the **mamillary bodies,** mamillothalamic tracts, midline thalamic nuclei, and the dorsomedial nucleus. Performance of such patients never approximates normal memory. (2) A milder form of memory deficit characterized by severe distractibility occurs in lesions of the intralaminar and medial thalamic nuclei. (3) Disturbances in verbal memory (retrieval, registration, and retention) occur in lesions of the left thalamus that include the ventrolateral and intralaminar nuclei and the mamillothalamic tract. Memory disturbances, which may be transient or permanent, are most common with bilateral thalamic lesions but do occur with unilateral lesions of either side.

Thalamus and Arousal

The essential role of the thalamus as the sole mechanism for cortical arousal has been challenged. It is now acknowledged that cortical activation is mediated by two mechanisms: (1) an indirect mechanism, via the thalamus, comprised of the ascending reticular activating system (ARAS), and (2) a direct mechanism (nonthalamic), via cholinergic, serotonergic, noradrenergic, and histaminergic arousal systems that originate in the brain stem, basal forebrain, or hypothalamus and do not pass through the thalamus.

The Cheiro-Oral Syndrome

This syndrome consists of sensory disturbances confined to one hand and to the ipsilateral mouth region. It is associated with focal lesions in the ventral posterior thalamic nucleus. A similar syndrome has been reported with lesions in the somatosensory cortex, border of the posterior limb of the internal capsule and corona radiata, midbrain, and pons. The involvement of the hand and mouth areas suggests that the sensory representation of these two areas is contiguous not only in the primary somatosensory cortex but also elsewhere in the neuraxis.

Language Deficits

Dominant hemisphere thalamic lesions may cause a transient deficit in language characterized by (1) reduction in spontaneous speech, (2) perseveration, (3) paraphasic errors, (4) impaired auditory comprehension, (5) impaired spontaneous writing and writing to dictation, and (6) word-production anomia.

KEY CONCEPTS

- Encoding memory defects, severe distractibility, and verbal memory disturbances have been described in thalamic lesions.
- The thalamus is one (indirect) of two mechanisms for cortical activation. The other (direct) mechanism is via cholinergic, serotonergic, noradrenergic, and histaminergic nonthalamic, systems.
- The cheiro-oral syndrome is not unique to the thalamus. It has been reported with lesions in cortical and subcortical sites.
- Language deficits occur with dominant thalamic lesions and are transient.

CLINICAL CORRELATES OF SUBTHALAMIC ANATOMY

Hemiballismus

Lesions in the subthalamic nucleus or in the pallidosubthalamic system are associated with violent, involuntary, flinging, ballistic movements of the contralateral half of the body. The abnormal movement involves primarily the extremities; the head and neck also may be involved.

Hemiballismus (Greek *hemi*, "half"; *ballismos*, "jumping about"). Violent flinging movement of one side of the body due to a lesion in the contralateral subthalamic nucleus.

KEY CONCEPTS

- A violent dyskinesia (hemiballismus) occurs with lesions in the subthalamic nucleus or its connections with globus pallidus.

SUGGESTED READINGS

Beric A: Central pain: "New" syndromes and their evaluation. *Muscle Nerve* 1993; 16:1017–1024.

Biller J, et al: Syndrome of the paramedian thalamic arteries: Clinical and neuroimaging correlation. *J Clin Neuro-Ophthalmol* 1985; 5:217–223.

Bogousslavsky J, et al: Thalamic infarcts: Clinical syndromes, etiology, and prognosis. *Neurology* 1988; 38:837–848.

Bogousslavsky J, et al: Loss of psychic self-activation with bithalamic infarction: Neurobehavioral, CT, MRI, and SPECT correlates. *Acta Neurol Scand* 1991; 83:309–316.

Caplan LR: "Top of the basilar" syndrome. *Neurology* 1980; 30:72–79.

Castaigne P, et al: Paramedian thalamic and midbrain infarcts: Clinical and neuropathological study. *Ann Neurol* 1981; 10:127–148.

Eslinger PJ, et al: "Frontal lobe" utilization behavior associated with paramedian thalamic infarction. *Neurology* 1991; 41:450–452.

Gentilini M, et al: Bilateral paramedian thalamic artery infarcts: Report of eight cases. *J Neurol Neurosurg Psychiatry* 1987; 50:900–909.

Graff-Radford NR, et al: Nonhemorrhagic thalamic infarction. *Brain* 1985; 108:485–516.

Guberman A, Stuss D: The syndrome of bilateral paramedian thalamic infarction. *Neurology* 1983; 33:540–545.

Isono O, et al: Cheiro-oral topography of sensory disturbances due to lesions of thalamocortical projections. *Neurology* 1993; 43:51–55.

Kinney HC, et al: Neuropathological findings in the brain of Karen Ann Quinlan: The role of the thalamus in the persistent vegetative state. *N Engl J Med* 1994; 330:1469–1475.

Mauguiere F, Desmedt JE: Thalamic pain syndrome of Dejerine-Roussy: Differentiation of four subtypes assisted by somatosensory evoked potentials data. *Arch Neurol* 1988; 45:1312–1320.

Mennemeier M, et al: Contributions of the left intralaminar and medial thalamic nuclei to memory. *Arch Neurol* 1992; 49:1050–1058.

Miwa H, et al: Thalamic tremor: Case reports and implications of the tremor-generating mechanism. *Neurology* 1996; 46:75–79.

Mori E, et al: Left thalamic infarction and disturbances of verbal memory: A clinicoanatomical study with a new method of computed tomographic stereotaxic lesion localization. *Ann Neurol* 1986; 20:671–676.

Nea JP, Bogousslavsky J: The syndrome of posterior choroidal artery territory infarction. *Ann Neurol* 1996; 39:779–788.

Reilly M, et al: Bilateral paramedian thalamic infarction: A distinct but poorly recognized stroke syndrome. *Q J Med* 1992; 29:63–70.

Wallesch CW, et al: Neuropsychological deficits associated with small unilateral thalamic lesions. *Brain* 1983; 106:141–152.

C H A P T E R 13

THE BASAL GANGLIA

The neural control of movement is the product of interactions within and among a number of cortical and subcortical neural structures (Fig. 13-1). Among the various subcortical structures, three are of particular significance. They are the basal ganglia, cerebellum, and the dopaminergic mesencephalic system. Whereas lesions in the motor cortex result in loss of movement, such as occurs in stroke, lesions in the basal ganglia or cerebellum result in incoordinated and disorganized movement, such as occurs in parkinsonism and Huntington's chorea. Recent experimental studies and clinical observations have focused on a new role for the basal ganglia in nonmotor functions, including cognition and behavior.

DEFINITION AND NOMENCLATURE

The term *basal ganglia* refers to the following nuclei: caudate, putamen, globus pallidus, nucleus accumbens septi, and olfactory tubercle (Table 13-1).

The term **corpus striatum** refers to the caudate, putamen, and globus pallidus. The terms *striatum, dorsal striatum,* and *neostriatum* refer to the caudate and putamen. The terms **pallidum** and **paleostriatum** refer to globus pallidus. The putamen and globus pallidus together compose the **lentiform nucleus.** The term *ventral striatum* refers to the ventral parts of caudate and putamen, the nucleus accumbens

Corpus striatum (Latin *corpus,* "body"; *striatus,* "striped"). Gray matter comprising caudate, putamen, and globus pallidus with striped appearance produced by myelinated fibers traversing the gray matter.

Pallidum (Latin *pallidus,* "pale"). The paler part of the basal ganglia comprises the globus pallidus.

Paleostriatum (Greek *palaios,* "ancient"; Latin *striatus,* "striped"). The phylogenetically older part of the corpus striatum comprises the globus pallidus.

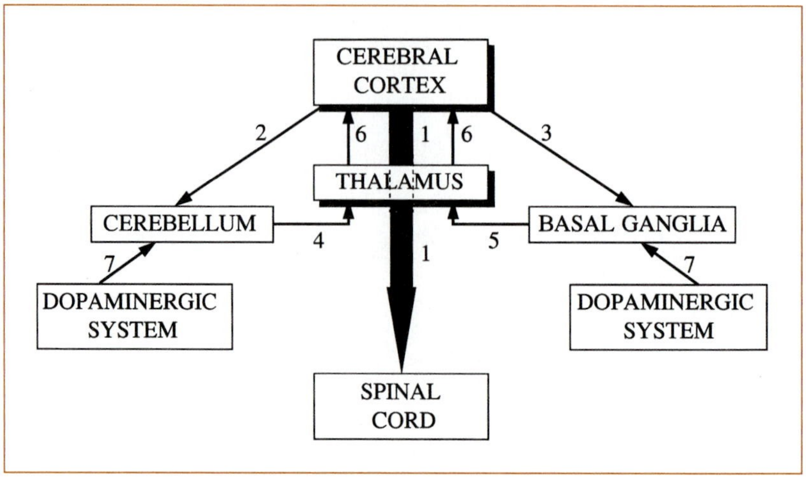

FIGURE 13-1

Schematic diagram of major cortical and subcortical neural structures involved in movement, behavior, and cognition. 1, corticospinal tract; 2, cerebrocerebellar pathways; 3, corticostriate pathways; 4, dentatothalamic pathways; 5, striatothalamic pathways; 6, thalamocortical pathways; and 7, dopaminergic pathways.

Lentiform nucleus (Latin *lens*, "lentil"; *forma*, "shape"). Lentiform nucleus (putamen and globus pallidus) so named because it is shaped like a lentil.

Extrapyramidal system. Vague term introduced but not defined by the British neurologist Kinnier Wilson. Currently used to refer to the basal ganglia and their connections.

septi, and the striatal part of the olfactory tubercle. The term **extrapyramidal system,** coined by British neurologist Kinnier Wilson, refers to the basal ganglia and an array of brain stem nuclei (red nucleus, subthalamic nucleus, substantia nigra, reticular formation) to which they are connected. This conglomerate of neural structures plays an important role in motor control.

Initially, the term *basal ganglia* was a descriptive term that included the thalamus and other subcortical structures. A major step in its definition was made when the thalamus was separated from the "striated body" by the French anatomist Felix Vic d'Azyr in 1786. The distinction between striatum and pallidum was made at the beginning of the twentieth century, and the importance of the corticostriatal

KEY CONCEPTS

- The basal ganglia consists of five subcortical nuclei.
- The extrapyramidal system refers to the basal ganglia and their connections.
- The terms *corpus striatum, striatum, neostriatum, pallidum, paleostriatum,* and *lentiform nucleus* refer to well-defined components of the basal ganglia.

TABLE 13-1

Basal Ganglia Nomenclature

	Corpus Striatum	Striatum, Dorsal Striatum, Neostriatum	Ventral Striatum	Pallidum, Paleo-striatum	Lentiform Nucleus
Caudate	+	+	+	−	−
Putamen	+	+	+	−	+
Globus pallidus	+	−	−	+	+
Nucleus accumbens	−	−	+	−	−
Olfactory tubercle	−	−	+	−	−

connections were recognized in the late 1960s. Since then, rapid advances have been made in our understanding of basal ganglia structure, internal organization, connectivity, and function.

NEURONAL POPULATION, SYNAPTIC RELATIONS, AND INTERNAL ORGANIZATION

Neostriatum (Striatum)

The terms **neostriatum** and **striatum** refer to the caudate nucleus and putamen. The **caudate nucleus** is a C-shaped structure with an expanded rostral extremity, the head, which tapers down in size to form a body and a tail. The head of the caudate nucleus bears a characteristic relationship to the anterior horn of the lateral ventricle. This part of the caudate characteristically bulges into the lateral ventricle. In degenerative central nervous diseases involving the caudate nucleus, such as Huntington's **chorea,** described by the American general practitioner George Huntington in 1872, the characteristic bulge of the caudate nucleus into the lateral ventricle is lost. While the head and body of the caudate nucleus maintain a relationship to the lateral wall of the anterior horn and body of the lateral ventricle, respectively, the tail of the caudate occupies a position in the roof of the inferior horn of the lateral ventricle.

The **putamen** is located lateral to the globus pallidus and medial to the external capsule. It is separated from the caudate nucleus by the internal capsule, except rostrally, where the head of the caudate and the putamen are continuous around the anterior limb of the internal capsule.

Neostriatal neurons are of two types: aspiny and spiny. Aspiny neurons are intrinsic neurons (interneurons). They are generally of two sizes. Large aspiny neurons use acetylcholine as neurotransmitter and are lost in Huntington's chorea, and small aspiny neurons use gamma-aminobutyric acid (GABA) as neurotransmitter.

Spiny neurons, the neostriatal projection (principal) neurons, constitute the great majority (90 percent) of neostriatal neurons. They contain GABA, taurine, and a number of neuropeptides, including substance P, enkephalin, neurotensin, dynorphin, and cholecystokinin. Spiny neurons are also lost in Huntington's chorea.

Molecular biology techniques have identified at least six dopamine receptor isoforms (D_1, D_2 long, D_2 short, D_3, D_4, and D_5) grouped into two subfamilies (D_1-like and D_2-like). D_1 and D_2 receptors are found in the striatum. D_2 receptors mediate the antipsychotic effects of neuroleptic drugs and exert feedback control on dopaminergic transmission. In Parkinson's disease, D_1 receptors are reduced, while D_2 receptors are significantly increased.

Axons from extrastriatal sites (cerebral cortex and substantia nigra) terminate on distal spines of projection neurons. Axons from intrastriatal sites (interneurons and other spiny neurons) terminate on proximal dendrites and cell bodies of projection neurons (Fig. 13-2). The convergence of cortical and nigral originating synapses on distal spines of projection neurons allows the dopaminergic input from the substantia nigra to modulate activity of cortical input to the striatum.

The adult neostriatum is made up of two compartments: The patches (striosomes) compartment contains cells that stain weakly for acetylcholine esterase and is inter-

Neostriatum (Greek *neos,* "new"; Latin *striatus,* "striped"). The phylogenetically newer part of the corpus striatum comprises the caudate and putamen nuclei.

Striatum (Latin *striatus,* "striped"). The caudate and putamen, so named because of their striped appearance in sections.

Caudate nucleus (Latin "having a tail"). The caudate nucleus is so named because it has a long extension or tail.

Chorea (Latin from Greek *choros,* "a dance"). Disorder of the neostriatum causing irregular, involuntary movements of the limbs or face, formerly called *St. Vitus dance.*

Putamen (Latin "shell"). Lateral part of the lentiform nucleus.

KEY CONCEPTS

- The striatum has compartmental organization, each with its well-defined inputs, outputs, neurotransmitters, and neuromodulators.

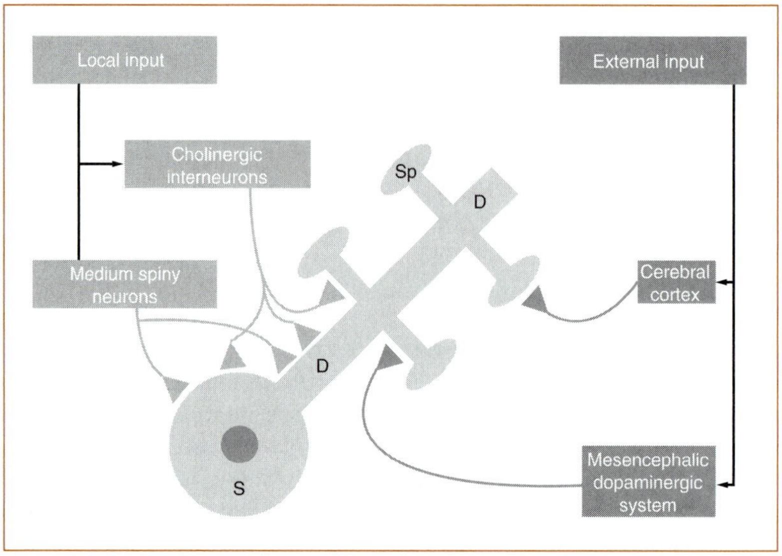

FIGURE 13-2

Schematic diagram of striatal medium spiny neuron showing the different patterns of termination of extrinsic (*right*) and local inputs (*left*) on dendrites and soma. S, soma; D, dendrite; Sp, dendritic spine. (*Modified from Trends in Neuroscience 13:259–265, 1990, figure 3, with permission from Elsevier Science Ltd.*)

spersed between strongly staining areas, the matrix compartment. Besides differences in acetylcholine esterase reactivity, the two compartments differ in their input, output, neurotransmitters, neuromodulators, sources of dopaminergic input, and distribution of dopaminergic receptor subtypes (Table 13-2).

TABLE 13-2

Characteristics of Striosome and Matrix Compartments

	Striosomes	Matrix
Acetylcholine esterase staining	Light	Heavy
Cell development	Early	Late
Input	Medial frontal cortex, limbic cortex, substantia nigra pars compacta, ventral substantia nigra pars reticulata	Sensorimotor cortex, supplementary motor cortex, association cortex, limbic cortex intralaminar thalamic nuclei, ventral tegmental area, dorsal substantia nigra pars compacta
Output	Substantia nigra pars compacta	Substantia nigra pars reticulata, globus pallidus
Neurotransmitter	GABA	GABA
Neuromodulators	Neurotensin, dynorphin, substance P	Somatostatin, enkephalin, substance P
Dopamine receptor	D_1	D_2

NOTE: GABA, gamma-aminobutyric acid.

Globus Pallidus and Substantia Nigra Pars Reticulata

The **globus pallidus** is a wedge-shaped nuclear mass located between the putamen and internal capsule. A lamina of fibers (external pallidal lamina) separates the globus pallidus from the putamen. Another lamina (internal pallidal lamina) divides the globus pallidus into a larger lateral (outer) and a smaller medial (inner) segment. The entopeduncular nucleus of nonprimate mammals is part of the medial pallidal segment in primate mammals.

The **substantia nigra** pars reticulata occupies the ventral zone of the substantia nigra and contains iron compounds.

Morphologically and chemically, the globus pallidus and the substantia nigra pars reticulata are similar. The latter is considered the part of the globus pallidus containing head and neck representation, whereas the internal segment of globus pallidus has arm and leg representation.

Most neurons in the globus pallidus and substantia nigra pars reticulata are large multipolar projection neurons. Interneurons are infrequent. All pallidal and nigral neurons use GABA as the inhibitory neurotransmitter.

Globus pallidus (Latin *globus,* "a ball or round mass," *pallidus,* "pale"). The paler inner part of the lentiform nucleus.

Substantia nigra (Latin "black substance"). Group of neurons between the cerebral peduncle and midbrain tegmentum. So named because of their melanin-containing neurons.

Neostriatal Input

Corticostriate Projection

Projections from the cerebral cortex to the striatum are both direct and indirect. Direct corticostriate projections reach the neostriatum via the internal and external capsules and via the subcallosal fasciculus. The indirect pathways include the corticothalamostriate pathway, collaterals of the corticoolivary pathway, and collaterals of the corticopontine pathway (Fig. 13-3).

The corticostriate projection comprises the most massive striatal afferents. Almost all cortical areas contribute to this projection. Cortical areas interconnected via corticocortical fibers tend to share common zones of termination in the neostriatum. Corticostriatal fibers are topographically organized into three distinct striatal territories: (1) sensorimotor, (2) associative, and (3) limbic. The sensorimotor territory receives its inputs from sensory and motor cortical areas. The associative territory receives fibers from the association cortices. The limbic territory receives input from limbic and paralimbic cortical areas.

Corticostriate pathways are also somatotopically organized such that cortical association areas project to the caudate nucleus, whereas sensorimotor cortical areas preferentially project to the putamen. Corticoputaminal projections are further organized in that the cortical arm, leg, and face areas project to corresponding areas within the putamen. The somatotopic organization of corticostriate projection is replicated throughout the basal ganglia. The excitatory neurotransmitter of corticostriate projections is glutamate.

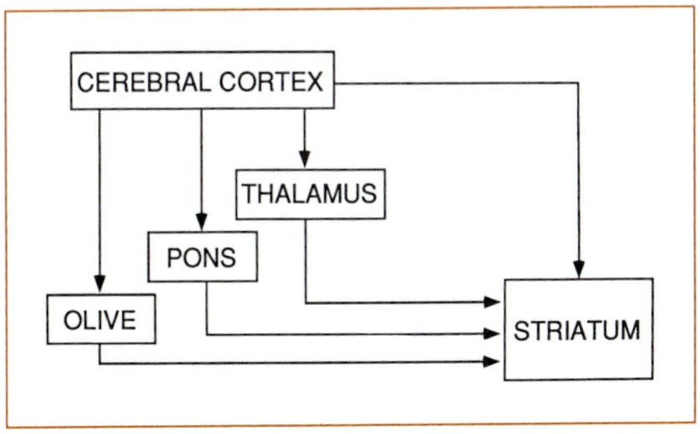

FIGURE 13-3

Schematic diagram of the direct and indirect corticostriate projections.

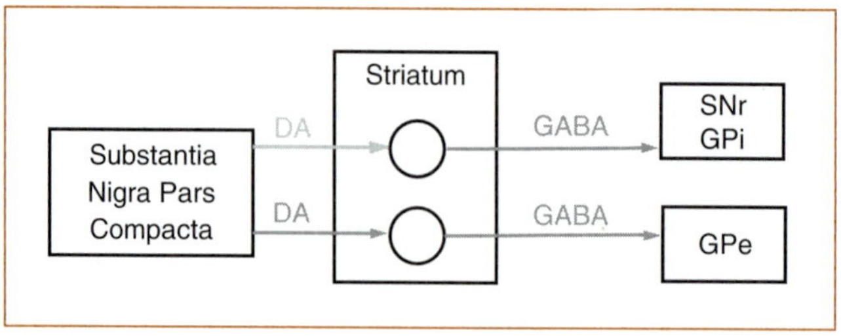

FIGURE 13-4

Schematic diagram of nigrostriatal pathway showing the facilitatory action of dopamine on striatal neurons that project to substantia nigra pars reticulata and internal segment of globus pallidus, and the inhibitory action of dopamine on striatal neurons that project to the external segment of globus pallidus. Dark gray denotes inhibitory transmission; light gray denotes excitatory transmission; DA, dopamine; GABA, gamma aminobytyric acid; GPe, external segment of globus pallidus; GPi, internal segment of globus pallidus; SNr, substantia nigra pars reticulata. (*Modified from J Child Neurol 9:249–260, 1994, figure 1 with permission from Decker Periodicals.*)

Mesencephalostriate Projection

The principal mesencephalostriate projection originates from dopamine-containing cells of the substantia nigra pars compacta. Dopamine has a net excitatory effect on striatal neurons that project to the internal segment of globus pallidus and substantia nigra pars reticulata and a net inhibitory effect on striatal neurons that project to the external segment of globus pallidus (Fig. 13-4).

In addition to the substantia nigra, the following mesencephalic dopaminergic nuclear groups project to the striatum: the ventral tegmental area of Tasi (area A10) and the retrorubral nucleus (substantia nigra pars dorsalis, area A8).

Thalamostriate Projections

Thalamostriate projections are the second most prominent afferents to the striatum. The centromedian nucleus projects mainly to the sensorimotor striatal territory, while the parafascicular nucleus projects to the associative and limbic striatal territories. Thalamostriate fibers are believed to be excitatory. The neurotransmitter is glutamate.

Other Projections

Other projections to the neostriatum include those from the raphe nuclei (serotoninergic) and the locus ceruleus (noradrenergic). Figure 13-5 is a schema of the major inputs to the neostriatum.

Neostriatal Output

The neostriatum projects to the substantia nigra pars reticulata, both segments of the globus pallidus, and the ventral pallidum. There is also a small projection from the neostriatum to the substantia nigra pars compacta.

The neostriatal projections to the different target areas, although containing one neurotransmitter (GABA), have different neuropeptides (Table 13-3).

KEY CONCEPTS

- Dopaminergic neurons in the substantia nigra excite some striatal neurons and inhibit others.
- The basal ganglia receive inputs from the cerebral cortex (major source) and subcortical structures.
- The basal ganglia project back to the cerebral cortex via the thalamus.

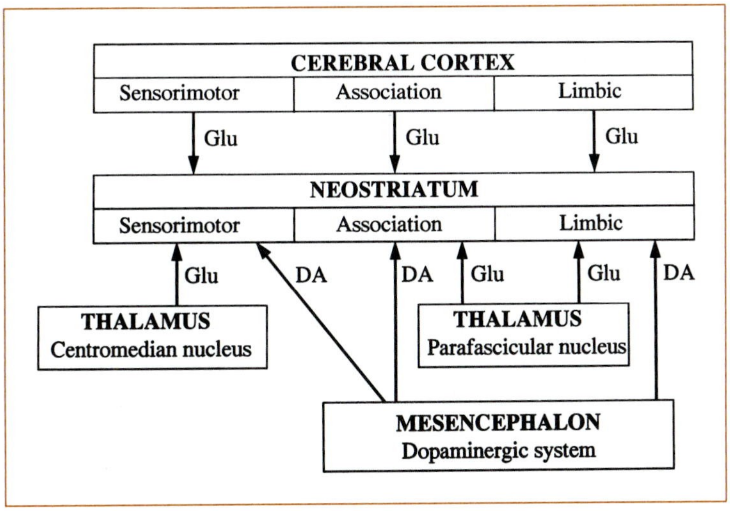

FIGURE 13-5

Schematic diagram of major sources of input to the sensorimotor, association, and limbic zones of the neostriatum. Glu, glutamine; DA, dopamine.

The striatal output to the globus pallidus and the substantia nigra is organized into direct and indirect projections (Fig. 13-6). The direct projection is from the neostriatum to the internal segment of the globus pallidus and the substantia nigra pars reticulata. The indirect projection is from the neostriatum to the external segment of the globus pallidus and via the subthalamic nucleus to the internal segment of the globus pallidus and the substantia nigra pars reticulata. Enhanced activity of the indirect pathway may be responsible for the poverty of movement (hypokinesia) of some basal ganglia disorders, whereas reduced activity in the direct pathway may result in excessive activity (hyperkinesia) of some basal ganglia disorders.

Pallidal and Nigral Inputs

Striatopallidal and Striatonigral Projections

The input to both segments of the globus pallidus is primarily from the putamen and the subthalamic nucleus, whereas the input to the substantia nigra pars reticulata is primarily from the caudate and the subthalamic nucleus. The input from the

TABLE 13-3

Neurotransmitters/Neuromodulators Involved in Striatal Output

	To GPi	To GPe	To SNr	To SNc
GABA	+	+	+	+
Substance P	+	−	+	−
Enkephalin	−	+	−	−
Dynorphin	+	−	+	+
Neurotensin	−	+	−	+

NOTE: Gpi, internal segment of globus pallidus; GPe, external segment of globus pallidus; SNr, substantia nigra pars reticulata; SNc, substantia nigra pars compacta; GABA, gamma-aminobutyric acid.

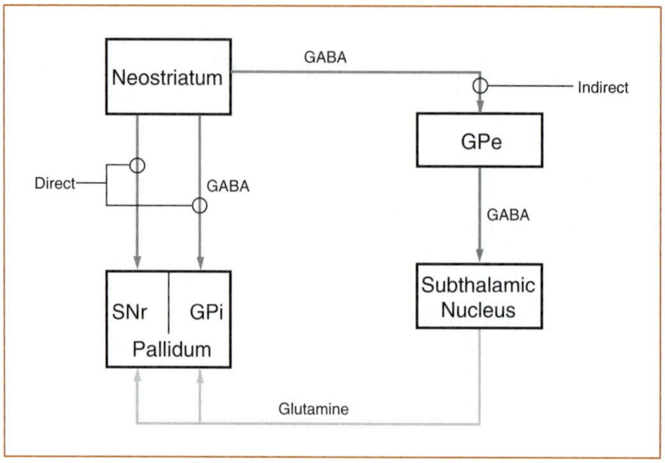

FIGURE 13-6

Schematic diagram of the direct and indirect striatopallidal pathways.

neostriatum is GABAergic (inhibitory). The input from the subthalamic nucleus is glutamatergic (excitatory).

Other Projections

Other, less significant pallidal afferents include those from dopaminergic and serotoninergic neurons of the brain stem.

Pallidal and Nigral Outputs (Fig. 13-7)

Major Output

The major output from the internal segment of the globus pallidus and the substantia nigra pars reticulata is to the thalamus. Pallidothalamic fibers follow one of two routes. Some traverse the internal capsule and gather dorsal to the subthalamic

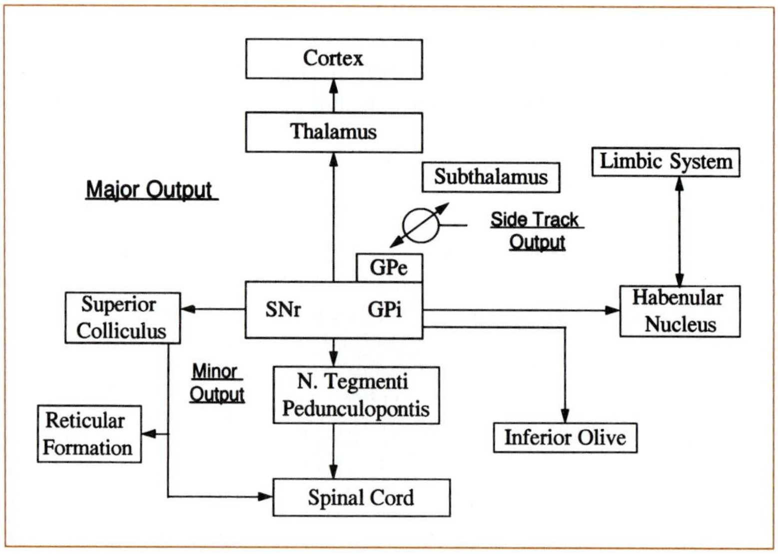

FIGURE 13-7

Schematic diagram of the efferent connections of internal segment of globus pallidus and substantia nigra pars reticulata. GPe, external segment of globus pallidus; GPi, internal segment of globus pallidus; SNr, substantia nigra pars reticulata. (*From J Child Neurol 9:249–260, 1994, figure 2 with permission from Decker Periodicals.*)

nucleus as the lenticular fasciculus (H_2 field of Forel, after the Swiss neuropsychiatrist August Henri Forel, who described these bundles); others pass around the internal capsule (ansa lenticularis). Both groups of fibers gather together to form the prerubral field (H field of Forel) and then join the thalamic fasciculus (H_1 field of Forel) to reach the target thalamic nuclei. The target thalamic nuclei are the ventral anterior, ventral lateral, dorsomedial, and intralaminar nuclei. The neurotransmitter is GABA. Pallidal output thus inhibits the excitatory thalamocortical loop. The pallidothalamic and nigrothalamic projections constitute the link between the neostriatum and the cerebral cortex.

The intralaminar nuclei (centromedian and parafascicular) are crucial elements in the striatothalamocortical circuitry. The centromedian nucleus forms a nodal point in sensorimotor and the parafascicular nucleus an important relay in the associative-limbic components of the circuit.

Minor Output

Minor outputs from the internal segment of the globus pallidus and the substantia nigra pars reticulata go to the following areas.

Nucleus Tegmenti Pedunculopontis This projection serves to link the basal ganglia and the spinal cord via the reticulospinal tract. The projection to the nucleus tegmenti pedunculopontis assumes particular significance because of the multiple connections and functions of this nucleus, the best known being motor function (mesencephalic locomotor center), arousal, and sleep. Others include motivation, attention, and learning.

Habenular Nucleus Via this connection, the basal ganglia are linked with the limbic system.

Superior Colliculus Through this pathway, the basal ganglia are linked (via the tectospinal tract) to the spinal cord and (via the tectoreticular tract) to brain stem nuclei related to head and eye movements.

Side Track Output

This output reciprocally relates the external segment of the globus pallidus with the subthalamic nucleus. The neurotransmitter is GABA.

The inputs and outputs of the basal ganglia are schematically summarized in Fig. 13-8.

The basal ganglia and its related neural systems may be viewed as composed of (1) a core and (2) regulators of the core. The core is composed of the striatum and its pallidal and nigral targets. The regulators of the core fall into two categories: (1) regulators of the striatum and (2) pallidonigral regulators (Fig. 13-9).

Subthalamic Nucleus

The subthalamic nucleus receives fibers from the following sources: (1) external segment of the globus pallidus, (2) cerebral cortex (areas 4 and 6), (3) reticular formation, and (4) thalamus. The outflow from the subthalamic nucleus is to both segments of the globus pallidus and to the substantia nigra pars reticulata. The

KEY CONCEPTS

- The striatum is the principal receptive structure and the globus pallidus is the principal output structure of the basal ganglia.

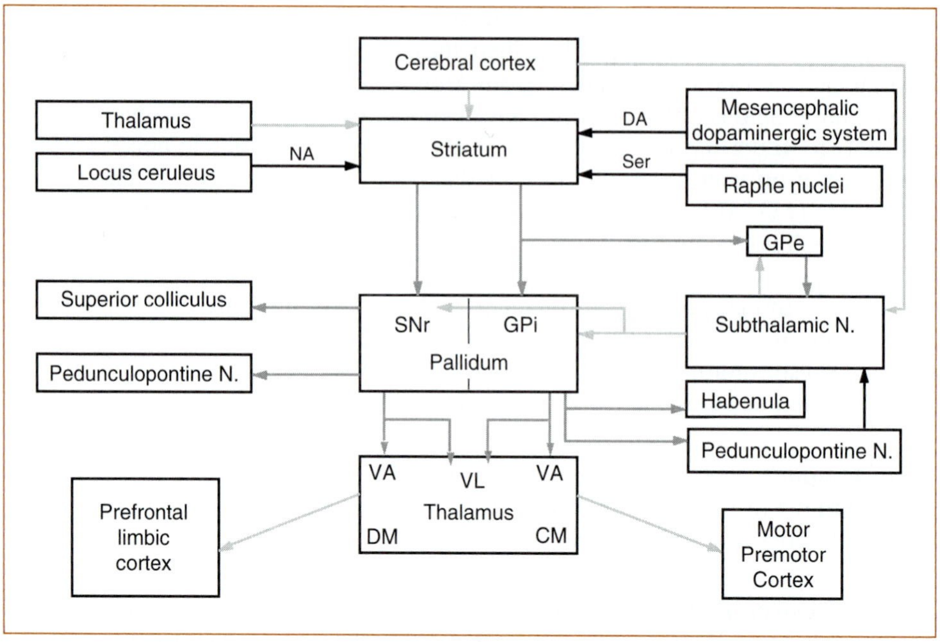

FIGURE 13-8

Simplified schematic summary diagram of afferent and efferent connections of the basal ganglia showing that the striatum is the major receiving area whereas the internal segment of globus pallidus and substantia nigra pars reticulata constitute the major output nuclei. Dark gray denotes inhibitory transmission; light gray denotes excitatory transmission; black denotes modulatory effect; DA, dopamine; Ser, serotonin; NA, noradrenaline; GPe, external segment of globus pallidus; GPi, internal segment of globus pallidus; SNr, substantia nigra pars reticulata; VA, ventral anterior nucleus; VL, ventrolateral nucleus; CM, centromedian nucleus; DM, dorsomedial nucleus. (*Modified from J Child Neurol 9:249–260, 1994, figure 3 with permission from Decker Periodicals.*)

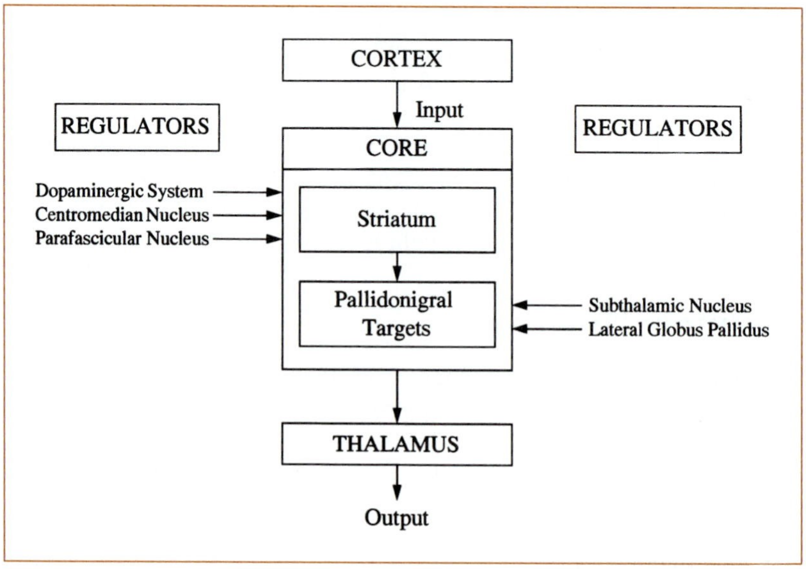

FIGURE 13-9

Schematic diagram showing the organization of the basal ganglia-associated neural system into a core made up of the striatum and its pallidonigral targets, and regulators acting either on the striatum or pallidonigral components of the core.

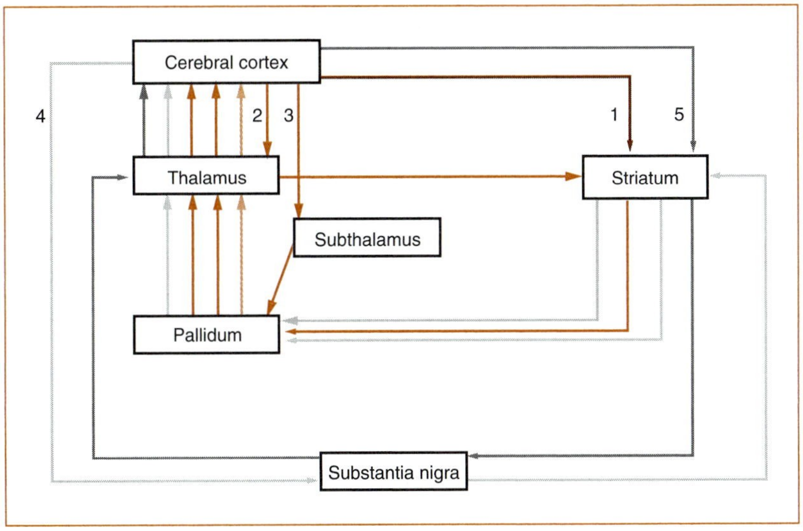

FIGURE 13-10

Schematic diagram of the five corticostriatocortical loops. (1) Cortex → striatum → pallidum → thalamus → cortex, in dark brown. (2) Cortex → thalamus → striatum → pallidum → thalamus → cortex, in medium brown. (3) Cortex → subthalamus → pallidum → thalamus → cortex, in light brown. (4) Cortex → substantia nigra → striatum → pallidum → thalamus → cortex, in light gray. (5) Cortex → striatum → substantia nigra → thalamus → cortex, in dark gray. (*Modified from J Child Neurol 9:352–361, 1994, figure 1 with permission from Decker Periodicals.*)

excitatory neurotransmitter in all these pathways is glutamate. Interruption of the subthalamopallidal pathway is responsible for the violent hyperkinesia of **ballism.**

Ballism (Greek *ballismos,* "jumping"). Violent involuntary movement due to a lesion in the subthalamic nucleus.

Ventral (Limbic) Striatum

Currently, the term *ventral striatum* refers to the following nuclei: nucleus accumbens septi, striatelike deep portions of the olfactory tubercle and ventral parts of the caudate nucleus, and the putamen (see Table 13-1). The ventral striatum receives fibers from the following sources: hippocampus, amygdala, entorhinal and perirhinal cortices (areas 28 and 35), anterior cingulate cortex (area 24), medial orbitofrontal cortex, and widespread sources within the temporal lobe. Dopaminergic input to the ventral striatum is substantial. The output from the ventral striatum is to the ventral pallidum. As is evident from its connections, the ventral striatum is related to the limbic system.

Corticostriatothalamocortical Loops

The corticostriatothalamocortical relationship may be defined in terms of five anatomic and five functional loops (circuits). The anatomic loops are illustrated in Fig. 13-10. The functional loops are made up of the following parallel and largely segregated pathways.

Motor Loop Pathway

The motor loop pathway is centered on the putamen and its connections (Fig. 13-11). The putamen of primates receives somatotopically organized (arm, leg, face) inputs from the primary motor, primary sensory, somatosensory association,

KEY CONCEPTS

- The basal ganglia contain diverse neurotransmitters and neuromodulators.

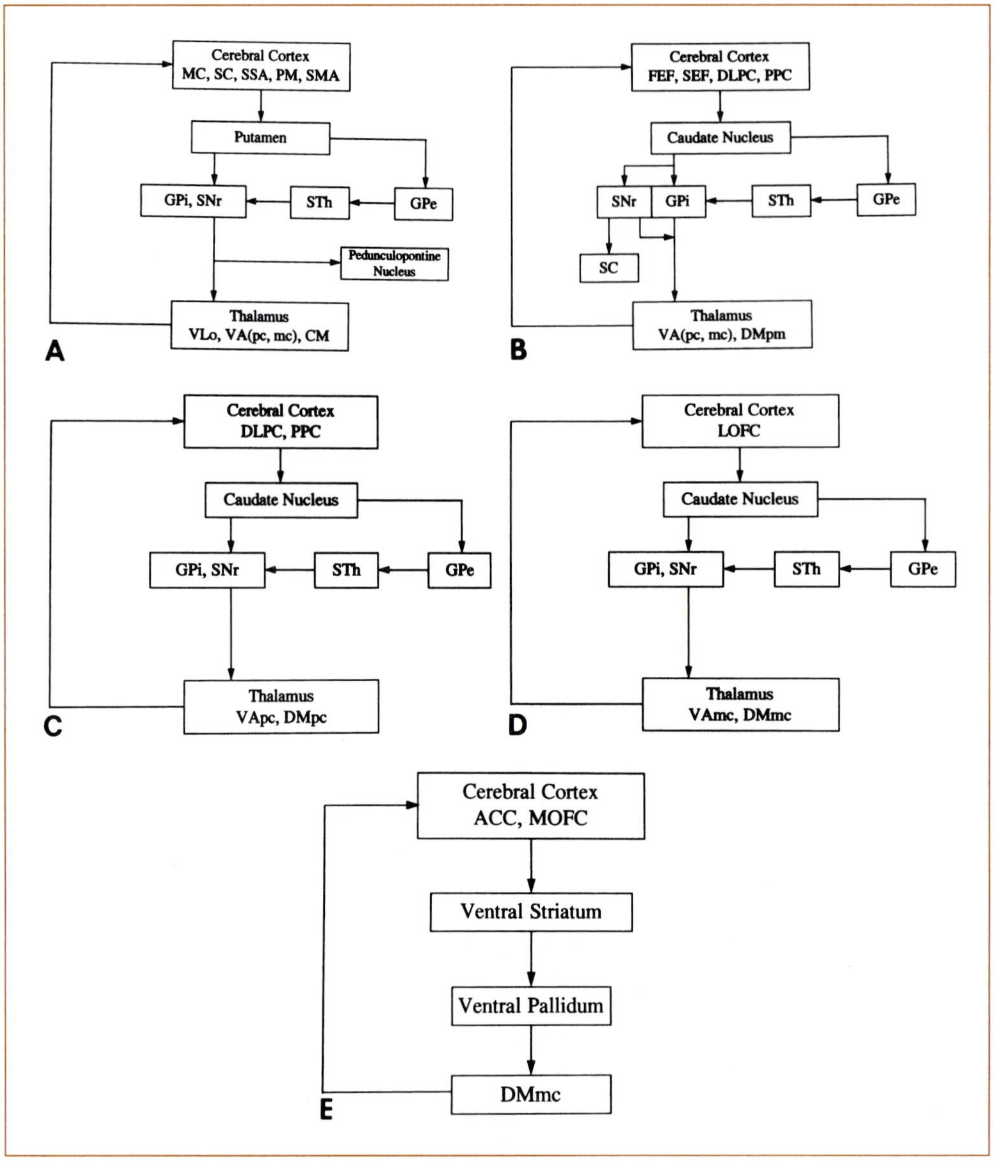

FIGURE 13-11

Schematic diagrams showing the anatomic substrates of the motor loop (A), oculomotor loop (B), dorsolateral prefrontal loop (C), lateral orbitofrontal loop (D), and the limbic loop (E). MC, primary motor cortex (area 4); SC, primary sensory cortex (areas 3, 1, and 2); SSA, somatory sensory association cortex (area 5); PM, premotor cortex; SMA, supplementary motor area; GPi, internal segment of globus pallidus; SNr, substantia nigra pars reticulata; STH, subthalamic nucleus; GPe, external segment of globus pallidus; VLo, ventrolateral nucleus of thalamus, pars oralis; VApc, ventral anterior nucleus of thalamus, pars parvicellularis; VAmc, ventral anterior nucleus of thalamus, pars magnocellularis; CM, centromedian nucleus of thalamus; FEF, frontal eye field (area 8); SEF, supplementary eye field; DLPC, dorsolateral prefrontal cortex (areas 9 and 10); PPC, posterior parietal cortex; DMpm, dorsomedial nucleus of thalamus, pars multiformis; SC, superior colliculus; LOFC, lateral orbitofrontal cortex; DMmc, dorsomedial nucleus of thalamus, pars magnocellularis; ACC, anterior cingulate cortex; MOFC, medial orbitofrontal cortex. (*From J. Child Neurology 9:352–361, 1994, figures 2 to 6 with permission from Decker Periodicals.*)

premotor, and supplementary motor cortices. Within each of these anatomic subchannels, further levels of functional organization exist pertaining to such behavioral variables as target location, limb kinematics, and muscle pattern. The putamen projects to both segments of the globus pallidus and to the substantia nigra pars reticulata. The internal pallidal segment projects to ventral lateral, ventral anterior, and centromedian nuclei of the thalamus, whereas the substantia nigra pars reticulata projects to the ventral anterior thalamic nucleus. The motor loop is completed by thalamocortical projections to the supplementary motor, premotor, and primary motor cortices.

An offshoot from the pallidothalamic component of the motor loop is a projection from the internal segment of the globus pallidus to the pedunculopontine nucleus.

A side loop in this motor pathway passes from the putamen to the external segment of the globus pallidus and from there to the subthalamic nucleus and back to the internal segment of the globus pallidus.

Oculomotor Loop Pathway

The oculomotor loop pathway (Fig. 13-11) is centered on the caudate nucleus. Cortical sources of input to the caudate nucleus include the frontal eye field, supplementary eye field, dorsolateral prefrontal cortex, and posterior parietal cortex. The caudate, in turn, projects to the internal segment of the globus pallidus and the substantia nigra pars reticulata. The thalamic targets of the oculomotor loop include the ventral anterior and dorsomedial nuclei. The oculomotor loop is completed by thalamocortical projections to frontal eye field and supplementary eye field.

Dorsolateral Prefrontal Loop Pathway

The dorsolateral prefrontal loop pathway (Fig. 13-11) is also centered on the caudate nucleus. Corticostriate input to this pathway originates from the dorsolateral prefrontal cortex and posterior parietal cortex. The caudate nucleus projects to the internal segment of the globus pallidus and the substantia nigra pars reticulata. The thalamic targets of this pathway are the ventral anterior and dorsomedial nuclei. The loop is completed by thalamic projections to the dorsolateral prefrontal cortex.

Lateral Orbitofrontal Prefrontal Loop Pathway

The lateral orbitofrontal prefrontal loop pathway (Fig. 13-11) is similarly centered on the caudate nucleus. The corticostriate projection originates from the lateral orbitofrontal cortex. The caudate nucleus projects to the internal segment of the globus pallidus and the substantia nigra pars reticulata. The thalamic targets of this pathway are the dorsomedial and ventral anterior nuclei. The loop is completed by thalamic projections to the lateral orbitofrontal cortex.

Limbic Loop Pathway

The limbic loop pathway (Fig. 13-11) is centered on the ventral striatum. Corticostriate projections originate from the anterior cingulate cortex, medial orbitofrontal cortex, and widespread areas in the temporal lobe. The ventral striatum projects to ventral pallidum. The thalamic target of this pathway is the dorsomedial nucleus. The loop is completed by thalamic projections to anterior cingulate and medial orbitofrontal cortices.

A role for the limbic circuit in the genesis of schizophrenia has been proposed.

Each of the five functional circuits has a direct and an indirect pathway from the striatum to the output nuclei (internal segment of the globus pallidus and substantia nigra pars reticulata). The direct pathway contains GABA and substance P and directly connects the striatum with the output nuclei (Fig. 13-12). The indirect pathway (Fig. 13-13) connects the striatum with the output nuclei via relays in the external segment of globus pallidus and the subthalamic nucleus. Activation of the direct pathway tends to disinhibit thalamocortical target neurons. Activation of the indirect system has a net effect of increasing the inhibition of thalamocortical target neurons.

Split Pathways

The preceding five circuits (loops) are characterized by parallel, segregated, and closed connections, in which little, if any, intercommunication takes place. An alternate model has been proposed that allows for cross-communication between

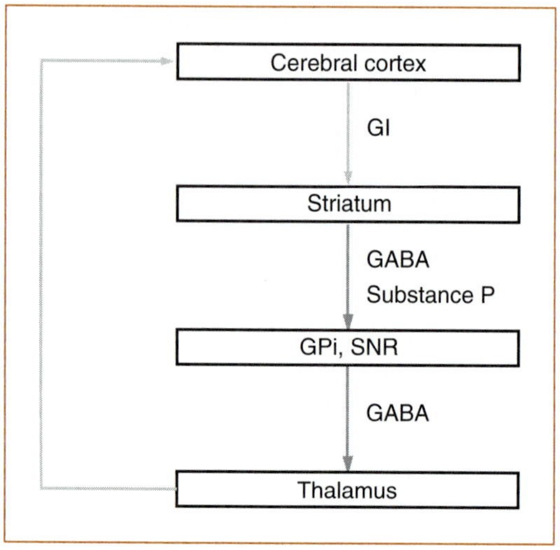

FIGURE 13-12

Schematic diagram showing the anatomic substrates of the direct striatopallidal pathway. Gl, glutamate; GABA, gamma aminobutyric acid; GPi, internal segment of globus pallidus; SNR, substantia nigra pars reticulata. Light gray denotes excitatory transmission; dark gray denotes inhibitory transmission. (*Modified from J Child Neurol 9:352–361, 1994, figure 7 with permission from Decker Periodicals.*)

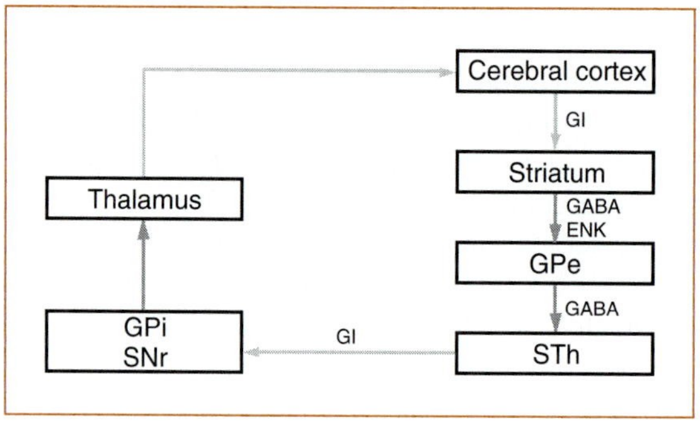

FIGURE 13-13

Schematic diagram showing the anatomic substrates of the direct striatopallidal pathway. Gl, glutamate; GABA, gamma aminobutyric acid; ENK, enkephalin; GPe, external segment of globus pallidus; GPi, internal segment of globus pallidus; SNr, substantia nigra pars reticulata; STh, subthalamic nucleus. Light gray denotes excitatory transmission; dark gray denotes inhibitory transmission. (*Modified from J Child Neurol 9:352–361, 1994, figure 8 with permission from Decker Periodicals.*)

circuits. In this model, three circuits are proposed: motor, associative, and limbic. Within each of these circuits, there are both closed and open loops (Figs. 13-14 to 13-16). The novel feature of the open and closed loops (split circuitry) model is that in each split circuit the engaged striatal area can influence, via its open loop, a cortical field that does not project to it. Interaction between split circuits can occur at two levels, the cerebral cortex and the substantia nigra.

KEY CONCEPTS

- Corticostriatothalamocortical connections are organized into five parallel and segregated loops and/or three split circuits.

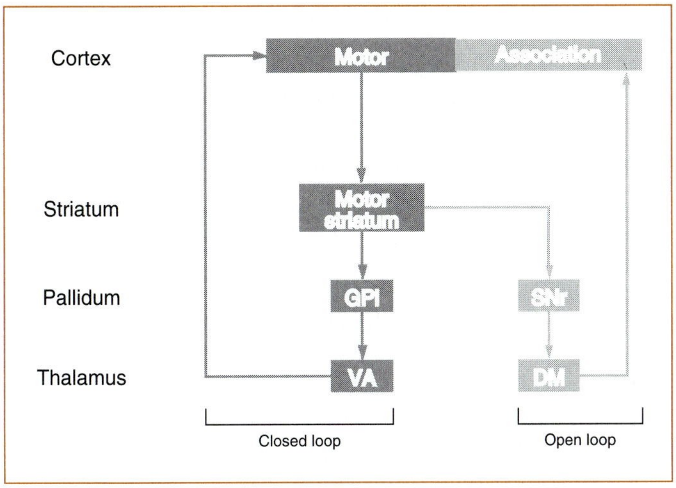

FIGURE 13-14

Schematic diagram of split motor circuit showing (dark gray) the closed loop and (light gray) the open loop of the circuit. (*Modified from Neuroscience 63:363–379, 1994, figure 3 with permission from Elsevier Science Ltd.*)

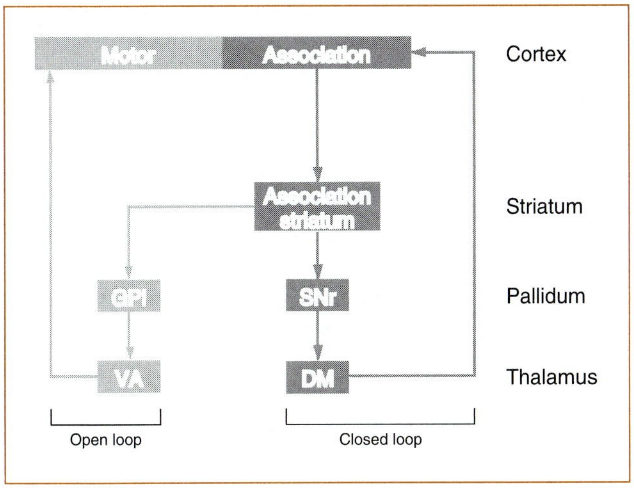

FIGURE 13-15

Schematic diagram of the split associative circuit showing (dark gray) the closed loop and (light gray) the open loop of the circuit. (*Modified from Neuroscience 63:363–379, 1994, figure 3 with permission from Elsevier Science Ltd.*)

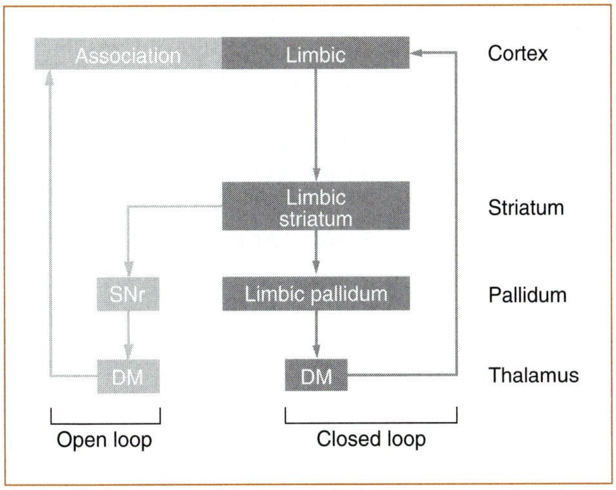

FIGURE 13-16

Schematic diagram of the split limbic circuit showing (dark gray) the closed loop and (light gray) the open loop of the circuit. (*Modified from Neuroscience 63:363–379, 1994, figure 4 with permission from Elsevier Science Ltd.*)

BASAL GANGLIA FUNCTION

Much of the available evidence suggests a role for the basal ganglia in motor control. There is also some recent evidence for possible roles in cognition and emotion. Motor function is subserved by the motor and oculomotor loops, cognitive function by the prefrontal loops, and emotion by the limbic loop.

Motor Function

Animal studies include stimulation, ablation, and single-unit recording. Effects of stimulation vary depending on the rate, strength, and pattern of stimulation. Reported abnormalities include contraversive head turning and circling, contralateral limb flexion, abrupt arrest of motor behavior, licking, chewing, or swallowing movements, and modification of cortically induced movements.

Effects of damage to the striatum suggest involvement in orientation to stimuli and the initiation and control of movement. Bilateral lesions in the lenticular nucleus in humans are associated with obsessive-compulsive motor behavior and elementary stereotyped movements. Unilateral pallidal ablation has little or no motor or behavioral effects. Bilateral pallidal ablation, however, produces a hypoactive, sleepy animal that seldom moves around or even changes position, simulating the hypokinesia of Parkinson's disease. This distinctive syndrome of massive decrease in spontaneous behavior has been referred to as the *athymhormic syndrome.*

Single-unit recordings confirm a nonmotor role for the caudate. In contrast, the putamen does respond to movement tasks. The external segment of the globus pallidus has low or no spontaneous activity. In contrast, the internal segment of the globus pallidus and the substantia nigra pars reticulata have sustained, high-frequency discharge rates with intermittent periods of silence. The subthalamus has high spontaneous discharge rates and responds to voluntary movement.

Contrary to the previously prevailing concept that the striatum is a hypnogenic (sleep-inducing) structure, recent studies have shown that the striatum promotes arousal of the motor system.

Studies that time neuronal discharge in relation to onset of stimulus-triggered movement suggest that activity within the basal ganglia is initiated at cortical levels. In the cortically initiated movement, information flow from the cortex to the basal ganglia (Fig. 13-17) begins with a command from the cortex to the striatum that initiates action of striatal neurons. The nigral input to the striatum provides a continuous damping effect so that cortical commands will be focused. The input from the thalamus and other sites informs and updates the striatum of the activity in other systems concerned with movement. The striatum integrates and feeds information to the globus pallidus and the substantia nigra pars reticulata. The globus pallidus and substantia nigra pars reticulata in turn influence activity of the thalamus and other targets (i.e., superior colliculus, reticular formation). According to Marsden, the basal ganglia are responsible for the automatic execution of a learned motor plan. As a motor skill is learned, the basal ganglia take over the role of automatically executing the learned strategy. When basal ganglia are damaged, the individual must revert to a slower, less automatic, and less accurate cortical mechanism for motor behavior.

Other roles for the basal ganglia in motor control include the preparation for movement. During both the preparation and execution of movement, separate populations of neurons within the motor loop discharge selectively in relation to

KEY CONCEPTS

- The role of the basal ganglia in motor control includes the preparation for and execution of cortically initiated movement.

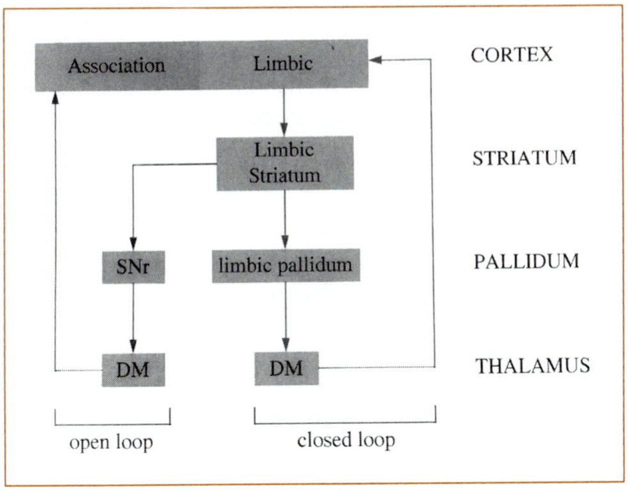

FIGURE 13-17

Schematic diagram of information flow in the basal ganglia (1) Command from cortex initiates action in striatum. (2) Nigral input from SNC to striatum provides continuous damping of static so that cortical command will be focused. (3) Input from thalamus and other sites updates and informs striatum of activity in other systems. (4) Striatum has an integrator role and feeds its results to GP and SNr. (5) GP and SNr influence (facilitate or inhibit) activity of thalamus and other targets (superior colliculus, reticular formation, etc). SNC, substantia nigra pars compacta; GP, globus pallidus; SNr, substantia nigra pars reticulata. (*Modified from J Child Neurol 9:352–361, 1994, figure 9 with permission from Decker Periodicals.*)

either target location in space, direction of limb movement, or muscle pattern. Similarly, in the oculomotor loop, populations of neurons have been described that discharge in relation to visual fixation, saccadic eye movement, or passive visual stimuli.

The recognition that basal ganglia neurons respond to stimuli colored by memory or significance indicates that this region of the brain is concerned with higher-order motor control.

Gating Function

Another possible function of the basal ganglia is gating of sensorimotor processing. According to the gating hypothesis, in normal subjects, dopamine (inhibitory) and cortical sensorimotor (excitatory) inputs to the striatum are in physiologic balance. The inhibitory output of the pallidum thus regulates sensorimotor access. In Parkinson's disease, the loss of dopamine (inhibitory) will allow cortical facilitation a free hand to stimulate the inhibitory basal ganglia output. This limits access of sensory information to the motor system and decreases motor activity (hypokinesia). In Huntington's chorea, loss of basal ganglia neurons results in a decrease in inhibitory output of the basal ganglia, with a resulting increase in access of sensory information to the motor system and increased activity.

Cognitive Function

In addition to their role in motor control, the basal ganglia subserve cognitive function. Lesions of the dorsolateral prefrontal circuit (loop) result in deficits on tasks that require spatial memory. Recent studies suggest that the basal ganglia

KEY CONCEPTS

- Loss of dopamine in the nigrostriatal system is associated with Parkinson's disease.

play a role in memory different from that mediated by the hippocampus and diencephalon. Lesions of the lateral orbitofrontal loop, on the other hand, interfere with the ability to make appropriate switches in behavior.

Lesions in the dorsolateral prefrontal circuit in humans have been linked to cognitive disturbances in schizophrenia, Huntington's chorea, and Parkinson's disease. Lesions in the lateral orbitofrontal circuit have been linked to obsessive-compulsive behavior.

Emotion and Motivation Function

The role of the basal ganglia in emotion and motivation is not as well defined as that of motor and cognitive function. The limbic loop conceivably may play a role in emotional and motivational processes and the genesis of Tourette syndrome, a chronic tic disorder described by the French neuropsychiatrist George Gilles de la Tourette in 1885.

COMPLEMENTARITY OF BASAL GANGLIA AND CEREBELLUM IN MOTOR FUNCTION

Review of basal ganglia and cerebellar structure, connectivity, and organization reveals many features in common. Both are components of the motor system, both influence cerebral cortical activity via the thalamus, both are linked with the cerebral cortex via recurrent loops, both have internal (local) circuitry that modulates loop activity, and both receive modulating inputs that influence their activities (climbing fibers in the cerebellum and dopaminergic input in the basal ganglia).

The emerging concept (Fig. 13-18) of the complementarity of basal ganglia and cerebellum in motor function suggests that the basal ganglia function as context encoders, providing to the cerebral cortex information that could be useful in planning and gating of action. The cerebellum, in contrast, functions as pattern generator and executor. According to this concept, the cerebral cortex, which receives diverse sensory information from the periphery via the different ascending tracts, as well as complex information already processed within the basal ganglia and cerebellum, serves two functions: a repository function to receive this diverse information, compute it, and share it with the basal ganglia and cerebellum and an executive function to implement the action emanating from its collective computation process.

BLOOD SUPPLY (Table 13-4)

The basal ganglia receive their blood supply from perforating (lenticulostriate) branches of the middle and anterior cerebral arteries and the anterior choroidal

KEY CONCEPTS

- Knowledge of connections and neurotransmitters of basal ganglia provides insight into their function in health and disease.
- The basal ganglia subserve roles in cognitive function, emotion, and motivation.
- Blood supply of the basal ganglia is derived from lenticulostriate branches of the middle and anterior cerebral arteries and the anterior choroidal branch of the internal carotid artery.

TABLE 13-4

Blood Supply of Basal Ganglia

	Middle Cerebral, Lateral Striate Branch	Anterior Cerebral, Medial Striate Branch	Internal Carotid, Anterior Choroidal
Caudate nucleus			
Head	+	+	
Body	+		
Tail			+
Putamen			
Rostral	+		
Caudal			+
Globus pallidus			
Lateral	+		+
Medial			+

branch of the internal carotid artery. The caudate and putamen nuclei (the striatum) are supplied mainly by the lateral striate branches of the middle cerebral artery. Rostromedial parts of the head of the caudate nucleus receive blood supply from the medial striate artery (of Huebner), a branch of the anterior cerebral artery. The tail of the caudate nucleus and caudal part of the putamen receive branches of the anterior choroidal artery. Most of the globus pallidus is supplied by the anterior choroidal branch of the internal carotid artery. The lateral (outer) segment of the globus pallidus receives blood supply also from the lateral striate branch of the middle cerebral artery.

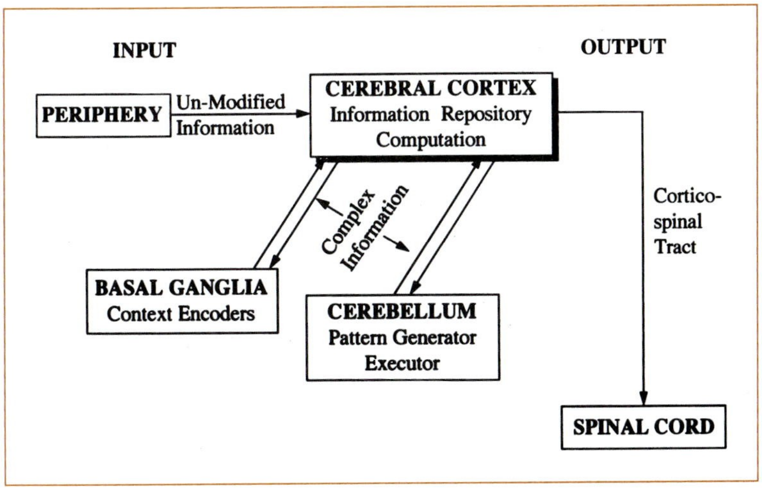

FIGURE 13-18

Simplified schematic diagram showing varied types of information received by the cerebral cortex, and the complimentarity of basal ganglia and cerebellar roles in motor function.

SUGGESTED READINGS

Albin RL, et al: The functional anatomy of basal ganglia disorders. *Trends Neurosci* 1989; 12:366–375.

Alexander GE, et al: Basal ganglia–thalamocortical circuits: Parallel substrates for motor, oculomotor, "prefrontal" and "limbic" functions. *Prog Brain Res* 1990; 85:119–146.

Butters N, et al: Specificity of the memory deficits associated with basal ganglia dysfunction. *Rev Neurol* 1994; 150:580–587.

Carpenter MB, et al: Connections of the subthalamic nucleus in the monkey. *Brain Res* 1981; 224:1–29.

Flaherty AW, Graybiel AM: Anatomy of basal ganglia. In Marsden CD, Fahn S (eds): *Movement Disorders.* Boston, Butterworth-Heinenemann, 1994:3.

Goldman-Rakic PS: Cytoarchitectonic heterogeneity of the primate neostriatum: Subdivision into island and matrix cellular compartments. *J Comp Neurol* 1982; 205:398–413.

Graybiel AM: Neurotransmitters and neuromodulators in the basal ganglia. *Trends Neurosci* 1990; 13: 244–254.

Houk JC, Wise SP: Distributed modular architectures linking basal ganglia, cerebellum, and cerebral cortex: Their role in planning and controlling action. *Cerebral Cortex* 1995; 2:95–110.

Joel D, Weiner I: The organization of the basal ganglia–thalamocortical circuits: Open interconnected rather than closed segregated. *Neuroscience* 1994; 63: 363–379.

Lynd-Balta E, Haber SN: The organization of midbrain projections to the striatum in the primate: Sensorimotor-related striatum versus ventral striatum. *Neuroscience* 1994; 59:625–640.

Marsden CD: Movement disorders and the basal ganglia. *Trends Neurosci* 1986; 9:512–515.

McGeer EG, et al: Neurotransmitters in the basal ganglia. *Can J Neurol Sci* 1984; 11:89–99.

Nauta HJW, Cole M: Efferent projections of the subthalamic nucleus: An autoradiographic study in monkey and cat. *J Comp Neurol* 1978; 180:1–16.

Parent A: Extrinsic connections of the basal ganglia. *Trends Neurosci* 1990; 13:254–258.

Penney JB, Young AB: GABA as the pallidothalamic neurotransmitter: Implications for basal ganglia function. *Brain Res* 1981; 207:195–199.

Rolls E: Neurophysiology and cognitive functions of the striatum. *Rev Neurol* 1994; 150:648–660.

Sadikot AF, et al: The center median and parafascicular thalamic nuclei project respectively to the sensorimotor and associative-limbic striatal territories in the squirrel monkey. *Brain Res* 1990; 510:161–165.

Schneider JS, et al: Deficits in orofacial sensorimotor function in Parkinson's disease. *Ann Neurol* 1986; 19:275–282.

Selemon LD, Goldman-Rakic PS: Common cortical and subcortical targets of the dorsolateral prefrontal and posterior parietal cortices in the rhesus monkey: Evidence for a distributed neural network subserving spatially guided behavior. *J Neurosci* 1988; 8:4049–4068.

Selemon LD, Goldman-Rakic PS: Longitudinal topography and interdigitations of corticostriatal projections in the rhesus monkey. *J Neurosci* 1985; 5:776–794.

Smith AD, Bolam JP: The neural network of the basal ganglia as revealed by the study of synaptic connections of identified neurones. *Trends Neurosci* 1990; 13:259–265.

Staines WA, et al: Neurotransmitters contained in the efferents of the striatum. *Brain Res* 1980; 194:391–402.

Steckler T, et al: The pedunculopontine tegmental nucleus: A role in cognitive processes? *Brain Res Rev* 1994; 19:298–318.

Stoetter B, et al: Functional neuroanatomy of Tourette syndrome: Limbic-motor interactions studied with FDG PET. *Adv Neurol* 1992; 58:213–226.

CHAPTER 14

BASAL GANGLIA: CLINICAL CORRELATES

HYPERKINETIC DISORDERS

Chorea

Athetosis

Ballism

Dystonia

Tourette Syndrome

HYPOKINETIC DISORDERS

Parkinsonism

Diseases of the basal ganglia are associated with abnormal involuntary movements that typically occur at rest and disappear in sleep. They are generally divided into two categories: *hyperkinetic,* characterized by excessive involuntary movement, and *hypokinetic,* characterized by slow movement (**bradykinesia**) or absence or difficulty in initiating movement (akinesia). The hyperkinetic variety is seen in such disorders as chorea, athetosis, ballism, dystonia, tremor, and **tics.** The hypokinetic variety is seen largely in Parkinson's disease. Despite voluminous literature on basal ganglia, clinicoanatomic correlations are not available for all basal ganglia disorders. However, the following anatomic loci for pathology are agreed on: substantia nigra in Parkinson's disease, caudate nucleus in chorea, and subthalamic nucleus in ballism. In a recent analysis of behavioral and motor consequences of focal lesions in the

Bradykinesia (Greek *brady,* "slow"; *kinesis,* "movement"). Abnormal slowness of movement as seen in Parkinson's disease.

Tics. Sudden, brief, repetitive involuntary movements that may be suppressed for a period by effort or will.

KEY CONCEPTS

- Diseases of the basal ganglia are characterized by abnormal involuntary movement at rest.
- Involuntary movements in basal ganglia diseases characteristically disappear in sleep.
- Movement disorders associated with basal ganglia lesions are of two categories: hyperkinetic and hypo- or akinetic.
- Involvement of central nervous system structures beyond the basal ganglia in most movement disorders precludes a one-to-one anatomic-clinical correlation in such disorders.

basal ganglia in humans, the following conclusions were made:

1. Dystonia was the most frequent movement disorder. It occurred in 36 percent of the patients. Chorea and **parkinsonism** were less frequent, occurring in 8 and 6 percent, respectively.
2. The most common behavioral disturbance was the syndrome of **abulia,** characterized by apathy, loss of initiative and of spontaneous thought and emotional response.
3. Lesions limited to the caudate nucleus rarely caused motor disturbances but were more likely to cause behavioral problems (abulia). Motor disturbances associated with caudate lesions were chorea and dystonia. The prominence of behavioral disturbances in caudate lesions is consistent with the known anatomic connections of this nucleus and emphasize the cognitive role of the nucleus.
4. Lesions of the lentiform nucleus (putamen and globus pallidus) commonly cause dystonia and rarely chorea. Lesions involving the putamen are more prone to cause dystonia than those involving the globus pallidus. Lesions of the **lentiform nucleus** infrequently cause behavioral disturbances such as abulia. The prominence of motor disturbances in lentiform nucleus lesions is consistent with known anatomic connections of the nucleus and emphasize the motor role of the nucleus.

HYPERKINETIC DISORDERS

Chorea

Chorea is a disorder of movement characterized by sudden, frequent, involuntary, purposeless, and quick jerks of the trunk, extremities, and head associated with facial grimaces. The term *chorea* is derived from the Greek word *choreia,* for "dance." The lesion producing chorea is believed to be in the caudate nucleus (Fig. 14-1), although the pathology is often diffuse and multiple involving other neural structures.

At the cellular level, reduced levels of the following neurotransmitters and neuropeptides have been reported: gamma-aminobutyric acid (GABA), acetylcholine, enkephalin, substance P, dynorphin, and cholecystokinin. Loss of noradrenergic neurons in the locus ceruleus also has been reported. Two varieties of chorea are known to occur. These are a benign, reversible variety (**Sydenham's chorea**) occurring in children as a complication of rheumatic fever and a malignant variety (**Huntington's chorea**) that is a hereditary (autosomal dominant) disorder linked to chromosome 4 and associated with mental deficiency and progressive mental and cognitive deterioration.

Appendicular musculature is predominantly involved in the Sydenham's variety, whereas truncal musculature is predominantly involved in the Huntington's variety.

KEY CONCEPTS

- In general, chorea, ballism, and parkinsonism are associated with lesions in the caudate nucleus, subthalamic nucleus, and the dopaminergic nigrostriatal system, respectively.
- Discrete lesions in the caudate nucleus are more likely to produce behavioral manifestations, whereas discrete lesions in the putamen are more likely to produce motor disturbances.

Parkinsonism. A chronic progressive degenerative disease characterized by tremor, rigidity, and akinesia. It was described initially by the English physician James Parkinson under the rubric "shaking palsy" published in 1817. Earlier descriptions were made by Galen, Boetius, and others.

Lentiform nucleus (Latin "lens"; *forma,* "shape"). Lens-shaped putamen and globus pallidus.

Abulia (Greek "without will"). A state in which the patient manifests lack of initiative and spontaneity, with preserved consciousness.

Chorea (Latin *choros,* "a dance"). Irregular involuntary movements of the limbs or face secondary to striatal lesion. The names of four saints (Vitus, Valentine, Modesti, and John) have been associated with chorea over the ages. The most used is *St. Vitus's dance.*

Sydenham chorea. An acute, benign, and self-limited chorea, a manifestation of rheumatic fever. Named after Thomas Sydenham, the English physician who first described the disorder in 1686.

Huntington's chorea. Progressive neurodegenerative disorder inherited as an autosomal dominant trait. The disease was imported to America from Suffolk in the United Kingdom by the emigrant wife of an Englishman in 1630. Her father was choreic, and his father disapproved of the match because of the bride's father's illness. The disorder is named after George Sumner Huntington, a general practitioner who described the disease.

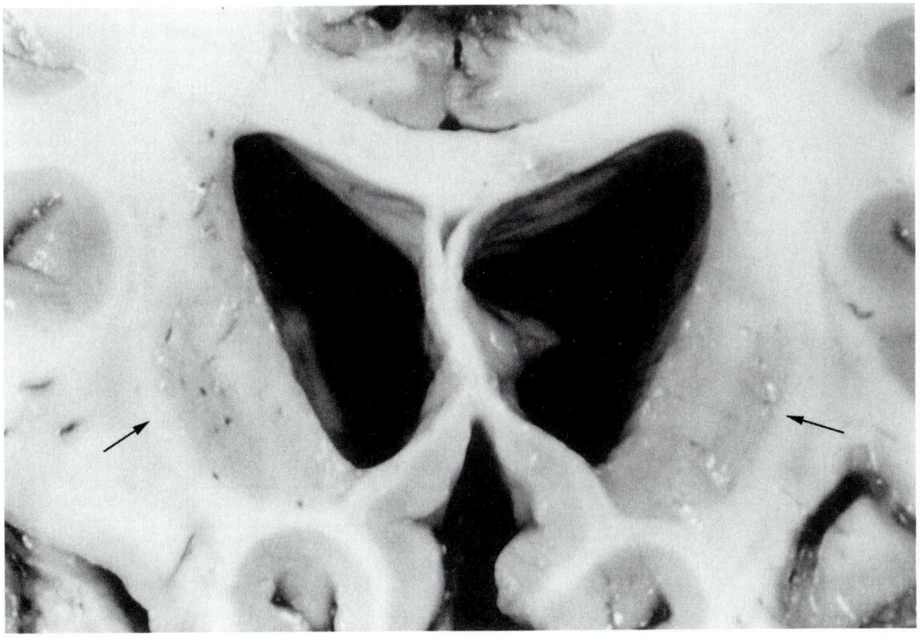

FIGURE 14-1

Coronal brain section from a patient with Huntington's chorea showing atrophy of the caudate nucleus.

Choreic patients are often unable to sustain a tight hand grip (**milkmaid's grip**) and cannot maintain a protruded tongue, which tends to dart in and out irregularly (**trombone tongue**). Figure 14-2 is a diagram showing how the striatal lesion in Huntington's chorea results in random expression of unwanted movement.

Athetosis

Athetosis is a disorder of movement characterized by slow, writhing, continuous, wormlike movements of the distal parts of the extremities, chiefly the fingers, which show bizarre posturing. The term *athetosis* is derived from the Greek word *athetos,* meaning "without position." The lesion producing athetosis is probably in the putamen. Differentiation of athetosis from chorea may at times be difficult because it is common to see patients with mixed choreoathetosis.

Ballism

Ballism is a disorder of movement usually caused by a vascular lesion in the subthalamic nucleus. The term *ballism* is derived from the Greek word *ballismos,* meaning "jump or throw." The movements of the limbs in this disorder are sudden, quick, continuous, unusually violent, and flinging in nature. The hyperkinesia is usually confined to one side of the body (hemiballismus) contralateral to the lesion in the subthalamic nucleus.

KEY CONCEPTS

- Hyperkinetic basal ganglia disorders include chorea, athetosis, ballism, tics, and dystonia.

Milkmaid's grip. Variability in the isometric force exerted by the wrist and by individual fingers during attempts to grasp an object. The sign is present in chorea.

Trombone tongue. Repetitive protrusion and replacement of the tongue seen characteristically in Huntington disease.

Athetosis (Greek *athetos,* "without position or place"). Involuntary movement disorder characterized by irregular, slow, writhing movements of distal parts of extremities. The condition was described by William Hammond in 1871.

Ballism (Greek *ballismos,* "jumping, throwing"). Violent flinging movements usually of one side of the body due to a lesion in the contralateral subthalamic nucleus.

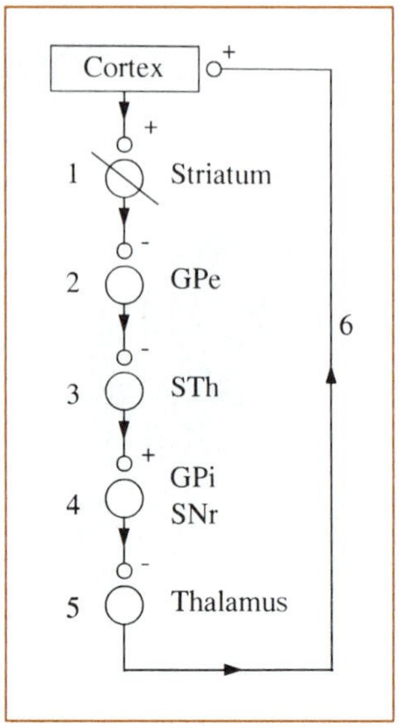

FIGURE 14-2

Schematic diagram showing how the striatal lesion in Huntington's chorea affects the indirect striatopallidal pathway and results in random expression of movement. (1) Loss of matrix neurons projecting to GPe. (2) Disinhibition of GPe. (3) Excess inhibition of STh. (4) Decreased excitation of GPi and SNr. (5) Less inhibition of thalamus. (6) Random expression of unwanted movement. GPe, external segment of globus pallidus; STh, subthalamic nucleus; GPi, internal segment of globus pallidus; SNr, substantia nigra pars reticulata. (*Modified from Adel K. Afifi: Basal ganglia: functional anatomy and physiology. Part II, J Child Neurol 9:352–361, 1994, Fig. 12, with kind permission from Decker Periodicals, Hamilton, Ontario, Canada.*)

Dystonia. Sustained and patterned muscle contractions of agonists and antagonist muscles leading to twisting involuntary movements. The clinical condition was first described by a German physician, Marcus Walter Schwalbe, in 1908.

Writer's cramp. A focal (hand) occupational dystonia precipitated by writing or typing. When first described by Bell in 1830 it was considered a psychiatric disorder.

Torticollis (Latin *tortere* "to twist"; *collis,* "neck"). A focal dystonia causing intermittent or persistent rotation of the neck.

Tourette syndrome. A dominantly inherited syndrome characterized by motor and vocal tics and a variety of behavioral symptoms and signs that include attention deficits and obsessive-compulsive behaviors. The syndrome is named after George-Edmond-Albert-Brutus Gilles de la Tourette, the French neuropsychiatrist who described the condition in 1885. The first recorded sufferer was the French prince of Condé, who had to stuff clothes into his mouth to stop himself from barking at King Louis XIV.

Dystonia

Dystonia is characterized by a twisting, slow, contorting, involuntary movement that, is somewhat sustained and often repetitive. The term *dystonia* is derived from the Greek words *dys* and *tonos,* for "bad tone." The affected body part may, with time, develop a fixed abnormal posture. Dystonia may be focal (involving a single body part such as the hand), segmental (involving two or more adjacent body parts such as the neck and arm), or generalized. **Writer's cramp,** an involuntary contraction of hand or finger muscles while writing, is an example of focal dystonia. **Torticollis** (involuntary turning or tilting of head) combined with facial dystonia constitutes segmental dystonia. Idiopathic torsion dystonia, a hereditary (autosomal dominant) disorder that begins in childhood, is an example of generalized dystonia.

No obvious specific pathology has been defined in the basal ganglia in hereditary idiopathic dystonia. However, discrete lesions in the striatum (Fig. 14-3) caused by stroke, tumor, or trauma have been associated with the development of dystonia.

Tourette Syndrome

Tourette syndrome is characterized by motor and vocal tics. Motor tics are sudden, brief involuntary movements involving muscles in different body parts such as eye

KEY CONCEPTS

- Dystonia is the most frequent basal ganglia disorder.

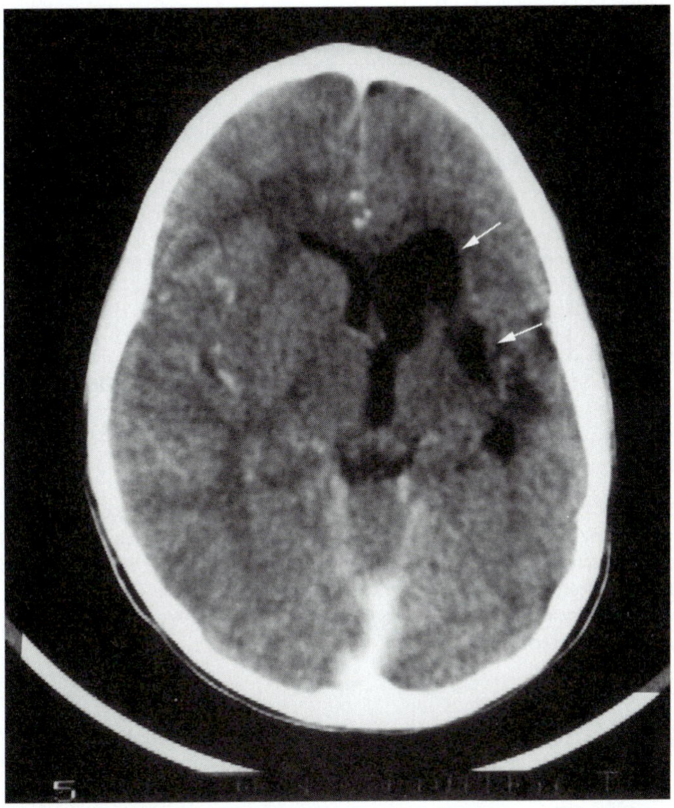

FIGURE 14-3

Computerized tomography (CT) of brain showing a lesion in the caudate nucleus and putamen in a patient with dystonia.

blinking and shoulder shrugging. Vocal tics consist of gutteral sounds, grunts, or verbalization of words and phrases. The motor manifestations are often associated with behavioral abnormalities such as attention deficits and compulsive ritualistic behaviors.

Previously considered a psychiatric or emotional disorder, Tourette syndrome is currently believed to have organic etiology.

Morphometric magnetic reasonance imaging (MRI) studies in Tourette syndrome reveal volume reduction in the caudate nucleus and the lenticular nucleus.

Postmortem studies in Tourette syndrome brains, although limited in number, report a decrease in overall volume of the striatum coupled with an increase in the number of small neurons and decreased dynorphin in striatopallidal axons. Based on the motor manifestations of Tourette syndrome (tics), the motor circuit of the basal ganglia or some subunits of it have been proposed as the primary site of pathology. The associated behavioral manifestations lend credence to involvement of the limbic basal ganglia circuit. An inhibitory limbic system drive acting on the motor cortex and motor striatum (Fig. 14-4) has been proposed as instrumental in the genesis of tics.

Tourette syndrome is named after Gilles de la Tourette, a French physician who described the syndrome in 1885. The first afflicted sufferer was reportedly the French prince of Condé, who had to stuff clothes into his mouth to stop himself from barking (vocal tics) at King Louis XIV.

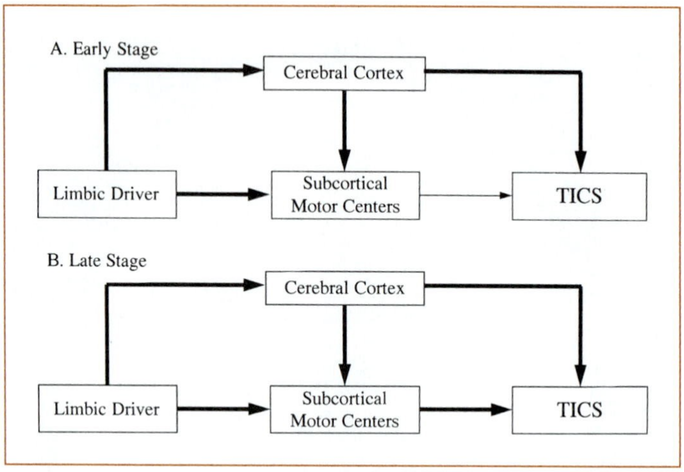

FIGURE 14-4

Schematic diagram depicting the roles of the limbic system drive, cerebral cortex, and subcortical motor centers in the genesis of tics. In early stages of tics (*A*), the cerebral cortex plays the major role in tic generation (thick arrow) while subcortical motor centers play a minor role (thin arrow). In late stages of tics (*B*), both the cortex and subcortical centers are equally capable of generating tics. (*From A. E. Lang et al.: "Signing tics"—insights into the pathophysiology of symptoms in Tourette's syndrome. Ann Neurol 33:212–215, 1993, Figs. A and B, with kind permission of Little, Brown, and Co., Boston, Massachusetts.)*

HYPOKINETIC DISORDERS

Parkinsonism

Parkinson's disease is a disorder characterized by tremor, rigidity, and hypo- or akinesia. The tremor of Parkinson's disease is rhythmic fine tremor recurring at the rate of 3 to 6 cycles per second and is best seen when the extremity is in a fixed posture rather than in motion (in contradistinction to cerebellar tremor, which is seen during movement of an extremity).

The rigidity is characterized by resistance to passive movement of a joint throughout the range of motion (**cogwheel rigidity**), resulting from an increase in tone of muscles with opposing action (agonists and antagonists).

Cogwheel rigidity. The arrhythmic, repetitive alteration of resistance to passive stretch occurring during passive movement of a joint; palpable tremor. A sign of basal ganglia disorder.

Hypokinesia. Poverty of willed movement.

Akinesia (Greek *a*, "negative, without"; *kinesis*, "movement"). Lack of spontaneous movement as seen in Parkinson's disease.

Hypokinesia or **akinesia** is manifested by a diminution or loss of associated movements, difficulty in initiating movement, and slow movement. The hypokinesia often causes difficulties for patients in getting dressed, feeding, and maintaining personal hygiene.

The coexistence of rigidity and hypokinesia in facial muscles accounts for decreased blinking rate and the expressionless mask facies.

The lesion producing Parkinson's disease is widespread in the central nervous system but affects the dopaminergic neurons in the substantia nigra most consistently. The lesion affects the dopaminergic nigrostriatal fiber system and depletes the striatal dopamine stores. The disease thus can be ameliorated by administration of L-dopa. Figure 14-5 is a diagram showing how dopamine depletion contributes to the poverty of movement and the difficulty in switching to new behaviors. In addition to the depletion of dopamine, reduction in concentration of the following neuropeptides occurs: enkephalin, somatostatin, neurotensin, substance P, and

KEY CONCEPTS

- Hypokinetic basal ganglia disorders include Parkinson's disease.

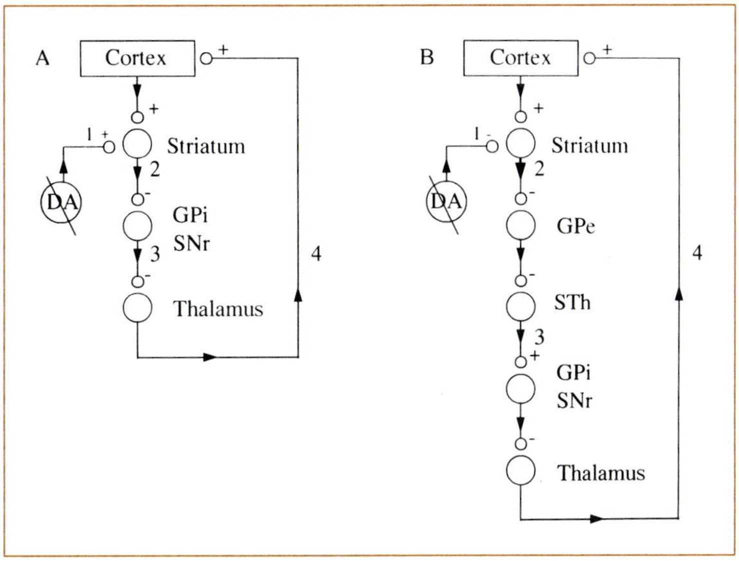

FIGURE 14-5

Schematic diagram showing how dopamine depletion in Parkinson's disease affects the direct and indirect striatopallidal pathways and movement. *A,* Slowness and poverty of movement. (1) Loss of excitatory DA input to striatal neurons projecting to GPi and SNr. (2) Decreased inhibition of GPi and SNr neurons. (3) Decreased disinhibition of thalamic neurons. (4) Slowness and poverty of movement. *B,* Inhibition of unwanted movement; difficulty switching to new behavior. (1) Loss of inhibitory DA input to striatal neurons projecting to GPe. (2) Increased inhibition of GPe neurons. (3) Disinhibition of STh input to GPi and SNr. (4) Reinforcing inhibition of unwanted movement. DA, dopamine; GPi, internal segment of globus pallidus; SNr, substantia nigra pars reticulata; GPe, external segment of globus pallidus; STh, subthalamic nucleus. (*Modified from Adel K. Afifi: Basal ganglia: functional anatomy and physiology. Part II. J Child Neurol 9:352–361, 1994, Fig. 11 with kind permission from Decker Periodicals, Hamilton, Ontario, Canada.*)

bombesin. Decrease in angiotensin II binding sites and loss of adrenergic neurons in the locus ceruleus also have been reported.

Prior to the discovery of the significance of L-dopa in parkinsonism, the tremor and rigidity of parkinsonism were treated by surgical lesions in the globus pallidus or thalamus. The former was more effective in the relief of rigidity and the latter in the relief of tremor.

Surgical approaches to treatment became less popular following the introduction of L-dopa therapy. Based on recent physiologic and anatomic data, lesions in the medial (internal) segment of the globus pallidus (posteroventral pallidotomy) are being used increasingly to treat selected drug-refractory patients.

SUGGESTED READINGS

Bhatia KP, Marsden CD: The behavioral and motor consequences of focal lesions of the basal ganglia in man. *Brain* 1994; 117:859–876.

Ceballos-Baumann AO, et al: Restoration of thalamocortical activity after posteroventral pallidotomy in Parkinson's disease. *Lancet* 1994; 344:814.

Dogali M, et al: Stereotactic ventral pallidotomy for Parkinson's disease. *Neurology* 1995; 45:753–761.

Koller WC: Chorea, hemichorea, hemiballismus, choreoathetosis and related disorders of movement. *Curr Opin Neurol Neurosurg* 1991; 4:350–353.

Lavoie B, et al: Immunohistochemical study of the basal ganglia in normal and parkinsonian monkeys. *Adv Neurol* 1992; 58:115–121.

Lozano AM, et al: Effect of GPi pallidotomy on motor function in Parkinson's disease. *Lancet* 1995; 346:1387–1388.

Peterson B, et al: Reduced basal ganglia volumes in Tourette's syndrome using three-dimensional reconstruction techniques from magnetic resonance images. *Neurology* 1993; 43:941–949.

Swedo SE, et al: Sydenham's chorea: Physical and psychological symptoms of St Vitus dance. *Pediatrics* 1993; 91:706–713.

Wilson SAK: Progressive lenticular degeneration: A familial nervous disease associated with cirrhosis of the liver. *Brain* 1912; 34:295–509.

Yoshida M: The neural mechanism underlying parkinsonism and dyskinesia: Differential roles of the putamen and caudate nucleus. *Neurosci Res* 1991; 12:31–40.

Young AB, Penney JB: Neurochemical anatomy of movement disorders. *Neurol Clin* 1984; 2:417–433.

CHAPTER 15

CEREBELLUM

GROSS FEATURES

The **cerebellum,** or "small brain," develops from the embryologic rhombic lip, a zone of cells between the alar and roof plates at the level of the pontine flexure. Although it develops from a "sensory" region (the rhombic lip), the cerebellum is concerned primarily (but not exclusively) with motor function.

The cerebellum is located in the posterior fossa of the skull, separated from the occipital lobes by a dural fold, the **tentorium cerebelli.** It overlies the dorsal surfaces of the pons and medulla oblongata and contributes to the formation of the roof of the fourth ventricle.

The cerebellum consists of a midline **vermis** and two laterally placed hemispheres.

KEY CONCEPTS

- The cerebellum, a derivative of sensory structure, has principally a motor function.

Cerebellum (Latin "little brain"). Erasistratus, a Greek physician and anatomist, divided the brain into cerebrum and cerebellum, and these terms were used by Galen. The term *cerebellum* appeared in English in 1565, but little was known of its function until Flourens published his experiments in 1822 to 1824 showing that the cerebellum was concerned with coordination of muscular movements. It was considered the seat of sexual appetite by Fraser in 1880.

Tentorium cerebelli (Latin *tentorium,* "a tent"). Horizontal dural fold between the cerebellum and cerebral hemisphere. The term was adopted about the end of the eighteenth century.

Vermis (Latin "a worm"). The midline portion of the cerebellum. The appearance of its folia bears a resemblance to the segmented body of a worm.

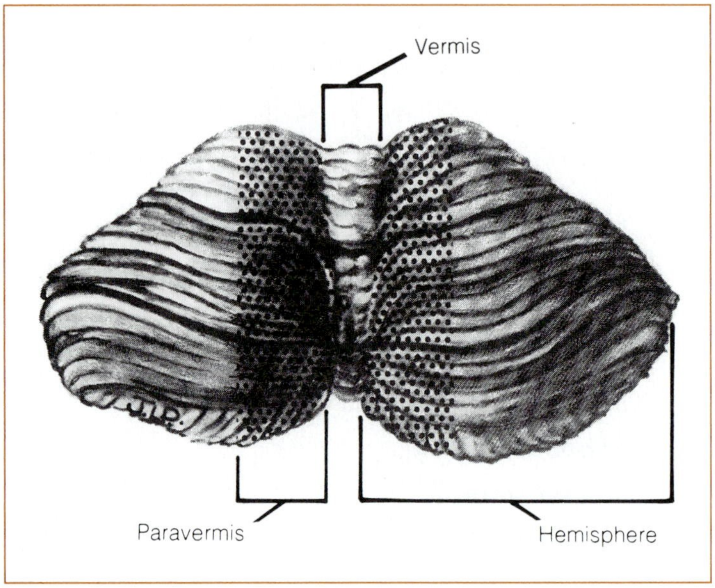

FIGURE 15-1

Schematic diagram of ventral surface of the cerebellum showing its subdivision into vermis, paravermis, and hemisphere.

The parts of the hemispheres adjacent to the vermis are known as the *paravermal* or *intermediate zones* (Fig. 15-1).

The dorsal cerebellar surface is rather flat; the demarcation of vermis and hemispheres is not evident on this surface (Fig. 15-2). The inferior surface is convex with a deep groove (vallecula) in the midline through which the vermis is apparent (Fig. 15-3).

The adult human cerebellum weighs approximately 150 g (10 percent of brain weight) and has a surface area of approximately 1000 cm^2 (40 percent of the cerebral cortex).

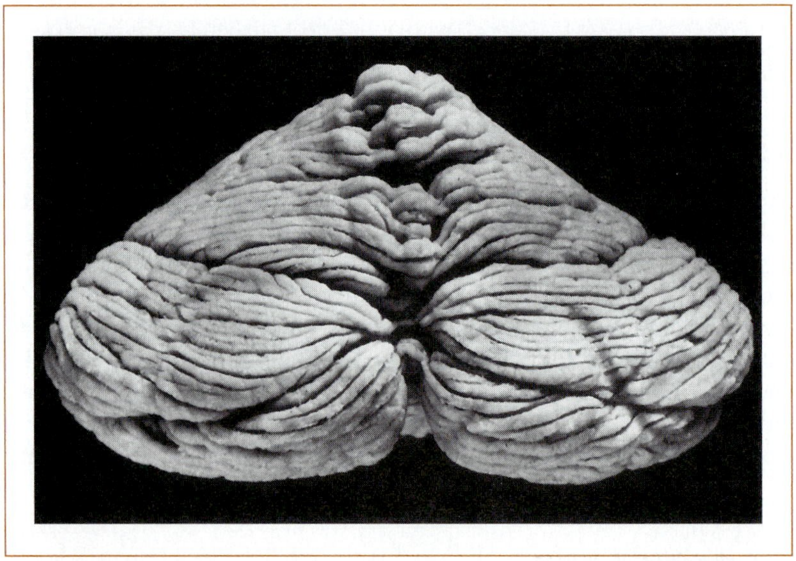

FIGURE 15-2

Photograph of dorsal surface of the cerebellum. (*From Gluhbegovic and Williams: The Human Brain, A Photographic Guide. Harper and Row Publishers, 1980, courtesy of the authors.*)

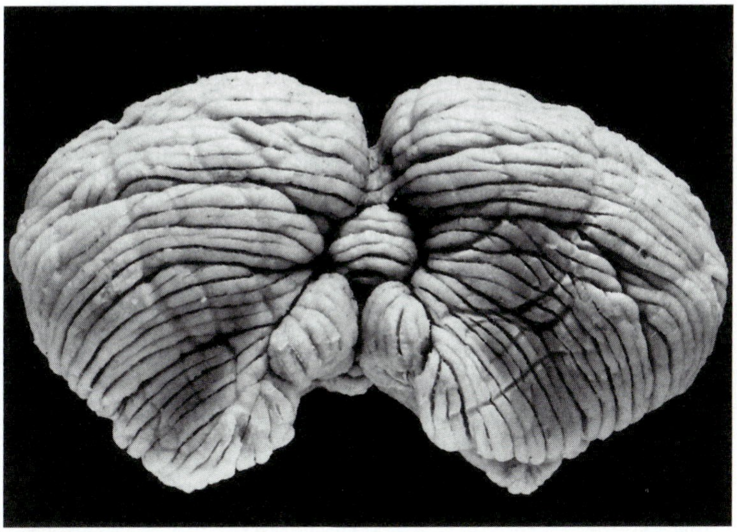

FIGURE 15-3

Photograph of ventral surface of the cerebellum. (*From Gluhbegovic and Williams: The Human Brain, A Photographic Guide. Harper and Row Publishers, 1980, courtesy of the authors.*)

The cerebellum is connected to the midbrain, pons, and medulla oblongata by three pairs of **peduncles.**

1. The superior cerebellar peduncle (**brachium** conjunctivum) connects the cerebellum with the midbrain.
2. The middle cerebellar peduncle (brachium pontis) connects the cerebellum with the pons.
3. The inferior cerebellar peduncle (**restiform** and juxtarestiform bodies) connects the cerebellum with the medulla oblongata.

The contents of each of these peduncles are discussed in the chapters on the mesencephalon (Chap. 9), pons (Chap. 7), and medulla oblongata (Chap. 5).

The cerebellum consists of a highly convoluted layer of gray matter, the cerebellar cortex, surrounding a core of white matter that contains the afferent and efferent tracts. Embedded in the white matter core are four pairs of deep cerebellar nuclei (Fig. 15-4):

1. **Fastigial nucleus**
2. **Globose nucleus**
3. **Emboliform nucleus**
4. **Dentate nucleus**

The globose and emboliform nuclei are referred to collectively as the *interposed nucleus.*

Lobes and Subdivisions (Table 15-1)

The cerebellum is divided anatomically by two transverse fissures (anterior and posterolateral or prenodular) into three lobes: anterior, posterior, and flocculo-

KEY CONCEPTS

- The cerebellum is organized into a cerebellar cortex and white matter core.

Peduncle (Latin *pedunculus,* "little foot"). Stemlike or stalklike process by which an anatomic part is joined to the main organ. The cerebellar peduncles connect the brain stem with the cerebellum.

Brachium (Latin "arm"). Denotes a discrete bundle of interconnecting fibers.

Restiform body (Latin *restis,* "cord or rope"; *forma,* "form or shape"). The inferior cerebellar peduncle has a cordlike appearance on the dorsolateral surface of the medulla. The restiform body was described and named by Humphrey Ridley (1653–1708), an English anatomist, in *Anatomy of the Brain* (London, 1695, p. 78).

Fastigial nucleus (Latin *fastigium,* "apex of a gabled, pointed roof"). The roof nucleus. The nucleus fastigi is located in the pointed roof of the fourth ventricle.

Globose nucleus (Latin *globus,* "a ball"). Rounded. The globose nucleus is rounded (spherical) in shape.

Emboliform nucleus (Greek *embolos,* "plug"; Latin *forma,* "form"). Plug-shaped. The emboliform nucleus plugs the opening of the dentate nucleus.

Dentate, nucleus (Latin *dentatus,* "toothed"). Like a tooth.

TABLE 15-1

Cerebellar Lobes and Subdivisions

Anatomic subdivisions			
Transverse plane	Anterior lobe	Posterior lobe	Flocculonodular lobe
Longitudinal plane	Vermis	Paravermis	Hemisphere
Functional subdivisions	Spino-cerebellum	Cerebro-cerebellum	Vestibulo-cerebellum
Phylogenetic subdivisions	Paleocerebellum	Neocerebellum	Archicerebellum

nodular. The demarcation of the three lobes is best seen in midsagittal sections (Fig. 15-5). Each of these lobes is further divided into lobules, which are in turn subdivided into leaflike folia by named *fissures* and *sulci* of no functional significance. The posterior lobe contains, on its inferior surface, the cerebellar tonsils. In cases of increased intracranial pressure such as occurs in brain tumors, intracranial hemorrhage, or severe head trauma, the cerebellar tonsils may herniate through the foramen magnum. This tonsillar herniation is a life-threatening neurologic emergency due to compromise of vital centers in the brain stem.

The cerebellum is also subdivided into three longitudinal zones, based on the arrangement of projections from the cerebellar cortex to deep cerebellar nuclei (see Fig. 15-1). These are the midline (vermis) zone, the intermediate (paravermal) zone, and the lateral (hemisphere) zone. The cortex of the vermis projects to the fastigial deep cerebellar nucleus, that of the paravermis to the interposed deep nuclei (emboliform and globose), and of the cerebellar hemisphere to the dentate nucleus (see Fig. 15-11). The borders that separate each of the transverse and longitudinal lobes and zones are far from precise. Clear functional subdivisions are

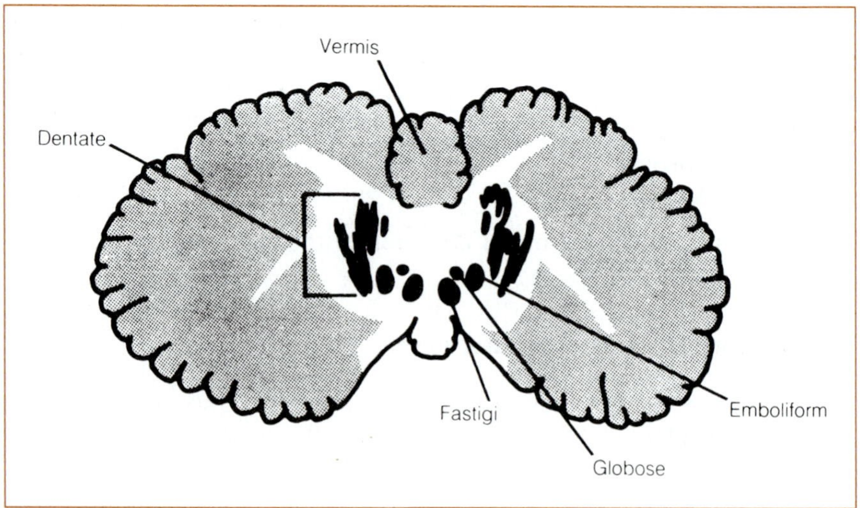

FIGURE 15-4

Schematic diagram of unfolded cerebellum showing the four cerebellar nuclei.

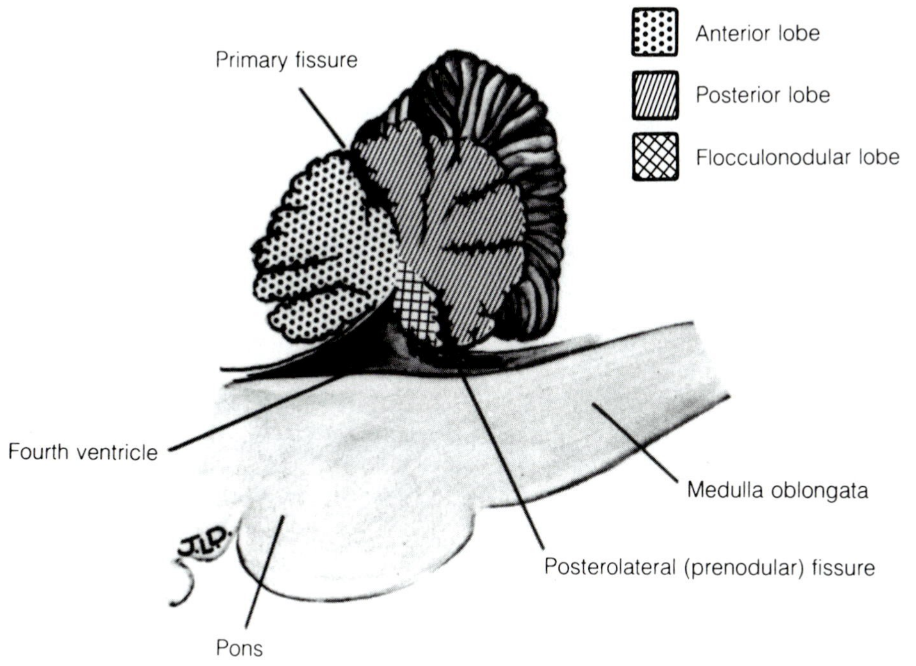
Anterior lobe
Posterior lobe
Flocculonodular lobe
Primary fissure
Fourth ventricle
Medulla oblongata
Posterolateral (prenodular) fissure
Pons

FIGURE 15-5

Schematic diagram of midsagittal view of the cerebellum and brain stem showing the three anatomic lobes of the cerebellum.

thus scarcely possible with reference to either the transversely oriented lobes or the longitudinally oriented zones.

Based on fiber connectivity, however, three functional subdivisions of the cerebellum have been delineated:

1. The vestibulocerebellum (corresponds best with the flocculonodular lobe) has reciprocal connections with vestibular and reticular nuclei and plays a role in control of body equilibrium and eye movement.
2. The spinocerebellum (corresponds best to the anterior lobe) has reciprocal connections with the spinal cord and plays a role in control of muscle tone as well as axial and limb movements.
3. The cerebrocerebellum or pontocerebellum (corresponds best to the posterior lobe) has reciprocal connections with the cerebral cortex and plays a role in planning and initiation of movements, as well as the regulation of discrete limb movements.

Phylogenetically, the cerebellum is divided into three zones: The **archicerebellum,** the oldest zone, corresponds to the flocculonodular lobe. The **paleocerebellum,** of more recent phylogenetic development than the archicerebellum, corresponds to the anterior lobe and a small part of the posterior lobe. The **neocerebellum,** the most recent phylogenetically, corresponds to the posterior lobe.

Archicerebellum (Greek *arche,* "beginning"). Phylogenetically old part of the cerebellum concerned with equilibrium and posture.

Paleocerebellum (Greek *palaios,* "ancient"; Latin *cerebellum,* "little brain"). Phylogenetically old part of the cerebellum.

Neocerebellum (Greek *neos,* "new"; Latin *cerebellum,* "small brain"). Phylogenetically new part of the cerebellum.

KEY CONCEPTS

- The cerebellum is divided into three imperfectly delineated lobes or zones based on morphology, connectivity, function, or phylogeny.

TABLE 15-2

Cerebellar Cortex Neurons

Neuron	Type	Layer	Projection	Synaptic Action
Purkinje	Principal (projection)	Purkinje	Deep cerebellar nuclei Lateral vestibular nucleus Other Purkinje cells Intrinsic neurons	Inhibitory
Basket	Interneuron	Molecular	Purkinje cell	Inhibitory
Stellate	Interneuron	Molecular	Purkinje cell	Inhibitory
Granule	Interneuron	Granule	Purkinje cell Basket cell Stellate cell Golgi cell	Excitatory
Golgi	Interneuron	Granule	Granule cell	Inhibitory

Somatotopic Representation

Somatotopic representation of body parts in the cerebellum was first described in 1943 by Adrian and later confirmed by others. In the anterior lobe, the body appears inverted, with hindlimbs represented rostral to the forelimbs and face. In the posterior lobe, the body appears noninverted and dually represented on each side of the midline, with face anteriorly and legs posteriorly represented. In general, the trunk is represented in the midline, and the extremities are represented more laterally in the hemispheres. Thus, in disorders predominantly affecting the midline cerebellum, disturbances of movement will be manifest primarily in trunk musculature and would affect body equilibrium. In contrast, in disorders primarily affecting the cerebellar hemispheres, disturbances of movement will manifest primarily in extremity movement.

MICROSCOPIC STRUCTURE

Cerebellar Cortex

The cerebellar cortex is made up of the following three layers.

1. Outer molecular layer (about 300 μm in thickness)
2. Middle Purkinje cell layer (about 100 μm in thickness)
3. Innermost granule cell layer (about 200 μm in thickness)

Five cells types (Table 15-2) are distributed in the different cortical layers. Basket and stellate cells are in the molecular layer, Purkinje cells are in the Purkinje cell layer, and granule and Golgi cells are in the granule cell layer.

KEY CONCEPTS

- Body parts are represented in the anterior and the posterior lobes.

Of these five cell types, the Purkinje cell constitutes the principal neuron of the cerebellum, since it is the only cerebellar neuron that sends its axons outside the cerebellum (projection neuron). All the other cells are intrinsic neurons and establish connections within the cerebellum.

Principal Neuron (see Table 15-2)

Cell bodies of Purkinje cells are arranged in a single sheet at the border zone between the molecular and granule cell layers. The cell is flask-shaped when viewed in the transverse plane and is narrow and vertical when viewed in longitudinal sections. The Purkinje cell measures approximately 30 to 35 μm in transverse diameter. Adjacent Purkinje cells are separated by 50 μm in the transverse plane and by 50 to 100 μm in the longitudinal plane. Each Purkinje cell has an elaborate dendritic tree that stretches throughout the extent of the molecular layer and is arranged at right angles to the long axis of the folium. The dendritic tree is made up of a sequence of primary, secondary, and tertiary branches, with the smaller dendritic branches profusely covered with dendritic spines or gemmules. It is estimated that each Purkinje cell has over 150,000 spines on its dendritic tree.

Each Purkinje cell has a single axon that courses through the granule cell layer and deep white matter to project on deep cerebellar nuclei. Some Purkinje cell axons (from the vermis) bypass the deep cerebellar nuclei to reach the lateral vestibular nucleus. Recurrent collateral axonal branches arise from Purkinje cell axons and project on adjacent Purkinje cells as well as on basket, stellate, and Golgi cells in neighboring or even distant folia. It is estimated that there are about 15 million Purkinje cells in the human cerebellum.

Intrinsic Neurons (see Table 15-2)

Basket Cell

Basket cells are situated in deeper parts of the molecular layer in close proximity to Purkinje cells. Dendritic arborizations of basket cells are disposed in the transverse plane of the folium in a manner similar to but less elaborate than the Purkinje cells. The axon courses in the molecular layer in the transverse plane of the folium just above the cell bodies of Purkinje cells. Each axon gives rise to several descending branches that surround Purkinje cell perikarya and initial segments of their axons in the form of a basket, hence their name. Each basket cell axon covers the territory of about 10 Purkinje cells. Basket formation, however, skips the Purkinje cell immediately adjacent to the basket cell and descends on the second Purkinje cell and onward in the row. In addition, axonal branches extend in the longitudinal plane of the folium to reach an additional three to six rows of Purkinje cells on both sides of the main axons. As a result of this, a single basket cell may reach as many as 200 Purkinje cells. More than one basket cell may contribute to a single basket formation around one Purkinje cell. While the descending branches of basket cell axons establish contact with Purkinje cell perikarya and initial segments of their axons, ascending branches of basket cell axons ascend in the molecular layer to reach the proximal dendrites of Purkinje cells. It is estimated that there are about 7 million basket cells in the human cerebellum.

Stellate Cell

Stellate cells are located in the superficial and deeper parts of the molecular layer. Axons of stellate cells are also disposed transversely in the folium and terminate on Purkinje cell dendrites. It is estimated that there are 12 million stellate cells in the human cerebellum.

The basket and stellate cells can be considered as belonging to the same class. Both receive the same input, and both act on Purkinje cells. The difference lies in the fact that stellate cells establish contact with the dendrites of Purkinje cells, whereas basket cells establish contact with dendrites, perikarya, and axons of Purkinje cells.

Granule Cell

Granule cells are among the smallest cells in the brain (6 to 9 μm) and fill the granule cell layer. Each cell gives rise to about three to five dendrites that establish synaptic contacts with axons in a synaptic zone (the glomerulus) within the granule cell layer. Axons of granule cells ascend in the granule cell layer, Purkinje layer, and molecular layer, where they bifurcate in a T fashion to form the parallel fiber system. Parallel fibers run horizontally in the molecular layer perpendicular to the plane of the Purkinje dendrites. Each parallel fiber branch is 1 to 1.5 mm in length; thus the axon of a single granule cell spans an area of approximately 3 mm. The parallel fibers establish contact with dendrites of Purkinje cells, Golgi cells, stellate cells, and basket cells. Generally, a parallel fiber comes in contact with a Purkinje cell only once or, rarely, twice. A single Purkinje cell, however, can receive up to 100,000 parallel fibers. The total number of granule cells is estimated to be on the order of 2.2 billion.

Golgi Type II Cell

Golgi neurons occupy the superficial part of the granule cell layer adjacent to the Purkinje cells. They are large neurons, about the same size as the Purkinje cell bodies. Dendrites of Golgi neurons arborize in either the molecular or the granule cell layer. Those which remain in the granule cell layer contribute to the glomeruli of that layer. Those which reach the molecular layer arborize widely and overlap the territories of three Purkinje cells in both the transverse and longitudinal planes. The Golgi neuron dendritic arborization is thus three times that of the Purkinje cell.

Glomerulus (Latin *glomero,* "to wind into a ball"). Small, rounded synaptic configuration around mossy fiber rosettes.

Axons of Golgi cells take part in the formation of the **glomerulus.** They are characterized by a dense arborization of short axonal branches that span the entire granule cell layer. The field of axonal arborization approaches that of dendritic arborization. The axonal arborization of the Golgi neurons is among the most unique in the brain. The Golgi neuron forms the central point of a functional hexagon that includes about 10 Purkinje cells. It is estimated that there are 4 million Golgi cells.

Cerebellar Glomerulus

In histologic sections of the cerebellar cortex there are islands between granule cells that stain lighter than the rest of the granule cell layer. These are the cerebellar glomeruli (Fig. 15-6). They are the sites of synaptic contact between the incoming cerebellar fibers (mossy fiber system) and processes of neurons within the granule cell layer. The elements that form a cerebellar glomerulus are

1. Cerebellar input via the mossy fiber system (origins of this system will be discussed later)
2. Dendrites of granule cells
3. Axon terminals of Golgi neurons
4. Proximal parts of Golgi dendrites

KEY CONCEPTS

- The cerebellar cortex has three layers and contains five cell types (one principal and four intrinsic).
- The white matter core contains incoming and outgoing fibers and four deep cerebellar nuclei.

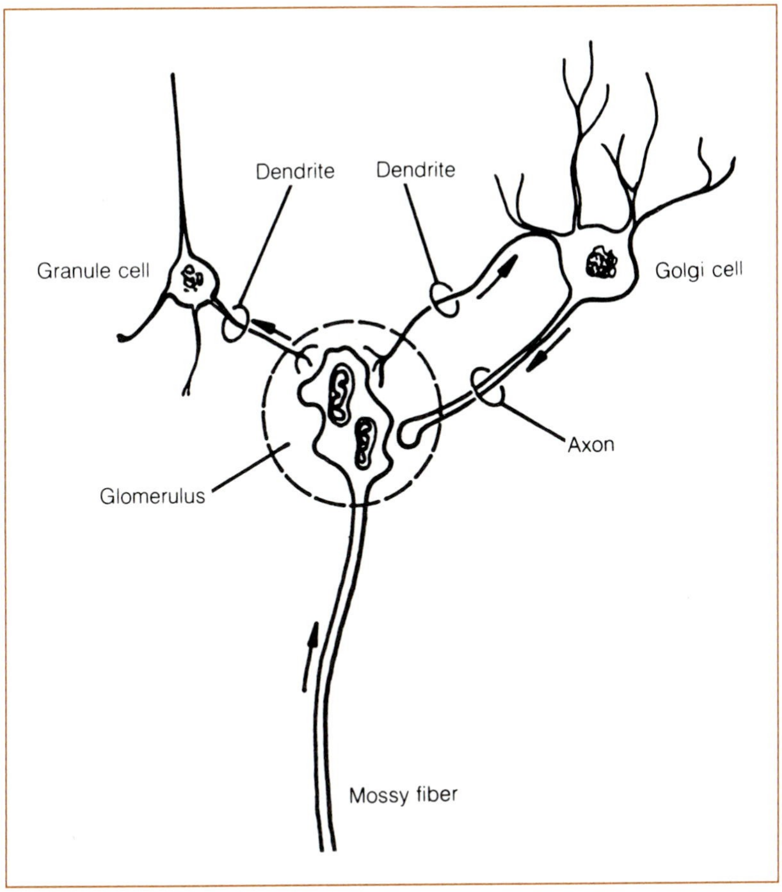

FIGURE 15-6

Schematic diagram of a cerebellar glomerulus showing the different sources of converging fibers.

Electron micrographs have shown that the mossy fiber axonal terminal is the central element in the glomerulus (terminal rosettes) around which are clustered dendrites of granule cells and axons of Golgi neurons. Both mossy fiber axons and Golgi axons act on the dendrites of granule cells. In addition, mossy fiber axons project on dendrites of Golgi neurons. The whole complex is surrounded by a glial envelope. It is estimated that a glomerulus contains about 100 to 300 dendritic terminals from some 20 granule cells.

CEREBELLAR INPUT

Containing more than half the neurons in the brain, the cerebellum is one of the busiest neuronal intersections in the brain, receiving input from and sending signals back to every major central nervous system. Input to the cerebellum originates from a variety of sources. The three major sources of afferents, however, are the spinal cord, vestibular system, and cerebral cortex (Fig. 15-7).

Inputs from the spinal cord are transmitted to the cerebellum via the dorsal and ventral spinocerebellar tracts and the rostral extension of the dorsal spinocerebellar tract, the cuneocerebellar tract. These tracts provide the cerebellum with information related to the position and condition of muscles, tendons, and joints.

Inputs from the vestibular system arise from the primary vestibular end organ in the vestibular labyrinth, as well as from vestibular nuclei in the brain stem. Vestibulocerebellar inputs provide information related to body equilibrium.

Cortical inputs to the cerebellum originate in neocortical as well as paleo- and archicortical areas. These include primary motor and sensory cortices as well as

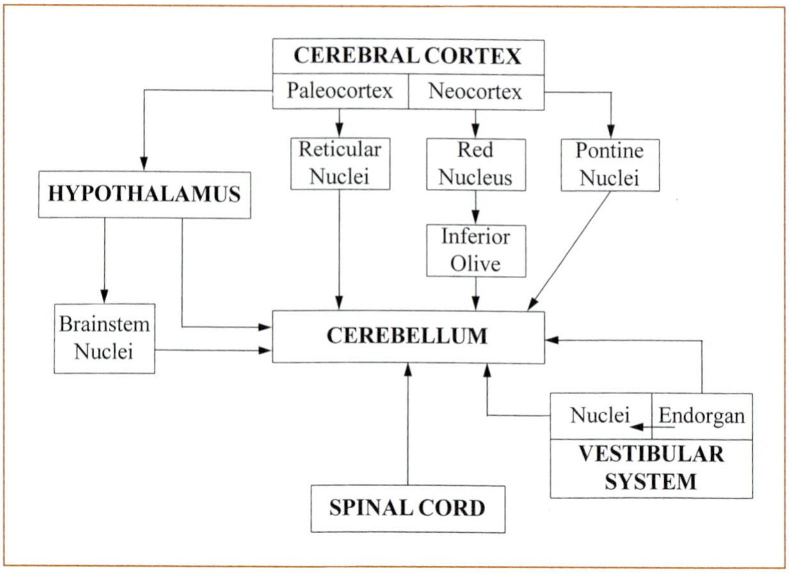

FIGURE 15-7

Schematic diagram showing major sources of input to the cerebellum.

association and limbic cortices. Inputs from neocortical areas reach the cerebellum after relays in the pontine nuclei (the vast majority), red nucleus, and inferior olive. Inputs from paleo- and archicortical areas establish relays in the reticular nuclei and hypothalamus prior to reaching the cerebellum. Corticocerebellar inputs provide information related to the planning and initiation of movement.

Other fiber inputs to the cerebellum include a noradrenergic projection from the locus ceruleus (A-6 cell group of primates), a dopaminergic projection from the ventral tegmental area of Tsai in the midbrain (A-10 cell group of primates), and a serotonergic projection from the raphe nuclei (B-5 and B-6 cell groups of primates) in the brain stem. The input from the locus ceruleus projects on Purkinje cell dendrites and exerts an inhibitory effect on Purkinje cell activity. It has been postulated that the input from the locus ceruleus plays a role in the development of Purkinje cells. The terminals from the locus ceruleus develop prior to Purkinje cell maturation. Destruction of the locus ceruleus results in immature development of Purkinje cells.

In the past few years, a series of investigations has revealed the existence of a complex network of direct and indirect pathways between the hypothalamus and the cerebellum. The projections are bilateral with ipsilateral preponderance. They originate from various hypothalamic nuclei and areas but principally from the lateral, dorsal, and posterior hypothalamic areas and the dorsal, ventromedial, supramamillary, and tuberomamillary nuclei. The indirect pathway reaches the cerebellum after relays in a number of brain stem nuclei. The hypothalamocerebellar network may provide the neuroanatomic substrate for the autonomic responses elicited from cerebellar stimulation.

Fiber inputs to the cerebellum from the preceding various sources arrive via three cerebellar peduncles: the inferior (restiform body), the middle (brachium pontis), and the superior (brachium conjunctivum).

KEY CONCEPTS

- The major inputs to the cerebellum are from three sources.

TABLE 15-3

Climbing and Mossy Fibers

	Projection Targets					
Fiber Type	Deep Nuclei	Purkinje	Basket	Stellate	Granule	Golgi
Climbing	+	+	+	+		+
Mossy	+				+	+

Inferior Cerebellar Peduncle

The fiber systems reaching the cerebellum via this peduncle are the following:

1. Dorsal spinocerebellar tract
2. Cuneocerebellar tract from the accessory cuneate nuclei
3. Olivocerebellar tract from the inferior olivary nuclei (major component)
4. Reticulocerebellar tract from the reticular nuclei of the brain stem
5. Vestibulocerebellar tract (both primary afferents from the vestibular end organ and secondary afferents from the vestibular nuclei)
6. Arcuatocerebellar tract from the arcuate nuclei of the medulla
7. Trigeminocerebellar tract from the spinal and main sensory nuclei of the trigeminal nerve

Middle Cerebellar Peduncle

The fiber systems reaching the cerebellum via this route are the following:

1. Pontocerebellar (corticopontocerebellar) tract from the pontine nuclei (major component)
2. Serotonergic fibers from the raphe nuclei

Superior Cerebellar Peduncle

The fiber input to the cerebellum via this route includes the following:

1. Ventral spinocerebellar tract
2. Trigeminocerebellar tract from the mesencephalic trigeminal nucleus
3. Cerulocerebellar tract from the nucleus ceruleus
4. Tectocerebellar tract from the superior and inferior colliculi

The various inputs to the cerebellum are segregated within the cerebellum into one of three fiber systems: climbing, mossy, and a recently described multilayered.

Climbing Fiber System (Fig. 15-8)
It is generally believed that the olivocerebellar tract is the major component of this system. Climbing fibers establish synapses on dendrites of the principal neuron of the cerebellum (the Purkinje cell), as well as on dendrites of intrinsic neurons (Golgi, basket, and stellate) (Table 15-3). The climbing fiber input is known to exert a powerful excitatory effect on a single Purkinje cell and a much less powerful

KEY CONCEPTS

- Inputs to the cerebellum arrive via one of the three cerebellar peduncles.

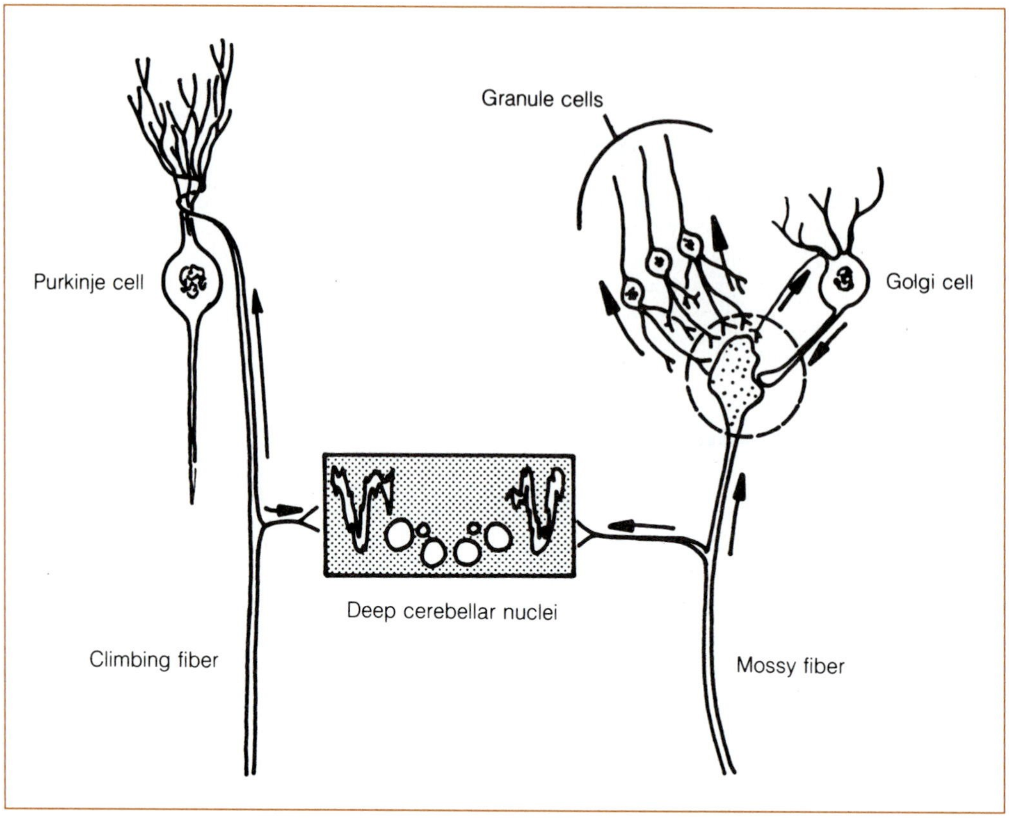

FIGURE 15-8

Schematic diagram comparing the climbing and mossy fiber systems within the cerebellum.

effect on intrinsic neurons. The relationship of climbing fibers to principal neurons is so intimate that one climbing fiber is restricted to one Purkinje cell and follows the branches of the Purkinje cell dendrites like a grapevine. The climbing fiber effect on a Purkinje cell is thus one-to-one, all-or-none excitation. It is estimated that one climbing fiber establishes 1000 to 2000 synaptic contacts with its Purkinje cell. Stimulation of the climbing fiber system elicits a prolonged burst of high-frequency action potentials from the Purkinje cell capable of overriding any ongoing activity in that cell.

Mossy Fiber System

The mossy fiber system includes all afferents to the cerebellum except those which contribute to the climbing fibers and the multilayered fiber system. Like the climbing fibers, mossy fibers enter the cerebellum via the core of deep white matter. They then diverge into the folia of the cerebellum, where they branch out into the granule cell layer. Within the granule cell layer, mossy fibers divide into several subbranches of terminal rosettes that occupy the center of each glomerulus, where they come in contact with dendrites of granule and Golgi neurons (see Fig. 15-8 and Table 15-3). It is estimated that each mossy fiber establishes contact with approximately 400 granule cell dendrites within a single folium and that each terminal mossy rosette contacts approximately 20 different granule cells. On the other hand, each granule cell receives synaptic contacts from four to five different mossy fiber terminals. The mossy fiber is believed to stimulate the largest number of cells to be activated by a single afferent fiber. Thus, in contrast to the climbing fiber input, which is highly specific and sharply focused on the Purkinje cell, the mossy fiber input is diffuse and complex (see Fig. 15-8). In addition to their contribution to the Purkinje and granule cells of the cerebellar cortex, both climbing and mossy fibers send collaterals to the deep cerebellar nuclei (see Fig. 15-8). These collaterals are excitatory in nature and help maintain a constant background discharge of these deep nuclei.

Multilayered Fiber System
This recently described fiber system includes afferents to the cerebellum from the hypothalamus, as well as the serotonergic input from the raphe nuclei, the noradrenergic input from the nucleus locus ceruleus, and the dopaminergic input from the mesencephalic dopaminergic neurons. Similar to the climbing and mossy fiber systems, the multilayered fiber system projects on neurons in the cerebellar cortex and the deep cerebellar nuclei.

INTERNAL CEREBELLAR CIRCUITRY

A mossy fiber input excites dendrites of a group of granule cells. The discharge from these granule cells will be transmitted through their axons (parallel fibers), which bifurcate in a T configuration in the molecular layer, coming in contact with the perpendicular orientation of dendrites of Purkinje, stellate, basket, and Golgi neurons. If the excited parallel fiber bundle is wide enough to cover the Purkinje cell dendritic field, activation will result in a single row of Purkinje cells parallel to the long axis of the folium and in the related basket and stellate cells. Golgi cells will not fire, however, because their dendritic fields are wider than those of the Purkinje cells. The activation of the basket and stellate cells, the axons of which are oriented perpendicular to those of the parallel fibers and Purkinje cells in the folium, will inhibit a wide zone of Purkinje cells on each side of the row of activated Purkinje cells. Thus the mossy fiber input will produce a row of activated Purkinje cells flanked on each side by a strip of inhibited Purkinje cells. The inhibited rows of Purkinje cells, by silencing surrounding activity, help the process of neural sharpening within the activated row of Purkinje cells.

If the activated bundle of parallel fibers becomes wide enough to span the dendritic field of a Golgi neuron, the Golgi cell is then excited and, through its axon in the glomerulus, will inhibit the granule cell. Thus a mossy fiber input is completely transferred into inhibition via one of two mechanisms:

1. Mossy fiber to granule cell dendrite (in the glomerulus) to granule cell axon (parallel fiber) to basket, stellate, and Golgi dendrites to basket, stellate, and Golgi axons to Purkinje cell or granule cell dendrite (Fig. 15-9)
2. Mossy fiber to Golgi dendrite within the glomerulus to Golgi axon to granule cell dendrite (see Fig. 15-9)

The mossy fiber input has both high divergence and convergence ratios. A single mossy fiber has 40 rosettes, each rosette connects with the dendritic terminals of 20 granule cells, and a single granule cell connects through the parallel fibers with 100 to 300 Purkinje cells. This gives a divergence ratio of about 1:100,000 to 1:300,000 from one mossy fiber to the Purkinje cell. On the other hand, each Purkinje cell has about 100,000 dendritic spines in synaptic contact with parallel fibers (granule cells) and hence a large ratio of convergence.

Similarly, a climbing fiber input will excite Purkinje cells as well as stellate, basket, and Golgi neurons. The effect on these different cells is similar to that described for the mossy fiber input and helps to focus on the activation of the

KEY CONCEPTS

- Within the cerebellum, various inputs are segregated into one of three fiber systems.

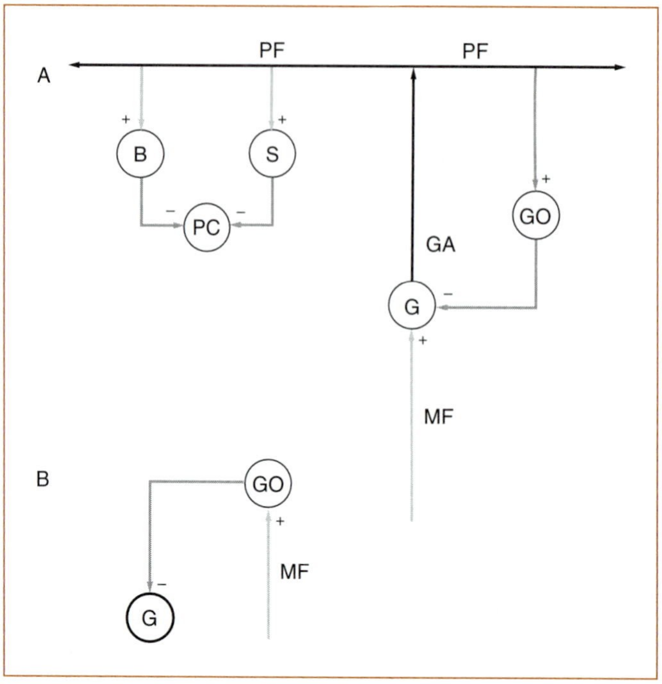

FIGURE 15-9

Schematic diagram showing how an excitatory mossy fiber input can be transformed into inhibition via granule cell axon (*A*), or Golgi cell axon (*B*). Light gray denotes excitation, dark gray denotes inhibition. MF, Mossy fiber; G, granule cell; GA, granule cell axion; PF, parallel fibers; GO, Golgi cell; S, stellate cell; B, basket cell; PC, Purkinje cell.

Purkinje cell amid a zone of inhibition induced by basket, stellate, and Golgi neurons. In contrast to the mossy fiber system, the convergence and divergence factors for the climbing fiber input are small (1:1).

Incoming fibers to the cerebellum thus excite Purkinje and granule cells of the cerebellar cortex, as well as the deep cerebellar nuclei (see Fig. 15-8). Purkinje cells are excited directly by climbing fibers and indirectly (via the granule cell) by mossy fibers. The excitation of Purkinje cells is modulated by several feedback circuits (via basket and stellate inhibitory interneurons) that inhibit Purkinje cell activity and supress transmission of impulses from Purkinje cells to deep cerebellar nuclei. The output of Purkinje cells to the deep cerebellar nuclei is thus a finely modulated inhibitory signal. The output of the deep cerebellar nuclei to extracerebellar targets is thus the product of excitatory input from climbing and mossy fibers and inhibitory projections from Purkinje cells (Fig. 15-10).

The mossy fiber pathways conduct faster than the climbing fiber pathways. However, the ultimate inhibitory potentials produced by the mossy fiber system develop slowly so that by the time the climbing fiber input arrives in the cerebellum, the full effect of the mossy fiber inhibitory potentials has not yet developed. This allows the climbing fiber system to act on the background activity of excitation and inhibition initiated by the mossy fiber input.

Thus, of all the cells of the cerebellar cortex, only the granule cell is excitatory; all others, including the Purkinje cells, are inhibitory. Recent studies on the cerebel-

KEY CONCEPTS

- Cerebellar inputs excite Purkinje cells directly via climbing fibers and indirectly via granule cell axons.
- Intrinsic cerebellar neurons are excited by cerebellar inputs and in turn inhibit Purkinje cells.

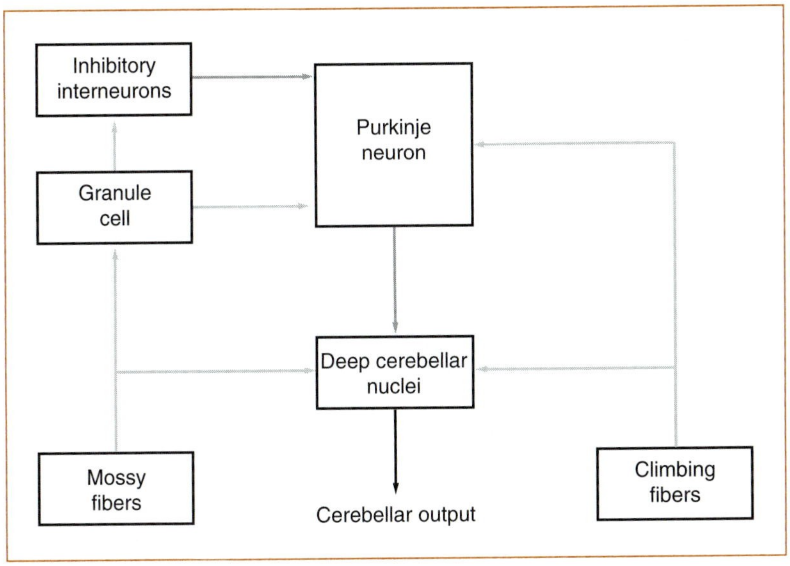

FIGURE 15-10

Schematic diagram of the intrinsic cerebellar circuitry. Light gray denotes excitation, dark gray denotes inhibition.

lum have given the Golgi neuron a central role in cerebellar organization. Through its contact with both the mossy fibers in the glomerulus and the climbing fiber collaterals, the Golgi neuron is able to select what input will reach the Purkinje cell at any one time.

CEREBELLAR OUTPUT

The cerebellar output system has two components: intracerebellar and extracerebellar. The intracerebellar component comprises the inhibitory projections of Purkinje cells to deep cerebellar nuclei. These projections are somatotopically organized (Fig. 15-11). Purkinje cells in the vermis project to the nucleus fastigi, while those in the paravermal and cerebellar hemisphere zones project, respectively, to the interposed nucleus (emboliform and globose) and the dentate nucleus. The vast majority of the extracerebellar component comprises the projections of deep cerebellar nuclei to extracerebellar targets. A smaller part of it originates from a group of Purkinje cells in the vestibulocerebellum whose axons bypass the deep cerebellar nuclei and project on the lateral vestibular nucleus in the brain stem. Extracerebellar targets of deep cerebellar nuclei (Figs. 15-12 to 15-14) include the vestibular and reticular nuclei of the brain stem (from the nucleus fastigi), the red nucleus in the midbrain and the inferior olivary nucleus in the medulla (from the interposed nucleus), the thalamus (from the dentate and interposed nuclei), and the hypothalamus (from all deep cerebellar nuclei).

Efferents from the cerebellum leave via the inferior and superior cerebellar peduncles. Cerebellovestibular and cerebelloreticular fibers travel via the inferior cerebellar peduncle, whereas the cerebellothalamic, cerebellorubral, and cerebelloolivary fibers travel via the superior cerebellar peduncle. The superior cerebellar peduncle crosses in the midbrain tegmentum (at the inferior colliculus level) and

KEY CONCEPTS

- Purkinje cell axons project on deep cerebellar nuclei in a topographic fashion.
- Deep cerebellar nuclei provide cerebellar output to extracerebellar targets.
- Extracerebellar targets include the vestibular and reticular nuclei, red nucleus, and thalamus.

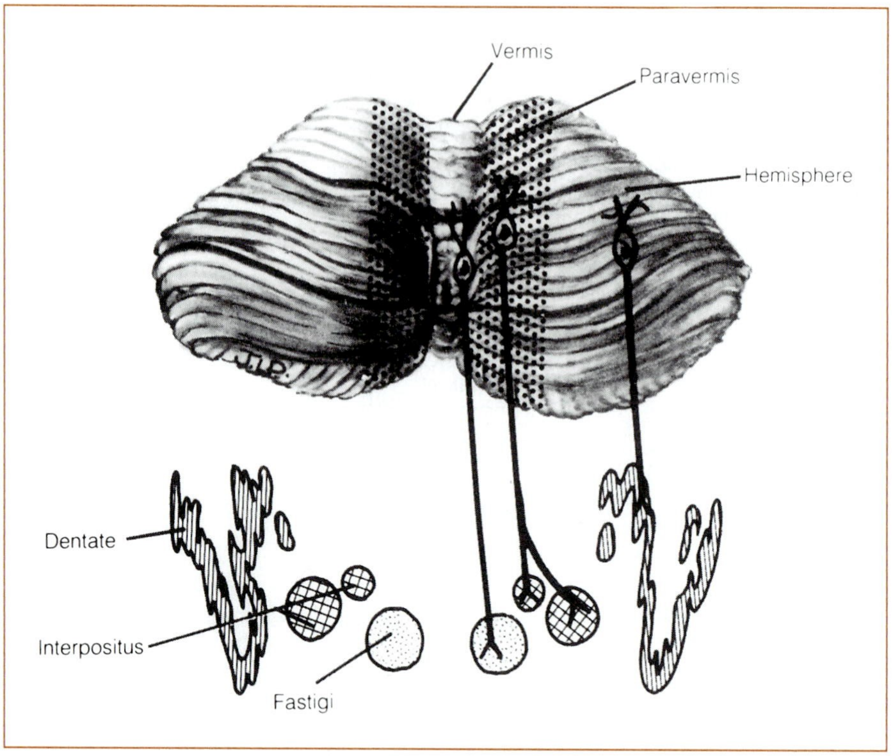

FIGURE 15-11

Schematic diagram showing topographic projections of Purkinje cells of different cerebellar zones into the respective deep cerebellar nuclei.

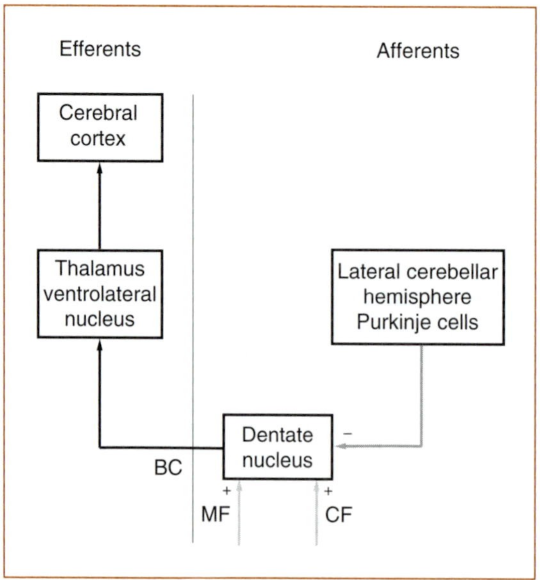

FIGURE 15-12

Schematic diagram showing the afferent and efferent connections of the dentate nucleus. Light gray denotes excitation, dark gray denotes inhibition. CF, Climbing fiber; MF, mossy fiber; BC, brachium conjunctivum.

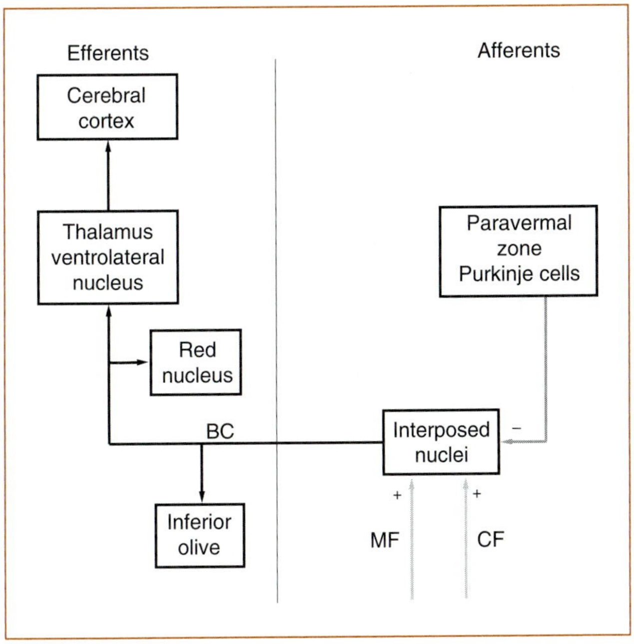

FIGURE 15-13

Schematic diagram showing the afferent and efferent connections of the interposed nuclei. Light gray denotes excitation, dark gray denotes inhibition. CF, Climbing fiber; MF, mossy fiber; BC, brachium conjunctivum.

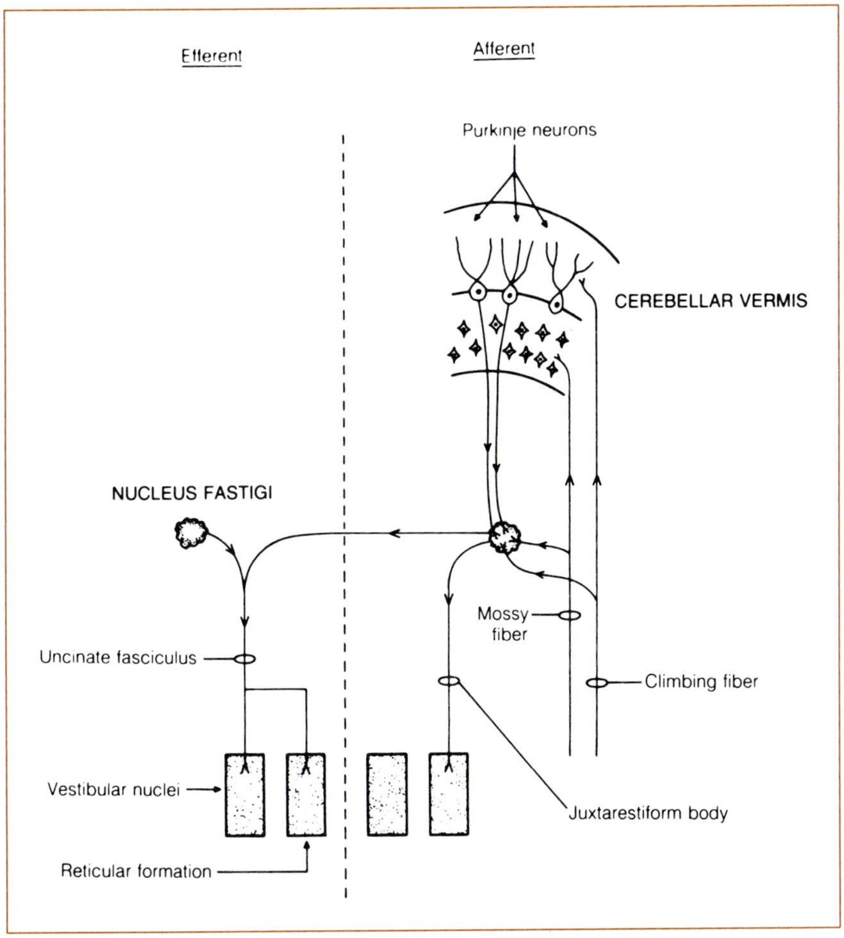

FIGURE 15-14

Schematic diagram showing the afferent and efferent connections of the nucleus fastigi.

projects on the contralateral red nucleus and ventrolateral nucleus of the thalamus. A small fascicle from this crossed system descends to the inferior olivary nucleus. The cerebellum exerts its most important influence on the motor and premotor cortices via the ventrolateral nucleus of the thalamus. Electrophysiologic studies show that pyramidal tract neurons in the motor and premotor cortices receive di- or trisynaptic excitatory inputs from the dentate and interposed nuclei after relays in the ventrolateral thalamic nucleus. Other corticofugal neurons in the motor and premotor cortices, such as those which project to the red nucleus, pontine nuclei, and spinal cord, also receive cerebellar fibers. In addition to the motor and premotor cortices, the cerebellum projects to the parietal and temporal association cortices.

DEEP CEREBELLAR NUCLEI

The deep cerebellar nuclei are embedded in the white matter core of the cerebellum. There are four pairs of nuclei arranged from lateral to medial as follows: dentate, emboliform, globose, and fastigi (see Fig. 15-4).

Dentate Nucleus

The dentate nucleus (see Fig. 15-12) is composed of multipolar neurons and resembles the inferior olive in configuration. It receives the axons of Purkinje cells located in the lateral part of the cerebellar hemispheres and collaterals of climbing and mossy fibers. The Purkinje cell input is inhibitory, whereas the inputs from climbing and mossy fibers are excitatory to the dentate nucleus.

The bulk of axons of the dentate nucleus project via the superior cerebellar peduncle to the contralateral ventrolateral nucleus of the thalamus. A relatively small number of axons project to the intralaminar nuclei of the thalamus (mainly the central lateral nucleus), to the rostral third of the red nucleus (origin of rubroolivary tract), and, via the descending limb of the brachium conjunctivum, to the reticulotegmental nucleus and inferior olive.

The expansion of the dentate nucleus and the lateral cerebellar hemisphere in the course of hominid evolution provided the neural basis for novel cerebellar trajectories and new functions. The phylogenetically older part of the dentate nucleus (the dorsomedial part) maintains connections with the motor cortex via the motor thalamus (ventrolateral nucleus) and with the spinal cord via the red nucleus, in line with the traditionally established role of the cerebellum in motor control. The phylogenetically newer part of the dentate nucleus (the ventrolateral part), in contrast, has connections, in addition to the motor cortex, with the prefrontal cortex, which has expanded in parallel with the dentate nucleus in the course of hominid evolution. Evidence is accumulating in favor of a nonmotor function of the neodentate nucleus.

Interposed Nuclei

These nuclei (see Fig. 15-13) include the emboliform nucleus, located medial to the hilum of the dentate nucleus, and the globose nucleus, located medial to the emboliform nucleus.

The interposed nuclei receive afferent fibers from the following sources:

1. Axons of Purkinje cells in the paravermal (intermediate) zone of the cerebellum that are inhibitory in function
2. Collaterals from climbing and mossy fiber systems that are excitatory in function

Axons of interposed nuclei leave the cerebellum via the superior cerebellar peduncle. The bulk projects on neurons in the caudal two-thirds of the red nucleus (the part that gives rise to the rubrospinal tract). A smaller number of axons project on the ventrolateral nucleus of the thalamus and, via the descending limb of the brachium conjunctivum, to the inferior olive.

Fastigial Nucleus

This nucleus (see Fig. 15-14) is located in the roof of the fourth ventricle medial to the globose nucleus; hence it is called the *roof nucleus.* It receives afferent fibers from the following sources:

1. Axons of Purkinje cells in the vermis of the cerebellum that are inhibitory in function
2. Collaterals of mossy and climbing fiber systems that are excitatory

In contrast to efferents from the dentate and the interposed nuclei, efferents of the fastigial nucleus do not travel via the brachium conjunctivum. A large number of fastigial efferents cross within the cerebellum and form the uncinate fasciculus. Uncrossed fastigial fibers join the juxtarestiform body. The bulk of fastigial efferents project on the vestibular nuclei (lateral and inferior) and several reticular nuclei of the brain stem. Fastigial projections to vestibular nuclei are bilateral. Fastigioreticular fibers are mainly crossed. A small number of fastigial efferents course rostrally in the brain stem to project on the superior colliculus, nuclei of the posterior commissure, and the ventrolateral thalamic nucleus.

In addition to the efferent projections of the deep cerebellar nuclei described above, all deep cerebellar nuclei have been shown to send axon collaterals to the areas of the cerebellar cortex from which they receive fibers; thus the nucleus fastigi sends axon collaterals to the cerebellar vermis, the interposed nuclei to the paravermal region, and the dentate nucleus to lateral parts of the cerebellar hemispheres. Although deep cerebellar nuclei receive axons of Purkinje cells, their axon collaterals do not project directly on Purkinje cells but on neuronal elements in the granule cell layer via the mossy fiber system. The exact cell type in the granule cell layer that receives these axon collaterals has not been identified with certainty.

Thus all the deep cerebellar nuclei receive a dual input; these are an excitatory input from extracerebellar sources (mossy and climbing fibers) and an inhibitory input from the cerebellar cortex (axons of Purkinje cells). In contrast, the output of the deep cerebellar nuclei is excitatory.

CEREBROCEREBELLAR AND CEREBELLOCEREBRAL CIRCUITRIES

The cerebral cortex communicates with the cerebellum via a multitude of pathways, of which the following are well recognized (Fig. 15-15):

1. Corticoolivocerebellar via the red nucleus and inferior olivary nucleus
2. Corticopontocerebellar via the pontine nuclei
3. Corticoreticulocerebellar via the reticular nuclei of the brain stem

The first two pathways convey to the cerebellum precisely localized and somatotopically organized information. Of these two, the pathway via the pontine nuclei is quantitatively more impressive. The pathway via the reticular nuclei is part of a system with diffuse input and output (reticular formation), in which information of cortical origin is integrated with information from other sources before transmission to the cerebellum.

The cerebellum influences the cerebrum mainly via the dentatothalamic system. The cerebellocerebral pathways are modest in number when compared with the cerebrocerebellar pathways (approximately 1 : 3). This is a reflection of the efficiency of the cerebellar machinery that makes it possible for the cerebellum to regulate cortically originating signals for movement. Corticocerebellar fibers originate from motor and nonmotor (associative and limbic) areas of the cerebral cortex. Similarly, cerebellar output fibers target both motor and nonmotor cerebral cortical areas.

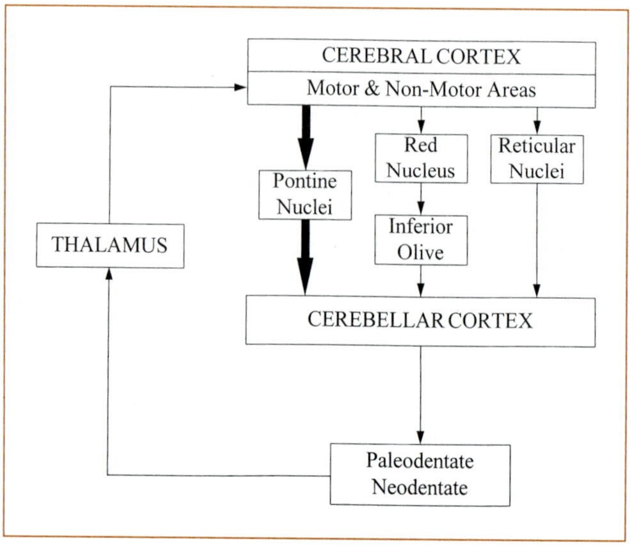

FIGURE 15-15

Schematic diagram of cerebrocerebellar and cerebellocerebral connections. Heavy arrows denote quantitatively significant pathway.

NEUROTRANSMITTERS

The following neurotransmitters have been identified in the cerebellum: gamma-aminobutyric acid (GABA), taurine, glutamate, aspartate, acetylcholine, norepinephrine, serotonin, and dopamine.

GABA is liberated from axons of Purkinje, basket, and Golgi neurons and exerts an inhibitory effect on target neurons. Taurine is believed to be the inhibitory neurotransmitter of the superficial stellate cells; taurine levels are high in the molecular layer and drop substantially when stellate cell development is blocked by x-irradiation. Glutamate is believed to be the excitatory neurotransmitter of granule cells; glutamate levels in the granule cell layer drop substantially in the agranular cerebellum of virus-infected and mutant mice. Aspartate is probably the neurotransmitter of the climbing fiber system; aspartate levels drop in cases of olivocerebellar atrophy, in which the inferior olive (major source of climbing fibers) is atrophied. Acetylcholine is probably the neurotransmitter of the mossy fiber system. Norepinephrine is the inhibitory neurotransmitter of the locus ceruleus projection on Purkinje cell dendrites. In addition to its presumed role in maturation of Purkinje neurons, norepinephrine seems to modulate Purkinje cell response to other cerebellar neurotransmitters. Stimulation of the locus ceruleus enhances sensitivity of Purkinje neurons to both glutamate and GABA. Serotonin and dopamine are released in terminals of projections from the raphe nuclei and midbrain dopamine neurons, respectively.

CEREBELLAR PHYSIOLOGY

Cerebellar Cortex

Cerebellar neurons are characterized by high rates of resting impulse discharge. Purkinje cells discharge at the rate of approximately 20 to 40 Hz, granule cells at 50 to 70 Hz, and inhibitory interneurons (basket, stellate, and Golgi) at 7 to 30 Hz. In the conscious monkey, the Purkinje cell has been found to discharge at rates varying between 3 and 125 Hz, with a mean discharge rate of 70 Hz. This high discharge rate of cerebellar neurons is derived from the nature of their synaptic drive. The activity of Purkinje cells correlates closely with the activity of mossy fibers, which also have high rates of resting discharge.

Stimulation of the mossy fiber system or of the parallel fibers (axons of granule cells) elicits in the Purkinje cell a brief excitatory postsynaptic potential (EPSP) (*simple spike*) lasting 5 to 10 ms, followed by a prolonged inhibitory postsynaptic potential (IPSP). The short EPSP is attributed to the activation of Purkinje cell dendrites by the parallel fibers. The IPSP, on the other hand, is attributed to the feedforward inhibition of Purkinje cells by stellate and basket cells that are activated simultaneously by the beam of parallel fibers. The prolonged time course of the IPSP implies a prolonged excitatory action on these cells by the parallel fiber input.

Stimulation of the climbing fiber system elicits in the Purkinje cell an intense and prolonged reaction characterized by an initial large spike followed by several small ones. This pattern is referred to as a *complex spike.* This complex EPSP is followed by a prolonged IPSP. The complex spike is explained on the basis of more than one mechanism. One mechanism for this complex spike in the Purkinje cell is the repetitive discharge emanating from inferior olive neurons because of axonal collaterals within the inferior olive. Another mechanism for the complex response of Purkinje cells lies in the intrinsic property of their membranes. The IPSP that follows the complex EPSP is attributed to simultaneous activation of stellate and basket cells by the climbing fibers, which in turn inhibit the Purkinje cell by a feedforward pathway. Both mossy and climbing fibers facilitate the Golgi cell, which in turn inhibits the granule cell and can thus contribute to Purkinje cell inhibition. After their initial activation by the mossy and climbing fiber input, intrinsic neurons (basket, stellate, and Golgi) ultimately are inhibited by Purkinje axon collaterals. The action of the recurrent Purkinje axon collaterals is thus to disinhibit the Purkinje cell.

It becomes evident from the preceding that the mossy and climbing input fibers are excitatory to the granule and Purkinje cells, whereas the action of all other cells within the cerebellum (except the granule cell) is inhibitory. It is thus not possible for cerebellar activity in response to an afferent input to be sustained.

Several investigators have studied the effects of cerebellar stimulation in humans. The results of such stimulation are similar to those described above.

Deep Cerebellar Nuclei

Like the Purkinje cells, deep nuclei of the cerebellum have high rates of impulse discharge at rest. Also like the Purkinje cells, the deep cerebellar nuclei receive both excitatory and inhibitory inputs, the former arriving via the climbing and mossy fibers and the latter by axons of Purkinje cells. Thus a mossy fiber input, for example, will cause first a high-frequency burst in the deep cerebellar nuclei followed by a lowering of the frequency as a result of inhibition arriving through the slower Purkinje cell loop. Purkinje cell inhibition is mediated by gamma-aminobutyric acid (GABA).

Motor Functions of the Cerebellum

The cerebellum traditionally has been relegated a motor function. Based on studies conducted by Gordon Holmes in the first quarter of the twentieth century on patients with wound injuries to the cerebellum, the Holmes motor triad of asthenia (easy fatigability), ataxia, and atonia became synonymous with cerebellar disease. Subsequent clinical and experimental studies confirmed a role for the cerebellum in control and integration of motor activity.

Neocerebellar Signs

The incoordination of movement noted in diseases of the neocerebellum is the result of disturbances in speed, range, force, or timing of movement. The smooth execution of voluntary acts requires a steady increase and decrease in force during

Asynergia (Greek *synergia,* "cooperation"). Lack of coordination among parts. Disturbance of proper association in the contraction of muscles that ensures that the different components of an act follow in proper sequence and at the proper moment so that the act is executed accurately.

Dysmetria (Greek *dys,* "difficult"; *metron,* "a measure"). Difficulty in accurately controlling (measuring) the range of movement. Occurrence of errors in judgment of distance when a limb is made to perform a precise movement.

movement. The lack of uniform velocity is responsible for the irregular and jerky movements (dyssynergia, **asynergia**) of cerebellar disease.

Proper timing in initiation and termination of movement is essential in the execution of smooth movement. A delay in the initiation of each successive movement will lead to the adiadochokinesis (disturbance in performance of rapid movement using antagonistic muscle groups) of cerebellar disease. A delay in the termination of movement produced by a delay in intervention of antagonistic muscles to check the movement results in **dysmetria** and overshooting. Thus adiadochokinesis and dysmetria are the result of an error in timing.

Intention (volitional) tremor is due to defective feedback control from the cerebellum on cortically initiated movement. Normally, cerebellar feedback mechanisms control the force and timing of cortically initiated movement. Failure of these mechanisms in cerebellar disease results in tremor.

The cerebellum is able to exert its corrective influence on cortically originating movement by virtue of the input it receives from the cerebral cortex and periphery. The cerebral cortex informs the cerebellum of intended movement via the cerebrocerebellar pathways described previously. During movement, the cerebellum receives also a constant flow of information, both proprioceptive and exteroceptive, from peripheral receptors (e.g., muscle spindle, Golgi tendon organ) concerning movement in progress. The cerebellum correlates peripheral information on movement in progress with central information on intended movement and corrects errors of movement accordingly. It has been proposed that the neuronal architecture of the cerebellar cortex serves to recognize complex states that are critical for the selection and control of actions, as well as for translation of this state information into spatiotemporal patterns of motor discharge appropriate for precise movement.

In addition to its role as "error detector" of cortically initiated movement, the cerebellum may be involved in motor learning and the initiation of movement. Long-lasting changes in synaptic efficacy may take place in the cerebellar cortex during motor learning, suggesting that the cerebellum may be capable of remembering what was done and thereby adapting its influence on motor neurons in accordance with the outcome of movement. Experimental evidence suggests that deep cerebellar nuclei fire simultaneously with pyramidal cortical neurons prior to movement.

The cerebellum also influences movement via its effects on the gamma system. The cerebellum normally increases the sensitivity of muscle spindles to stretch. Cerebellar lesions are associated with a depression of gamma motor neuron activity that leads to erroneous information in the gamma system about the degree of muscle stretch. The erroneous information conveyed by the muscle spindle to the alpha motor neuron results in disturbances in discharge of the alpha motor neuron and is manifested by a disturbance in force and timing of movement.

The depression of tonic activity of gamma motor neurons in cerebellar disease is the basis of the hypotonia associated with neocerebellar syndromes.

Archi- and Paleocerebellar Signs

The archicerebellum and paleocerebellum influence spinal activity via the vestibulospinal and reticulospinal tracts. The increase in myotatic and postural reflexes associated with the anterior lobe syndrome is due to an increase in motor signals to the alpha motor neurons and a simultaneous decrease in signals to the gamma system. Thus the rigidity of cerebellar disease is an alpha type of rigidity.

KEY CONCEPTS

- Motor functions of the cerebellum include error detection and correction of cortically initiated movement, motor learning, and the initiation of movement.

Disturbances in Equilibrium and Gait

Disturbances in gait may be seen following involvement of all divisions of the cerebellum. When accompanied by disturbances in equilibrium, such as inability to assume upright posture, gait disturbance is indicative of lesions in the posterior part of the vermis and flocculonodular lobe. Abnormalities of gait secondary to lesions in the anterior lobe are usually not associated with equilibrium disturbances. In humans, unsteadiness of gait (gait **ataxia**) may be the only manifestation of the anterior lobe syndrome.

Ataxia (Greek *taxis,* "order"). Want of order, lack of coordination, resulting in unsteadiness of movement. The term was used by Hippocrates and Galen for any morbid state, especially one with disordered or irregular action of any part such as irregularity of the pulse.

Ocular Motor Signs

Several ocular motor abnormalities have been described in cerebellar disorders. **Nystagmus** has been reported in disorders of the cerebellum without concomitant brain stem involvement. Two types of cerebellar nystagmus have been described, the spontaneous and the positional.

Spontaneous horizontal nystagmus with a quick component toward the side of the lesion occurs with asymmetric (unilateral) lesions in the posterior vermis, flocculonodular lobe, and nucleus fastigi. It is believed to represent the release of the vestibular nuclei from the posterior vermis.

Positional nystagmus also has been reported following lesions in the same sites that produce spontaneous nystagmus. It is best seen in the supine position with a quick component in the direction of gaze.

Complete cerebellectomy in humans is associated with inability to maintain eccentric gaze, defective smooth pursuit movements, failure to suppress optokinetic nystagmus by visual fixation, and a moderate increase in the vestibuloocular reflex (adjustment of eye position in response to head movement). In unilateral cerebellar lesions, the preceding signs appear **ipsilateral** to the lesion.

Nystagmus (Greek *nystagmos,* "nodding in sleep"). Rhythmic involuntary oscillatory movements of the eyes. The term is said to have been first used by Plenck. The association of these eye movements with vertigo was first noted by Purkinje and further investigated by Flourens.

Ipsilateral (Latin *ipse,* "self"; *lateralis* from *latus,* "side"). Situated in or with reference to the same side of the body.

Cerebellum and Epilepsy

Cerebellar stimulation has been shown to have beneficial effects on both experimentally induced epilepsy and human epilepsy. Cerebellar stimulators are used to treat intractable epilepsy in humans. The results of such investigations are variable, and more study is needed before the role of the cerebellum in the control of epilepsy can be defined clearly.

Complementarity of Basal Ganglia and Cerebellum in Motor Function

Review of basal ganglia and cerebellar structure, connectivity, and organization reveals many features in common. Both are components of the motor system, influence cerebral cortical activity via the thalamus, are linked with the cerebral cortex via recurrent loops, have internal (local) circuitry that modulates loop activity, receive modulating inputs that influence their activities (climbing fibers in the cerebellum and dopaminergic input in the basal ganglia), have a high convergence ratio of inputs on their principal neurons (spiny neuron in the basal ganglia and Purkinje cell in the cerebellum), and play a role in pattern recognition.

KEY CONCEPTS

- Cerebellar diseases in humans manifest as three syndromes: midline, cerebellar hemisphere, and pancerebellar.
- Signs and symptoms of cerebellar disease are manifested ipsilateral to the cerebellar lesion.

The emerging concept (see Fig. 13-18) of the complementarity of basal ganglia and cerebellar roles in motor function suggests that the basal ganglia function as detectors of specific contexts, providing to the cerebral cortex information that could be useful in planning and gating of action. The cerebellum, in contrast, functions in programming, execution, and termination of actions. According to this concept, the cerebral cortex, which receives diverse sensory information from the periphery via the different ascending tracts as well as complex information already processed within the basal ganglia and cerebellum, serves two functions: a repository function to receive this diverse information, compute it, and share it with the basal ganglia and cerebellum and an executive function to implement the action emanating from its collective computation process.

Nonmotor Functions of the Cerebellum

A growing body of data suggest a nontraditional role for the cerebellum in the regulation of autonomic function, behavior, and cognition. Following cerebellar ablation or stimulation, a multitude of visceral and affective responses has been reported, including cardiovascular and endocrine changes; altered respiration, intestinal motility, and bladder tone; reduced aggressiveness; mood changes; and alerting reactions. These visceral and affective responses were believed to be mediated through cerebellar connections with brain stem reticular nuclei. Recent evidence for a complex network of pathways between the hypothalamus and cerebellum suggests an alternate mechanism for these responses.

The possibility that the cerebellum may be involved in nonmotor function was first suggested by phrenologists in the eighteenth and nineteenth centuries and by later studies dating back almost half a century. The founder of phrenology, Franz Gall, considered the primary function of the cerebellum to be a locus of the emotion of love.

Reports of neuropsychological dysfunction in patients with developmental and acquired cerebellar pathology and neuroimaging studies in normal adults have given credence to the proposed involvement of the cerebellum in "higher order" nonmotor processes. Psychiatric disorders (schizophrenia, manic depression, and dementia) have been reported in association with cerebellar agenesis or hypoplasia. Damage to the cerebellum has been shown to impair rapid and accurate mental shifts of attention between and within sensory modalities. Increased planning and word-retrieval time have been described in patients with cortical cerebellar atrophy, and transient mutism has been reported following posterior fossa craniectomy for cerebellar tumors and following bilateral stereotactic lesions of the dentate nucleus. Recent data from positron-emission tomography (PET) and single photon emission computed tomography (SPECT) seem to confirm a role for the cerebellum in nonmotor function. Neocerebellar areas are metabolically active during language and cognitive processes such as the association of verbs to nouns, mental imagery, mental arithmetic, motor ideation, and learning to recognize complicated figures, whereas vermal and paravermal structures are metabolically active during panic and anxiety states.

Stimulation of the fastigial nucleus in animals has been reported to produce an alerting reaction, grooming response, savage predatory attack, and outbursts of sham rage, suggesting that the fastigial nucleus may serve a modulatory role for emotional reactions. Following lesions in the cerebellar vermis, aggressive monkeys are reported to have become docile, and chronic cerebellar stimulation in humans has been reported to reduce anxiety, tension, and aggression.

The reported association between cerebellar disorders and cognition and behavior does not necessarily imply causality, however. Whether the cognitive and behavioral manifestations reported in cerebellar disorders are due to the cerebellar lesion

TABLE 15-4

Functions of Cerebellum

Region	Motor Function (Established)	Nonmotor Function (Proposed)
Archicerebellum	Equilibrium and posture	Primitive autonomic responses, emotion, affect, sexuality, affectively important memory ("limbic" cerebellum)
Neocerebellum	Coordination of extremity movement	Modulation of thought, planning, strategy formation, spatial and temporal parameters, learning, memory, language

itself or are secondary to associated cerebral hemisphere dysfunction remains unsettled. The cerebellum and cerebral cortex are closely related anatomically and functionally.

The reciprocal anatomic connections between the cerebral cortex and cerebellum may thus provide the anatomic basis for the potentially reversible functional hypometabolism between a cerebral hemisphere and the contralateral cerebellum.

Based on the available behavioral and cognitive data, a new concept of cerebellar function has evolved that assigns to each cerebellar lobe a role in behavior and cognition (Table 15-4). Thus the archicerebellum may be concerned not only with control of equilibrium and posture but also with primitive defense mechanism such as the "fight or flight" response, emotion, affect, and sexuality, whereas the neocerebellum may be concerned, in addition to coordination of rapid movement of the extremities, with modulation of thought, planning, strategy formation, spatial and temporal parameters, learning, memory, and language.

SENSORY SYSTEMS AND CEREBELLUM

Although the cerebellum is generally regarded as a motor center, recent studies suggest that it has a role in sensory mechanisms. The cerebellum has been shown to receive tactile, visual, and auditory impulses. Furthermore, reciprocal connections have been demonstrated between the cerebral and cerebellar tactile, visual, and auditory areas.

KEY CONCEPTS

- Nonmotor roles for the cerebellum in autonomic regulation, behavior, cognition, and learning are being explored.

BLOOD SUPPLY

The cerebellum is supplied by three long circumferential arteries arising from the vertebral basilar system: (1) the posterior inferior cerebellar artery (PICA), (2) the anterior inferior cerebellar artery (AICA), and (3) the superior cerebellar artery (SCA).

The posterior inferior cerebellar artery (PICA) arises from the rostral end of the vertebral artery and reaches the caudal part of the cerebellar hemisphere and vermis. It also gives rise to branches to the dorsal and sometimes the lateral aspects of the medulla oblongata. Two areas may be distinguished in the PICA territory: a dorsomedial area, supplied by the medial branch of the PICA, whose territory includes the dorsolateral portion of the medulla oblongata, and an anterolateral area, supplied by the lateral branch of the PICA, which does not supply the medulla oblongata.

The anterior inferior cerebellar artery (AICA) arises from the caudal third of the basilar artery. Because of its usual small size, it supplies a small area of the anterior and medial cerebellum (the middle cerebellar peduncle and the flocculus). Proximal branches of the artery usually supply the lateral portion of the pons, including the facial, trigeminal, vestibular, and cochlear nuclei, the roots of the facial and cochleovestibular cranial nerves, and the spinothalamic tract. When there is a large AICA, the ipsilateral PICA is usually hypoplastic, and the AICA territory then encompasses the whole anteroinferior aspect of the cerebellum.

The superior cerebellar artery (SCA) is the most constant in caliber and territory of supply. It arises from the rostral basilar artery. The SCA supplies the rostral half of the cerebellar hemisphere and vermis as well as the dentate nucleus. Along its course, branches of the SCA supply the lateral tegmentum of the rostral pons, including the superior cerebellar peduncle, spinothalamic tract, lateral lemniscus, descending sympathetics, and more dorsally, the root of the contralateral trochlear nerve.

The three circumferential arteries and their branches are connected by numerous free cortical anastomoses that help limit the size of the infarct with cerebellar, vertebral, or basilar artery occlusions.

KEY CONCEPTS

- Blood supply of the cerebellum is provided by three arteries from the vertebral-basilar arterial system.

SUGGESTED READINGS

Ackermann H, et al: Speech deficits in ischaemic cerebellar lesions. *J Neurol* 1992; 239:223–227.

Amarenco P: The spectrum of cerebellar infarctions. *Neurology* 1991; 41:973–979.

Appollonio IM, et al: Memory in patients with cerebellar degeneration. *Neurology* 1993; 43:1536–1544.

Brown-Gould B: The organization of afferents to the cerebellar cortex in the cat: Projections from the deep cerebellar nuclei. *J Comp Neurol* 1979; 184:27–42.

Chaves CJ, et al: Cerebellar infarcts. *Curr Neurol* 1994; 14:143–177.

Cody FWJ, Richardson HC: Mossy and climbing fiber projections of trigeminal inputs to the cerebellar cortex in the cat. *Brain Res* 1978; 153:352–356.

Courville J, Faraco-Cantin F: On the origin of the climbing fibers of the cerebellum: An experimental study in the cat with an autoradiographic tracing method. *Neuroscience* 1978; 3:797–809.

Daum I, Ackermann H: Cerebellar contributions to cognition. *Behav Brain Res* 1995; 67:201–210.

Dietrichs E, et al: Hypothalamocerebellar and cerebellohypothalamic projections: Circuits for regulating nonsomatic cerebellar activity? *Histol Histopathol* 1994; 9:603–614.

Estanol B, et al: Effect of cerebellectomy on eye movements in man. *Arch Neurol* 1979; 36:281–284.

Houk JC, Wise SP: Distributed modular architectures linking basal ganglia, cerebellum, and cerebral cortex: Their role in planning and controlling action. *Cerebral Cortex* 1995; 2:95–110.

Ito M: Recent advances in cerebellar physiology and pathology. In Kark RAP, et al (eds): *Advances in Neurology,* vol 21. New York, Raven Press, 1978:59.

Itoh K, Mizuno N: A cerebello-pulvinar projection in the cat as visualized by the use of anterograde transport of horseradish peroxidase. *Brain Res* 1979; 171:131–134.

Jueptner M, et al: Localization of a cerebellar timing process using PET. *Neurology* 1995; 45:1540–1545.

Leiner HC, et al: Reappraising the cerebellum: What does the hindbrain contribute to the forebrain? *Behav Neurosci* 1989; 103:998–1008.

Leiner HC, et al: The human cerebro-cerebellar system: Its computing, cognitive, and language skills. *Behav Brain Res* 1991; 44:113–128.

Leiner HC, et al: The role of the cerebellum in the human brain. *TINS* 1993; 16:453–454.

Leiner HC, et al: Cognitive and language functions of the human cerebellum. *TINS* 1993; 16:444–447.

Macklis RM, Macklis JD: Historical and phrenologic reflections on the nonmotor functions of the cerebellum: Love under the tent? *Neurology* 1992; 42: 928–932.

Middleton FA, Strick PL: Anatomical evidence for cerebellar and basal ganglia involvement in higher cognitive function. *Science* 1994; 266:458–461.

Nadvornik P, et al: Experiences with dentatomy. *Confin Neurol* 1972; 34:320–324.

ReKate HL, et al: Muteness of cerebellar origin. *Arch Neurol* 1985; 42:697–698.

Roland PE: Partition of the human cerebellum in sensory-motor activities, learning and cognition. *Can J Neurol Sci* 1993; 20(suppl 3):S75–S77.

Ryding E, et al: Motor imagery activates the cerebellum regionally: A SPECT rCBF study with T_c-HMPAO. *Cogn Brain Res* 1993; 1:94–99.

Sasaki K, et al: Projections of the cerebellar dentate nucleus onto the frontal association cortex in monkeys. *Exp Brain Res* 1979; 37:193–198.

Schmahmann JD: An emerging concept: The cerebellar contribution to higher function. *Arch Neurol* 1991; 48:1178–1187.

Shinoda Y, et al: Thalamocortical organization in the cerebello-thalamo-cortical system. *Cerebral Cortex* 1993; 3:421–429.

van Dongen HR, et al: The syndrome of "cerebellar" mutism and subsequent dysarthria. *Neurology* 1994; 44:2040–2046.

Voogd J: The morphology of the cerebellum: The last 25 years. *Eur J Morphol* 1992; 30:81–96.

CHAPTER 16

CEREBELLUM: CLINICAL CORRELATES

The cerebellum has fascinated neuroscientists since its description by Aristotle and Galen. Early observers attributed to the cerebellum roles in memory, movement, and sexual activity. Early descriptions of cerebellar clinical symptoms and signs came from studies of patients with heredofamilial (e.g., **Friedreich's ataxia**) and demyelinating (e.g., multiple sclerosis) disorders, both of which involve, in addition to the cerebellum, many extracerebellar areas in the brain stem and spinal cord. In the first quarter of the twentieth century, Gordon Holmes established the triad of cerebellar signs of asthenia (fatigability), **ataxia** (incoordination, unsteadiness), and atonia (decreased muscle tone). He derived his triad from observation of patients with cerebellar injuries during World War I. Early attempts at anatomicoclinical correlations of cerebellar signs utilizing patients with cerebellar strokes were not rewarding. Localizing signs could not be elicited in unconscious stroke patients and were present in less than half the conscious patients. Findings in such patients included inability to walk, vomiting, headache, gaze palsy, and vertigo without hemiparesis. The introduction in the mid-1970s of computed tomography (CT) scans and in the 1980s of magnetic resonance imaging (MRI) and magnetic resonance arteriography (MRA), coupled with better definition of cerebellar vascular territories, permitted a more accurate anatomicoclinical correlation in cerebellar disorders.

Friedreich's Ataxia. Progressive hereditary degenerative central nervous system disorder characterized by combination of posterior column, lateral corticospinal, and spinocerebellar tract signs. Described in 1863 by Nikolaus Friedreich, the German pathologist.

Ataxia (Greek *taxis*, "order"). Want of order, lack of coordination, resulting in unsteadiness of movement. The term was used by Hippocrates and Galen for any morbid state, especially one with disordered or irregular action of any part such as irregularity of the pulse.

CLINICAL MANIFESTATIONS

Clinical cerebellar disorders are associated with a variety of etiologies: congenital malformations, hereditary, metabolic, infectious, toxic, vascular, demyelinating, and neoplastic. Cerebellar disorders share the following clinical characteristics:

1. Ipsilateral signs
2. Abnormalities in limb movements associated with lateral cerebellar hemisphere lesions
3. Abnormalities in trunk movements associated with midline vermis lesions
4. Lesions in deep cerebellar nuclei or the superior cerebellar peduncle producing more severe signs than lesions in the cerebellar cortex
5. Signs of cerebellar disease tending to improve with time, especially when the lesion occurs in childhood and the underlying disease is nonprogressive

CEREBELLAR SYNDROMES

The classically described archi-, paleo-, and neocerebellar syndromes in experimental animals following ablation of the respective lobes of the cerebellum are not ordinarily observed in humans. Instead, in humans, two cerebellar syndromes are clearly delineated: midline (archi- and paleocerebellar) and lateral cerebellar hemisphere (neocerebellar).

Experimental Animals

Archicerebellar Syndrome

The archicerebellum (flocculonodular lobe) is related to the vestibular system. It receives fibers from the vestibular nuclei and nerve and projects to the vestibular and reticular nuclei, which in turn project to the spinal cord (via the vestibulospinal and reticulospinal tracts) and ocular motor system (via the medial longitudinal fasciculus). The function of this system is the control of body equilibrium and eye movements. Ablation of the flocculonodular lobe in experimental animals produces **nystagmus** and disturbances in body equilibrium.

Nystagmus (Greek *nystagmos*, "nodding in sleep"). Rhythmic involuntary oscillatory movements of the eyes. The term is said to have been first used by Plenck. The association of these eye movements with vertigo was first noted by Purkinje and further investigated by Flourens.

Paleocerebellar Syndrome

The paleocerebellum is functionally related to the spinal cord and is concerned with posture, muscle tone, and gait. Ablation of the paleocerebellum in animals produces decerebrate rigidity and an increase in myotatic and postural reflexes.

Neocerebellar Syndrome

The neocerebellum is functionally related to the cerebral cortex and plays a role in planning and initiation of movement as well as the regulation of discrete limb movements.

Humans

Midline Syndrome

A picture corresponding to the archicerebellar (flocculonodular lobe) syndrome is often seen in children with a special type of tumor, the medulloblastoma. This

KEY CONCEPTS

- Signs of cerebellar disease are ipsilateral to the side of the cerebellar lesion.
- Lesions of the vermis are manifested by abnormalities in trunk movements, whereas lesions of the cerebellar hemispheres are manifested by abnormalities of movement in the extremities.
- Two cerebellar syndromes are well defined in humans: midline (archi- and paleocerebellar) syndrome, and lateral (neocerebellar syndrome).

tumor almost always arises in the most posterior part of the vermis and is manifested by unsteadiness of gait and nystagmus.

The paleocerebellar syndrome as described in experimental animals is usually not encountered in humans. However, some patients with atrophy of the cerebellum demonstrate unsteadiness of gait and increased myotatic reflexes in the lower extremities. It is believed that in such patients the anterior lobe is affected primarily by the atrophy.

Cerebellar Hemisphere Syndrome
Lesions of the cerebellar hemispheres (neocerebellum) produce the following manifestations:

Ataxia: A drunken, unsteady gait.
Dysmetria: Inability to estimate the range of voluntary movement. In attempting to touch the tip of the finger to the tip of the nose, a patient will overshoot the finger past the nose to the cheek or ear.
Decomposition of movement (**dyssynergia**): Jerky and tremulous voluntary movements. In attempting to touch the nose with the finger or to move the heel over the shin, the patient's movements are uneven and jerky throughout the range of motion.
Adiadochokinesia (dysdiadochokinesia): Inability to perform rapid successive movements such as tapping one hand on the other in an alternating supination and pronation sequence.
Intention tremor: Terminal tremor as the moving limb approaches its target.
Muscular hypotonia: Decrease in muscular tone and in the resistance to passive stretching of muscles.
Dysarthria: Slurred, hesitating type of speech.
Nystagmus: Nystagmus is frequently observed in cerebellar hemisphere lesions with the fast component to the side of the cerebellar lesion.

Pancerebellar Syndrome
This syndrome is a combination of the preceding two syndromes and is characterized by bilateral signs of cerebellar dysfunction involving the trunk, extremities, and eyes.

The cerebellum is well known for its ability to compensate for its deficits. The compensation is especially marked in children. The mechanisms underlying this ability to compensate are not known; the assumption of lost cerebellar functions by other noncerebellar structures or by remaining parts of the cerebellum are two explanations for this compensation.

VASCULAR SYNDROMES

Superior Cerebellar Artery (SCA) Syndrome (Fig. 16-1)

This is the most frequently encountered vascular syndrome of the cerebellum. Clinical signs include ipsilateral dysmetria, limb ataxia, and Horner's syndrome,

Dysmetria (Greek *dys*, "difficult"; *metron*, "a measure"). Difficulty in accurately controlling (measuring) the range of movement. Occurrence of errors in judgment of distance when a limb is made to perform a precise movement.

Dyssynergia (Greek *dys*, "difficult"; *synergia*, "cooperation"). Disturbance of muscular coordination between contraction and relaxation of muscles which normally act together in a group to produce smooth movement.

Dysdiadochokinesia (Greek *dys*, "difficult"; *diadochos*, "succeeding"; *kinesis*, "motion"). Impairment of the ability to perform rapid alternating movements, such as sequential pronation and supination of the arm.

Dysarthria (Greek *dys*, "difficult"; *arthroun*, "to articulate"). The indistinct pronunciation of words usually resulting from disturbances in the muscular control of the speech mechanism.

KEY CONCEPTS

- Midline cerebellar syndrome is manifested by unsteadiness of gait and nystagmus.
- Lateral (hemispheral, neocerebellar) syndrome is manifested by ataxia, dysmetria, dyssynergia, dysdiadochokinesia, intention tremor, muscular hypotonia, dysarthria, and nystagmus.

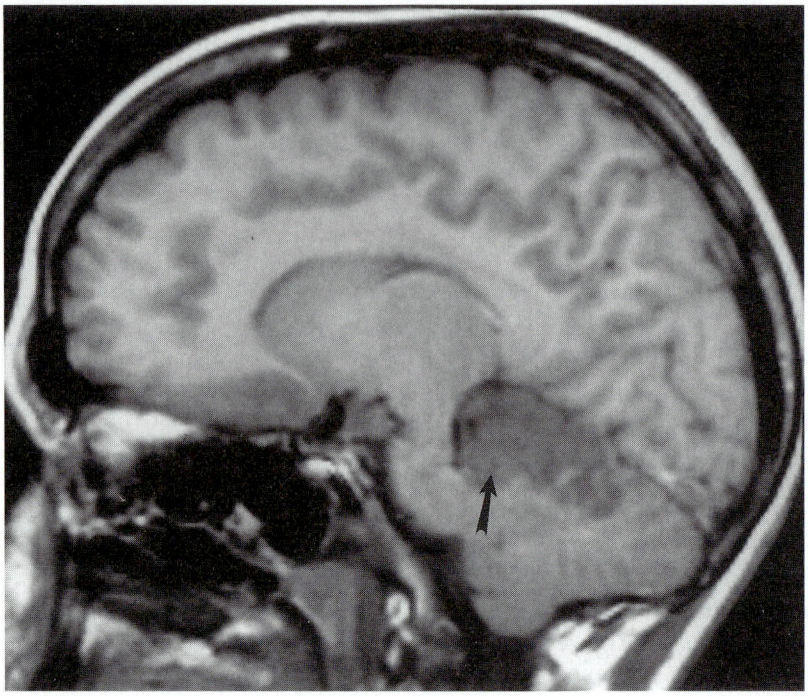

FIGURE 16-1

T1-weighted parasagittal MR image showing a cerebellar infarct (*arrow*) in the distribution of the superior cerebellar artery (SCA).

contralateral pain and thermal sensory loss, and contralateral trochlear nerve palsy. Horner's syndrome, the pain and thermal sensory deficits, and trochlear nerve palsy are due to involvement of the brain stem tegmentum. Dysarthria is common and is characteristic of rostral cerebellar lesions, whereas vertigo is not as common in SCA infarcts and is more characteristic of the posterior inferior cerebellar artery (PICA) syndrome. Isolated dysarthria (without other cerebellar signs) has been reported in occlusion of the medial branch of the superior cerebellar artery with an infarct limited to the paravermal area. Prognosis for recovery in SCA syndrome is usually good.

Anterior Inferior Cerebellar Artery (AICA) Syndrome

Occlusion of the anterior inferior cerebellar artery (AICA) is uncommon, and often is misdiagnosed as the lateral medullary syndrome (PICA syndrome). It is

KEY CONCEPTS

- Three vascular cerebellar syndromes are well defined: superior cerebellar artery (SCA) syndrome, anterior inferior cerebellar artery (AICA) syndrome, and posterior inferior cerebellar artery syndrome (PICA). The SCA and PICA syndromes are more frequently encountered than the AICA syndrome.

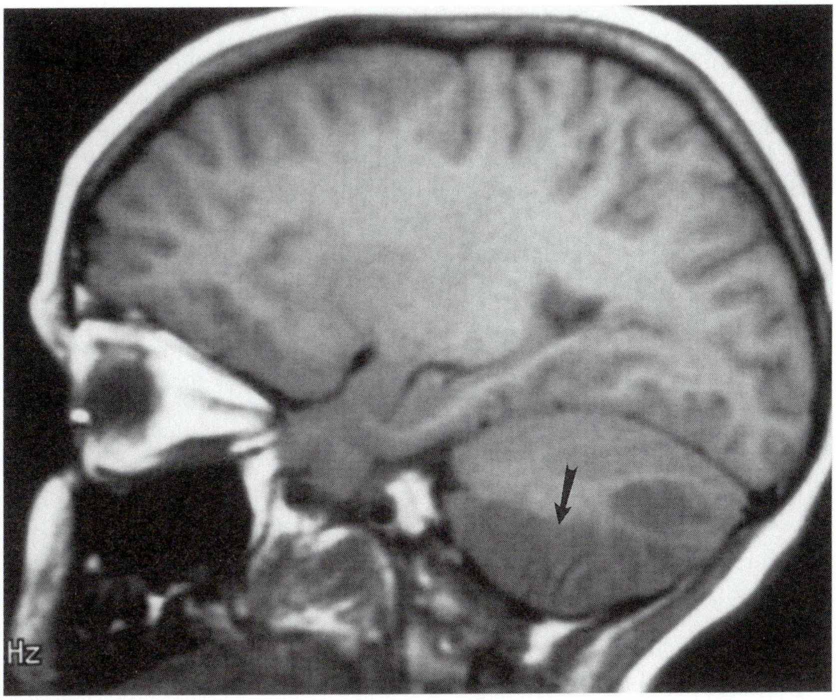

FIGURE 16-2

T1-weighted parasagittal MR image showing a cerebellar infarct (*arrow*) in the distribution of the posterior inferior cerebellar artery (PICA).

characterized by ipsilateral dysmetria, vestibular signs, Horner's syndrome, facial sensory impairment, contralateral pain and thermal sensory loss in the limbs, and at times, dysphagia. Other signs seen in this syndrome and unusual in the lateral medullary syndrome include ipsilateral severe facial motor palsy, deafness, lateral gaze palsy, and multimodal sensory impairment over the face due to involvement of facial, cochleovestibular, abducens, and trigeminal nerves and/or nuclei, respectively. AICA occlusion also can be manifested by purely cerebellar signs.

Posterior Inferior Cerebellar Artery (PICA) Syndrome (Fig. 16-2)

This syndrome is as frequent as the superior cerebellar artery (SCA) syndrome. Clinical features of the syndrome are described in the chapter on clinical correlates of the medulla oblongata (Chap. 6).

Occlusion of the medial branch of the PICA may be clinically silent or may present with one of the following three patterns: (1) isolated vertigo often misdiagnosed as inner ear disease (labyrinthitis), (2) vertigo, ipsilateral axial lateropulsion (involuntary tendency to go to one side while in motion), and dysmetria or unsteadiness, or (3) classic lateral medullary syndrome when the medulla is also involved in the lesion.

Clinical manifestations of occlusion of the lateral branch of the PICA are unknown, since reported cases have been chance autopsy findings with no available clinical information.

SUGGESTED READINGS

Amarenco P: The spectrum of cerebellar infarctions. *Neurology* 1991; 41:973–979.

Amarenco P, et al: Infarction in the anterior rostral cerebellum (the territory of the lateral branch of the superior cerebellar artery). *Neurology* 1991; 41: 253–258.

Amarenco P, et al: Paravermal infarct and isolated cerebellar dysarthria. *Ann Neurol* 1991; 30:211–213.

Amarenco P, et al: Anterior inferior cerebellar artery territory infarcts: Mechanisms and clinical features. *Arch Neurol* 1993; 50:154–161.

Barth A, et al: The clinical and topographic spectrum of cerebellar infarcts: A clinical–magnetic resonance imaging correlation study. *Ann Neurol* 1993; 33: 451–456.

Chaves CJ, et al: Cerebellar infarcts. *Curr Neurol* 1994; 14:143–177.

CHAPTER 17

CEREBRAL CORTEX

CORTICAL ELECTROPHYSIOLOGY

Evoked Potentials

Somatosensory, Visual, and Auditory Evoked Responses

ELECTROENCEPHALOGRAPHY

BLOOD SUPPLY

Arterial Supply

Venous Drainage

Cortex (Latin "bark"). External gray layer of the cerebrum.

Neocortex (Greek *neos*, "new"; Latin *cortex*, "bark"). The most recent phylogenetic development of the cerebral cortex.

Isocortex (Greek *isos*, "equal"; Latin *cortex*, "bark"). Six-layered cerebral cortex.

Homotypical cortex (Greek *homos*, "same"; *typos*, "pattern"). Association areas of the neocortex all have a similar six-layered structure.

Heterotypical cortex (Greek *heteros*, "different"; *typos*, "pattern"). The isocortex (neocortex) in which some of the six layers are obscured, as in motor cortex and visual cortex.

Koniocortex (Greek *konis*, "dust"; Latin *cortex*, "bark"). Areas of cerebral cortex with large number of small neurons.

Allocortex (Greek *allos*, "other"; Latin *cortex*, "bark"). Phylogenetically old, three-layered cerebral cortex. Divided into paleocortex and archicortex.

Paleocortex (Greek *palaios*, "ancient"; Latin *cortex*, "bark"). Phylogenetically old, three-layered cortex. The cortex found in rostral insular cortex, piri-

The cerebral **cortex** is the layer of gray matter capping the white matter core of the cerebral hemispheres. Its thickness varies from 1.5 to 4.5 mm, with an average thickness of 2.5 mm. The cerebral cortex is thickest in the primary motor area (4.5 mm thick) and thinnest in the primary visual cortex (1.5 mm thick). The cortex is irregularly convoluted, forming gyri separated by sulci or fissures. The outer layer of the human cerebral cortex is around 0.2 m^2, but only one-third of this area is exposed to the surface. The number of neurons in the cerebral cortex is estimated at between 10 and 20 billion. A relatively small area of the cerebral cortex in humans is specialized for receiving sensory input from the eyes, ears, and skin and for projecting motor output down the pyramidal tract to bring about movement. Over 80 percent of the cortex in humans serves an association function specially related to integrative and cognitive activities such as language, calculation, planning, and abstract reasoning.

TYPES OF CORTEX

On the basis of phylogenetic development and microscopic structure, the following three types of cortices are recognized.

Isocortex (Neocortex or Homogenetic Cortex)

This cortex is six layered and of recent phylogenetic development. It is characteristic of mammalian species, increases in size in higher mammals, and comprises 90 percent of the cerebral cortex in humans.

Isocortex in which the six layers are clearly evident (such as the primary sensory cortex) is termed **homotypical cortex**. Isocortex in which some of the six layers are obscured (such as the motor cortex and visual cortex) is termed **heterotypical cortex**. The visual cortex is also known as *granular cortex* or **koniocortex** (from the Greek *konis*, meaning "dust"). The motor cortex, in contrast, is known as *agranular cortex* because of the predominance of large pyramidal neurons.

Allocortex (Paleocortex, Archicortex, or Heterogenetic Cortex)

The **allocortex** is three layered and phylogenetically older. It is subdivided into **paleocortex** (rostral insular cortex, piriform cortex, and primary olfactory cortex) and **archicortex** (hippocampal formation).

Mesocortex

This type of cortex is found in much of the cingulate gyrus, entorhinal, parahippocampal, and orbital cortices and is intermediate in histology between the isocortex and allocortex. The terms *periallocortex* and *periarchicortex* are used to refer to this cortex to denote its transitional nature between neocortex and allocortex.

MICROSCOPIC STRUCTURE

Cell Types

Attempts to make a comprehensive inventory of types of cortical neurons started with Ramon y Cajal in 1911 and have continued until today. The neurons of the cerebral cortex are of two functional categories: (1) principal (projection) neurons and (2) interneurons. The principal neurons provide corticocortical and corticosubcortical outputs. Interneurons are concerned with local information processing. The cerebral cortex has its full complement of neurons (10 to 20 billion) by the eighteenth week of intrauterine life.

form cortex, and primary olfactory cortex.

Archicortex (Greek *arche*, "beginning"; Latin *cortex*, "bark"). Phylogenetically old, three-layered cortex seen in the hippocampal formation. A variety of paleo- or allocortex.

Mesocortex. Intermediate cortex (in histology) between the isocortex and allocortex. Also known as ***periallocortex* and *periarchicortex*.**

Principal (Projection) Neurons

Two types of cortical neurons belong to the principal category. They are the pyramidal neurons and the **fusiform** neurons. The excitatory neurotransmitter in both is glutamate or aspartate. Principal neurons constitute more than half of all cortical neurons.

Fusiform (Latin *fusus*, "spindle";*forma*, "shape"). A cell that is widest in the middle and tapering at both ends.

Pyramidal Neurons

These neurons derive their name from their shape. The apex of the pyramid is directed toward the cortical surface. Each pyramidal neuron has an apical dendrite directed toward the surface of the cortex and several horizontally oriented basal dendrites that arise from the base of the pyramid. Branches of all dendrites contain numerous spines that increase the size of the synaptic area. A slender axon leaves the base of the pyramidal neuron and projects on other neurons in the same or contralateral hemisphere or else leaves the cortex to project on subcortical regions. The axon gives rise within the cortex to two types of axon collaterals. These are the recurrent axon collaterals (RACs), which project back on neurons in more superficial layers, and the horizontal axon collaterals (HACs), which extend horizontally to synapse on neurons in the vicinity.

Pyramidal neurons are found in all cortical layers except layer I. They vary in size; most are between 10 and 50 μm in height. The largest are the giant pyramidal cells of Betz, which measure about 100 μm in height and are found in layer V of the motor cortex.

Fusiform, Spindle Neurons

These are small neurons with elongated perikarya in which the long axis is oriented perpendicular to the cortical surface. A short dendrite arises from the lower pole of the perikaryon and arborizes in the vicinity. A longer dendrite arises from the upper pole of the perikaryon and extends to more superficial layers. The axon enters the deep white matter. Fusiform neurons are found in the deepest cortical laminae.

KEY CONCEPTS

- Based on phylogenetic development and microscopic structure, the cerebral cortex is divided into three types: a six-layered isocortex of recent phylogenetic development, a three-layered phylogenetically older allocortex, and a transitional mesocortex.
- Principal neurons are of two types: pyramidal and fusiform.

Interneurons

Several types of cortical interneurons are recognized on the basis of dendritic architecture. They include the stellate neurons, the horizontal cells of Cajal, and the cells of Martinotti.

Stellate (Latin *stella*, "star"). Stellate neurons have many short dendrites that radiate in all directions like a star.

Stellate or Granule Neurons

These are small (4 to 8 μm) star-shaped neurons with short, extensively branched, spiny dendrites and short axons. They are most numerous in lamina IV. Stellate cells are the only type of excitatory interneurons in the cortex. The neurotransmitter is glutamate. All other interneurons exert inhibitory influence by gamma-aminobutyric acid (GABA).

Horizontal Cells of Cajal

These are small fusiform neurons with their long axes directed parallel to the cortical surface. A branching dendrite arises from each pole of the perikaryon, and an axon arises from one pole. The dendrites and axon are oriented parallel to the cortical surface. The horizontal cells of Cajal are found only in lamina I and disappear or are rare after the neonatal period.

Martinotti, Giovanni. Italian physician who described the Martinotti neuron in the cerebral cortex.

Myeloarchitectonics. The arrangement of nerve fibers in the cerebral and cerebellar cortex that varies in different regions and allows mapping of the brain.

Agyria (Greek *a*, "negative"; *gyros*, "ring"). A malformation in which the convolutions of the cerebral cortex are not normally developed. Also called *lissencephaly* (smooth brain).

Pachygyria (Greek *pachys*, "thick"; *gyros*, "convolutions"). A developmental disorder of neuronal migration in which there are few, thickened, and wide cerebral gyri.

Micropolygyria (polymicrogyria) (Greek *mikros*, "small"; *gyros*, "convolutions"). A malformation of the brain characterized by the development of numerous small convolutions.

Heterotopia (Greek *heteros*, "other, different"; *topos*, "place"). The presence of cortical tissue in an abnormal location during development.

Cells of Marinotti

Giovanni Marinotti in 1890 first described cells whose axons ascend toward the surface of the cortex. Martinotti neurons are multipolar with short branching dendrites and an axon that projects to more superficial layers, giving out horizontal axon collaterals en route. The Martinotti neurons are found in deeper cortical laminae.

Layers

The division of the neocortex into layers has been the outcome of extensive cytoarchitectonic (organization based on studies of stained cells) and **myeloarchitectonic** (organization based on studies of myelinated fiber preparations) studies. Although several such studies are available, the most widely used are the cytoarchitectonic classification of Brodmann and the myeloarchitectonic classification of the Vogts. According to these two classifications, the neocortex is divided into six layers (Table 17-1).

The six layers of the neocortex are recognizable by about the seventh month of intrauterine life. The neurons in the six cortical layers develop in waves from the periventricular germinal matrix. Successive waves of migrating neuroblasts become situated progressively farther away from the germinal matrix (inside-out gradient of cortical histogenesis) (see Table 17-2). Interruption of the normal process of migration or its arrest is associated with cortical gyral malformations such as **agyria, pachygyria, micropolygyria,** and **heterotopia**. Many of these are associated with mental retardation, seizures, and other neurologic deficits.

Layer I (Molecular, Plexiform)

Layer I consists primarily of a dense network of nerve cell processes among which are scattered sparse interneurons (horizontal cells of Cajal) and neuroglia. The

KEY CONCEPTS

- Cortical neurons are of two types: principal (projection) neurons and interneurons.
- Several types of interneurons are recognized on the basis of dendritic architecture, including stellate, horizontal cells of Cajal and cells of Martinotti.

TABLE 17-1

Cortical Layers

Layer Number	Cytoarchitectonic Name	Myeloarchitectonic Name
I	Molecular	Tangential
II	External granular	Dysfibrous
III	Pyramidal	Suprastriatal
IV	Internal granular	External of Baillarger
V	Ganglionic	Internal of Baillarger and interstriatal
VI	Multiform	Infrastriatal

nerve cell processes in this layer comprise projection axons from extracortical sites as well as axons and dendrites of neurons in other cortical areas. This layer of the cortex is primarily a synaptic area.

Layer II (External Granular)
Layer II consists of a dense packing of small and medium-sized pyramidal neurons and interneurons intermingled with axons from other cortical layers of the same and opposite hemispheres (association and commissural fibers), as well as axons and dendrites passing through this layer from deeper layers. The dendrites of pyramidal neurons in this layer project to layer I, while their axons project to deeper layers. This layer of the cortex contributes to the complexity of intracortical circuitry.

Layer III (External Pyramidal)
Layer III consists of pyramidal neurons that increase in size in deeper parts of the layer. The dendrites of neurons in this layer extend to layer I, while the axons project to other layers within the same and contralateral hemisphere (association and commissural fibers) or leave the hemisphere as projection fibers to more distant extracortical sites. This layer receives primarily axons of neurons in other cortical areas (association and commissural fibers), as well as axons of neurons in extracortical regions such as the thalamus.

TABLE 17-2

Chronologic Age of Cortical Layers

Layer	Order of Migration
I	Oldest (acellular)
II	Fifth wave of neuroblast migration
III	Fourth wave of neuroblast migration
IV	Third wave of neuroblast migration
V	Second wave of neuroblast migration
VI	First wave of neuroblast migration

Layer IV (Internal Granular)

Layer IV consists of pyramidal cells and densely packed small stellate cells with processes that terminate within the same layer, either on axons of other stellate cells or on axons of cortical or subcortical origin passing through this layer. The cell packing density in layer IV is the greatest of all cortical layers. Few of the larger stellate cells in this layer project their axons to deeper cortical layers. Layer IV is especially well developed in primary sensory cortical areas. In the primary visual (striate) cortex, this layer is traversed by a dense band of horizontally oriented nerve fibers known as the *external band of Baillarger* or the *stripe of Gennari.* The band of Baillarger was described by the nineteenth-century French neurologist and psychiatrist **Jean-Gabriel-François Baillarger**. The stripe of Gennari was first described in 1782 by **Francesco Gennari**, an eighteenth-century Italian medical student, and independently by Vic d'Azyr in 1786. Because of the presence of this stripe, the primary visual cortex is known as the *striate cortex*. The internal granular layer is the major recipient of thalamocortical fibers from modality-specific sensory relay nuclei.

Baillarger, Jules Gabriel Francois. French psychiatrist who described the lines of Baillarger in the cerebral cortex.

Gennari, Francesco. Italian physician who, as a medical student, described the lines of Gennari that characterize lamina IV of the visual cortex.

Layer V (Internal Pyramidal)

Layer V consists of large and medium-sized pyramidal cells, stellate cells, and cells of Martinotti. The cell packing density in this layer is the lowest of all cortical layers. The largest pyramidal cells in the cerebral cortex (cells of Betz) are found in this layer (hence the name *ganglionic layer*). Dendrites of neurons in this layer project to the more superficial layers. Axons project on neurons in other cortical areas but mainly to subcortical sites (projection fibers) except the thalamus, which receives fibers from layer VI. This layer receives axons and dendrites arising in other cortical sites or in subcortical sites. It is also traversed by a dense band of horizontally oriented fibers; this is the *internal band of Baillarger*. Fibers originating in thalamic sensory nuclei contribute heavily to the lines of Baillarger, especially the outer one in lamina IV. The lines of Baillarger are thus prominent in primary cortical sensory areas.

Layer VI (Multiform)

Layer VI consists of cells of varying shapes and sizes, including fusiform cells and the cells of Martinotti, which are prominent in this layer. Dendrites of smaller cells arborize locally or in adjacent layers, while those of large neurons reach the molecular layer. Axons of neurons in this layer project to other cortical laminae or to subcortical regions.

Layers I, V, and VI are present in all types of cortex (neo-, paleo-, and archicortex). Layers II, III, and IV, however, are present only in neocortex and thus are considered of more recent phylogenetic development. In general, layers I to IV are considered receptive. The somata of the majority of cells that establish intracortical connections (ipsilaterally and contralaterally) lie in layers II and III. Layers V and VI are efferent. Neurons in lamina V give rise to corticofugal fibers that target subcortical areas (brain stem and spinal cord). Neurons in **lamina** VI give rise to corticofugal fibers to the thalamus.

Lamina (Latin "a thin plate or layer").

KEY CONCEPTS

- On the basis of cytoarchitectonic and myeloarchitectonics, the cerebral cortex is organized into six horizontal layers.
- The stripe of Gennari, a dense band of horizontally oriented nerve fibers in layer IV, is prominent in the primary visual cortex and gives it its characteristic striate appearance.

In contrast to the horizontal anatomic lamination, the vertical lamination described by Mountcastle seems to be the more functionally appropriate. The studies of Lorente de Nó, Mountcastle, Szentágothai, and others have shown that the functional unit of cortical activity is a column of neurons oriented vertically to the surface of the cortex. Each such column or module is 300 to 500 μm in diameter, with its height the thickness of the cortex, and contains 4000 neurons, 2000 of which are pyramidal neurons. All neurons in a column are activated selectively by the same peripheral stimulus. There are approximately 3 million such modules in the human neocortex. Each module sends pyramidal cell axons to other modules within the same hemisphere or to modules in the other hemisphere. Of interest is the fact that activation of a module tends to inhibit neuronal activity in adjacent modules. The columnar organization of the neocortex is established in fetal life, but the synaptic connections increase in number in the postnatal period in response to stimulation from the external environment. Lack of external stimuli during a critical period of cortical maturation, usually in the first year of life, will adversely affect normal cortical development.

INPUT TO CEREBRAL CORTEX

The input to the cerebral cortex originates in four sites (Fig. 17-1):

1. Thalamus
2. Extrathalamic modulatory
3. Cortex of the same hemisphere (association fibers)
4. Cortex of the contralateral hemisphere (commissural fibers)

Thalamocortical Input

The input from the thalamus travels via two systems. (1) The modality-specific thalamocortical system originates in modality-specific thalamic nuclei (e.g., ventral anterior, ventral lateral, ventral posterior) and projects on specific cortical areas (primary motor, premotor, and somesthetic cortex). This fiber system reaches the cortex as an ascending component of the internal capsule. The majority of fibers in this system project on neurons in lamina IV, with some projecting on neurons in lamina III and lamina VI. (2) The nonspecific thalamocortical system is related to the reticular system and originates in nonspecific thalamic nuclei (intralaminar, midline, and reticular nuclei). In the cortex, fibers of this system project diffusely on all laminae and establish mostly axodendritic types of synapses. This fiber system is intimately involved in the arousal response and wakefulness.

Extrathalamic Modulatory Input

Until recently, it was commonly assumed that essentially all afferents to the cortex arose from the thalamus. With the development of methods to visualize monoaminergic and cholinergic processes, it is now clear that there are at least four substantial extrathalamic projections to the cortex.

KEY CONCEPTS

- Cortical neurons in the different horizontal layers are also organized into vertical functional columns or laminae. All neurons in a vertical column are activated selectively by the same peripheral stimulus.

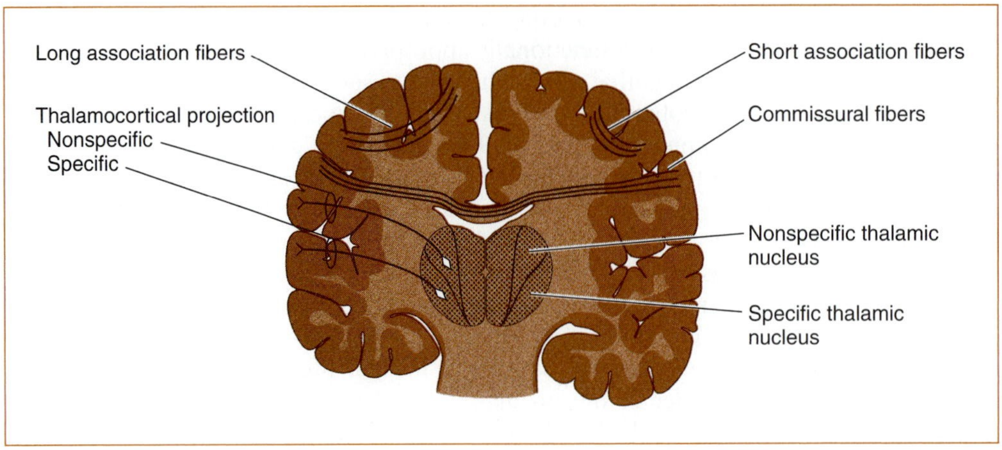

FIGURE 17-1

Schematic diagram showing sources of fiber input to the cerebral cortex.

Monoaminergic and cholinergic pathways reach the cerebral cortex directly without passing through the thalamus. They arise from nuclei in the brain stem, caudal hypothalamus, the diagonal band of Broca, and the nucleus basalis of Meynert.

Monoaminergic Input

Serotonergic Input The serotonergic input to the cerebral cortex originates from the raphe nuclei in the mesencephalon and rostral pons. It terminates in the same cortical layers that receive the thalamocortical input (layers III, IV, and VI). The function of the serotonergic pathway to the cortex is not well understood. Serotonergic pathways elsewhere have been related to a variety of functions, including pain control and sleep. The serotonergic input to the cortex is believed to alter cortical neuronal responses to afferent input in response to change in state.

Dopaminergic Input The dopaminergic input to the cerebral cortex originates from dopaminergic neurons in the mesencephalon (ventral tegmental area of Tsai and substantia nigra pars compacta). It terminates in all areas of the cortex, but especially in the motor, prefrontal, and temporal association areas. The dopaminergic input to the cortex is believed to play a role in orienting behavior. The laminar and regional pattern of termination of this system suggests that it influences activities of corticocortical rather than thalamocortical circuits and higher-order integrative processes than the more analytic aspects of sensory processing. In addition, it may influence cortical regulation of motor control.

Noradrenergic Input The noradrenergic input to the cerebral cortex originates from cells in the locus ceruleus in the rostral pons. It terminates in cortical layers that give rise to corticofugal fibers. The noradrenergic input is implicated in higher-order information processing and the state of arousal. It is believed to enhance the selectivity and vigor of cortical responses to sensory stimuli or other synaptic inputs to the target neurons in the cortex.

Histaminergic Input The histaminergic input to the cerebral cortex originates from the tuberomamillary nucleus in the posterolateral hypothalamus. The function of this system is not known.

Cholinergic Input

The cholinergic input to the cerebral cortex originates from the nucleus basalis of Meynert. This input terminates in all areas of the cortex. It is the most important system for cortical arousal and motivation. It has been implicated in the genesis of memory deficit in Alzheimer's disease.

GABAergic Input

The GABAergic input to the cerebral cortex originates from cells in the septum and the diagonal band of Broca. It terminates primarily in the **hippocampus**.

Hippocampus (Greek *hippokampos*, "sea horse"). In coronal sections, the hippocampus resembles a sea horse.

Association Fiber System (Fig. 17-2)

The association fibers arise from nearby (short association u-fibers) and distant (long association fibers) regions of the same hemisphere. They too project diffusely in all laminae but mostly in laminae I to III.

The long association fiber system includes such bundles as the **cingulum**, superior longitudinal **fasciculus**, arcuate fasciculus, inferior longitudinal fasciculus, occipitofrontal fasciculus, and the uncinate fasciculus. The *cingulum* is the white matter core of the cingulate **gyrus**. It connects the anterior perforated substance and the parahippocampal gyrus. The *superior longitudinal fasciculus*, located in the lateral part of the hemisphere above the insula, connects portions of the frontal lobe with parietal, occipital, and temporal lobes. The *arcuate fasciculus* is the part of the superior longitudinal fasciculus that sweeps around the insula (island of Reil) to connect the speech areas in the inferior frontal lobe (Broca's area) and superior temporal lobe (Wernicke's area). The *inferior longitudinal fasciculus* is a thin sheet of fibers that runs superficially beneath the lateral and ventral surfaces of the temporal and occipital lobes. This fiber bundle is difficult to demonstrate by dissection and to separate from other fiber systems running in its vicinity. The existence of the inferior longitudinal fasciculus in humans has been questioned. The only long fiber bundle common to both the occipital and temporal lobes in humans is the optic radiation (geniculostriate pathway). In addition, the two lobes are interconnected by a series of u-fibers (short association fibers) that connect adjacent regions of occipital and temporal cortices. Based on this, it has been proposed that the term *inferior longitudinal fasciculus* be replaced by the term *occipitotemporal projection system*. The *occipitofrontal fasciculus* extends backwards from the frontal lobe, radiating into the temporal and occipital lobes. Two subdivisions of the occipitofrontal fasciculus are recognized. The *superior (subcallosal) bundle* is located deep in the hemisphere, dorsolateral to the lateral ventricle, sandwiched between the corpus callosum, internal capsule, and caudate nucleus. The *inferior bundle* is located lateral to the temporal horn of the lateral ventricle and below the insular cortex and lentiform nucleus. The **uncinate fasciculus** is the component of the inferior occipitofrontal fasciculus that courses at the bottom of the Sylvian fissure to connect the inferior frontal gyrus with the anterior temporal lobe.

Cingulum (Latin "a girdle"). A bundle of association fibers within the cingulate gyrus.

Fasciculus (Latin "a small bundle"). A small bundle of nerve fibers.

Gyrus (Greek *gyros*, "circle"). Cerebral convolution.

Uncinate (Latin "hook-shaped"). Uncinate fasciculus connects the cortex of the ventral surface of the frontal lobe with that of the temporal pole.

Commissural Fiber System

The commissural fibers arise from corresponding and noncorresponding regions in the contralateral hemisphere, travel via the **corpus callosum**, and project on neurons in all laminae but mostly laminae I, II, and III.

Commissure (Latin *commissura*, "a joining together"). A bundle of nerve fibers connecting like structures in the two hemispheres.

Corpus callosum (Latin *corpus*, "body"; *callosus*, "hard"). The commissural fiber bundle connecting corresponding parts of the cerebral hemispheres.

KEY CONCEPTS

- Association fibers are of two types: short connecting contiguous gyri and long connecting distant gyri within the same hemisphere.
- Long association fiber bundles: the cingulum and the superior longitudinal, arcuate, inferior longitudinal, occipitofrontal, and uncinate fasciculi.

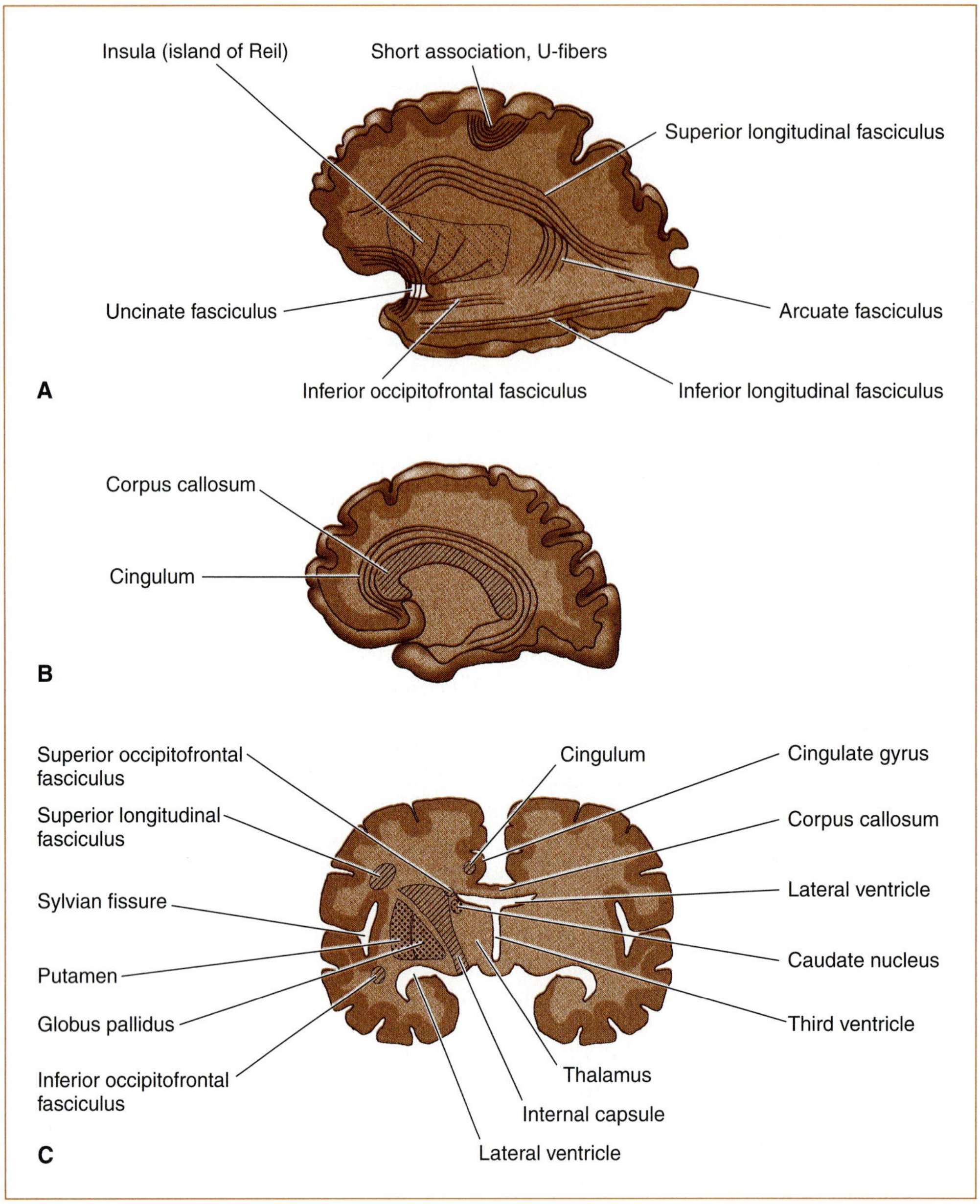

FIGURE 17-2

Schematic diagram showing the long association fiber bundles.

Studies on the topographic distribution of interhemispheric projections in the corpus callosum have shown that the genu interconnects the prefrontal cortex, the rostral part of the body interconnects the premotor and supplementary motor

KEY CONCEPTS

- The cerebral cortex receives fibers from internal and external sources. Internal sources include the cortex of the same hemisphere via association fiber bundles and the contralateral hemisphere via commissural fibers. External sources of input include the thalamus and nonthalamic subcortical sources.
- The corpus callosum is the major commissural fiber bundle. Different parts of the corpus callosum interconnect specific corresponding areas in the two hemispheres.

cortices, the middle part of the body interconnects the primary motor and primary and secondary somatic sensory areas, the caudal part of the body interconnects the posterior parietal cortex, and the **splenium** interconnects temporal and occipital cortices.

Splenium (Greek *splenion*, "bandage"). Thickened posterior extremity of the corpus callosum.

OUTPUT OF CEREBRAL CORTEX

Efferent outflow from the cerebral cortex is grouped into three categories (Fig. 17-3). These are (1) the association fiber system, (2) the commissural fiber system, and (3) the corticofugal fiber system. The association and commissural fiber systems have been described in the section on input to the cortex. Essentially, they represent intrahemispheric and interhemispheric connections.

The corticofugal fiber system includes all fiber tracts that leave the cerebral cortex to project on various subcortical structures. They include the following pathways.

Corticospinal Pathway (Fig. 17-4)

This corticofugal fiber tract connects the cerebral cortex directly with motor neurons in the spinal cord and is concerned with highly skilled volitional movement. It arises from pyramidal neurons in layer V from wide areas of the cerebral cortex but principally from the somatic motor, premotor, and somatosensory cortices. It contains, on each side, roughly 1 million fibers of various sizes (9 to 22 μm), about 3 percent of which are large in size and arise from the giant cells of Betz in layer V of the motor cortex. The fibers of this system descend in the internal capsule, the middle part of the cerebral peduncle, the basis points, and the pyramids before gathering in the spinal cord as the lateral and anterior corticospinal tracts. The former (lateral corticospinal) constitutes the majority of the descending corticospinal fibers and decussates in the pyramids (motor decussation); the latter (anterior corticospinal) is smaller and crosses at segmental levels in the spinal cord. The classic notion that the corticospinal tract is of particular importance for skilled and delicate voluntary movement is in essence correct, but it is obvious that a number of other indirect tracts passing through the brain stem nuclei, reticular formation, and cerebellum are also involved. The direct corticospinal tract most likely superimposes speed and agility on the motor mechanisms subserved by other descending indirect pathways. The component of the corticospinal pathway from the somatosen-

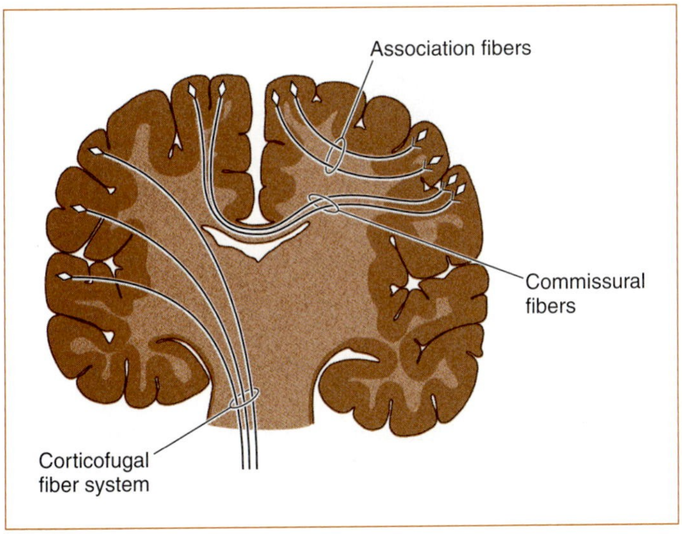

FIGURE 17-3

Schematic diagram of the major groups of cortical output.

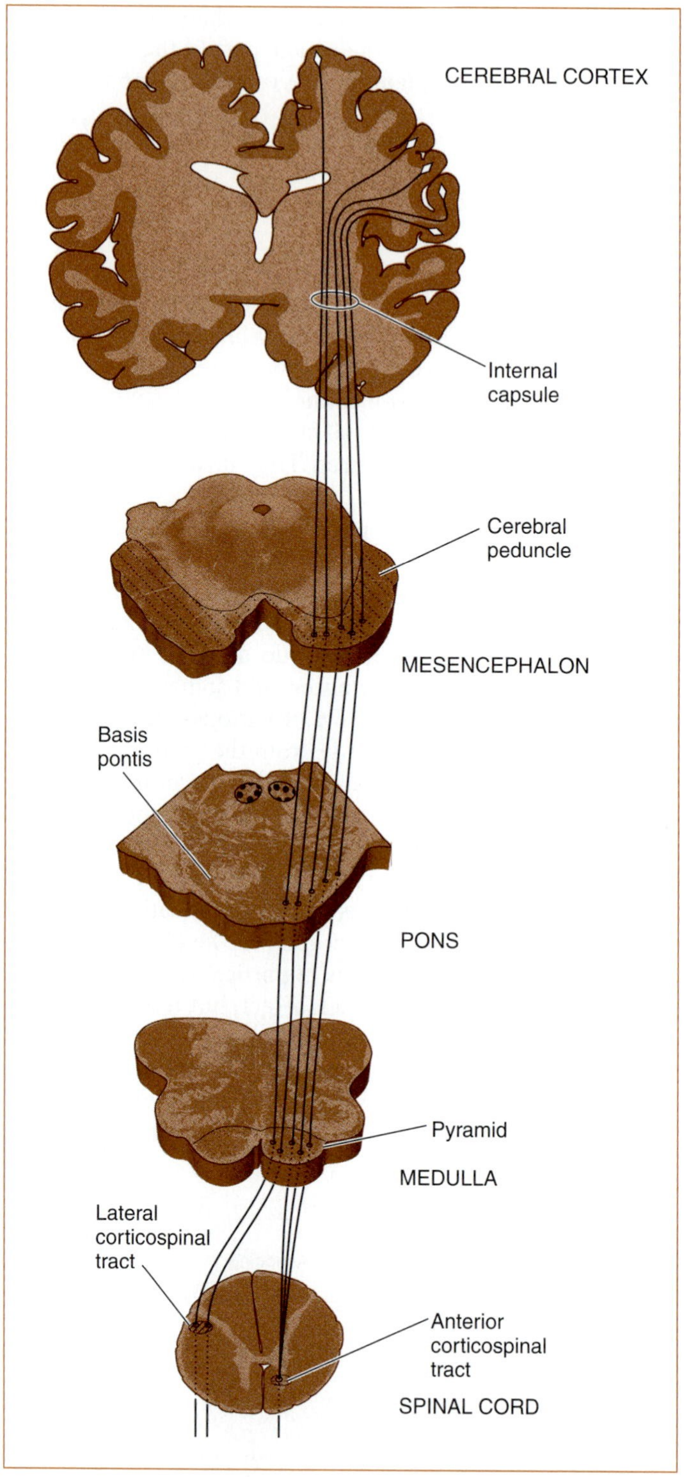
CEREBRAL CORTEX
Internal capsule
Cerebral peduncle
MESENCEPHALON
Basis pontis
PONS
Pyramid
MEDULLA
Lateral corticospinal tract
Anterior corticospinal tract
SPINAL CORD

FIGURE 17-4

Schematic diagram of the corticospinal pathway.

sory cortex terminates on sensory neurons in the dorsal horn of the spinal cord and is concerned with somatosensory function possibly related to ongoing movement. A fairly large proportion of the sensory component of the corticospinal pathway originates from area 3a, which adjoins the primary motor cortex and receives sensory input from proprioceptors.

Corticoreticular Pathway

This fiber tract arises from most if not all parts of the cerebral cortex but primarily from motor, premotor, and somatosensory cortices and accompanies the corticospinal fiber system, leaving it at different levels of the neuraxis to project on reticular neurons in the brain stem. The corticoreticular fibers arising from one cerebral hemisphere project roughly equally to both sides of the brain stem reticular formation. Many of these fibers ultimately project on cranial nerve nuclei in the brain stem, thus forming the corticoreticulobulbar pathway.

Corticobulbar Pathway

Corticobulbar fibers originate from the face area of the motor cortex. They project on motor nuclei of the trigeminal, facial, glossopharyngeal, vagus, accessory, and hypoglossal nerves.

Direct corticobulbar fibers (without intermediate synapses on reticular neurons) are known to project from the cerebral cortex to nuclei of trigeminal (CN V), facial (CN VII), and hypoglossal (CN XII) cranial nerves. Corticobulbar fibers descend in the genu of the internal capsule and occupy a dorsolateral corner of the corticospinal segment of the cerebral peduncle, as well as a small area in the medial part of the base of the cerebral peduncle. In the pons, corticobulbar fibers are intermixed with the corticospinal fibers within the basis pontis. The corticobulbar input to nuclei of trigeminal and hypoglossal cranial nerves is bilateral. The input to that part of the facial nucleus which supplies upper facial muscles is also bilateral. The input to that part of the facial nucleus which supplies lower facial muscles is mainly from the contralateral hemisphere. Bilateral interruption of the corticobulbar or corticoreticulobulbar fiber system results in **paresis** (weakness) but not **paralysis** of the muscles supplied by the corresponding cranial nerve nucleus. This condition is known as *pseudobulbar palsy* to distinguish it from bulbar palsy, which is a condition characterized by complete paralysis of muscles supplied by a cranial nerve nucleus as a result of a lesion of the nucleus.

Paresis (Greek *parienai*, "to relax"). Partial paralysis.

Paralysis (Greek *para*, "beside"; *lyein*, "to loosen"). Loss of power of motion.

Corticopontine Pathway (Fig. 17-5)

Fibers comprising this pathway arise from all parts of the cerebral cortex but primarily from the frontal, parietal, and occipital lobes. Most fibers, however, arise from the primary motor (precentral gyrus) and primary sensory (postcentral gyrus) cortices, with relatively substantial contribution from the premotor, supplementary motor, and posterior parietal cortices and few from the temporal and prefrontal cortices. These fibers descend in the internal capsule and occupy the most medial and lateral parts of the cerebral peduncle before reaching the basis pontis, where they project on pontine nuclei. The corticopontine fibers constitute by far the largest component of the corticofugal fiber system. It is estimated that each corticopontine pathway contains approximately 19 million fibers. With approximately the same number of pontine neurons on each side of the basis pontis, the ratio of corticopontine fibers to pontine neurons becomes 1:1. Corticopontine fibers terminate in sharply delineated lamellae extending rostrocaudally. Various cortical regions project to separate parts of the pontine nuclei, although considerable overlap takes place between some projection areas. Pontine neurons that receive corticopontine fibers give rise to the pontocerebellar pathway discussed in the chapter on the pons (Chap. 7). The corticopontine pathway is thus one of several pathways that link the cerebral crotex with the cerebellum for the coordination and regulation of movement. Lesions of the corticopontine pathway at its sites of origin in the cortex or along its course will result in incoordinated movement (ataxia) contralateral to the lesion. The ataxia observed in some patients with frontal or temporal lobe pathology is thus explained as an interruption of the corticopontine pathway.

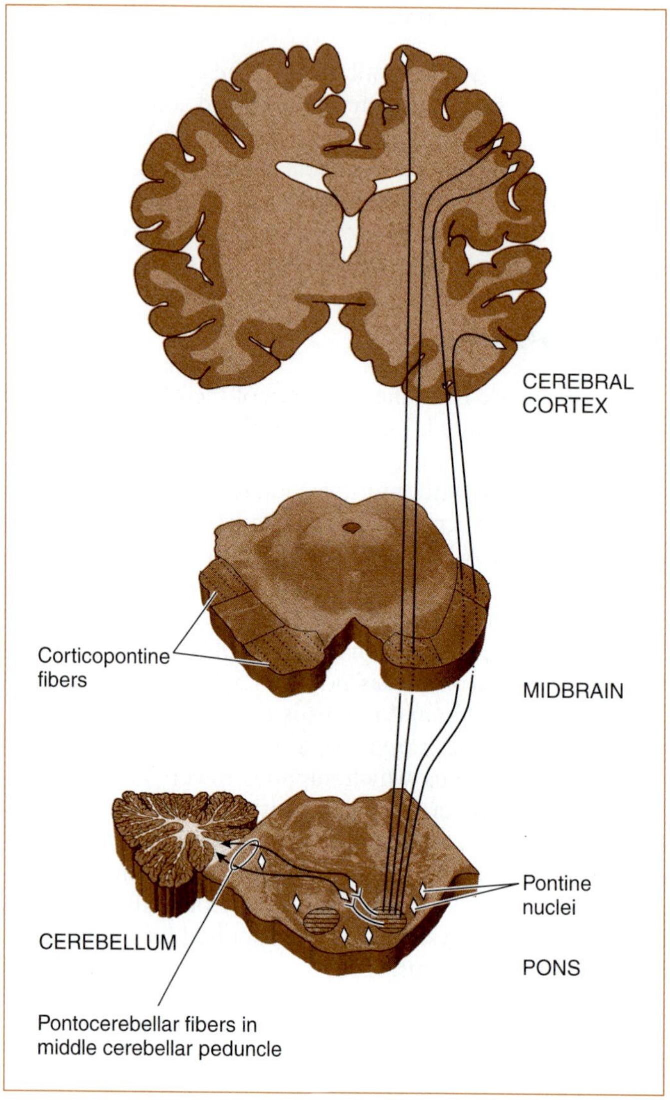
CEREBRAL
CORTEX
Corticopontine
fibers
MIDBRAIN
Pontine
nuclei
CEREBELLUM
PONS
Pontocerebellar fibers in
middle cerebellar peduncle

FIGURE 17-5

Schematic diagram of the corticopontine and pontocerebellar pathways.

Corticothalamic Pathway

The corticothalamic pathway arises from cortical areas that receive thalamic projections and thus constitutes a feedback mechanism by which the cerebral cortex influences thalamic activity. The thalamocortical relationship is such that a thalamic nucleus that projects to a cortical area receives in turn a projection from that area. Examples of such reciprocal connections (Fig. 17-6) include the dorsomedial thalamic nucleus and prefrontal cortex, anterior thalamic nucleus and cingulate cortex, ventrolateral thalamic nucleus and motor cortex, posteroventral thalamic nucleus and postcentral gyrus, medial geniculate nucleus and auditory cortex, and lateral geniculate nucleus and visual cortex. The corticothalamic input to the reticular thalamic nucleus, however, is not reciprocal. The reticular nucleus receives afferents from almost all cortical areas but does not project back to the cerebral cortex. The reticular nucleus receives collaterals from all thalamocortical and all corticothalamic projections. Thus the reticular nucleus is informed of activities passing in both directions between the thalamus and cerebral cortex.

Corticothalamic fibers descend in various parts of the internal capsule and enter

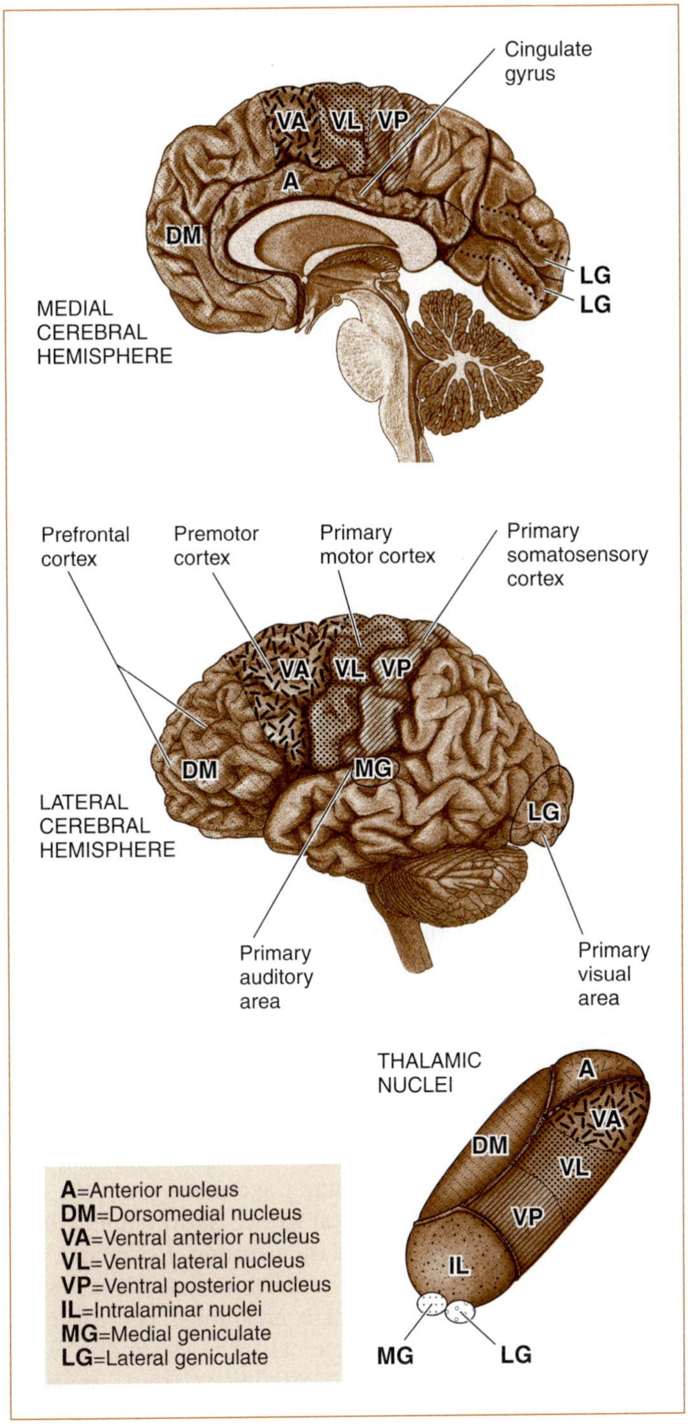

FIGURE 17-6

Schematic diagram of thalamocortical relationships.

the thalamus in one bundle known as the *thalamic radiation*, which also includes the reciprocal thalamocortical fibers.

Corticohypothalamic Pathway

The corticohypothalamic fibers arise from prefrontal cortex, cingulate gyrus, amygdala, olfactory cortex, hippocampus, and septal area.

Corticostriate Pathway

Projections from the cerebral cortex to the striatum are both direct and indirect. Direct corticostriate projections reach the neostriatum via the internal and external capsules and via the subcallosal fasciculus. The indirect pathways include the corticothalamostriate pathway, collaterals of the corticoolivary pathway, and collaterals of the corticopontine pathway.

The corticostriate projection comprises the most massive striatal afferents. Almost all cortical areas contribute to this projection. Cortical areas interconnected via corticocortical fibers tend to share common zones of termination in the neostriatum. Corticostriatal fibers are organized topographically into three distinct striatal territories: (1) sensorimotor, (2) associative, and (3) limbic. The sensorimotor territory receives its inputs from sensory and motor cortical areas. The associative territory receives fibers from the association cortices. The limbic territory receives input from limbic and paralimbic cortical areas.

Corticostriate pathways are also organized somatotopiocally such that cortical association areas project to the caudate nucleus, whereas sensorimotor cortical areas preferentially project to the putamen. Corticoputaminal projections are further organized in that the cortical arm, leg, and face areas project to corresponding areas within the putamen.

Other Corticofugal Pathways

These include cortical projections to several sensory brain stem nuclei, such as the nuclei gracilis and cuneatus, trigeminal nuclei, and others. Most of these fibers serve a feedback purpose. Corticosubthalamic projections originate from the primary motor and premotor cortical areas. A corticotectal projection has been described arising from the frontal eyefields (area 8 of the frontal cortex) in addition to an already established origin from the occipital cortex. Corticorubral fibers originate from the same cortical areas as the corticospinal tract and terminate on the red nucleus in the midbrain.

INTRACORTICAL CIRCUITRY

Cortical neurons may have descending, ascending, horizontal, or short axons. The descending axons contribute to the association and the corticofugal fiber systems outlined above. The ascending, horizontal, and short axons play important roles in intracortical circuitry. Neurons with ascending axons are the cells of Martinotti. The horizontal cells of Cajal have horizontal axons. Short axons arborizing in the vicinity of the cell body are seen in stellate neurons. Pyramidal neurons have horizontal and recurrent axon collaterals that terminate at all levels of the cortex and contribute significantly to intracortical connections. The axon collaterals of pyramidal neurons may project on a stellate cell or a Martinotti cell that in turn may influence other cortical neurons and thus provide for rapid dispersion of activity throughout a population of neurons. This fact was recognized by Cajal, who referred to it as *avalanche conduction*. A simplified account of intracortical circuitry is illustrated diagrammatically in Fig. 17-7. A thalamocortical input (Fig. 17-7) will (1) excite pyramidal (projection) neurons in layer VI and interneurons (excitatory and inhibitory) in layer IV. (2) Inhibitory interneurons in layer IV inhibit other

KEY CONCEPTS

- Corticofugal fiber system includes the corticospinal, corticoreticular, corticobulbar, corticopontine, corticothalamic, corticohypothalamic, corticostriate, and others.

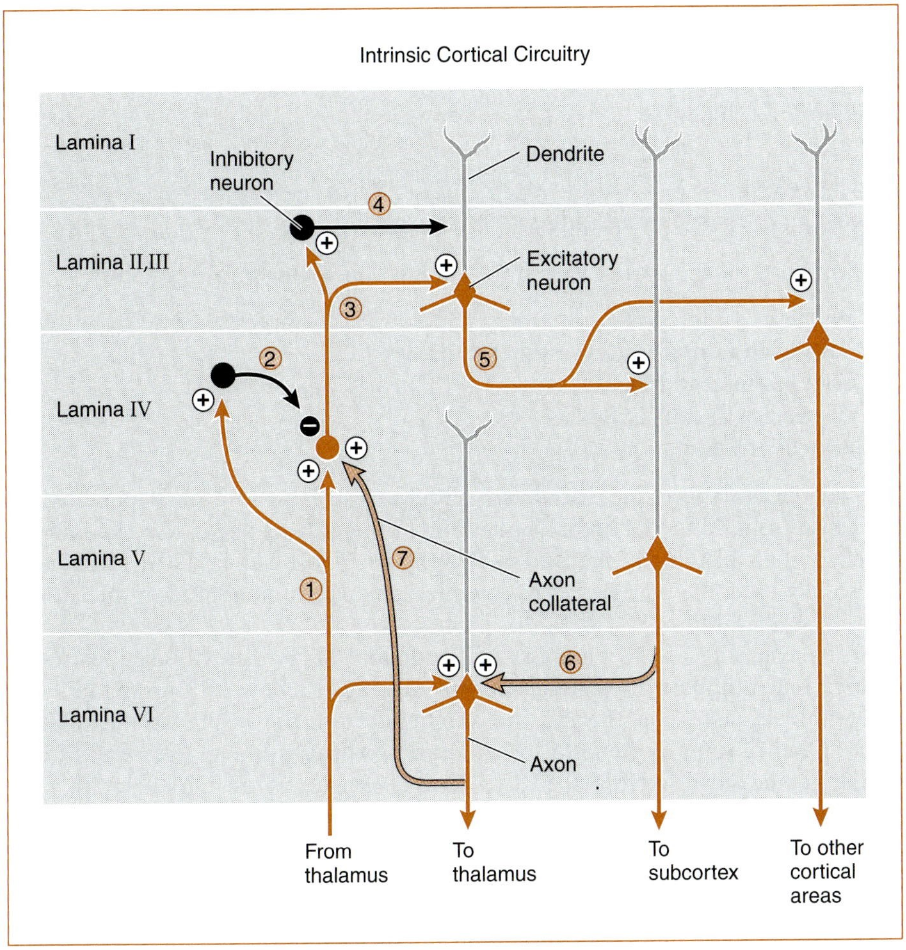

FIGURE 17-7

Schematic diagram showing intrinsic cortical circuitry.

interneurons in the same layer. (3) Excitatory interneurons in layer IV excite pyramidal neurons and inhibitory interneurons in layers II and III. (4) Inhibitory interneurons in layers II and III inhibit pyramidal neurons in the same layers. (5) Pyramidal neurons in layers II and III excite projection neurons in layers IV and V. (6) Axon collaterals of projection neurons in layer V excite corticothalamic projection neurons in layer VI. (7) Axon collaterals of corticothalamic projection neurons in layer VI project back to the excitatory interneurons in layer IV, thus closing the loop. Interneurons in deep cortical layers (cells of Martinotti) and in superficial cortical layers (horizontal cells of Cajal) contribute to intracortical circuitry by vertical and horizontal spread of impulses. Martinotti cells, excited by axon collaterals of pyramidal neurons, in turn excite either a pyramidal neuron or another interneuron. Similarly, the horizontally oriented axons of the horizontal cells of Cajal influence the vertically oriented processes of pyramidal neurons or interneurons. Because of their paucity or absence in the post-neonatal period, the horizontal cells of Cajal play a minimal role in intracortical circuitry in the adult.

KEY CONCEPTS

- Input to the cerebral cortex is spread horizontally and vertically via various intracortical connections comprising a complex intracortical circuitry.

From the preceding it can be seen that an input to the cortex is spread both horizontally and vertically via the various intracortical connections. The complexity of these interconnections is far from clear definition and is the basis of the complexity of human brain function.

CORTICAL CYTOARCHITECTONIC AREAS

Cytoarchitectonic. The design of the cellular characteristics of the cortex, which varies in different regions of the brain and allows mapping of the brain.

Different parts of the cortex vary in relation to the following parameters:

1. Thickness of the cortex
2. Width of the different layers of the cortex
3. Cell types in each layer
4. Cell density in each layer
5. Nerve fiber lamination

Brodmann, Korbinian. German neuropsychiatrist who developed the most commonly used cytoarchitectonic map of the cerebral cortex.

Reil, Johann Christian. Danish physiologist, anatomist, and psychiatrist who was the first to describe the insula or island of Reil in 1796.

Based on the preceding variations, different investigators have parceled the cortex into from 20 to 200 areas depending on the criteria used. The classification of the German histologist **Korbinian Brodmann**, published in 1909, remains the most widely used. It contains 52 cytoarchitectonic areas numbered in the order in which he studied them.

Careful counting of the numbers of Brodmann areas in textbook illustrations indicates that numbers 13 through 16 are missing. Review of Brodmann's 1909 monograph revealed that the missing numbers are in the insula (island of **Reil**). Areas 13 and 14 refer to the anteriorly placed two insulae breves, and areas 15 and 16 refer to the posteriorly placed two insulae longes. More important than the cytoarchitectonic classification is the functional classification of the cortex into several motor and sensory areas. The account that follows will focus on functional areas of the cortex. Brodmann's terminology will be used because it is the most frequently cited. The commonly used classification of cortical areas into purely sensory and motor is somewhat misleading and inaccurate. There is ample evidence to suggest that motor responses can be elicited from so-called sensory areas. This has prompted the use of the term *sensory motor cortex* to refer to previously designated sensory and motor areas.

However, for didactic purposes, the motor and sensory areas of the cortex will be discussed separately.

CORTICAL SENSORY AREAS

Sensory function in the cortex is localized mainly in three lobes: parietal, occipital, and temporal. There are six primary sensory areas in the cortex:

Somesthetic (Greek *soma*, "body"; *aisthesis*, "perception"). Somesthetic sensations are those of pain, temperature, touch, pressure, position, movement, and vibration.

1. Primary **somesthetic** (general sensory, somatosensory) area in the postcentral gyrus of the parietal lobe
2. Primary visual area in the calcarine gyrus of the occipital lobe

KEY CONCEPTS

- Based on thickness of cortex, width of the different cortical layers, cell types within each layer, and nerve fiber lamination patterns, the cerebral cortex has been divided into between 20 and 200 cytoarchitectonic areas. The most widely used classification is that of Brodmann, which contains 52 areas numbered in the order in which they were studied.
- The cerebral cortex is also divided into several sensory and motor areas based on function.

3. Primary auditory area in the transverse gyri of Heschl of the temporal lobe
4. Primary gustatory (taste) area in the most ventral part of the postcentral gyrus of the parietal lobe
5. Primary olfactory (smell) area in the piriform and periamygdaloid regions of the temporal lobe
6. Primary vestibular area in the temporal lobe

Each of these areas receives a specific sensory modality (i.e., pain, touch, vibration, vision, audition, taste, smell). Sensory modalities reaching each of these areas (except olfaction) pass through the thalamus (modality-specific thalamic nucleus) prior to reaching the cortex. Each of the preceding sensory areas is designated as a primary sensory area. Primary sensory cortices have restricted receptive fields. Adjacent to the primary somesthetic, visual, and auditory areas are secondary sensory areas. The secondary sensory areas are found by recording evoked potentials in the respective areas following an appropriate peripheral stimulus (sound, light, etc.). In general, the secondary sensory areas are smaller in size than the primary areas, and their ablation is without effect on the specific sensory modality.

Primary Somesthetic (General Sensory, Somatosensory) Area (SI)

This area (Fig. 17-8) corresponds to the postcentral gyrus of the parietal lobe (areas 1, 2, and 3 of Brodmann) and the posterior part of the paracentral lobule. Area 3 is divided into two parts: 3b on the posterior wall of the central **sulcus** and 3a in the depth of the sulcus. In 1916, Dusser de Barenne applied strychnine, a central stimulant drug, to the postcentral gyrus of monkeys and noted that the animals scratched their skin. Subsequent work by Head on World War I soldiers with head injuries and by the neurosurgeons Cushing and Penfield has added tremendously to knowledge about the function of this area.

Sulcus (Latin "groove, furrow").

Although the primary somesthetic area is concerned basically with sensory modalities, it is possible to elicit motor responses following its stimulation. The primary somesthetic area receives nerve fibers from the ventral posterolateral and ventral posteromedial nuclei of the thalamus. These fibers convey general sensory (touch, pain, and temperature) as well as proprioceptive sensory modalities (position, vibration, and two-point discrimination).

In addition to thalamic afferents, the primary somesthetic cortex receives commissural fibers through the corpus callosum from the contralateral primary somesthetic cortex and short association fibers from the adjacent primary motor cortex. Efferents from the primary somesthetic cortex project to the motor cortex, the opposite primary somesthetic cortex, and the association somatosensory cortex (area 5) in the posterior parietal cortex. In addition, projection fibers descend within the internal capsule to the ventral posterior nuclei of the thalamus, posterior column nuclei of the medulla oblongata, and dorsal horn of the spinal cord. The contralateral half of the body is represented in a precise but disproportionate manner (sensory homunculus) in each of the three areas (1, 2, and 3) of the somesthetic cortex (Fig.

KEY CONCEPTS

- There are six primary sensory cortical areas: somesthetic, visual, auditory, gustatory, olfactory, and vestibular.
- Each primary sensory area subserves a specific sensory modality (i.e., pain, touch, vibration, vision, audition, taste, smell).
- Adjacent to some of the primary sensory areas are secondary sensory areas.

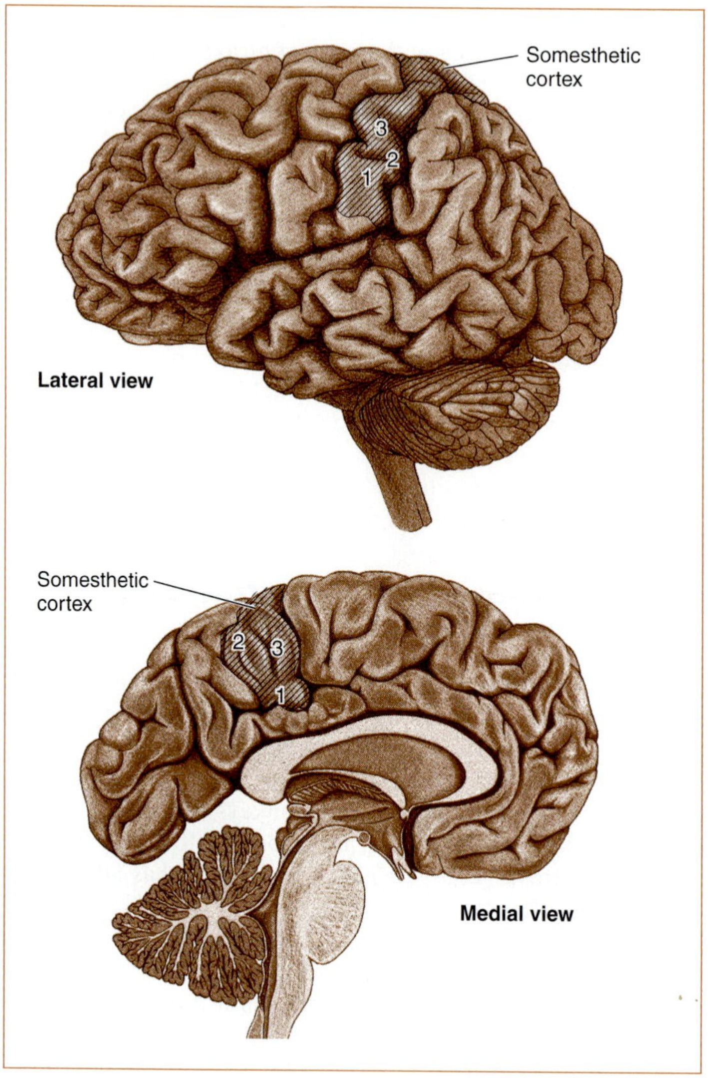

FIGURE 17-8

Schematic diagram of the primary somesthetic cortex.

17-9). The pharynx, tongue, and jaw are represented in the most ventral portion of the lateral surface of the somesthetic area, followed in ascending order by the face, hand, arm, trunk, and thigh. The leg and foot are represented on the medial surface of this area. The anal and genital regions are represented in the most ventral portion of the medial surface just above the cingulate gyrus. The representation of the face, lips, hand, thumb, and index fingers is disproportionately large in comparison with their relative size in the body. This is a reflection of the functional importance of these parts in sensory function.

Stimulation of the primary somesthetic cortex in conscious patients elicits sensations of numbness and tingling, a feeling of electricity, and a feeling of movement without actual movement. These sensations are referred to the contralateral half

KEY CONCEPTS

- Stimulation of the primary somesthetic area elicits sensations of numbness and tingling, a feeling of electricity, and a feeling of movement without actual movement.

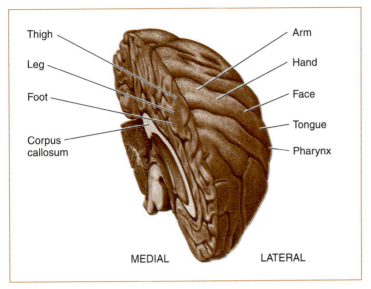

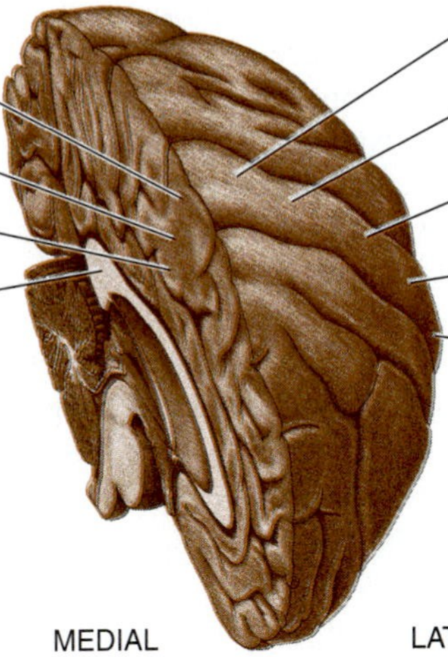
Thigh
Leg
Foot
Corpus callosum
Arm
Hand
Face
Tongue
Pharynx
MEDIAL
LATERAL

FIGURE 17-9

Schematic diagram of the sensory homunculus.

of the body, except when the face area is stimulated. The face and tongue are represented bilaterally.

Ablation of the postcentral gyrus will result, in the immediate postoperative period, in loss of all modalities of sensation (touch, pressure, pain, and temperature). Soon, however, pain and temperature sensations will return. It is believed that pain and temperature sensations are determined at the thalamic level, whereas the source, severity, and quality of such sensations are perceived in the postcentral gyrus. Thus the effects of postcentral gyrus lesions would be (1) complete loss of discriminative touch and proprioception and (2) crude awareness of pain, temperature, and light touch.

Neurophysiologic studies of the somesthetic cortex have revealed the following information: (1) The functional cortical unit appears to be associated with a vertical column of cells that is modality specific. Neurons within a cortical unit are activated by the same peripheral stimulus and are related to the same peripheral receptive field. (2) Area 3b is activated by cutaneous stimuli and areas 2 and 3a by proprioceptive impulses, whereas area 1 is activated by either cutaneous or proprioceptive impulses. (3) Somatosensory neurons responding to joint movement show a marked degree of specificity in that they respond to displacement in one direction. (4) Fast- and slow-adapting neuronal pools have been identified in response to hair displacement or cutaneous deformation. (5) Fibers mediating cutaneous sensations terminate rostrally, while those mediating proprioceptive sensations terminate more caudally in the somesthetic area.

Secondary Somesthetic Area (SII)

A secondary somesthetic area has been described in humans and primates. It is located on the most inferior aspect of the postcentral gyrus and in the superior

KEY CONCEPTS

- Lesions in the primary somesthetic area result in loss of discriminative touch and proprioception and in the crude awareness of pain, temperature, and light touch.

bank and depth of the lateral sulcus (parietal operculum). Body representation in this area is bilateral, with contralateral predominance, and is the reverse of that in the primary area so that the two face areas are adjacent to each other.

The secondary sensory area contains neurons with receptive fields that are large, poorly demarcated, overlap extensively, and often have bilateral representation. **Lesions** of the secondary somesthetic area and the insula produce **asymbolia** for pain, suggesting that the secondary somesthetic area is an important cortical locus for the conscious perception of noxious stimuli. Recent positron-emission tomographic (PET) studies in human volunteers subjected to noxious stimuli have demonstrated increased metabolic activity in the secondary somesthetic area as well as in the postcentral and cingulate gyri. The secondary somesthetic area contains no cells sensitive to joint movement or joint position. The secondary somesthetic area has been shown to have reciprocal connections with ventral posteromedial and centrolateral nuclei of the thalamus. It also receives inputs from the ipsi- and contralateral primary somesthetic cortices. Efferent connections project to the primary somesthetic and primary motor areas within the same hemisphere. Lesions interrupting connections between the secondary somesthetic area, posterior parietal cortex, and ventral posteromedial and centrolateral thalamic nuclei have been associated with pseudothalamic pain syndrome. The pain is spontaneous and characterized as burning or icelike and is associated with impairment of pain and temperature appreciation.

Lesion (Latin *laesum*, "hurt"). A lesion in the nervous system may be destructive (infarct, hemorrhage, tumor) or may stimulate neurons (epilepsy).

Asymbolia (Greek *a*, "negative"; *symbolon*, "symbol"). Loss of power to comprehend symbols as words, figures, gestures, and signs. Asymbolia of pain is the absence of psychic reaction to painful sensations. The term *asymbolia* for pain was first described by Schilder and Stengel in 1938.

Supplementary Sensory Area (SSA)

This area was defined originally by Penfield and Jasper with intraoperative stimulation studies in humans. The supplementary sensory area lacks Brodmann's numeric designation, but it encompasses medial area 5 of Brodmann and probably the anterior part of medial area 7. Neurons in the supplementary sensory area have large receptive fields, and some neurons are sensitive to pain.

Somatosensory (Somesthetic) Association Areas

The somatosensory association areas encompass areas 5 and 7 in the superior parietal lobe. They receive their inputs mainly from the primary somatosensory areas but also have reciprocal connections with the pulvinar nucleus of the thalamus. Neuronal responses in the somatosensory association areas are complex and involve the integration of a number of cortical and thalamic inputs. The processing of multisensory somatosensory inputs in these areas allows for the perception of shape, size, and texture and the identification of objects by contact (stereognosis). The somatosensory association areas project to multimodal association areas (areas 39 and 40) in the inferior parietal lobule that receive inputs from more than one sensory modality and serve intermodal integration and multisensory perceptions.

Single-cell recordings in area 5 in monkeys suggest that this area is essential for the proper use of somatosensory information, for goal-directed voluntary movements, and for the manipulation of objects.

KEY CONCEPTS

- Lesions of the secondary sensory area produce asymbolia for pain.
- Lesions that interrupt connections between the secondary sensory area, posterior parietal cortex, and the thalamus produce pseudothalamic pain syndrome.
- The somatosensory association areas are concerned with the perception of shape, size, and texture and the identification of objects by contact (stereognosis).

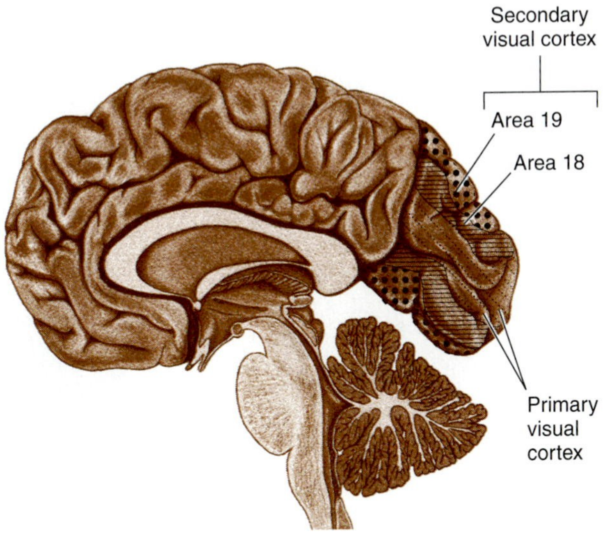

FIGURE 17-10

Schematic diagram of the primary and secondary visual cortices.

Single-cell recordings in area 7 indicate that this area plays an important role in the integration of visual and somatosensory stimuli, which is essential for coordination of eyes and hands in visually guided movements.

Bilateral lesions in the somatosensory association areas in humans are associated with inability to move the hand toward an object that is clearly seen (optic ataxia). Such patients are unable to pour water from a bottle into a glass and repeatedly pour the water outside the glass. Unilateral lesions in the somatosensory association areas in the nondominant hemisphere produce neglect of the contralateral half of the body and visual space.

Primary Visual Cortex (V_1)

This area (Fig. 17-10) corresponds to the calcarine gyrus on the medial surface of the occipital lobe on each side of the calcarine sulcus (area 17 of Brodmann). In sections of fresh cortex, this area is characterized by the appearance of a prominent band of white matter that can be identified by the naked eye and is named the *band of Gennari*, after the Italian medical student who described it in 1782. The band of Gennari represents a thickened external band of Baillarger in layer IV of the cortex. In myelin preparations, the band of Gennari appears as a prominent dark band in the visual cortex, also known as the *striate cortex*. The term *striate* refers to the presence in unstained preparations of the thick white band of Gennari.

The primary visual area receives fibers from the lateral geniculate nucleus. These fibers originate in the retina, synapse in the lateral geniculate nucleus, and reach

KEY CONCEPTS

- Bilateral lesions in the somatosensory association areas are associated with optic ataxia.
- Unilateral lesions in the somatosensory association areas in the nondominant hemisphere result in neglect of the contralateral half of the body and visual space.

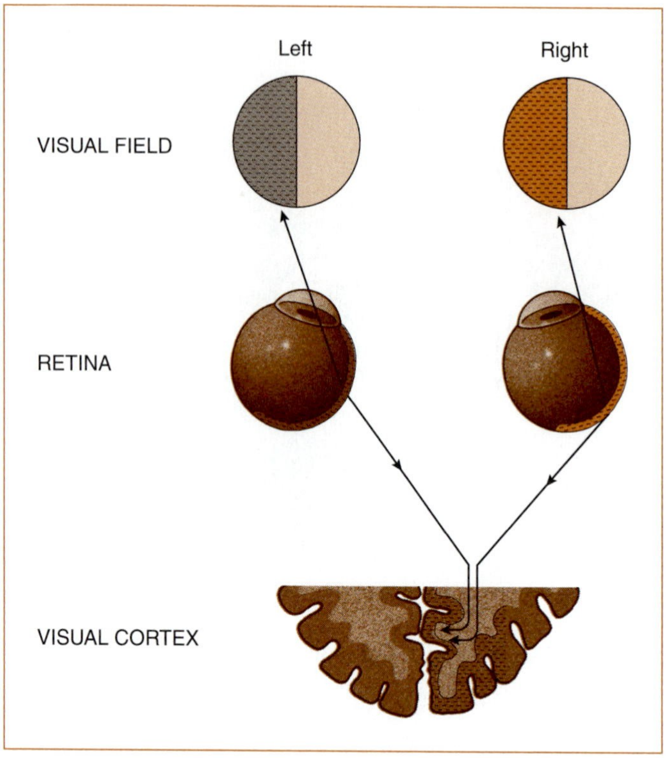

FIGURE 17-11

Schematic diagram of retinal representation in the primary visual cortex.

the visual cortex via the optic (geniculocalcarine) radiation. Each visual cortex receives fibers from the ipsilateral half of each retina (Fig. 17-11) that convey information about the contralateral half of the visual field. Thus lesions of one visual cortex are manifested by loss of vision in the contralateral half of the visual field (homonymous hemianopsia). The projections from the retina into the visual cortex are organized spatially in such a way that macular fibers occupy the posterior part of the visual cortex, while peripheral retinal fibers occupy the anterior part (Fig. 17-12). Fibers originating from the superior half of the retina terminate in the superior part of the visual cortex; those from the inferior half of the retina terminate in the inferior part (Fig. 17-13). Thus lesions involving portions of the visual cortex, such as the inferior calcarcine cortex, produce an upper contralateral **quadrantanopsia** in which blindness is limited to the contralateral upper quadrant of the visual field. Similarly, lesions limited to the upper calcarine cortex produce a lower contralateral quadrantanopsia in which blindness is limited to the contralateral lower quadrant of the visual field. The representation of the macula in the visual cortex is disproportionately large in comparison with its relative size in the retina. This is a reflection of its important function as the retinal area of keenest vision.

Quadrantanopsia (quadrantanopsia). Loss of vision in one-quarter of the visual field. This occurs with parietal (inferior quadrant loss) or temporal (superior quadrant loss) lobe lesions.

Stimulation of the visual cortex elicits a crude sensation of bright flashes of light; patients with irritative lesions (such as tumors) of the visual cortex experience visual

KEY CONCEPTS

- Stimulation of the primary visual cortex produces contralateral crude sensation of bright flashes of light.
- Lesions in the primary visual area produce loss of vision in the contralateral visual field.

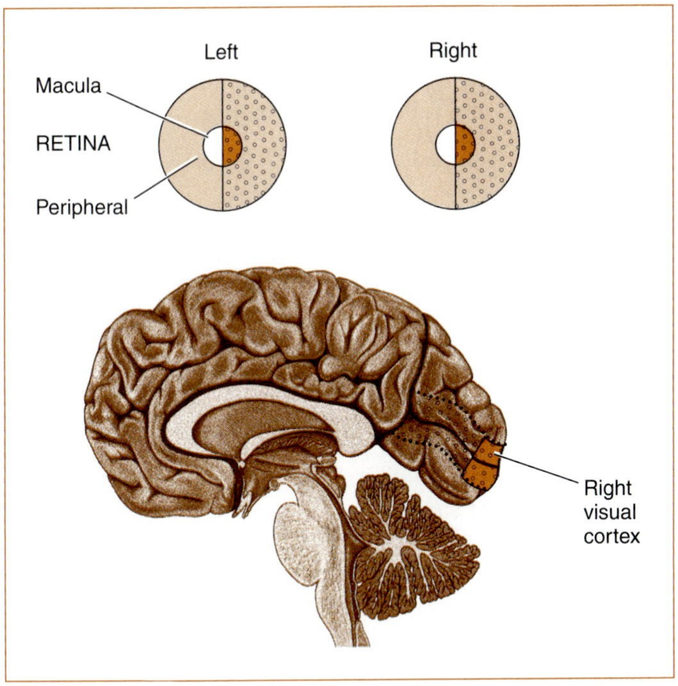

FIGURE 17-12

Schematic diagram of retinal representation in the primary visual cortex.

hallucinations that consist of bright light. Conversely, lesions that destroy the visual cortex of one hemisphere result in loss of vision in the contralateral half of the visual field. If the destructive lesion is of vascular origin, such as occurs in occlusions of the posterior cerebral artery, central (macular) vision in the affected visual field is spared. This phenomenon is known clinically as *macular sparing* and is attributed

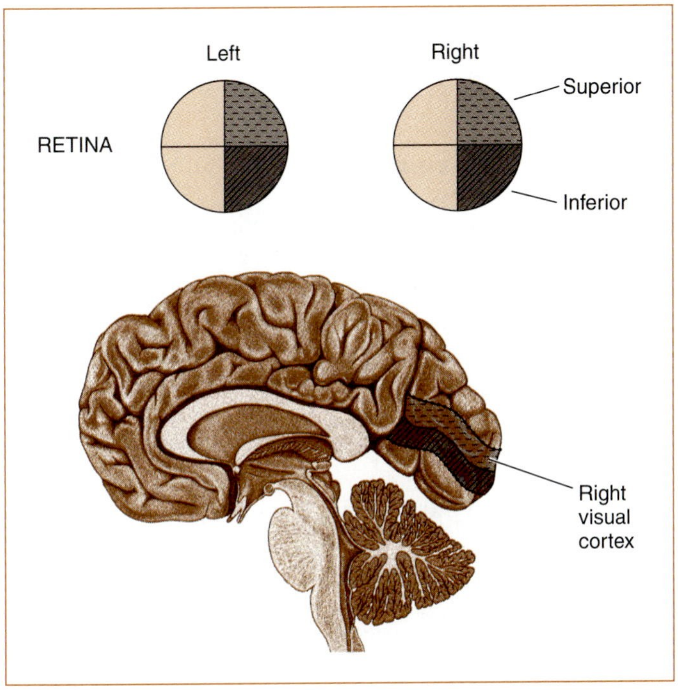

FIGURE 17-13

Schematic diagram of retinal representation in the primary visual cortex.

to the collateral arterial supply of the posterior visual cortex (macular area) from the patent middle cerebral artery.

In the last decade, elegant neurophysiologic studies of single neurons in the visual cortex have revealed the following information:

1. The visual cortex is organized into units that correspond to specific areas in the retina.
2. These units respond to linear stripe (straight-line) configurations.
3. For each unit, a particular orientation of the stimulus is most effective. Some units respond only to vertically oriented stripes, while others respond only to horizontally oriented stripes. Some units respond at onset of illumination, while others respond at cessation of illumination.
4. Units are of two varieties, simple and complex. Simple units react only to stimuli in corresponding fixed retinal receptive fields. Complex units are connected to several simple cortical units. It is presumed that the complex units represent an advanced stage in cortical integration.
5. Units that respond to the same stimulus pattern and orientation are grouped together in repeating units referred to as *columns*, similar to those described for the somesthetic cortex. Two general varieties of functional columns have been described: ocular dominance and orientation columns. Ocular dominance columns are parallel columns arranged perpendicular to the cortical surface and reflect eye preference (right versus left) of cortical neurons. Alternating ocular dominance columns are dominated by inputs from the left and right eyes. Orientation columns comprise a sequence of cells that have the same receptive field axis orientation.
6. Visual columns respond poorly, if at all, to diffuse retinal illumination.
7. Visual units respond optimally to moving stimuli.
8. Most cortical units receive fibers from corresponding receptive fields in both retinas, thus allowing for single-image vision of corresponding points in the two retinas.
9. The striate cortex is organized into vertical and horizontal systems. The vertical (columnar) system is concerned with retinal position, line orientation, and ocular dominance. The horizontal system segregates cells of different orders of complexity. Simple cells located in layer IV are driven monocularly, while complex and hypercomplex cells, located in other layers, are driven by impulses from both eyes.

Secondary Visual Areas

Adjacent to the primary visual area are the secondary visual (association, extrastriate, prestriate) areas. They include areas 18 and 19 of Brodmann (Fig. 17-10). Area 18 corresponds to the second (V_2) and area 19 to the third (V_3) visual areas. V_4, in humans, is probably located in the inferior occipitotemporal area, in the region of the lingual or fusiform gyrus. V_5 in humans is probably located in area 19 of Brodmann. V_2, like V_1, is retinotopically organized. Visual areas beyond V_2 are associated with varying visual functions. V_3 is associated with form, V_4 with color, and V_5 with motion. Units in the secondary visual areas are of the complex or hypercomplex types.

Afferents to areas 18 and 19 are mainly from the primary visual area (area 17)

KEY CONCEPTS

- The secondary (association) visual areas are concerned with form, color, and motion.

but include some direct thalamic projections from the lateral geniculate nucleus and pulvinar nucleus. The primary visual area projects bilaterally and reciprocally to areas 18 and 19. The projections from the pulvinar nucleus constitute important extrageniculate links to the visual cortex.

Outputs from areas 18 and 19 project to the posterior parietal cortex (area 7) and to the inferotemporal cortex (areas 20 and 21). The projection to area 7 is concerned with **stereopsis** (depth perception) and movement. The inferotemporal projection is concerned with analysis of form and color. The inferotemporal cortex represents highest visual function. Electrical stimulation of area 21 evokes lifelike visual hallucinations. Area 37, behind area 21, at the occipitotemporal junction contains modules devoted to recognition of faces. Bilateral lesions in this area result in failure to recognize familiar faces **(prosopagnosia)**. Color vision is localized inferiorly in the inferior occipitotemporal cortex (V_4). No color representation is found in the superior association visual cortex. Thus in unilateral inferior association visual cortex lesions the patient loses color vision in the contralateral half field (central **hemiachromatopsia**). Loss of color vision and face recognition usually coexist because of the proximity of the areas responsible for them. Connections of the association visual cortex to the angular gyrus (area 39) play a role in recognition of visual stimuli. Lesions interrupting this connection result in visual agnosia, inability to recognize objects in the visual field. Bilateral lesions of visual area 5 (V_5) are associated with a defect in visual motion perception **(akinetopsia)**.

Projections from areas 18 and 19 also reach the frontal eye fields (area 8 of Brodmann) in the frontal lobe, as well as the superior colliculus and motor nuclei of extraocular muscles. These projections play a key role in conjugate eye movement induced by visual stimuli (visual pursuit).

Stereopsis (Greek *stereos*, "solid, having three dimensions"; *opsis*, "vision"). The ability to discriminate depth; stereoscopic vision.

Prosopagnosia (Greek *prosopon*, "face"; *gnosis*, "to know"). Inability to recognize familiar faces.

Hemiachromatopsia. Loss of color vision in one-half the visual field.

Akinetopsia. Cerebral motion blindness, a syndrome in which a patient loses specifically the ability to perceive visual motion as a result of cortical lesions outside the striate cortex.

Primary Auditory Cortex

David Ferrier, a British physician, is credited with localizing the primary auditory cortex of monkeys to the superior temporal gyrus during the latter half of the nineteenth century. This localization was not accepted by his contemporaries. Subsequent studies in animals and humans, however, have confirmed his early observations.

The primary auditory cortex (Fig. 17-14) corresponds to the transverse temporal gyri of **Heschl** (areas 41 and 42 of Brodmann) located in the temporal lobe within the lateral fissure. Recording of primary evoked responses to auditory stimuli during surgery for epilepsy provides evidence for a restricted portion of Heschl's gyrus (its posteromedial part) as the primary auditory area.

The primary auditory cortex receives fibers (auditory radiation) from the medial geniculate nucleus. These fibers reach the auditory cortex via the sublenticular part of the internal capsule. Auditory fibers originate in the peripheral organ of Corti and establish several synapses in the neuraxis, both homolateral and contralateral to their side of origin, before reaching the medial geniculate nucleus of the thalamus. The primary auditory cortex, therefore, receives fibers originating from both organs of Cotri, predominantly from the contralateral side. Stimulation of the primary auditory cortex produces crude auditory sensations such as buzzing, humming, or

Ferrier, David. Scottish neurophysiologist and neurologist who is credited with localization of the primary auditory cortex in the superior temporal gyrus.

Heschl, Richard. Austrian anatomist and pathologist who described the anterior transverse temporal gyri (Heschl's convolutions), which serve as the primary auditory area.

KEY CONCEPTS

- Stimulation of the inferotemporal association visual cortex evokes lifelike visual hallucinations.
- Bilateral lesions in area 37 at the occipitotemporal junction result in loss of face recognition (prosopognosia).

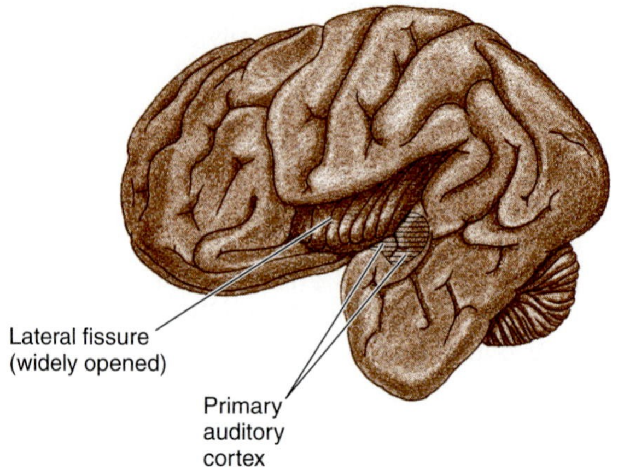

FIGURE 17-14

Schematic diagram of the primary auditory cortex.

knocking. Such sensations are referred to clinically as *tinnitis*. Lesions of the auditory cortex result in (1) impairment in sound localization in space and (2) diminution of hearing bilaterally but mostly contralaterally. The functional organization of the auditory cortex is similar to that of the somesthetic and visual cortices. Column cells in the auditory cortex share the same functional properties. Columnar organization is thus based on isofrequency stripes, each stripe responding to a particular tonal frequency.

The primary auditory cortex is connected with the association auditory cortex. Other important connections include the auditory cortex of the contralateral hemisphere, the primary somesthetic cortex, frontal eye fields, Broca's area of speech in the frontal lobe, and the medial geniculate nucleus. Via its projection to the medial geniculate body in the thalamus, the primary auditory cortex controls its own input by changing the excitability of medial geniculate neurons. Responses of some auditory cortex neurons to sound stimuli depend on whether the type of these sounds was anticipated. A similar anticipatory response to sound stimuli exists in some medial geniculate neurons, suggesting that transmission of information through the auditory thalamus (medial geniculate nucleus) and on to the auditory cortex is controlled by behavioral contingencies.

Physiologic studies of the primary auditory cortex have revealed that it does not play a major role in sound frequency discrimination but rather in the temporal pattern of acoustic stimuli. Frequency discrimination of sound is a function of subcortical acoustic structures. The optimal stimulus that fires auditory cortical units seems to be a changing frequency of sound stimuli rather than a steady-frequency stimulus.

KEY CONCEPTS

- Stimulation of the primary auditory cortex produces crude auditory sensations of buzzing, humming, or knocking.
- Lesions of the primary auditory cortex result in diminution of hearing bilaterally but mostly contralaterally.

Association Auditory Cortex

Adjacent to the primary auditory cortex is the association auditory cortex (areas 22 and 24 of Brodmann). This area is concerned with the comprehension of spoken sound. Area 22 in the dominant hemisphere is known as *Wernicke's area.* Lesions of this area are associated with a receptive type of aphasia, a disorder of communication characterized by the inability of the patient to comprehend spoken words. The association auditory cortex is connected via the anterior commissure with the prefrontal cortex and via the corpus callosum with the prefrontal, premotor, parietal, and cingulate cortices.

Primary Gustatory Cortex

Gustatory (Latin *gustatorius,* "pertaining to the sense of taste").

The cortical receptive area for taste is located in the parietal operculum, ventral to the primary somesthetic area and in close proximity to the cortical areas receiving sensory afferents from the tongue and pharynx. It corresponds to area 43 of Brodmann. Irritative lesions in this area in humans have been shown to give rise to hallucinations of taste, usually preceding the onset of an epileptic attack. Such a prodromal symptom preceding an epileptic fit focuses attention on the site of the irritative lesion. Conversely, ablation of this area produces impairment of taste contralateral to the site of the lesion. The gustatory cortex receives fibers from the posteroventral medial nucleus of the thalamus, upon which converge sensory fibers from the face and mouth, including taste fibers. Although crude taste sensations can be perceived at the thalamic level, discrimination among different taste sensations is a cortical function.

Primary Olfactory Cortex

The primary olfactory cortex is located in the tip of the temporal lobe and consists of the **piriform** cortex and the periamygdaloid area. The primary olfactory cortex receives fibers from the lateral olfactory stria and has an intimate relationship with adjacent cortical regions comprising part of the limbic system. Such relationships, as well as the role of olfaction in emotion and behavior, are discussed in the chapter on the limbic system (Chap. 21). Adjacent to the primary olfactory cortex is the entorhinal cortex (area 28), which is considered the *association* or *secondary olfactory cortical area.*

Piriform (Latin *pyrum,* "pear"; *forma,* "form"). Pear-shaped. The piriform cortex is a region of the olfactory cortex.

Irritative lesions in the region of the olfactory cortex give rise to olfactory hallucinations that are usually disagreeable. As in the case of taste, such hallucinations frequently precede an epileptic fit. Since olfactory hallucinations frequently occur in association with lesions in the uncus of the temporal lobe (including the olfactory cortex), they are referred to clinically as *uncinate fits.*

The olfactory system is the only sensory system in which fibers reach the cortex

KEY CONCEPTS

- The association auditory cortex is concerned with comprehension of speech.
- Stimulation of the primary gustatory area results in hallucinations of taste.
- Lesions of the primary gustatory area result in impairment of taste contralateral to the side of the lesion.
- Stimulation of the primary olfactory cortex results in olfactory hallucinations, usually disagreeable smells.

without passing through the thalamus. Basic olfactory functions needed for reflex action reside in subcortical structures. The discrimination of different odors, however, is a function of the olfactory cortex.

Primary Vestibular Cortex

Data are scant about the anatomic location as well as the physiologic properties of the primary vestibular cortex. Several distinct and separate areas of the parietal and temporal cortex have been identified in animal studies as receiving vestibular afferents. Knowledge about vestibular cortex function in humans is less precise. There is ample evidence to suggest, however, that the posterior insular cortex is the site of vestibular function in humans. Evidence in support of this localization include the following: (1) this area corresponds to the region in which electrical stimulation in humans produce sensations of rotation and motion, (2) it is the area where epileptic foci have been recorded in patients who report strong illusions of rotation during a seizure, (3) it is the area where increased cerebral blood flow is detected during caloric stimulation of the auditory end organ, and (4) lesions in this area in humans impair perceptual judgments about body orientation and movement. Such lesions, however, do not impair brain stem vestibular reflexes such as the vestibuloocular reflex.

CORTICAL MOTOR AREAS

There are three major cerebral cortical areas involved in motor control:

1. Primary motor area (MI)
2. Supplementary motor area (MII)
3. Premotor area

The primary motor area is coextensive with area 4 of Brodmann, and the supplementary motor and premotor areas are coextensive with area 6 of Brodmann. The supplementary motor and premotor areas together represent the nonprimary motor cortex. The three motor areas differ in their electrical excitability, functional neuronal properties, and connectivity. They receive inputs from different thalamic nuclei and have different corticocortical connections and different output projections.

Primary Motor Area (MI)

The primary motor area (Fig. 17-15) corresponds to the precentral gyrus (area 4 of Brodmann). On the medial surface of the hemisphere, the primary motor area

KEY CONCEPTS

- Stimulation of the primary vestibular area produces sensations of rotation and motion.
- Lesions in the primary vestibular area impair perceptual judgment about body orientation and movement.
- Three motor areas have been defined: primary motor, supplementary motor, and premotor.
- The supplementary motor and premotor areas are collectively known as the *nonprimary motor cortex.*

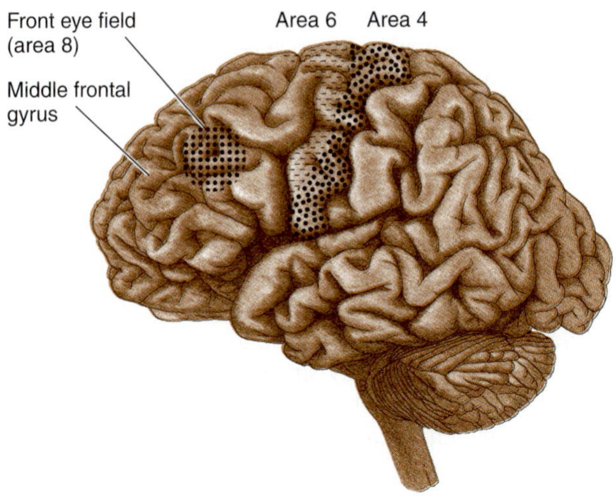
Front eye field
(area 8)
Middle frontal
gyrus
Area 6
Area 4

FIGURE 17-15

Schematic diagram of the primary motor area (area 4), premotor area (area 6), and the frontal eye field (area 8).

comprises the anterior part of the paracentral lobule. The contralateral half of the body is represented in the primary motor area in a precise but disproportionate manner, giving rise to the motor homunculus in the same way as that described for the primary somesthetic cortex. Stimulation of the motor cortex in conscious humans gives rise to discrete and isolated contralateral movement limited to a single joint or a single muscle. Bilateral responses are seen in extraocular muscles and muscles of the face, tongue, jaw, larynx, and pharynx. The primary motor cortex thus functions in the initiation of highly skilled fine movements, such as buttoning one's shirt or sewing.

The representation of bodily regions in the contralateral motor cortex does not seem to be rigidly fixed. Thus repetitive stimulation of the thumb area will produce movement of the thumb, followed after a while by immobility of the thumb and movement at the index finger or even the wrist. This has been interpreted to mean that in the thumb area of the cortex the motor units controlling the index finger and wrist have a higher threshold for stimulation than those controlling the thumb.

The motor area receives fibers from the ventrolateral nucleus of the thalamus, the main projection area of the cerebellum. The motor are also receives fibers from the somesthetic cortex (areas 1, 2, and 5) and the supplementary motor cortex. The connections between the primary motor and somesthetic cortices are reciprocal. The output contributes to the association, commissural, and corticofugal fiber systems discussed earlier. The primary motor cortex is the site of origin of about 30 to 40 percent of the fibers in the pyramidal tract. Furthermore, all the large-diameter axons (approximately 3 percent of the pyramidal fibers) originate from the giant motor neurons (of **Betz**) in the primary motor cortex. Most of the neurons contributing fibers to the corticospinal tract have glutamate or aspartate as their excitatory neurotransmitter. Ablation of the primary motor cortex results in flaccid (hypotonic) paralysis in the contralateral half of the body associated with loss of all reflexes. With time, there is recovery of stereotyped movement at proximal joints, but the function of distal muscles concerned with skilled movement remains impaired. Exaggerated myotatic reflexes and a Babinski sign also appear.

Betz, Vladimir A. Russian anatomist who described the giant pyramidal cells in the motor area of the cerebral cortex.

Although the primary motor cortex is not the sole area from which movement can be elicited, it is nevertheless characterized by initiating highly skilled movement at a lower threshold of stimulation than the other motor areas. Epileptic patients with a lesion in the primary motor cortex frequently manifest a seizure (epileptic) pattern that consists of progression of the epileptic movement from one part of the body to another in a characteristic sequence corresponding to body representation in the motor cortex. Such a phenomenon is known clinically as a **Jacksonian march**, after the English neurologist Hughlings Jackson.

Jacksonian march (Jacksonian epilepsy, Bravais-Jackson epilepsy). The spread of tonic-clonic epileptic activity through contiguous body parts on one side of the body due to spread of epileptic activity in the corresponding motor areas of the cortex. Named after Hughlings Jackson (1835–1911), one of the greatest figures in the history of neurology. Bravais described the same pattern of epileptic spread in his graduation thesis in 1827 but did not elaborate on the etiology.

Neurophysiologic studies of motor cortex neurons reveal that action potentials can be recorded from motor neurons in the cortex about 60 to 80 ms before muscle movement. Furthermore, two types of neurons in the motor cortex have been identified. These are a larger neuron with a phasic pattern of firing and a smaller neuron that fires in a tonic pattern. From experiments on conscious animals performing specific tasks, it has been shown that the frequency of firing is highly correlated with the force exerted to perform a specific movement. Motor neurons supplying a given muscle are usually grouped together in a columnar fashion. Although some motor neurons can be stimulated from a wide area, each has a so-called best point from which it can be stimulated most easily. Such best points usually are confined to a cylindric area of cortex about 1 mm in diameter.

Supplementary Motor Area (MII)

The supplementary motor area is located on the medial surface of the frontal lobe, anterior to the medial extension of the primary motor cortex (area 4). It corresponds roughly to the medial extensions of area 6 of Brodmann. Although the existence of a motor area in the medial aspect of the frontal cortex rostral to the precentral leg area of primates has long been known, **Penfield** and Welch were the first to call this portion of the cortex the *supplementary motor area* in 1949 and 1951. A homunculus has been defined for the supplementary motor area in which face and upper limbs are represented rostral to the lower limbs and trunk. Stimulation in humans gives rise to complex movement in preparation for the assumption of characteristic postures.

Penfield, Wilder Graves. Canadian neurosurgeon who made major contributions to localization of function in the cerebral cortex, speech mechanisms, and epilepsy.

Although simple motor tasks are elicited from stimulation of the supplementary motor area, the role of this area in simple motor tasks is much less significant and is likely to be subsidiary to that of the primary motor area. On the other hand, the supplementary motor area assumes more significance in executing simple motor tasks as a compensatory mechanism when the primary motor area is destroyed. The supplementary motor area seems crucial in the temporal organization of movement, especially in sequential performance of multiple movements, and in motor tasks that demand retrieval of motor memory. Cells were identified in the supplementary motor area in response to movements of both proximal and distal extremity muscles, ipsi- and contralateral. Supplementary motor area neurons differ from primary motor area neurons in that only a small percentage (5 percent) of supplementary motor area neurons contribute axons to the pyramidal tract and these neurons have insignificant input from the periphery and are activated bilaterally.

The supplementary motor cortex is connected reciprocally with the ipsilateral primary motor (area 4), premotor (area 6), and somatosensory (areas 5, 7) cortices and the contralateral supplementary motor cortex. Subcortical projections to the supplementary motor area are predominantly from the basal ganglia via the thalamus. An input from the cerebellum via the basal ganglia also has been shown to exist. Subcortical projections of the supplementary motor cortex are profuse to parts of the caudate nucleus and putamen and to the ventral anterior, ventral

KEY CONCEPTS

- Simple motor tasks are elicited from stimulation of the primary motor area but also from stimulation of the supplementary motor area.

lateral, and dorsomedial thalamic nuclei. Approximately 5 percent of neurons in the supplementary motor cortex contribute fibers to the corticospinal tract. Available anatomic and physiologic data suggest that the supplementary motor area could be the site where external inputs and commands are matched with internal needs and drives to facilitate formulation (programming) of a strategy of voluntary movement. The threshold of stimulation of the supplementary motor area is higher than that of the primary motor cortex and the responses elicited are ipsi- or bilateral.

In contrast to the evidence from physiologic studies, few clinical case reports have described persistent effects on motor behavior of damage to the supplementary motor area. In the acute phase, patients have global reduction in movement **(akinesia)** that is particularly pronounced on the side contralateral to the lesion and a grasp reflex. Lesions in the supplementary motor area of the dominant hemisphere are associated with severe impairment of spontaneous speech with preserved repetition. These manifestations are mostly transient and resolve within a few weeks. The lasting disorder of motor behavior reported to occur in humans after supplementary motor area lesions has been a disturbance of alternating movements of the two hands. Other clinical manifestations, of uncertain etiology, associated with lesions in the supplementary motor area include hypertonia, increase in myotatic reflexes, clonus, and the Babinski sign.

Akinesia (Greek *a*, "negative"; *kinesis*, "motion"). Absence or poverty of movement.

Recent data suggest that the traditionally defined supplementary motor area includes two separate regions: a caudal region (supplementary motor area proper) that has reciprocal connections with the primary motor area and projects to the spinal cord and a rostral region (presupplementary motor area) that receives projections from the prefrontal and cingulate cortices. Basal ganglia input reaches the caudal region, whereas cerebellar input reaches the rostral region. Neuronal responses to visual stimuli prevail in the rostral region, whereas somatosensory responses prevail in the caudal region. The urge to initiate movement in humans is elicited only from the rostral region.

Premotor Area

The concept of a premotor cortex was first proposed in 1905 by Campbell, who called it the *intermediate precentral cortex*. The term *premotor cortex* was first used by Hines in 1929. The premotor cortex has undergone a strong phylogenetic development. Whereas in monkeys the premotor area is equally large as the primary motor area, in humans the premotor area is about six times larger than the primary motor area.

The premotor area (Fig. 17-15) is located in the frontal lobe just anterior to the primary motor area. It corresponds to area 6 of Brodmann. The premotor area is concerned with voluntary motor function dependent on sensory inputs (visual, auditory, somatosensory). Stimulation of the premotor area elicits a stereotyped gross movement that requires coordination among many muscles, such as turning movements of the head, eyes, and trunk toward the opposite side, elevation of the arm, elbow flexion, and pronation of the hand. The threshold of stimuli that elicit responses from this area is higher than that required for the primary motor cortex.

In normal subjects, the premotor area shows increased activity when motor routines are run in response to visual, auditory, or somatosensory cues such as reaching for an object in space, obeying a spoken command, or identifying an object

KEY CONCEPTS

- The supplementary motor area is crucial in the temporal organization of movement, especially in sequential performance of multiple movements, and in motor tasks that demand retrieval of motor memory.

by manipulation. The premotor area exerts influence on movement via the primary motor area or directly through its projections to the pyramidal and extrapyramidal systems. Approximately 30 percent of pyramidal fibers originate from the premotor area. The premotor area is activated when a new motor program is established or when the motor program is changed on the basis of sensory information received, for example, when the subject is exploring the environment or objects. Ablation of the premotor cortex in humans may produce a deficit in the execution of skilled, sequential, and complex movement such as walking. Such a deficit is known clinically as **apraxia**. In such a syndrome, the patient has difficulty in walking, although there is no voluntary motor paralysis. The grasp reflex attributed to lesions of the premotor area in the older literature is now believed to be due to involvement of the supplementary motor cortex.

Apraxia (Greek *a*, "negative"; *pratto*, "to do"). Inability to perform complex purposeful movements, although muscles are not paralyzed.

Some neuroscientists consider the separation of the motor cortex into primary motor and nonprimary motor areas somewhat artificial. However, closer consideration of this issue justifies this separation on the basis of the threshold of stimuli that elicit motor responses (much lower in the primary motor area) as well as the type of movement elicited from stimulation (simple from the primary motor area versus coordinated, complex movement from the nonprimary areas).

Although neural activity in relation to each of many aspects of motor control seems to be distributed in multiple cortical areas, an individual motor area (primary motor, premotor, supplementary motor) is used preferentially under specific circumstances requiring a certain variety of motor behavior.

In clinical situations, however, all areas are more often than not involved together in disease processes, be it vascular occlusion or hemorrhage leading to stroke or a tumor invading this region of the cortex. In such situations, the clinical manifestations can be classified into those seen immediately after the onset of the pathology and those which follow after a few days or weeks. The former consist of loss of all reflexes and hypotonia of affected muscles. Within hours or days, however, stereotyped movement, particularly in proximal muscles, returns, hypotonia changes to hypertonia and areflexia to hyperactive myotatic reflexes, and a Babinski sign appears. The discrete movements in distal muscles, however, remain impaired. Such a clinical picture is seen often following a stroke involving this region of the cortex.

Cortical Eye Fields

Saccadic Eye Movements

Saccadic movements are fast eye movements with rapid refixation of vision from point to point with no interest in the points in between. Three cortical areas are capable of triggering saccadic eye movements: (1) frontal eye field, (2) supplementary eye field, and (3) parietooccipital eye field. Three other areas, the prefrontal cortex, the inferior parietal lobule, and the hippocampus seem involved in planning, integration, and chronologic ordering of saccadic eye movements.

Saccadic (French *saccader*, "to jerk"). Quick movements of the eyes.

Frontal Eye Field The frontal eye field (Fig. 17-15) is located in the middle frontal gyrus anterior to or in the anterior portion of the motor strip. It corresponds to area 8 of Brodmann and the immediately adjacent cortex. The frontal eye field triggers intentional (voluntary) saccades to visible targets in the visual environment, to remembered target locations, or to the location where it is predicted that the

KEY CONCEPTS

- The premotor area is concerned with voluntary motor function dependent on sensory inputs (visual, auditory, somatosensory).

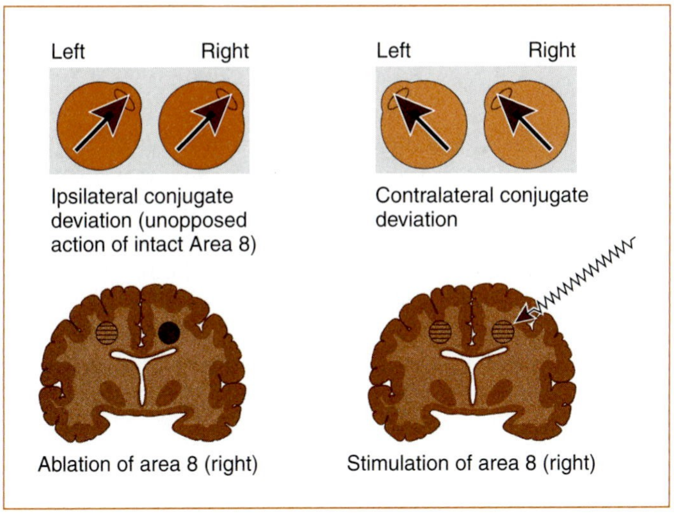

FIGURE 17-16

Schematic diagram of the effects of stimulation and lesions in the frontal eye fields on conjugate eye movements.

target will appear. These movements subserve intentional exploration of the visual environment. The frontal eye field receives multiple cortical inputs, in particular from the parietooccipital eye field, supplementary eye field, and the prefrontal cortex (area 46 of Brodmann). The frontal eye field elicits intentional (voluntary) saccades through connections to nuclei of extraocular muscles in the brain stem. The pathway from the frontal eye field to the nuclei of extraocular movement is not direct but involves multiple brain stem reticular nuclei, including the superior colliculus, the interstitial nucleus of the medial longitudinal fasciculus (RiMLF), and the paramedian pontine reticular formation (PPRF). Irritating lesions in the frontal eye field, as in an epileptic focus, will deviate both eyes in a direction contralateral to the irritative lesion (Fig. 17-16). Conversely, ablation of the frontal eye field will result in deviation of the eyes to the side of ablation (Fig. 17-16) as a result of the unopposed action of the intact frontal eye field. Such a condition is encountered in patients with occlusion of the middle cerebral artery, which supplies the bulk of the lateral surface of the hemisphere, including the frontal eye field. As a result of the arterial occlusion, infarction (death) of cortical tissue will ensue. Such patients manifest paralysis of face and extremities (upper more than lower) contralateral to the side of arterial occlusion and conjugate deviation of the eyes toward the cortical lesion.

In humans, conjugate eye deviations occur more frequently after lesions in the right hemisphere than after lesions in the left hemisphere. There is no explanation for this other than that it may be related to the neglect syndrome associated more frequently with right hemisphere lesions. Conjugate eye deviations also have been

KEY CONCEPTS

- Three cortical areas are capable of triggering saccadic eye movements: the frontal eye field, the supplementary eye field, and the parietooccipital eye field.
- The cortical eye fields project to nuclei of extraocular movement indirectly via the superior colliculus and the brain stem pulse generators for extraocular movement in the pons for horizontal saccades and the midbrain for vertical saccades.
- Stimulation of the frontal eye field produces conjugate deviation of the eyes to the contralateral side.

observed with lesions that spare the frontal eye field but that interrupt the connections between the parietooccipital and frontal eye fields or their subcortical projections.

Supplementary Eye Field An oculomotor area in the frontal cortex, separate from the frontal eye field, was first defined by Schlag in 1985. It is located rostral to the supplementary motor area (MII) on the medial surface of the hemisphere. The supplementary eye field receives multiple cortical inputs, in particular from the prefrontal cortex and the posterior part of the cerebral hemisphere. The supplementary eye field projects to the frontal eye field and to subcortical nuclei involved in eye movements (superior colliculus and reticular formation). The supplementary eye field plays a role in triggering sequences of saccades and in the control of saccades concerned with complex motor programming such as those made during head or body movements (spatiotopic saccades).

Parietooccipital Eye Field The parietooccipital eye field corresponds to areas 39, 40, and 19 of Brodmann. This area triggers reflexive, visually guided saccades. The parietooccipital eye field exerts its influence on saccadic eye movements via its connections to the frontal eye field or directly to the superior colliculus. Patients with lesions in the parietooccipital eye field lose reflexive visually guided saccades but are able to move their eyes in response to command (intentional saccades).

Cortical Areas Preparing Saccades

Three cortical areas not involved directly in triggering of saccades play important roles in planning, integration, and chronologic ordering of saccades. The prefrontal cortex (area 46 of Brodmann) plays a role in planning saccades to remembered target locations. The inferior parietal lobule is involved in visuospatial integration. Bilateral lesions in this area result in **Balint syndrome**, named after the Hungarian neurologist Rudolph Balint (optic ataxia, ocular apraxia, psychic paralysis of visual fixation), a rare syndrome characterized by the inability to direct the eyes to a certain point in the visual field despite retention of intact vision and eye movements. The hippocampus appears to control the temporal working memory required for chronologic order of saccade sequences.

Balint syndrome. Also known as ***Balint-Holmes syndrome, ocular apraxia, optic ataxia.*** A rare syndrome resulting from bilateral parieto-occipital disease and characterized by inability to direct the eyes to a certain point in the visual field despite intact eye movements. Named after Rudolph Balint, a Hungarian neurologist.

KEY CONCEPTS

- Lesions that destroy the frontal eye field result in conjugate deviation of the eyes to the side of the lesion.
- The frontal eye field is concerned with intentional (voluntary) saccades.
- The parietooccipital eye field is concerned with reflexive, visually guided saccades.
- The supplementary eye field plays a role in triggering sequences of saccades and in the control of saccades concerned with complex motor programming.
- Three cortical areas are involved in planning, integration, and chronologic ordering of saccadic eye movement: the prefrontal cortex, the inferior parietal lobule, and the hippocampus.
- The prefrontal cortex plays a role in planning saccades to remembered target locations.
- The inferior parietal lobule is involved in visuospatial integration. Bilateral lesions in this area result in an inability to direct the eyes to a certain point in the visual field (Balint syndrome, optic ataxia).
- The hippocampus controls the temporal working memory required for chronologic ordering of saccadic sequences.

Smooth-Pursuit Eye Movements

Smooth-pursuit movements are slow eye movements initiated by a moving object. Each hemisphere has been shown to mediate smooth-pursuit eye movements to the ipsilateral side. Cortical areas involved in smooth pursuit are not as well delineated as those involved in saccadic eye movements but probably include the posterior parietal cortex or the temporooccipital region. The pathogenesis of pursuit deficits and pathways involved in smooth pursuit eye movements are not completely understood. Specific lesions in the temporooccipitoparietal cortex in humans associated with smooth-pursuit deficits correspond to Brodmann areas 19, 37, and 39. Lesions in the frontal eye field also have been associated with deficits in smooth pursuit. The corticofugal pathways for smooth-pursuit movements remain controversial. Two pathways have been described. The first courses from the temporooccipitoparietal cortex through the posterior limb of the internal capsule to the dorsolateral pontine nucleus in the midpons. The second courses from the frontal eye field to the dorsolateral pontine nucleus and nucleus reticularis tegmenti pontis. Pursuit pathways from the brain stem (dorsolateral pontine nucleus) to the cerebellum are less well defined, although the dorsolateral pontine nucleus and the cerebellar flocculus are important in the monkey. Cerebral hemisphere lesions impair ocular pursuit ipsilaterally or bilaterally, whereas posterior fossa lesions impair ocular pursuit either contralaterally or ipsilaterally. This variability probably reflects involvement of a presumed pursuit pathway that crosses from the pontine nuclei to the cerebellum and then consists of a unilateral projection from the cerebellum to vestibular nuclei.

CORTICAL LANGUAGE AREAS

Language is an arbitrary and abstract way to represent thought processes by means of sentences and to present concepts or ideas by means of words. The neural system for language is made up of many components in several areas of the brain. Most components of the language system are located in the left hemisphere. Hence the left hemisphere is the dominant hemisphere for language. Nearly all right-handers and about two-thirds of left-handers have such dominance. A disorder in language function (**aphasia** or **dysphasia**) includes disturbances in the ability to comprehend (decoding) and/or program (coding) the symbols necessary for communication. The cortical area of the left hemisphere invariably involved in aphasia is a central core surrounding the sylvian fissure, which includes Wernicke's area, the arcuate fasciculus, the angular gyrus, and Broca's area. This perisylvian core area is surrounded by a larger region in which aphasia occurs less frequently.

Traditionally, a distinction has been made between two major cortical language areas: (1) Wernicke's area and (2) Broca's area. The two areas are connected via a long association fiber bundle, the arcuate fasciculus.

Aphasia (Greek *a*, "negative"; *phasis*, "speech"). Impairment of language function, inability either to speak (motor aphasia) or to comprehend (sensory aphasia).

Dysphasia (Greek *dys*, "difficult"; *phasis*, "speech"). Difficulty in the understanding or expression of language.

Sylvius, Francis de la Boe. French anatomist who gave the first description of the lateral sulcus of the cerebral hemisphere.

Wernicke, Karl. German neuropsychiatrist who conceived that sensory aphasia was due to damage to the left temporal lobe.

Wernicke's Area

Wernicke's area, named after the German neurologist **Karl Wernicke**, comprises an extensive region that includes the posterior part of the superior temporal gyrus

KEY CONCEPTS

- Cortical areas for smooth pursuit movement include the posterior parietal cortex or the temporooccipitoparietal region.
- Pathways involved in smooth pursuit are not well defined but probably involve the dorsolateral pontine nucleus and cerebellar flocculus.

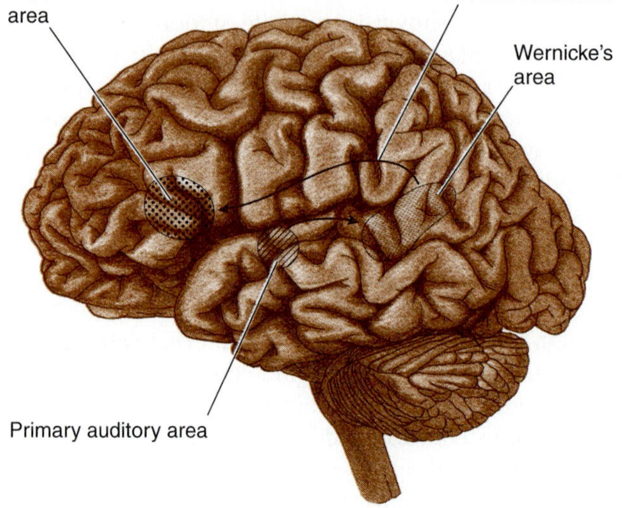

FIGURE 17-17

Schematic diagram showing transmission of auditory symbols from the primary auditory cortex to Wernicke's area for comprehension, and via the arcuate fasciculus to Broca's area of speech.

(Brodmann area 22) and the parietooccipitotemporal junction area including the angular gyrus (Brodmann area 39). The latter component is a recent addition to Wernicke's area not included in the area originally described by Wernicke. The upper surface of area 22, the planum temporale, is distinctly longer on the left side (dominant hemisphere for language) in most people. Wernicke's area is concerned with the comprehension of language. The superior temporal gyrus component of Wernicke's area (area 22) is concerned with comprehension of spoken language, whereas the angular gyrus (area 39) and adjacent regions are concerned with comprehension of written language. Spoken language is perceived in the primary auditory area (Heschl's gyrus, areas 41 and 42) in the superior temporal gyrus and transmitted to the adjacently located Wernicke's area where it is comprehended (Fig. 17-17). Lesions in Wernicke's area are associated with a type of aphasia (sensory, receptive, posterior, fluent) in which patients have difficulty comprehending spoken language.

Broca's Area

Broca, Pierre Paul. French pathologist and anthropologist. Broca localized the cortical motor speech area in the inferior frontal gyrus. He also described the diagonal band of Broca in the anterior perforated substance.

Operculum (Latin *opertum*, "covered"). The frontal, temporal, and parietal opercula cover the insular cortex.

Broca's area, named after the French pathologist **Pierre Paul Broca** who defined this area in 1861, comprises the posterior part of the triangular gyrus (Brodmann area 45) and the adjacent opercular gyrus (Brodmann area 44) in the inferior frontal gyrus of the dominant hemisphere (Fig. 17-18). Broca's area receives inputs from Wernicke's area via the arcuate fasciculus (Fig. 17-17). Within Broca's area, a coordination program for vocalization is formulated. The elements of the program are transmitted to the face, tongue, vocal cords, and pharynx areas of the motor cortex for execution of speech. Broca's area is also connected to the supplementary

KEY CONCEPTS

- Two cortical areas traditionally have been associated with language function: Wernicke's and Broca's areas in the left hemisphere.

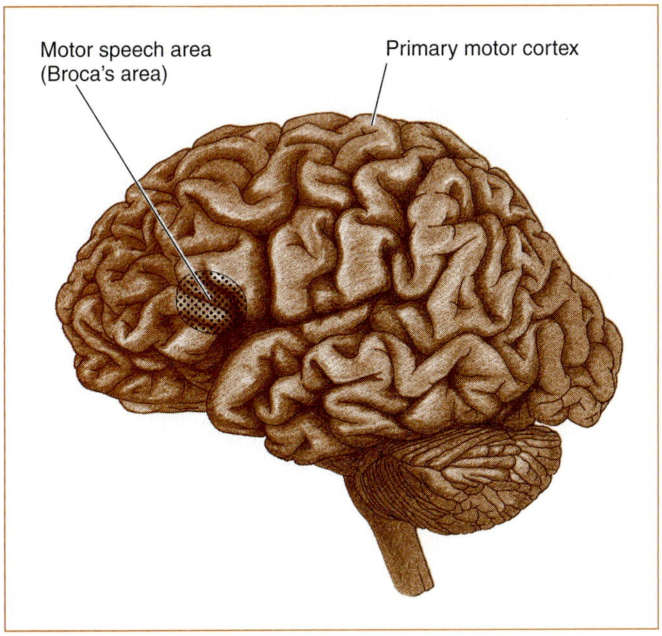

FIGURE 17-18

Schematic diagram of Broca's area of speech.

motor area, which is concerned with the initiation of speech. Lesions is Broca's area are associated with a type of aphasia (motor, anterior, expressive, nonfluent) characterized by inability of the patient to express himself or herself by speech. Such patients are able to comprehend language (intact Wernicke's area).

Electrophysiologic studies and cerebral blood flow studies have confirmed the role of Broca's area in speech expression. Records made from scalp electrodes placed over Broca's area have revealed a slow negative potential of several seconds in duration appearing over Broca's area 1 to 2 s prior to uttering of words. Stimulation of Broca's area in conscious patients may inhibit speech or may result in utterance of vowel sounds. Studies on cerebral blood flow have shown a marked increase in flow in Broca's area during speech.

The Arcuate Fasciculus

The **arcuate** fasciculus (Fig. 17-17) is a long association fiber bundle that links Wernicke's and Broca's areas of speech. Damage to the arcuate fasciculus is associated with impairment of repetition of spoken language.

Arcuate (Latin *arcuatus*, "bow-shaped"). Shaped like an arc. The arcuate fasciculus arches around the sylvian fissure to connect Wernicke's area in the temporal lobe with Broca's area in the frontal lobe.

KEY CONCEPTS

- Wernicke's area in the left temporal lobe and adjacent parietal cortex is concerned with speech comprehension.
- Broca's area in the left inferior frontal gyrus is concerned with the formulation of a coordinated program for vocalization.
- Lesions in Wernicke's area result in an inability to comprehend spoken language (sensory, receptive aphasia).
- Lesions in Broca's area result in an inability to express oneself by language (motor, expressive aphasia).
- Wernicke's and Broca's areas are interconnected by the arcuate fasciculus.

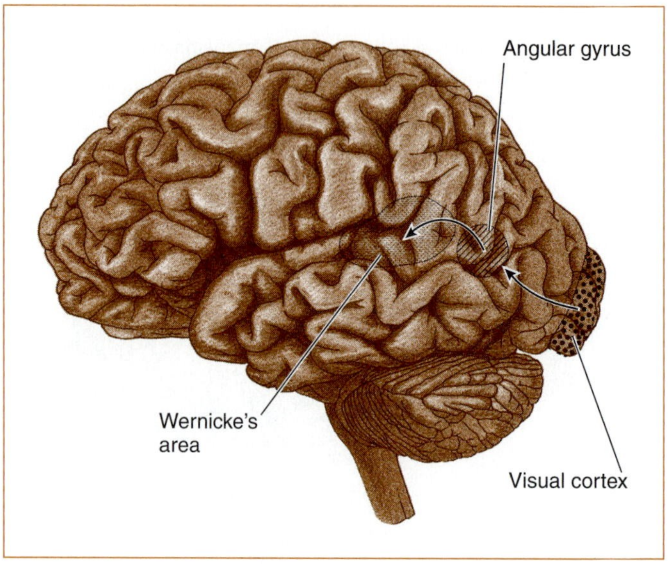

FIGURE 17-19

Schematic diagram showing transmission of output from the primary visual area to the angular gyrus where the auditory form of the word is elicited from Wernicke's area.

Sequence of Cortical Activities during Language Processing

The sequence of the complex cortical activities during the production of language may be summarized as follows: When a word is heard, the output from the primary auditory area (Heschl's gyrus) is conveyed to the adjacent Wernicke's area, where the word is comprehended (Fig. 17-17). If the word is to be spoken, the comprehended pattern is transmitted via the arcuate fasciculus from Wernicke's area to Broca's area in the inferior frontal gyrus (Fig. 17-17). If the word is to be read, representations visualized as words or images are conveyed from the visual cortex (areas 17, 18, and 19) to the angular gyrus (area 39), which in turn arouses the corresponding auditory form of the word in Wernicke's area (Fig. 17-19). From Wernicke's area, the information is relayed via the arcuate fasciculus to Broca's area.

The Right Hemisphere and Language

Although several areas in the left hemisphere are dominant in the reception, programming, and production of language function, corresponding areas in the right hemisphere are metabolically active during speech. These areas are believed to be concerned with melodic function of speech **(prosody)**. Lesions in such areas of the right hemisphere render speech amelodic (aprosodic). Lesions in area 44 on the right side, for example, result in a dull monotonic speech. Lesions in area 22 on the right side, on the other hand, may lead to inability of the patient to detect inflection of speech. Such patients may be unable to differentiate whether a particular remark is intended as a statement of fact or as a question.

Prosody (Greek *prosodos*, "a solemn procession"). The variation in stress, pitch, and rhythm of speech by which different shades of meaning are conveyed.

Aprosodia (Greek *a*, "negative"; *prosodos*, "a solemn procession"). The variation in stress, pitch, and rhythm of speech by which different shades of meaning are conveyed; the affective component of language.

KEY CONCEPTS

- The right hemisphere is concerned with melodic function (prosody) of speech.
- Lesions in the right hemisphere result in amelodic monotonous (aprosodic) speech.

CORTICAL LOCALIZATION OF MUSIC

With the allocation of specific functions to each hemisphere, the question has arisen as to which hemisphere is specialized for music. In this context, one should separate musical perception from musical execution by the naive, casual listener and the music professional. Whereas a naive listener perceives music in its overall melodic contour, the professional perceives music as a relation between musical elements and symbols (language). With this type of analysis, it is conceivable that the naive listener perceives music in the right hemisphere, whereas the professional perceives music in the left hemisphere. Musical execution (singing), on the other hand, seems to be a function of the right hemisphere irrespective of musical knowledge and training.

OTHER CORTICAL AREAS

In addition to the previously discussed cortical areas, the cerebral cortex contains other functionally important areas. These include the prefrontal cortex and the major association cortex.

Prefrontal Cortex

The *prefrontal cortex* (Fig. 17-20) refers to the area of the cortex comprising the pole of the frontal lobe. It corresponds to areas 9, 10, and 11 of Brodmann. Motor responses are as a rule not elicited by stimulation of this area of the frontal lobe. The prefrontal cortex is well developed only in primates and especially so in humans. It is believed to play a role in affective behavior and judgment. Clues about the functions of the prefrontal cortex have been gained by studying patients with frontal lobe damage, such as Phineas Gage, the New England railroad worker who was struck by a thick iron bar that penetrated his prefrontal cortex. Miraculously, he survived but with a striking change in his personality. Whereas prior to the injury he was an efficient and capable supervisor, following the accident he was unfit to perform such work. He became fitful and engaged in profanity. Thus lesions in the prefrontal cortex result in inappropriate judgmental behavior and emotional lability. More dramatic effects are seen after bilateral lesions. Such patients usually neglect their appearance, laugh or cry inappropriately, and have no appreciation of norms of social behavior and conduct. They are uninhibited and highly distractable. Apathy and lack of initiative are more pronounced in lesions of the dorsolateral parts of the frontal lobe, whereas orbitofrontal lesions are more apt to produce changes in mood and affect, including impulsive and inappropriate behavior. A characteristic symptom in humans with prefrontal lobe lesions is perseveration, the inability to alter responses when the stimulus changes. Such patients continue to make the same response even though it is no longer adequate. Surgical ablation of the prefrontal cortex (prefrontal lobotomy) was resorted to in the past to treat patients with mental disorders such as schizophrenia and intractable pain. In the latter group,

KEY CONCEPTS

- Music appreciation is perceived in different hemispheres by the naive listener and the music professional.
- Musical execution (singing) is a function of the right hemisphere.
- The prefrontal cortex comprises the frontal pole (areas 9, 10, 11 of Brodmann).
- The prefrontal cortex plays a role in affective behavior and judgment.

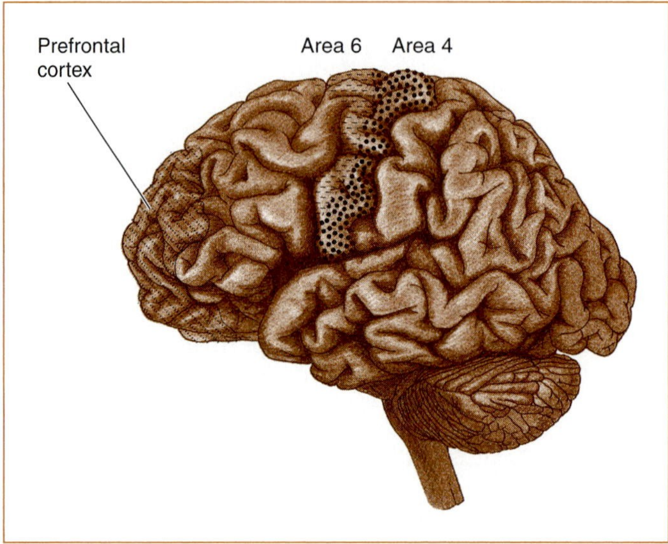
Prefrontal cortex
Area 6
Area 4

FIGURE 17-20

Schematic diagram of the prefrontal cortex.

Agraphia (Greek *a*, "negative"; *graphein*, "to write"). Inability to express thoughts in writing. The first modern descriptions were those of Jean Pitres in 1884 and Dejerine in 1891.

Agnosia (Greek *a*, "negative"; *gnosis*, "knowledge"). Inability to recognize and interpret sensory information.

Acalculia (Greek *a*, "negative"; Latin *calculare*, "to reckon"). Difficulty in calculating. Usually associated with inability to copy (acopia). The condition was described and named by Henschen in 1919.

Gerstmann syndrome. A clinical syndrome characterized by right-left disorientation, acalculia, agraphia, and finger agnosia due to a lesion in the left angular gyrus. Josef Gerstmann, Austrian neuropsychiatrist, developed the concept of a body image with visual, tactile, and somesthetic components in 1924 and considered cortical representation for these in the angular gyrus. The syndrome is also known as *angular gyrus syndrome* and the *Badal-Gerstmann syndrome.* Jules Badal's description of the syndrome in 1888 was less complete.

Syndrome (Greek *syndromos*, "a running together"). A group of symptoms and signs that characterize a disease.

the effect of the operation was not to relieve the sensation of pain but rather to alter the affective reaction (suffering) of the patient to pain. Such patients continue to feel pain but become indifferent to it. The ablation of the prefrontal area in patients with mental illness has been replaced largely by administration of psychopharmacologic drugs. Through its interconnections with association cortices of other lobes and with the hypothalamus, medial thalamus, and amygdala, the prefrontal cortex receives information about all sensory modalities as well as about motivational and emotional states.

Major Association Cortex

The *major association cortex* (Fig. 17-21) refers to the supramarginal and angular gyri in the inferior parietal lobule. It corresponds to areas 39 and 40 of Brodmann. The major association cortex is connected with all the sensory cortical areas and thus functions in higher-order and complex multisensory perception. Its relation to the speech areas in the temporal and frontal lobes gives it an important role in communication skills. Patients with lesions in the major association cortex of the dominant hemisphere present a conglomerate of manifestations that include receptive and expressive aphasia, inability to write **(agraphia)**, inability to synthesize, correlate, and recognize multisensory perceptions **(agnosia)**, left-right confusion, difficulty in recognizing the different fingers (finger agnosia), and inability to calculate **(acalculia)**. These symptoms and signs are grouped together under the term **Gerstmann's syndrome**.

Involvement of the major association cortex in the nondominant hemisphere is usually manifested by disturbances in drawing (constructional apraxia) and in the awareness of body image. Such patients have difficulty in drawing a square or circle

KEY CONCEPTS

- The major association cortex is interconnected with all the sensory cortical areas and thus functions in higher-order, complex, multisensory perception.

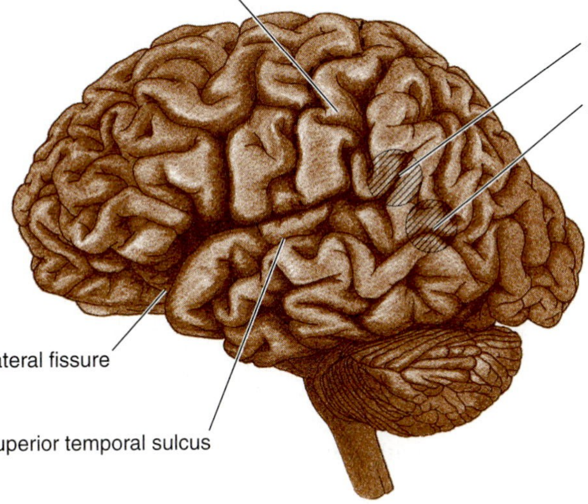
Primary somesthetic cortex
MAJOR ASSOCIATION CORTEX
Supramarginal gyrus
Angular gyrus
Lateral fissure
Superior temporal sulcus

FIGURE 17-21

Schematic diagram of the major association cortex.

or copying a complex figure. They often are unaware of a body part and thus neglect to shave one-half the face or dress one-half the body.

CORTICAL ELECTROPHYSIOLOGY

Evoked Potentials

Evoked potentials represent the electrical responses recorded from a population of neurons in a particular cortical area following stimulation of the input to that area. The most studied of the evoked potentials is the primary response recorded from the cortical surface and elicited by a single shock to a major thalamocortical pathway. This response is characterized by a diphasic, positive-negative wave and is generated primarily by synaptic currents in cortical neurons.

Evoked potentials elicited by a volley of impulses in thalamocortical pathways are of two varieties, recruiting responses and augmenting responses.

Recruiting responses are recorded following 6- to 12-cps (cycles per second) stimulation of a nonspecific thalamocortical pathway (e.g., from intralaminar nuclei). They are characterized by a long latency (multisynaptic pathway), a predominantly surface negative response that increases in amplitude to a maximum by the fourth to the sixth stimulus of a repetitive train. This is followed by a decrease in amplitude (waxing and waning). Such a response has a diffuse cortical distribution. This pattern of response is generally attributed to an oscillator network at cortical as well as thalamic levels in which cortical and thalamic elements provide both positive and negative feedback.

KEY CONCEPTS

- Lesions in the major association cortex of the dominant hemisphere result in Gerstmann's syndrome.

Augmenting responses are recorded following low-frequency (6- to 12-cps) stimulation of a specific thalamocortical pathway (e.g., from ventrolateral thalamic nucleus). They are characterized by a short latency (monosynaptic pathway), a diphasic, positive-negative configuration that increases in amplitude and latency during the initial four to six stimuli of the train. The response to subsequent stimuli remains augmented but waxes and wanes in amplitude. This type of response is localized in the primary cortical area to which the stimulated specific thalamocortical pathway projects.

Somatosensory, Visual, and Auditory Evoked Responses

Recording of cortical evoked potentials following somatosensory (skin), visual (flashes or patterns of light), and auditory (sound) stimuli has been used to study pathology along each of these pathways in humans. The determination of latency and amplitude of the evoked potential frequently can aid in localizing the site of pathology in the respective pathway.

ELECTROENCEPHALOGRAPHY

Electroencephalography (Fig. 17-22) is the recording of spontaneous cortical activity from the surface of the scalp. This procedure is used very commonly in the investigation of diseases of the brain. Its usefulness is mainly in the diagnoses of epilepsy and localized (focal) brain pathology (e.g., brain tumors). In recent years and with the advent of the concept of brain death, the electroencephalogram (EEG) has been used to confirm a state of electrical brain silence (brain death). In such a condition, electroencephalographic tracings will show no evidence of cortical potentials (flat EEG).

The spontaneous rhythmic activity of the cortex is classified into four types:

1. Alpha rhythm with a range of frequency from 8 to 13 cps. This type is most developed over the posterior part of the hemisphere.
2. Beta rhythm with a range of frequency faster than 13 cps (17 to 30 cps). This activity can be seen over wide regions of the cortex and is especially apparent in records from patients receiving sedative drugs.
3. Theta rhythm with a range of frequency from 3 to 7 cps.
4. Delta rhythm with a range of frequency from 0.5 to 3 cps.

The EEG pattern varies in different age groups. The EEG is dominated by slow activity (theta and delta) in childhood. The alpha rhythm increases in amount with the advent of puberty. In the adult, delta activity and excessive theta activity usually denote cerebral abnormality.

The EEG of unconscious patients is dominated by generalized slow frequencies. The EEG in epileptic patients is characterized by the presence of spike potentials. Two EEG patterns have been associated with sleep. The first is a slow pattern

KEY CONCEPTS

- Cortical evoked potentials elicited after thalamic stimulation are of two types: recruiting responses and augmenting responses.
- Electroencephalography (EEG) records spontaneous cortical activity by means of scalp electrodes.
- Four types of spontaneous rhythmic activity are recorded by EEG: alpha, beta, theta, and delta.

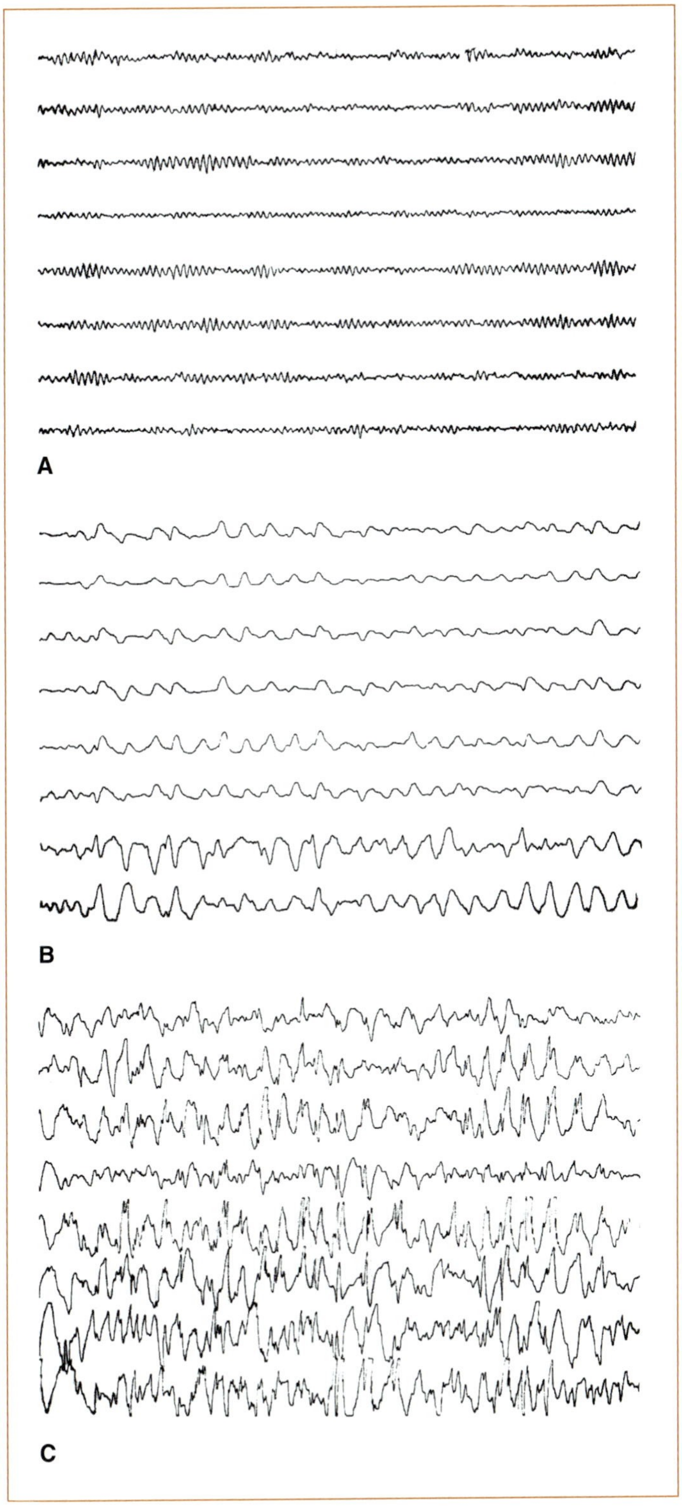

FIGURE 17-22

Electroencephalograms showing the normal alpha pattern (*A*), slow delta pattern (*B*), and spike potentials (*C*).

(delta and theta) associated with the early phase of sleep. The second is a fast pattern (beta) associated with a later and deeper stage of sleep. This second pattern is associated with rapid eye movements (REM) and dreaming; hence this stage of sleep has been called *REM sleep* or *D-sleep* (dreaming).

BLOOD SUPPLY

Arterial Supply

The blood supply to the cerebral cortex is provided by the anterior and middle cerebral arteries (branches of the internal carotid artery) and the posterior cerebral artery (branch of the basilar artery). The *anterior cerebral artery* runs through the interhemispheric fissure, giving off five major branches: orbitofrontal, frontopolar, pericallosal, callosomarginal, and paracentral. These branches supply the medial surface of the frontal and parietal lobes as far back as the parieto-occipital fissure (Fig. 17-23). All branches cross the convexity of the frontal and parietal lobes to supply a strip of marginal cortex on the lateral surface of the hemisphere. Occlusion of the anterior cerebral artery results in paralysis and sensory deficits in the contralateral leg due to interruption of blood supply to the leg area in the medial surface of the motor and sensory cortices.

The *middle cerebral artery* is a continuation or the main branch of the internal carotid artery. It courses within the lateral (sylvian) fissure and divides into a number of branches (frontal, rolandic, temporal, parietal) that supply most of the lateral surface of the hemisphere (Fig. 17-24).

The *posterior cerebral artery* constitutes the terminal branch of the basilar artery. Several branches (temporal, occipital, parietooccipital) supply the medial surfaces of the occipital lobe, temporal lobe, and caudal parietal lobe.

Rolando, Luigi. Italian anatomist. The central sulcus of the cerebral hemisphere is named after him and so is the substantia gelatinosa of the spinal cord.

Venous Drainage

Three groups of cerebral veins drain the lateral and inferior surfaces of the cerebral hemisphere: superior, middle, and inferior (Fig. 17-25). The *superior cerebral group* drains the dorsolateral and dorsomedial surfaces of the hemisphere and opens into the superior sagittal sinus. Conventionally, the most prominent of these veins in the central sulcus is called the *superior anastomotic vein of Trolard*, which connects the superior and middle groups of veins.

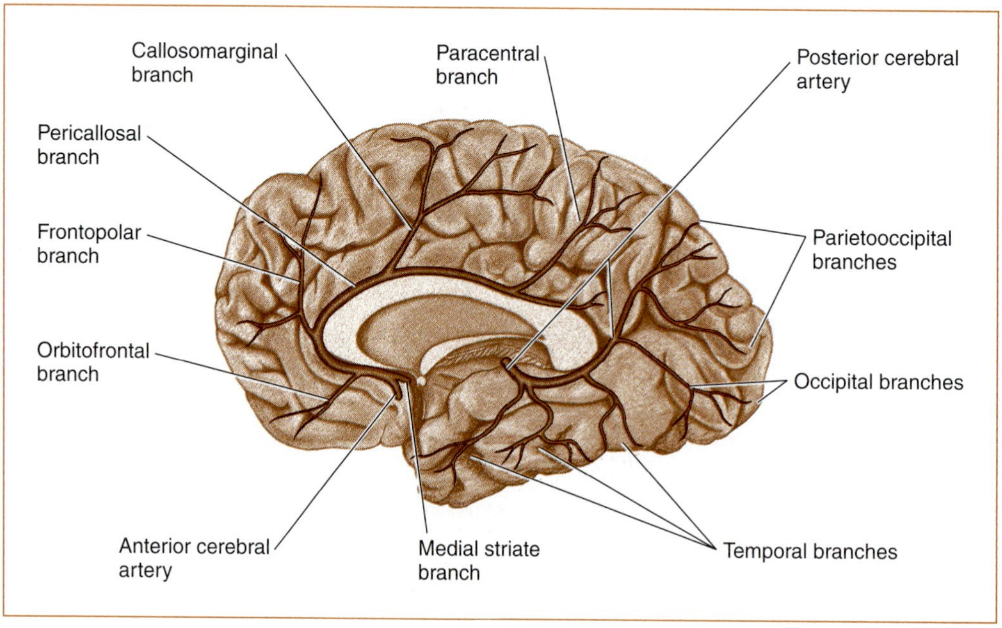

FIGURE 17-23

Schematic diagram of the major branches of the anterior cerebral and posterior cerebral arteries and the areas they supply.

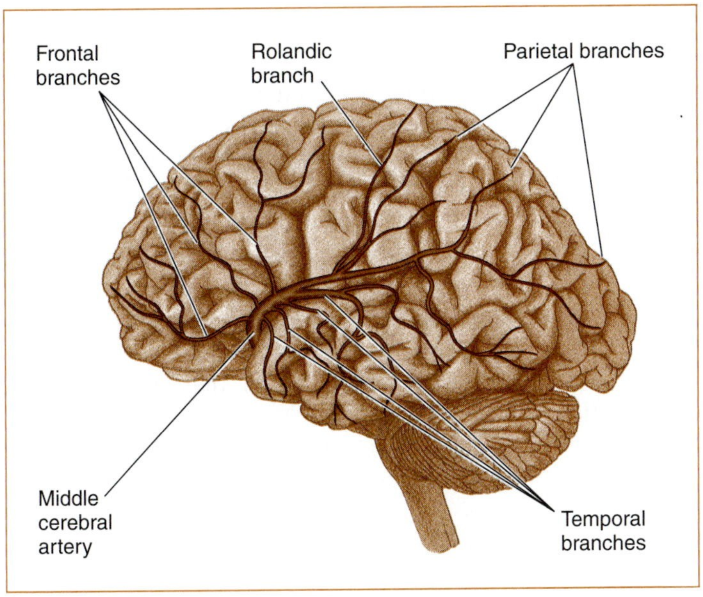

FIGURE 17-24

Schematic diagram of the major branches of the middle cerebral artery and the areas they supply.

The *middle cerebral group* runs along the sylvian fissure, drains the inferolateral surface of the hemisphere, and opens into the cavernous sinus. The *inferior cerebral group* drains the inferior surface of the hemisphere and opens into the cavernous and transverse sinuses. The anastomic vein of Labbé interconnects the middle and inferior groups of cerebral veins.

The medial surface of the hemisphere is drained by a number of veins that open into the superior and inferior sagittal sinuses, as well as into the basal vein and the great cerebral vein of Galen.

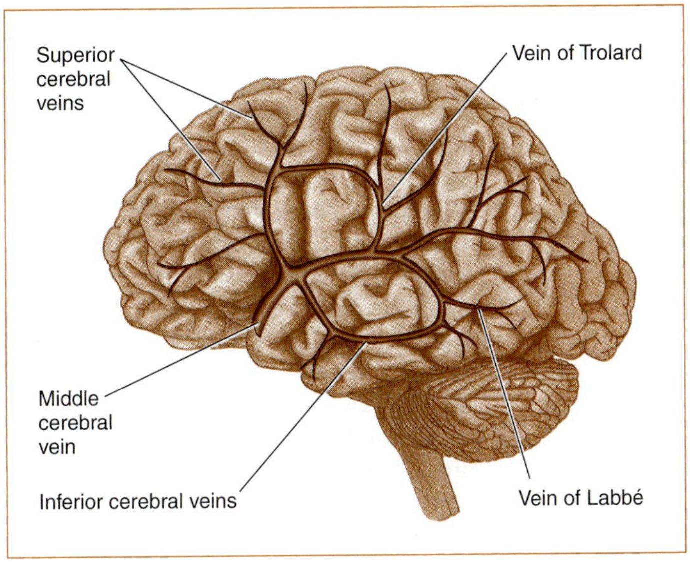

FIGURE 17-25

Schematic diagram of the superficial system of venous drainage of the brain.

SUGGESTED READINGS

Brandt Th, et al: Vestibular cortex lesions affect the perception of verticality. *Ann Neurol* 1994; 35:403–412.

Brinkman C, Porter R: Supplementary motor area in the monkey: Activity of neurons during performance of a learned motor task. *J Neurophysiols* 1979; 42:681–709.

Brodal P: The corticopontine projection in the rhesus monkey: Origin and principles of organization. *Brain* 1978; 101:251–283.

Brouwer B, Ashby P: Altered corticospinal projections to lower limb motoneurons in subjects with cerebral palsy. *Brain* 1991; 114:1395–1407.

Caselli RJ: Ventrolateral and dorsomedial somatosensory association cortex damage produces distinct somesthetic syndromes in humans. *Neurology* 1993; 43:762–771.

Cherubini E, et al: Caudate neuronal responses evoked by cortical stimulation: Contribution of an indirect corticothalamic pathway. *Brain Res* 1979; 173: 331–336.

Damasio A, et al: Central achromatosia: Behavioral, anatomic and physiologic aspects. *Neurology* 1980; 30:1064–1071.

Damasio H, et al: The return of Phineas Gage: Clues about the brain from the skull of a famous patient. *Science* 1994; 264:1102–1105.

Divac I, et al: Vertical ascending connections in the isocortex. *Anat Embryol* 1987; 175:443–455.

Eccles JC: The modular operation of the cerebral neocortex considered as the material basis of mental events. *Neuroscience* 1981; 6:1839–1856.

Fallon JH, Ziegler BTS: The crossed cortico-caudate projection in the rhesus monkey. *Neurosci Lett* 1979; 15:29–32.

Foote SL: Extrathalamic modulation of cortical function. *Ann Rev Neurosci* 1987; 10:67–95.

Freund H-J, Hummelsheim H: Lesions of premotor cortex in man. *Brain* 1985; 108:697–733.

Gallese V, et al: Action recognition in the premotor cortex. *Brain* 1996; 119:593–609.

Gaymard B, et al: Role of the left and right supplementary motor areas in memory-guided saccade sequences. *Ann Neurol* 1993; 34:404–406.

Godoy J, et al: Versive eye movements elicited by cortical stimulation of the human brain. *Neurology* 1990; 40:296–299.

Gorman DG, Unützer J: Brodmann's "missing" numbers. *Neurology* 1993; 43:226–227.

Green JR: The beginning of cerebral localization and neurological surgery. *BNI Quart* 1985; 1:12–28.

Heffner HE: Ferrier and the study of auditory cortex. *Arch Neurol* 1987; 44:218–221.

Hocherman S, Yirmiya R: Neuronal activity in the medial geniculate nucleus and in the auditory cortex of the rhesus monkey reflects signal anticipation. *Brain* 1990; 113:1707–1720.

Iwatsubo T, et al: Corticofugal projections to the motor nuclei of the brain stem and spinal cord in humans. *Neurology* 1990; 40:309–312.

Jinnai K, Matsuda Y: Neurons of the motor cortex projecting commonly on the caudate nucleus and the lower brain stem in the cat. *Neurosci Lett* 1979; 13:121–126.

Karbe H, et al: Planum temporale and Brodmann's area 22: Magnetic resonance imaging and high resolution positron emission tomography demonstrate functional left-right asymmetry. *Arch Neurol* 1995; 52:869–874.

Leichnetz GR, et al: The prefrontal corticotectal projection in the monkey: An anterograde and retrograde horseradish peroxidase study. *Neuroscience* 1981; 6:1023–1041.

Leigh RJ: Human vestibular cortex. *Ann Neurol* 1994; 35:383–384.

Lekwuwa GU, Barnes GR: Cerebral control of eye movements: I. The relationship between cerebral lesion sites and smooth pursuit deficits. *Brain* 1996; 119:473–490.

Liegeois-Chauvel C, et al: Localization of the primary auditory area in man. *Brain* 1994; 114:139–153.

Lüders H, et al: The second sensory area in humans: Evoked potential and electrical stimulation studies. *Ann Neurol* 1985; 17:177–184.

Markowitsch HJ, et al: Cortical afferents to the prefrontal cortex of the cat: A study with the horseradish peroxidase technique. *Neurosci Lett* 1979; 11: 115–120.

Morrow MJ, Sharpe JA: Cerebral hemispheric localization of smooth pursuit asymmetry. *Neurology* 1990; 40:284–292.

Meyer BU, et al: Inhibitory and excitatory interhemispheric transfers between motor cortical areas in normal humans and patients with abnormalities of the corpus callosum. *Brain* 1995; 118:429–440.

Orgogozo JM, Larsen B: Activation of supplementary motor area during voluntary movements in man suggests it works as a supramotor area. *Science* 1979; 206:847–850.

Pierrot-Deseilligny C, Gaymard B: Eye movement disorders and ocular motor organization. *Curr Opin Neurol Neurosurg* 1990; 3:796–801.

Pierrot-Deseilligny C, et al: Cortical control of saccades. *Ann Neurol* 1995; 37:557–567.

Roland PE, et al: Different cortical areas in man in

organization of voluntary movement in extrapersonal space. *J Neurophysiol* 1980; 43:137–150.

Romansky KV, et al: Corticosubthalamic projection in the cat: An electron microscopic study. *Brain Res* 1979; 163:319–322.

Rumeau C, et al: Location of hand function in the sensorimotor cortex: MR and functional correlation. *AJNR* 1994; 15:567–572.

Schmahmann JD, Leifer D: Parietal pseudothalamic pain syndrome: Clinical features and anatomic correlates. *Arch Neurol* 1992; 49:1032–1037.

Shatz CJ: Dividing up the neocortex. *Science* 1992; 258:237–238.

Sutherling WW, et al: Cortical sensory representation of the human hand: Size of finger regions and nonoverlapping digit somatotopy. *Neurology* 1992; 42:1020–1028.

Tanji J, Kurata K: Changing concepts of motor areas of the cerebral cortex. *Brain Dev* 1989; 11:374–377.

Tanji J: The supplementary motor area in the cerebral cortex. *Neurosci Res* 1994; 19:251–268.

Tijssen CC, et al: Conjugate eye deviation: Side, site, and size of hemispheric lesion. *Neurology* 1991; 41:846–850.

Tusa RJ, Ungerleider LG: The inferior longitudinal fasciculus: A reexamination in humans and monkeys. *Ann Neurol* 1985; 18:583–591.

Urasaki E, et al: Cortical tongue area studied by chronically implanted subdural electrodes: With special reference to parietal motor and frontal sensory responses. *Brain* 1994; 117:117–132.

Van Hoesen GW, et al: Widespread corticostriate projections from temporal cortex of the rhesus monkey. *J Comp Neurol* 1981; 199:205–219.

Verfaellie M, Heilman KM: Response preparation and response inhibition after lesions of the medial frontal lobe. *Arch Neurol* 1987; 44:1265–1271.

Wise SP: The primate premotor cortex: Past, present, and preparatory. *Ann Rev Neurosci* 1985; 8:1–19.

Yeterian EH, Van Hoesen GW: Cortico-striate projections in the rhesus monkey: The organization of certain cortico-caudate connections. *Brain Res* 1978; 139:43–63.

Zeki S, Lamb M: The neurology of kinetic art. *Brain* 1994; 117:607–636.

CHAPTER 18

CEREBRAL CORTEX: CLINICAL CORRELATES

EPILEPTIC SEIZURES

Epilepsy is a common clinical condition characterized by recurrent paroxysmal attacks of motor, sensory, autonomic, or psychic symptoms and signs depending on the area of the brain involved. Epileptic seizures are triggered by synchronized discharges of a group of neurons in the cerebral cortex as a result of developmental abnormality, infection, trauma, tumor, metabolic derangement, or stroke. Epileptic

KEY CONCEPTS

- Epileptic seizures are manifestations of synchronized discharges of groups of neurons.

seizures may be focal or generalized. When generalized, they are usually associated with loss of consciousness. The most common generalized seizure type is the tonic-clonic seizure type known as *grand mal seizure.* Focal seizures are manifestations of the function of the cortical area from which epileptic discharges emanate. Epileptic discharges in the region of the central sulcus may give rise to motor and sensory symptoms. Spreading of the epileptic discharge along the motor or sensory homunculus produces the so-called **Jacksonian seizures** or Jacksonian march. In such a patient, a focal motor seizure may start by shaking of the side of the face contralateral to the cortical lesion in the precentral gyrus and spread to involve the thumb, hand, arm, and leg in this order in a pattern consistent with the location of these body parts in the motor homunculus. A similar pattern of sensory march is associated with lesions in the postcentral gyrus. An epileptic discharge in the frontal eye field produces attacks consisting of contralateral turning of eyes and head (**adversive seizures**). Occipital discharges are associated with visual hallucinations. Discharges in the primary visual cortex produce contralateral flashes of light, whereas discharges in the association visual cortex produce well-formed images. Epileptic discharges from the uncus and adjacent regions of the temporal lobe (**uncinate** fits) produce a combination of complex motor and autonomic symptoms (psychomotor seizures). The epileptic attack in such patients consists of a dreamy state, olfactory hallucinations (usually of "bad" odors), gustatory hallucinations, oral movements of chewing, swallowing, or smacking of lips, visual hallucinations (**déjà vu** experiences), and possibly aggressive behavior. Complex acts and movements such as walking and fastening or unfastening buttons may occur.

Jacksonian seizures. The spread of tonic-clonic seizure activity through contiguous body parts on one side of the body secondary to excitation of adjacent cortical areas within the motor or sensory homunculus. Also known as *Jacksonian march* and *Bravais-Jackson epilepsy*. L. Bravais described this phenomenon in his graduation thesis in 1827 from the University of Paris but did not analyze the etiology, which John Hughlings Jackson did.

Adversive seizures. A variety of seizures in which there is deviation of eyes and/or head to one side secondary to a stimulating lesion in the contralateral frontal eye field region.

Uncinate (Latin *uncinus*, "hook-shaped"). Pertaining to the uncus of the temporal lobe. Uncinate seizures are temporal lobe seizures in which olfactory and gustatory hallucinations occur as part of the seizure. The name *uncinate fits* was applied by Jackson in 1899.

Déjà vu (French "already seen"). An illusion in which a new situation is incorrectly viewed as a repetition of a previous situation. Usually an aura of a temporal lobe seizure.

HEMISPHERE SPECIALIZATION

The concept of cerebral dominance has undergone significant modification in recent years, primarily because of studies on patients with unilateral brain damage. The older concept, introduced by Gustav Dax and Paul Broca in 1865, which assigned to the left hemisphere a dominant role in higher cerebral function, with the right hemisphere being subordinate to the dominant hemisphere, has been replaced by a new concept of hemisphere specialization that implies that each hemisphere is in some way dominant for the execution of specific tasks. According to this concept, the left hemisphere is dominant or specialized for comprehension and expression of language, arithmetic, and analytic functions, whereas the right hemisphere is specialized for complex nonverbal perceptual tasks and for some aspects of visual and spatial perception. Language is localized to the left hemisphere in 99 percent

KEY CONCEPTS

- Focal seizures are manifestations of the function(s) of the cortical area from which epileptic discharges emanate.
- Jacksonian march is a focal motor or sensory seizure in which epileptic discharges emanate from the motor or sensory homunculi.
- Adversive seizures are focal motor seizures in which epileptic discharges emanate from the frontal eye field region.
- Uncinate fits are focal seizures in which epileptic discharges emanate from the uncus and adjacent areas of the temporal lobe.
- The left hemisphere is specialized or dominant for comprehension and expression of language, arithmetic, and analytic functions.
- The right hemisphere is specialized or dominant for complex nonverbal perceptual tasks and some aspects of visual and spatial perception.

of right-handed people and two-thirds of left-handers. Thus lesions of the left hemisphere are associated with disorders of language (**aphasia** or **dysphasia**), whereas lesions of the right hemisphere are associated with impairment of visuospatial and visuoconstructive skills. Patients with right hemisphere lesions are more likely to show such manifestations as constructional **apraxia** (inability to construct or to draw figures and shapes), dressing apraxia, denial of the left side of the body (denial that their left side is part of their body), and hemineglect (visual and spatial neglect of the left side of their space, including their own body parts). **Idiographic** (pictographic) language (Japanese Kanji) may be processed by the right hemisphere because of its pictorial features.

Aphasia (dysphasia) (Greek *a*, "negative"; *phasis*, "speech"). Language impairment following cortical lesion in the left hemisphere. Either inability to speak or to comprehend language or both.

Dysphasia (Greek *dys*, "difficult"; *phasis*, "speech"). Disturbance in communication involving language.

Apraxia (Greek *a*, "negative"; *praxis*, "action"). Inability to carry out learned skilled movements on command despite intact motor and sensory systems and good comprehension.

Idiographic language. Pictographic language such as Japanese Kanji.

APHASIA

A disorder in language function (*aphasia* or *dysphasia*) includes disturbances in the ability to comprehend (decoding) and/or program (coding) the symbols necessary for communication. Aphasia is encountered most frequently in cortical lesions in the left hemisphere, although it may occur in subcortical lesions. The cortical area of the left hemisphere invariably involved in aphasia is a central core surrounding the sylvian fissure. The perisylvian core area is surrounded by a larger region in which aphasia occurs less frequently.

The brain processes language by means of three interacting neural processes: (1) concept processing and formation, (2) word-form implementation (generation of words and sentences), and (3) a mediation process that links or mediates between the other two processes. The mediation process selects the correct words to express a particular concept and directs the generation of sentence structures that express relations among concepts. Neural structures that are concerned with concept formation are distributed across both hemispheres in many sensory and motor areas. The word-form implementation and mediation neural structures are located in the left hemisphere. Word-form implementation neural structures are in the perisylvian region of the left hemisphere, whereas mediation neural structures are in the inferior frontal gyrus for verb mediation and the middle temporal and inferior parietal regions for noun mediation.

The sequence of complex cortical activities during the production of language may be simplified as follows: When a word is heard, the output from the primary auditory area (Heschl's gyrus) is conveyed to an adjacent cortical area (Wernicke's area), where the speech sounds are processed into word form and the word is comprehended (see Fig. 17-17). If the word is to be spoken, the comprehended pattern is transmitted via the arcuate fasciculus from Wernicke's area to Broca's area of speech in the inferior frontal gyrus (see Fig. 17-17). If the word is to be read, the output from the primary visual area in the occipital cortex is transmitted to the angular gyrus, which in turn arouses the corresponding auditory form of the word in Wernicke's area (see Fig. 17-19).

For didactic purposes, aphasia is classified into Broca's, Wernicke's, conduction, transcortical, anomic, and global. The different varieties of aphasia can be classified into those with impaired repetition (Broca's, Wernicke's, conduction, and global

KEY CONCEPTS

- Aphasia is a disorder in comprehending or programming the symbols necessary for language communication.
- The brain processes language by means of three interacting neural systems: (1) concepts formation, (2) word-form implementation, and (3) mediation between the two other systems.

TABLE 18-1

Aphasias

Type	Repetition	Fluency	Auditory Comprehension	Localization
Broca's	−	−	+	Lower posterior frontal
Wernicke's	−	+	−	Posterior and superior temporal
Conduction	−	+	+	Usually supramarginal gyrus; often extends to insula and primary auditory cortex
Global	−	−	−	Massive perisylvian or separate Broca's and Wernicke's areas
Transcortical Motor	+	−	+	Anterior or superior to Broca's area; may involve part of Broca's area
Sensory	+	+	−	Surrounding Wernicke's area
Mixed	+	−	−	Border zone, watershed area of middle and anterior cerebral arteries
Anomic	+	+	+	Variable sequela of any type of aphasia

NOTE: +, intact; −, impaired.

aphasias) and those in which repetition is preserved (transcortical and anomic aphasias) (Table 18-1).

Broca's aphasia is also known as *nonfluent, anterior, motor,* or *expressive aphasia.* This type of aphasia is characterized by a decreased and labored language output

KEY CONCEPTS

- Aphasias are classified into two major categories based on whether repetition is intact or not.
- Aphasias with intact repetition include transcortical and anomic aphasias.
- Aphasias with impaired repetition include Broca's, Wernicke's, conduction, and global aphasias.

of 10 words or less per minute, during which the patient utilizes facial grimaces, body posturing, deep breaths, and hand gestures to aid output; characteristically, small grammatical words and the endings of nouns and verbs are omitted, resulting in telegraphic speech. The speech output is thus unmelodic and dysrhythmic (**dysprosody**). Despite the preceding limitations in verbal output, the speech often conveys considerable information. These patients are unable to repeat what has been said to them. Although Broca's aphasia is usually attributed to a lesion in Broca's area of the frontal lobe, recent correlations of aphasic speech with lesions seen on computed tomography (CT scan) have shown that the lesion is frequently larger than Broca's area and involves the insula and the insulolenticular area. Since the temporal lobe is intact in these patients, auditory comprehension is usually intact.

Dysprosody (Greek *dys*, "difficult"; *prosodos*, "a solemn procession"). Disturbance in stress, pitch, and rhythm of speech. A feature of all types of aphasia, but especially of Broca's aphasia.

Broca's aphasia occurs often as a result of stroke (infarcts) most commonly affecting the middle cerebral artery territory. Such infarcts often involve the motor cortex; thus patients with Broca's aphasia are often hemiplegic with the arm (middle cerebral artery territory) more affected than the leg (anterior cerebral artery territory). Broca's aphasia is named after Paul Broca, the French anthropologist-physician who studied patient Leborgne (nicknamed "Tan" because the only word he could utter was *tan*) with aphasia and localized the lesion to the posterior part of the left inferior frontal convolutions. Pierre Marie, in 1906, examined Leborgne's brain and found that the lesion was much more extensive.

Wernicke's aphasia is also known as *fluent, posterior, sensory,* or *receptive aphasia.* In contrast to Broca's aphasia, the quantity of output in this type ranges from low normal to supernormal, with an output in most patients of 100 to 150 words per minute. Speech is produced with little or no effort, articulation and phrase length are normal, and the output is melodic. Pauses to search for a meaningful word are frequent, and substitution without language (**paraphasia**) is common; this may be substitution of a syllable (literal paraphasia) (*wellow* for *yellow*), phonemic substitution of a word (*kench* for *wrench*) (verbal paraphasia), semantic substitution (*knife* for *fork*), or substitution of a meaningless nonsense word (**neologism**). If a word is not readily available, the patient may attempt to describe it, and the description may necessitate yet another description, resulting in a meaningless output (**circumlocution**). Paraphasias also may occur in Broca's aphasia, but these are articulatory errors, in contrast to those in Wernicke's aphasia, which are true substitutions. Despite the fluent nature of speech output in Wernicke's aphasia, little information is conveyed (empty speech). As in Broca's aphasia, patients with Wernicke's aphasia are unable to repeat what is said to them. Wernicke's aphasia is attributed to a lesion in Wernicke's area in the posterior part of the superior temporal gyrus.

Paraphasia (Greek *para*, "to, at, from the side of"; *phasis*, "speech"). An aphasic phenomenon in which the patient employs wrong words or uses words in wrong combinations.

Neologism (Greek *neos*, "new"; *logos*, "word"). A newly coined word either in response to a communicative need or as a result of brain disorder. In the latter case, the newly coined word is a replacement of a desired word but without meaning.

Circumlocution. Convoluted, meaningless speech output, providing information rather than defining the objects to be communicated. Characteristic of Wernicke's aphasia.

Wernicke's aphasia is named after Karl Wernicke, a German neurologist who designated the posterior part of the superior temporal gyrus (area 22) of the left hemisphere as an area concerned with the understanding of the spoken word.

Conduction aphasia is characterized by fluent paraphasic speech, intact comprehension, poor naming, and repetition. Classically, patients with conduction aphasia cannot read out loud because of paraphasic intervention. Writing usually involves the use of incorrect letters in words. Pathology in these patients is usually located in the posterior perisylvian region and interrupts the output from Wernicke's area to Broca's area via the arcuate fasciculus. Recent reports suggest that conduction aphasia may result from lesions deep to the insula affecting the extreme capsule.

KEY CONCEPTS

- The right hemisphere contributes to the prosody of speech. Lesions in the right hemisphere result in aprosodic (dysprosodic) speech.

Global aphasia is a severe form of aphasia in which all the major functions of language (verbal output, comprehension, repetition, naming, reading, and writing) are severely impaired. Pathology is invariably extensive, involving much of the dominant hemisphere in the middle cerebral artery territory.

Transcortical aphasia has been subdivided into motor, sensory, and mixed types. All are characterized by preserved repetition. In transcortical motor aphasia, verbal output is nonfluent and comprehension is intact, but writing is invariably abnormal. Pathology in this type of aphasia is located in the dominant frontal lobe in the neighborhood of Broca's area. In transcortical sensory aphasia, speech output is fluent and paraphasic, comprehension is poor, and there are associated difficulties in reading and writing. Pathology in such cases is usually in the border zone between the temporal and parietal lobes in the neighborhood of Wernicke's area. Mixed transcortical aphasia, also known as *isolation* of the speech area, is characterized by nonfluent speech output, poor comprehension, and inability to name, read, or write. Pathology in these patients usually spares the perisylvian core region but involves the surrounding border zone or watershed area, which is supplied by the most distal tributaries of the middle cerebral artery.

Anomia (Greek *a*, "negative"; *onoma*, "name"). Inability to name objects or of recognizing and recalling their names.

Anomic aphasia, also known as *amnestic* or *nominal aphasia*, is characterized primarily by word-finding difficulty. Verbal output is fluent and empty with little or no paraphasia, comprehension is relatively normal, and repetition is intact. Anomic aphasia is often a sequela of any type of recovering aphasia. Although common, this type of aphasia is the most difficult to localize.

Pure word deafness, also known as *verbal auditory agnosia*, is characterized by poor comprehension of spoken language and by poor repetition with intact comprehension of written language, naming, writing, and spontaneous speech. The lesion in this type of disorder either affects the primary auditory area or disconnects this area from Wernicke's area. This syndrome is "pure" in the sense that it is not associated with other aphasic symptoms.

Apraxia (Greek *a*, "negative"; *praxis*, "action"). Inability to carry out learned skilled movements on command despite intact motor and sensory systems and good comprehension.

Ideomotor apraxia (motor apraxia). The inability to perform a motor act on command that can be performed spontaneously.

APRAXIA

Apraxia is the inability to perform skilled, learned, purposeful motor acts correctly despite intact relevant motor and sensory neural structures, attention, and comprehension. There are several types of apraxia: ideomotor, ideational, and visuoconstructive.

Ideomotor Apraxia

Ideomotor apraxia is the inability to carry out, on verbal command, an activity that can be performed perfectly well spontaneously. It is implied that this "inability" is not due to comprehension, motor, or sensory defects. Thus a patient with ideomotor apraxia will not be able to carry out a verbal command to walk, stop, salute, open a door, stick out the tongue, etc.

To appreciate the pathophysiology of ideomotor apraxia, it should be understood that for a skilled task to be performed, several events must take place. For example, the command to walk, if oral, reaches the primary auditory area and is relayed to the left auditory association cortex (Wernicke's area) for comprehension. Wer-

KEY CONCEPTS

- Apraxia is the inability to perform skilled, learned, purposeful motor acts correctly.
- Ideomotor apraxia pertains to the inability to carry out, on verbal command, an activity that can be performed spontaneously.

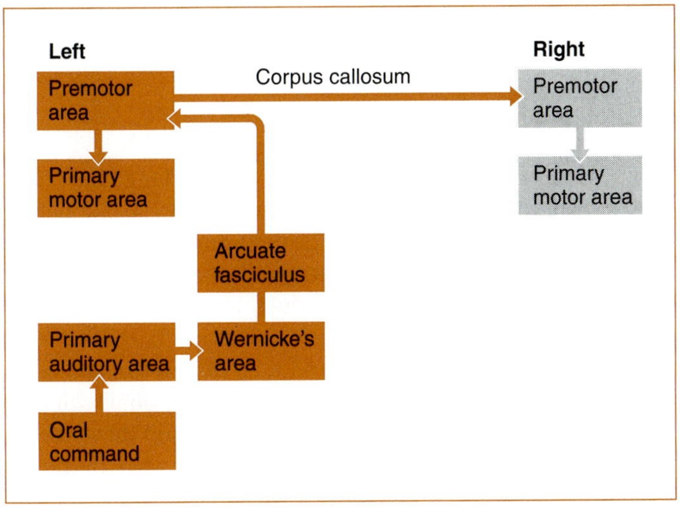

FIGURE 18-1

Schematic diagram showing the pathways involved in carrying out a motor skill in response to an oral command.

nicke's area is connected to the ipsilateral premotor area (motor association cortex, area 6) via the arcuate fasciculus. The motor association area on the left side is connected to the primary motor cortex (area 4) on the left side. When the person is asked to carry out a command with the left hand, the information is relayed from the left premotor area to the right premotor area (via the anterior part of the corpus callosum) and from there to the right primary motor area, which controls movements of the left side of the body (Fig. 18-1). Based on the preceding anatomic connections, three clinical varieties of ideomotor apraxia have been recognized: parietal, in which the lesion is in the anteroinferior parietal lobe of the dominant hemisphere; sympathetic, in which the lesion is in the left premotor area; and callosal, in which the lesion is in the anterior part of the corpus callosum.

Ideational Apraxia

Ideational apraxia is an abnormality in the conception of movement so that the patient may have difficulty sequencing the different components of a complex motor act. The lesion in ideational apraxia is in the dominant temporoparietooccipital area.

Ideational apraxia. A defect in the actual handling of common objects or a loss of conceptual knowledge relating to the use of tools.

Visuoconstructive Apraxia

Visuoconstructive apraxia, also known as *constructional apraxia*, is the inability of the individual to put together or articulate component parts to form a single shape or figure, such as assembling blocks to form a design or drawing four lines to form a shape. It implies a defect in perceiving spatial relationships among the component parts. Visuoconstructive apraxia was described originally in lesions of the left (domi-

KEY CONCEPTS

- Ideational apraxia pertains to an abnormality in the conception and sequencing of movement.
- Visuoconstructive apraxia pertains to the inability of the individual to put together component parts to make a whole.

nant) posterior parietal area. Subsequently, it was shown that this type of apraxia is more prevalent and severe in right hemisphere parietal lesions.

Alexia (Greek *a*, "negative"; *lexis*, "word"). Inability to comprehend the meaning of written or printed words and sentences.

Dyslexia (Greek *dys*, "difficult"; *lexis*, "word"). Impaired reading ability.

Agraphia (Greek *a*, "negative"; *grapho*, "to write"). Inability to express thoughts in writing due to a cerebral lesion. The first modern descriptions of agraphia are those of Jean Pitres in 1884 and of Joseph-Jules Dejerine in 1891.

ALEXIA (DYSLEXIA)

Alexia (**dyslexia**) is the inability to comprehend written language (reading disability). It may be acquired (acquired alexia or **dyslexia**), as in stroke patients who lose the ability to read, or developmental (developmental dyslexia), in which there is an inability to learn to read normally from childhood. Acquired alexia is of two types: pure alexia (alexia without **agraphia**, pure word blindness) and alexia with agraphia (parietal alexia).

In *pure alexia*, the defect in comprehension may manifest as an inability to read letters (literal alexia) or words (verbal alexia) or may be global with a total inability to read either letters or words (global alexia). The anatomic substrate of pure alexia is usually a lesion in the left primary visual area coupled with another lesion in the splenium of the corpus callosum (Fig. 18-2). The lesion in the left visual area prevents visual stimuli entering the left hemisphere from reaching the left (dominant) angular gyrus, which is necessary for comprehension of written language. The lesion in the splenium of the corpus callosum prevents visual stimuli entering the intact right visual area from reaching the left angular gyrus. Writing is normal in this type of alexia, but the patient cannot read what he or she writes. Cases have been described of pure alexia without a splenial lesion. In such cases, one deep lesion in the left occipitotemporal region isolates both occipital cortices from the left speech area in the angular gyrus.

Most commonly, alexia without agraphia occurs as a result of infarction in the territory of the left posterior cerebral artery that supplies neural structures involved. Usually, a right homonymous visual field defect is present.

Agnosia (Greek *a*, "negative"; *gnosis*, "knowledge"). Impairment of the ability to recognize stimuli that were recognized formerly despite intact perception, intellect, and language. The term was coined by Sigmund Freud in 1891. The lesion is usually in the posterior parietal region.

Prosopagnosia (Greek *prosopon*, "face"; *gnosis*, "knowledge"). Inability to recognize familiar faces. The word was coined by Bodamer in 1947, although the phenomenon had been recognized by Jackson and Charcot at the end of the nineteenth century.

Simultanagnosia. The inability to comprehend more than one element of a visual scene at the same time or to integrate the parts into a whole.

In *alexia with agraphia*, there is a defect in both reading comprehension and writing. The reading disorder is usually verbal (inability to read words). The writing difficulty is usually severe. The anatomic substrate of this type of alexia is a lesion in the dominant angular gyrus, hence the name *parietal alexia.*

AGNOSIA

Agnosia is the inability of the individual to recognize perceived sensory information. Implied in this definition is an intact sensory processing of the input, clear mental state, and intact naming ability.

Agnosia is often modality specific: visual, auditory, and tactile. Visual agnosias include visual object agnosia (inability to recognize objects presented visually), visual color agnosia (inability to recognize colors), **prosopagnosia** (i.e., inability to recognize faces, including one's own face, cars, types of trees), picture agnosia, and **simultanagnosia** (inability to recognize the whole, although parts of the whole are appreciated correctly).

KEY CONCEPTS

- Alexia pertains to the inability to comprehend written language (reading disability). Two forms are recognized: pure alexia (without agraphia) and alexia with agraphia.
- Agnosia pertains to the inability to recognize stimuli that were recognized formerly. Agnosia is modality specific: visual, auditory, and tactile.
- Visual agnosias include agnosias of objects (object agnosia), color (color agnosia), faces (prosopagnosia), and simultanagnosia (inability to recognize the whole).

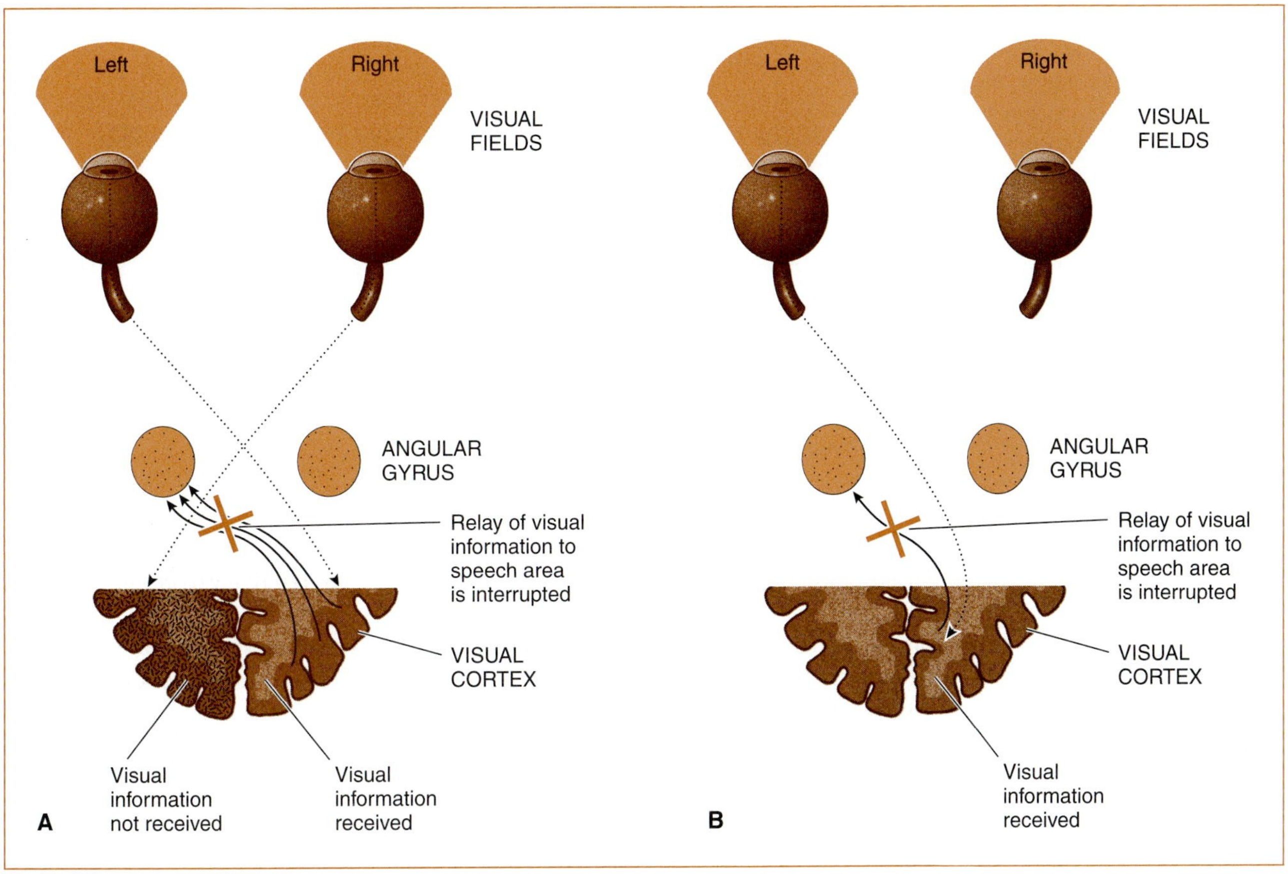

FIGURE 18-2

Schematic diagram showing the neural substrate of the syndrome of pure alexia without agraphia (*A*) and of hemialexia (*B*).

Auditory agnosia is the inability to recognize sounds in the presence of otherwise adequate hearing. It includes auditory verbal agnosia (inability to recognize spoken language or pure word deafness), auditory sound agnosia (i.e., inability to recognize nonverbal sounds such as animal sounds, sound of running water, sound of a bell), and sensory amusia (inability to recognize music).

Tactile agnosia is the inability to recognize objects by touch. It is usually associated with parietal lobe lesions of the contralateral hemisphere. **Astereognosia** is the loss of ability to judge the form of an object by touch. It includes **amorphognosia** (impaired recognition of size and shape of objects), **ahylognosia** (impaired discrimination of quality of objects, such as weight, texture, density), and **asymbolia** (impaired recognition of the identity of an object in the absence of amorphognosia and ahylognosia). *Asymbolia* is used by some authors to refer to tactile agnosia.

KEY CONCEPTS

- Auditory agnosias include agnosias of words (verbal agnosia), sounds (sound agnosia), and music (amusia).
- Tactile agnosias include agnosias of form (astereognosia), size and shape (amorphognosia), weight and texture (ahylognosia), and identity (asymoblia).

Astereognosis (Greek *a*, "negative"; *stereos*, "solid;" *gnosis*, "knowledge"). Inability to recognize familiar objects by feeling them.

Amorphognosia. A variety of tactile recognition disorders (astereognosis) characterized by impaired recognition of the size and shape of objects.

Ahylognosia. A variety of tactile recognition disorders (astereognosis) characterized by impairment in the discrimination of distinctive qualities of objects such as density, weight, texture, and thermal properties.

Asymbolia (Greek *a*, "negative"; *symbolon*, "sym-

bol"). Inability to comprehend symbols as words, figures, gestures, signs, etc. Asymbolia for pain denotes absence of psychic reaction to pain. The term *asymbolia* was suggested by Finkelberg as more encompassing than aphasia.

CALLOSAL SYNDROME

The disconnection of the right from the left hemisphere by lesions in the corpus callosum results in the isolation of each hemisphere in such a way that each has its own learning processes and memories that are inaccessible to the other hemisphere. The following are some of the effects of callosal disconnection seen in such patients. The effects of callosal transection are considerably less in younger children compared with adults because of the continued reliance in this age group on ipsilateral pathways.

Visual Effects

Each hemisphere retains its own visual images and memories, but only the left hemisphere is able to communicate, because of the callosal disconnection, what it sees through speech or writing.

Hemialexia

Patients are unable to read material presented in the left hemifield. This occurs when the splenium of the corpus callosum is involved in the lesion. Such visually presented material reaches the right occipital cortex but cannot be comprehended because the splenial lesion interferes with transmission of the visual image to the left (dominant) angular gyrus (Fig. 18-2).

Unilateral (Left) Ideomotor Apraxia

In response to verbal commands, patients are unable to carry out with the left hand some behavior that is readily carried out with the right hand. The verbal command is adequately received by the left (dominant) hemisphere but, because of the callosal disconnection, cannot reach the right hemisphere, which controls left hand movement.

Unilateral (Left) Agraphia

Patients with callosal lesions are unable to write using their left hand (Fig. 18-3).

Unilateral (Left) Tactile Anomia

Patients with callosal disconnection are unable, with eyes closed, to name or describe an object placed in the left hand, although they readily name the same object in the right hand. The object placed in the left hand is perceived correctly in the right somatosensory cortex but cannot be identified because of the callosal lesion that disconnects the right parietal cortex from the left (dominant) hemisphere (Fig. 18-3).

Left Ear Extinction

Patients with callosal lesions show left ear extinction when sounds are presented simultaneously to both ears (dichotic listening). Sounds presented to the left ear

KEY CONCEPTS

- Callosal syndromes include hemialexia, unilateral (left) ideomotor apraxia, unilateral (left) agraphia, unilateral (left) tactile anomia, and left ear extinction.

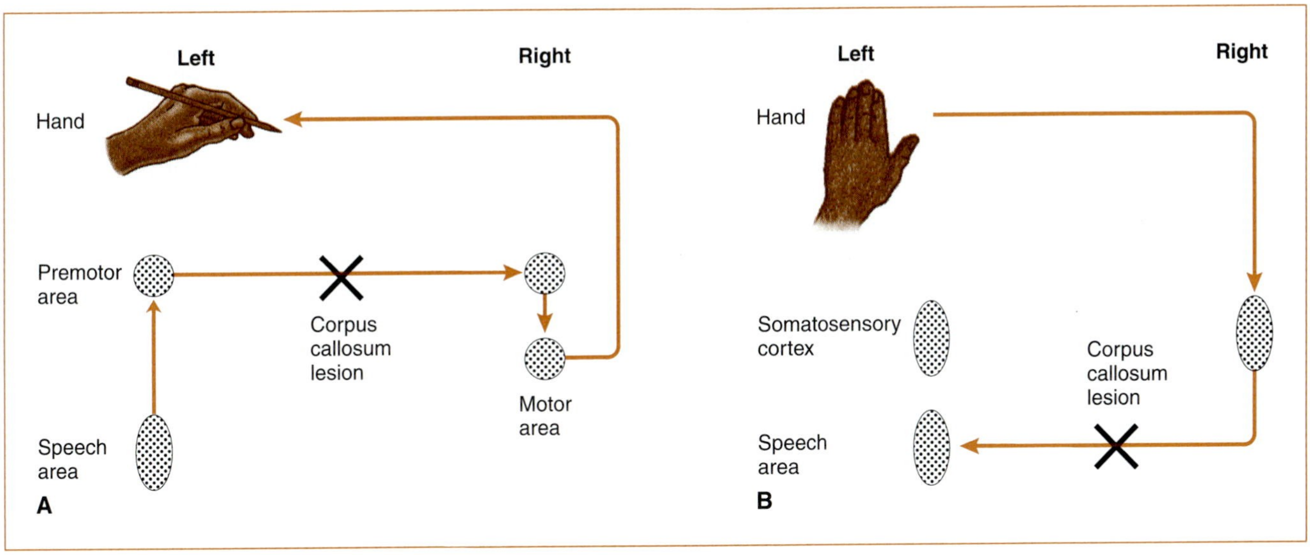

FIGURE 18-3

Schematic diagram illustrating the mechanism of unilateral (left) ideomotor apraxia (*A*) and of unilateral (left) tactile anomia (*B*).

reach the right temporal cortex but, because of the callosal disconnection, are not related to the left temporal cortex (dominant) for comprehension.

There is evidence to suggest functional specialization of different segments of the corpus callosum. Thus lesions in the posterior part of the corpus callosum (splenium) are associated with hemialexia, lesions in the anterior part are associated with left ideomotor apraxia, and lesions in the middle part are associated with left-hand agraphia; lesions in the middle and posterior parts result in left-hand tactile anomia.

PREFRONTAL LOBE SYNDROME

The prefrontal lobe syndrome occurs in association with tumors, trauma, or degenerative disease in the prefrontal and orbitofrontal cortices. The syndrome is characterized by a conglomerate of signs and symptoms that include impairments in decision making, ability to plan, social judgment, conduct, modulation of affect and of emotional response, and creativity. Such patients lose spontaneity in motor as well as mental activities. They do not appear to realize that they are neglecting themselves and their responsibilities at home and work. Affected patients may sit for hours looking at objects in front of them or staring out a window. They manifest loss of inhibition in social behavior and are usually euphoric and unconcerned. They may become incontinent of stools and urine because of the lack of spontaneity.

KEY CONCEPTS

- Prefrontal lobe syndrome pertains to a conglomerate set of signs and symptoms that includes impairments in decision making, ability to plan, social judgment, conduct, modulation of affect and of emotional response, and creativity.

THE GRASP REFLEX

Some brain-damaged patients show, in response to tactile stimulation of their hands or to the mere presentation of an object, a tendency to grasp at the object without any apparent intention to use it in a purposeful manner. Two types of grasp phenomena have been described: (1) the grasp reflex and (2) the instinctive grasp reaction.

The grasp reflex is generally considered an index of frontal lobe pathology, although the evidence in support of this localization is not so compelling. The grasp reflex has been reported with pathology in the basal ganglia, temporal lobe, parietal lobe, and parieto-occipital region. In the majority of cases, however, pathology is either in the frontal lobe or in subcortical structures. Unilateral lesions usually result in bilateral grasping.

In contrast, the instinctive grasp reaction is usually ipsilateral to the focal cerebral lesion and is seen more often with retrorolandic lesions of the right hemisphere, suggesting that it is one of the right hemisphere behavioral syndromes caused by disturbances of selective attention.

ALZHEIMER'S DISEASE

Alzheimer's disease is the example par excellence of cortical dementia. It is characterized by global loss of memory. In some cases, remote memory may be less severely affected than immediate or intermediate memory. The memory loss is progressive. With advance in the disease, patients will be unable to recognize their family members or their familiar surroundings. Neuronal loss in Alzheimer's patients is most marked in the hippocampus and in the nucleus basalis of Meynert. The pathologic hallmarks are neurofibrillary tangles and senile plaques. The former are intracellular aggregates of cytoskeletal filaments, whereas the latter are extracellular deposits of B-amyloid.

BALINT'S SYNDROME

This rare syndrome is named after the Hungarian neurologist Rudolph Balint. The syndrome is also known as *Balint-Holmes syndrome, optic ataxia, ocular apraxia,* and *psychic paralysis of visual fixation.* It is characterized by the inability to direct the eyes to a certain point in the visual field despite intact vision and eye movements. Patients are unable to pour water from a bottle into a glass and repeatedly pour the water outside the glass. The associated cortical lesion is bilateral parieto-occipital.

GERSTMANN'S SYNDROME

This syndrome is named after Josef Gerstmann, an Austrian neuropsychiatrist who described the syndrome in 1930. The syndrome is also known as the *Badal-*

KEY CONCEPTS

- The grasp phenomenon is of two types: (1) grasp reflex and (2) instinctive grasp reaction.
- The grasp reflex is associated with frontal lobe pathology, whereas the instinctive grasp reaction is associated with retrorolandic pathology.
- Alzheimer's disease is the example par excellence of cortical dementia.
- The Balint syndrome is the inability to direct the eyes to a certain point in the visual field despite intact vision and eye movements.

Gerstmann syndrome and the *angular gyrus syndrome.* Antoine-Jules Badal, a French ophthalmologist, had reported some features of the syndrome in 1888. The syndrome consists of the combination of right-left disorientation, acalculia (reduced ability to perform simple calculations), agraphia (inability to write), and finger agnosia (inability to recognize various fingers) due to a lesion in the left angular gyrus. Asymbolia for pain and constructional apraxia are added features in some cases.

ANOSOGNOSIA (DENIAL SYNDROME, ANTON-BABINSKI SYNDROME)

The term **anosognosia** was introduced by Josef Babinski in 1912 for unawareness of physical deficits or disease. This is seen most often with lesions of the nondominant (right) parietal lobe, with unawareness of deficits of the left side of the body. The denial syndrome may include denial that the paretic limbs belong to the patient. Hemispatial neglect often co-occurs with anosognosia. In hemispatial neglect, the contralateral side of the body and visual space are ignored but can be used if attention is drawn to them. Hemispatial neglect occurs after damage to either hemisphere but is typically more common and severe after right hemisphere lesions.

Anosognosia (Greek *a*, "negative"; *nosos*, "disease;" *gnosis*, "knowledge"). Unawareness or denial of a neurologic deficit such as hemiplegia. The term was introduced in 1912 by Josef Babinski. Anosognosia is most often with lesions of the right parietal lobe.

ANTON'S SYNDROME

Anton's syndrome traditionally refers to the clinical phenomenon of denial of blindness (anosognosia for blindness) in a patient who has suffered acquired cortical blindness. The most common setting is acute bilateral occipital cortex ischemia secondary to posterior circulation insufficiency. Although classically a manifestation of cortical blindness, Anton's syndrome has been reported in patients with blindness from peripheral visual pathway lesions (optic nerve, chiasm). The syndrome is named after Gabrial Anton, an Austrian neurologist who described the syndrome in 1899.

KLUVER-BUCY SYNDROME

The Kluver-Bucy syndrome was first described in 1939 in monkeys after bilateral temporal lobectomy. The human counterpart was described by Terzian and Dalle Ore in 1955 after bilateral removal of the temporal lobes. The syndrome consists of six main elements: (1) blunted affect with apathy, (2) psychic blindness or visual agnosia with inability to distinguish between friends, relatives, and strangers, (3) hypermetamorphosis with a marked tendency to take notice and attend to fine and minute visual stimuli, (4) hyperorality, placing all items in the mouth, (5) bulimia or unusual dietary habits, and (6) alteration in sexual behavior.

KEY CONCEPTS

- Gerstmann's syndrome pertains to a conglomerate set of signs and symptoms that includes right-left disorientation, acalculia, agraphia, and finger agnosia.
- Anosognosia is the denial of impairment in one-half the body, usually the left.
- Anton's syndrome is denial of blindness.
- Kluver-Bucy syndrome consists of blunted affect, psychic blindness, hypermetamorphosis, hyperorality, hypersexuality, and bulimia.

SIMULTANAGNOSIA

Simultanagnosia is the inability to appreciate more than one aspect of the visual panorama at any single time. Affected patients cannot experience a spatially coherent visual field. Objects in the visual field of affected patients appear and disappear erratically. Affected patients fail to see a match flame held several inches away when their attention is focused on the tip of a cigarette held between their lips. This condition is associated with bilateral or right posterior parietal cortex lesion in the watershed region. The term *simultanagnosia* was introduced by Wolpert in 1924 to refer to a condition in which the patient is unable to recognize or abstract the meaning of the whole (pictures or series of pictures) even though the details are appreciated correctly.

THE ALIEN HAND SYNDROME

The alien hand syndrome is characterized by the unwilled and uncontrolled actions of an upper limb on either the dominant or nondominant side. The alien hand performs autonomous activity that the subject cannot inhibit and then often contrasts with voluntary actions performed by the other hand. Patients often state that the alien hand has a mind of its own. The alien hand syndrome was first described in 1908 by Goldstein. Two forms of alien hand exist: (1) an acute, transient condition due to callosal lesion and (2) a chronic condition resulting from additional medial frontal lesions involving the supplementary motor area. The combined callosal and medial frontal lesions presumably release the lateral frontal motor system responsible for environmentally driven activity.

KEY CONCEPTS

- The alien hand syndrome is the unwilled and uncontrolled action of one upper extremity secondary to callosal or medial frontal lesions.

SUGGESTED READINGS

Absher RR, Benson DF: Disconnection syndromes: An overview of Geschwind's contributions. *Neurology* 1993; 43:862–867.

Albert ML: Alexia. In Heilman KM, Valenstein E (eds): *Clinical Neuropsychology*. New York, Oxford University Press, 1979:59.

Alexander MP, et al: Broca's area aphasias: Aphasia after lesions including the frontal operculum. *Neurology* 1990; 40:353–362.

Banks G, et al: The alien hand syndrome: Clinical and postmortem findings. *Arch Neurol* 1989; 46:456–459.

Benson DF: Aphasia. In Heilman KM, Valenstein E (eds): *Clinical Neuropsychology*. New York, Oxford University Press, 1979:22.

Benson DF: Aphasia, alexia, and agraphia. In Glaser GH (ed): *Clinical Neurology and Neurosurgery Monographs*, vol 1. New York, Churchill-Livingstone, 1979:1–205.

Benton A: Visuoperceptive, visuospatial, and visuoconstructive disorders. In Heilman KM, Valenstein E (eds): *Clinical Neuropsychology*. New York, Oxford University Press, 1979:186.

Benton A: Gerstmann's syndrome. *Arch Neurol* 1992; 49:445–447.

Boeri R, Salmaggi A: Prosopagnosia (commentary). *Curr Opin Neurol* 1994; 7:61–64.

Boegn JE: The callosal syndrome. In Heilman KM, Valenstein E (eds): *Clinical Neuropsychology*. New York, Oxford University Press, 1979:308.

Branch Coslett H, et al: Pure word deafness after bilateral primary auditory cortex infarcts. *Neurology* 1984; 34:347–352.

Butters N: Amnesic disorders. In Heilman KM, Valenstein E (eds): *Clinical Neuropsychology*. New York, Oxford University Press, 1979:439.

Damasio AR: Notes on the anatomical basis of pure

alexia and of color anomia. In Taylor M, Höök S (eds): *Aphasia: Assessment and Treatment.* Stockholm, Almqvist & Wiksell, 1978:126.

Damasio AR: The neural basis of language. *Ann Rev. Neurosci* 1984; 7:127–147.

Damasio AR: Prosopagnosia. *TINS* 1985; 8:132–135.

Damasio AR: The nature of aphasias: Signs and syndromes. In Taylor Sarno M (ed): *Acquired Aphasia.* New York, Academic Press, 1981:51.

Damasio H: Cerebral localization of the aphasias. In Taylor Sarno M (ed): *Acquired Aphasia.* New York, Academic Press, 1981:27.

Damasio AR, Damasio H: The anatomic basis of pure alexia. *Neurology* 1983; 33:1573–1583.

Damasio AR, Damasio H: Brain and language: A large set of neural structures serves to represent concepts; a smaller set forms words and sentences; between the two lies a crucial layer of mediation. *Sci Am* Sept. 1992; 89–95.

Damasio H, Damasio AR: *Lesion Analysis in Neuropsychology.* New York, Oxford University Press, 1989.

Damasio H, Damasio AR: The anatomical basis of conduction aphasia. *Brain* 1980; 103:337–350.

Damasio AR, et al: Face agnosia and the neural substrates of memory. *Annu Rev Neurosci* 1990; 13: 89–109.

DeRenzi E, Barbieri C: The incidence of the grasp reflex following hemispheric lesions and its relation to frontal damage. *Brain* 1992; 115:293–313.

Feinberg TE, et al: Two alien hand syndromes. *Neurology* 1992; 42:19–24.

Feinberg TE, et al: Anosognosia and visuoverbal confabulation. *Arch Neurol* 1994; 51:468–473.

Finger S, Roe D: Gustave Dax and the early history of cerebral dominance. *Arch Neurol* 1996; 53:806–813.

Funkenstein HH: Approaches to hemispheric asymmetries. In Tyler HR, Dawson DM (eds): *Current Neurology*, vol 1. Boston, Houghton Mifflin Medical Division, 1978:336.

Heilman KM: Apraxia. In Heilman KM, Valenstein E (eds): *Clinical Neuropsychology.* New York, Oxford University Press, 1979:159.

Kertesz A, et al: Computer tomographic localization, lesion size and prognosis in aphasia and nonverbal impairment. *Brain Language* 1979; 8:34–50.

Lassonde M, et al: Effects of early and late transection of the corpus callosum in children: A study of tactile and tactuomotor transfer and integration. *Brain* 1986; 109:953–967.

Mazzochi F, Vignolo LA: Localization of lesions in aphasia: Clinical–CT scan correlations in stroke patients. *Cortex* 1979; 15:627–654.

McDaniel KD, McDaniel LD: Anton's syndrome in a patient with posttraumatic optic neuropathy and bifrontal contusions. *Arch Neurol* 1991; 48:101–105.

Mori E, Yamadori A: Unilateral hemispheric injury and ipsilateral instinctive grasp reaction. *Arch Neurol* 1985; 42:485–488.

Rizzo M, Hurtig R: Looking but not seeing: Attention, perception, and eye movements in simultanagnosis. *Neurology* 1987; 37:1642–1648.

Rizzo M, Robin DA: Simultanagnosia: A defect of sustained attention yields insights on visual information processing. *Neurology* 1990; 40:447–455.

Rubens AB: Agnosia. In Heilman KM, Valenstein E (eds): *Clinical Neuropsychology*. New York, Oxford University Press, 1979:233.

Schäffler L, et al: Comprehension deficits elicited by electrical stimulation of Broca's area. *Brain* 1993; 116:695–715.

Schlaug G, et al: In vivo evidence of structural brain asymmetry in musicians. *Science* 1995; 267:699–701.

Smith Doody R, Jankovic J: The alien hand and related signs. *J Neurol Neurosurg Psychiatry* 1992; 55: 806–810.

Trojano L, et al: How many alien hand syndromes? Follow-up of a case. *Neurology* 1993; 43:2710–2712.

Warrington EK, Shallice T: Word-form dyslexia. *Brain* 1980; 103:99–112.

Watson RT, et al: Posterior neocortical systems subserving awareness and neglect: Neglect associated with superior temporal sulcus but not area 7 lesions. *Arch Neurol* 1994; 51:1014–1021.

Weintraub S, Mesulam MM: Right cerebral dominance in spatial attention: Further evidence based on ipsilateral neglect. *Arch Neurol* 1987; 44:621–625.

Yamadori A, et al: Left unilateral agraphia and tactile anomia: Disturbances seen after occlusion of the anterior cerebral artery. *Arch Neurol* 1980; 37:88–91.

CHAPTER 19

HYPOTHALAMUS

BOUNDARIES AND DIVISIONS

The hypothalamus is the area of the diencephalon ventral to the hypothalamic sulcus (see Fig. 11-1). It weighs about 4 g and comprises 0.3 to 0.5 percent of brain volume. It is limited anteriorly by the lamina terminalis and is continuous posteriorly with the mesencephalon. On its ventral surface, caudal to the optic chiasma, the hypothalamus narrows to a small neck, the tuber cinereum. The ventral-most portion of the tuber cinereum constitutes the median eminence. The median eminence blends into the infundibular stalk, which is continuous with the posterior lobe of the **pituitary** gland. In coronal sections, the hypothalamus is seen to be bordered medially by the third ventricle and laterally by the subthalamus (see Fig. 11-2). The fornix divides the hypothalamus into medial and lateral regions. The lateral region contains mainly longitudinally oriented fibers of the medial forebrain bundle (which

Infundibulum (Latin "funnel"). Andreas Vesalius, the Belgian anatomist, used this term to describe the attachment of the pituitary gland of the brain.

Pituitary (Latin *pituita*, "phlegm or mucus"). Pituitary gland. Jacob Berengarius, the Italian anatomist and surgeon, noted the presence of the pituitary gland in 1524. Andreas Vesalius, the Belgian anatomist, called it "glandula pituitam cerebri excipiens" and thought that the gland secreted mucus into the nose, an opinion held until the seventeenth century.

KEY CONCEPTS

- The hypothalamus is part of the diencephalon.
- The following landmarks delineate the topography of the hypothalamus: lamina terminalis rostrally, hypothalamic sulcus dorsally, third ventricle medially, subthalamus laterally, and mesencephalic-diencephalic junction caudally.
- The hypothalamus is divided by the fornix into medial and lateral zones.

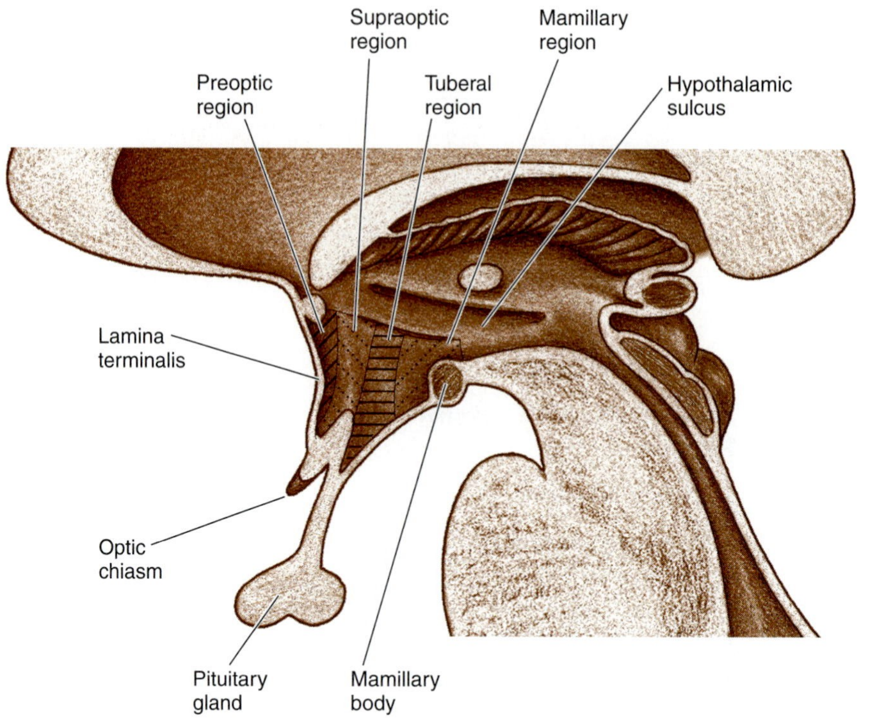

FIGURE 19-1

Schematic diagram showing the four regions of the medial hypothalamus.

connects the septal area, hypothalamus, and midbrain tegmentum), among which are scattered neurons of the lateral hypothalamic nucleus. The medial region has a cluster of nuclei organized into four major groups. In a rostrocaudal orientation (Fig. 19-1), these nuclear groups are as follows:

1. Preoptic
2. Suprachiasmatic (supraoptic)
3. Tuberal
4. Mamillary

Preoptic Region (Fig. 19-2)

The gray matter in the most rostral part of the hypothalamus, just caudal to the lamina terminalis, is the preoptic region. It contains medial and lateral preoptic nuclei and the preoptic periventricular nucleus.

Suprachiasmatic (Supraoptic) Region (See Fig. 19-2)

This nuclear group contains the supraoptic, paraventricular, anterior hypothalamic, and suprachiasmatic nuclei. The supraoptic nucleus is located above the optic tract,

KEY CONCEPTS

- The hypothalamus contains the following nuclear groupings: preoptic, suprachiasmatic (supraoptic), tuberal, and mamillary.

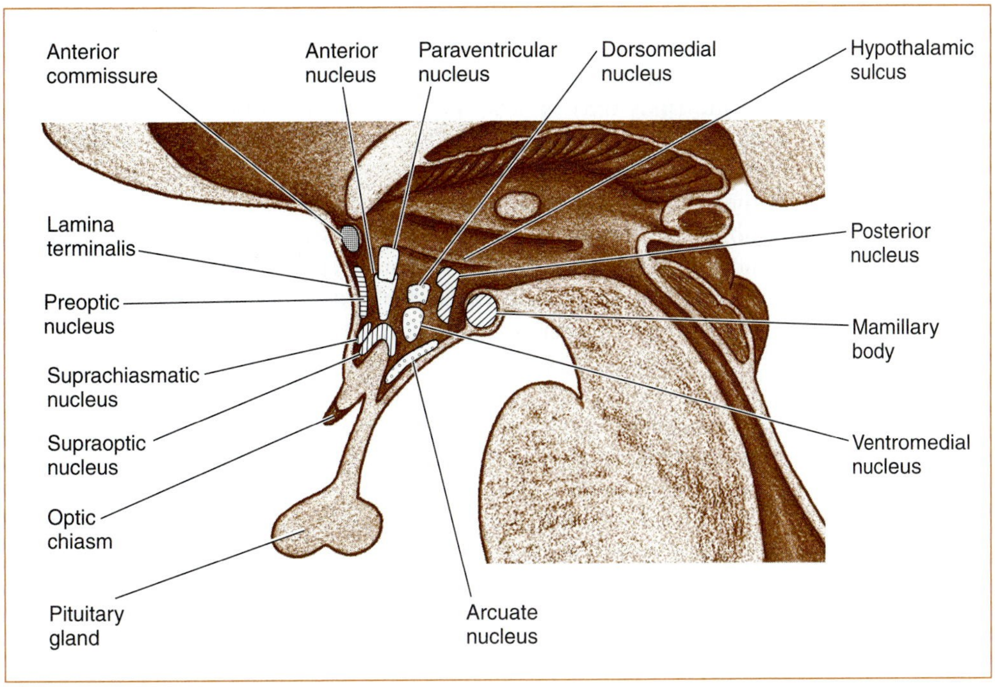

FIGURE 19-2

Schematic diagram showing nuclei within each of the regions of the medial hypothalamus.

whereas the paraventricular nucleus is dorsal to it, lateral to the third ventricle (see Fig. 19-3). Axons of both nuclei course in the pituitary stalk to reach the posterior lobe of the pituitary (hypothalamoneurohypophysial system), transporting neurosecretory material elaborated in these nuclei and stored in axonal swellings within the posterior lobe. The neurosecretory material consists of vasopressin [antidiuretic hormone (ADH)] and oxytocin. There is evidence to suggest that the supraoptic nucleus elaborates mainly ADH, whereas the paraventricular nucleus elaborates

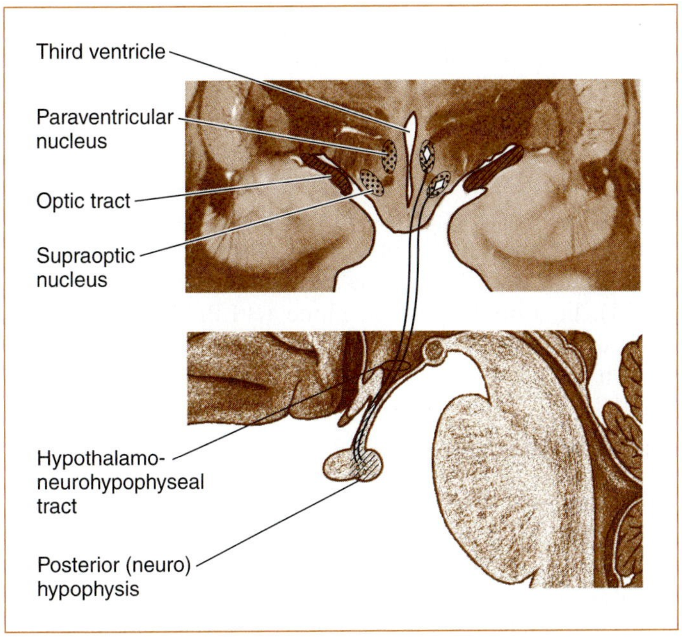

FIGURE 19-3

Schematic diagram showing the hypothalamo-neurohypophyseal system.

mainly oxytocin. ADH acts on the distal convoluted tubules of the kidney to increase reabsorption of water. Lesions of the supraoptic nucleus, the hypothalamoneurohypophysial system, or the posterior lobe of the pituitary result in excessive excretion of urine (**polyuria**) of low specific gravity. This condition is known as **diabetes insipidus**. Another symptom of this condition is excessive intake of water (**polydipsia**). Unlike **diabetes mellitus**, diabetes insipidus is not associated with alterations in the sugar content of blood or of urine. Production of ADH is controlled by the osmolarity of the blood that bathes the supraoptic nucleus. An increase in blood osmolarity, as occurs in dehydration, increases ADH production, whereas the reverse occurs in states of lowered blood osmolarity, such as excessive hydration. ADH secretion is increased by pain, stress, and such drugs as morphine, nicotine, and barbiturates; it is decreased by alcohol intake.

Oxytocin causes contraction of uterine smooth musculature and promotes milk ejection from the lactating mammary glands by stimulating contraction of its myoepithelial cells. Commercially produced oxytocin is used to induce labor. The function of oxytocin in males is not yet known.

The anterior nucleus merges with the preoptic region. Stimulation of the anterior part of the hypothalamus in animals results in excessive intake of water, suggesting that a center for thirst is located in this region. Tumors in this region in children are associated with refusal of patients to drink despite severe dehydration.

The suprachiasmatic nucleus, poorly developed in humans, overlies the optic chiasma. It receives bilateral inputs from ganglion cells of the retina and plays a role in circadian rhythm. Lesions of the nucleus in experimental animals will disturb the cyclic variations of a number of bodily functions (e.g., temperature cycle, sleep-wake cycle, circadian changes of hormones).

Polyuria (Greek *polys*, "many"; *ouron*, "urine"). The passage of a very large volume of urine, characteristic of diabetes.

Diabetes insipidus (Greek *diabetes*, "a syphon"). A condition of excessive production of urine from deficiency of the antidiuretic hormone. The condition was distinguished from diabetes mellitus by Thomas Willis, the English physician in 1674. The relation of the condition to lesions in the neurohypophysis is attributed to the German physiologist Alfred Frank.

Polydipsia (Greek *polys*, "many"; *dipsa*, "thirst"). Chronic excessive thirst as in diabetes insipidus and mellitus.

Diabetes mellitus (Greek *diabetes*, "a syphon"; L. *mellitus*, "honey sweet"). A disorder of carbohydrate metabolism with high levels of glucose in blood and urine. Thomas Willis in 1674 differentiated sweet urine (diabetes mellitus) from clear, insipid urine (diabetes insipidus).

Arcuate (Latin *arcuatus*, "bow-shaped"). The arcuate nucleus of the hypothalamus has an arcuate shape in coronal sections.

Tuberal Region (see Fig. 19-2)

This is the widest region of the hypothalamus and the one in which the division of the hypothalamus into medial and lateral areas by the fornix is best illustrated. The tuberal region contains the ventromedial hypothalamic, dorsomedial hypothalamic, and **arcuate** (infundibular) nuclei.

The ventromedial nucleus, a poorly delineated area of small neurons, is concerned with satiety. Bilateral lesions in the ventromedial nucleus in animals produce a voracious appetite, obesity, and savage behavior. Lesions in the lateral hypothalamus at this level produce loss of appetite. Thus a center for satiety is believed to be associated with the ventromedial nucleus and a feeding center with the lateral hypothalamus.

The dorsomedial nucleus is a poorly delineated mass of small neurons dorsal to the ventromedial nucleus. The arcuate nucleus consists of small neurons located ventral to the third ventricle near the infundibular recess. The arcuate nucleus contains dopamine, which controls prolactin and growth hormone secretions. In addition, neurons of the arcuate nucleus stain positively for adrenocorticotrophic hormone (ACTH), beta-lipotrophic hormone (β-LPH), and beta-endorphin (β-END). The arcuate nucleus is believed to play a role in emotional behavior and endocrine function.

Mamillary Region (see Fig. 19-2)

The most caudal region of the hypothalamus is the mamillary region; it contains mamillary and posterior hypothalamic nuclei. The mamillary nuclei (bodies) are two spherical masses protruding from the ventral surface of the hypothalamus in the interpeduncular fossa.

The posterior hypothalamic nucleus is a mass of large neurons located dorsal to the mamillary bodies. It is the main source of descending hypothalamic fibers to the brain stem.

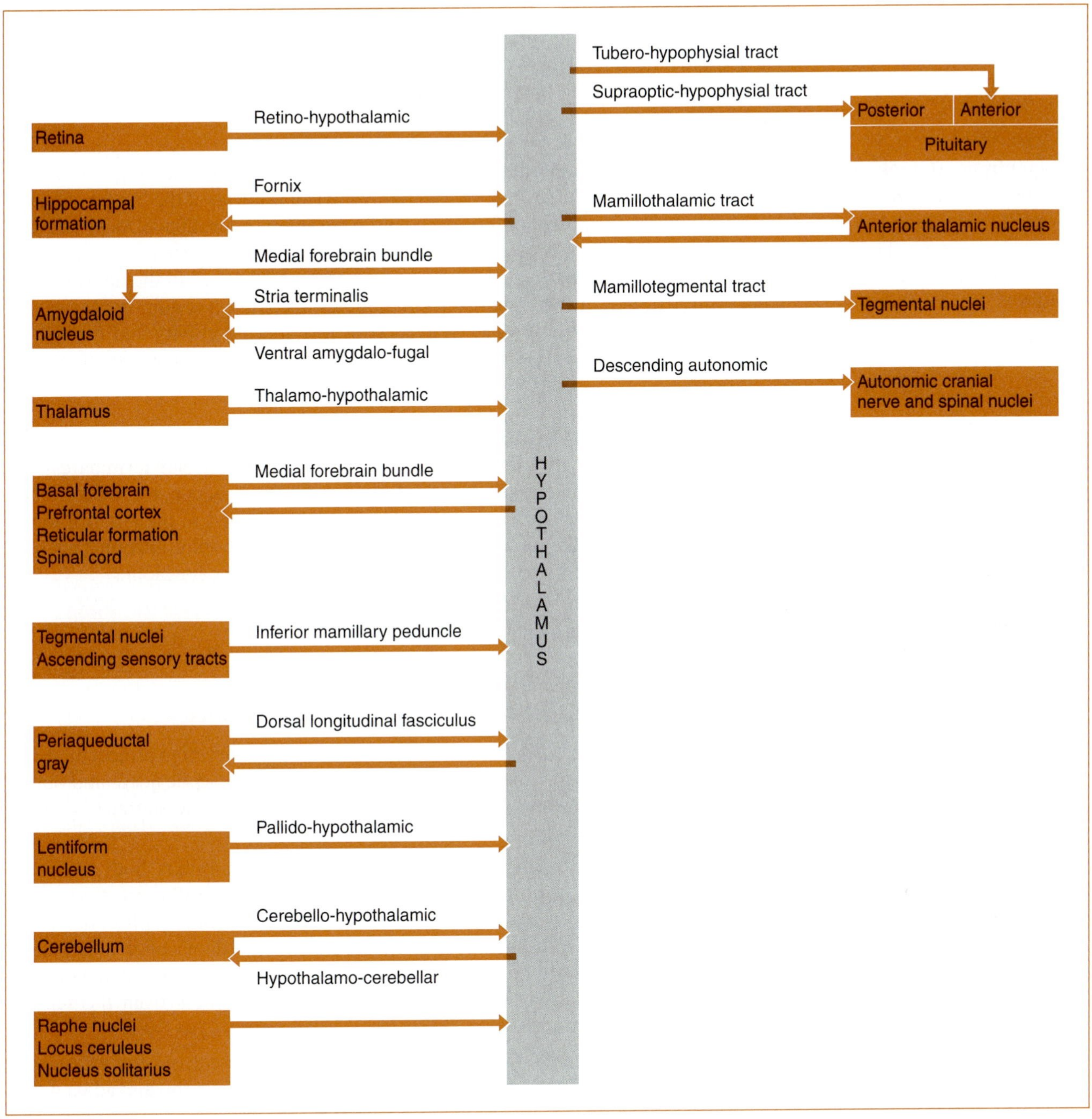

FIGURE 19-4

Schematic diagram showing the main sources of hypothalamic input and output targets.

CONNECTIONS (Figs. 19-3 and 19-4)

The hypothalamus has extensive connections reflecting its roles in endocrine, autonomic, and somatic integration.

KEY CONCEPTS

- Hypothalamic connections are divided into local (efferent) and extrinsic (afferent and efferent).

Local Connections

The hypothalamus influences pituitary function via two pathways: the hypothalamo-hypophysial (supraoptic-hypophysial) tract and the tuberohypophysial (tuberoinfundibular) tract.

Hypophysis (Greek *hypo*, "under"; *phyein*, "to grow"). Anything growing under or beneath. The pituitary gland is under the brain.

The Hypothalamohypophysial (Supraoptic-Hypophysial) Tract (see Fig. 19-3)
This tract arises from the supraoptic and paraventricular nuclei of the hypothalamus and terminates in the posterior lobe of the pituitary gland (neurohypophysis). Axons in this tract transport vasopressin (ADH) from the supraoptic nucleus and oxytocin from the paraventricular nucleus to the fenestrated capillary bed in the neurohypophysis. Interruption of this tract results in diabetes insipidus, a condition characterized by excessive urine excretion (polyuria) of low specific gravity and excessive intake of water (polydipsia) without alterations in the glucose content of blood or urine.

The Tuberohypophysial (Tuberoinfundibular) Tract
This tract arises from the arcuate and periventricular nuclei and terminates on capillaries in the median eminence and infundibular stem. Fibers in this tract transmit hypothalamic releasing factors (hypophysiotrophic agents) to the anterior lobe of the pituitary gland via the hypophysial portal system. Hypophysiotrophic agents stimulate or inhibit secretion of anterior lobe of the pituitary hormones.

Extrinsic Connections (see Fig. 19-4)

Afferent Extrinsic Connections
The following hypothalamic extrinsic inputs have been reported:

1. *Retinohypothalamic tract.* Fibers from ganglion cells of the retina project bilaterally to the suprachiasmatic nuclei of the hypothalamus via the optic nerve and optic chiasma. This tract transmits light periodicity information to the suprachiasmatic nucleus, which plays a role in the circadian rhythm.

Fornix (Latin "arch"). The fornix is an archlike cerebral structure that connects the hippocampal formation with the mamillary body. The fornix was noted by Galen and described by Andreas Vesalius, the sixteenth-century Belgian anatomist. Thomas Willis introduced the name *fornix cerebri.*

2. *Fornix.* The **fornix** comprises the major input to the mamillary body. Arising from the hippocampal formation and subiculum, the fornix follows a C-shaped course underneath the corpus callosum as far forward as the interventricular foramen of Monro, where it disappears in the substance of the diencephalon to reach the mamillary bodies. Although the major component of the fornix comes from the hippocampal formation and subiculum, it also carries fibers from the septal area to the mamillary bodies.

3. *Amygdalohypothalamic tract.* Inputs to the hypothalamus from the amygdala follow two pathways. One is via the stria terminalis, which links the amygdala with

KEY CONCEPTS

- Local hypothalamic connections consist of the hypothalamohypophysial tract and the tuberohypophysial (tuberoinfundibular) tract.
- The hypothalamohypophysial tract links the supraoptic and paraventricular nuclei of the hypothalamus and the posterior lobe of the pituitary gland (neurohypophysis).
- The tuberohypophysial tract links the arcuate and periventricular nuclei of the hypothalamus with the anterior lobe of the pituitary gland via the hypophysial portal system.
- Extrinsic hypothalamic connections are afferent and efferent.

the medial preoptic, anterior hypothalamic, ventromedial, and arcuate nuclei of the hypothalamus. The other is via the ventral amygdalofugal fiber system, which links the amygdala with the lateral hypothalamic nucleus.

4. *Thalamohypothalamic fibers.* These fibers run from dorsomedial and midline thalamic nuclei to the lateral and posterior hypothalamus and are sparse. Fibers from the anterior thalamic nuclei reach the mamillary bodies via the mamillothalamic tract and provide a feedback mechanism to the mamillary bodies.

5. *Medial forebrain bundle.* This fiber bundle runs in the lateral hypothalamus. It conveys to the hypothalamus inputs from a variety of sources, including the basal forebrain (olfactory cortex, septal area, nucleus accumbens septi), amygdala, premotor frontal cortex, brain stem reticular formation, and spinal cord.

6. *Inferior mamillary peduncle.* This fiber bundle links the dorsal and ventral tegmental nuclei of the midbrain and the mamillary body. It also contains indirect inputs from ascending sensory pathways.

7. *Dorsal longitudinal fasciculus of Schütz.* Afferent fibers in this fasciculus link the periaqueductal (central) gray matter of the midbrain with the hypothalamus.

8. *Pallidohypothalamic fibers.* This fiber bundle originates from the lentiform nucleus and projects on neurons in the ventromedial hypothalamic nucleus.

9. *Cerebellohypothalamic fibers.* This fiber bundle originates from all deep cerebellar nuclei and relates the cerebellum to autonomic function.

10. *Other inputs.* Other afferents to the hypothalamus from the brain stem include those from the raphe nuclei, locus ceruleus, and nucleus solitarius. These fibers enter the hypothalamus via the medial forebrain bundle.

Efferent Extrinsic Connections

The hypothalamus sends fibers to most areas from which it receives inputs. The following hypothalamic extrinsic efferent connections have been reported:

1. *Mamillothalamic tract (tract of* **Vicq d'Azyr***)* (see Fig. 11-4). This is a two-way fiber system connecting the mamillary bodies with the anterior thalamic nucleus.

2. *Mamillotegmental tract* (see Fig. 11-4). Fibers from the mamillary bodies course caudally to terminate on dorsal and ventral tegmental nuclei and secondarily on autonomic cranial (dorsal motor nucleus of vagus, nucleus solitarius, nucleus ambiguus) and spinal nuclei (intermediolateral cell column).

3. *Fornix.* Reciprocal fibers travel in the fornix from the mamillary body to the hippocampal formation.

4. *Medial forebrain bundle.* This bundle conveys impulses from the lateral hypothalamus rostrally to the septal nuclei and caudally to tegmental nuclei and periaqueductal (central) gray of the midbrain.

5. *Dorsal longitudinal fasciculus of Schütz.* Fibers in this fasciculus link the medial hypothalamus with the periaqueductal gray matter of the midbrain.

Vicq d'Azyr. Felix Vicq d'Azyr (1748–1794), a French anatomist and physician to Queen Marie Antoinette who described the mamillothalamic tract (tract of Vicq d'Azyr) in 1781, although his observation was not published until 1805.

KEY CONCEPTS

- Afferent extrinsic connections include the retinohypothalamic, fornix, amygdalohypothalamic, thalamohypothalamic, medial forebrain bundle, inferior mamillary peduncle, dorsal longitudinal fasciculus (of Schütz), and pallidohypothalamic.
- Efferent extrinsic connections include the mamillothalamic, mamillotegmental, fornix, medial forebrain bundle, dorsal longitudinal fasciculus (of Schütz), hypothalamoamygdaloid, descending autonomic, and hypothalamocerebellar.

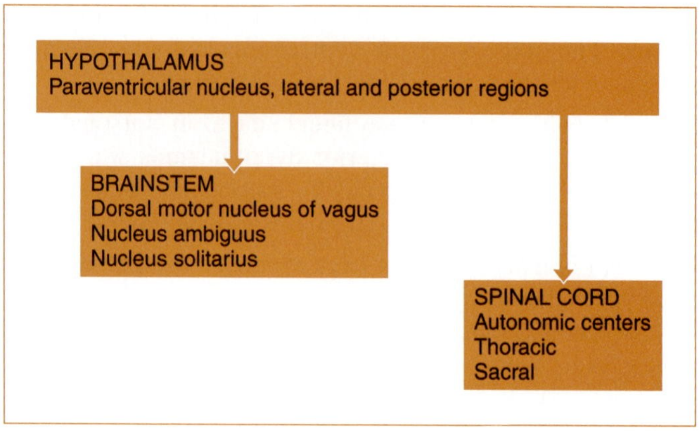

FIGURE 19-5

Schematic diagram showing descending autonomic projections of the hypothalamus.

6. *Hypothalamoamygdaloid fibers.* These fibers travel via the stria terminalis and ventral amygdalofugal fiber system and provide feedback information to the amygdaloid nucleus.

7. *Descending autonomic fibers* (Fig. 19-5). Axons of neurons in the paraventricular nucleus, the lateral hypothalamic area, and the posterior hypothalamus project into autonomic cranial nerve nuclei in the brain stem (dorsal motor nucleus of the vagus, nucleus ambiguus, nucleus solitarius) and autonomic spinal cord nuclei in the intermediolateral cell column and the sacral autonomic cell column. Via these connections, the hypothalamus exerts control over central autonomic processes related to blood pressure, heart rate, temperature regulation, and digestion. Many of these fibers are components of the dorsal longitudinal fasciculus of Schütz.

8. *Hypothalamocerebellar fibers.* In the past few years, a series of investigations has revealed the existence of a complex network of direct and indirect pathways between the hypothalamus and cerebellum. The projections are bilateral with ipsilateral preponderance. They originate from various hypothalamic nuclei and areas but principally from the lateral and posterior hypothalamic areas. The indirect pathway reaches the cerebellum after relays in a number of brain stem nuclei. The hypothalamocerebellar pathway may provide the neuroanatomic substrate for the autonomic responses elicited from cerebellar stimulation.

Table 19-1 is a summary of the afferent and efferent connections of the hypothalamus.

FUNCTIONS OF THE HYPOTHALAMUS

The functions of the hypothalamus, mediated through its varied and complex connections, involve several important bodily activities. The following is a listing of some of the most important and best known.

Control of Posterior Pituitary (Neurohypophysis)

This is served through the hypothalamoneurohypophysial system discussed earlier. Approximately 100,000 unmyelinated fibers extend from the supraoptic and paraventricular nuclei of the hypothalamus to the fenestrated capillary bed of the neurohypophysis. These fibers convey two peptide hormones: vasopressin (ADH) and oxytocin. Vasopressin promotes reabsorption of water from the kidney. In lesions of the neurohypophysis, urine output of low specific gravity reaches 10 to

Connections of the Hypothalamus

Pathway	Afferent	Efferent	Origin	Termination
Hypothalamohypophysial tract		+	Supraoptic and paraventricular nuclei	Neurohypophysis
Tuberohypophysial tract		+	Arcuate and periventricular nuclei	Median eminence and infundibular stalk
Retinohypothalamic tract	+		Ganglion cells of retina	Suprachiasmatic nucleus
Fornix	+		Hippocampal formation, subiculum	Mamillary body
		+	Mamillary body	Hippocampal formation
Stria terminalis	+		Amygdaloid nucleus	Preoptic and arcuate nuclei
		+	Preoptic and arcuate nuclei	Amygdaloid nucleus
Ventral amygdalofugal tract	+		Amygdaloid nucleus	Lateral hypothalamic nucleus
		+	Lateral hypothalamic nucleus	Amygdaloid nucleus
Thalamohypothalamic	+		Dorsomedial and midline thalamic nuclei	Lateral and posterior hypothalamus
Medial forebrain bundle	+		Basal forebrain, amygdala, premotor frontal cortex, brainstem reticular formation (raphe nuclei, locus ceruleus, nucleus solitarius), spinal cord	Lateral hypothalamus
		+	Lateral hypothalamus	Septal nuclei, tegmental nuclei, and periaqueductal gray matter of midbrain
Inferior mamillary peduncle	+		Tegmental nuclei of midbrain, ascending sensory pathways	Mamillary body
Dorsal longitudinal fasciculus (of Schütz)	+		Periaqueductal gray matter of midbrain	Medial hypothalamus
		+	Medial hypothalamus	Periaqueductal gray matter of midbrain
Pallidohypothalamic	+		Lentiform nucleus	Ventromedial hypothalamic nucleus
Cerebellohypothalamic fibers	+		Deep nuclei of cerebellum	Lateral and posterior hypothalamus
Hypothalamocerebellar fibers		+	Lateral and posterior hypothalamus	Deep cerebellar nuclei and cerebellar cortex
Mamillothalamic tract		+	Mamillary body	Anterior thalamic nucleus
Mamillotegmental tract		+	Mamillary body	Tegmental nuclei of midbrain
Descending autonomic fibers		+	Paraventricular nucleus, lateral hypothalamic area, posterior hypothalamus	Autonomic cranial nerve and spinal cord nuclei

15 liters per day, a condition known as *diabetes insipidus.* Oxytocin stimulates contraction of smooth muscles of the uterus and promotes ejection of milk from the lactating mammary gland.

Control of Anterior Pituitary

Several trophic factors (hypophysiotropins, hypothalamic releasing factors) are produced in the hypothalamus and influence production of hormones in the anterior pituitary. Trophic factors are released into capillaries of the median eminence, from which they reach the anterior pituitary via the hypophysial portal circulation. In the anterior lobe, trophic factors act on the appropriate chromophil cell to release or inhibit the appropriate trophic hormone. The anterior pituitary trophic hormones then act on the appropriate target gland. The serum hormone level of the target gland has a feedback effect on hypothalamic trophic factors. The known hypothalamic trophic factors include corticotropin-releasing factor (CRF), which influences production of adrenocorticotropic hormone (ACTH) and beta-lipotropin (precursor of ACTH and of endorphins) by the pituitary basophils; thyrotropin-releasing factor (TRF), which influences secretion of thyroid-stimulating hormone (TSH) from the basophils; gonadotropin-releasing factor (GnRF), which influences production of follicle-stimulating (FSH) and luteinizing hormones (LH) from the basophils; growth hormone–releasing factor (GHRF), which influences growth hormone (somatostatin, GH) secretion from the acidophils; melanocyte-stimulating hormone–releasing factor (MSHRF), which influences melanocyte-stimulating hormone (MSH) production; prolactin-inhibiting factor (PIF), which inhibits production of prolactin from the acidophils; somatic inhibiting–releasing factor (SIRF), also known as somatostatin (SS); growth hormone–inhibiting factor (GHIF) or somatotropin release–inhibiting factor (SRIF), which inhibits release of growth hormone (GH) and thyrotropin (TSH); and melanocyte-stimulating hormone release–inhibiting factor (MIF), which inhibits the release of melanocyte-stimulating hormone (MSH).

Secretion of growth hormone–releasing factor (GHRF) and growth hormone–inhibiting factor (GHIF) is stimulated by dopamine, norepinephrine, and serotonin. The prolactin-inhibiting factor (PIF) is dopamine.

Autonomic Regulation

The hypothalamus is known to control brain stem and spinal cord autonomic centers. Stimulation or ablation of the hypothalamus influences cardiovascular, respiratory, and gastrointestinal functions. Autonomic influences are mediated via the dorsal longitudinal fasciculus and the mamillotegmental tract. Although definite delineation within the hypothalamus of sympathetic and parasympathetic centers is not feasible, it is generally held that the rostral and medial hypothalamus is concerned with parasympathetic control, whereas the caudal and lateral hypothalamus is concerned with sympathetic control mechanisms.

Stimulation of the rostral and medial hypothalamus (preoptic and supraoptic areas) results in parasympathetic activation, characterized by a slowing of heart rate, decrease in blood pressure, vasodilatation, pupillary constriction, increased sweating, and increased motility and secretions of the alimentary tract. In contrast, stimulation of the posterior and lateral hypothalamus (particularly the posterior) results in sympathetic activation, characterized by an increase in heart rate and blood pressure, vasoconstriction, pupillary dilatation, piloerection, decreased motility and secretion of the alimentary tract, bladder inhibition, and heightened somatic reactions of shivering and running.

Temperature Regulation

Some regions of the hypothalamus contain thermal receptors that are sensitive to changes in the temperature of blood perfusing these regions. Anterior regions of the hypothalamus are sensitive to a rise in blood temperature and trigger mechanisms for heat dissipation, which include sweating and cutaneous vascular dilatation in humans. Bilateral damage to this region, through surgery or by tumors or vascular lesions, results in elevation of body temperature (hyperthermia). In contrast, the posterior hypothalamic region is sensitive to the lowering of blood temperature and triggers the mechanisms for heat conservation, which include cessation of sweating, shivering, and vascular constriction. Bilateral damage to this region results in **poikilothermia**, in which body temperature fluctuates with environmental temperature.

Poikilothermia (Greek *poikilos*, "varied"; *therme*, "heat"). Variation of body temperature with environmental temperature.

Emotional Behavior

The hypothalamus is a major component of the central autonomic nervous system and as such plays a role in emotional behavior. Lesions of the ventromedial hypothalamic nuclei in animals are associated with a rage reaction, characterized by hissing, snarling, biting, piloerection, arching of the back, and pupillary dilatation. In contrast, stimulation of lateral regions of the anterior hypothalamus elicits a flight response. Stimulation of some hypothalamic regions elicits a pleasurable response. Stimulation of other regions produces unpleasant responses. The role of the hypothalamus in behavior and emotion is intimately related to that of the limbic system.

Feeding Behavior

As detailed earlier, bilateral lesions in the ventromedial nucleus elicit hyperphagia (excessive feeding), whereas similar lesions in the lateral hypothalamic nucleus produce loss of hunger, suggesting the presence of a **satiety** center and feeding center, respectively, in these regions.

Satiety (Latin *satis*, "sufficient"; *ety*, "state or condition of"). Sufficiency or satisfaction or gratification of thirst or appetite.

Drinking and Thirst

In addition to the control of body water by ADH, stimulation of the lateral and anterior regions of the hypothalamus elicits drinking behavior that persists despite overhydration. Lesions of the same area abolish thirst.

Sleep and Wakefulness

The hypothalamus is believed to play a role in the daily sleep-wakefulness cycle. A sleep center is proposed to be in the anterior part of the hypothalamus and a waking center in the posterior part. The posterior waking center may be part of the ascending reticular activating system.

Circadian Rhythm

Through the connections of the suprachiasmatic nucleus with the retina and brain regions related to circadian rhythm, the hypothalamus plays an important role as an internal clock regulating cyclic variations of a number of bodily functions such as temperature cycle, sleep-wake cycle, and hormonal cyclic variations.

Memory

Through its connections with the hippocampal formation and anterior thalamic nucleus, the mamillary body of the hypothalamus plays a role in memory.

KEY CONCEPTS

- The hypothalamus is involved in a variety of functions that include (1) control of water reabsorption in the kidney through secretion of the antidiuretic hormone (ADH) or vasopressin, (2) contraction of uterine smooth muscle and ejection of milk from the lactating nipple through secretion of oxytocin, (3) control of anterior pituitary function through secretion of hypothalamic releasing factors, (4) control of brain stem and spinal cord autonomic centers related to cardiovascular, respiratory, and gastrointestinal functions, (5) control of body temperature through thermoreceptors that are sensitive to changes in temperature of blood perfusing the hypothalamus, (6) emotional behavior and the "fight or flight" reaction, (7) regulation of feeding behavior through the hypothalamic satiety and feeding centers, (8) regulation of drinking and thirst, (9) wakefulness and sleep through the hypothalamic centers for wakefulness and sleep, (10) circadian rhythm through the connections of the suprachiasmatic nucleus, and (11) memory through connections to the anterior thalamic nucleus and hippocampal formation.

SUGGESTED READINGS

Braak H, Braak E: The hypothalamus of the human adult: Chiasmatic region. *Anat Embryol* 1987; 175:315–330.

Dietrichs E, et al: Hypothalamocerebellar and cerebellohypothalamic projection circuits for regulating nonsomatic cerebellar activity? *Histol Histopathol* 1994; 9:603–614.

Hatton GL: Emerging concepts of structure-function dynamics in adult brain: The hypothalamo-neurohypophysial system. *Prog Neurobiol* 1990; 34:337–504.

Holstege G: Some anatomical observations on the projections from the hypothalamus to brain stem and spinal cord: An HRP and autoradiographic tracing study in the cat. *J Comp Neurol* 1987; 260:98–126.

Kordon C: Neural mechanisms involved in pituitary control. *Neurochem Int* 1985; 7:917–925.

Nauta WJH, Haymaker W: Hypothalamic nuclei and fiber connections. In Haymaker W, et al (eds): *The Hypothalamus.* Springfield, IL, Charles C Thomas, 1969:136.

Pickard GE, Silverman AJ: Direct retinal projections to the hypothalamus, piriform cortex, and accessory optic nuclei in the golden hamster as demonstrated by a sensitive anterograde horseradish peroxidase technique. *J Comp Neurol* 1981; 196:155–172.

Rafols JA, et al: A Golgi study of the monkey paraventricular nucleus: Neuronal types, afferent and efferent fibers. *J Comp Neurol* 1987; 257:595–613.

Saper CB, et al: Direct hypothalamo-autonomic connections. *Brain Res* 1976; 117:305–312.

CHAPTER 20

HYPOTHALAMUS: CLINICAL CORRELATES

A large number of clinical signs and symptoms have been reported in association with hypothalamic dysfunction. They include disturbances in (1) water balance, (2) thermoregulation, (3) caloric balance, (4) emotional behavior, (5) sleep, and (6) memory.

DISORDERS OF WATER BALANCE

Diabetes Insipidus

Diabetes insipidus results from lesions that destroy the majority of neurons of the supraoptic and paraventricular nuclei [sites of antidiuretic hormone (ADH)

Diabetes insipidus (Greek *diabetes*, "a syphon"). A condition of excessive production of urine from deficiency of the antidiuretic hormone.

KEY CONCEPTS

- A number of clinical signs and symptoms have been associated with lesions of the hypothalamus. They are related to disorders of water balance, temperature regulation, caloric balance, alertness and sleep, memory, and emotional behavior.

Polyuria (Greek *polys*, "many"; *ouron*, "urine"). The passage of a very large volume of urine, characteristic of diabetes.

Polydipsia (Greek *polys*, "many"; *dipsa*, "thirst"). Chronic excessive thirst, as in diabetes insipidus and mellitus.

secretion] or that interrupt the supraoptic-neurohypophysial tract. Affected patients pass large volumes of dilute urine (**polyuria**). Because the thirst mechanism is intact, patients drink large amounts of fluid (**polydipsia**). Such patients drink over 10 liters of water per day and excrete a similar amount of urine. In contrast to diabetes mellitus, values for glucose in blood and urine are normal in diabetes insipidus. The two types of diabetes were differentiated by Thomas Willis in 1674. The relation of diabetes insipidus to the neurohypophysis was recognized by the German physiologist Alfred Frank. Diabetes insipidus can be caused by a variety of disease processes, including hypothalamic tumors, trauma, storage diseases, and infection. A familial variety of diabetes insipidus may be due to a defect in the neurophysin gene precluding normal production of ADH. Treatment of diabetes insipidus consists of intranasal administration of a long-acting vasopressin analogue, desmopressin acetate (desamino-D-arginine vasopressin, DDAVP).

Syndrome of Inappropriate Secretion of ADH (SIADH)

This syndrome is due to lesions in the region of the supraoptic and paraventricular nuclei that impair hypothalamic osmoreceptors and that result in elevated ADH release. The syndrome is characterized by (1) hyponatremia, (2) low serum osmolarity, (3) normal renal excretion of sodium, (4) elevated urine osmolarity, and (5) absence of volume depletion.

DISORDERS OF THERMOREGULATION

Hypothermia

Shapiro syndrome. A hypothalamic syndrome characterized by recurrent hypothermia and agenesis of the corpus callosum. Named after W. R. Shapiro, who described the syndrome in 1969.

Hypothermia of hypothalamic origin may be chronic or periodic (episodic). Chronic hypothermia is associated with posterior hypothalamic injury from trauma, tumor, infection, or metabolic or vascular disease. Episodic hypothermia (**Shapiro syndrome,** diencephalic epilepsy) is characterized by spontaneous episodic hypothermia lasting minutes to days occurring at variable intervals (daily or decades). The condition may respond to antiepileptic drug therapy. The lesion in the hypothalamus may involve the arcuate nucleus and the premamillary area. Agenesis of the corpus callosum is often present.

Hyperthermia

Hyperthermia of hypothalamic origin may be sustained or episodic (periodic). Sustained hyperthermia usually is associated with head trauma or with surgery adjacent to the anterior hypothalamus. It usually lasts 1 to 2 days but may last up to

KEY CONCEPTS

- Two syndromes are related to disorders of water balance: diabetes insipidus and the syndrome of inappropriate antidiuretic hormone (ADH) secretion (SIADH). The lesion in the former is in the supraoptic and paraventricular nuclei or the supraopticohypophysial tract. The lesion in SIADH involves hypothalamic osmoreceptors in the region of the supraoptic and paraventricular nuclei.
- Disturbances in hypothalamic thermoregulation may result in hypothermia, hyperthermia, or poikilothermia related to pathology in different regions of the hypothalamus. In general, chronic hypothermia and poikilothermia are related to posterior hypothalamic pathology, whereas sustained hyperthermia is related to pathology in the anterior hypothalamus.

2 weeks. Episodic hyperthermia has been associated with lesions in the ventromedial hypothalamus.

Poikilothermia

Fluctuations in body temperature with changes in environmental temperature are associated with bilateral posterior hypothalamic lesions.

Poikilothermia (Greek *poikilos*, "varied"; *therme*, "heat"). Variation of body temperature with environmental temperature.

DISORDERS OF CALORIC BALANCE

Diencephalic Syndrome of Infancy

This condition is characterized by progressive emaciation during the first year of life despite a reasonable food intake. Despite their emaciation, such children are characteristically happy and active. Other associated clinical signs include poor temperature regulation, vomiting, and nystagmus. Growth hormone may be normal or elevated. The etiology of this syndrome is usually a slowly growing tumor of the anterior hypothalamus. Other lesions interrupting projections from or to the anterior hypothalamus can produce the syndrome.

Fröhlich Syndrome (Babinski-Fröhlich Syndrome, Dystrophia-Adiposogenitalis)

Fröhlich syndrome is characterized by obesity, genital hypoplasia, and stunted growth as a result of hypothalamic or pituitary lesion. Obesity in this syndrome is attributed to damage to the ventromedial nucleus of the thalamus (satiety center) and hypogonadism to the involvement of the adjacent infundibulum.

Fröhlich syndrome. A hypothalamic syndrome characterized by obesity, genital hypoplasia, and stunted growth. Named after Alfred Fröhlich (1871–1953), the Viennese neurologist and pharmacologist. Also known as *Babinski-Fröhlich syndrome.*

DISORDERS OF EMOTIONAL BEHAVIOR

Lesions in the ventromedial region of the hypothalamus have been associated with rage, whereas lesions in the posterior hypothalamus have been associated with fear and apathy.

DISORDERS OF SLEEP

Sleep disturbances associated with hypothalamic lesions were attributed previously to concomitant involvement of the ascending reticular pathways. Accumulating evidence, however, points to the existence of a waking center in the posterior hypothalamus. Lesions of the posterior hypothalamus provoke lethargy and hypersomnia, whereas lesions in the anterior hypothalamus cause insomnia.

KEY CONCEPTS

- Disturbances in hypothalamic caloric balance are associated with two syndromes: emaciation (diencephalic syndrome) and obesity (Fröhlich syndrome). The former is related to pathology in the anterior hypothalamus or its connections; the latter is related to pathology in the ventromedial nucleus.
- Disorders of emotional behavior include rage reaction after ventromedial region pathology and fear and apathy after posterior hypothalamic pathology.
- Disturbances in sleep are associated with hypersomnolence (posterior hypothalamus), insomnia (anterior hypothalamus), and the Kleine-Levin syndrome.

Kleine-Levin Syndrome

Kleine-Levin syndrome. A hypothalamic syndrome occurring in adolescent males and, less frequently, in females characterized by episodic hypersomnolence, hypersexuality, and compulsive eating. The syndrome was described by Willi Kleine, the German neuropsychiatrist, in 1925. Max Levin, the American neurologist, reported another case in 1929 and summarized the features of the syndrome in 1936.

Hypothalamic lesions have been associated with **Kleine-Levin syndrome** which is characterized by episodic compulsive eating (**bulimia**), hypersomnolence, and hypersexuality in adolescent males and, rarely, in females. A similar syndrome occurs with lesions in the medial thalamus. Each episode lasts 1 to 2 weeks at intervals of 3 to 6 months between episodes. The episodes decrease in frequency with age and usually disappear by the fourth decade. Some evidence indicates that the dopaminergic tone of the hypothalamus is reduced during the symptomatic phase of the syndrome.

DISORDERS OF MEMORY

Hypothalamic lesions in the posterior hypothalamus involving the mamillary bodies or the fornix are associated with inability to establish (encode) new memories for personally experienced, context- and time-specific events (episodic memory) such as the memory of eating a specific dish at a specific restaurant. The connections of the mamillary bodies with the hippocampus (via the fornix) and with the anterior

TABLE 20-1

Hypothalamic Disorders

Hypothalamic Function	Hypothalamic Disorder	Site of Pathology
Water balance	Diabetes insipidus	Supraoptic and paraventricular nuclei
	Syndrome of inappropriate secretion of ADH (SIADH)	Supraoptic and paraventricular nuclei or neighborhood
Thermoregulation	Hypothermia	
	Chronic	Posterior hypothalamus
	Episodic	Arcuate nucleus, premamillary area
	Hyperthermia	
	Sustained	Anterior hypothalamus
	Episodic	Ventromedial hypothalamus
	Poikilothermia	Posterior hypothalamus
Caloric balance	Diencephalic syndrome of infancy	Anterior hypothalamus
	Fröhlich syndrome	Ventromedial nucleus, infundibulum
Emotional behavior	Rage	Ventromedial nucleus
	Fear, apathy	Posterior hypothalamus
Sleep	Hypersomnolence	Posterior hypothalamus
	Insomnia	Anterior hypothalamus
Memory	Loss of episodic memory	Mamillary bodies, fornix

thalamic nucleus (via the mamillothalamic tract) make them crucial to the process of acquisition of recent memory.

The different hypothalamic disorders discussed herein and corresponding sites of hypothalamic pathology are summarized in Table 20-1.

Bulimia (Greek *bous*, "ox"; *limos*, "hunger"). A disorder of eating occurring predominantly in adolescent females characterized by morbid hunger and binge eating that continue until terminated by abdominal pain, vomiting, or sleep.

KEY CONCEPTS

- Disturbances in episodic memory are associated with lesions in the mammillary body or fornix.

SUGGESTED READINGS

Arroyo HA, et al: A syndrome of hyperhidrosis, hypothermia, and bradycardia possibly due to central monoaminergic dysfunction. *Neurology* 1990; 40:556–557.

Bartter FC, Schwartz WB: The syndrome of inappropriate secretion of antidiuretic hormone. *Am J Med* 1967; 42:790–806.

Bauer HG: Endocrine and other clinical manifestations of hypothalamic disease. *J Clin Endocrinol Metab* 1954; 14:13–31.

Burr IM, et al: Diencephalic syndrome revisited. *J Pediatr* 1976; 88:439–444.

Chesson AL, et al: Neuroendocrine evaluation in Kleine-Levin syndrome: Evidence of reduced dopaminergic tone during periods of hypersomnolence. *Sleep* 1991; 14:226–232.

Culebras A: Neuroanatomic and neurologic correlates of sleep disturbances. *Neurology* 1992; 42(suppl 6):19–27.

Gaffan EA, et al: Amnesia following damage to the left fornix and to other sites. *Brain* 1991; 114:1297–1313.

Gamstorp I, et al: Diencephalic syndrome of infancy. *J Pediatr* 1967; 70:383–390.

Gillberg C: Kleine-Levin syndrome: Unrecognized diagnosis in adolescent psychiatry. *J Am Acad Child Adolesc Psychiatry* 1987; 26:793–794.

Harris AS: Clinical experience with desmopressin: Efficacy and safety in central diabetes insipidus and other conditions. *J Pediatr* 1989; 114:711–718.

LeWitt PA, et al: Episodic hyperhidrosis, hypothermia, and agenesis of the corpus callosum. *Neurology* 1983; 33:1122–1129.

Maghnie M, et al: Correlation between magnetic resonance imaging of posterior pituitary and neurohypophysial function in children with diabetes insipidus. *J Clin Endocrinol Metab* 1992; 74:795–800.

Perry RJ, Hodges JR: Spectrum of memory dysfunction in degenerative disease. *Curr Opin Neurol* 1996; 9:281–285.

Reeves AG, Plum F: Hyperphagia, rage, and dementia accompanying a ventromedial hypothalamic neoplasm. *Arch Neurol* 1969; 20:616–624.

Russel A: A diencephalic syndrome of emaciation in infancy and childhood. *Arch Dis Child* 1951; 26:274.

Shapiro WR, et al: Spontaneous recurrent hypothermia accompanying agenesis of the corpus callosum. *Brain* 1969; 92:423–436.

CHAPTER 21

LIMBIC SYSTEM

DEFINITION OF TERMS: LIMBIC LOBE, LIMBIC SYSTEM, AND RHINENCEPHALON

The concept of the limbic system is derived from the limbic lobe. The term *limbic lobe,* coined by Broca in 1878, refers to a number of structures on the medial and basal surfaces of the hemisphere that form a limbus (border or ring) around the brain stem. The limbic lobe and all lthe structures connected to it constitute the limbic system, which plays a major role in visceral function, emotional behavior, and memory.

Because of the large size of the limbic lobe in phylogenetically lower animals, Broca postulated that it might have an olfactory function; hence, the terms *limbic lobe* and *smell brain* (rhinencephalon) were used synonymously. In humans, the limbic lobe has very little if any primary olfactory function. The rhinencephalon, by contrast, is primarily concerned with olfaction but has some reciprocal relationships with parts of other limbic system regions.

RHINENCEPHALON (SMELL BRAIN)

The **rhinencephalon** (Fig. 21-1) consists of the following structures:

Rhinencephalon (Greek *rhin,* "nose"; *enkephalos,* "brain"). The smell brain. The part of the brain concerned with the olfactory system.

1. Olfactory nerve rootlets
2. Olfactory bulb
3. Olfactory tract

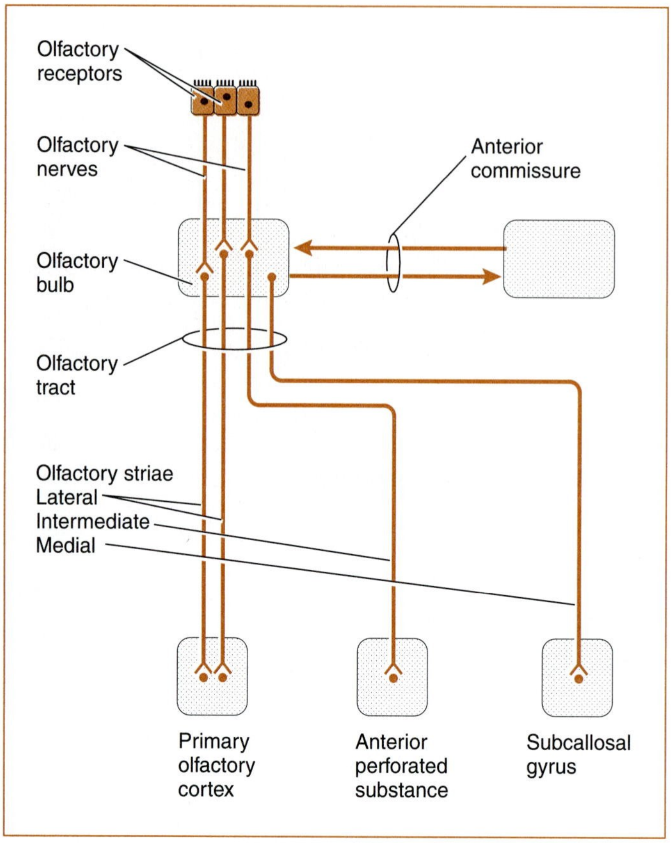

FIGURE 21-1

Schematic diagram of olfactory pathways.

4. Olfactory striae
5. Primary olfactory cortex

Olfactory Nerve Rootlets

The olfactory nerve is composed of unmyelinated thin processes (rootlets) of the olfactory hair cells (receptors) in the nasal mucosa. Fascicles of the olfactory nerve pierce the cribriform plate of the ethmoid bone, enter the cranial cavity, and terminate on neurons in the olfactory bulb.

Olfactory Bulb

The olfactory bulb is the main relay station in the olfactory pathways.

Lamination and Cell Types

In histologic sections (Fig. 21-2), the olfactory bulb appears to be laminated into the following layers:

1. The olfactory nerve layer is composed of incoming olfactory nerve fibers.
2. In the glomerular layer synaptic formations occur between the olfactory nerve axons and the dendrites of olfactory bulb neurons (mitral and tufted neurons).
3. The external plexiform layer consists of tufted neurons, some granule cells, and a few mitral cells with their processes.
4. The **mitral cell** layer is composed of large neurons (mitral neurons).
5. The granule layer is composed of small granule neurons and processes of granule and mitral cells; it also contains incoming fibers from other cortical regions.

Mitral cells (Latin *mitra,* "a cap"). Mitral cells in the olfactory bulb have a cap-like shape.

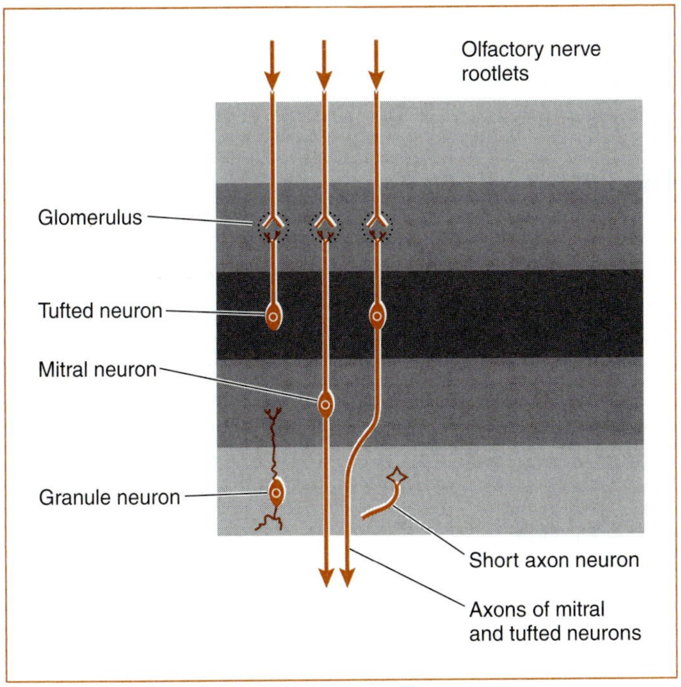

FIGURE 21-2

Schematic diagram of olfactory bulb showing laminae and types of cells.

The mitral cells and tufted cells are considered the principal neurons of the olfactory bulb. Their dendrites establish synaptic relationships with olfactory nerve fibers within the glomeruli.

The granule cells are considered the intrinsic neurons of the olfactory bulb. These cells have vertically oriented dendrites but no axon and exert their action on other cells solely by means of dendrites. Another type of intrinsic neuron, the short axon neuron, is found in the glomerular layer (periglomerular short axon neuron) and the granular layer.

The olfactory bulb receives fibers (input) from the following sources:

1. Olfactory hair cells in the nasal mucosa
2. Contralateral olfactory bulb
3. Primary olfactory cortex
4. Diagonal band of Broca
5. Anterior olfactory nucleus

The output from the olfactory bulb is composed of axons of the mitral cells and tufted cells (principal neurons), which project to the following areas:

1. Contralateral olfactory bulb
2. Subcallosal gyrus
3. Anterior perforated substance
4. Primary olfactory cortex
5. Anterior entorhinal cortex

Neuronal Population

Quantitative studies in the rabbit have revealed that there are 50 million olfactory hair cells in the nasal mucosa. Since there is a 1 : 1 ratio between olfactory receptor cells and olfactory nerve fibers, it follows that 50 million olfactory nerve fibers enter the olfactory bulb. The number of principal neurons in the olfactory bulb is estimated to be 50,000 (48,000 tufted cells and 2000 mitral cells), suggesting a convergence ratio of 1000 olfactory nerve fibers on a single principal neuron. There are more intrinsic neurons than principal neurons in the olfactory bulb. The ratio varies from 25 periglomerular cells per 1 principal neuron to 200 granule cells per 1 principal neuron.

Olfactory Tract

The olfactory tract is the outflow pathway of the olfactory bulb. It is composed of the axons of principal neurons (mitral cells and tufted cells) of the olfactory bulb and centrifugal axons originating from central brain regions. The olfactory tract also contains the scattered neurons of the anterior olfactory nucleus, the axons of which travel in the olfactory tract, cross in the anterior commissure, and project on the contralateral anterior olfactory nucleus and the olfactory bulb. At its caudal extremity, just anterior to the anterior perforated substance, the olfactory tract divides into the olfactory striae.

Olfactory Striae

At its caudal extremity, just rostral to the anterior perforated substance, the olfactory tract divides into three striae:

1. Lateral olfactory stria
2. Medial olfactory stria
3. Intermediate olfactory stria.

Each stria is covered by a thin layer of gray matter known as an olfactory gyrus.

The lateral olfactory stria projects to the primary olfactory cortex in the temporal lobe. The medial olfactory stria projects on the medial olfactory area, which also is known as the septal area, on the medial surface of the frontal lobe, ventral to the genu and rostrum of the corpus callosum and anterior to the lamina terminalis. The medial olfactory area is closely related to the limbic system and thus is concerned with emotional responses elicited by olfactory stimuli. It does not play a role in the perception of olfactory stimuli. The medial and intermediate striae are poorly developed in humans. The intermediate stria blends with the anterior perforated substance. The thin cortex at this site is designated the intermediate olfactory area. The three areas of olfactory cortex are interconnected by the diagonal band of Broca, a bundle of subcortical fibers in front of the optic tract.

Olfactory Cortex

Pyriform (Latin *pirum,* "a pear"; *forma,* "shape"). Pear-shaped. The pyriform gyrus of the temporal lobe is pear-shaped.

The olfactory cortex is located within the temporal lobe and is composed of the **pyriform** cortex, the periamygdaloid area, and part of the entorhinal area. The pyriform cortex is the region on each side of and beneath the lateral olfactory stria; hence, it is also called the lateral olfactory gyrus. The periamygdaloid area is dorsal and rostral to the amygdaloid nuclear complex. The pyriform cortex and the periamygdaloid area constitute the primary olfactory cortex. The entorhinal area, which is situated in the rostral part of the parahippocampal gyrus, corresponds to Brodmann's area 28. It constitutes the secondary olfactory cortex. The olfactory

KEY CONCEPTS

- The term *rhinencephalon* refers to the structures concerned with olfaction. These structures include the olfactory receptor organ and the olfactory nerve, bulb, striae, and cortex.

cortex is relatively large in some animals, such as the rabbit, but in humans it occupies a small area. The primary olfactory cortex in humans is concerned with the conscious perception of olfactory stimuli. In contrast to all other primary sensory cortices (vision, audition, taste, and somatic sensibility), the primary olfactory cortex is unique in that afferent fibers from the receptors reach it directly without passing through a relay in the thalamus.

The primary olfactory cortex contains two types of neurons: (1) principal neurons (pyramidal cells) with axons which leave the olfactory cortex and project to nearby or distant regions and (2) intrinsic neurons (stellate cells) with axons which remain within the olfactory cortex.

The major input to the primary olfactory cortex is from (1) the olfactory bulb via the lateral olfactory stria and (2) other central brain regions.

The output from the primary olfactory cortex is via axons of principal neurons which project to (1) the secondary olfactory cortex in the entorhinal area, (2) the amygdaloid nucleus, and (3) the dorsomedial nucleus of the thalamus.

The output of the secondary olfactory cortex, the entorhinal area, is to the (1) hippocampal formation and (2) the anterior insular and frontal cortices.

The connections of the olfactory cortex with the thalamus, the amygdaloid nucleus, the hippocampal formation, and the insular and frontal cortices provide the anatomic basis for a role of olfaction in emotional behavior, visceral function, and memory.

Quantitative studies of the primary olfactory cortex have revealed that (1) there is a predominance of principal neurons (compared with the intrinsic variety) and (2) the number of principal neurons far exceeds the number of fibers in the lateral olfactory stria. Thus, in contrast to the olfactory bulb, in which there is a high convergence ratio, the ratio of intput to output in the primary olfactory cortex is low. This is similar to the pattern in the neocortex and the climbing fiber system of the cerebellar cortex.

LIMBIC LOBE

As described by Broca in 1878, the **limbic** lobe refers to the gray matter in the medial and basal parts of the hemisphere that forms a limbus (border) around the brain stem. The limbic lobe is a synthetic lobe whose component parts are derived from different lobes of the brain (frontal, parietal, temporal). There is no general agreement on all the parts that enter into the formation of the limbic lobe. The following, however, are generally accepted as limbic lobe components (see Fig. 2-11):

1. Subcallosal gyrus, inferior to the genu and rostrum of the corpus callosum, just anterior to the lamina terminalis
2. **Cingulate gyrus**
3. **Isthmus** of the cingulate gyrus, posterior and inferior to the splenium of the corpus callosum
4. Parahippocampal gyrus (and the underlying hippocampal formation and dentate gyrus)
5. **Uncus**

Limbic (Latin *limbus*, "fringe, border, margin"). The limbic lobe forms a margin around the brain stem.

Cingulate gyrus (Latin, "belt or girdle"). A four-layered paleocortex above the corpus callosum. Part of the limbic lobe.

Isthmus (Greek *isthmos*, "a narrow connection between two larger bodies or parts"). The isthmus of the cingulate gyrus is its constricted portion between the cingulate and parahippocampal gyri.

Uncus (Latin, "hook"). The medially curved anterior end of the parahippocampal gyrus.

KEY CONCEPTS

- The term *limbic lobe* refers to the structures that form a limbus (ring or border) around the brain stem. These structures include the subcallosal gyrus, cingulate gyrus, isthmus, parahippocampal gyrus, and uncus.

The limbic lobe is formed of archicortex (hippocampal formation and dentate gyrus), paleocortex (rostral parahippocampal gyrus and uncus), and juxtallocortex or mesocortex (cingulate gyrus).

Originally, the limbic lobe was assigned a purely olfactory function. Recently, it has been established that only a minor part of the limbic lobe has an olfactory function. The rest of the limbic lobe, which forms part of the limbic system, plays a role in emotional behavior and memory.

Papez circuit. A circuit connecting the hippocampus with the hypothalamus, thalamus, and cingulate gyrus. Described by James Papez, an American neuroanatomist, in 1937. The circuit subsequently laid the basis for the concept of the limbic lobe.

THE PAPEZ CIRCUIT

In 1937, James Papez, an American neuroanatomist, described a closed circuit of connections starting and ending in the hippocampus that later became known as Papez circuit. It was suggested that the structures connected by this circuit play a role in emotional reactions. The circuit consisted of outflow of impulses from the hippocampus via the fornix to the mamillary bodies of the hypothalamus; from there, via the mamillothalamic tract, to the anterior thalamic nucleus; and, via the thalamocortical fiber system, to the cingulate gyrus, from which impulses returned to the hippocampus via the entorhinal area. The circuit which has been modified since its introduction, provided the basis for the concept of the limbic system introduced in the early 1950s.

LIMBIC SYSTEM

The limbic system is defined as the limbic lobe and all the cortical and subcortical structures related to it. These include the following structures:

1. Septal nuclei
2. Amygdala
3. Hypothalamus (particularly the mamillary body)
4. Thalamus (particularly the anterior and medial thalamic nuclei)
5. Brain stem reticular formation
6. Epithalamus
7. Neocortical areas in the basal frontotemporal region
8. Olfactory cortex
9. Ventral parts of the striatum

This conglomerate of neural structures, which constitute the old part of the brain and are highly interconnected, seems to play a role in the following processes:

1. Emotional behavior
2. Memory
3. Integration of homeostatic responses such as those related to preservation of the species, securing food, and the fight or flight response.
4. Sexual behavior
5. Motivation

The underlying mechanisms for these different functions are very complex and are inadequately understood. Furthermore, it has become difficult to define the

KEY CONCEPTS

- The term *Papez circuit* refers to a closed circuit of connections that begins and ends in the hippocampus.
- The term *limbic system* refers to the limbic lobe and the structures connected to it.
- Limbic system structures play important roles in emotional behavior, memory, homeostatic responses, sexual behavior, and motivation.

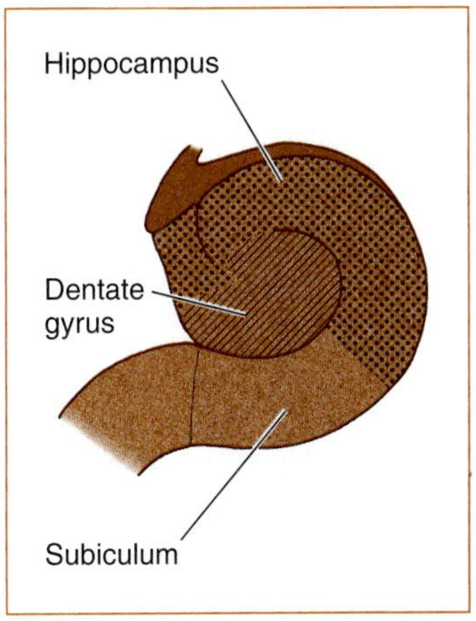

FIGURE 21-3

Schematic diagram showing the components of the hippocampal formation.

extent of the limbic system with precision and to attribute common connections and functions to its individual components. Some researchers have advocated the theory that the limbic system is not useful as a scientific or clinical concept.

The presentation of the limbic system in this chapter focuses on the following components: hippocampal formation, amygdala, and septal area. These are the regions that are most closely related to the limbic lobe.

Hippocampal Formation

The hippocampal formation (Fig. 21-3) is an infolding of the parahippocampal gyrus into the inferior (temporal) horn of the lateral ventricle and consists of three regions: **hippocampus**, **dentate gyrus**, and **subiculum**. The dentate gyrus occupies the interval between the hippocampus and the parahippocampal gyrus. Its name is derived from its toothed or beaded surface. The subiculum is the part of the parahippocampal gyrus that is in direct continuity with the hippocampus.

Of the three components of the hippocampal formation, the hippocampus is the largest in and the best studied in humans. Therefore, it is presented in this chapter as the prototype of this segment of the limbic system.

The hippocampus appears as a C-shaped structure in coronal sections, bulging into the inferior horn of the lateral ventricle. The hippocampus is closely associated with the adjacent dentate gyrus (Fig. 21-4), and together they form an S-shaped structure.

Hippocampal Terminology

In the late 1500s, the anatomist Arantius exposed a convoluted structure in the floor of the temporal horn of the lateral ventricle. He called this structure the hippocampus because of its resemblance to a sea horse. A century later the term

Hippocampus (Greek, "sea horse"). Part of the hippocampal formation. The inferiomesial part of the parahippocampal gyrus. So named because of its resemblance to a sea horse. The structure was first observed by Achillini and named by Arantius.

Dentate gyrus (Latin *dentatus,* "having teeth"; Greek *gyros,* "circle"). The three-layered archicortex of the temporal lobe. A component of the hippocampal formation.

Subiculum (Latin *subicere,* "to raise or lift"). An underlying or supporting structure.

KEY CONCEPTS

- The limbic system structures most closely related to the limbic lobe are the hippocampal formation, amygdala, and septal area.
- The term *hippocampal formation* refers to the hippocampus, dentate gyrus, and subiculum.

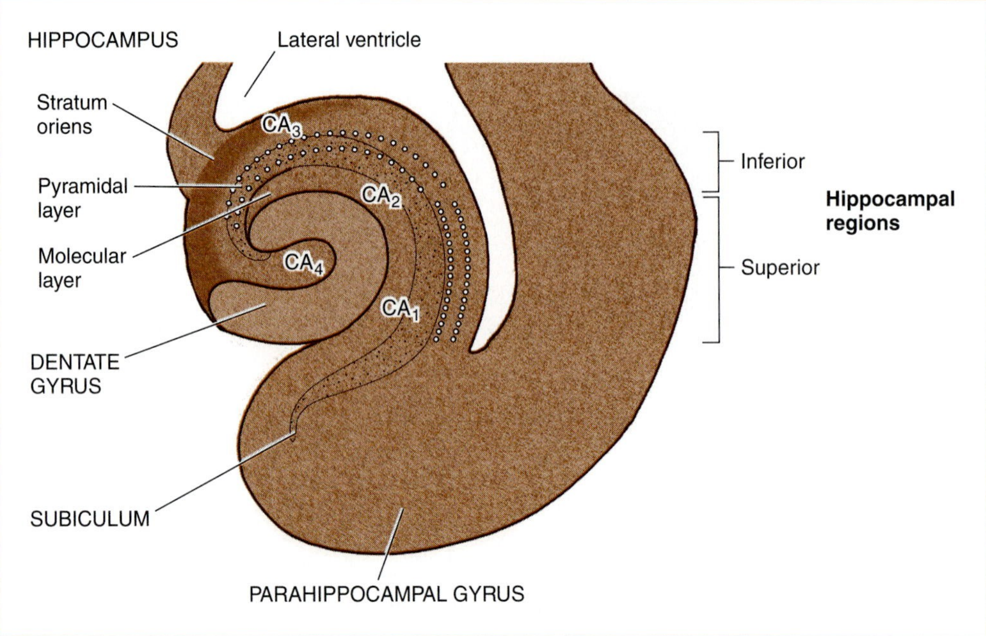

FIGURE 21-4

Schematic diagram showing layers of the hippocampus and the division of the hippocampus into superior and inferior regions, and four fields (CA_1 to CA_4).

Cornu Ammonis. Ammon's horn. Anatomists likened the hippocampus to a ram's horn or to the horns of the ancient Egyptian deity Ammon, who had a ram's head.

pes hippocampus was used to describe the same structure, and two centuries later anatomists likened the structure to a ram's horn or the horns of the ancient Egyptian deity Ammon, who had a ram's head, hence the name *Ammon's horn* or **cornu Ammonis.** Terminology over the years became abundant and often confusing. Table 21-1 lists the preferred terminology and synonyms used for hippocampal structures.

Lamination and Divisions

Although Ramon y Cajal described seven laminae in the hippocampus, it is customary to combine the different laminae into three major layers (Fig. 21-4): the molecular layer, the pyramidal cell layer, and the stratum oriens (polymorphic layer).

The pyramidal cell layer is divided into a zone in which the pyramidal cells are compact and a zone (rostral to the compact zone) in which the pyramidal cells are less compact. The boundary between the compact and less compact zones of the pyramidal layer separates the two divisions of the hippocampus (Fig. 21-4) into the superior division (compact zone) and the inferior division (less compact zone).

The hippocampus has been subdivided further into fields (Fig. 21-4) designated as cornu Ammonis 1, 2, 3, and 4 (CA_1 through CA_4). CA_1, the largest hippocampal field in humans, is located in the superior division at the interface between the hippocampus and the subiculum. CA_2 and CA_3 are in the inferior division within the hippocampus. CA_4 constitutes the transition zone between the hippocampus and the dentate gyrus. Field CA_1 (also known as **Sommer's sector** and the vulnerable

Sommer's sector. Field CA_1 of the hippocampus. Also known as the vulnerable sector because of its sensitivity to anoxia and ischemia. Named after Wilhelm Sommer, a German physician.

KEY CONCEPTS

- The hippocampus is divided into four fields designated cornu Ammonis (CA) 1 to 4. The CA_1 field, also known as Sommer's sector, is highly vulnerable to anoxia and ischemia and is the trigger zone for some forms of temporal lobe epilepsy.

TABLE 21-1

Terminology of Hippocampal Structures

Structure	Preferred Terminology	Synonyms
Hippocampus	Hippocampus	Hippocampal formation Ram's horn Ammon's horn Cornu Ammonis Pes hippocampus Pes hippocampus major
Cornu Ammonis	Cornu Ammonis	Ammon's horn Hippocampus proper Hippocampus
Cornu Ammonis 1 (CA_1)	CA_1	Sommer's sector Vulnerable sector
Cornu Ammonis 2 (CA_2)	CA_2	
Cornu Ammonis 3 (CA_3)	CA_3	Resistent sector Spielmeyer sector
Cornu Ammonis 4 (CA_4)	CA_4	Hilus of fascia dentata End folium Bratz sector
Dentate gyrus	Dentate gyrus	Gyrus dentatus Fascia dentata
Commissure of fornix	Hippocampal commissure	Psalterium Lyre of David

sector) is of interest to neuropathologists because its pyramidal neurons are highly sensitive to anoxia and ischemia and because it is the trigger zone for some forms of temporal lobe epilepsy. CA_2 and CA_3 have been referred to as resistant sectors because they are less sensitive to anoxia. CA_4 (the **Bratz sector**) is also called the medium vulnerability sector because of its medium sensitivity to hypoxia.

Bratz sector. Cornu Ammonis field CA_4. Also known as the medium vulnerability (to anoxia) sector.

Neuronal Population

There are basically two types of neurons in the hippocampus: the principal neurons (pyramidal cell) and the intrinsic neurons (polymorphic cell, basket cell) (Fig. 21-5).

Principal Neurons The pyramidal neurons in the pyramidal cell layer are the principal neurons of the hippocampus. They are the only neurons with axons which contribute to the outflow tract from the hippocampus. Pyramidal neurons vary in size and density in different regions of the hippocampus. They are smaller and more densely packed in the superior region than in the inferior region. The largest neurons in the inferior region are referred to as the giant pyramidal cells of the hippocampus.

Basal dendrites of pyramidal neurons are oriented toward the ventricular surface; apical dendrites are oriented toward the molecular layer. Both types of dendrites arborize extensively and are rich in dendritic spines.

Axons of pyramidal cells are directed toward the ventricular surface, where they gather to form the alverus and fimbria and finally join the fornix as the outflow

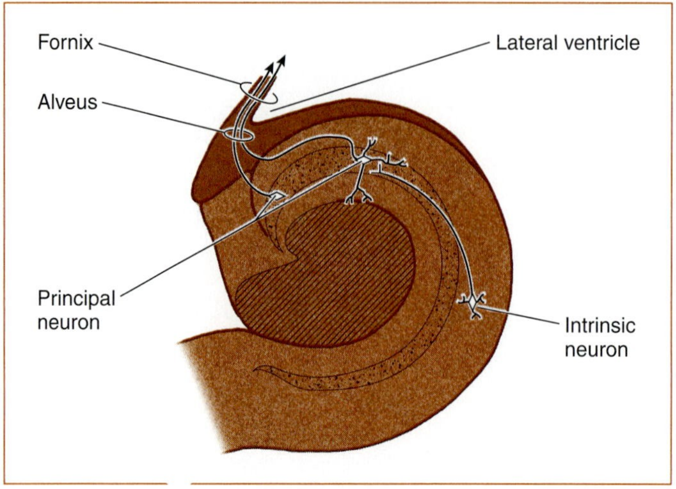

FIGURE 21-5

Schematic diagram showing the major types of neurons in the hippocampus and their interrelationships.

tract from the hippocampus. Recurrent axon collaterals terminate within the stratum oriens or reach the molecular layer. They exert a facilitatory influence.

It is estimated that the hippocampus of humans contains 1.2 million principal neurons on each side, a figure close to the number of pyramidal tract fibers.

Intrinsic Neurons Intrinsic neurons have axons which remain within the hippocampus. Because of the irregularity of their perikarya and dendrites, they are referred to as polymorphic neurons. They are situated in the stratum oriens (Fig. 21-5). Their irregularly oriented dendrites arborize locally, while their axons ramify between pyramidal neurons and arborize around the perikarya of pyramidal neurons in a basket formation (hence the term *basket cells*). They are inhibitory (GABAergic) to pyramidal cell activity. There are no estimates of the exact number of intrinsic neurons in the hippocampus. It has been estimated, however, that one basket cell is related to about 200 to 500 pyramidal cells. Thus, it is believed that the intrinsic neurons are much fewer in number than are the principal neurons.

Like the hippocampus, the dentate gyrus is a three-layered structure composed of a molecular layer, a granular cell layer, and a polymorphic layer. The molecular layer is continuous with that of the hippocampus. The granular layer is made up of small, densely packed granular cells whose axons form the mossy fiber system which links the dentate gyrus and the hippocampus. The cells in the polymorphic layer are varied and include pyramidal and basket cells. Unlike the hippocampus, the output of the dentate gyrus does not leave the hippocampal formation.

In cross sections, the subiculum appears as a wing-shaped magnicellular structure. Like the hippocampus and the dentate gyrus, the subiculum is composed of three layers: a molecular layer, a pyramidal layer, and a polymorphic layer. The polymorphic layer originates in the adjoining entorhinal cortex. Axons of pyramidal neurons in the subiculum, like those in the hippocampus, contribute to the output of the hippocampal formation.

Entorhinal cortex. The rostral part of the parahippocampal gyrus in the temporal lobe. It corresponds to Brodmann's area 28.

Afferent Pathways

The bulk of extrinsic input to the hippocampal formation comes from the **entorhinal** area (Brodmann's area 28) of the parahippocampal gyrus and, to a lesser extent, the septal area (Fig. 21-6). Other inputs include those from the contralateral hippo-

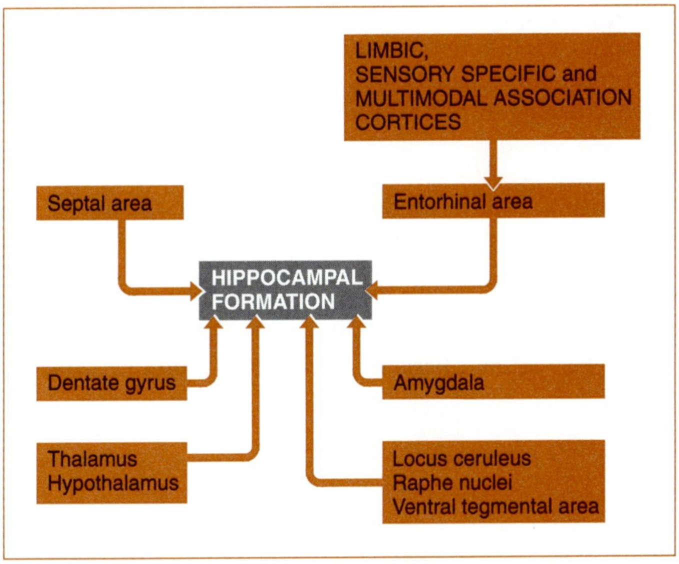

FIGURE 21-6

Schematic diagram showing the major afferents to the hippocampal formation.

campus, hypothalamus, amygdala, thalamus, locus ceruleus, raphe nuclei, and ventral tegmental area of Tsai.

Parahippocampal Gyrus

Fibers from the parahippocampal gyrus arise mainly from its rostral part, the entorhinal area (Brodmann's area 28). They constitute the major input to the hippocampus, dentate gyrus, and subiculum, which they reach by two routes. The main input travels through (perforates) the adjacent subicular area en route to the hippocampus and dentate gyrus and is therefore called the perforant path. A smaller input arrives in the hippocampus at the ventricular surface, where the alveus (axons of hippocampal pyramidal neurons) is formed, and is therefore called the alvear path. The existence of an alvear path has been questioned. The entorhinal area serves as an important gateway between the cerebral cortex and the hippocampus. Information from many cortical areas (limbic, modality sensory-specific, and multimodal association cortices) in the frontal, temporal, parietal, and occipital lobes converges on the entorhinal cortex and the posterior parahippocampal gyrus. The entorhinal cortex in turn conveys this cortical information to the hippocampus.

Septal Area

Fibers from the septal nuclei reach the hippocampus via the fornix. Compared with the input from the entorhinal area, the septal input is modest.

Dentate Gyrus

Axons of small pyramidal neurons (granule cells) in the dentate gyrus reach the hippocampus via the mossy fiber pathway.

KEY CONCEPTS

- The bulk of extrinsic input to the hippocampal formation comes from the entorhinal area and the septal area.

Contralateral Hippocampus

The two hippocampi are in communication via the hippocampal commissure (commissure of the fornix). Interhippocampal communication in humans is minimal, and the hippocampal commissure is thus rudimentary.

Hypothalamus

Fibers from the hypothalamus originate from cell groups in the vicinity of the mamillary body and exert a strong inhibitory influence on the hippocampus.

Amygdala

Amygdalohippocampal connections travel in the adjacent temporal lobe white matter and may form the anatomic basis for the effect of emotion on memory function.

Thalamus

Thalamic input to the hippocampus has been shown to originate in the anterior thalamic nucleus.

Locus Ceruleus

Noradrenergic fibers from the locus ceruleus have been traced to the hippocampus and the dentate gyrus.

Raphe Nuclei

Serotonergic fibers from the raphe nuclei also have been traced to the hippocampus.

Ventral Tegmental Area

Dopaminergic fibers from the ventral tegmental area of Tsai in the midbrain have been traced to the hippocampus.

The noradrenergic, serotoninergic, and dopaminergic inputs exert a modulatory effect on memory function in the hippocampus.

Efferent Pathways

The output from the hippocampal formation consists of axons of pyramidal neurons in the hippocampus and subicultum (Fig. 21-7). Axons of granule neurons in the dentate gyrus have no extrinsic connections but terminate locally as mossy fibers on hippocampal pyramidal neurons. Both the hippocampus and the subiculum project on the entorhinal cortex. From there, impulses are mediated to limbic, sensory-specific, and multimodal association cortical areas. Another major output from the hippocampus is to the subiculum. Both the hippocampus and the subiculum contribute fibers to the fornix, the output tract of the hippocampal formation. Subiculum-originating fibers constitute the major component of the fornix and are distributed, via its postcommissural division, to the mamillary bodies of the hypothalamus and the anterior nucleus of the thalamus. Hippocampal originating

KEY CONCEPTS

- Pyramidal neurons in the hippocampus receive excitatory inputs from the dentate gyrus (via the mossy fiber system) and from the entorhinal area (via the perforant path) as well as local input from inhibitory hippocampal basket cells. The axons of hippocampal pyramidal neurons constitute the only output pathway of the hippocampus.
- The output of the hippocampal formation is composed of axons of pyramidal neurons in the hippocampus and subiculum.
- The major targets of the hippocampal formation's output are the entorhinal cortex, the hypothalamus, and the septal area.

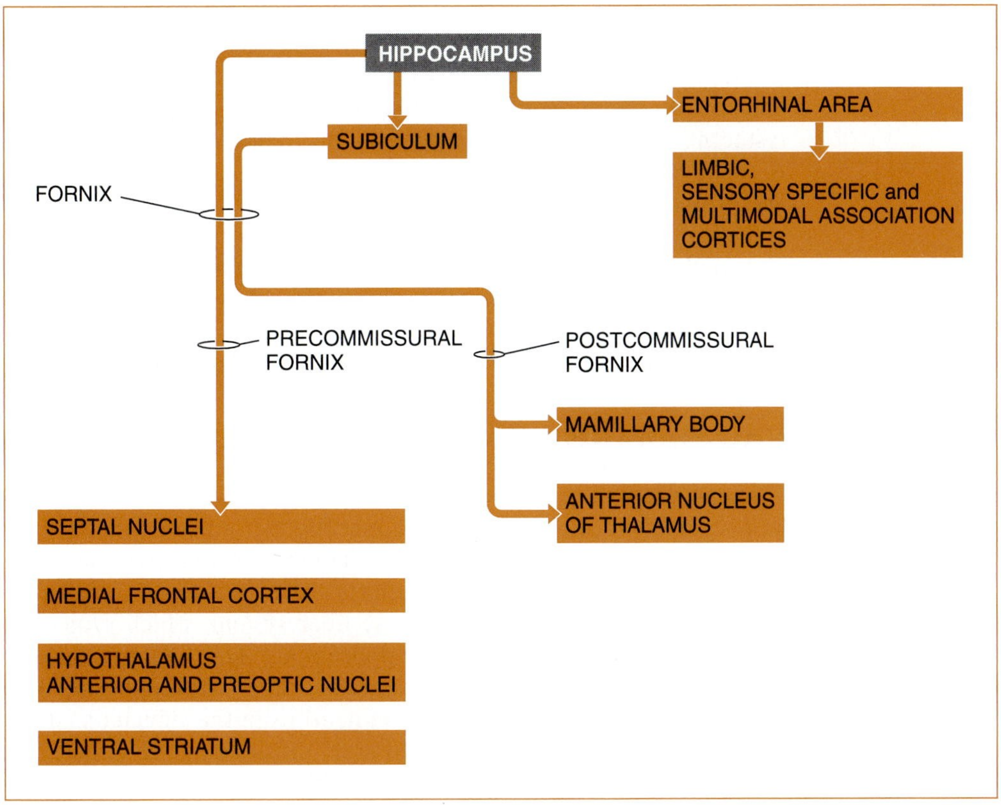

FIGURE 21-7

Schematic diagram showing the major efferents of the hippocampus.

fibers in the fornix constitute its smaller precommissural division and are distributed to the septal nuclei, the medial area of the frontal cortex, the anterior and preoptic hypothalamic nuclei, and the ventral striatum.

Fornix

The **fornix** is a fiber bundle that reciprocally connects the hippocampal formation with a number of subcortical areas, including the thalamus, the hypothalamus, and the septal region. It thus has both hippocampofugal and hippocampopetal fibers. The hippocampofugal fibers are axons of pyramidal neurons in the subiculum and hippocampus which gather at the ventricular surface of the hippocampus as the **alveus**. Fibers in the alveus converge farther on to form a flattened ribbon of white matter, the **fimbria**. Traced posteriorly on the floor of the inferior horn of the lateral ventricle, the fimbria, at the posterior limit of the hippocampus, arches under the splenium of the corpus callosum to form the **crus** of the **fornix**. The two crura converge to form the body of the fornix, which is attached to the inferior surface of the septum pellucidum to the level of the rostral thalamus. As the crura converge to form the body, a small number of fibers cross to the other side (hippocampal commissure, fornical commissure, **psalterium**). The hippocampal commissure is rudimentary in humans. Just above the interventricular foramen of Monro, the

KEY CONCEPTS

- The fornix is composed of the axons of pyramidal neurons in the subiculum and hippocampus.

Fornix (Latin, "arch"). The outflow tract of the hippocampal formation is arch-like. Noted by Galen and first described by Vesalius. Thomas Willis named it the fornix cerebri.

Alveus (Latin, "a trough or canal"). The alveus of the hippocampus is the thin layer of white matter that covers the ventricular surface of the hippocampus.

Fimbria (Latin, "fringe, border, edge"). The band of white matter along the medial edge of the ventricular surface of the hippocampus. Part of the fornix.

Crus fornix (Latin, "leg or shin, arch"). The flattened band of white beneath the splenium of the corpus callosum. The two crura join to form the body of the fornix.

Psalterium (Greek *psalterion*, "harp"). The hippocampal commissure or fornical commimssure is called the psalterium.

body of the fornix splits to form the two anterior columns of the fornix, which arch ventrally. Most of the fibers (75 percent) in each anterior column descend caudal to the anterior commissure to form the postcommissural fornix. The majority of fibers in this component of the fornix terminate in the mamillary body, and the rest terminate in the anterior nucleus of the thalamus and the midbrain tegmentum. A small component (25 percent) of each anterior column descends rostral to the anterior commissure to form the precommissural fornix. Fibers in this component of the fornix terminate in the septal nuclei, medial frontal cortex, anterior hypothalamus, and ventral striatum. Fibers in the postcommissural fornix originate in the subiculum, whereas those in the precommissural fornix originate in both the hippocampus and the subiculum.

Each fornix contains 1.2 million axons of pyramidal neurons in humans.

Entorhinal-Hippocampal Circuitry

Using a variety of neuroanatomic and neurophysiologic techniques, the entorhinal-hippocampal-entorhinal circuit of connections has been defined. The circuit starts in the entorhinal area, which projects via the perforant pathway to granule cells in the dentate gyrus and pyramidal cells in the hippocampus. Axons of granule cells in the dentate gyrus form the mossy fiber system, which projects on pyramidal neurons in the CA_3 field of the hippocampus. The CA_3 pyramidal neurons send **Schaffer collaterals** to the pyramidal cells of the CA_1 hippocampal field. Axons of pyramidal neurons in CA_1 project on neurons in the subiculum. The subiculum in turn projects back to the entorhinal area, thus closing the circuit. The synapses in this circuit are all excitatory; the only inhibitory synapses are those from hippocampal basket neurons in the stratum oriens whose axons terminate on the perikarya of pyramidal neurons.

Schaffer collaterals. Collaterals of axons of pyramidal neurons in the CA_3 field of the hippocampus that project on pyramidal cells in the CA_1 field.

Functional Considerations

In considering the functions of the hippocampus, it is important to emphasize the complex relationships of the hippocampus with other brain regions, as was outlined above. The effects of stimulation or ablation of the hippocampus cannot be evaluated in isolation from the elaborate systems of hippocampal communication.

The hippocampus is no longer believed to play a role in olfaction. The hippocampus is very well developed in humans, who are microsmatic; it is also present in the whale, which is anosmatic. No direct pathways from the primary olfactory cortex can be traced to the hippocampus, although a multisynaptic pathway through the primary olfactory cortex and the parahippocampal gyrus (entorhinal area) exists. Olfactory bulb stimulation results in excitatory postsynaptic potential (EPSP) activity but no action potential firing in the hippocampus. This is consistent with a polysynaptic pathway from the olfactory bulb to the hippocampus. It has been suggested that this subthreshold EPSP activity may be comparable to a conditional stimulus that plays a role in memory and learning.

Action potentials, in contrast, have been recorded in the hippocampus after stimulation of various areas, both centrally and peripherally. Hippocampal responses have been elicited after visual, acoustic, gustatory, and somatosensory stimulation as well as after stimulation of various cortical and subcortical areas. Such responses are characteristically labile and are easily modified by a variety of factors.

KEY CONCEPTS

- The entorhinal area is reciprocally connected with the hippocampus and serves as a gateway between the cerebral cortex and the hippocampus.

Stimulation and ablation of the hippocampus give rise to changes in behavioral, endocrine, and visceral functions. The same effects may follow either ablation or stimulation.

The hippocampus has been implicated in the processes of attention and alertness. Stimulation of the hippocampus in animals produces glancing and searching movements that are associated with bewilderment and anxiety.

Bilateral ablation of the hippocampus in humans (usually involving adjacent regions as well) results in a loss of recent memory and the inability to store newly learned facts (anterograde **amnesia**). Past memories, however, remain intact. Unilateral ablation of the hippocampus in humans does not affect memory to a significant degree. Studies of humans with brain lesions indicate that the hippocampus is important for the memory of events, objects, and words (**declarative** or **associative** memory).

The hippocampus has a low threshold for seizure (epileptic) activity; however, the spread of such epileptic activity to the nonspecific thalamic system, and hence all over the cortex, is not usual. This may explain why temporal lobe epilepsy (psychomotor epilepsy) in humans does not become generalized and usually is not associated with the loss of consciousness encountered in generalized epilepsy.

Amnesia (Greek, "forgetfulness"). Lack or loss of memory. *Amnesia* was an old term for loss of memory. The modern use of the word dates from about 1861 and the work of Broca, who divided disorders of speech caused by central lesions into aphemia and verbal amnesia. The term first appeared in English in 1862. Broca's use of the term *verbal amnesia* (impaired word finding) is no longer current.

Declarative memory. The conscious recollection of specific events and facts. Also known as associative memory and database memory.

Associative memory. The conscious recollection of specific events and facts. Also known as declarative memory and database memory.

Amygdala (Greek *amygdale,* "almond"). The amygdaloid nucleus is an almond-shaped nuclear mass in front of the tail of the caudate nucleus.

Amygdala

The amygdalar (from the Greek *amygdala,* "almonds") nuclei, a major component of the limbic system, resemble almonds in shape and are located in the tip of the temporal lobe beneath the cortex of the uncus and rostral to the hippocampus and the inferior horn of the lateral ventricle. There are two main groups of these nuclei: the corticomedial and central and the basolateral. The corticomedial-central group is relatively small and is phylogenetically older. It maintains connections with the phylogenetically older regions of the central nervous system, such as the olfactory bulb, hypothalamus, and brain stem. The basolateral group is larger and phylogenetically more recent. It has extensive connections with the cerebral cortex. Several neurotransmitters have been demonstrated in the amygdala, including acetylcholine, gamma-aminobutyric acid (GABA), noradrenaline, serotonin, dopamine, substance P, and enkephalin.

Afferent Pathways

The amygdala receives a broad range of exteroceptive afferents (olfactory, somatosensory, auditory, and visual) for integration with interoceptive stimuli from a variety of autonomic areas (Fig. 21-8). Most of the amygdalar connections are reciprocal.

KEY CONCEPTS

- The hippocampus plays a role in declarative or associative memory, attention and alertness, and behavioral, endocrine, and visceral functions.
- The amygdala is composed of two main cell groups: a phylogenetically older corticomedial and central group and a phylogenetically more recent basolateral group.
- The corticomedial-central nuclear group of the amygdala has connections with phylogenetically older regions such as the olfactory system, hypothalamus, and brain stem.
- The basolateral nuclear group of the amygdala has connections with the cerebral cortex.

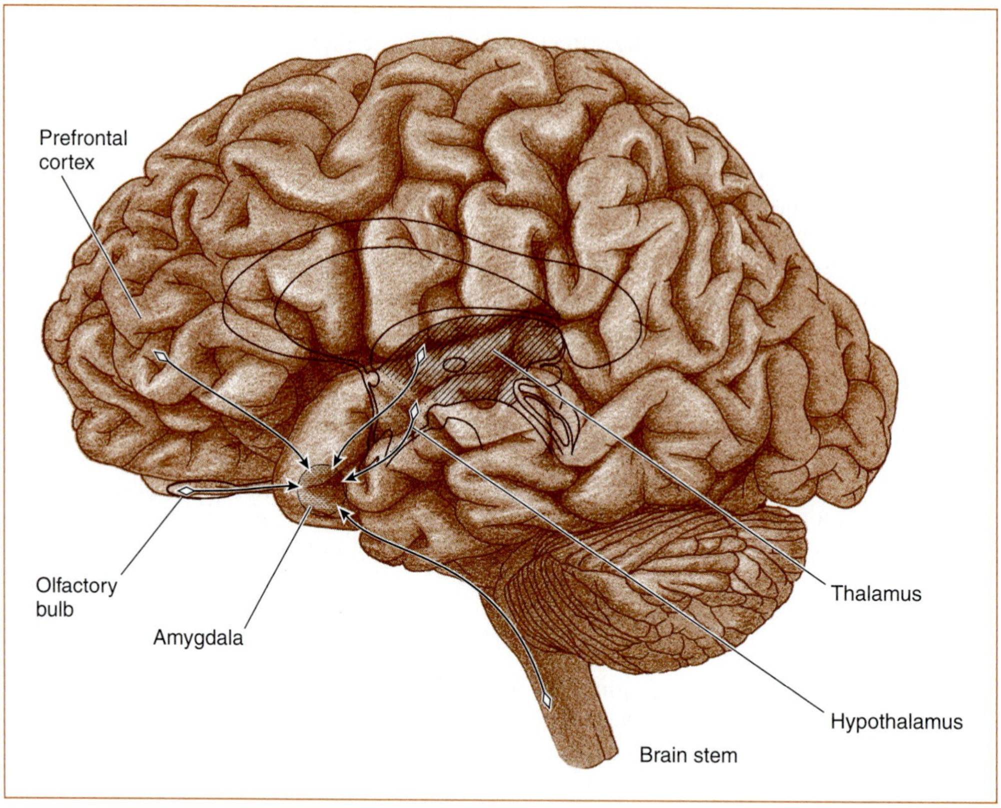

FIGURE 21-8

Schematic diagram of the major afferent connections of the amygdala.

Uncinate (Latin, "hook"). The uncinate fasciculus is like a hook connecting the frontal and temporal lobes.

The basolateral nuclear group, the largest in humans, receives inputs from the following cortical and subcortical sources: (1) cortical input from the prefrontal, temporal, occipital, and insular cortices, which convey to the amygdala highly processed somatosensory, auditory, and visual sensory information from modality-specific and multimodal association areas as well as visceral information, (2) the thalamus (dorsomedial nucleus), and (3) the olfactory cortex. The basolateral nuclear group is intimately and reciprocally connected with the prefrontal cortex via the **uncinate** fasciculus.

The corticomedial and central nuclear complex receives inputs from the following sources: (1) olfactory bulb (directly via the lateral olfactory stria and indirectly via the olfactory cortex), (2) thalamus (dorsomedial nucleus), (3) hypothalamus (ventromedial nucleus and lateral hypothalamic area), (4) septal area, and (5) brain stem nuclear groups concerned with visceral function (periaqueductal gray matter, parabrachial nucleus, nucleus of the solitary tract).

Efferent Pathways

A large number of amygdalar efferents terminate in nuclei that regulate endocrine and autonomic function, and others are directed to the neocortex. Output from the amygdala is conveyed via two main pathways: (1) stria terminalis (dorsal amygdalofugal pathway) and (2) ventral amygdalofugal pathway (ventrofugal bundle).

Stria Terminalis The stria terminalis (Fig. 21-9) is the main outflow tract of the amygdala. It arises predominantly from the corticomedial group of amygdalar nuclei. From its sites of origin, it follows a C-shaped course caudally, dorsally, anteriorly,

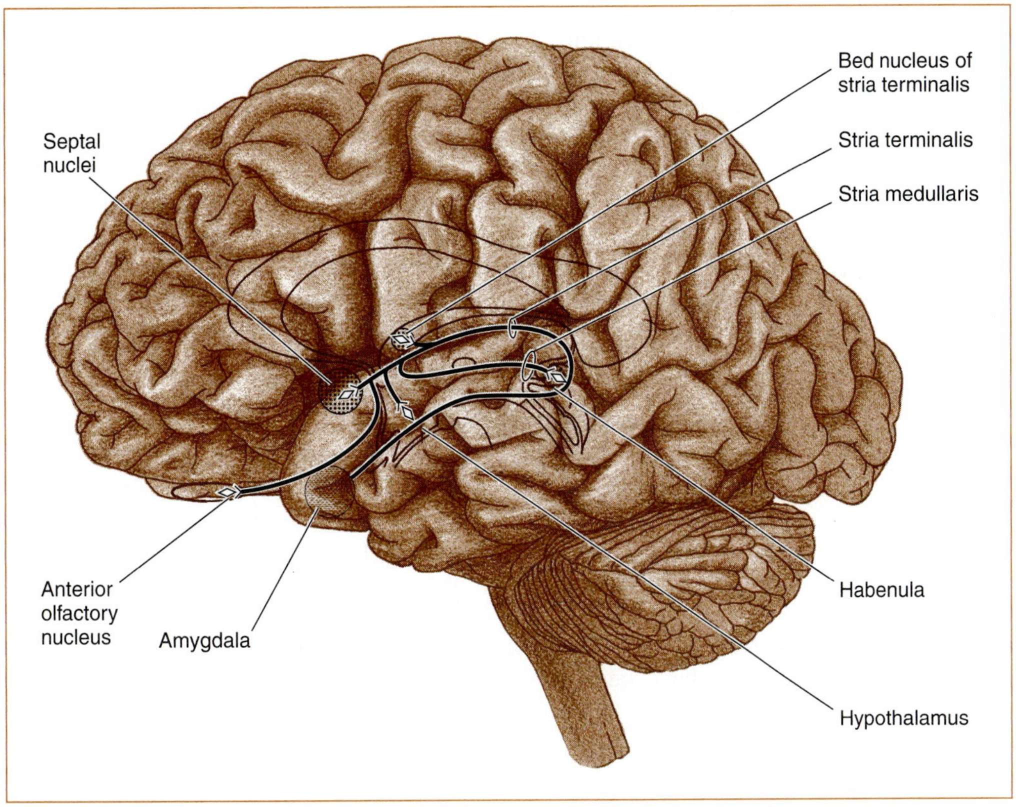

FIGURE 21-9

Schematic diagram of the major efferent connections of the amygdala.

and ventrally along the medial surface of the caudate nucleus to reach the region of the anterior commissure, where it branches out to supply the following areas: (1) septal nuclei, (2) anterior, preoptic, and ventromedial nuclei of the hypothalamus and the lateral hypothalamic area, and (3) bed nucleus of the stria terminalis (a scattered group of nuclei at the rostral extremity of the stria terminalis).

Ventral Amygdalofugal Pathway The ventral amygdalofugal pathway is a ventral outflow tract that originates from the basolateral and central amygdalar nuclei. It proceeds along the base of the brain beneath the lentiform nucleus and distributes fibers to the following areas. Fibers originating from the basolateral amygdalar nucleus project to the following cortical and subcortical areas: (1) prefrontal, inferior temporal (entorhinal area and subiculum), insular, cingulate, and occipital cortices, (2) ventral striatum, (3) thalamus (dorsomedial nucleus), (4) hypothalamus (preoptic and lateral hypothalamic areas), (5) septal area, and (6) substantia innominata,

KEY CONCEPTS

- Output from the amygdala is carried in two pathways: the stria terminalis (dorsal amygdalofugal pathway) and the ventral amygdalofugal pathway (ventrofugal bundle).

from which a diffuse cholinergic system activates the cerebral cortex in response to significant stimuli.

Fibers in the ventral amygdalofugal pathway originating in the central amygdalar nucleus are distributed to brain stem nuclei concerned with visceral function (dorsal motor nucleus of the vagus, raphe nuclei, locus ceruleus, parabrachial nucleus, and periaqueductal gray matter).

The two amygdala communicate with each other through the stria terminalis and the anterior commissure. Fibers leave one amygdaloid nuclear complex and travel via the stria terminalis to the level of the anterior commissure, where they cross and join the other stria terminalis and return to the contralateral amygaloid nuclear complex. Nuclear groups within each amygdaloid nuclear complex communicate with each other via short fiber systems.

Functional Considerations

The functions of the amygdala are somewhat elusive. Stimulation and ablation experiments usually involve adjacent neural structures. The intricate neural connectivity of the amygdala makes it difficult to ascribe an observed behavior purely to the amygdala. The following manifestations, however, have been noted to occur after stimulation or ablation of the amygdala.

Autonomic Effects Changes in heart rate, respiration, blood pressure, and gastric motility have been observed after amygdalar stimulation. Both an increase and a decrease in these functions have been observed, depending on the area that is stimulated.

Orienting Response Stimulation of the amygdala enhances the orienting response to novel events. Such animals arrest ongoing activity and orient their bodies to the novel situation. Animals with amygdalar lesions manifest reduced responsiveness to novel events in the visual environment. Their responsiveness, however, is improved if they are rewarded for the response.

Emotional Behavior and Food Intake There seem to be two regions in the amygdala that are antagonistic to each other with regard to emotional behavior and eating. Lesions in the corticomedial nuclear group of the amygdala result in aphagia, decreased emotional tone, fear, sadness, and aggression. Lesions of the basolateral nuclear group, by contrast, produce hyperphagia, happiness, and pleasure reactions. Stimulation of the basolateral nuclear group of the amygdala is associated with fear and flight. Stimulation of the corticomedial nuclear group produces a defensive and aggressive reaction. The attack behavior elicited by amygdalar stimulation differs from that elicited by hypothalamic stimlation in its gradual buildup and gradual subsidence upon the onset and cessation of stimulation. Attack behavior elicited from the hypothalamus, in contrast, begins and subsides almost immediately after the onset and cessation of the stimulus. Of interest also is the fact that prior septal stimulation prevents the occurrence of aggressive behavior elicited from both the amygdala and the hypothalamus.

Arousal Response Stimulation of the basolateral nuclear group of the amygdala produces an arousal response that is similar to but independent of the arousal

KEY CONCEPTS

- The amygdala plays an important role in a variety of functions, including autonomic and orienting responses, emotional behavior, food intake, arousal, sexual activity, and motor activity.

response that follows stimulation of the reticular activating system of the brain stem. The amygdalar response is independent of the reticular activating system response, since it can be elicited after lesions have been made in the reticular formation of the brain stem. Stimulation of the corticomedial nuclear group of the amygdala, by contrast, produces the reverse effect (a decrease in arousal and sleep). The net total effect of the amygdala, however, is facilitatory, since ablation of the amygdala results in a sluggish, hypoactive animal which is placid and tame. Such animals avoid social interaction and may become social isolates.

Sexual Activity The amygdala contains the highest density of receptors for sex hormones. Stimulation of the amygdala has been associated with a variety of sexual behaviors, including erection, ejaculation, copulatory movements, and ovulation. Bilateral lesions of the amygdala produce hypersexuality and perverted sexual behavior.

Motor Activity Stimulation of the corticomedial nuclear group of the amygdala produces complex rhythmic movements related to eating, such as chewing, smacking of the lips, licking, and swallowing.

Animal experiments support the importance of the amygdala in the organization of fear-related behavior. Bilateral removal of the amygdala abolishes naturally occurring fear-related responses in animals. Electric stimulation of the amygdala elicits defensive or fear-related behavior. The amygdaloid projections to the hypothalamus via the ventral amygdalofugal pathway seem to be essential for fear-related behavior.

Stimulation of the amygdala during brain surgery in humans is associated with a variety of autonomic and emotional reactions and a feeling of fear and anxiety. Some of these patients report a memorylike delusion of recognition known as the **déjà vu** phenomenon (a French term meaning "already seen"). The déjà vu phenomenon, as well as olfactory and gustatory hallucinations, is frequently experienced as auras in patients who experience temporal lobe seizures.

Déjà vu (French, "already seen"). An illusion in which a new situation is incorrectly viewed as a repetition of a previous situation. Usually an aura of a temporal lobe seizure.

Destruction of both amygdalas in humans has been done to relieve intractable epilepsy and treat violent behavior. Such patients usually become complacent and sedate and show significant changes in emotional behavior.

It should be pointed out that many, if not all, of these functions can be observed after stimulation or ablation of other brain regions, notably the hypothalamus and the septal regions. It has been proposed that the amygdala plays an integrative role in all these functions.

Septal Area

The septal area has two divisions: the septum pellucidum and the septum verum. The septum pellucidum is a thin leaf that separates the lateral ventricles. It is made up of glia and lined by ependyma. The septum verum (Fig. 21-10) is ventral to the septum pellucidum, between the subcallosal gyrus rostrally and the anterior commisure and the anterior hypothalamus caudally. Most authors include the fol-

KEY CONCEPTS

- Disorders of the amygdala in humans are associated with olfactory and gustatory hallucinations as well as the "déjà vu" phenomenon.
- The term *septal area* refers to the septum pellucidum and the septum verum. The septum pellucidum is a thin glial partition between the lateral ventricles; the septum verum is a group of basal nuclei that includes the septal nuclei.

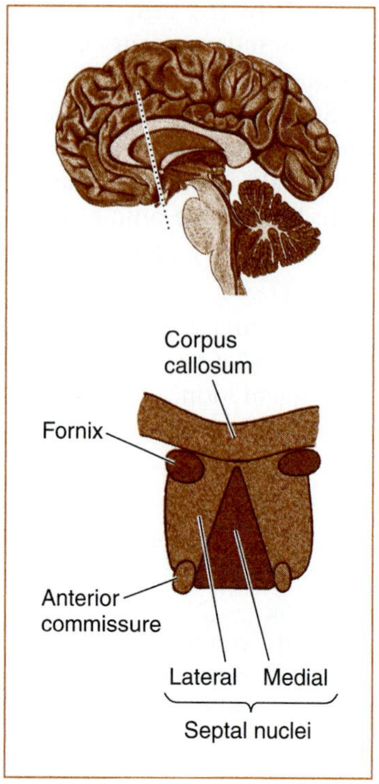

FIGURE 21-10

Schematic diagram of the location and divisions of the septal nuclei.

lowing structures in the septum verum: the septal nuclei, the diagonal band of Broca, the bed nucleus of the stria terminalis, and the nucleus accumbens septi.

The septal nuclei are made up of medium-size neurons which are grouped into medial, lateral, and posterior groups. The lateral group receives most of the septal afferents and projects to the medial septal group. The medial group gives rise to most of the septal efferents. The posterior group receives input from the hippocampus and directs its output to the habenular nuclei. The septal nuclei are poorly developed in humans.

Connections

The septal area has reciprocal connections (Fig. 21-11) with the following areas: (1) hippocampus, (2) amygdala, (3) hypothalamus, (4) midbrain, (5) habenular nucleus, (6) cingulate gyrus, and (7) thalamus.

The reciprocal connections between the septal area and the hippocampus constitute the major connection of the septal area and travel via the fornix. The hippocampal-septal relationship is topographically organized so that specific areas of the hippocampus project on specific regions of the septum (CA_1 of the hippocampus to the medial septal region; CA_3 and CA_4 of the hippocampus to the lateral septal region). The hippocampal-septal relationship assumes more importance when one considers that septal projection to the hippocampus is from the medial septal region to CA_3 and CA_4 of the hippocampus. When one adds to this the intrinsic connection between the medial and lateral septal regions and between CA_1 and CA_3–CA_4 of the hippocampus, it becomes evident that a neural circuit is established connecting these two limbic regions.

The reciprocal connections between the septal area and the amygdala travel via the stria terminalis and the ventral amygdalofugal pathway.

Reciprocal connections with the hypothalamus travel via the medial forebrain

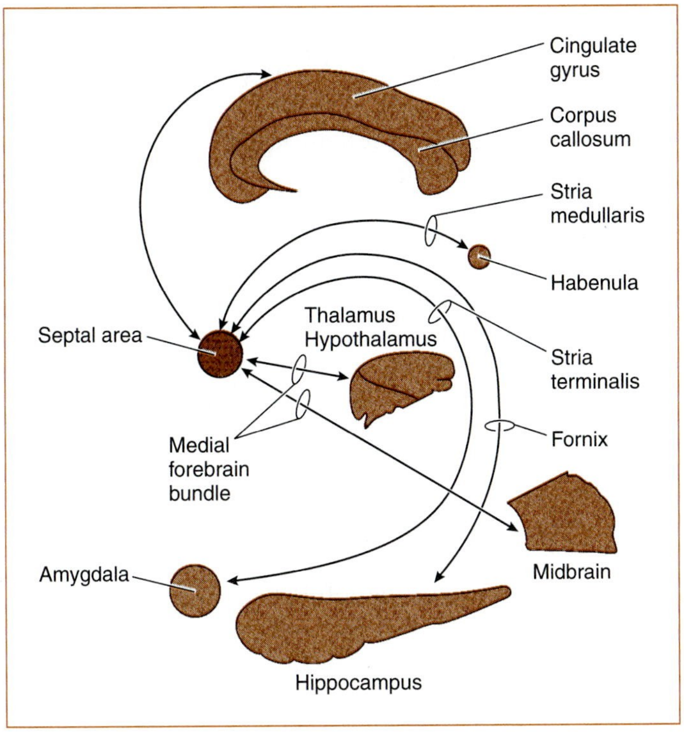

FIGURE 21-11

Schematic diagram showing afferent and efferent connections of the septal area.

bundle. The hypothalamic nuclei involved include the preoptic, anterior, paraventricular, and lateral. The medial forebrain bundle is an ill-defined bundle of short nerve fibers that courses through the lateral hypothalamus, interconnecting nuclei located close together and extending from the septal area into the midbrain.

Fibers between the septal area and the midbrain travel via the medial forebrain bundle. The periaqueductal gray region and the ventral tegmental area are the primary brain stem areas involved in this connection.

The stria medullaris thalami reciprocally connects the septal area and the habenular nuclei. From the habenular nuclei, the habenulointerpeduncular tract connects the septal area indirectly with the interpeduncular nucleus of the midbrain.

The thalamic nuclei involved in the septothalamic connection are the dorsomedial and the anterior nuclei.

Functional Considerations

The functional importance of the septal area lies in providing a site of interaction between limbic and diencephalic structures. The connection of the hippocampus with the hypothalamus via the septal region is an illustration of this.

Stimulation and ablation experiments have provided the following information about the role of the septal region.

KEY CONCEPTS

- Reciprocal connections with the hippocampus (via the fornix) constitute the major connection of the septal area. Other connections include those with the amygdala, hypothalamus, thalamus, brain stem, and cingulate gyrus.

Emotional Behavior Lesions of the septal area in animal species such as rats and mice produce rage reactions and hyperemotionality. These behavioral alterations usually are transitory and disappear 2 to 4 weeks after the lesion.

Water Consumption Animals with lesions in the septal area tend to consume increased amounts of water. There is evidence to suggest that this is a primary effect of the lesion and is caused by disruption of a neural system concerned with water balance in response to changes in total fluid volume. Chronic stimulation of the septal area tends to decrease spontaneous drinking even in animals that have been deprived of water for a long time.

Activity Animals with septal lesions demonstrate a high initial state of activity in response to a novel situation. This heightened activity, however, rapidly declines almost to immobility.

Learning Animals with septal lesions tend to learn tasks quickly and perform them effectively once they have been learned.

Reward Stimulation of several regions of the septal area gives rise to pleasure or rewarding effects.

Autonomic Effects Stimulation of the septal region has an inhibitory effect on autonomic function. Cardiac deceleration ensues after septal stimulation and is reversed by the drug atropine, suggesting that septal effects are mediated via the cholinergic fibers of the vagus nerve.

Septal Syndrome Destruction of the septal nuclei gives rise to behavioral overreaction to most environmental stimuli. Behavioral changes occur in sexual and reproductive behavior, feeding, drinking, and the rage reaction.

Relatively few discrete septal lesions or stimulations have been reported in humans. Chemical stimulation in the septal area using acetylcholine results in euphoria and sexual orgasm. Recordings from the septal area during sexual intercourse have shown spike and wave activity during orgasm. Markedly increased sexual activity has been reported in humans after septal damage.

OVERVIEW OF THE LIMBIC SYSTEM

It is evident that the limbic system is a highly complex system that is interconnected by a multiplicity of pathways and reciprocal circuits among its component parts, notably the hypothalamus.

The main components of the limbic system (hippocampal formation, amygdala, entorhinal cortex) are densely interconnected and are connected with neural systems that subserve somatosensory, somatomotor, and autonomic and endocrine func-

KEY CONCEPTS

- The septal area plays an important role in emotional behavior, learning, reward, autonomic responses, drinking and feeding, and sexual behavior.
- The limbic system plays a major role in integrating exteroceptive and interoceptive information by serving as a link between cortical sensory association areas, the subcortical autonomic and endocrine centers, and the prefrontal association cortex. It thus mediates the effects of emotion on motor function.

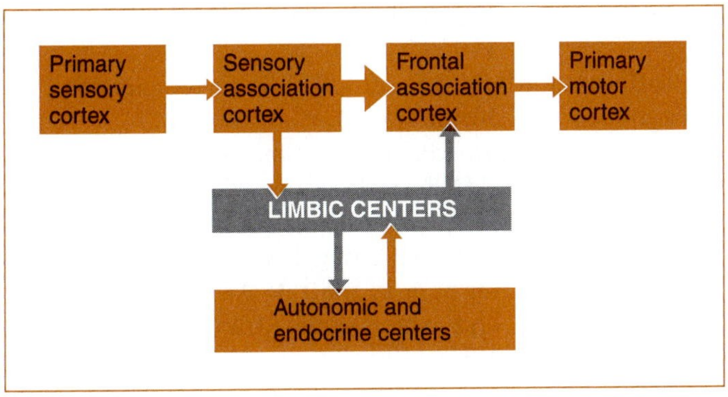

FIGURE 21-12

Schematic diagram showing the anatomic substrate for the integrative function of the limbic system (the limbic loop).

tions. They are thus in a unique position to integrate exteroceptive and interoceptive information and are essential for the maintenance of emotional stability, learning ability, and memory function. A limbic loop (Fig. 21-12) has been proposed as the anatomic substrate for the integrative role of the limbic system. The afferent limb of the loop consists of collaterals to the limbic system from the pathway connecting neocortical association cortices with the prefontal cortex. Autonomic and endocrine centers are reciprocally connected with the same limbic system centers that receive cortical collaterals. The efferent limb of the loop consists of projections from the limbic centers to the prefrontal assocation cortex. The prefrontal cortex plays a role in guiding behavior and is indirectly involved in the initiation of movement. The input from the limbic centers into the prefrontal cortex subserves the effects of emotion on motor function. At best, one can define the overall functions of the limbic system in the most general terms as subserving the following:

1. Homeostatic mechanisms for preservation of the individual (flight or defensive response, eating, drinking) and preservation of the species (sexual and social behavior)
2. Emotional behavior (including fear, rage, pleasure, and sadness)
3. Memory
4. Matching up sensory input with autonomic-endocrine drives and putting it into the context of the situation

KEY CONCEPTS

- Other important functions of the limbic system include the regulation of homeostatic mechanisms used for preservation of the individual and the species, emotional behavior, and memory.

SUGGESTED READINGS

Baleydier C, Mauguiere F: The duality of the cingulate gyrus in monkey: Neuroanatomical study and functional hypothesis. *Brain* 1980; 103:525–554.

Ben-Ari Y, et al: Regional distribution of choline acetyltransferase and acetylcholinesterase within the amygdaloid complex and stria terminalis system. *Brain Res* 1977; 120:435–445.

Braak H, et al: Functional anatomy of human hippocampal formation and related structures. *J Child Neurol* 1996; 11:265–275.

Brodal P: *The Central Nervous System,* 5th ed. New York, Oxford University Press, 1992:383–397.

Bronen RA: Hippocampal and limbic terminology. *AJNR* 1992; 13:943–945.

Brumback RA, Leech RW: Memories of a sea horse. *J Child Neurol* 1996; 11:263–264.

Emson PC, et al: Contributions of different afferent pathways to the catecholamine and 5-hydroxytryptamine-innervation of the amygdala: A neurochemical and histochemical study. *Neuroscience* 1979; 4:1347–1357.

Girgis M: Kindling as a model for limbic epilepsy. *Neuroscience* 1981; 6:1695–1706.

Gorman DG, Cummings JL: Hypersexuality following septal injury. *Arch Neurol* 1992; 49:308–310.

Hopkins DA, Holstege G: Amygdaloid projections to the mesencephalon, pons and medulla oblongata in the cat. *Exp Brain Res* 1978; 32:529–547.

Horel JA: The neuroanatomy of amnesia: A critique of the hippocampal memory hypothesis. *Brain* 1978; 101:403–445.

Kosel KC, et al: Olfactory bulb projections to the parahippocampal area of the rat. *J Comp Neurol* 1981; 198:467–482.

Lopes da Silva FH, Arnolds DEAT: Physiology of the hippocampus and related structures. *Annu Rev Physiol* 1978; 40:185–216.

Mark LP, et al: The fornix. *AJNR* 1993; 14:1355–1358.

Mark LP, et al: The hippocampus. *AJNR* 1993; 14:709–712.

Mark LP, et al: Hippocampal anatomy and pathologic alterations on conventional MR images. *AJNR* 1993; 14:1237–1240.

Mark LP, et al: Limbic connections. *AJNR* 1995; 16:1303–1306.

Mark LP, et al: Limbic system anatomy: An overview. *AJNR* 1993; 14:349–352.

Mark LP, et al: The septal area. *AJNR* 1994; 15:273–276.

Meibach RC, Siegel A: Efferent connections of the septal area in the rat: An analysis utilizing retrograde and anterograde transport methods. *Brain Res* 1977; 119:1–20.

Ottersen OP, Ben-Ari Y: Afferent connections to the amygdaloid complex of the rat and cat: I. Projections from the thalamus. *J Comp Neurol* 1979; 187: 401–424.

Swanson LW, Cowan WM: An autoradiographic study of the organization of the efferent connections of the hippocampal formation in the rat. *J Comp Neurol* 1977; 172:49–84.

Tranel D, Hyman BT: Neuropsychological correlates of bilateral amygdala damage. *Arch Neurol* 1990; 47:349–355.

Van Hoesen GW: The parahippocampal gyrus: New observations regarding its cortical connections in the monkey. *Trends Neurosci* 1982; 5:345–350.

Van Hoesen GW: Anatomy of the medial temporal lobe. *Magn Reson Imaging* 1995; 13:1047–1055.

CHAPTER 22

LIMBIC SYSTEM: CLINICAL CORRELATES

ABNORMALITIES OF OLFACTION

Rhinencephalic structures can be affected in several sites, resulting in derangement of the sense of smell.

Olfactory receptors in the nose are involved in common colds, resulting in bilateral diminution or loss of smell (**anosmia**). Olfactory nerve fibers may be affected in their course through the **cribriform** plate of the ethmoid bone after fractures of the plate and severe falls. The anosmia in such cases is postulated to result from the shearing of the fine olfactory nerve fibers as they pass through the cribriform plate. The olfactory bulb and tract may be involved in inflammatory processes of the meninges (meningitis) or tumors (meningiomas) in the inferior surface of the frontal lobe or the anterior cranial fossa. Unilateral loss of smell may be the earliest clinical manifestation of a subfrontal meningioma. Pathologic processes in the region of the primary olfactory cortex (uncus of the temporal lobe) usually give rise to hallucinations of smell (**uncinate fits**). The odor experienced in such cases often is described as unpleasant. Such hallucinations may herald an epileptic seizure or be part of it.

Rhinencephalon (Greek *rhin,* "nose"; *enkephalos,* "brain"). The smell brain.

Anosmia (Greek *an,* "negative"; *osme,* "smell"). Absence of the sense of smell. The condition was first mentioned by Galen.

Cribriform (Latin *cribrum,* "sieve"; *forma,* "form"). The cribriform plate of the ethmoid bone is perforated with small apertures, resembling a sieve. Ancient anatomists were especially interested in the perforations of the ethmoid bone because of their theory that pituita (mucous brain secretions) entered the nose through these channels.

KEY CONCEPTS

- Anosmia (loss of smell) can result from lesions in the olfactory receptors, nerve rootlets, bulb, or cortex.
- Anosmia may be the earliest clinical sign of a subfrontal meningioma.

MEMORY

The role of the nervous system in memory has been studied by using neurosurgical techniques (ablation of selective areas of the brain), electrophysiologic methods (neural pathways and mechanisms), biochemical studies (the role of RNA and other proteins), a neuropharmacologic approach (the effect of drugs on synaptic transmission and intracellular processes), and studies of humans with a memory deficit (**amnesia**). Memory seems to depend on two distinct changes: an electric membrane event of a temporary nature and a more stable, permanent change in the chemistry of the nervous system. The discovery that DNA and RNA can act as codes for synaptic transmission has led to the theory that those substances are responsible for transforming short-term memories into permanent stores.

Uncinate fits (Latin, "hook"). Uncinate fits arise from the area of the uncus, the medially curved (like a hook) anterior end of the parahippocampal gyrus.

Amnesia (Greek, "forgetfulness"). Lack of or loss of memory. *Amnesia* was an old term for loss of memory. The modern use of the word dates from about 1861 and the work of Broca, who divided disorders of speech caused by central lesions into aphemia and verbal amnesia. The term first appeared in English in 1862. Broca's use of the term *verbal amnesia* (impaired word finding) is no longer current.

Types of Memory

It is generally acknowledged that there are two types of memory: (1) short-term and (2) long-term.

Short-Term (Immediate, Recent, Working) Memory

Short-term memory refers to the memory of a limited amount of information (e.g., a seven-digit telephone number) for a short period (less than 60 s). This type of memory decays in seconds if it is not refreshed continuously. Current models of short-term memory point to two separate subsystems that handle verbal and spatial information: the articulatory loop system and the visuospatial sketchpad, respectively. Positron emission tomography scan has shown that verbal short-term memory is localized to the left perisylvian region. Spatial short-term memory is localized to the posterior region of the right hemisphere.

Long-Term (Remote) Memory

Long-term memory refers to the memory of an unlimited amount of memoranda for a variable period (minutes to years). Long-term memory includes two memory systems: (1) **explicit memory** and (2) implicit memory.

Explicit memory. A type of memory that requires the conscious recall of specific facts. Also known as declarative memory.

Declarative memory. A type of memory that requires the conscious recall of specific facts. Also known as explicit memory.

Episodic memory. Memory of personally experienced facts and events with special spatial and temporal localization. Also known as unique memory.

Semantic memory. The memory of culturally and educationally acquired knowledge. Also known as generic memory. A subtype of explicit (declarative) memory.

Explicit (Declarative) Memory Explicit memory supports the learning and retention of facts and the conscious recollection of prior events (knowing that). Thus, it is consciously accessed. There are two subtypes of explicit memory: (1) episodic and (2) semantic. **Episodic** (unique) **memory** is the memory of personally experienced facts and events with special spatial and temporal localization, such as the memory of eating a specific type of food in a restaurant. Episodic memory is localized to the circuitry that links the medial temporal cortex (hippocampus, parahippocampal gyrus, entorhinal cortex) and the diencephalon. **Semantic** (nonunique, generic) **memory** refers to the memory of culturally and educationally acquired

KEY CONCEPTS

- There are two types of memory: immediate (short-term) and remote (long-term).
- Short-term memory entails the memory of a limited amount of information for less than 60 s.
- Long-term memory entails the memory of an unlimited amount of information for more than 60 s, usually for minutes to years.
- There are two types of long-term memory: explicit (declarative) and implicit (procedural).

encyclopedic knowledge such as the meaning of words, arithmetical facts, and geographic and historical information, for example, that Paris is the capital of France and that *bistro* is French for "restaurant." Semantic memory is localized to the left temporal cortex, the frontal association cortex, and the cingulate area.

The cholinergic system seems to be necessary for an intact explicit memory. Central cholinergic blockage (Alzheimer's disease, bilateral medial temporal lobectomy, Korsakoff's syndrome) results in disruption of function in the cholinergic projection system to the neocortex and hippocampus and causes a striking reduction in the acquisition of explicit (declarative) knowledge.

Implicit (Procedural) Memory Implicit memory supports the learning and retention of skills (knowing how). It is the memory of experience-affected behaviors that are performed unconsciously. It includes (1) skill learning, such as driving or riding a bike, (2) simple conditioning, such as salivating on hearing a dinner bell, and (3) **priming,** such as completing a three-letter stem with a word that has been presented previously or recognizing a word or a picture faster or more accurately because of prior exposure. Implicit memory for skill learning is localized to the cerebellum, basal ganglia, and frontal association cortex bilaterally. Priming is localized to the left parietal cortex. Lesions in these sites may have substantial effects on procedural learning and memory.

Priming. A subtype of implicit (procedural) memory which includes completing a three-letter stem with a word that has been presented previously or recognizing a word or picture faster because of prior exposure.

Immediate memory may be explained as a transient electric alteration at the synapse; longer-lasting memory may be explained as an actual physical or chemical alteration of the synapse. Several of these alterations have been described in different experimental situations, including changes in the number and size of synaptic terminals as well as their chemical composition. Changes in postsynaptic neurons also have been described. Such changes in the pre- or postsynaptic components of the synapse have been thought to facilitate the transmission of impulses at the synapse and thus establish a memory code, or ingram.

Several biochemical studies have suggested a role for protein and RNA in memory mechanisms. Evidence for this role has been obtained from (1) experiments in which protein and RNA syntheses were increased or blocked by drugs, (2) measurement of the protein and RNA content of stimulated neuronal systems, and (3) experiments in which learned tasks were presumably transferred from a trained animal to an untrained animal after the injection of RNA or protein from the brain of the trained subject.

Types of Memory Loss (Amnesia)

Several types of amnesia are recognized: (1) retrograde, (2) anterograde, (3) global, (4) modality-specific, (5) permanent, and (6) transient.

Retrograde amnesia is amnesia for information learned before the onset of an illness. **Anterograde amnesia** is amnesia for information that should have been

Retrograde amnesia. Memory loss for events that occurred before the onset of an illness.

Anterograde amnesia. Loss of the capacity to learn new material.

KEY CONCEPTS

- Explicit memory is the memory of specific facts (knowing that). Implicit memory is the memory of skills (knowing how).
- There are two types of explicit memory: episodic (unique) and semantic (generic).
- Episodic memory is the memory of personally experienced facts and events. Semantic memory is the memory of culturally and educationally acquired knowledge.
- Amnesia (memory loss) may be anterograde, retrograde, global, or modality-specific. It may be transient or permanent.

acquired after the onset of an illness. Global amnesia is amnesia in which information cannot be retrieved through any sensory channel. Modality-specific amnesia is the inability to retrieve information through a specific channel, such as vision. Amnesia may be permanent, as in Alzheimer's disease, or transient, as in posttraumatic amnesia.

Much of our knowledge about memory loss has come from careful observations of patients with amnesia. Although a relationship between the temporal lobe and loss of memory was recognized at around the turn of the century by the Russian neuropathologist Vladimir Bekhterev, it was William Scoville in 1953 who established a precise relationship between bilateral anterior temporal lobe lesions and anterograde amnesia. Scoville's patient underwent bilateral anterior temporal lobectomies for the treatment of intractable seizures. The lesion included the anterior hippocampal formation and parahippocampal gyrus and the amygdala. While the seizures responded favorably, the patient was left with severe declarative memory loss and anterograde memory loss. His retrograde memory and implicit (procedural) memory were not affected.

Subsequent observations on patients with memory loss have confirmed the following observations.

1. The hippocampus and adjacent limbic areas (entorhinal cortex areas 28, 35, and 36) are not involved in short-term (immediate) memory or retrograde memory. They are, however, involved in the acquisition of new knowledge of the declarative type (anterograde memory).
2. The left hippocampus is essential for the acquisition of new verbal knowledge, whereas the right hippocampus is essential for the acquisition of new nonverbal knowledge (faces).
3. Bilateral lesions in the fornix (the major outflow pathway of the hippocampal formation) result in anterograde amnesia.
4. The lateral temporal cortex is critical for the retrieval of knowledge.
5. The basal ganglia, cerebellum, and sensorimotor cortices are essential for skill learning.

Pathologic processes in the brain may affect one type of memory and spare others. Older people lose the ability to recall what they ate earlier in the day but can recall, in the minutest detail, experiences they had many years earlier. People who suffer head trauma in a car accident are unable to recall what transpired for minutes to hours before the accident, but the recall of older memories remains intact.

Severe impairment of episodic memory (a type of explicit long-term memory) is the hallmark of Alzheimer's disease. However, other types of memory are affected in this disease, including semantic memory (another type of explicit long-term memory), some aspects of implicit memory, and short-term memory.

In global amnesia, there is selective impairment of episodic memory.

KEY CONCEPTS

- The hippocampus and the adjacent limbic areas are key structures in anterograde memory (acquisition of knowledge).
- The left hippocampus is involved in the acquisition of new verbal knowledge, and the right hippocampus is involved in the acquisition of new nonverbal knowledge.
- The lateral temporal cortex is important for the retrieval of knowledge.
- The basal ganglia, cerebellum, and sensorimotor cortices are essential for the acquisition of mental and physical skills.

WERNICKE-KORSAKOFF SYNDROME

The Wernicke-Korsakoff syndrome, which was described by Wernicke in 1881 and Korsakoff in 1887, is characterized by severe anterograde and retrograde amnesia and confabulation. The cause of this syndrome is vitamin B_1 (thiamine) deficiency resulting from malnutrition associated with chronic alcohol intake. The lesion in **Korsakoff's syndrome** involves the dorsomedial and midline nuclei of the thalamus, mamillary body, and frontal cerebral cortex.

Korsakoff's syndrome (Wernicke-Korsakoff syndrome). A syndrome of thiamine deficiency in chronic alcoholics that is characterized by loss of memory and confabulation. The syndrome was first described by Magnus Huss, a Swedish physician. Strumpell in 1883 and Charcot in 1884 called attention to this syndrome. Charles Gayet described the pathology in 1875. Karl Wernicke, a German neuropsychiatrist, described three cases in 1881 and named the disorder *acute superior hemorrhagic polioencephalitis.* Sergi Korsakoff, a Russian neuropsychiatrist, summarized the syndrome and described it as an entity between 1887 and 1889.

TRANSIENT GLOBAL AMNESIA

Transient global amnesia is a short-term neurologic condition that is characterized by sudden memory loss of recent events, transient inability to retain new information (anterograde amnesia), and retrograde amnesia of variable extension. Immediate and very remote memories are unaffected. Complete recovery usually occurs within a few hours. The term *transient global amnesia* was coined by Fisher and Adams in 1964. The exact mechanism of transient global amnesia remains controversial. This type of amnesia has been associated with epilepsy, migraine headache, and tumor. Most reports emphasize bilateral transient ischemia in the territory of the posterior cerebral circulation affecting medial temporal lobe structures that are important for memory. The episodes of transient amnesia may be preceded by characteristic events or activities such as exertion, intense emotion, sexual intercourse, temperature extremes, and bathing.

KLÜVER-BUCY SYNDROME

The Klüver-Bucy syndrome is a clinical syndrome observed in humans and other animals after bilateral lesions in the temporal lobe that involve the amygdala, hippocampal formation, and adjacent neural structures. The syndrome was first described by Klüver and Bucy in 1939 in monkeys after bilateral temporal lobectomy. The human counterpart was described by Terzian and Dalle Ore in 1955 and by Marlowe in 1975. The syndrome is manifested by the following symptoms:

1. Visual agnosia or **psychic blindness** (inability to differentiate between friends, relatives, and strangers).
2. Hyperorality (tendency to examine all objects by mouth).
3. Hypersexuality (normal as well as perverted sexual activity). Such patients and animals manifest heightened sexual drives toward either sex of their own or other species and even inanimate objects.
4. Docility.
5. Lack of emotional response, blunted affect, and apathy.

Klüver-Bucy syndrome. A clinical syndrome characterized by visual agnosia, hyperorality, hypersexuality, docility, blunted affect, bulimia, and memory deficit. First described in monkeys by H. Klüver, and P. C. Bucy in 1937.

Psychic blindness (visual agnosia). A disorder in which patients with normal vision fail to comprehend the nature or meaning of nonverbal visual stimuli.

KEY CONCEPTS

- Korsakoff's syndrome, a thiamine deficiency syndrome seen in chronic alcoholics, is characterized by amnesia (anterograde and retrograde) and confabulation.
- Transient global amnesia is caused by ischemia in memory structures in the medial temporal lobe.
- Various manifestations of the Klüver-Bucy syndrome can be explained as defects in relating sensory information to past experience or in evaluating sensory stimuli in terms of their biologic significance.

Bulimia (Greek *bous,* "ox"; *limos,* "hunger"). An eating disorder characterized by episodes of binge eating that continue until they are terminated by abdominal pain, sleep, or self-induced vomiting.

Déjà vu (French, "already seen"). An illusion in which a new situation is incorrectly viewed as a repetition of a previous situation. Usually an aura of temporal lobe seizures.

6. Increased appetite, **bulimia**.
7. Memory deficit.

The various manifestations of this syndrome reflect a defect in relating sensory information to past experience or evaluating sensory stimuli in terms of their biologic significance.

TEMPORAL LOBE EPILEPSY

Another manifestation of limbic lesions in humans is temporal lobe epilepsy, which also is known as psychomotor seizures, uncinate fits, and complex partial seizures. During the seizure, the patient may manifest one or more of the following symptoms:

1. Olfactory hallucinations consisting of transient and recurrent episodes of unpleasant olfactory experiences such as smelling burning rubber.
2. Gustatory hallucinations consisting of a transient unpleasant taste sensation.
3. Auditory hallucinations.
4. Visual hallucinations (**déjà vu**).
5. Rhythmic movements related to feeding (chewing, licking, swallowing).
6. Complex motor acts such as walking, undressing, and twisting movements of trunk and extremities.
7. Amnesia, which may last several hours or days.
8. Aggressive behavior. During the seizure, such patients may commit violent or even criminal acts.

The pathology in temporal lobe seizures involves the hippocampus, entorhinal cortex, and amygdala. Magnetic resonance imaging (MRI) is useful in identifying temporal lobe pathology, such as mesial temporal lobe sclerosis and tumor (Fig. 22-1). Unexplained death has been reported in patients with temporal lobe epilepsy. This has been attributed to autonomic changes in cardiovascular function during a seizure. Autonomic cardiovascular responses have been elicited on stimulation of the insular cortex in humans. Stimulation of the right insular cortex produces sympathetic effects on cardiovascular function (tachycardia and pressor effects). Stimulation of the left insular cortex, in contrast, produces parasympathetic effects (bradycardia and depressor effects).

SCHIZOPHRENIA

Schizophrenia is a severe mental illness characterized by disorganized thought processes, hallucinations, delusions, and cognitive deficits. Although the definitive neuropathology of schizophrenia has not been defined, some studies have pointed to the temporal and frontal cortices and the limbic subcortical nuclei as likely sites of the pathology. Abnormalities in these sites include a decrease in the size of ventromedial temporal lobe structures, a decrease in the thickness of the parahippocampal cortex, and a decrease in neuronal density and size in the limbic, temporal, and frontal regions. Numerous pathologic mechanisms have been proposed for schizophrenia. The currently predominant hypothesis is abnormal neurodevelopment that becomes manifest in adolescence. The alternative hypothesis is a neurode-

KEY CONCEPTS

- Temporal lobe epilepsy is characterized by a combination of psychological and motor manifestations.
- Schizophrenia is a mental illness with undefined neuropathology. Cortical and subcortical limbic structures are likely sites of the neuropathology.

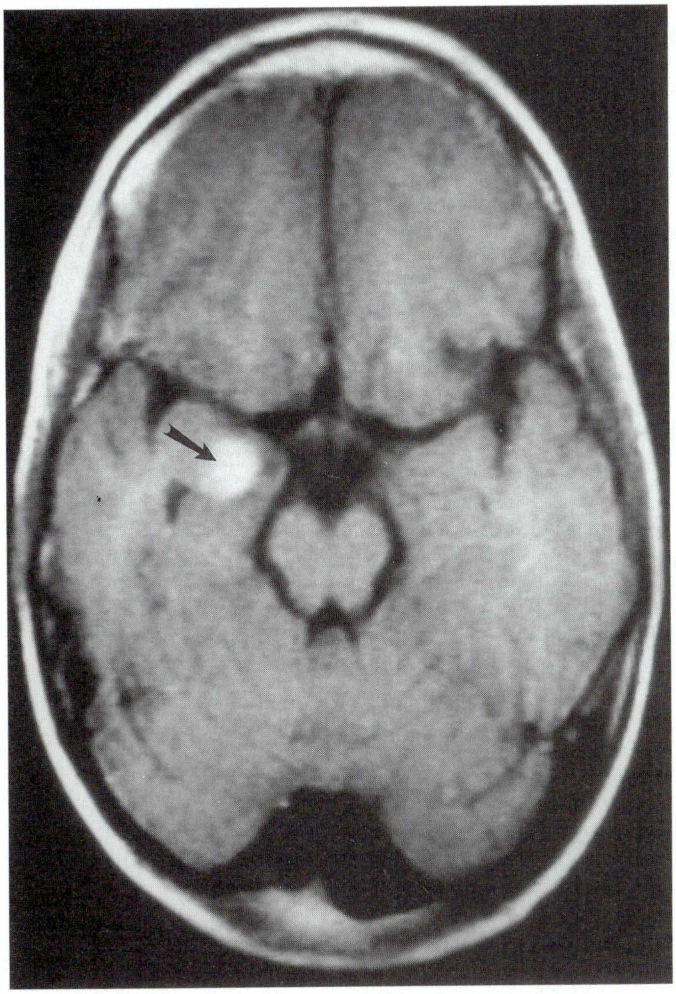

FIGURE 22-1

Gadolinium-enhanced T1-weighted magnetic resonance image of the brain showing an enhancing lesion (tumor) (*arrow*) in the temporal lobe.

generative one. Cytoarchitectural studies in schizophrenic brains point to abnormal laminar organization in limbic structures that are suggestive of abnormal neuronal migration during brain development. Findings from different studies suggest a "miswiring" of neural connections in the schizophrenic brain.

ALZHEIMER'S DISEASE

Alzheimer's disease. A progressive degenerative brain disorder characterized by severe loss of memory, disorientation, and behavioral changes. Named after Alois Alzheimer, a German neuropsychiatrist and pathologist who described the disorder verbally in 1906 and in writing in 1907.

Alzheimer's disease is a degenerative brain disorder that is characterized by memory loss severe enough to impair everyday activities; disorientation to time, place, and person; and behavioral changes such as depression, paranoia, and aggressiveness. The gross neuropathologic hallmarks of Alzheimer's disease consist of atrophic gyri and widened sulci (Fig. 22-2) most prominent in the superior frontal lobule, the inferior parietal lobes, the temporal lobe, and the limbic lobe. Microscopically, the neuropathologic hallmarks of the disease consist of neurofibrillary tangles and senile plaques. Neurochemical studies have demonstrated abnormal accumulation in senile plaques of a breakdown product of amyloid precursor protein known as beta-amyloid or A4 amyloid as well as accumulation of tau protein in neurons

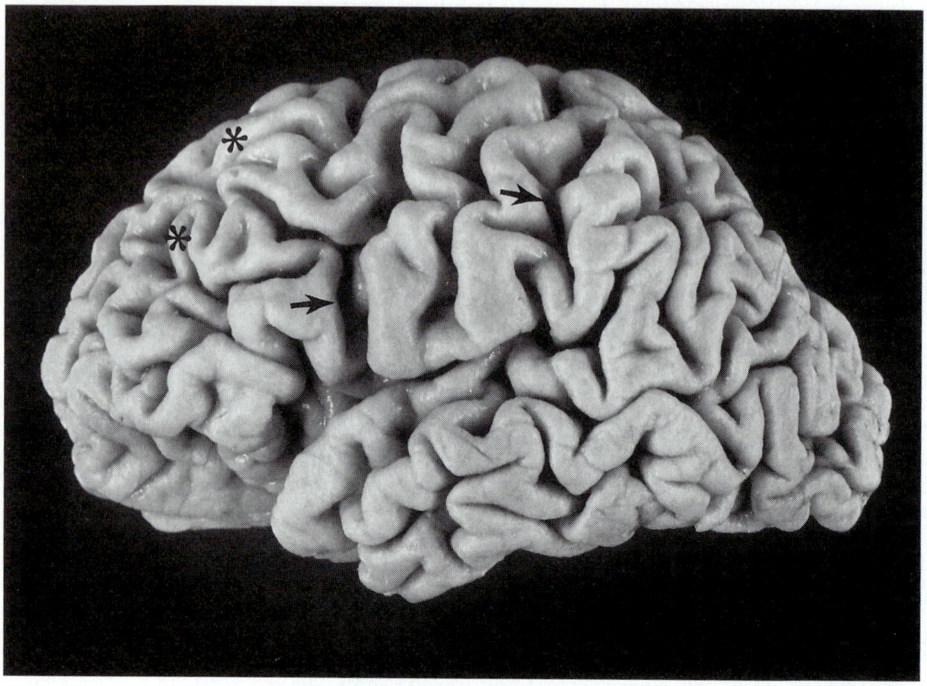

FIGURE 22-2

Lateral view of the brain showing prominence of sulci (*arrows*) and atrophy of gyri (*star*) in Alzheimer's disease.

destined to have neurofibrillary tangles. The cognitive deficit in Alzheimer's disease has been attributed to an abnormality in the cholinergic system. In support of this hypothesis are the loss in Alzheimer's brains of cholinergic projection neurons in the **nucleus basalis of Meynert** and the loss throughout the cerebral cortex of choline acetyltransferase activity.

Nucleus basalis of Meynert. A group of neurons in the substantia innominata below the globus pallidus. This nucleus is the source of cholinergic innervation of the cerebral cortex. Loss of neurons in the nucleus occurs in patients with Alzheimer's disease. Named after Theodor Hermann Meynert, an Austrian psychiatrist.

Careful studies on the distribution of neurofibrillary tangles in Alzheimer's brains have shown a preponderance of these tangles in limbic and multimodal association cortices compared with primary association, primary sensory, and primary motor cortices. The temporal lobe contains more tangles than do all the other lobes, and the entorhinal cortex has the greatest density of neurofibrillary tangles. It is well established that the entorhinal cortex serves as a link between the hippocampal formation (important for memory) and the rest of the cerebral cortex. Severe neuropathology in the entorhinal cortex, as occurs in Alzheimer's disease, thus isolates or disconnects the hippocampal formation from the remainder of the cortex and results in severe memory loss.

KEY CONCEPTS

- Alzheimer's disease is a degenerative brain disease characterized by severe memory loss, disorientation, and behavioral changes. The brunt of the pathology is in the entorhinal cortex, which isolates the hippocampal formation from the rest of the cerebral cortex.

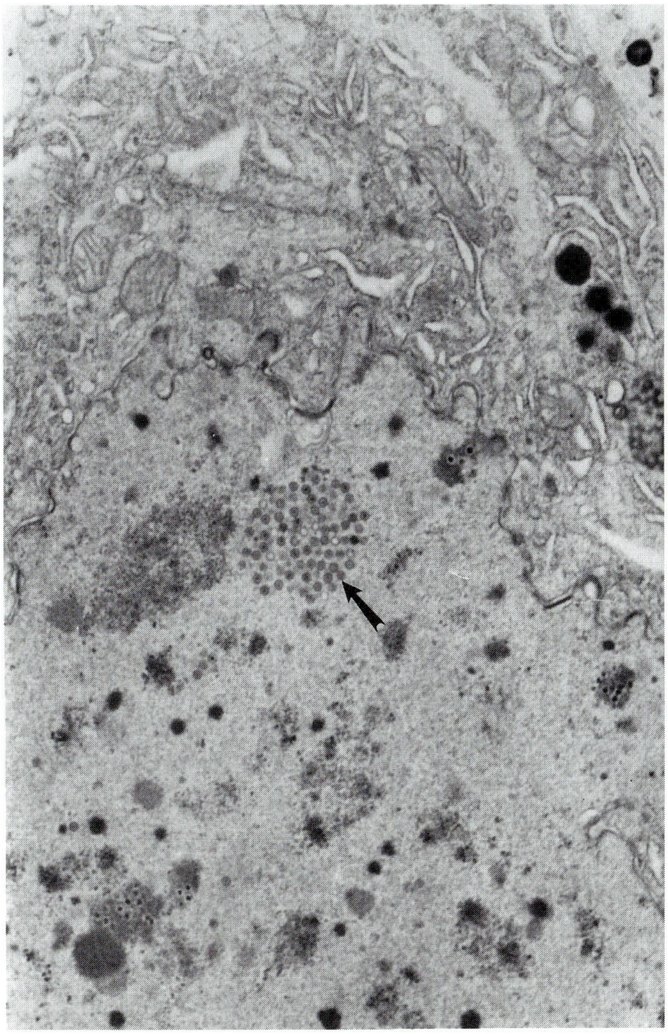

FIGURE 22-3

Electron micrograph showing intranuclear viral inclusions (Cowdry type A) (*arrow*) in brain biopsy of a patient with herpes simplex encephalitis.

HERPES SIMPLEX ENCEPHALITIS

Herpes simplex encephalitis is a viral encephalitis caused by herpesvirus and characterized by focal seizures, focal neurologic signs, and progressive deterioration of consciousness. It is the single most important cause of fatal sporadic encephalitis in the United States. The neuropathology consists of a severe focal necrotizing process with a predilection for the limbic system. A brain biopsy is diagnostic in showing characteristic intranuclear viral inclusions (Fig. 22-3) (Cowdry type A inclusions) and inflammation. MRI is the most sensitive noninvasive test for the early diagnosis of herpes simplex encephalitis and the demonstration of pathology in the limbic system (Fig. 22-4). Early diagnosis is crucial because there is an effective antiviral treatment for this type of encephalitis.

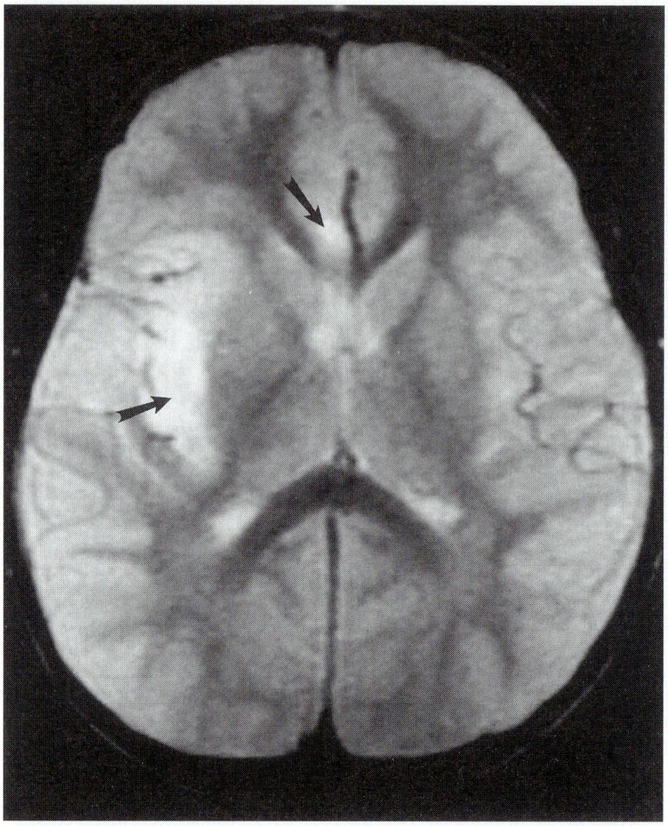

FIGURE 22-4

T2-weighted magnetic resonance image of the brain showing increased signal intensity (*arrows*) in components of the limbic system in a patient with herpes simplex encephalitis.

SUGGESTED READINGS

Arnold SE, Trojanowski JQ: Recent advances in defining the neuropathology of schizophrenia. *Acta Neuropathol* (*Berl*) 1996; 92:217–231.

Blass JP, Gibson GE: Abnormality of a thiamine-requiring enzyme in patients with Wernicke-Korsakoff syndrome. *N Engl J Med* 1977; 297:1367–1370.

Bossi L, et al: Somatomotor manifestations of temporal lobe seizures. *Epilepsia* 1984; 25:70–76.

Braak H, et al: Functional anatomy of human hippocampal formation and related structures. *J Child Neurol* 1996; 11:265–275.

D'Esposito M, et al: Amnesia following traumatic bilateral fornix transection. *Neurology* 1995; 45:1546–1550.

Eichenbaum H, et al: Selective olfactory deficits in case H.M. *Brain* 1983; 106:459–472.

Freeman R, Schachter SC: Autonomic epilepsy. *Semin Neurol* 1995; 15:158–166.

Gabrieli JDE: Disorders of memory in humans. *Curr Opin Neurol Neurosurg* 1993; 6:93–97.

Gaffan D, Gaffan EA: Amnesia in man following transection of the fornix. *Brain* 1991; 114:2611–2618.

Gaffan EA, et al: Amnesia following damage to the left fornix and to other sites: A comparative study. *Brain* 1991; 114:1297–1313.

Horel JA: The neuroanatomy of amnesia: A critique of the hippocampal memory hypothesis. *Brain* 1978; 101:403–445.

Jafek BW, et al: Post-traumatic anosmia: Ultrastructural correlates. *Arch Neurol* 1989; 46:300–304.

Klüver H, Bucy PC: Preliminary analysis of functions of the temporal lobes in monkeys. *Arch Neurol Psychiatry* 1939; 42:979–1000.

Kritchevsky M, et al: Transient global amnesia: Characterization of anterograde and retrograde amnesia. *Neurology* 1988; 38:213–219.

Laloux P, et al: Technetium-99m HM-PAO single photon emission computed tomography imaging in transient global amnesia. *Arch Neurol* 1992; 49:543–546.

Marlow WB, et al: Complete Klüver Bucy syndrome in man. *Cortex* 1975; 11:53–59.

Mesulam MM: Large-scale neurocognitive networks and distributed processing for attention, language, and memory. *Ann Neurol* 1990; 28:597–613.

Miller JW, et al: Transient global amnesia: Clinical characteristics and prognosis. *Neurology* 1987; 37:733–737.

Miller JW, et al: Transient global amnesia and epilepsy: Electroencephalographic distinction. *Arch Neurol* 1987; 44:629–633.

Nissen, MJ, et al: Neurochemical dissociation of memory systems. *Neurology* 1987; 37:789–794.

Perani D, et al: Evidence of multiple memory systems in the human brain: A [^{18}F] FDG PET metabolic study. *Brain* 1993; 116:903–919.

Perry RJ, Hodges JR: Spectrum of memory dysfunction in degenerative disease. *Curr Opin Neurol* 1996; 9: 281–285.

Rapp PR, Heindel WC: Memory systems in normal and pathological aging. *Curr Opin Neurol* 1994; 7:294–298.

Scoville WB, Milner B: Loss of recent memory after bilateral hippocampal lesions. *J Neurol Neurosurg Psychiatry* 1957; 20:11–21.

Terzian H, Dalle Ore G: Syndrome of Klüver and Bucy reproduced in man by bilateral removal of the temporal lobes. *Neurology* 1955; 5:373–380.

Van Hoesen GW, Solodkin A: Cellular and systems neuroanatomical changes in Alzheimer's disease. In Distenhoff JE, et al (eds): *Calcium Hypothesis of Aging and Dementia. Ann NY Acad Sci* 1994; 747:12–35.

Winocur G, et al: Amnesia in a patient with bilateral lesions to the thalamus. *Neuropsychologia* 1984; 22:123–143.

Yanker B, Mesulam M-M: β-Amyloid and the pathogenesis of Alzheimer's disease. *N Engl J Med* 1991; 325:1849–1857.

CHAPTER 23

SPECIAL SENSES

The different sensations perceived by the human body are grouped into two major categories: those concerned with general sensations (touch, pressure, pain, and temperature) and those concerned with special sensations (olfaction, taste, vision, audition, and sense of position and movement). This chapter is devoted to a consideration of the organs of special senses. Whereas nerve endings concerned with general sensibility are distributed widely, those concerned with special sensations are limited to specific areas of the body.

OLFACTION

Olfactory stimuli are received by receptors of the olfactory epithelium in the nasal wall and are conveyed via olfactory nerve fibers through the cribriform plate of the ethmoid bone to the olfactory bulb inside the cranial cavity. Within the olfactory bulb, axons of the olfactory nerve synapse with mitral and tufted cells in a complex

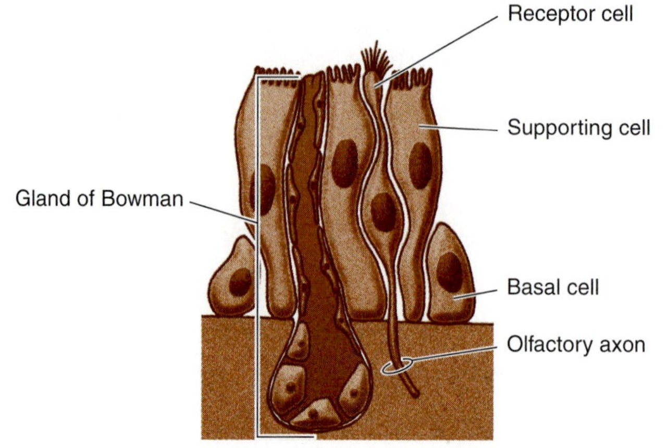
Receptor cell
Supporting cell
Gland of Bowman
Basal cell
Olfactory axon

FIGURE 23-1

Schematic diagram of the cellular components of the olfactory mucosa.

structure known as the *olfactory glomerulus.* Axons of mitral and tufted neurons form the olfactory tract, which lies in the olfactory sulcus on the undersurface of the frontal lobe. Close to the anterior perforated substance, the olfactory tract divides into the lateral, intermediate, and medial olfactory striae. The lateral olfactory stria terminates in the primary olfactory cortex, where olfaction is perceived. The medial olfactory stria joins the anterior commissure to reach the contralateral olfactory tract and bulb. It also projects on limbic system structures. The intermediate olfactory stria blends with the anterior perforated substance. The medial and intermediate olfactory striae are not well developed in humans and do not play a role in perception of olfactory stimuli.

Olfactory (Latin *olfacere,* "to smell"). Pertaining to the sense of smell. The olfactory nerve, the first cranial nerve in today's classification, was proposed by Sömmerring (1755–1830), the German anatomist, although it was not included as a cranial nerve by Galen. The olfactory nerves were first noted by Theophilus Protospatharius, physician to the Emperor Heraclius in the seventh century A.D. The function of the olfactory nerve was correctly stated by Achillini, and its relationship to the neuroepithelium of the nasal mucosa was demonstrated by Max Schultze in 1856.

Olfactory Epithelium

The olfactory epithelium is located in the mucous membrane lining the uppermost part of the roof of the nasal cavity. From the roof, the olfactory epithelium extends down both sides of the nasal cavity to cover most of the superior concha laterally and 1 cm of nasal septum medially. Humans are microsmatic animals in whom the surface area of olfactory mucous membrane in both nostrils is small (approximately 5 cm^2).

The olfactory epithelium contains three types of epithelial cells: receptor cells, supporting cells, and basal cells (Fig. 23-1). Interspersed among epithelial cells are ducts of Bowman's glands.

Receptor Cells

Olfactory receptor cells are bipolar sensory neurons. Their perikarya are located in the lower part of the olfactory epithelium. Each cell has a single dendrite that reaches the surface of the epithelium and forms a knoblike expansion that extends beyond the epithelial surface. From this expansion, 10 to 20 cilia project into a

KEY CONCEPTS

- The olfactory sense organ is located in the roof of the nose and the upper part of the lateral wall and septum.

layer of fluid covering the epithelium. From the basal part of the perikaryon, a nonmyelinated axon emerges and joins with axons of adjacent receptor cells to form the olfactory nerve (first cranial nerve). Olfactory nerve bundles penetrate the **cribriform** plate of the ethmoid bone to reach the olfactory bulb.

Cribriform (Latin *cribrum*, "a sieve"; *forma*, "form"). The cribriform plate of the ethmoid bone is so named because of the numerous perforations.

It is estimated that there are more than 100 million receptor cells in the olfactory mucosa. The specialized nerve cells of the olfactory epithelium are highly sensitive to different odors. Olfactory neurons are produced continuously from basal cells of the olfactory epithelium and are lost continuously by normal wear and tear. The presence of these nerve cells at the surface exposes them unduly to damage; it is estimated that 1 percent of the fibers of the olfactory nerves (axons of olfactory neurons) are lost each year of life because of injury to the perikarya. The sense of smell thus diminishes in the elderly as a result of exposure of the olfactory epithelium to repeated infections and trauma in life. The presence of olfactory neurons at the surface represents the only exception to the evolutionary rule by which nerve cell bodies of afferent neurons migrate along their axons to take up more central and well-protected positions. The surface of the olfactory epithelium is moistened constantly by secretions of Bowman's glands. This moistening helps dissolve the gaseous substances, facilitating stimulation of the olfactory epithelium. The continuous secretion also cleanses the receptors of accumulated odorous substances and prevents their retention.

It is believed that different basic odors stimulate different olfactory neurons. Stimulation of different combinations of receptors for basic odors is believed to be the basis for humans' ability to recognize all the varieties of odors to which they are exposed.

Supporting (Sustentacular) Cells

Supporting cells are columnar epithelial cells that separate the olfactory receptor cells. The surface of supporting cells is specialized into microvilli that project into the fluid layer covering the epithelium.

Basal Cells

Basal cells are polygonal cells limited to the basal part of the epithelium. They are the source of new epithelial cells. Mitotic activity persists in these cells through maturity.

Bowman's Glands

Bowman's glands contain serous and mucous cells and are located beneath the epithelium. They send their ducts in between epithelial cells to pour their secretion onto the surface of the epithelium, bathing the cilia of receptor cells and the microvilli of supporting cells. The secretion of Bowman's glands plays an important role in dissolving odorous substances and diffusing them to receptor cells.

Bowman's gland. Branched and tubuloalveolar glands located beneath the olfactory epithelium. Secretions of the glands are important in dissolving odorous substances and diffusing them to olfactory receptor cells. Named after Sir William Bowman (1816–1892), an English ophthalmologic surgeon and anatomist.

Olfactory Nerve

The olfactory nerve (see Fig. 21-1) is composed of unmyelinated thin processes (rootlets) of the olfactory hair cells in the nasal mucosa. Fascicles of the olfactory nerve pierce the cribriform plate of the ethmoid bone, enter the cranial cavity, and terminate on neurons in the olfactory bulb.

KEY CONCEPTS

- Olfactory epithelium contains three types of cells: receptor, supporting, and basal.
- Axons of receptor cells form the olfactory nerve.

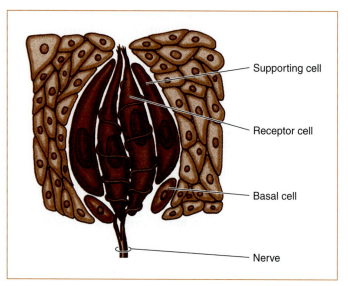

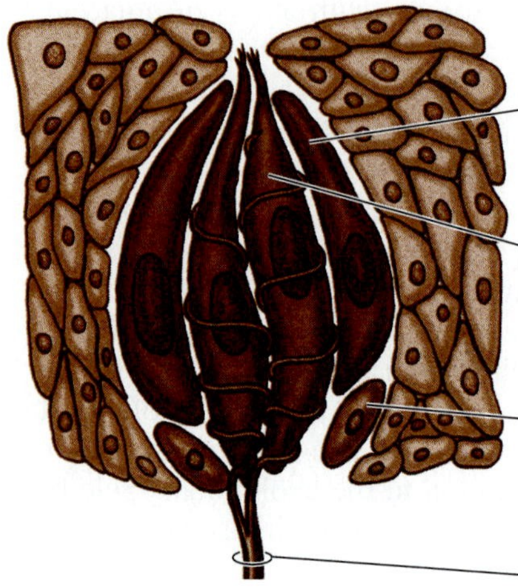
Supporting cell
Receptor cell
Basal cell
Nerve

FIGURE 23-2

Schematic diagram of the cellular components of the taste bud.

Olfactory Bulb

The olfactory bulb (see Fig. 21-1) is the main relay station in the olfactory pathways.

Lamination and Cell Types (Fig. 21-2)
In histologic sections, the olfactory bulb appears laminated into the following layers (see Fig. 21-2):

Mitral (Latin *mitra,* "a kind of a hat with two cusps, a turban, or head band").

Olfactory nerve layer. This layer is composed of incoming olfactory nerve fibers.
Glomerular layer. In this layer, synaptic formations occur between olfactory nerve axons and dendrites of olfactory bulb neurons (**mitral** and tufted neurons).
Plexiform layer. This layer consists of tufted neurons, some granule cells, and a few mitral cells with their processes.
Mitral cell layer. This layer is composed of large neurons (mitral neurons).
Granule layer. Composed of small granule neurons and processes of granule and mitral cells, this layer also contains incoming fibers from other cortical regions.

The mitral and tufted cells are considered the principal neurons of the olfactory bulb. Their dendrites establish synaptic relationships with the olfactory nerve fibers within the glomeruli.

The granule cells are considered to be the intrinsic neurons of the olfactory bulb. These cells have vertically oriented dendrites but no axon and exert their action on other cells solely by dendrites. The olfactory bulb contains two other varieties of intrinsic neurons. These are the periglomerular short axon cells in close proximity to the glomeruli in the glomerular layer and the deep short axon cells located in the granule layer.

The olfactory bulb receives fibers (input) from the following sources:

1. Olfactory hair cells in the nasal mucosa
2. Contralateral olfactory bulb

KEY CONCEPTS

- Olfactory nerve fibers synapse on mitral and tufted neurons of the olfactory bulb.

3. Primary olfactory cortex
4. Diagonal band of Broca
5. Anterior olfactory nucleus

The output from the olfactory bulb is the olfactory tract.

Olfactory Tract

The olfactory tract (see Fig. 21-1) is the outflow pathway of the olfactory bulb. It is composed of the axons of principal neurons (mitral and tufted cells) of the olfactory bulb and centrifugal axons originating from the contralateral olfactory bulb, as well as from central brain regions. The olfactory tract also contains the scattered neurons of the anterior olfactory nucleus, the axons of which contribute to the olfactory tract. At its caudal extremity, just anterior to the anterior perforated substance, the olfactory tract divides into the olfactory striae (see Fig. 21-1).

Olfactory Striae

At its caudal extremity, just rostral to the anterior perforated substance, the olfactory tract divides into three striae:

1. Lateral olfactory stria
2. Medial olfactory stria
3. Intermediate olfactory stria.

Each of the striae is covered by a thin layer of gray matter, the olfactory gyri.

The lateral olfactory stria projects to the primary olfactory cortex in the temporal lobe. The medial olfactory stria projects on the medial olfactory area, also known as the *septal area,* located on the medial surface of the frontal lobe, ventral to the genu and rostrum of the corpus callosum (subcallosal gyrus) and anterior to the lamina terminalis. The medial olfactory area is closely related to the limbic system and hence is concerned with emotional responses elicited by olfactory stimuli. It does not play a role in the perception of olfactory stimuli. The medial and intermediate striae are poorly developed in humans. The intermediate stria blends with the anterior perforated substance. The thin cortex at this site is designated the *intermediate olfactory area.* The primary terminal stations of the three olfactory striae (olfactory cortices) are interconnected by the diagonal band of Broca, a bundle of subcortical fibers in front of the optic tract, and with a number of cortical and subcortical areas concerned with visceral function and emotion (hippocampus, thalamus, hypothalamus, epithalamus, and brain stem reticular formation). Through these connections, the olfactory system exerts influence on visceral function (salivation, nausea) and behavioral reactions.

Primary Olfactory Cortex

The primary olfactory cortex is located within the uncus of the temporal lobe and is composed of the prepiriform cortex, periamygdaloid area, and part of the

KEY CONCEPTS

- Axons of mitral and tufted neurons form the olfactory tract.
- The olfactory tract subdivides into three striae.
- The lateral olfactory stria terminates in the primary olfactory cortex.
- The medial and intermediate striae link the olfactory system with the limbic system.

entorhinal area. The prepiriform cortex is the region on each side of and beneath the lateral olfactory stria; hence it is also called the *lateral olfactory gyrus.* It is considered the major part of the primary olfactory cortex. The primary olfactory cortex is relatively large in some animals, such as the rabbit, but in humans it occupies a small area. The primary olfactory cortex in humans is concerned with the conscious perception of olfactory stimuli. In contrast to all other primary sensory cortices (vision, audition, taste, and somatic sensibility), the primary olfactory cortex is unique in that afferent fibers from the receptors reach it directly without passing through a relay in the thalamus.

The primary olfactory cortex contains two types of neurons. These are (1) principal neurons (pyramidal cells) with axons that leave the olfactory cortex and project to nearby or distant regions and (2) intrinsic neurons (stellate cells) with axons that remain within the olfactory cortex.

The major input to the primary olfactory cortex is from (1) the olfactory bulb via the lateral olfactory stria and (2) other central brain regions. The output from the olfactory cortex is via axons of principal neurons that project to nearby areas surrounding the primary olfactory cortex, as well as to more distant areas, such as the thalamus and hypothalamus, which play important roles in behavior and emotion.

Olfactory Mechanisms

Olfaction is a chemical sense. For a substance to be detected, it should have the following physical properties:

- *Volatility,* so that it can be sniffed
- *Water solubility,* so that it can diffuse through the olfactory epithelium
- *Lipid solubility,* so that it will interact with the lipids of the membranes of olfactory receptors

After an odorous substance is dissolved in the fluid bathing the surface of the olfactory mucosa, it interacts with receptor sites located on the cilia of receptor cells. The binding of a single appropriate molecule to one receptor site causes a change in membrane permeability. The ion flux that ensues gives rise to a slow surface negative wave (receptor or generator potential) that can be detected at the surface of the receptor cell. An all-or-none action potential, however, can be detected in the axons of receptor cells.

The olfactory receptors show a marked variability in sensitivity to different odors. They can detect methyl mercaptan (garlic odor) in a concentration of less than one-millionth of a milligram per liter of air but ethyl ether in a concentration of 5.8 mg per liter of air.

Olfactory receptors adapt rather quickly to a continuous stimulus. Although the olfactory mucosa can discriminate among a large number of different odors, its ability to detect changes in concentration of an odorous substance is rather poor. It is estimated that the concentration of an odorous substance must change by 30 percent before it can be detected by receptor cells. The mechanism of discrimination

KEY CONCEPTS

- Olfaction is a chemical sense.
- The sense of taste is a chemical sense.
- Interaction of an odorous substance with olfactory receptor cells gives rise to a receptor or generator potential.
- Receptor potentials are transformed into action potentials in the olfactory nerve.

is poorly understood but is probably related to a spatial pattern of stimulation of the receptor cells.

TASTE

The **gustatory** (taste) sense organs in higher vertebrates are limited to the cavity of the mouth. Taste receptors are located within taste buds in the tongue (**circumvallate** and **fungiform** papillae), as well as in the soft palate, oropharynx, and epiglottis. There are about 2000 taste buds in the human tongue. This number decreases progressively with age. Taste sensations are conveyed centrally via three cranial nerves: the facial (CN VII), glossopharyngeal (CN IX), and vagus (CN X) cranial nerves.

Gustatory (Latin *gustatorius,* "pertaining to the sense of taste").
Circumvallate (Latin *circum,* "around"; *vallare,* "to wall"). Surrounded by a trench or wall.
Fungiform. Shaped like a fungus or mushroom.

Taste Buds

Taste buds (Fig. 23-2) are barrel-like structures distributed in the epithelium of the tongue, soft palate, oropharynx, and epiglottis. Each taste bud is composed of receptor (neuroepithelial), supporting, and basal cells, and nerve fibers.

Receptor Cells

Two types of receptor cells can be identified in taste buds, clear receptor cells and dense receptor cells. Clear receptor cells contain clear vesicles; dense receptor cells contain dense-core vesicles that store glycosaminoglycans. Both cell types presumably function as receptors. They are believed to represent two stages in the development of receptor elements, the dense cell being the more mature. The apex of each receptor cell is modified into microvilli, which increase the receptor surface area and project into an opening, the taste pore. Approximately 4 to 20 receptor cells are located in the center of each taste bud. Receptor elements decrease in number with age. Receptor cells are stimulated by substances in solution.

Supporting Cells

These are spindle-shaped cells that surround the receptor cells. They are located at the periphery of the taste bud. They have both an insulating function and a secretory function. They are believed to secrete the substance that bathes the microvilli in the taste pore.

Basal Cells

Basal cells are located at the base of the taste bud and, by division, replenish the receptor cells that are lost continually.

Nerve Fibers

The nerve fibers in the taste bud are terminal nerve fibers of the facial, glossopharyngeal, and vagus nerves. They are peripheral processes of sensory neurons in the geniculate ganglion of the facial nerve and in the inferior ganglia of the glossopharyngeal and vagus nerves. They enter the taste bud at its base and wind themselves around the receptor cells in close apposition to receptor cell membranes. Synaptic vesicles cluster on the inner surfaces of receptor cell membranes at sites of apposition to nerve terminals.

KEY CONCEPTS

- The gustatory (taste) sense organs (taste buds) are distributed in the tongue, soft palate, oropharynx, and epiglottis.
- Taste buds are composed of three types of cells: receptor, supporting, and basal.

Physiology of Taste

Although all taste buds look alike histologically, sensitivity to the four basic taste modalities is different in different regions of the tongue. Like olfaction, the sense of taste is a chemical sense. Although humans can taste a large number of substances, only four primary taste sensations are identified:

- Sour
- Salty
- Sweet
- Bitter

Most taste receptors respond to all four primary taste modalities at varying thresholds but respond preferentially at a very low threshold to only one or two. Thus taste buds at the tip of the tongue respond best to sweet and salty substances, and those at the lateral margins and posterior part of the tongue respond best to sour and bitter substances, respectively.

The ability of taste buds to detect changes in concentration of a substance is poor, similar to the response of olfactory receptors. A difference in taste intensity remains undetected until the concentration of a substance has changed by 30 percent. The mechanism by which a substance is tasted is not well understood. Substances in solution enter the pore of the taste bud and come in contact with the surface of taste receptors. This contact induces a change in the electrical potential of the membrane of the receptor cells (receptor or generator potential). The receptor potential in turn generates an action potential in nerve terminals in apposition to the receptor cell surface.

Central Transmission of Taste Sensations (Fig. 23-3)

Taste sensations from the anterior two-thirds of the tongue are mediated to the central nervous system via the chorda tympani of the seventh (facial) cranial nerve, those from the posterior one-third of the tongue via the ninth (glossopharyngeal) cranial nerve, and those from the epiglottis and lower pharynx via the tenth (vagus) cranial nerve. These nerves contain the peripheral processes of pseudounipolar sensory nerve cells located in the geniculate ganglion (seventh nerve), petrous ganglion (ninth nerve), and nodose ganglion (tenth nerve). These peripheral processes enter the deep ends of the taste buds and establish intimate contact with the neuroepithelial cells of the buds.

The central processes of these sensory neurons project to the nucleus of the tractus solitarius in the brain stem. Axons of neurons in the nucleus solitarius

KEY CONCEPTS

- Four basic taste sensations are identified: sour, salty, sweet, and bitter.
- Taste buds in different locations of the tongue respond best to different tastes. Those at the tip of the tongue respond best to sweet and salty substances; those at the margins and posterior part of the tongue respond best to sour and bitter substances.
- Taste sensations are transmitted centrally via three cranial nerves: facial, glossopharyngeal, and vagus.
- Central taste pathways establish synapses in several brain stem nuclei (nucleus solitarius, reticular nuclei, ventral posterior medial) before reaching the primary gustatory cortex in the inferior part of the somesthetic cortex.

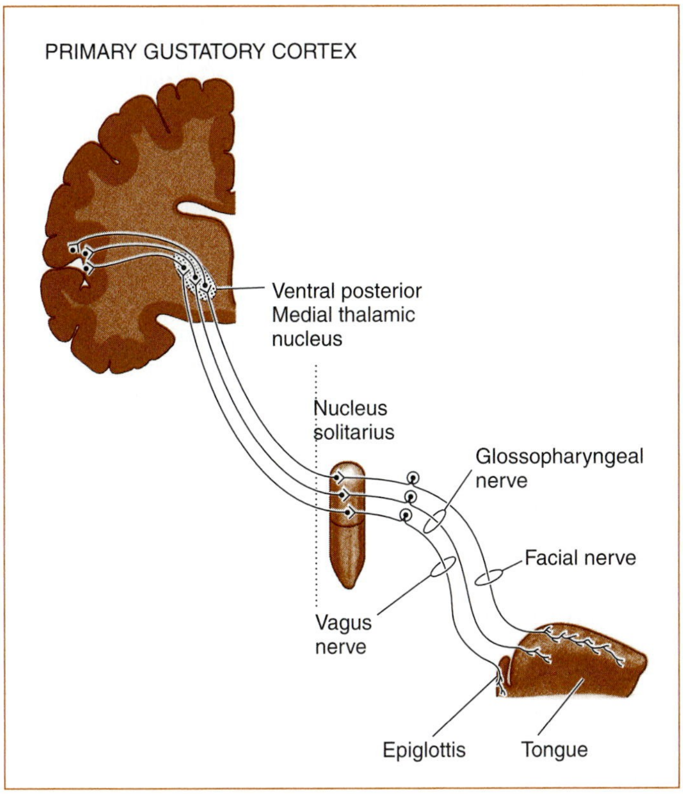
PRIMARY GUSTATORY CORTEX
Ventral posterior
Medial thalamic
nucleus
Nucleus
solitarius
Glossopharyngeal
nerve
Facial nerve
Vagus
nerve
Epiglottis
Tongue

FIGURE 23-3

Schematic diagram of the gustatory pathways.

project on a number of reticular nuclei before crossing the midline to reach the ventral posterior medial (VPM) nucleus of the thalamus, giving on their way collateral branches to such nuclei as the nucleus ambiguus and salivatory nuclei for reflex activity. From the VPM nucleus, axons project to the cerebral cortex to terminate on neurons in the inferior part of the somesthetic cortex, just anterior to the face area (primary gustatory cortex).

VISION

Vision is by far the most important of the human senses. Most of our perception of the environment around us comes through our eyes. Our visual system is capable of adapting to extreme changes in light intensity to allow us to see clearly; it is also capable of color discrimination and depth perception. The organ of vision is the eye; accessory structures are the eyelids, lacrimal glands, and extrinsic eye muscles.

The eye has been compared with a camera. Although structurally the two are similar, the camera lacks the intricate automatic control mechanism involved in vision. As an optic instrument, the eye has four functional components: a protective coat, a nourishing lightproof coat, a dioptric system, and a receptive integrating layer. The protective coat is the tough, opaque **sclera**, which covers the posterior five-sixths of the eyeball; it is continuous with the dura mater around the optic nerve. The anterior one-sixth is covered by a transparent cornea, which belongs to the dioptric system. The nourishing coat is made up of the vascular choroid, which supplies nutrients to the retina and, because of its rich content of melanocytes, acts as a light-absorbing layer. It corresponds to the pia-arachnoid layer of the nervous system. Anteriorly, this coat becomes the ciliary body and iris. The iris ends at a circular opening, the pupil.

Sclera (Greek *skleros,* "hard"). The outermost, tough, fibrous coat of the eyeball. The term was first used to refer to the whole white outer layer by Salomon Albertus, professor of anatomy in Wittenburg in 1585.

Cornea (Latin *corneus,* "horny"). The transparent structure forming the anterior part of the fibrous tunic of the eye.

Lens (Latin *lentil,* "a bean"). The lens of the eye resembles a lentil.

Ciliary muscle (Latin *cilium,* "eyelid or eyelash"). Smooth muscles of the ciliary body; the circumferential fibers were described by Heinrich Müller in 1858 and the radial fibers by William Bowman in 1847. Together they control the aperture of the pupil and the degree of curvature of the lens.

The dioptric system comprises the **cornea**, the **lens**, the aqueous humor within the anterior eye chamber, and the vitreous body. The dioptric system helps focus the image on the retina. The greatest refraction of incoming light takes place at the air-cornea interface. The lens is supported by the suspensory ligament from the ciliary body, and changes in its shape permit change of focus. This is a function of the **ciliary muscle**, which is supplied by the parasympathetic nervous system. In late middle age, the lens loses its elastic properties, and a condition known as *presbyopia* results, wherein accommodative power is diminished, especially for near vision. The amount of light entering the eye is regulated by the size of the pupil. Pupillary size is controlled by the action of the constrictor and dilator smooth muscles of the iris. The constrictor muscle is supplied by the parasympathetic nervous system and the dilator muscle by the sympathetic nervous system.

The receptive integrating layer of the eye is the retina, which is an extension of the brain, to which it is connected by the optic nerve. The rods and cones are the sensory retinal receptors.

The Retina

Light rays falling on the eye pass through its refractive media (cornea, lens, and anterior and posterior chambers) before reaching the visual receptor cells (the rods and cones) in the retina. The refractive media help focus the image on the retina.

The retina (Fig. 23-4), an ectodermal derivative, is an outward extension of the brain, to which it is connected by the optic nerve. The human retina is made up of the following ten layers, starting with the outermost:

- Layer of pigment epithelium
- Layer of rods and cones
- External limiting membrane
- Outer nuclear layer
- Outer plexiform layer
- Inner nuclear layer
- Inner plexiform layer
- Layer of ganglion cells
- Optic nerve layer
- Internal limiting membrane

Five types of neurons are distributed throughout these layers:

- Receptor cells
- Bipolar cells
- Ganglion cells
- Horizontal cells
- **Amacrine** cells

Amacrine (Greek *a,* "negative"; *makros,* "long"). Having no long processes. The amacrine cells of the retina have no long processes.

KEY CONCEPTS

- Light rays pass through the dioptric system of the eye (cornea, lens, aqueous humor, vitreous body) before reaching the visual receptors in the retina.
- The visual receptor cells are located in the retina.
- The retina is an outward extension of the brain.

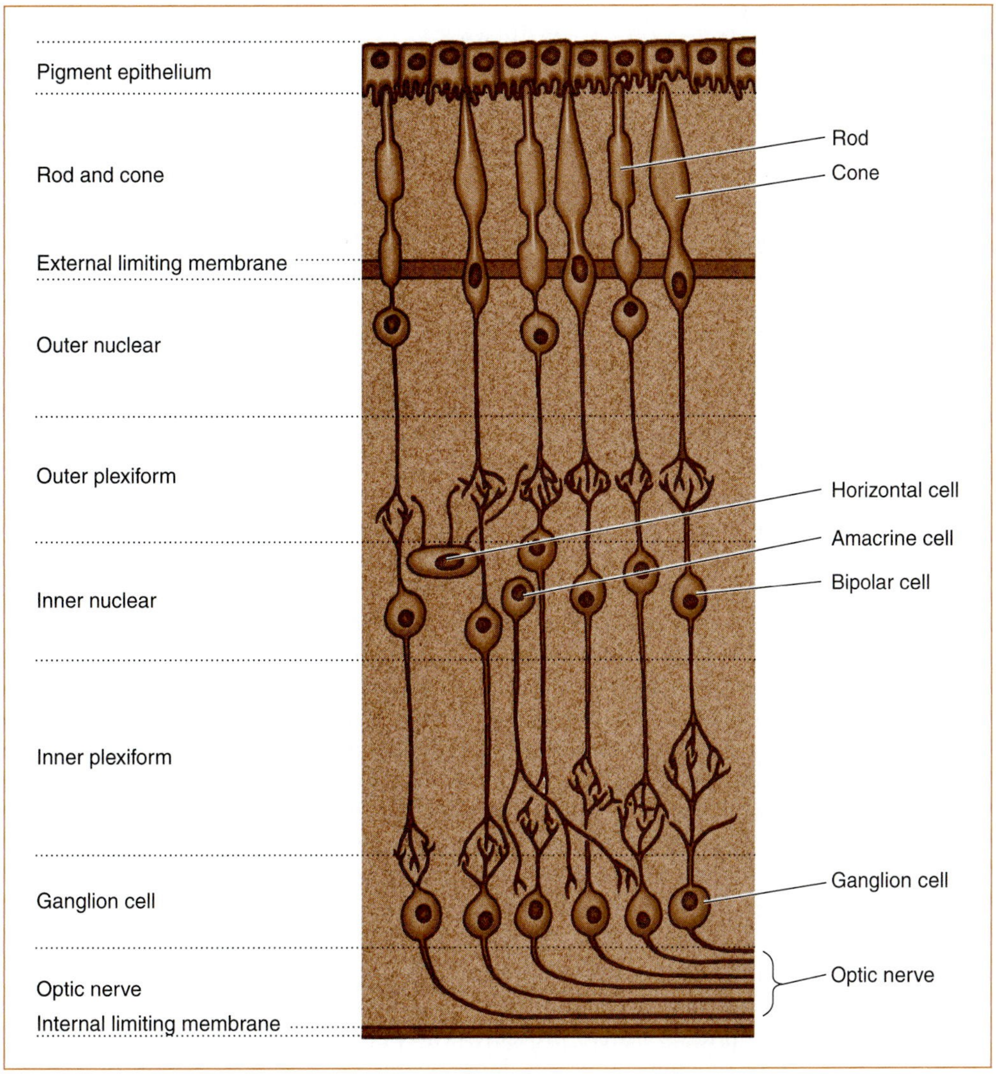

FIGURE 23-4

Schematic diagram of the layers of the retina and their cellular components.

Layer of Pigment Epithelium

The pigment epithelium is a single layer of melanin-containing, pigmented cuboidal cells firmly bound at their bases to the choroid layer. The cell membrane at the apices of these epithelial cells is specialized into slender microvilli that interdigitate with the outer segments of photoreceptor cells. The lateral walls show conspicuous zonulae occludentes and zonulae adherentes as well as desmosomes and gap junctions. The function of this layer is not well understood; it probably plays a role in light absorption. Retinal detachment, essentially a splitting of this layer from the other retinal layers, is nowadays treated with laser surgery.

Layer of Rods and Cones

The rods and cones are the light-sensitive parts of the photoreceptors. The human retina contains approximately 100 million rods and 6 to 7 million cones. The rods and cones differ in their distribution along the retina. In humans, a modified region called the **fovea** contains only cones and is adapted for high visual acuity. At all other points along the retina, rods greatly outnumber cones.

Fovea (Latin "a pit, a small hollow"). The part of the macula that receives light from the central part of the visual field and which contains high concentration of cones.

Rods

The rod photoreceptor cell is a modified neuron having as components the cell body, axonal process, and photosensitive process. The cell body contains the nucleus. This part of the rod is located in the outer nuclear layer. The axonal process is located in the outer plexiform layer. The photosensitive process is located in the layer of rods and cones. The photosensitive process of the rod is made up of two segments, outer and inner, connected by a narrow neck containing cilia. The outer segment has been shown by electron microscopy to be filled with stacks of double-membrane disks containing the visual pigment rhodopsin. The disks are not continuous with the cell membrane. The function of the outer segment is to trap the light that reaches the retina. The visual pigment molecules are positioned within the disk membranes in such a way as to maximize the probability of their interacting with the path of incident light. The extensive invagination of the disk membranes increases the total surface area available for visual pigment. Rhodopsin is composed of a vitamin A aldehyde (retinal) combined with the protein scotopsin. Exposure to light breaks the bond between retinal and the protein. This chemical change triggers a change in the electric potential and produces a generator (receptor) potential. The stacked disks in the outer segment are shed continually and are replaced by the infolding of the cell membrane. The outer segments are separated and supported by processes from the layer of pigment epithelium.

The inner segment of the rod's photosensitive process contains mitochondria, glycogen, endoplasmic reticulum, and Golgi apparatus. It is the site of formation of the protein scotopsin, which subsequently moves to the outer segment. The inner segment is connected to the cell body of the rod fiber, which traverses the external limiting membrane. The outer segment of rods is the photosensitive part, where the receptor potential is generated, whereas the inner segment is the site of metabolic activity, where protein and phospholipids are synthesized and energy is produced. Extremely sensitive to light, rods are the receptors used when low levels of light are available, such as at night.

Cones

Cones have the same structural components as the rods (cell body, axonal process, and photosensitive process). The photosensitive processes of cones, like those of rods, contain outer and inner segments. The disks in the outer segments, unlike those of rods, are attached to the cell membrane and are not shed. They contain iodopsin, an unstable, light-sensitive visual pigment composed of vitamin A aldehyde conjugated to a specific protein (cone opsin). Cones are sensitive to light of higher intensity than that required for rod vision.

External Limiting Membrane

A sievelike sheet, the external limiting membrane, is fenestrated to allow the passage of processes that connect the photosensitive processes of rods and cones with their cell bodies. It also contains the outer processes of Müller's (supporting) cells.

Outer Nuclear Layer

The outer nuclear layer of the retina contains the cell bodies of rods and cones with their nuclei. Cone nuclei are ovoid and limited to a single row close to the

KEY CONCEPTS

- There are two types of visual receptor cells: rods and cones.
- Other cell types in the retina are bipolar, ganglion, horizontal, and amacrine.
- The human retina contains 6 to 7 million cones and 100 million rods.

external limiting membrane. Rod nuclei are rounded and distributed in several layers.

Outer Plexiform Layer
Also known as the *outer synaptic layer,* the outer plexiform layer contains axonal processes of rods and cones, as well as dendrites of bipolar cells and processes of horizontal cells.

Inner Nuclear Layer
The inner nuclear layer contains cell bodies and nuclei of bipolar cells and association cells (horizontal and amacrine) as well as supporting (Müller's) cells. The layer has three zones: an outer zone containing horizontal cells, an intermediate zone containing bipolar cells, and an inner zone containing amacrine cells.

Three types of bipolar cells are recognized. Rod bipolar cells are related to several rod axons, midget bipolar cells are related to one cone axon, and flat bipolar cells are related to several cone axons.

The horizontal association cells are larger than bipolar cells. Their axons and dendrites are located in the outer plexiform layer. Their axons establish synapses with rod and cone axons, whereas their dendrites establish relationships with cone axons. Thus they connect cones of one area with cones and rods of another area.

The amacrine association cells are pear shaped. Each has a single process that terminates on a bipolar or ganglion cell process in the inner plexiform layer. Müller's supporting cells send their processes to the outer plexiform layer.

Inner Plexiform Layer
The inner plexiform, also called *synaptic,* layer contains axons of bipolar cells, dendrites of ganglion cells, and processes of the association (amacrine) cells.

Layer of Ganglion Cells
The perikarya of multipolar ganglion cells constitute the eighth layer of the retina. Two types of ganglion cells are recognized on the basis of their dendritic connections: a monosynaptic (midget) ganglion cell related to a single bipolar midget cell and a diffuse (polysynaptic) ganglion cell related to several bipolar cells. The axons of ganglion cells traverse the inner surface of the retina and collect at the papilla, where they penetrate the sclera to form the optic nerve. This part of the retina contains no receptor cells and is called the *blind spot.* In humans, the number of ganglion cells is estimated to be 1 million.

Optic Nerve Layer
The optic nerve layer is composed of axons of ganglion cells that form the optic nerve, as well as some Müller's fibers and neuroglial cells. Axons of ganglion cells in this layer are unmyelinated but have a glial sheath around them. They run toward the posterior pole of the eye, where they form the optic disk and penetrate the sclera to form the optic nerve.

Internal Limiting Membrane
The expanded inner ends of the processes of Müller's cells form the internal limiting membrane. Müller's cells, the cell bodies of which are located in the inner nuclear layer, send processes both outward to the external limiting membrane and inward to the internal limiting membrane. They are thus homologous to glial cells of the central nervous system.

Variations in Retinal Structure

The retinal structure just described is maintained throughout the retina except at two sites, the fovea centralis in the central area of the retina and the ora serrata at the periphery of the retina. In both sites, the ganglion cell layer, inner plexiform layer, and bipolar cell layer are absent.

The fovea centralis represents the area of greatest visual acuity, and its center contains only cones arranged in multiple rows. The cones of the fovea are slender and resemble rods. The thinning of the retina at the fovea centralis reduces to a minimum tissue through which light passes, hence improving visual acuity. Cones in this area function for sharp vision and color perception.

Near the ora serrata, at the periphery of the retina, rods predominate, increase in thickness, and become shorter. The cones decrease in number and also become shorter.

The retina receives its vascular supply from two sources. The outer retina is vascularized by the choriocapillaris layer of the choroid. The inner retina receives its blood supply from the central artery of the retina and its branches. The foveal area, the area of most acute vision, is vascularized mostly by the underlying choriocapillaries of the choroid. If the retina surrounding the fovea becomes semiopaque, as in occlusion of the central retinal artery or in some of the lipid storage diseases (e.g., Tay-Sachs disease), the choroid underlying the thin avascular fovea appears as a bright red circle called a *cherry red spot.*

Synaptic Organization of the Retina (Fig. 23-5)

The human retina is considered to be a simple retina in which there is relatively little processing of information, compared with complex retinas, such as the frog's, in which information processing is more extensive. The different types of cells encountered in the retina can be divided into three categories:

- Input elements (rods and cones)
- Output elements (ganglion cells)
- Intrinsic elements (bipolar, horizontal, and amacrine cells)

It is estimated that the human retina contains 100 million rods, 6 to 7 million cones, and 1 million ganglion cells. This provides input-to-output ratios of 100:1 for rods and 5:1 for cones. This difference correlates well with the function of cones, namely, high-acuity vision. The input-to-output ratio is lowest (approximately 1:1) in the fovea centralis, where visual acuity is highest.

Synaptic interaction in the retina takes place in two layers, the outer plexiform layer and the inner plexiform layer.

Synaptic Interaction in the Outer Plexiform Layer

In the outer plexiform layer, synaptic interaction occurs both vertically and horizontally. The vertical interaction is represented by the rod and cone terminals on bipolar cell dendrites. The horizontal interaction is represented by the interaction of horizontal cell processes with both rod and cone axons. Axon terminals of rods (rod spherules) are smaller than cone terminals; the latter are flat or pyramidal and large (cone pedicles).

Receptor–Bipolar Cell Interaction

As stated previously, there are three varieties of bipolar cells. A rod bipolar cell forms synapses with several rod spherules. A midget bipolar cell forms

KEY CONCEPTS

- The fovea centralis (retinal area of greatest visual acuity) contains only cones. In all other areas of the retina, rods outnumber cones.
- Retinal receptor cells synapse with bipolar and horizontal cells.

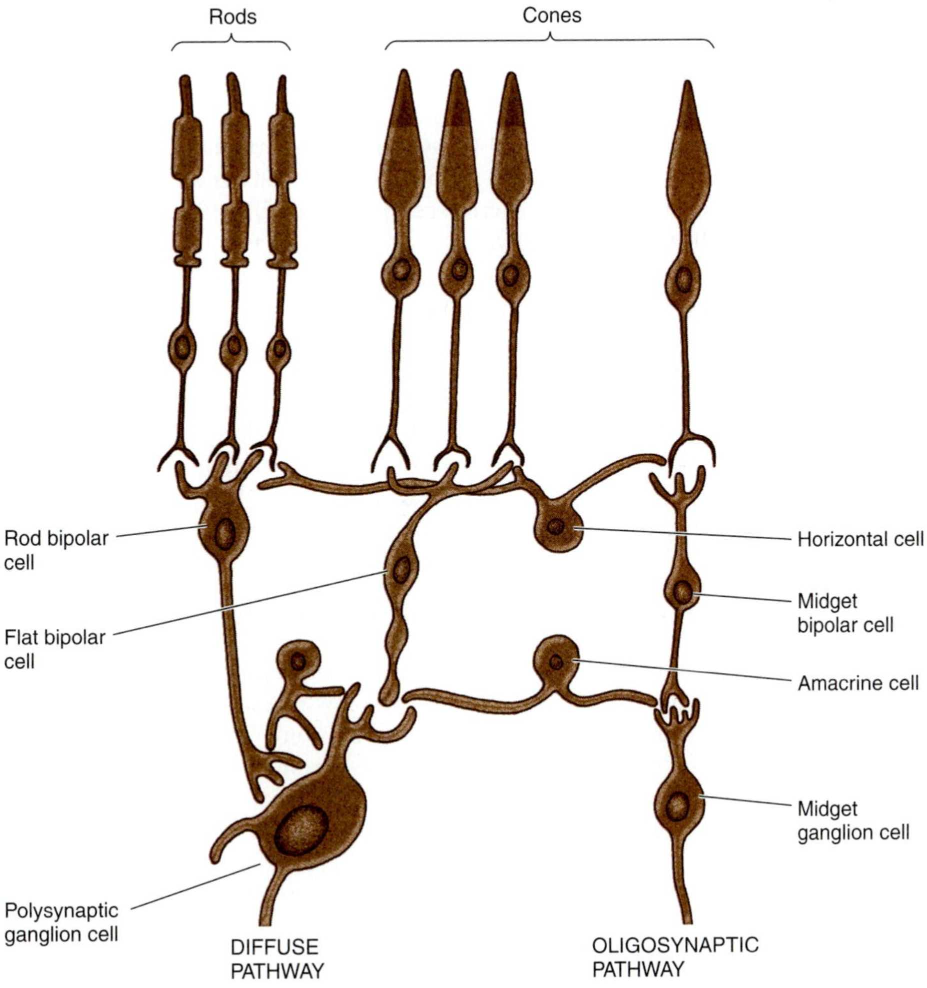

FIGURE 23-5

Schematic diagram of the types of synaptic activity within the retina.

synapses with one cone pedicle. A flat bipolar cell forms synapses with several cone pedicles.

Horizontal Cell–Receptor Interaction

Horizontal cell processes form synapses with several cones or rods, relating cones of one area to rods and cones of another area. Processes of horizontal cells are not classified as either axons or dendrites and possibly transmit bidirectionally.

Synaptic Interaction in the Inner Plexiform Layer

In the inner plexiform layer, synaptic interaction occurs vertically, between bipolar and ganglion cells, as well as horizontally, among amacrine, bipolar, and ganglion cells.

KEY CONCEPTS

- Bipolar cells synapse with ganglion and amacrine cells.

Bipolar Cell–Ganglion Cell Interaction
Rod bipolar cells project on several ganglion cells. Midget bipolar cells relate to one ganglion cell (midget ganglion cell). Flat bipolar cells relate to several ganglion cells.

Amacrine, Bipolar, and Ganglion Cell Interaction
Amacrine cells relate to axons of bipolar cells as well as to dendrites and perikarya of ganglion cells. Amacrine cell processes, like horizontal cell processes, probably conduct bidirectionally.

Characteristics of Synaptic Interaction
It is apparent, from the preceding description, that synaptic activity in the retina has the following characteristics:

- It is oriented both vertically (receptor-bipolar-ganglion cell axis) and horizontally (via horizontal and amacrine cell connections).
- It is carried out by both diffuse (flat bipolar– or rod bipolar–polysynaptic ganglion cell) and oligosynaptic (midget bipolar–midget ganglion cell) pathways (Fig. 23-5).

Photochemistry and Physiology of the Retina

The retina contains two types of photoreceptors, the rods and the cones. The rods are highly sensitive to light, have a low threshold of stimulation, and are thus best suited for dim-light vision (scotopic vision). Such vision, however, is poor in detail and does not differentiate colors (achromatic). The cones, however, have a high threshold of stimulation and function best in strong illumination (daylight) (photopic vision). They provide the substrate for acute vision as well as color vision.

On exposure to light, the visual pigments in the outer segments of the rods and cones (rhodopsin and cone opsin, respectively) break down into two components, retinal (colorless pigment) and the protein opsin. The degradation of visual pigment triggers a change in the electric potential of the photoreceptors (receptor or generator potential). The generator potential of rods and cones (unlike similar potentials in other receptors) is in the hyperpolarizing direction. This unique response of the photoreceptors has been attributed to the fact that the photoreceptor membrane is depolarized in the resting state (darkness) by a constant entry of sodium ions into the outer segment through cyclic guanosine monophosphate (cGMP)–gated ionophores. Exposure to light closes the cGMP-gated ionophores and reduces the permeability of the membrane to sodium ions, lowers the electric current, and hyperpolarizes the membrane. Thus hyperpolarizing currents in photoreceptors are produced by turning off depolarizing sodium ion conductance, whereas the orthodox hyperpolarization—inhibitory postsynaptic potential (IPSP)—seen in other neurons is produced by turning on hyperpolarizing potassium ion conductance in the neuronal membrane.

KEY CONCEPTS

- Rods are best adapted for low-intensity light, cones for high-intensity light and color vision.
- The electrical potential of the rods and cones (receptor or generator potential) is a hyperpolarizing state triggered by the breakdown of visual pigment on exposure to light.
- Action potentials are recorded in the optic nerve.

The generator potential of photoreceptors leads to hyperpolarization or depolarization of the bipolar and horizontal cells. Neither of these cell types, however, is capable of triggering a propagated action potential.

On the basis of their hyperpolarizing or depolarizing response, two types of bipolar cells are identified. One type responds by hyperpolarization to a light spot in the center of its receptive field and by depolarization to a light spot in the area surrounding the center (the surround). The other type responds in a reverse fashion by depolarization to a light spot in the center of its receptive field and by hyperpolarization to the surround. The bipolar cell is the first of the retinal elements to show this variation of response in relation to the spatial position of the stimulus in its receptive field.

The amacrine cell responds to a light stimulus by a propagated, all-or-none action potential. It is the first cell of the retinal elements to generate a propagated action potential.

Ganglion cells discharge continuously at a slow rate in the absence of any stimulus. On superimposition of a circular beam of light, ganglion cells may behave in a variety of ways. Some cells increase their discharge in response to the superimposed stimulus ("on" cells). Others inhibit their discharge in response to the superimposed stimulus but discharge again with a burst when the stimulus is turned off ("off" cells). Still others increase their discharge when the stimulus is turned both on and off ("on-off" cells). Furthermore, the behavior of ganglion cells, like that of bipolar cells, is regulated by the spatial position of the stimulus in their receptive field. "On" cells, which increase their discharge in reponse to a spot of light in the center of their receptive field, inhibit their discharge when light is shone in the area surrounding the center. The same principle applies to "off" cells, which inhibit their discharge in response to a light stimulus in the center of the receptive field but increase their discharge when the stimulus is shone in the surround.

Furthermore, some ganglion cells respond only to a steady stimulus of light in their receptive field, whereas others respond only to a change in intensity of illumination; still others respond only to a stimulus moving in a particular direction.

Dark and Light Adaptation

When an individual moves from an environment of bright light to dim light or darkness, the retina adapts and becomes more sensitive to light. This process, called *dark adaptation,* takes about 20 min to become maximally effective. The time required for maximal adaptation to darkness can be shortened by wearing red glasses. Light waves in the red end of the spectrum do not effectively stimulate the rods, which remain dark-adapted. Nor do red light waves interfere with cone stimulation, so the individual can still see in bright light. The process of dark adaptation has two components, a fast one attributed to adaptation of cones and a slower one attributed to adaptation of rods.

Conversely, when an individual moves from a dark environment to a bright one, it takes time to adapt to the bright environment. This process, called *light adaptation,* takes about 5 min to be effective.

Night Blindness

Night blindness (**nyctalopia**) is encountered in individuals with vitamin A deficiency. As mentioned previously, photoreceptor pigment is formed of two substances, vitamin A aldehyde (retinal) and the protein opsin. In vitamin A deficiency, the total amount of visual pigment is reduced, thus decreasing the sensitivity to light of both rods and cones. Although this reduction does not interfere with bright-light (daylight) vision, it does significantly affect dim-light (night) vision, because the amount of light is not enough to excite the depleted visual pigment. This condition is treatable by administration of vitamin A.

Nyctalopia (Greek *nyx,* "night"; *alaos,* "blind"; *opia,* "eye"). Night blindness.

Color Vision

Color vision is a function of the retina, lateral geniculate nucleus, and cerebral cortex. In the retina, the cone receptors and the horizontal cells as well as ganglion cells take part in the integration of color vision. According to the Young-Helmholtz theory of color vision, there are three varieties of retinal cone receptors: those which respond maximally to wavelengths in the red end of the spectrum, those which respond maximally to wavelengths in the green end of the spectrum, and those which respond maximally to wavelengths in the blue range of the spectrum. A monochromatic color (red, green, or blue) stimulates one variety of cones maximally and the other varieties of cones to a variable but lesser degree. Blue light, for example, stimulates blue cones maximally, green cones much less so, and red cones not at all. This pattern is interpreted centrally as blue color. Two monochromatic colors stimulating two types of cones equally and simultaneously are interpreted as a different color; thus, if green and red lights stimulate green and red cones simultaneously and equally, they are interpreted as yellow. Simultaneous and equal stimulation by red, green, and blue lights is interpreted as white.

The horizontal cells respond to a particular monochromatic color by either depolarization or hyperpolarization. A red-green horizontal cell responds by depolarization to red light and by hyperpolarization to green light. Such a cell is turned off by equal and simultaneous stimulation by red and green light. There are also yellow-blue horizontal cells, accounting for the four hues—red, green, blue, and yellow. The depolarization and hyperpolarization responses of horizontal cells also explain why red with green and blue with yellow are complementary colors, which, when mixed together in proper amounts, result in the cancellation of color.

Ganglion cells of the retina respond in an "on-off" manner to monochromatic light. Thus there are green "on" and red "off" ganglion cells, blue "on" and yellow "off" ganglion cells, and so on.

Furthermore, there are color-sensitive neurons in the lateral geniculate nucleus and occipital cortex that respond maximally to color in one part of the spectrum. They also play a role in color discrimination. The color-contrast cells in the striate cortex form a distinct population separate from cells concerned with brightness contrast. As with cells concerned with brightness discrimination, the color-contrast cells can be divided into simple, complex, and hypercomplex cells.

Color Blindness

Some people have a deficiency in or lack of a particular color cone. Such people have color weakness or color blindness, respectively. Most color-blind persons are red-green blind; a minority are blue blind. Among the group blind to red-green, there is a preponderance of green color blindness.

Color blindness for red and green is inherited by an X-linked recessive gene; thus there are more males with red-green color blindness than females. Color blindness for blue is inherited through an autosomal gene.

Visual Pathways

Axons of ganglion cells in the retina gather together at the optic disk in the posterior pole of the eye, penetrate the sclera, and form the optic nerve. At the point of exit of ganglion cell axons from the retina the optic disk is devoid of receptor elements (blind spot). There are approximately 1 million axons in the optic nerve. Outside

KEY CONCEPTS

- Axons of ganglion cells form the optic nerve.

the sclera, the optic nerve is covered by extensions of the meninges that ensheathe the brain. Marked increase in intracranial pressure from tumors or bleeding inside the cranial cavity or an increase in cerebrospinal fluid pressure around the nerve sufficient to interfere with venous return from the retina results in swelling of the optic disk (papilledema). This swelling can be seen using a special instrument, an ophthalmoscope, that views the retina through the pupil. The optic nerve enters the cranial cavity through the optic foramen. Thus tumors of the optic nerve (optic glioma) may be diagnosed by taking radiographs of the optic foramen, which appears enlarged in such conditions. Lesions of the optic nerve produce unilateral blindness on the side of the lesion (Fig. 23-6).

The two optic nerves come together at the optic **chiasma**, where partial crossing of optic nerve fibers takes place. Optic nerve fibers from the nasal half of each retina cross at the optic chiasma. Fibers from the temporal halves remain uncrossed. The optic chiasma is related to the hypothalamus above and pituitary gland below. Thus tumors in the pituitary gland encroaching (as they do initially) on the crossing fibers of the optic nerve cause degeneration of optic nerve fibers arising in the nasal halves of both retinae. This results in loss of vision in both temporal fields of vision (bitemporal hemianopia) (Fig. 23-6).

The crossed and uncrossed fibers from both optic nerves join caudal to the optic chiasma to form the optic tract. Lesions of the optic tracts, therefore, cause degeneration of optic nerve fibers from the temporal half of the ipsilateral retina and nasal half of the contralateral retina. This produces loss of vision in the contralateral half of the visual field (**homonymous hemianopia**) (Fig. 23-6).

The lateral geniculate nucleus is laminated into six layers. Not all parts of the retina are represented equally in the lateral geniculate nucleus. Proportionally much more of the nucleus is devoted to the representation of the central area than of the periphery of the retina.

Axons of neurons in the lateral geniculate nucleus project to the visual cortex in the occipital lobe via the geniculocalcarine tract (optic radiation). Geniculocalcarine fibers from the upper halves of both retinae course directly backwards around the lateral ventricle in the inferior part of the parietal lobe to reach the visual cortex. Geniculocalcarine fibers from the lower halves of both retinae course foward toward the tip of the temporal horn of the lateral ventricle and then loop backward (Meyer's loop, Flechsig's loop, Archambault's loop) in the temporal lobe to reach the visual cortex. Lesions of the geniculocalcarine tract give rise to a contralateral homonymous hemianopia similar to that occurring with lesions of the optic tract (Fig. 23-6). Because of the spread of geniculocalcarine fibers in the parietal and temporal lobes, a lesion involving part of this fiber system at these sites produces a contralateral quadrantic visual field defect (upper if the temporal fibers are affected and lower if the parietal fibers are affected) (Fig. 23-7).

The geniculocalcarine fibers project on neurons in the primary visual cortex (area 17 of Brodmann). As described in the chapter on cerebral cortex (Chap. 17),

Chiasma (Greek *chiasma*, "two-crossing line," from the shape of the letter *chi*, "X"). The decussation of the fibers of the optic nerve. The decussation was described by Galen without naming it. It was named by Rufus of Ephesus.

Homonymous (Greek *homos*, "same"; *onoma*, "name"). Pertaining to the corresponding halves of the visual fields.

Hemianopia (Greek *hemi*, "half"; *a*, "without"; *opia*, "eye"). Loss of vision in one-half the visual field.

KEY CONCEPTS

- Partial crossing of optic nerve fibers occurs in the optic chiasma.
- Crossed and uncrossed optic nerve fibers join caudal to the optic chiasma to form the optic tract.
- Optic tract fibers synapse in the lateral geniculate nucleus.
- Axons of neurons in the lateral geniculate nucleus form the geniculocalcarine tract (optic radiation).
- Geniculocalcarine fibers that course forward toward the tip of the temporal horn before turning back to reach the occipital cortex comprise Meyer's loop.

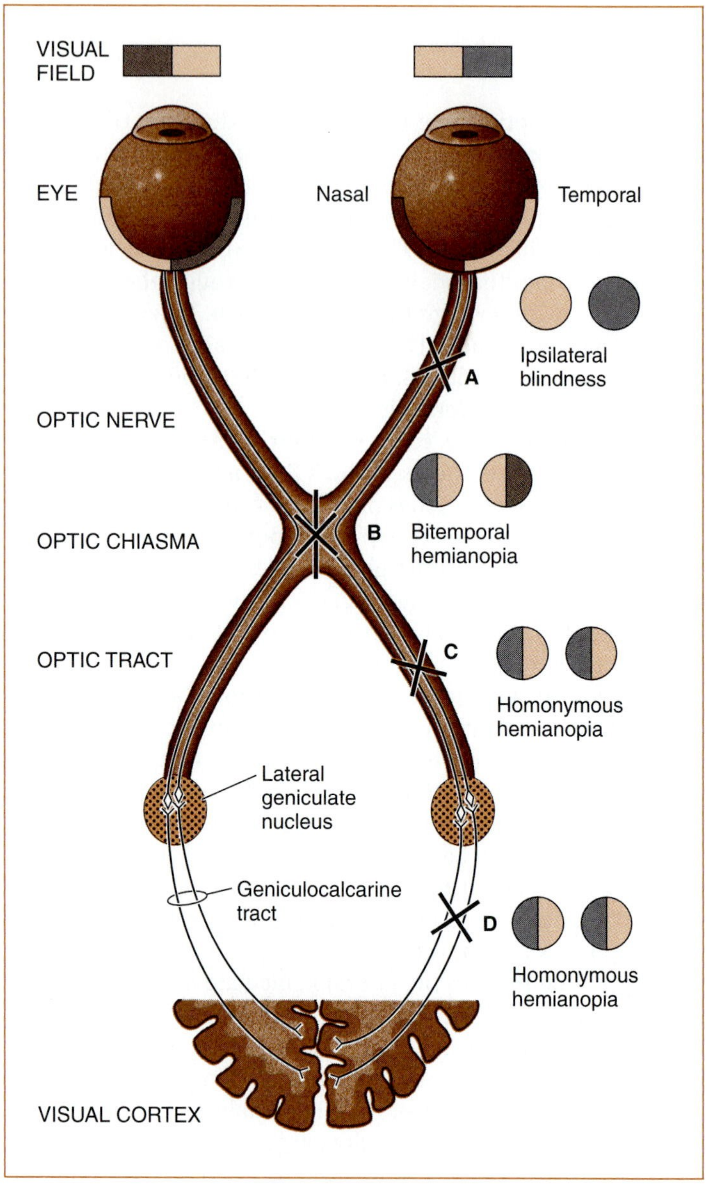

FIGURE 23-6

Schematic diagram of the visual pathways showing clinical manifestations of lesions in various sites.

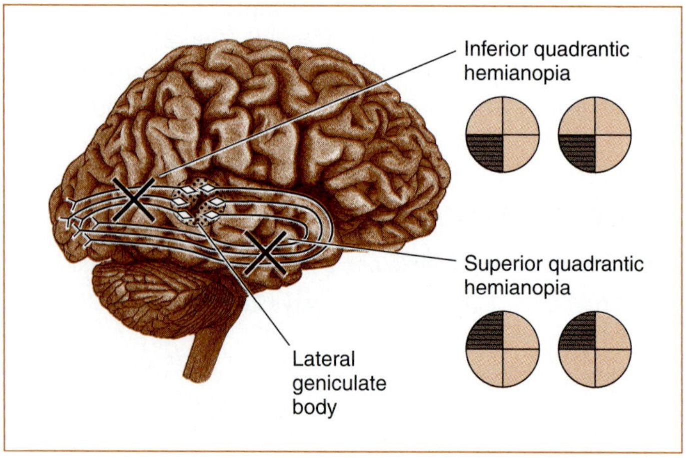

FIGURE 23-7

Schematic diagram showing the clinical manifestations of lesions in the optic radiation in the temporal and par
lobes.

fibers from the upper retina terminate in the upper calcarine gyrus, those from the lower retina in the lower calcarine gyrus, those from the macular area of the retina posteriorly, and those from the peripheral retina anteriorly in the visual cortex. Thus a lesion destroying the whole of the visual cortex on one side produces contralateral homonymous hemianopia, whereas a lesion destroying the upper or lower calcarine gyrus will produce only a contralateral lower or an upper quadrantic visual field defect. As stated in the chapter on cerebral cortex (Chap. 17), vascular lesions in the occipital cortex tend to spare the macular area because of its two sources of blood supply (posterior and middle cerebral arteries).

In addition to the classic geniculostriate visual pathway that terminates in the primary visual (striate) cortex, a second visual pathway has been described; this is the retinocolliculopulvinar-cortical pathway, which terminates in extrastriate cortical areas, including areas 18 and 19 and the temporal lobe. The classic geniculostriate pathway is concerned with the identification of objects, whereas the second visual pathway is important for processing highly abstracted visual perceptions.

HEARING

The Ear

The ear has three compartments: external, middle, and internal. Each component plays a specific role in the hearing process. The organs of hearing and equilibrium are located within the internal compartment of the ear.

External Ear

The external ear is formed of the auricle or **pinna**, external auditory canal, and tympanic membrane. The auricle collects sound and funnels it into the external auditory **meatus**. The external auditory canal is a narrow tube through the temporal bone.

The tympanic membrane (eardrum) delimits the external auditory canal medially. The core of the tympanic membrane is tough connective tissue made up of collagen and elastic fibers and fibroblasts.

Pinna (Latin "a feather"). The part of the external ear that projects from the side of the head. So named by Rufus of Ephesus.

Meatus (Latin *meo,* "passage"). The external auditory meatus is a path or a way for sound waves.

Middle Ear

The middle ear (tympanic cavity) is located within the temporal bone. It communicates with the nasopharynx anteriorly via the **eustachian** (auditory) **tube** and with the mastoid air cells posteriorly. The tympanic membrane separates the middle ear medially from the external ear laterally. Two windows (oval and round) separate the middle ear from the inner ear. The middle ear cavity is traversed by three bony

Eustachian tube. The auditory tube, a connection between the middle ear and nasopharynx. Named after Bartolommeo Eustachio, the Italian anatomist who provided the classic description of this structure in 1563. The term *eustachian tube* was coined by Val Salva in 1704. The eustachian tube was known to the ancients. Alcmaeon (500 B.C.) had dissected it. It was described by Aristotle and other early writers.

KEY CONCEPTS

- Geniculocalcarine fibers terminate, in a retinotopic fashion, in the primary visual (striate) cortex in the occipital lobe.
- The geniculocalcarine visual pathway is concerned with the identification of objects (perception of visual stimuli).
- A second visual pathway, the retinocolliculopulvinar-cortical pathway, terminates in extrastriate visual cortex and is important in the processing of highly abstracted visual perceptions.
- The ear has three compartments: external, middle, and internal.
- The sense organs for hearing and equilibrium are in the inner ear.
- The external ear collects sounds and transmits them to the middle ear.

Malleus (Latin *malleus,* "a hammer"). One of the bones of the middle ear. So named by Vesalius but probably seen much earlier.
Stapes (Latin "a stirrup"). The stapes of the middle ear resembles a stirrup. So named by Ingrassias in 1546.
Incus (Latin *anvil,* "one of the bones in the middle ear"). So named by Vesalius, although probably seen much earlier.
Labyrinth (Greek *labyrinthos,* "a system of interconnecting cavities or canals," as in the inner ear).

ossicles. The **malleus** is attached to the tympanic membrane, the **stapes** fits into the foramen ovale (oval window), and the **incus** is in between. The three ossicles transmit sound vibrations from the tympanic membrane to the oval window. The cavity also contains two muscles, the tensor tympani and stapedius. The tensor tympani muscle inserts into the malleus and the stapedius muscle into the stapes.

Inner Ear

The inner ear, located within the petrous portion of the temporal bone, contains two systems of canals or cavities, the osseous **labyrinth** and the membranous labyrinth. Both systems contain fluids, perilymph in the osseous labyrinth and endolymph in the membranous labyrinth. The osseous labyrinth has a large central cavity, the vestibule, located medial to the tympanic cavity. Three semicircular canals open into the vestibule posteriorly, and a coiled winding tube, the cochlea, communicates with the vestibule anteriorly.

The membranous labyrinth, located within the osseous labyrinth, maintains a similar configuration. The central cavity of the membranous labyrinth (within the vestibule of the osseous labyrinth) contains two cavities. The utricle, the posterior cavity, communicates with the membranous labyrinth of the semicircular canals (semicircular ducts). The saccule, the anterior cavity, communicates with the membranous labyrinth of the cochlea (cochlear duct). At the junction of the membranous semicircular canals (semicircular ducts) with the utricle, the epithelium of the semicircular ducts becomes specialized to form a receptive sensory area (neuroepithelium) for equilibrium, the crista ampullaris. Similar sensory receptive areas in the utricle and saccule are the macula utriculi and the macula sacculi. The macula sacculi is located in the floor of the saccule, whereas the macula utriculi is in the lateral wall of the utricle at right angles to the saccule. The sensory receptive organ for hearing is the organ of Corti within the cochlear duct.

Sound Transmission

Sound waves traverse the external ear and middle ear before reaching the inner ear, where the auditory end organ (organ of Corti) is located. The tympanic membrane between the external ear and middle ear vibrates in response to pressure changes produced by the incoming sound waves. Vibrations of the tympanic membrane are transmitted to the bony ossicles of the middle ear (malleus, incus, and stapes). The handle of the malleus is attached to the tympanic membrane, and the footplate of the stapes is attached to the oval window between the middle ear and inner ear. Vibrations of the footplate of the stapes are then transmitted to the membrane of the oval window and subsequently to the fluid medium (perilymph) of the inner ear.

The tensor tympani muscle, attached to the handle of the malleus, and the stapedius muscle, attached to the neck of the stapes, have a damping effect on

KEY CONCEPTS

- Three bony ossicles in the middle ear (malleus, incus, and stapes) conduct sound from the tympanic membrane to the oval window.
- Two muscles in the middle ear (tensor tympani and stapedius) exert a damping effect on sound waves.
- Loss of damping effect as occurs in lesions of the facial nerve (which supplies the stapedius muscle) results in unpleasant augmentation of sound stimuli (hyperacusis).
- The inner ear contains two cavities: an osseous labyrinth containing perilymph and a membranous labyrinth containing endolymph.

sound waves. Loud sounds cause these muscles to contract reflexively, to prevent strong sound waves from excessively stimulating the hair cells of the organ of Corti; this is the *tympanic reflex.* When this damping effect is lost, as in lesions of the facial nerve (which supplies the stapedius muscle), sound stimuli are augmented unpleasantly (hyperacusis).

Because of the marked difference in elasticity and density between air and fluid, almost 99 percent of acoustic energy is reflected back at the air-fluid interface between the middle ear and inner ear. This is, however, counteracted by two mechanisms. First, the ratio between the surface areas of the tympanic membrane and the footplate of the stapes is approximately 25:1. However, because the tympanic membrane is not a piston but a stretched membrane attached around its edge, its effective area is 60 to 75 percent of its actual area. Thus the ratio between the effective area of the tympanic membrane and the area of the footplate of the stapes is only 14:1. Second, the lever effect counteracts energy lost at the air-fluid interface. The movements of the tympanic membrane are transmitted to the malleus and incus, which move as one unit. The manubrium of the malleus is a longer lever than the long process of the incus. The force exerted at the footplate of the stapes is thus greater than that at the tympanic membrane by a ratio of 1.3:1.

The total pressure amplification via the two mechanisms just described thus counteracts the energy lost at the air-fluid interface. The total gain in force per unit area achieved by conductance in the middle ear is a factor of about 18.

Cochlea

The cochlea is a snail-shaped structure consisting of two and one-half spirals filled with fluid. It has three compartments, the **scala** vestibuli, scala tympani, and scala media (cochlear duct). The three compartments wind together in a circular pattern around a central core, the modiolus. The scala vestibuli and scala tympani are separated by a bony shelf (osseous spiral lamina) projecting from the **modiolus** across the osseous canal of the cochlea.

The scala media, lying between the scala vestibuli (above) and the scala tympani (below), contains the auditory end organ (organ of Corti). The scala vestibuli and scala tympani are continuous through the **helicotrema** at the apex of the coil. The oval window and round window separate, respectively, the scala vestibuli and scala tympani from the middle ear (Fig. 23-8).

Vibrations of the oval window are transmitted to the perilymph in the scala vestibuli and, subsequently, via **Reissner's membrane** (which separates the scala vestibuli from the scala media), to the endolymph of the scala media. Vibrations in the endolymph are then transmitted via the basilar membrane (which separates the scala media from the scala tympani) to the perilymph of the scala tympani and out through the round window.

KEY CONCEPTS

- The cochlea has three compartments: scala vestibuli, scala tympani, and scala media (cochlear duct). The scalae vestibuli and tympani contain perilymph; the scala media contains endolymph.
- The scala media contains the auditory end organ (organ of Corti).
- Sound vibrations are transmitted, via the oval window, to the perilymph of the scala vestibuli.
- Oscillations of the perilymph in the scala vestibuli are transmitted, via Reissner's membrane, to the endolymph of the scala media, and via the basilar membrane, to the perilymph of the scala tympani and the round window.

Cochlea (Latin "snail shell," from Greek "a winding staircase"). The coiled winding tube of the cochlea in the inner ear resembles a snail shell. It was first described by Eustachius (1552) and named *cochlea* by Fallopius about 1561.

Scala (Latin "stairway or ladder"). The scala tympani and scala vestibuli are so named because of their circular staircase appearance.

Modiolus (Latin "the hub of a wheel"). The central pillar of the cochlea. Described and so named by Eustachius in 1563. Its structure suggests the hub of the wheel with radiating spokes (lamina spiralis) attached to it.

Helicotrema (Greek *helix,* "a spiral"; *trema,* "a hole"). The passage or hole that connects the scala vestibuli at the apex of the cochlea with the scala tympani. First described in 1761 by Cotugno and so named by Breschet.

Reissner's membrane. The membrane that separates the scalae vestibuli and media. Described in 1851 by Ernst Reissner (1824–1878), a German anatomist.

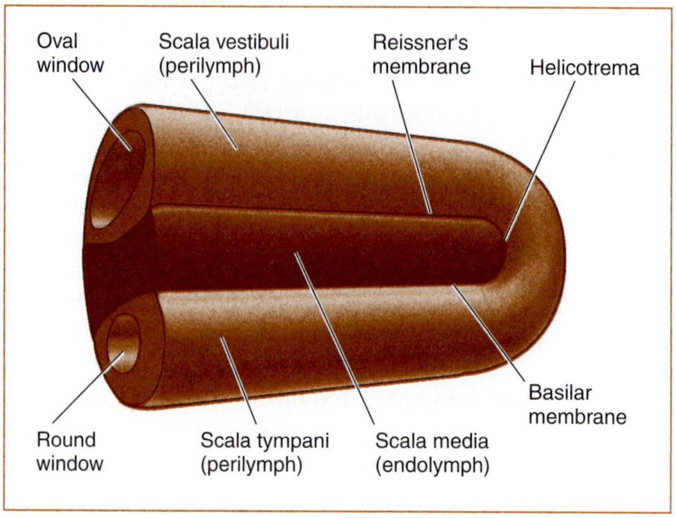

FIGURE 23-8

Schematic diagram showing the three components of the cochlea and their interrelationships.

Organ of Corti. Auditory end organ in the inner ear. Named after Marchese Alfonso Corti (1822–1888), the Italian histologist who is known for his investigations of the mammalian cochlea in 1851.

Auditory End Organ (Organ of Corti)

The organ of Corti (Fig. 23-9) is located in the scala media (cochlear duct), which is separated from the underlying scala tympani by the basilar membrane and from the scala vestibuli by Reissner's (vestibular) membrane. The cochlear duct is part of the endolymphatic system and contains endolymph. The basilar membrane forms the base of the cochlear duct and gives support to the organ of Corti (Fig. 23-9). The organ of Corti contains the following cellular elements (Fig. 23-10).

Hair Cells

The auditory receptor cells, the hair cells, are of two types: inner hair cells, which number approximately 3500 arranged in a single row, and outer hair cells, which number approximately 20,000 arranged in three to four rows. The "hairs" of the hair cells are in contact with the tectorial membrane, which transmits to them vibrations from the endolymph. The hair cells are columnar or flask shaped, with a basally located nucleus and about 50 to 100 hairlike projections (microvilli) emanating from their apical surfaces. Cochlear nerve fibers establish synapses with their basal membranes.

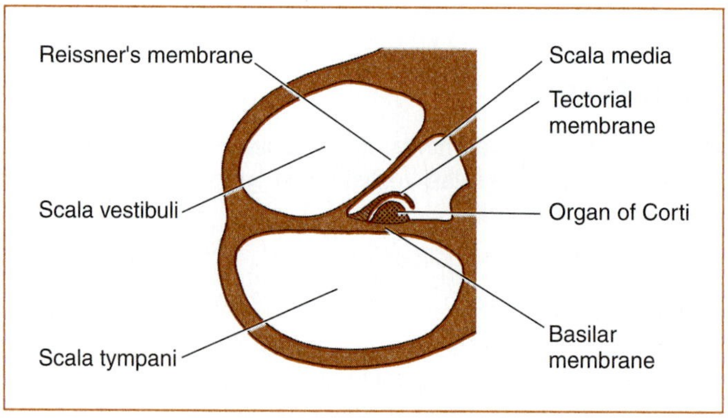

FIGURE 23-9

Schematic diagram of the cochlear compartments showing the organ of Corti in the scala media.

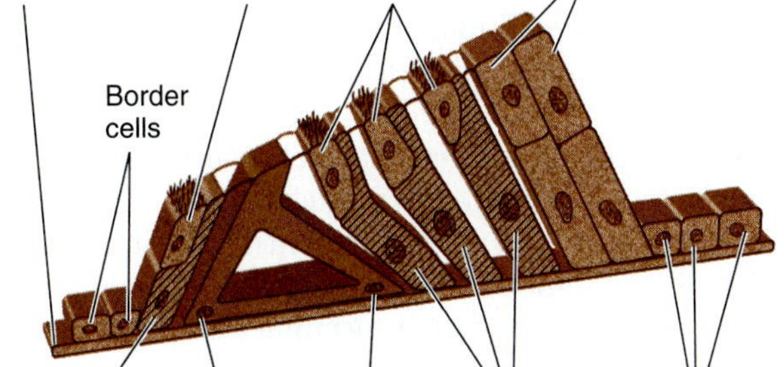

FIGURE 23-10

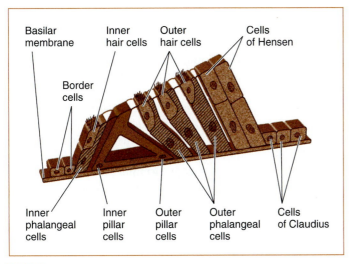

Simplified schematic diagram of the cellular components of the organ of Corti.

Supporting Cells

Supporting cells are tall, slender cells extending from the basilar membrane to the free surface of the organ of Corti. They include the following cell types: pillar or rod cells (outer and inner), phalangeal (**Deiter's**) cells (outer and inner), and cells of Hensen.

Deiters cells. Also known as *phalangeal cells.* One type of cells in the organ of Corti. Described by Otto Friedrich Karl Deiters (1834–1863), a German anatomist.

Pillar Cells Pillar cells are filled with tonofibrils. The apices of the inner and outer pillar cells converge at the free surface of the organ of Corti and fan out as a cuticle to form, along with a similar formation of Deiter's cells, a thin plate through which the apices of the inner and outer hair cells pass.

Phalangeal (Deiter's) Cells Arranged in three to four outer rows and one inner row, Deiter's cells give support to the outer and inner hair cells, respectively. They extend from the basilar membrane, like all supporting cells, to the free surface of the organ of Corti, where they contribute to the formation of the cuticular plate through which the hairs of the hair cells pass. Phalangeal cells are flask shaped and contain tonofibrils. Some of the tonofibrils support the base of the hair cells; others extend along their sides to the free surface of the organ.

Cells of Hensen Cells of Hensen are columnar cells located adjacent to the outermost row of outer phalangeal cells. They constitute the outer border of the organ of Corti. They merge laterally with cuboidal cells (cells of Claudius). Similar (cuboidal) cells adjacent to the inner phalangeal cells, known as *border cells,* constitute the inner border of the organ.

Cells of Hensen. Type of cells in the organ of Corti. Named after Viktor Hensen (1835–1924), a German physiologist.

Tectorial Membrane

The tectorial membrane is a gelatinous structure in which filamentous elements are embedded. It extends over the free surface of the organ of Corti. The hairs of the hair cells are attached to the tectorial membrane. Vibrations in the endolymph are transmitted to the tectorial membrane, resulting in deformation of the hairs attached to it. Such deformation initiates an impulse in the afferent nerve fibers in contact with the basal part of the hair cells.

Tectorial membrane (Latin *tego,* "a covering"). The part of the cochlea in which the cilia of hair cells are embedded.

Nerve Supply

The hair cells of the organ of Corti receive two types of nerve supply, afferent and efferent. The afferent fibers are peripheral processes of bipolar neurons in the spiral ganglion located in the bony core of the cochlear spiral. There are about 30,000 bipolar neurons in the spiral ganglion, 90 percent of which innervate the inner hair cells. Each inner hair cell receives contacts from about ten fibers; each fiber contacts only one inner hair cell. The remaining 10 percent of the peripheral processes of bipolar neurons innervate the outer hair cells; each fiber diverges to innervate many outer hair cells.

The efferent fibers originate in the contralateral superior olive in the pons. These fibers form the olivocochlear bundle of Rasmussen, which leaves the brain stem via the vestibular component of the vestibulocochlear (eighth cranial) nerve, joins the cochlear component (vestibulocochlear anastomosis), and terminates peripherally on the outer hair cells and the afferent terminal boutons innervating inner hair cells. These fibers have an inhibitory effect on auditory stimuli.

Auditory Physiology

Conduction of Sound Waves

Sound waves may reach the inner ear via three routes:

- Ossicular route
- Air route
- Bone route

Ossicular Route The ossicular route normally conducts sound. Sound waves entering the external auditory meatus produce vibrations in the tympanic membrane, which are transmitted to the bony ossicles of the middle ear and through them to the footplate of the stapes. The energy lost at the air-fluid interface in the oval window is counteracted by the factors outlined previously.

Air Route An alternate route, the air route, is used when the orthodox ossicular route is not operative owing to disease of the ossicles. In this situation, vibrations of the tympanic membrane are transmitted through air in the middle ear to the round window. This route is not effective in sound conduction.

Bone Route Sound waves also may be conducted via the bones of the skull directly to the perilymph of the inner ear. This route plays a minor role in sound conduction in normal individuals but is utilized by deaf people who can use hearing aids.

Fluid Vibration

Vibrations of the footplate of the stapes are transmitted to the perilymph of the scala vestibuli. Pressure waves in the perilymph are transmitted via Reissner's membrane to the endolymph of the scala media and, through the helicotrema, to the perilymph of the scala tympani.

Vibrations of Basilar Membrane

Pressure waves in the endolymph of the scala media produce traveling waves in the basilar membrane of the organ of Corti. The basilar membrane varies in width and degree of stiffness in different regions. It is widest and stiffest at its apex and thinnest and least stiff at its base.

KEY CONCEPTS

- Efferent nerves originating from the superior olivary complex modulate activity in hair cells.

Pressure waves in the endolymph initiate a traveling wave in the basilar membrane that proceeds from the base toward the apex of the membrane. The amplitude of the traveling waves varies at different sites on the membrane depending on the frequency of sound waves. High-frequency sounds elicit waves with highest amplitude toward the base of the membrane. With low-frequency sounds, the waves with highest amplitude occur toward the apex of the membrane. Similarly, each sound frequency has a site of maximum amplitude wave on the basilar membrane. The frequency of the wave, measured in cycles per second or hertz (Hz), determines its pitch. The amplitude of the wave is correlated with its loudness; a special scale, the decibel (dB) scale, is used to measure this aspect of sound. Thus the basilar membrane exhibits the phenomenon of tonotopic localization seen along the central auditory pathways all the way to the cortex.

Receptor Potential

Vibrations of the basilar membrane produce displacement of the hair cells, the hairs of which are attached to the tectorial membrane. The shearing force produced on the hairs by the displacement of hair cells is the adequate stimulus for the receptor nonpropagated potential of the hair cells. This receptor potential is also known as the *cochlear microphonic potential.* It can be recorded from the hair cells and their immediate neighborhood and is a faithful replica of the mechanical events of sound waves described previously. The genesis of receptor potentials is not fully understood. It is believed, however, to be due to a change in membrane potential between the hair cells and the surrounding endolymph induced by the bending of the hairs of hair cells.

Action Potential

The receptor potential initiates an action potential in the afferent nerves in contact with hair cells. The exact mechanism by which receptor potentials initiate action potentials is not fully understood. Records of afferent nerve activity reveal that the afferent nerves have a constant background activity (background noise) that is modified by an incoming sound stimulus.

Increasing the intensity of sound of a particular frequency raises the number of hair cells stimulated, the number of afferent nerve fibers activated, and the rate of discharge of impulses. A single nerve fiber responds to a range of frequencies but is most sensitive to a particular frequency, called its *characteristic frequency;* this is related to the region of the basilar membrane that the fiber innervates. Fibers innervating the part of the basilar membrane near the oval window have high characteristic frequencies, whereas those innervating the part of the basilar membrane near the apex of the cochlea have low characteristic frequencies.

Central Transmission

Action potentials generated in the afferent nerve fibers travel via the central components (axons) of bipolar neurons in the spiral ganglion to reach the cochlear nuclei in the pons. The cochlear nuclei contain a variety of physiologic cell types. In

KEY CONCEPTS

- Vibrations of the basilar membrane produce displacement of the hair cells of the organ of Corti and the generation of a receptor potential (cochlear microphonic potential).
- Action potentials are recorded from afferent nerves in contact with hair cells.
- Central auditory pathways synapse in several brain stem nuclei before terminating in the primary auditory cortex (transverse gyri of Heschl) in the temporal lobe.

addition to cells that respond to tone bursts in a manner similar to primary eighth nerve fibers, there are cells that respond only to the onset of the stimulus, some in which the rate of firing builds up slowly during the course of the stimulus and others that pause, showing no response to the onset of the stimulus. Axons of cochlear nuclei synapse in some or all of several brain stem nuclei (nucleus of the trapezoid body, superior olive, nucleus of the lateral lemniscus, inferior colliculus, reticular nuclei of the brain stem, medial geniculate nucleus) before terminating in the primary auditory cortex (transverse gyri of Heschl) in the temporal lobe. The central auditory pathways are organized into two systems: core pathways, and belt pathways. Core pathways are direct, fast conducting, and tonotopically organized. Belt pathways are less tonotopically organized.

Audiometry

The quantitative clinical assessment of hearing acuity is known as *audiometry;* the resulting record is the *audiogram.* In audiometry, pure tones of known frequency and varying intensity are presented via earphones to the individual, who is asked to signal a response when he or she hears a tone. The examiner records the audible frequencies and intensities on a chart. The record is then examined to compare the audible range of the individual with that of normal individuals.

Deafness

The range of audible frequencies in the normal adult is 20 to 20,000 Hz. With advancing age, there is a decrease in perception of high frequencies (high-frequency deafness). This loss correlates with the loss of hair cells in the basal turns of the cochlea. Similar high-frequency deafness is encountered in individuals intoxicated by the antibiotic streptomycin. Rock band performers, on the other hand, develop middle-frequency deafness.

Deafness disorders generally are separated into two groups, conductive deafness and sensorineural deafness. The first group includes deafness due to obstruction of the external auditory meatus by wax, as well as middle ear diseases, such as chronic otitis media and ossicle sclerosis. The second group includes conditions in which hair cells are affected (advancing age, streptomycin toxicity), as well as diseases of the auditory nerve, such as nerve tumors (acoustic neuroma).

The two types of deafness can be identified clinically by use of the tuning fork. A vibrating tuning fork is placed in front of the ear and then on a bony prominence over the skull. A person with normal hearing can hear the tuning fork better when it is placed in front of the ear. A subject with conductive deafness hears the tuning fork better when it is placed over a bony prominence, because sound waves bypass the site of obstruction in the external auditory meatus or the middle ear and reach the auditory end organ via the round window or directly through skull bones to the perilymph.

In patients with unilateral sensorineural deafness, a tuning fork placed over the forehead will be heard best in the healthy ear, since air conduction in such patients is better than bone conduction.

KEY CONCEPTS

- Disorders of deafness are generally categorized as conductive (due to disorders in the external or middle ears) and sensorineural (due to disorders of the hair cells or auditory nerve).

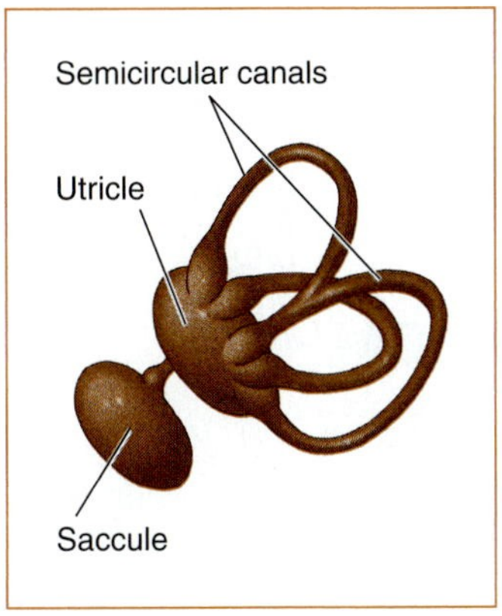

FIGURE 23-11

Schematic diagram of the vestibular end organ.

VESTIBULAR SENSATION

The receptors of the vestibular sense organ are located in the semicircular canals, utricle, and saccule in the inner ear. The utricle and saccule are located in the main cavity of the bony labyrinth, the vestibule; the semicircular canals, three in number, are extensions of the utricle (Fig. 23-11). Vestibular sensory receptors are located in the floor of the utricle, wall of the saccule, and dilated portions (ampullae) of each of the three semicircular canals. The optimal stimulus for receptors in the utricle and saccule is linear acceleration of the body, whereas receptors in the semicircular canals respond to angular acceleration.

The vestibular receptor in the semicircular canal (crista ampullaris) is composed of hair cells and supporting cells (Fig. 23-12). The hair cells are of two types. The type I hair cell is flask shaped and is surrounded by a nerve terminal (calyx). The type II hair cell is cylindrical and is not surrounded by a calyx. Both types of hair cells show on their free surfaces about 40 to 100 short stereocilia (modified microvilli) and one long kinocilium attached to one border of the cell. The short stereocilia increase progressively in length toward the kinocilium. The stereocilia are nonmotile; the kinocilium is motile.

Supporting cells are slender columnar cells that reach the basal lamina; their free surfaces are specialized into microvilli. The subapical parts of supporting cells are related to adjacent hair cells by junctional complexes.

The apical processes of hair and supporting cells are embedded in a dome-shaped, gelatinous protein-polysaccharide mass, the cupula. The cupula swings from side to side in response to currents in the endolymph that bathes it.

KEY CONCEPTS

- Receptors of the vestibular sense organ are located in the inner ear (semicircular canals, utricle, saccule).
- The optimal stimulus for receptors in the utricle and saccule is linear acceleration of the body and for those in the semicircular canals is angular acceleration.
- Hair cells (receptors) of the vestibular end organ have several nonmotile stereocilia and a single motile kinocilium on their free apical surface. The stereocilia and kinocilium are embedded in a gelatinous mass that swings sideways in response to currents in the endolymph.

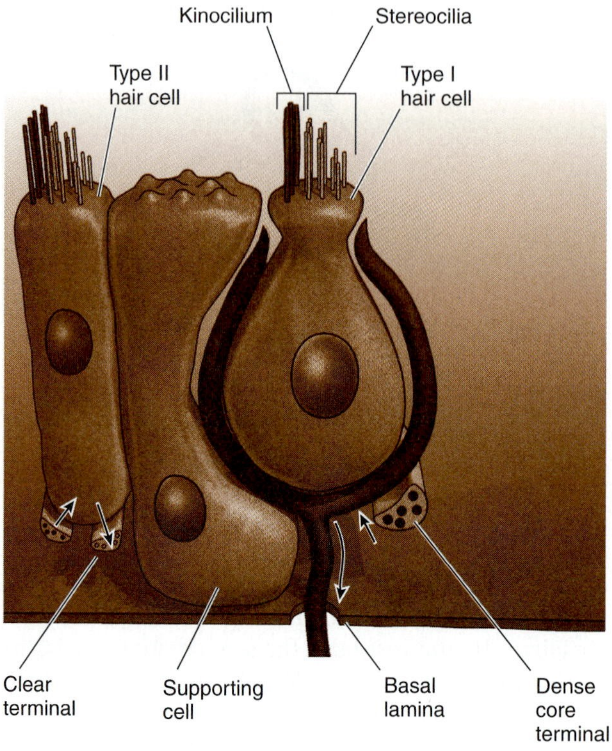
Kinocilium
Stereocilia
Type II hair cell
Type I hair cell
Clear terminal
Supporting cell
Basal lamina
Dense core terminal

FIGURE 23-12

Schematic diagram of the vestibular sensory receptor.

The vestibular receptor organ of the utricle and saccule (macula) is similar in structure to that of the semicircular canals. The gelatinous mass into which the apical processes of hair and supporting cells project is the otolithic membrane. It is flat and contains numerous small crystalline bodies, the otoliths or otoconia, composed of calcium carbonate and protein.

The hair cells of the semicircular canals, utricle, and saccule receive both afferent and efferent nerve terminals (Fig. 23-12). The afferent terminals contain clear vesicles, whereas efferent terminals contain dense-core vesicles. In type II hair cells, both afferent and efferent terminals are related to the cell body and are sites of neurochemical transmission. In type I hair cells, the calyx that surrounds the hair cell is regarded as the afferent nerve terminal. The efferent terminals in type I hair cells are applied to the external surface of the calyx.

Type I hair cells receive vestibular nerve fibers that are large in diameter and fast conducting. Each vestibular nerve fiber innervates a small number of type I hair cells. Thus type I hair cells are regarded as more discriminative than type II hair cells, which receive small-diameter, slow-conducting vestibular nerve fibers projecting on a large number of hair cells.

Cupula (Latin "a small inverted cup or dome-shaped cap").

The stimulus adequate to discharge hair cells is movement of the **cupula** or otolithic membrane, which bends or deforms the stereocilia. The manner in which this deformation triggers ionic conductance in hair cells is uncertain. The resting vestibular end organ has a constant discharge of impulses detected in afferent vestibular nerve fibers. This resting activity is modified by mechanical deformation of the stereocilia. Bending the stereocilia toward the kinocilium increases the frequency of resting discharge, whereas bending the stereocilia away from the kinocilium lowers the frequency. The signals emitted by hair cells of the vestibular end organ are transmitted to the central nervous system via processes of bipolar cells in Scarpa's ganglion that terminate on neurons in the four vestibular nuclei in the pons. Output of vestibular nuclei is directed to several central nervous system regions, including the spinal cord, cerebellum, thalamus, and nuclei of extraocular movements. The pathway to the primary vestibular cortex in the temporal lobe is not well defined but most likely passes through the thalamus.

Although we are normally not aware of the vestibular component of our sensory experience, this component is essential for the coordination of motor responses, eye movements, and posture.

KEY CONCEPTS

- Movements of the gelatinous mass (cupula in semicircular canals and otolithic membrane in utricle and saccule) bend stereocilia toward or away from the kinocilium, thus increasing or decreasing resting potential of the hair cells.
- Central vestibular pathways are directed to several neural structures: spinal cord, cerebellum, thalamus, nuclei of extraocular movement, and the cerebral cortex.
- The vestibular system is essential for the coordination of motor responses, eye movement, and posture.

SUGGESTED READINGS

Barbur JL, et al: Human visual responses in the absence of the geniculo-calcarine projection. *Brain* 1980; 103:905–928.

Brown KT: Physiology of the retina. In Mountcastle VB (ed): *Medical Physiology,* 14th ed, vol 1. St. Louis, Mosby, 1980:504.

Goldstein MH: The auditory periphery. In Mountcastle VB (ed): *Medical Physiology,* 14th ed, vol 1. St. Louis, Mosby, 1980:428.

Hubel DH, Wiesel TN: Functional architecture of macaque monkey visual cortex. *Proc R Soc Lond [B]* 1977; 198:1–59.

Hubel DH, Wiesel TN: Brain mechanisms of vision. *Sci Am* 1979; 241(3):150–162.

Hudspeth AJ: The hair cells of the inner ear. *Sci Am* 1983; 248:54–64.

Kaneko A: Physiology of the retina. *Annu Rev Neurosci* 1979; 2:169–191.

Lim DJ: Functional structure of the organ of Corti: A review. *Hear Res* 1986; 22:117–146.

Merigan WH, Maunsell JHR: How parallel are the primate visual pathways: *Annu Rev Neurosci* 1993; 16: 369–402.

Shepherd GM: Synaptic organization of the mammalian olfactory bulb. *Physiol Rev* 1972; 52:864–917.

Zeki S: The representation of colours in the cerebral cortex. *Nature* 1980; 284:412–418.

Zihl J, von Cramon D: The contribution of the "second" visual system to directed visual attention in man. *Brain* 1979; 102:835–856.

CHAPTER 24

SPECIAL SENSES: CLINICAL CORRELATES

DISORDERS OF OLFACTION
ABNORMALITIES IN TASTE
DISORDERS OF VISION
DISORDERS OF HEARING
VESTIBULAR DISORDERS

DISORDERS OF OLFACTION

The olfactory system can be affected in several sites with resulting derangements in the sense of smell. Olfactory receptors are involved in common colds, resulting in bilateral diminution or loss of smell (**anosmia**). Olfactory nerve fibers may be affected in their course through the **cribriform plate** of the ethmoid bone in fractures of the plate.

The olfactory bulb and tracts may be involved in inflammatory processes of the meninges (meningitis) or tumors in the frontal lobe or the anterior cranial fossa. Unilateral loss of smell may be the earliest clinical manifestation in such processes.

Pathologic processes in the region of the primary olfactory cortex (the uncus of the temporal lobe) usually give rise to hallucinations of smell (**uncinate** fits). The odor experienced in such cases is often described as unpleasant. Such hallucinations may herald an epileptic seizure or be part of it. They also may be a manifestation of a tumor in that region.

Anosmia (Greek *a*, "negative"; *osme*, "smell"). Loss of sense of smell.

Cribriform plate (Latin *cribrum*, "a sieve"; *forma*, "form"). The cribriform plate of the ethmoid bone has many holes (like a sieve) through which olfactory nerve fibers pass.

Uncinate (Latin "hooked"). Pertaining to the uncus. Uncinate fits are complex partial seizures in which olfactory or gustatory hallucinations occur. The term was used by Hughlings-Jackson, a British neurologist in 1899.

ABNORMALITIES IN TASTE

Taste sensations are impaired ipsilateral to lesions of the following cranial nerves: facial in the anterior two-thirds of the tongue, glossopharyngeal in the posterior third of the tongue, and vagus in the epiglottis. Abnormal taste sensations (usually unpleasant sensations) occur preceding a temporal lobe seizure or as part of the

KEY CONCEPTS

- The olfactory system may be involved in disease processes at the olfactory receptors (common cold), olfactory nerve (fractures of the cribriform plate of the ethmoid), olfactory bulb and tract (inflammation, tumors), and olfactory cortex (tumor, epilepsy).

seizure, especially if the epileptic focus is close to the uncus of the temporal lobe (uncinate seizures) or to the primary **gustatory** cortex in the inferior part of the somesthetic cortex.

Gustatory (Latin *gustatorius,* "pertaining to the sense of taste"). Relating to the sense of taste.

DISORDERS OF VISION

The visual system can be affected in several sites. Alterations in length of the eyeball result in refraction errors. Normally, distant objects are brought to focus on the retina. In persons with elongated eyeballs, distant objects are brought to focus in front of the retina (myopic eyes). In such persons, only near objects can be brought to focus on the retina (nearsightedness). In persons with flattened eyeballs, distant objects are brought to focus behind the retina (hyperopic eyes). Both conditions can be corrected by use of appropriate lenses.

Night blindness (**nyctalopia**) is encountered in individuals with vitamin A deficiency. Photoreceptor pigment is formed of vitamin A aldehyde and a protein. Thus, in vitamin A deficiency states, the total amount of visual pigment is reduced, decreasing the sensitivity to light of both rods and cones. This reduction in visual pigment, while not affecting bright-light (daylight) vision, does significantly interfere with dim-light (night) vision. This condition is treatable by vitamin A administration.

Color blindness is associated with deficiency or lack of a particular color cone. Most color blind persons are red-green blind; a minority are blue blind. Color blindness for red and green is inherited by X-linked recessive gene; hence it is more prevalent in males. Color blindness for blue is inherited by autosomal recessive gene.

Lesions of the optic nerve (tumor, demyelination) result in monocular blindness (blindness in one eye). Lesions of the optic chiasma, where partial crossing of optic nerve fibers occurs, result in bitemporal hemianopsia (blindness in both temporal visual fields) due to involvement of the crossing fibers. Such a visual defect is seen in association with lesions in the pituitary gland (pituitary adenoma) or tumors in the hypothalamus. Lesions in the optic tract result in **homonymous** hemianopia contralateral to the lesion in the optic tract due to involvement of crossed fibers from the contralateral retina and uncrossed fibers from the ipsilateral retina. Lesions of the direct path of the optic radiation in the parietal lobe or of the indirect path of the optic radiation (**Meyer's loop**) in the temporal lobe result in quadrantic **hemianopia**. The inferior quadrants of the visual field will be affected in parietal lobe lesions and the superior quadrants in temporal lobe lesions. Similarly, lesions

Myopia (Greek *myein,* "to shut"; *opia,* "eye"). An error of refraction (shortsightedness) in which light rays fall in front of the retina as a result of a too long eyeball from front to back.

Hyperopia (Greek *hyper,* "above"; *opia,* "eye"). An error of refraction (farsightedness) in which the entering light rays are focused behind the retina as a result of a short eyeball from front to back.

Nyctalopia (Greek *nyx,* "night"; *alaos,* "blind"; *opia,* "eye"). Impairment of night vision. The original Greek usage referred to the ability to see by night only. Galen changed the meaning to impairment of night vision.

Homonymous (Greek *homo,* "same"; *onoma,* "name"). Pertaining to the corresponding halves of the visual field.

Meyer's loop. Also known as *Fleschig loop.* The part of the optic radiation that loops around the tip of the temporal horn before reaching the primary visual cotex in the occipital lobe. Named after Adolph Meyer (1866–1950), a Swiss-American neurologist and psychiatrist who described this loop.

Hemianopia (Greek *hemi,* "half"; *an,* "negative"; *opia,* "eye"). Loss of vision in one-half the visual field of each eye.

KEY CONCEPTS

- Taste may be affected in lesions of the facial, glossopharyngeal, and vagus cranial nerves and in lesions of or near the primary gustatory cortex.
- Alterations in the length of the eyeball result in refraction errors. Elongated eyeballs are associated with myopia and flattened eyeballs with hyperopia.
- Nyctalopia (night blindness) occurs in persons with vitamin A deficiency.
- Color blindness is associated with deficiency or lack of a particular color cone.
- Color blindness for red and green (most common) is inherited by X-linked recessive gene and is more prevalent in males.
- Color blindness for blue is inherited by autosomal recessive gene.
- Lesions of the optic nerve are associated with monocular blindness.
- Lesions of the optic chiasma are associated with bitemporal hemianopia.
- Lesions of the optic tract are associated with contralateral homonymous hemianopia.

of the upper or lower banks of the **calcarine** sulcus will result in a quadrantic visual field defect, inferior in upper bank lesions and superior in lower bank lesions. Lesions of the primary visual cortex (upper and lower banks) result in contralateral homonymous hemianopia. If the lesion is vascular (occlusion of posterior cerebral or calcarine arteries), there will be macular sparing due to collateral supply of the macular area from the middle cerebral artery.

Calcarine (Latin *calcarinus*, "spur-shaped"). Pertaining to the calcar, a structure resembling a spur.

DISORDERS OF HEARING

Disorders of hearing are generally of two types: conductive and sensorineural. Conductive hearing loss is associated with processes that interfere with conduction of sound waves in the external and middle ears. Such processes include wax (cerumen) accumulations in the external auditory meatus, chronic otitis media, and ossicle sclerosis (**otosclerosis**).

Otosclerosis (Greek *otos*, "ear"; *sklerosis*, "hardening"). Conductive hearing loss due to sclerosis of the ossicles in the middle ear.

Sensorineural hearing loss is associated with lesions of the hair cells in the organ of Corti, the cochlear nerve (tumors of the nerve, such as in cerebellopontine angle tumors, labyrinthine artery occlusion), cochlear nuclei in the pons, or the central auditory pathways. Hearing loss is ipsilateral to the lesion in disorders of the hair cells, cochlear nerve, and cochlear nuclei. Lesions of the central auditory pathways (lateral lemniscus, medial geniculate body, auditory cortex) result in a bilateral decrease in hearing more marked contralateral to the lesion. Ringing, buzzing, hissing, or paper crushing noises (**tinnitus**) in the ear are early signs of diseases of the cochlea.

Tinnitus (Latin "ringing"). Hallucinatory sound associated with cochlear disorders.

The two types of hearing disorders (conductive and sensorineural) are differentiated by placing a vibrating tuning fork on the vertex in the midline of the skull (**Weber test**) or alternately on the mastoid process and next to the auricle (**Rinne test**). Using the Weber test, a person with normal hearing will hear the sound of the vibrating tuning fork equally well in both ears. A person with conductive deafness in one ear will hear the sound louder in the deaf ear because the masking effect of environmental noises is absent on the affected side. A person with sensorineural deafness will hear the sound louder in the normal ear. With the Rinne test, a person with normal hearing will continue to hear the sound of the vibrating tuning fork placed next to the ear (air conduction) after he or she stops hearing the sound of the tuning fork placed on the mastoid process (bone conduction). A person with

Weber test. A hearing test to differentiate conductive and sensorineural deafness by placing a vibrating tuning fork on the vertex of the skull. Named after Ernest Heinrich Weber, a German anatomist who described the test in 1834.

Rinne test. Hearing test to compare air and bone conduction of sound by placing a vibrating tuning fork on the mastoid process and in front of the ear. Named after H. A. Rinne (1819–1868), a German otolaryngologist who described the test.

KEY CONCEPTS

- Lesions of the optic radiation in the temporal and parietal lobes are associated with contralateral quadrantanopsia.
- Lesions of the upper or the lower bank of the calcarine sulcus are associated with contralateral quadrantaposia.
- Lesions of the primary visual cortex (both banks of the calcarine sulcus) are associated with contralateral homonymous hemianopia.
- In vascular lesions of the primary visual cortex (occlusion of posterior cerebral artery), macular (central) vision is preserved (macular sparing).
- There are two types of deafness: conductive and sensorineural.
- Conductive deafness results from disorders that interfere with conduction of sound through the external and middle ears.
- Sensorineural deafness results from disorders that interfere with function of the auditory end organ, cochlear nerve, cochlear nuclei, or central auditory pathways.
- The two types of deafness are differentiated clinically by the use of a vibrating tuning fork (Weber and Rinne tests).

conductive deafness will not hear the vibrations of the tuning fork in air after bone conduction is over. A person with sensorineural deafness will continue to hear vibrations in air after bone conduction is over.

VESTIBULAR DISORDERS

Vertigo (Latin *vertigo,* "turning or whirling around"). Hallucination of movement, a sign of peripheral or central vestibular system disorders.

Nystagmus (Greek *nystagmos,* "drowsiness," from *nystazein,* "to nod"). Involuntary, rapid rhythmic oscillations of the eyes.

The vestibular system can be affected in several sites, including the peripheral end organ in the inner ear, vestibular nerve, vestibular nuclei, and central vestibular pathway, and by a variety of disease processes, including infection, demyelination, vascular disorders, and tumor. Disorders of the vestibular system are manifested by an illusory sensation of motion (**vertigo**), oscillatory involuntary eye movements (**nystagmus**), and postural disequilibrium (truncal ataxia).

Lesions of the semicircular canals induce rotatory vertigo, whereas disease of the utricle or saccule produces sensations of tilt or levitation. An example of end-organ vertigo is sea sickness, which is caused by irregular continuous movement of endolymph in susceptible individuals. Vertigo also may occur with disease of vestibular structures in the brain stem. This is usually associated with other signs of brain stem damage such as hemiparesis, hemisensory loss, and cranial nerve signs.

Both central and peripheral vestibular lesions induce nystagmus, an involuntary back-and-forth movement of the eyes in horizontal, vertical, or rotatory pattern. Peripheral and central nystagmus are differentiated from each other by the following: (1) fixation of the eyes suppresses peripheral but not central nystagmus, and (2) pure vertical or torsional nystagmus is usually central.

Truncal (vestibular) ataxia occurs in association with peripheral and central vestibular disease. A dramatic feature of such patients is the inability to stand upright without support and a staggering gait with a tendency to fall toward the side of the lesion.

KEY CONCEPTS

- Vestibular disorders (peripheral and central) are associated with vertigo, nystagmus, and truncal ataxia.

SUGGESTED READINGS

Brandt T: Man in motion: Historical and clinical aspects of vestibular function. *Brain* 1991; 114:2159–2174.

Brandt T, Daroff RB: The multisensory physiological and pathological vertigo syndromes. *Ann Neurol* 1980; 7:195–203.

Borruat FX, et al: Congruous quadrantanopia and optic radiation lesion. *Neurology* 1993; 43:1430–1432.

Collard M, Chevalier Y: Vertigo. *Curr Opin Neurol* 1994; 7:88–92.

D'Amico DJ: Disease of the retina. *N Engl J Med* 1994; 331:95–106.

Luxon LM: Disorders of hearing. In Asbury AK, et al (eds): *Diseases of the Nervous System: Clinical Neurobiology.* Philadelphia, Saunders, 1992:434.

Masdeu JC: The localization of lesions in the oculomotor system. In Brazis PW, et al (eds): *Localization in Clinical Neurology.* Boston, Little, Brown, 1985:118.

Newman NJ: Neuro-ophthalmology: The afferent visual system. *Curr Opin Neurol* 1993; 6:738–746.

Sharpe JA, Johnston JL: Vertigo and nystagmus. *Curr Opin Neurol Neurosurg* 1990; 3:789–795.

Troost BT: Nystagmus: A clinical review. *Rev Neurol* 1989; 145:417–428.

Zeki S: The visual image in mind and brain. *Sci Am* 1992; 267(September):69–76.

CHAPTER 25

CENTRAL NERVOUS SYSTEM DEVELOPMENT

DEVELOPMENT

The development of the central nervous system occurs in two stages: (1) embryogenesis and (2) histogenesis.

Embryogenesis

Embryogenesis includes the following developmental events: (1) induction, (2) neurulation, and (3) vesicle formation.

Induction

Induction is a process of cell-to-cell signaling by which the underlying mesoderm induces the ectoderm to become neuroectoderm and form the neural plate, which

KEY CONCEPTS

- Embryogenesis includes three developmental events: induction, neurulation, and vesicle formation.
- During induction, ectoderm becomes neuroectoderm.

Embryogenesis (Greek *embryo,* "seed that develops into an individual"; *genesis,* "production, generation"). The process of embryo formation.

Induction (Latin *inductio,* "the process of inducing or causing to occur through the influence of organizers"). The formation of the neural plate is induced by the underlying mesoderm.

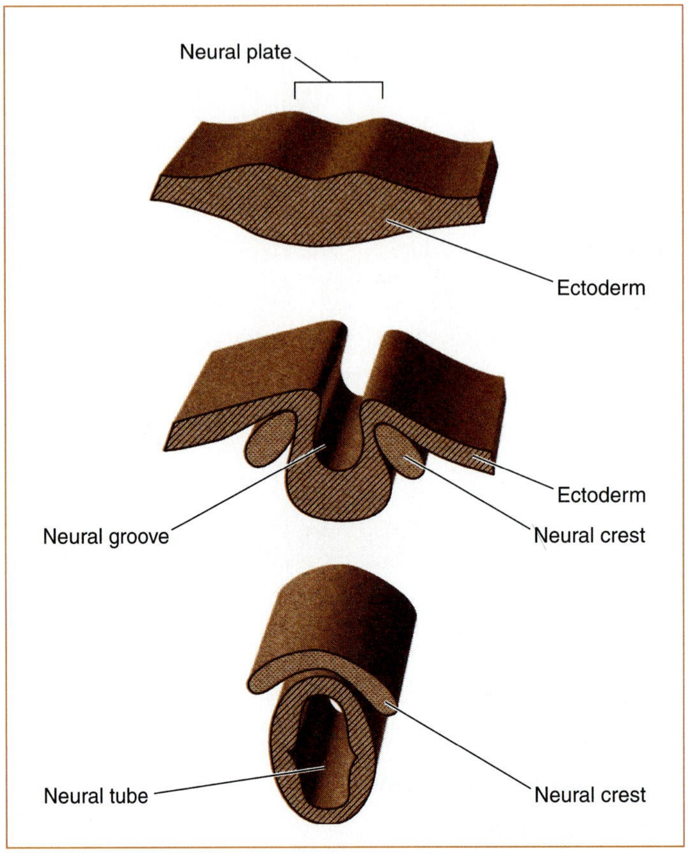

FIGURE 25-1

Schematic diagram showing the stages of formation of the neural tube.

gives rise to most of the nervous system. Neuroectodermal induction is believed to be due to the actions of hormones, neurotransmitters, and growth factors. The specific biochemical mechanisms are unknown. The process of induction takes place in the ectoderm of the head process overlying the notochord at about the seventeenth day of intrauterine life.

Neurulation. A stage of embryogenesis that includes the formation and closure of the neural tube.

Neurulation

The process by which the neural plate folds to become a neural tube is known as neurulation (Fig. 25-1). There are two neurulation processes: (1) primary, by which most of the neural tube is formed, and (2) secondary, by which the most caudal part of the neural tube is formed.

Primary Neurulation Primary neurulation is the process by which the brain and most of the spinal cord form. On about the eighteenth day of intrauterine life, the neural plate begins to thicken at its lateral margins. Rapid growth at these margins results in elevation of the margins and formation of neural folds as well as invagi-

KEY CONCEPTS

- Neurulation is the process by which the neural plate of neuroectoderm becomes the neural tube.
- Almost all of the central nervous system develops by primary neurulation. The sacral and coccygeal spinal cord segments develop by secondary neurulation.

nation of the neural plate to form the neural groove. The elevated lateral margins of the neural tube (the neural folds) then approximate each other in the midline and fuse to form the neural tube.

In the human embryo, fusion of the margins of the neural groove begins on the twenty-first day in the region of the fourth somite (middle of the embryo, presumptive cervical region) and proceeds in both directions; it is completed by the twenty-fifth day. Two orifices delimit the completed neural tube, one at its rostral end (anterior neuropore) and the other at its posterior end (posterior neuropore).

Through these orifices, the lumen of the neural tube (the neural canal) communicates with the amniotic cavity. The anterior neuropore closes on about the twenty-fourth day of intrauterine life, and the posterior neuropore closes 2 days later. The neural canal persists as the future ventricular system.

Secondary Neurulation Secondary neurulation is the process by which the caudal parts of the spinal cord (sacral and coccygeal segments) are formed. Secondary neurulation begins on about the twenty-sixth day of intrauterine life as the posterior neuropore is closing. At about that time a mass of cells, the caudal eminence, develops caudal to the neural tube. The caudal eminence then enlarges and develops a cavity within itself. Eventually, the caudal eminence joins the neural tube and its cavity becomes continuous with that of the neural tube.

Defective primary neurulation leads to a group of congenital central nervous system malformations known as **dysraphic defects**. They include **anencephaly**, in which the brain fails to form; **encephalocele**, in which the intracranial contents, including the brain, herniate through a defect in the cranium; and spina bifida cystica, in which the contents of the spinal canal, including the spinal cord, herniate through a defect in the vertebral column. Defects associated with secondary neurulation (**myelodysplasias**) include the **tethered cord** syndrome, in which the conus medullaris and the filum terminale are abnormally fixed to the vertebral column.

Neural Crest As the neural tube is being formed, a cluster of ectodermal cells that originally were at the margins of the neural groove separate to form the neural crest. The neural crest gives rise to the dorsal root (spinal) ganglia, including their satellite cells; the sensory ganglia of cranial nerves V, VII, VIII, IX, and X; the parasympathetic ganglia of cranial nerves VII, IX, and X; the autonomic ganglia (paravertebral, prevertebral, enteric); the Schwann cells; the melanocytes; the chromaffin cells of the adrenal medulla; and the pia and arachnoid layers of the meninges.

Vesicle Formation

After closure of the anterior neuropore at about the twenty-fourth day of intrauterine development, the rostral, larger portion of the neural tube subdivides into three vesicles (Fig. 25-2): the **prosencephalon** (forebrain), **mesencephalon** (midbrain), and **rhombencephalon** (hindbrain).

At about the thirty-second day, the prosencephalon and rhombencephalon subdivide further into two parts each, while the mesencephalon remains undivided. The prosencephalon divides into an anterior **telencephalon** and a posterior diencephalon. The telencephalon differentiates further into two telencephalic vesicles which

KEY CONCEPTS

- Dysraphic defects result from defective neurulation.
- Neural crest derivatives are both neural and nonneural.
- The rostral neural tube develops into three vesicles: prosencephalon, mesencephalon, and rhombencephalon.
- From the three vesicles, a five-vesicle structure develops.

Dysraphic defects (Greek *dys,* "abnormal, disordered"; *raphe,* "seam"). Defects caused by incomplete closure of the neural tube, such as anencephaly and spina bifida cystica.

Anencephaly (Greek *an,* "negative"; *enkephalos,* "brain"). Congenital absence of the cranial vault with failure of the cerebral hemispheres to develop as a result of a defect in the development of the rostral neural tube. A condition incompatible with life.

Encephalocele (Latin *encephalon,* "brain"; Greek *kele,* "hernia"). A congenital developmental defect characterized by extracranial herniation of part of the cerebral hemisphere through a midline skull defect.

Myelodysplasia (Greek *myelos,* "medulla, marrow"; *dys,* "abnormal"; *plassein,* "to form"). Defective development of the caudal spinal cord and vertebral column.

Tethered cord. A developmental defect of the caudal spinal cord in which the conus medullaris is low in the vertebral canal and is anchored to the sacrum.

Prosencephalon (Greek *prosos,* "before"; *enkephalos,* "brain"). The most anterior of the three primary brain vesicles of the embryologic neural tube. Gives rise to the diencephalon and the cerebral hemispheres.

Mesencephalon (Greek *mesos,* "middle"; *enkephalos,* "brain"). The midbrain. Developed from the middle of the three primary brain vesicles of the embryologic neural tube.

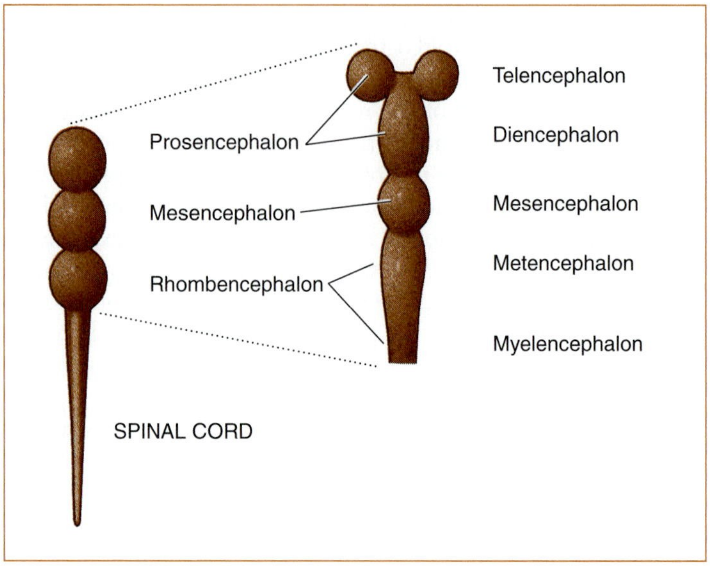

FIGURE 25-2

Schematic diagram showing the vesicle stages of brain development.

Rhombencephalon (Greek *rhombos,* "rhomb"; *enkephalos,* "brain"). The most caudal of the three primary brain vesicles. Gives rise to the medulla oblongata, pons, and cerebellum.

Telencephalon (Greek *telos,* "end"; *enkephalos,* "brain"). The anterior of the two vesicles that develop from the prosencephalon. Gives rise to the cerebral hemispheres.

Metencephalon (Greek *meta,* "after, beyond, over"; *enkephalos,* "brain"). The anterior portion of the most caudal primary vesicle of the embryologic neural tube (the rhombencephalon). Develops into the pons and the cerebellum.

Myelencephalon (Greek *myelos,* "medulla, marrow"; *enkephalos,* "brain"). The caudal part of the rhombencephalon. Develops into the medulla oblongata.

extend beyond the anterior limit of the original neural tube (lamina terminalis) and eventually become the cerebral hemispheres. From the diencephalon, two secondary bulges (the optic vesicles) appear, one on each side. These structures differentiate to form the optic nerves and retinas. The rhombencephalon divides into an anterior **metencephalon** and a posterior **myelencephalon**. The metencephalon eventually becomes the pons and cerebellum, and the myelencephalon is differentiated into the medulla oblongata.

Thus, the five vesicles that develop from the rostral part of the neural tube eventually give rise to the whole brain. Table 25-1 summarizes the sequence of events leading to the development of the various regions of the brain.

As a result of the unequal growth of the different parts of the developing brain, three flexures appear (Fig. 25-3).

Midbrain Flexure The midbrain flexure develops in the region of the midbrain; as a result, the forebrain (prosencephalon) bends ventrally until its floor lies almost parallel to the floor of the hindbrain (rhombencephalon).

Cervical Flexure The cervical flexure appears at the junction of the hindbrain (rhombencephalon) and the spinal cord.

Pontine Flexure The pontine flexure appears in the region of the developing pons.

The midbrain and cervical flexures are concave ventrally, whereas the pontine flexure is convex ventrally.

KEY CONCEPTS

- The prosencephalon develops into a midline diencephalon and two lateral telencephalic vesicles, the precursors of the cerebral hemispheres.
- The mesencephalic vesicle remains undivided.
- The rhombencephalic vesicle develops into the metencephalon (future pons and cerebellum) and the myelencephalon (future medulla oblongata).

TABLE 25-1

Developmental Sequence of Brain Regions

Three-Vesicle Stage	Five-Vesicle Stage	Brain Region
Prosencephalon	Telencephalon	Cerebral hemisphere
	Diencephalon	Diencephalon
		Optic nerve and retina
Mesencephalon	Mesencephalon	Mesencephalon
Rhombencephalon	Metencephalon	Pons
		Cerebellum
	Myelencephalon	Medulla Oblongata

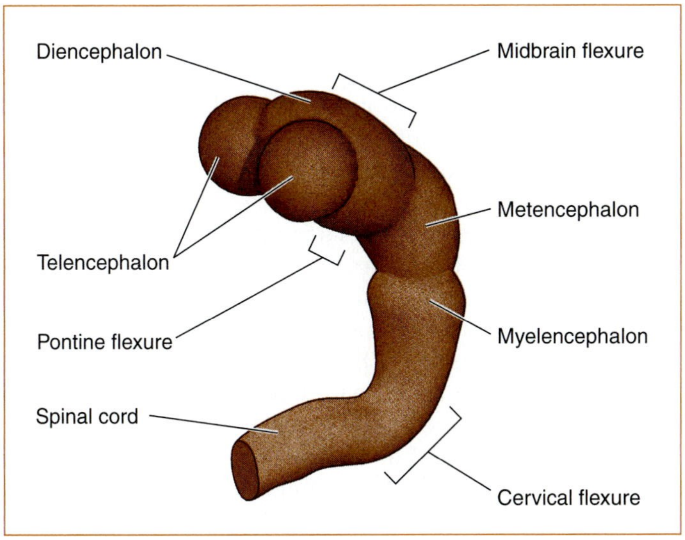

FIGURE 25-3

Schematic diagram showing the formation of flexures in brain development.

Ventricular System

After the appearance of the three vesicles in the rostral part of the neural tube, cavities develop within the vesicles. Initially, three cavities are visible, corresponding to the three vesicles: (1) the **prosocele**, the cavity of the prosencephalon, (2) the **mesocele**, the cavity of the mesencephalon, and (3) the **rhombocele**, the cavity of the rhombencephalon.

Simultaneous with the division of the prosencephalon into the two telencephalic vesicles and the diencephalic vesicle, the prosocele undergoes corresponding divisions (Fig. 25-4), resulting in the formation of the following structures:

1. Two telencephalic cavities, one on each side (lateral **teloceles**)
2. A midline cavity between the telencephalic vesicles (median telocele)
3. A diencephalic cavity (**diocele**)

KEY CONCEPTS

- The neural canal, the cavity within the neural tube, develops into the ventricular system.

Prosocele (Greek *prosos,* "before"; *koilos,* "hollow"). The foremost cavity of the brain. The ventricular cavity of the prosencephalon.

Mesocele (Greek *mesos,* "middle"; *koilos,* "hollow"). The cavity of the mesencephalon, the aqueduct of Sylvius.

Rhombocele (Greek *rhombos,* "rhomb"; *koilos,* "hollow"). The cavity of the rhombencephalon.

Telocele (Greek *telos,* "end"; *koilos,* "hollow"). The cavity of the telencephalon. The lateral ventricles.

Diocele (Greek *dis,* "twice"; *koilos,* "hollow"). The cavity of the diencephalon, the third ventricle.

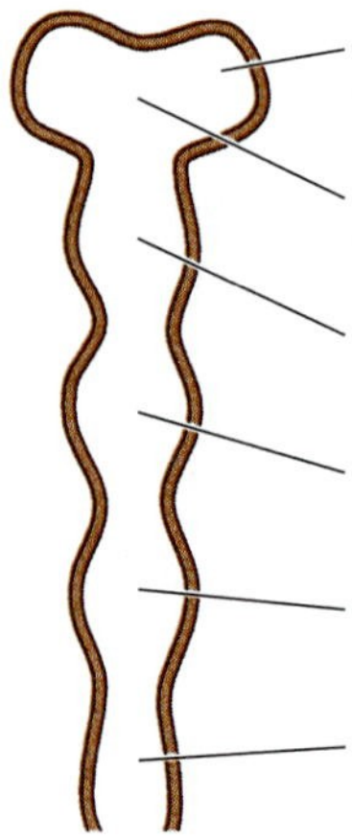

FIGURE 25-4

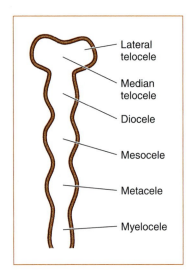

Schematic diagram showing the formation of brain cavities.

Aqueduct of Sylvius (Latin *aqua,* "water"; *ductus,* "canal"). The narrow passage in the midbrain linking the third and fourth ventricles. Described by Jacques Dubois (Sylvius) in 1555.

Metacele (Greek *meta,* "after, beyond, over"; *koilos,* "hollow"). The cavity of the metencephalon.

Myelocele (Greek *myelos,* "medulla, marrow"; *koilos,* "hollow"). The cavity of the myelencephalon. The fourth ventricle.

Histogenesis (Greek *histos,* "web"; *genesis,* "production, generation"). The formation of tissues from undifferentiated germinal cells in the embryo.

The two lateral teloceles develop into the two lateral ventricles. The median telocele and the diocele develop into the third ventricle. The cavity of the mesencephalon (mesocele) remains undivided (Fig. 25-4) and eventually becomes the **aqueduct of Sylvius**.

After the division of the rhombencephalon into a metencephalon and a myelencephalon, its cavity (rhombocele) divides into the **metacele**, the cavity of the metencephalon, and the **myelocele**, the cavity of the myelencephalon (Fig. 25-4). The metacele and myelocele become the fourth ventricle.

As the different parts of the brain change shape, corresponding changes in the cavities follow. The connections between the lateral ventricles and the third ventricle become smaller and constitute the interventricular foramina of Monro. The median aperture (of Magendie) in the roof of the fourth ventricle appears during the third month of intrauterine life, followed by the appearance of the lateral apertures (of Luschka). Table 25-2 summarizes the sequence of events leading to the formation of the various ventricles.

Histogenesis

Neurons and macroglia arise from a single precursor cell from which two lineage cells arise: the neuroblast, which gives rise to neurons, and the glioblast, from which macroglia (astrocytes and oligodendroglia) develop. Microglia are derived not from neuroectoderm but from mesoderm-derived monocytes. Histogenesis includes two main processes: (1) cellular differentiation and (2) cellular maturation.

Cellular Differentiation

Once it has been determined that a region will become part of the nervous system, its cells begin to differentiate. Differentiation involves three phases: cellular proliferation, migration of cells to characteristic positions, and maturation of cells with specific interconnections.

KEY CONCEPTS

- Histogenesis includes two processes: cellular differentiation and cellular maturation.

TABLE 25-2

Developmental Sequence of Ventricular Cavities

Three-Vesicle Stage	Five-Vesicle Stage	Adult Structure
Prosocele	Lateral telocele Median telocele Diocele	Lateral ventricle Third ventricle
Mesocele	Mesocele	Aqueduct of Sylvius
Rhombocele	Metacele Myelocele	Fourth ventricle

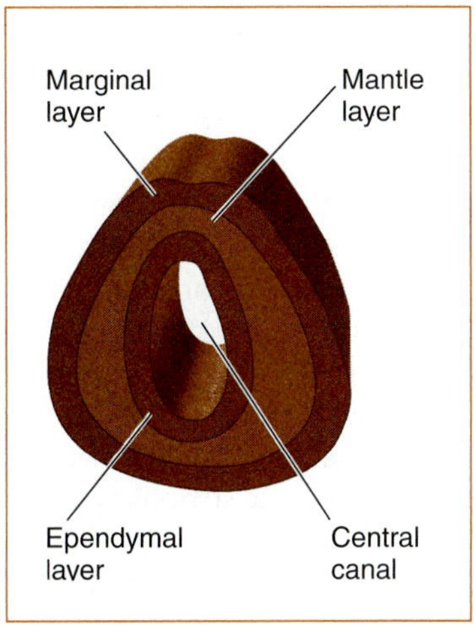

FIGURE 25-5

Schematic diagram of the three basic layers of the neural tube.

When the neural tube is formed, the cells of the germinating epithelium around the lumen of the tube (ventricular zone) proliferate actively to form an ependymal layer of columnar cells lining the cavity of the neural tube. Some of these cells migrate peripherally to form the intermediate (mantle) layer. Processes of cells in the mantle layer extend to the periphery to form the marginal layer. Cell migration from the periventricular zone to the periphery of the neural tube utilizes transient glial cell guides (radial glia). Radial glia subsequently disappear and may be transformed into astrocytes. As development continues, the central cavity diminishes in size, the mitotic activity of the ependymal cells decreases, and three distinct layers are established (Fig. 25-5): the ependymal, intermediate (mantle), and marginal. The intermediate (mantle) and marginal layers are the primordia of the future gray and white matter, respectively.

KEY CONCEPTS

- The neural tube has three layers: ventricular, intermediate (mantle), and marginal.
- Cells migrate from the ventricular zone to other zones of the neural tube by using glial cell guides (radial glia).

A full-term fetus is born with a full complement of neurons. It has been estimated that roughly 20,000 neurons are formed each minute during the period of prenatal development. The rate varies in different growth periods. In general, there are two growth spurts in the human embryo. The first extends from the tenth week to the eighteenth week of gestation. The second begins in the thirtieth week of gestation and extends through the second year of life. The first growth spurt is vulnerable to irradiation, chromosomal anomalies, and viral infections; these factors may leave the fetus with serious defects. Congenital infection with toxoplasma, rubella, cytomegalovirus (CMV), and herpes simplex at this stage may damage the developing heart, brain, and eyes of the fetus, resulting in a newborn with congenital heart disease, mental retardation, and blindness. The second growth spurt is sensitive to factors such as malnutrition. Within any given neural region, different cell types are generated during specific periods. In general, large nerve cells develop before small cells do, motor neurons develop before sensory neurons do, and interneurons are the last to develop. Glial cells proliferate after the neurons and continue to grow rapidly after birth.

During histogenesis, one and a half to two times more neurons are produced than are present in the mature brain. The excess neurons are disposed of during development by a genetically determined process of cell death (**apoptosis**).

Apoptosis (Greek *apo*, "off"; *ptosis*, "fall"). A genetically determined process of cell death. The fragmentation of a cell into membrane-bound particles that are then eliminated by phagocytosis.

Cellular Maturation

Neuronal maturation consists of four stages: (1) outgrowth and elongation of axons, (2) elaboration of dendritic processes, (3) expression of appropriate biochemical properties, and (4) formation of synaptic connections.

Axons grow out before any other sign of neuronal maturation occurs. Axonal growth is guided by specialized structures that are rich in actin filaments important for motility at the tip of the growing process (growth cones) and is influenced by factors that guide the neuron toward its target (tropic factors) and factors that maintain the metabolism of the neuron (trophic factors). Axonal growth is not random but is aimed toward a specific target.

Dendrites grow after axons have developed. Unlike axons, which have few branches if any, dendrites may form elaborate branches.

When axonal growth cones arrive at their targets, they undergo biochemical and morphologic changes to establish synapses. Similarly, the target cells undergo changes to enhance synaptic interaction involving neurotransmitter receptors and second messenger molecules. Normally, more synapses are produced than are needed. Subsequently, many synapses are lost. The use and disuse of synapses are important factors in their growth and regression.

Regional Development

Alar and Basal Plates

During the formation of the neural tube, a longitudinal groove appears on each side of the lumen. This groove, which is known as the sulcus limitans, divides the neural tube into a dorsal area, the alar plate, and a ventral area, the basal plate (Fig. 25-6). Alar and basal plates give rise to all the elements destined to make up the spinal cord, medulla oblongata, pons, and mesencephalon. The regions of the brain rostral to the mesencephalon (diencephalon and cerebral cortex) develop

KEY CONCEPTS

- Exposure of a fetus to radiation or infection early in development leaves the fetus with serious defects.
- Cellular maturation involves the growth of processes (axons and dendrites) and the formation of synapses.

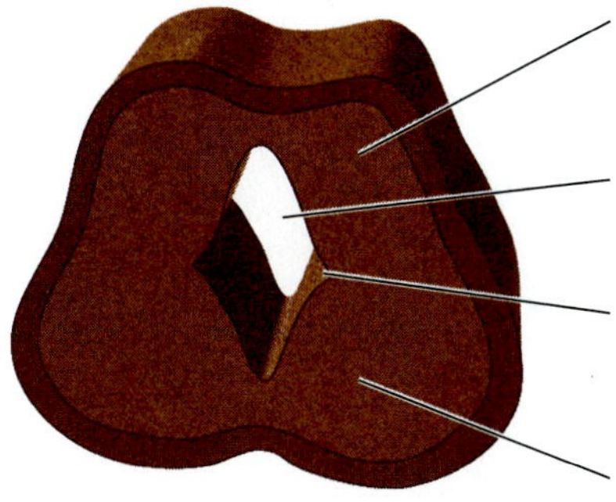
Alar plate
Central canal
Sulcus limitans
Basal plate

FIGURE 25-6

Schematic diagram showing the stage of plate formation in central nervous system development.

from the alar plate, as does the cerebellum. The mantle layer of the alar plate generally gives rise to sensory neurons and interneurons, whereas that of the basal plate gives rise to motor neurons and interneurons.

Spinal Cord

The adult spinal cord maintains the organizational pattern of the embryologic neural tube, with a central canal (neural canal), the ependyma (ventricular zone), and central gray matter (intermediate, or mantle, zone) surrounded by white matter (marginal zone). The cervical, thoracic, and lumbar segments develop from the neural tube by the process of primary neurulation. The sacral and coccygeal segments develop from the caudal eminence by the process of secondary neurulation. The cord matures from the cervical region caudally. The basal and alar plates give rise to the ventral (motor) and dorsal (sensory) horns of the adult spinal cord, respectively. The intermediate zone of the adult spinal cord develops from the interface of the alar and basal plates. By the fourteenth week of gestation all the cell groups in the central gray matter can be recognized. Axons of motor neurons in the ventral horn develop in the fourth week of gestation and form the ventral root. Later in the fourth week, axons from the dorsal root ganglia grow into the dorsal horn.

Early in development, the spinal cord and the vertebral column which develops from the surrounding mesoderm grow at the same rate. At the end of the first trimester of pregnancy, the spinal cord occupies the entire length of the vertebral column and the spinal nerves travel at right angles to exit at their corresponding intervertebral foramina. In the fourth month of gestation, however, growth of the spinal cord slows in comparison with that of the vertebral column. By term, the tip of the spinal cord lies at the level of the third lumbar vertebra, and in the adult it lies at the lower border of the first or second lumbar vertebra. As a result, the spinal roots, which originally were horizontal, become oblique, being dragged down by the growth of the vertebral column. The degree of obliquity increases from the lower cervical segment caudally, particularly in the lumbar and sacral segments, where the roots form the **cauda equina**, extending well below the end of the cord.

Cauda equina (Latin, "horse's tail"). A bundle of lumbosacral nerve roots beyond the tip of the spinal cord that form a cluster in the spinal canal which resembles the tail of a horse.

Medulla Oblongata and Pons

The medulla oblongata and the pons are derivatives of the embryologic myelencephalon and metencephalon, respectively. At the junction of the spinal cord and the

KEY CONCEPTS

- The alar plate of the neural tube gives rise to sensory structures in the spinal cord and brain stem. The basal plate gives rise to motor structures.

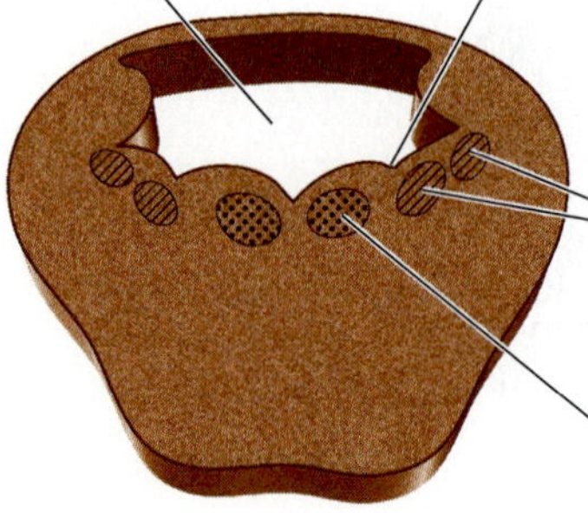

FIGURE 25-7

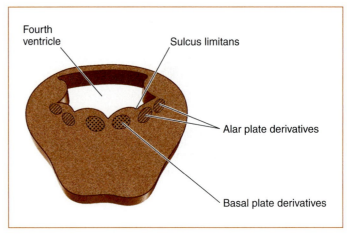

Schematic diagram showing reorganization of basal and alar plate derivatives induced by formation of the fourth ventricle.

Tela choroidea (Latin *tela,* "a web"; *chorion,* "membrane"; *epidos,* "form"). A membrane of pia and ependyma that includes the choroid plexus. Found in the lateral ventricles, the roof of the third ventricle, and the posterior roof of the fourth ventricle.

medulla oblongata, the central canal opens to form the fourth ventricle. This forces the alar plate to rotate dorsolaterally. Thus, sensory neurons of the alar plate come to lie lateral or dorsolateral to motor neurons of the basal plate (Fig. 25-7). A thin single cell layer of ependyma (roof plate) also is formed, supported by a richly vascularized mesenchymal tissue (**tela choroidea**). The sulcus limitans, which disappears in the spinal cord during development, is retained in the floor of the fourth ventricle between alar plate and basal plate neuronal derivatives. The same pattern of organization is maintained in the pons. The alar plate gives rise to the following cranial nerve nuclei in the medulla and pons: spinal trigeminal nucleus, principal (main) sensory trigeminal nucleus, nucleus solitarius, and vestibular and cochlear nuclei. The alar plate also gives rise to the following structures in the medulla and pons: the inferior olivary nucleus of the medulla and the pontine nuclei in the basis pontis. The basal plate gives rise to the following cranial nerve nuclei in the medulla and pons: hypoglossal nucleus, nucleus ambiguus, dorsal motor nucleus of the vagus, inferior salivatory nucleus, abducens nucleus, superior salivatory nucleus, trigeminal motor nucleus, and facial motor nucleus.

Cerebellum

Rhombic lip. Part of the alar plate in the dorsolateral wall of the fourth ventricle. Gives rise to the cerebellum.

The cerebellum, like the pons, is a derivative of the metencephalon. It arises from an alar plate structure (the **rhombic lip**) in the dorsolateral wall of the fourth ventricle, which also gives rise to the inferior olive, cochlear, and vestibular nuclei. The cerebellar primordia in each rhombic lip grow outward to form the cerebellar hemispheres and inward toward the midline, where they meet to form the cerebellar vermis in the roof of the fourth ventricle.

Neurons of the cerebellum are derived from neuroblasts in the ventricular zone of the cerebellar primordium. Some of these neuroblasts migrate outward along radial glia to form the deep cerebellar nuclei (dentate, emboliform, globose, and fastigii) and the Purkinje and Golgi cells. Another group of periventricular neuroblasts from the lateral edges of the rhombic lip move across the rhombic lip to the

KEY CONCEPTS

- Reorganization of sensory and motor nuclei occurs in the medulla oblongata as a result of the opening of the central canal of the spinal cord into the fourth ventricle.
- Cells of the cerebellum develop from two areas: the ventricular zone and the external granular layer.

subpial zone and from there to the external surface of the cerebellum to form the external granular layer. These neuroblasts retain their proliferative potential and give rise to cells that migrate inward to form the granule, basket, and stellate cells of the adult cerebellum. Some external granular layer cells (those destined to form granule cells of the internal granular layer) develop tangentially oriented axonal processes (future parallel fibers of granule cells) before migrating inward along radial glial guides to form the granule cells of the internal granular cell layer in the adult cerebellum. The external granular layer generates neurons throughout the last 7 months of gestation and the first 7 months of postnatal life. The cerebellum remains relatively small during development; the main growth spurt in humans occurs from 30 weeks of gestation through the first year of postnatal life.

Mesencephalon (Midbrain)

The midbrain is a derivative of the embryologic mesencephalic vesicle. The tectum (superior and inferior colliculi) and the central (periaqueductal) gray matter are derivatives of the alar plate; the tegmentum, which contains the oculomotor and trochlear nuclei, the red nucleus, and the substantia nigra, is a derivative of the basal plate. Thickening of the walls of the embryologic mesencephalon reduces the central ventricular space into a narrow passage, the aqueduct of Sylvius.

Diencephalon

The diencephalon develops solely from the alar plate. Three swellings in the wall of the central cavity (future third ventricle) develop into the future epithalamus, thalamus, and hypothalamus. After further development, the area of the epithalamus diminishes in size, whereas the thalamus and hypothalamus grow. The two thalami are connected across the midline (massa intermedia) in about 80 percent of individuals. The hypothalamic sulcus separates the thalamus and hypothalamus. This sulcus is not a rostral continuation of the sulcus limitans, which terminates at the rostral mesencephalon. Within the thalamus, laterally placed nuclei (lateral and medial geniculate, ventral lateral, ventral anterior, and ventral posterior) develop before the medially placed nuclei (dorsomedial, anterior) do.

Basal Ganglia

The caudate and putamen nuclei develop from a ventral telencephalic swelling, the **ganglionic eminence**, in the floor of the future cerebral hemispheres. In addition to the caudate and the putamen, the ganglionic eminence contributes cells to the amygdaloid nucleus and the bed nucleus of the stria terminalis. Initially, the caudate and putamen appear as a single cellular mass. With the development of the internal capsule, which connects the cerebral hemispheres with subcortical structures, the single cell mass is divided into a medial caudate nucleus and a lateral putamen.

Ganglionic eminence. A swelling in the ventral telencephalon from which the basal ganglia develop.

The derivation of the globus pallidus is controversial. It is probably derived from telancephalic anlage as well as diencephalic anlage. The external (lateral) segment of the globus pallidus is derived partly from the telencephalic ganglionic eminence and partly from the diencephalon, whereas the internal segment of the globus pallidus is derived from the diencephalon. The portions of the globus pallidus that are derived from the diencephalon are subsequently incorporated in the telencephalon.

KEY CONCEPTS

- The diencephalon develops solely from the alar plate.
- The basal ganglia develop from the ganglionic eminence.
- The globus pallidus develops from two areas: diencephalic anlage and telencephalic anlage.

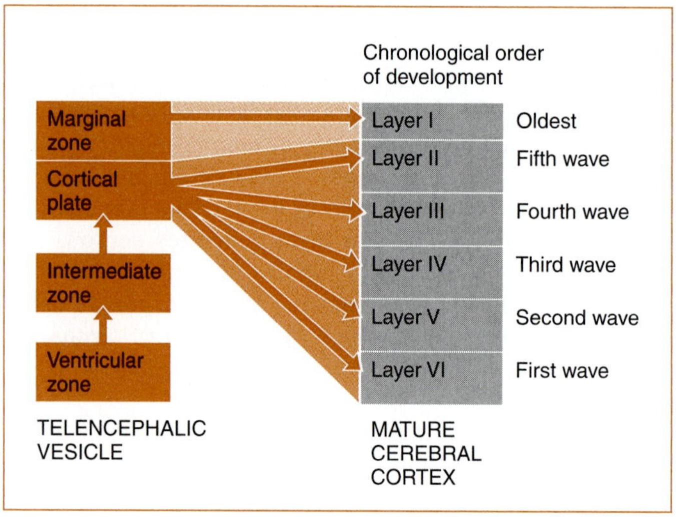

FIGURE 25-8

Schematic diagram showing origin of mature cerebral cortical layers from the telencephalic vesicle.

Cortical plate. The part of the intermediate (mantle) zone of the telencephalic vesicle that gives rise to layers II to VI of the cerebral hemispheres.

Heterotopia (Greek *heteros,* "other, different"; *topos,* "place"). Displacement of parts; the presence of tissue in an abnormal location. Neuronal heterotopia refers to the presence of gray matter within white matter as a result of abnormal neuronal migration during histogenesis.

Lissencephaly (Greek *lissos,* "smooth"; *enkephalos,* "brain"). A developmental brain anomaly characterized by a smooth brain surface devoid of gyral convolutions or a paucity of convolutions. Also known as agyria. A defect of neuronal migration.

Schizencephaly (Greek *schizein,* "to divide"; *enkephalos,* "brain"). A developmental brain anomaly characterized by the presence of unilateral or bilateral clefts in the cerebral hemisphere. A neuronal migration defect.

Cerebral Hemisphere

The cerebral hemispheres develop from the telencephalic vesicles. Early in development, each telencephalic vesicle is composed of three zones: ventricular, intermediate (mantle), and marginal. The marginal zone develops into the acellular, most superficial layer I of the mature cerebral cortex. Layers II to VI develop from the **cortical plate**, a group of cells that migrate from the ventricular zone to the outer part of the intermediate (mantle) zone (Fig. 25-8). The development of layers II to VI from the cortical plate is accomplished by an "inside-out" sequence in which newly arrived cells migrate outward past their predecessors in the cortical plate. Thus, in the mature adult cerebral cortex, acellular layer I is the oldest; cellular layer VI is formed by the first wave of neuroblast migration, followed in chronologic sequence by cellular layers V, IV, III, and II (Table 25-3). Unlike the spinal cord, where gray matter is centrally placed compared with white matter, the reverse is true in the cerebral cortex, where gray matter is superficial to the white matter core. Defects in the inside-out migration sequence result in a variety of developmental brain disorders, such as **heterotopias**, **lissencephaly**, and **schizencephaly**. Because of the rapid accumulation of cells, the telencephalic vesicles grow rapidly forward, upward, and backward to form the frontal, parietal, occipital, and temporal lobes. In the process of rapid growth, the newly formed cortex covers cortical and subcortical structures such as the insula and the diencephalon. Local variations in the rate of growth result in the formation of the gyri, sulci, and fissures that demarcate different cortical convolutions and lobes. The sylvian fissure is the first to develop, at about the fourteenth week of gestation. The central (rolandic) and calcarine sulci appear between 24 and 26 weeks of gestation. The formation of the cortical gyri proceeds rapidly near the thirtieth week of gestation, and the entire hemisphere surface is gyrated by the thirty-second week of gestation.

KEY CONCEPTS

- The cellular layers of the cerebral hemispheres are developed from two sites: the ventricular zone and the cortical plate.
- Layers II to VI of the cerebral hemisphere develop from the cortical plate by an "inside-out" process.

TABLE 25-3

Development of Cortical Layers: The Inside-Out Process

Layer	Origin	Chronologic Age
I	Periventricular layer	Oldest
II	Cortical plate	Fifth wave of neuroblast migration
III	Cortical plate	Fourth wave of neuroblast migration
IV	Cortical plate	Third wave of neuroblast migration
V	Cortical plate	Second wave of neuroblast migration
VI	Cortical plate	First wave of neuroblast migration

Cerebral Commissures

At about the sixth week of gestation, the dorsal part of the lamina terminalis (site of the embryologic anterior neuropore) thickens to form a densely cellular cell mass, the **lamina reuniens** (lamina of His). The lamina reuniens increases rapidly in size to form the commissural plate, from which the cerebral commissures and the septum pellucidum develop. Pioneer cerebral commissure fibers cross the midline with the help of early glial cells and are guided either by cell surface markers or by chemotactic substances that are expressed into the extracellular space. The anterior commissure is the first to form at about the sixth gestational week and the first to cross in the anterior portion of the commissural plate at about the tenth week of gestation. The hippocampal commissure is the next structure to form. It crosses further dorsally in the commissural plate at about the eleventh week of gestation. The first fibers of the corpus callosum begin to cross at approximately the twelfth gestational week. Growth of the corpus callosum continues over the next 5 to 7 weeks in an anterior to posterior direction with the formation of the callosal body and splenium. The corpus callosum also grows anteriorly to form the rostral part of the genu and the rostrum. Because the posterior growth of the corpus callosum occurs more rapidly than does the anterior growth, the rostrum is the last part of the corpus callosum to form after the genu, body, and splenium. This sequence of callosal growth is reflected in patients with callosal hypogenesis, who may manifest the presence of the early formed portions of the corpus callosum (genu, body, splenium) and the absence of the portions that form later (rostrum).

The septum pellucidum, another derivative of the commissural plate, is a thin structure that separates the anterior horns of the lateral ventricles. At about 8 weeks of gestation, the central part of the commissural plate undergoes cystic

Lamina reuniens (lamina of His). The dorsal part of the lamina terminalis, from which the cerebral commissures develop. Described by Wilhelm His (1831–1904), a Swiss anatomist.

KEY CONCEPTS

- Cerebral commissures develop from the commissural plate, a specialized area in the lamina terminalis.
- The anterior commissure is the first commissure to form, followed by the hippocampal commissure and the corpus callosum.
- The rostrum of the corpus callosum develops after the genu, body, and splenium.
- The septum pellucidum develops from the commissural plate.

necrosis and forms the thin leaves of the septum pellucidum with the cavum septum pellucidum between them.

Congenital absence of the corpus callosum and septum pellucidum is at times associated with hypothalamic abnormalities. This can be explained by the fact that the septal nuclei, which are related anatomically and functionally to the anterior hypothalamus, arise from an area of the anterior diencephalon just ventral to the lamina reuniens.

Myelination

In the central nervous system, myelin is formed by oligodendrocytes. Myelin formation in the central nervous system begins at about the sixth month of gestation and continues into adulthood. The factors that initiate myelin formation have not been fully elucidated. It is known, however, that myelination is retarded when the conduction of nerve impulses through axons is interrupted and that myelin production by oligodendrocytes is enhanced when neural cell extracts are added to cultures. It appears that both neural impulses and some unknown cellular communication between neurons and oligodendrocytes (surface markers, chemotactic factors) stimulate the process of myelination. Different fiber systems myelinate at different developmental periods. In general, motor and sensory tracts myelinate before association tracts do. Myelination proceeds in a caudal-to-rostral order. The spinal cord and spinal nerve roots begin to myelinate during the second trimester in utero. Toward the end of the second trimester and the beginning of the third trimester, myelination begins in the brain stem. No myelin is detectable in the cerebral hemisphere until the first postnatal month.

Myelination undergoes dramatic changes in the first 2 postnatal years. Multiple rules govern the chronologic and topographic sequences of central nervous system myelination during this period. These rules include the following: (1) Sensory pathways myelinate before motor pathways, (2) projection pathways myelinate before association pathways, (3) central telencephalic sites myelinate before telencephalic poles, (4) occipital poles myelinate before frontal and temporal poles, (5) the posterior limb of the internal capsule myelinates earlier and faster than the anterior limb, (6) the body and splenium of the corpus callosum myelinate earlier and faster than the rostrum, and (7) the central segment of the cerebral peduncle myelinates earlier than both the lateral and medial segments. The lateral segment (from posterior cerebral hemisphere sites) myelinates before the medial segment (from anterior cerebral hemisphere sites) does.

PRENATAL BRAIN PERFORMANCE

The cardiovascular and nervous systems are the first systems to function in an embryo. The heart begins to beat 3 weeks after conception. The earliest detectable reflex in the nervous system appears in about the eighth week of intrauterine life. If a stimulus is applied to the lip region at this time, the hand region exhibits a withdrawal reflex. Touching the lips at 11 weeks of gestation elicits swallowing

KEY CONCEPTS

- Myelin begins to form in the last trimester of pregnancy and continues forming to adulthood.
- Myelination follows a caudal-rostral sequence in which motor and sensory systems myelinate before association systems do.

movements. At 14 weeks of gestation, the reflexogenic zones spread so that touching the face of the embryo results in a complex sequence of movements consisting of head rotation, grimacing, stretching of the body, and extension of the extremities. At 22 weeks of gestation, the embryo manifests stretching out movements and pursing of the lips; at 29 weeks, sucking movements become apparent. At birth almost all reflexes are of brain stem origin; cortical control of these reflexes is minimal.

POSTNATAL DEVELOPMENT AND GROWTH

The brain of a human newborn weighs 350 g, which is approximately 10 percent of its body weight; in contrast, the brain of an adult weighs about 1400 g (roughly 2 percent of body weight). This difference in weight between the adult brain and the newborn brain is accounted for by the laying down of myelin, which occurs mainly in the first 2 years of life, as well as by an increase in the size of neurons, the number of glial elements, and the complexity of neuronal processes. Virtually no neurons are added after birth, since the human newborn has the full complement of neurons. Structurally, in the brain of a newborn all the lobes are clearly distinguishable. The central lobe (insula, island of Reil) is not covered by the frontal and temporal opercula. The color of the cortex at birth is pale, approximating that of white matter. Histologically, a newborn brain shows the six-layered cytoarchitectonic lamination of the adult cerebral cortex. In contrast to the adult cortex, however, the cells of the newborn cortex are tightly packed together with few if any processes to separate them. Nissl substance is sparse in cortical neurons and abundant in brain stem and spinal cord neurons. Dendritic development in the newborn cortex is poor, and this correlates with the absence of alpha activity in the electroencephalogram of a newborn. At birth, most of the synapses are of the axodendritic variety; axosomatic synapses develop later.

At 3 months of age, the brain weighs approximately 500 g. The island of Reil is completely covered by the frontal and temporal opercula. Although the gray matter and white matter remain poorly demarcated and the cortical Nissl substance remains scanty, the neurons are not as closely packed as they are in the newborn brain.

At 6 months of age, the brain weighs approximately 660 g. The cytoplasm of neurons is more abundant. Nissl material is more prominent, and the distinction between gray matter and white matter can be made easily.

At 1 year of age, the brain weighs approximately 925 g. The density of cortical neurons is reduced as a result of an increase in neuronal and glial processes between neuronal perikarya; Nissl substance within the cell bodies is well developed.

By the third postnatal year, average brain weight (1080 g) triples compared to birth weight, and by 6 to 14 years, average brain weight (1350 g) approximates that of an adult. Even when adult brain weight has been reached, maturational changes continue to occur in the brain. Although active myelination in the human brain continues throughout the first decade, remodeling of myelin continues throughout life. The electroencephalogram and stimulus-evoked potentials undergo maturational changes that continue into the second decade of life.

KEY CONCEPTS

- The weight of the brain triples from birth to the third postnatal year and approximates adult weight by age 6 to 14 years.
- The increase in brain weight in the postnatal period is attributed to myelination, an increase in glia, and the complexity of neuronal processes.

FUNCTIONAL MATURATION

Cerebral Oxygen Consumption

Oxygen consumption is relatively low in the newborn brain and increases gradually with maturation. It reaches approximately 5 ml/100 g of brain tissue per minute, which is equivalent to about 50 percent of the child's total oxygen consumption. With further development, cerebral oxygen consumption decreases to reach the adult level of 3.5 ml/100 g of brain tissue per minute. The low cerebral oxygen consumption of the brain at birth explains the ability of a newborn brain to tolerate states of anoxia. This tolerance to anoxia also may be explained by the dependence of the brain before birth on anaerobic glycolysis as a source of energy. Just before birth, the level of enzymes needed for aerobic glycolysis (succinodehydrogenase, succinooxidase, adenylphosphatase, etc.) increases in preparation for the change in brain metabolism from anaerobic to aerobic processes.

Cerebral Blood Flow

Cerebral blood flow in a newborn brain is low. It increases with age to reach a maximum of 105 ml/100 g per minute between the ages of 3 and 5 years. It then decreases to reach the adult rate of 54 ml/100 g per minute.

Cerebral Metabolic Rate for Glucose

Studies using positron emission tomography to study local cerebral metabolic rates for glucose in infants and children have shown a pattern of glucose utilization in the neonatal brain that is markedly different from that in the adult brain. Typically, four brain regions are metabolically prominent: sensorimotor cortex, thalamus, brain stem, and cerebellar vermis. By 1 year of age, local cerebral metabolic rates for glucose resemble qualitatively those of young adults. Quantitatively, however, glucose metabolic rates mature slowly. In a neonate, the local cerebral metabolic rate for glucose is 70 percent that of an adult. It increases and exceeds the adult rate by 2 to 3 years of life. It remains at these high levels until 9 or 10 years of life, and then it declines to reach the adult rate by 16 to 18 years. The stage of decline in the cerebral metabolic rate for glucose between 9 and 18 years of age corresponds to the stage of a notable decrease in brain plasticity after injury.

POSTNATAL BRAIN PERFORMANCE

Brain performance after birth proceeds through several stages of increasing complexity.

The first stage spans the first 2 years of life. During this stage, the infant changes from a baby with no awareness of the environment to a child who is aware of the environment and is able to discriminate among varying environmental stimuli.

The second stage occurs between 2 and 5 years of age. This is a stage of preconceptual representation in which the child develops picture images as symbols and begins to use language as a system of symbol signs.

KEY CONCEPTS

- Oxygen consumption and cerebral blood flow are relatively low in a newborn, increase with maturation to levels higher than adult values, and then decrease to reach adult values.

TABLE 25-4

Brain Development: Anatomic, Functional, and Behavioral Correlations

Age, Months	Brain Weight, g	Local Cerebral Metabolic Rate for Glucose	Behavior
Neonate	350	Primary sensorimotor cortex, thalamus, brain stem, cerebellar vermis	Subcortical reflexes (**Moro's, grasp, rooting**)
2–3	500	Parietal cortex, temporal cortex, primary visual cortex, basal ganglia, cerebellar hemispheres	Visuospatial and visuosensorimotor integrative functions
6–8	660	Lateral frontal cortex	Higher cortical and cognitive functions, interaction with surroundings, phenomenon of stranger anxiety
8–12	925	Prefrontal cortex	

The third stage is noted between 5 and 8 years of age. This is a stage of conditional representation in which the child becomes aware that he or she is not alone in the universe and begins to interact with other features and forces of the universe.

The fourth stage, which extends from 7 to 12 years of age, is a stage of operational thinking in which the child begins to recognize the relationships between objects and appreciate their relative values, such as more or less, heavier or lighter, and longer or shorter.

Along with these stages of behavioral development, the child proceeds through stages of motor and sensory development of increasing complexity. In general, motor development precedes sensory development. Starting as a subcortical creature at 1 month of age, the child proceeds to grasp, raise its head, smile, focus its eyes, hear, roll over, crawl, pick up small objects, stand, and walk.

As these behavioral, motor, and sensory developments proceed, the central nervous system develops nerve processes, synapses, and myelinated pathways. It is difficult, however, to match each of these developmental stages with a definitive structural change.

Table 25-4 presents a simplified summary correlating anatomic, functional, and behavioral developments in the first year of life.

AGING

Aging in the nervous system is associated with characteristic morphologic and functional alterations.

KEY CONCEPTS

- Concomitant with the development of myelin, nerve processes, and synapses, a child undergoes the development of increasingly complex behavioral, motor, and sensory skills.

Moro's reflex. Abduction and extension of the arms and opening of the hands followed by adduction of the arms in response to sudden withdrawal of support of the head. Normally present from birth to 5 months of age. Named after E. Moro, an Austrian pediatrician who described it in 1918.

Grasp reflex. Flexion of the fingers when an object is placed gently in the palm. Normally present in infants from birth to about 6 months of age.

Rooting reflex. Mouth opening and head turning in response to stroking of the corner of the mouth. An exploratory reflex of the mother's skin to locate the nipple. A normal reflex from birth to 6 months of life.

Corpora amylacea (Latin *corpus*, "body"; *amylaceus*, "starchy"). Starchlike bodies. Basophilic structures found in astrocytic processes with advancing age and in various degenerative diseases. The name was applied by Virchow to certain "amyloid" bodies in the central nervous system which had been noted by Purkinje.

Morphologic Alterations

The following structural alterations have been described in the aging nervous system.

1. Cortical atrophy manifested by broadening of sulci, a decrease in the size of gyri, and widening of ventricular cavities.
2. A reduction in the number and size of neurons. This is best seen in larger neurons such as the pyramidal cells of Betz and Purkinje neurons.
3. A reduction in the amount of Nissl material.
4. Thickening and clumping together of neurofibrils.
5. An increase in the number of amyloid bodies (**corpora amylacea**), particularly around the ventricular surface. The origin of amyloid bodies has not been established with certainty, but they are believed to represent products of neuronal degeneration.
6. An increase in lipofuscin pigment in both neurons and glia. Among the glia, the astrocytes are particularly affected, whereas the oligodendroglia and microglia are relatively spared. The predominant involvement of astrocytes in this aging process has a deleterious effect on neuronal function.
7. Thickening of the walls of cerebral blood vessels.

Functional Alterations

The following functional alterations are believed to contribute to some of these structural alterations or result from such structural modifications.

1. A decrease in cerebral blood flow. The reduction in cerebral blood flow can be the end product of the thickening of blood vessel walls, which in turn can lead to ischemia and dropout of neuronal elements.
2. A reduction in oxygen utilization by cerebral tissues.
3. A reduction in glucose utilization by cerebral tissues.
4. An increase in cerebrovascular resistance.

KEY CONCEPTS

- Aging of the brain is associated with characteristic morphologic and functional alterations.

SUGGESTED READINGS

Barkovich AJ, et al: Formation, maturation, and disorders of white matter. *AJNR* 1992; 13:447–461.

Chugani HT: Functional maturation of the brain. *Int Pediatr* 1992; 7:111–117.

Cowan WM: The development of the brain. *Sci Am* 1979; 241:112–133.

Crelin ES: Development of the nervous system. *Ciba Clin Symp* 1974; 26:2–32.

Dorovini-Zis K, Dolman CL: Gestational development of the brain. *Arch Pathol Lab Med* 1977; 101:192–195.

Friede RL: Gross and microscopic development of the central nervous system. In Friede RL (ed): *Developmental Neuropathology.* Berlin, Springer-Verlag, 1989; 2–20.

Hayflick L: The cell biology of human aging. *Sci Am* 1980; 242:58–65.

Leech RW: Normal development of central nervous system. In Leech RW, Brumback RA (eds): *Hydrocephalus, Current Clinical Concepts.* St. Louis, Mosby Year Book, 1991:9–17.

Marin-Padilla M: Prenatal development of human cerebral cortex: An overview. *Int Pediatr* 1995; 10 (suppl):6–15.

Moore K: The nervous system. In Moore K (ed): *The Developing Human.* Philadelphia, Saunders, 1982: 375–412.

Naidich TP: Normal brain maturation. *Int Pediatr* 1990; 5:81–86.

Norman MG, et al: Embryology of the central nervous system. In Norman MG, et al (eds): *Congenital Malformations of the Brain: Pathological, Embryological, Clinical, Radiological, and Genetic Aspects.* New York, Oxford University Press, 1995:9–50.

O'Rahilly R, Müller F: *The Embryonic Human Brain: An Atlas of Developmental Stages.* New York, Wiley-Liss, 1994.

Rockstein M: *Development and Aging in the Nervous System.* New York, Academic Press, 1973.

Yakovlev PI, Lecours AR: The myelogenetic cycles of regional maturation of the brain. In Mikowski A (ed): *Regional Development of the Brain in Early Life.* Philadelphia, Davis, 1967:3–70.

CHAPTER 26

CENTRAL NERVOUS SYSTEM DEVELOPMENT: CLINICAL CORRELATES

Congenital malformations of the brain occur in approximately 0.5 percent of live births and 3 percent of stillbirths. They are generally attributed to one of two causes: exogenous and endogenous. Exogenous causes include nutritional factors, radiation, viral infections, chemicals, ischemic insults, and medications. Endogenous causes are mainly genetic. The different etiologic factors affect the embryo adversely during specific periods of development. Since the same malformation may be produced

KEY CONCEPTS

- Congenital malformations of the brain have exogenous and endogenous causes and occur in 0.5 percent of live births.
- Congenital malformations of the brain are classified with reference to the stages of development at which they occur.

by both exogenous and endogenous causes, it is customary to classify the different malformations according to the developmental stage at which they occur.

Neurulation. A stage of embryogenesis that includes the formation and closure of the neural tube.

NEURULATION (NEURAL TUBE) DEFECTS

Congenital malformations associated with defective neurulation are among the most commonly encountered malformations in humans. They include (1) anencephaly, (2) encephalocele, (3) myelomeningocele, (4) diastematomyelia, and (5) tethered cord. The first three are associated with primary neurulation defects, and the last two with secondary neurulation defects.

Two features of human neural tube defects point to failure of closure of the neural tube as the more likely cause of malformations: (1) Pathologic studies show that the neural tube is open at the area of the defect, with continuity of the neural epithelium and surface epithelium, suggesting failure of fusion of the neural tube, and (2) neural tube malformations occur mostly at the rostral and caudal regions of the neural tube just proximal to the areas of final neural tube fusion, suggesting that the malformations result from a defect in neural tube closure.

Teratogenic (Greek *teratos,* "monster"; *genesis,* "production"). Tending to produce anomalies of formation.

In experimental animals, neural tube defects can be produced by introducing a variety of **teratogens** during the stage of closure of the anterior and posterior neuropores.

Early prenatal detection of neural tube defects is possible by the determination of alpha-fetoprotein (AFP) and acetylcholinesterase in amniotic fluid. AFP is synthesized in fetal liver and excreted in urine. It increases in amount in the amniotic fluid in patients with various malformations, in particular those resulting from neural tube defects. AFP elevation in maternal serum is not as reliable as similar elevations in amniotic fluid. Acetylcholinesterase is produced in nervous tissue, is excreted in cerebrospinal fluid, and passes into the amniotic fluid only in cases of neural tube defects. Neural tube defects also can be detected early by ultrasonography.

The risk of neural tube malformation can be reduced by daily intake of folic acid.

Primary Neurulation Defects

Primary neurulation refers to the formation of the neural tube from approximately the caudal lumbar level to the cranial end of the embryo. Most of the central nervous system is thus developed by primary neurulation, which occurs during the third and fourth weeks of gestation. Three malformations are generally associated with defective primary neurulation: (1) anencephaly, (2) encephalocele, and (3) myelinomeningocele.

Anencephaly (Greek *an,* "negative"; *enkephalos,* "brain"). Congenital absence of the cranial vault with failure of the cerebral hemispheres to develop as a result of a defect in the development of the rostral neural tube. A condition incompatible with life.

Anencephaly

Anencephaly (Fig. 26-1) is characterized by the absence or underdevelopment of the cranial vault, maldevelopment of the skull base, and a constant anomaly of the sphenoid bone that resembles "a bat with folded wings." The orbits are shallow,

KEY CONCEPTS

- There are two major groups of brain malformations: those caused by neurulation (neural tube) defects and those caused by neuroblast migration defects.
- Malformations associated with defective neurulation include anencephaly, encephalocele, myelomeningocele, diastematomyelia, and tethered cord.
- Neural tube defects can be detected prenatally by examining alpha-fetoprotein and acetylcholinesterase in the amniotic fluid and by ultrasonography.

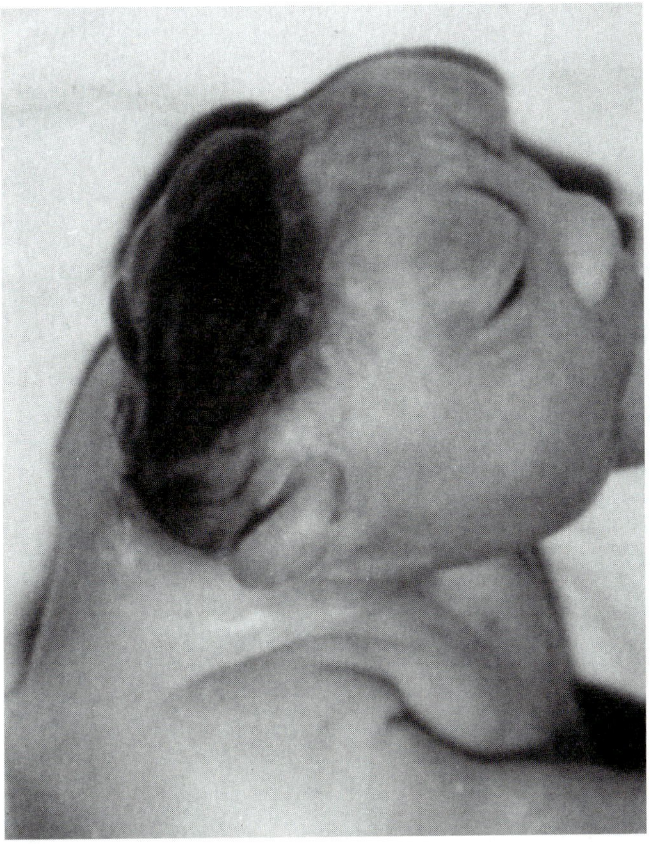

FIGURE 26-1

Photograph of a neonate with anencephaly.

causing protrusion of the eyes. The anomaly of the skull imparts a froglike appearance to the patient when viewed face on. The forebrain is absent and is replaced by a reddish irregular mass of vascular tissue with multiple cavities containing cerebrospinal fluid. The primary defect is failure of closure of the rostral part of the neural tube. The onset of the malformation is estimated to occur no later than at 24 days of gestation. Anencephaly was known in Egyptian antiquity. Affected infants are stillborn or die early (a few days) in the neonatal period. The incidence of anencephaly varies from 0.5 to 2.0 per 1000 live births, and anencephaly accounts for approximately 30 percent of all major abnormal live births. Females are affected more frequently than are males, and white infants more than nonwhite infants. Epidemiologic studies have shown a high incidence (1 to 6 per 1000 live births) of anencephaly in Ireland and Wales. Both environmental and genetic factors operate

KEY CONCEPTS

- Anencephaly is due to failure of closure of the rostral part of the neural tube. The cranial vault is absent or deficient, and the forebrain is absent. This malformation is incompatible with life.
- The incidence of anencephaly is higher in women, whites, and the Irish and Welsh populations.

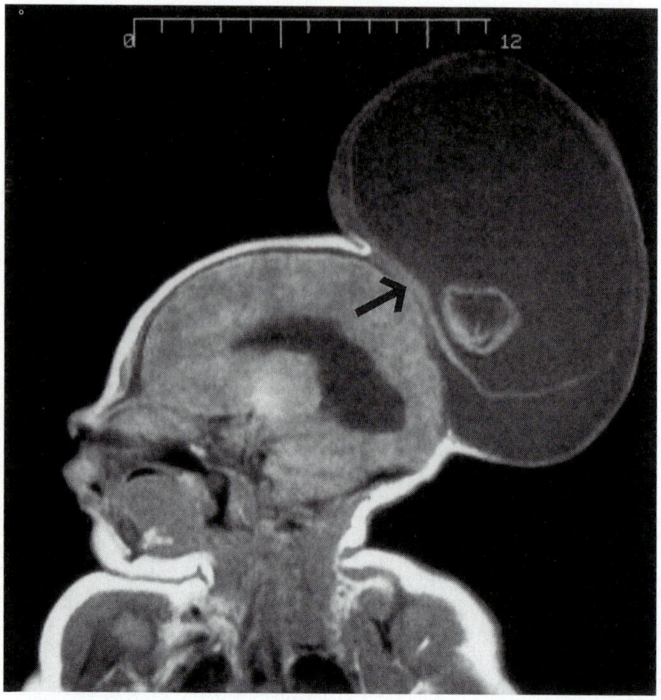

FIGURE 26-2

Magnetic resonance image (MRI) of the brain showing an occipital encephalomeningocele (*arrow*).

in the genesis of the malformation. Familial cases have been reported; the mode of transmission, however, is poorly understood.

The incidence of anencephaly has been declining. This has been attributed to early detection by ultrasonography, AFP, and acetylcholinesterase determination, and elective termination of pregnancy when the fetus is found to have anencephaly.

Encephalocele (Latin *encephalon,* "brain"; Greek *kela,* "hernia"). A congenital developmental defect characterized by extracranial herniation of part of the cerebral hemisphere through a midline skull defect.

Encephalocele (Encephalomeningocele)

An encephalocele (Fig. 26-2) consists of a protrusion of brain and meninges through a skull defect. Rarely, only the meninges (meningocele) protrude through the skull defect (Fig. 26-3). Encephaloceles may occur in the occipital, parietal, frontal, nasal, and nasopharyngeal sites but are most common (75 to 85 percent) in the occipital area. The incidence of encephaloceles is approximately 0.8 to 3.0 per 10,000 births. They account for 0.07 percent of all pediatric admissions and about 10 percent of all craniospinal malformations. Occipital encephaloceles are more common in females, whereas encephaloceles in other sites occur more frequently in males. Most encephaloceles occur sporadically. They typically present at birth and usually come to medical attention within the first days or weeks of life. Encephaloceles typically have an intact skin cover but are variable in size, shape, and consistency. Occipital encephaloceles are usually large. The outcome is poor. Seventy-five per-

KEY CONCEPTS

- An encephalocele (encephalomeningocele) is a protrusion of the brain and meninges through a defect in the skull, most often in the occipital region. The large majority of infants with encephalocele die or are severely retarded.

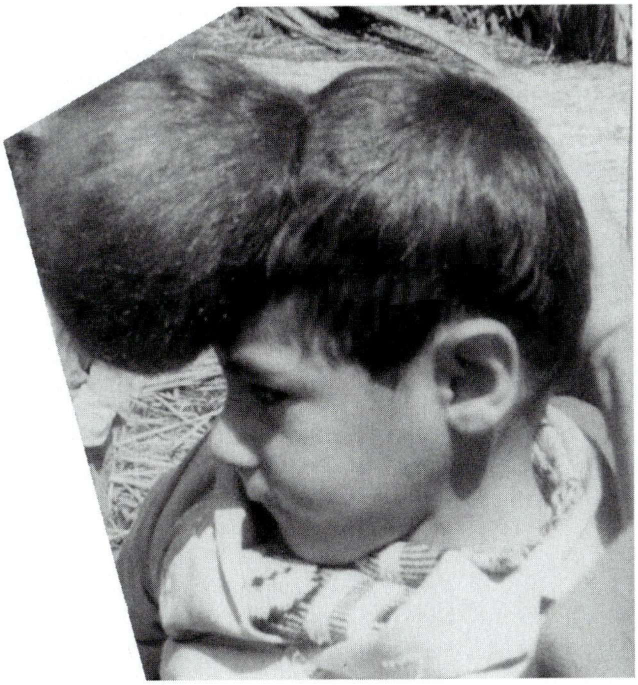

FIGURE 26-3

Photograph of a child with frontal meningocele.

cent of occipital encephalocele and 100 percent of parietal encephalocele infants die or are severely retarded.

Myelomeningocele

A myelomeningocele (Fig. 26-4) is characterized by herniation of the lower spinal cord and overlying meninges through a large midline defect in the vertebral column. The protruding mass consists of a distended meningeal sac filled with cerebrospinal fluid containing spinal cord tissue. The sac is covered by a thin membrane or skin. The malformation results from a defect in closure of the caudal neural tube. Approximately 80 percent of myelomeningoceles are in the lumbar region, the last region of the neural tube to close.

The onset of the malformation occurs not later than the twenty-sixth day of gestation. The incidence is approximately 2 to 3 per 1000 births. As with anencephaly, the incidence is higher in Ireland and Wales. Most cases are sporadic. There is increased risk of the malformation in families with a history of neural tube defects. Females are affected about twice as often as are males. Other frequently associated malformations include the **Arnold-Chiari malformation,** hydrocephalus, **syringohydromyelia,** and diastematomyelia. The clinical picture is characterized by sensorimotor deficits in the lower extremities. IQ is normal in 90 percent of patients. Recent advances in the care of children with myelomeningocele have resulted in increased

KEY CONCEPTS

- A myelinomeningocele is a herniation of the spinal cord and meninges through a defect in the vertebral column. Early surgical repair of the malformation improves the chance of survival.

Myelomeningocele (Greek *myelos,* "marrow"; *meninx,* "*membrane*"; *koilos,* "hollow"). A severe defect of neural tube closure in which the spinal cord and meninges herniate through a midline defect in the vertebral column.

Arnold-Chiari malformation. A brain malformation characterized by cerebellar and brain stem elongation and protrusion through the foramen magnum. This malformation was first observed by Cleland in 1883 but was more definitively described by Hans Chiari, an Austrian pathologist, in 1891 and by Julius Arnold, a German physician, in 1894.

Syringohydromyelia (Greek *syrinx,* "pipe or tube"; *hydor,* "water"; *myelos,* "marrow"). A cavitation within the spinal cord filled with cerebrospinal fluid.

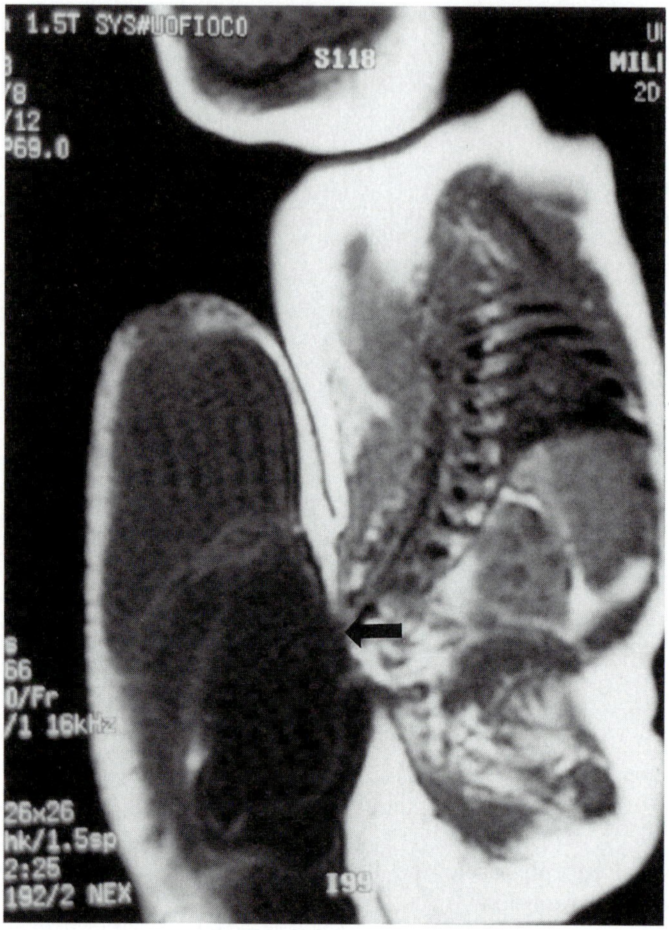

FIGURE 26-4

MRI of the spinal canal showing a myelomeningocele (*arrow*).

survival. Early surgery involves closure of the spinal lesion and frequently the placement of a shunt.

Secondary Neurulation Defects

Secondary neurulation refers to the process by which the sacral and coccygeal segments of the spinal cord are developed. Two malformations are generally associated with defective secondary neurulation: diastematomyelia and tethered cord.

Diastematomyelia (Greek *diastema,* "cleft"; *myelos,* "marrow, cord"). Splitting of the spinal cord by a connective tissue septum or bony septum.

Diastematomyelia

Diastematomyelia is characterized by the presence of two hemicords within a single dural sac separated by a vascular mass of connective tissue or in two separate dural sacs between which there may be a bony septum. The term is derived from the Greek *diastema,* meaning "cleft," and *myelos,* meaning "spinal cord." The malformation usually occurs in the lower thoracic or lumbar cord segments but may occur at any

KEY CONCEPTS

- Diastematomyelia refers to splitting of the spinal cord into two hemicords separated by connective tissue or a bony septum.

spinal level. Seventy percent of cases occur between the first and fifth lumbar cord segments. The cord is normal above and below the level of the split. The central canal bifurcates to extend into each hemicord and reunites below the split. Similarly, the anterior cerebral artery divides at the level of the split so that each hemicord has an independent arterial supply. This condition may be asymptomatic in neonates and become symptomatic later in childhood, between 2 and 10 years of age. Females are affected more than males are. Although not an inherited disorder, diastematomyelia has been reported to occur in members of the same family. The malformation frequently is associated with spina bifida.

On imaging studies, diastematomyelia may be difficult to distinguish from **diplomyelia,** a rare condition characterized by a duplicated spinal cord instead of two facing hemicords, as in diastematomyelia.

Diplomyelia (Greek *diploos,* "double"; *myelos,* "marrow"). Doubling of the spinal cord.

The oldest known specimen of diastematomyelia, dating back to the Roman period, approximately A.D. 100, was recovered from a burial site in the Negev desert in Palestine. The term *diastematomyelia* was coined by Ollivier, a French neurologist, in 1837.

Tethered Cord

The tethered cord malformation (Fig. 26-5) is characterized by an abnormally low conus medullaris tethered (anchored) by one or more forms of intradural abnormalities, such as a short thickened filum terminale, fibrous bands, or adhesions,

Tethered cord. A type of spinal dysraphism in which the lower part of the spinal cord (conus medullaris) is anchored to the sacrum.

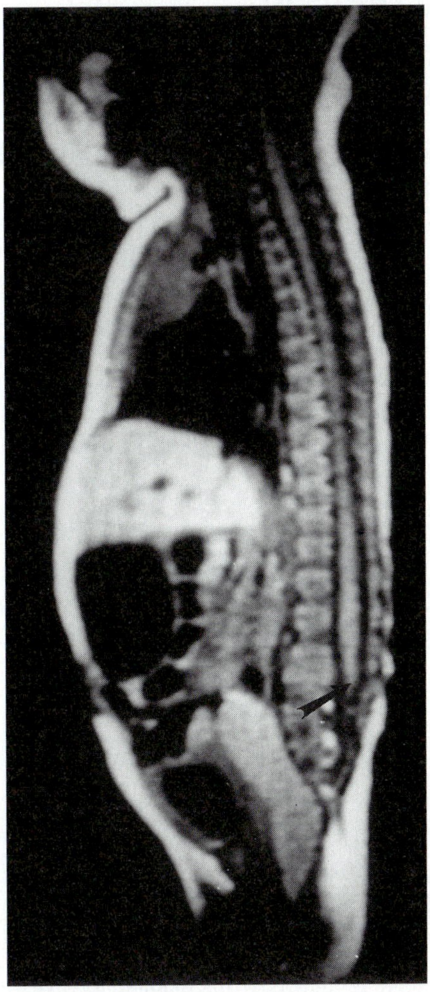

FIGURE 26-5

MRI of the spinal canal showing a low-lying conus medullaris (*arrow*) in a tethered cord.

or a totally intradural lipoma. The underlying pathologic anomaly is a dural defect through which the spinal cord comes in contact with the subcutaneous tissue early in embryonic development. The spinal cord thus is anchored to subcutaneous tissue, preventing its upward displacement. The clinical picture is characterized by progressive motor and sensory deficits in the lower extremities, scoliosis, back pain, and a neurogenic bladder. Associated cutaneous signs in the lumbosacral region include a hairy skin patch, a hemangioma, and a dimple.

NEUROBLAST MIGRATION DEFECTS

Neuroblast migration is a critical stage in normal histogenesis in which neuroblasts migrate, guided by radial glial processes, from the ventricular or periventricular zone to their proper position. In many regions, the migratory pathway is long and migration occurs over a protracted period. The time involved is the third month to the sixth month of gestation.

Congenital malformations associated with defective neuroblast migration include (1) lissencephaly (agyria), (2) pachygyria, (3) polymicrogyria, (4) cortical heterotopias, and (5) schizencephaly. The causes of these malformations are varied and include genetic maternal, and environmental factors. Many are associated with agenesis or hypoplasia of the corpus callosum.

Lissencephaly (Greek *lissos,* "smooth"; *enkephalos,* "brain"). A developmental brain anomaly characterized by a smooth brain surface devoid of gyral convolutions or a paucity of convolutions. Also known as agyria. A defect of neuronal migration.

Agyria (Greek *a,* "negative"; *gyros,* "ring"). A malformation in which the brain surface is devoid of gyri and has a smooth appearance. Also known as lissencephaly.

Miller-Dieker syndrome. The association of lissencephaly (smooth brain) with dysmorphic facial features, renal anomalies, polydactyly, seizures, and microcephaly. Described by J. Q. Miller in 1963 and H. Dieker in 1969. The term was introduced by Jones in 1980.

Walker-Warburg syndrome. A lethal autosomal recessive congenital syndrome with brain, eye, and muscle abnormalities. The majority of these children die in the neonatal period secondary to defects in brain development. Those who survive are severely mentally retarded.

Pachygyria (Greek *pachys,* "thick"; *gyros,* "ring"). Thick, broad, shallow gyral convolutions in the cerebral hemisphere.

Lissencephaly (Agyria)

Lissencephaly (Fig. 26-6) is characterized by a smooth brain surface resulting from the absence or paucity of gyri and sulci. The cerebral cortex is composed of four layers, similar to that of a 3-month fetus: (1) an outermost, relatively accellular molecular layer, (2) a thick, richly cellular intermediate (mantle) zone, (3) an innermost thin band of white matter, and (4) a layer of periventricular gray matter. The migratory defect of this malformation occurs between 12 and 16 weeks of gestation. It has been proposed that late-migrating neuroblasts that are destined to become cortical layers II and IV are arrested by a deep cortical and subcortical laminar necrosis at about the fourth fetal month. Neurologic abnormalities are evident at birth or shortly afterward. Affected infants are hypotonic and microcephalic and have intractable seizures. Neurologic development is severely impaired. Most cases of lissencephaly are sporadic; some are associated with genetic syndromes such as the **Miller-Dieker** and **Walker-Warburg** syndromes.

Pachygyria

Pachygyria (Fig. 26-7) is characterized by a reduced number of coarse, broad, shallow gyri and sulci. The gyral malformation differs from lissencephaly only in degree. Both malformations may be found in different areas of the same hemisphere.

KEY CONCEPTS

- Tethered cord is a malformation in which the conus medullaris is abnormally low and is anchored by one or more types of intradural abnormalities.
- Malformations associated with neuroblast migration include lissencephaly (agyria), pachygyria, polymicrogyria, cortical heterotopias, and schizencephaly.
- Lissencephaly (agyria) refers to a smooth brain surface devoid of gyri and sulci.
- Pachygyria refers to a reduction in the number of gyri, which are also broad and shallow.

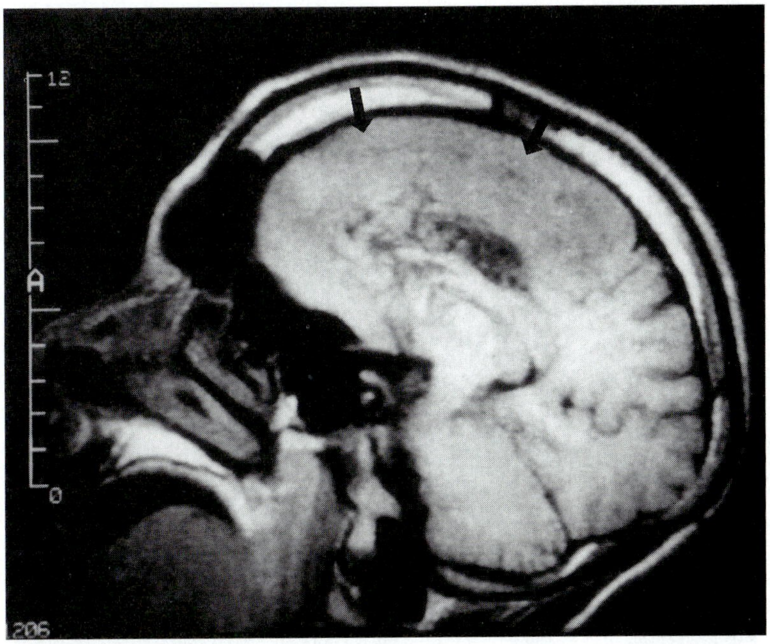

FIGURE 26-6

MRI of the brain showing the smooth surface of the cerebral hemisphere (*arrows*) in a patient with lissencephaly.

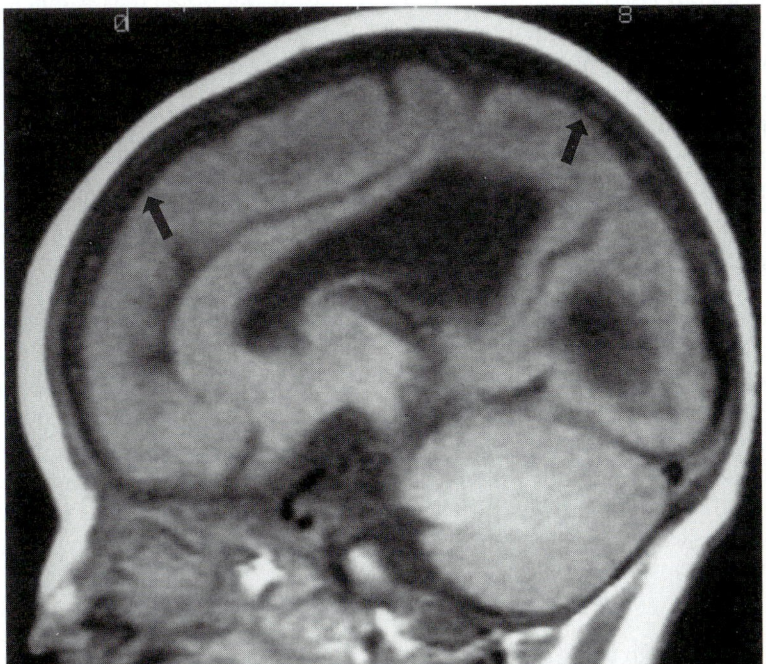

FIGURE 26-7

MRI of the brain showing wide gyri (*arrows*) in pachygyria.

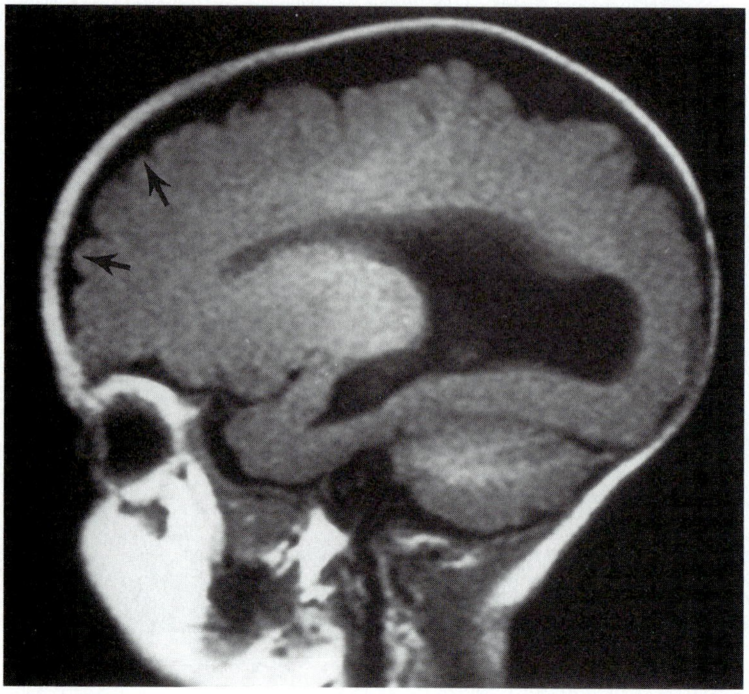

FIGURE 26-8

MRI of the brain showing small gyri (*arrows*) in polymicrogyria.

The pachygyric cortex is made up of four layers: (1) an outermost normal-appearing molecular layer, (2) a layer of neurons of decreased population which has not received its full complement of neurons by radial migration, (3) a much thicker layer of neurons, usually poorly organized and arranged in broad columns, which represent heterotopic neurons arrested in their migration, and (4) a relatively thin layer of white matter encroached on by heterotopic neurons. The migration defect resulting in pachygyria occurs at a slightly later stage of development than is the case in lissencephaly. Affected infants are hypotonic at birth, develop seizures within the first year of life, and are severely neurologically retarded.

Polymicrogyria (Greek *polys,* "many"; *mikros,* "small"; *gyros,* "ring or circle, convolution"). A malformation of the brain characterized by numerous small gyri.

Polymicrogyria

Polymicrogyria (Fig. 26-8) is characterized by a large number of very small gyri without intervening sulci or with shallow sulci bridged by the overlying molecular layers of adjacent gyri. The appearance of the polymicrogyric cortex has been compared to that of a cauliflower. The polymicrogyric malformation may cover the entire surface of the hemisphere or occur in limited areas of one or both hemispheres. On imaging studies, polymicrogyria may mimic pachygyria. In general, the cerebral cortex in polymicrogyria (5 to 7 mm) is not as thick as it is in pachygyria (approximately 8 mm). The migration defect that leads to polymicrogyria is attrib-

KEY CONCEPTS

- Polymicrogyria refers to a large number of very small gyri without intervening sulci or with shallow sulci.

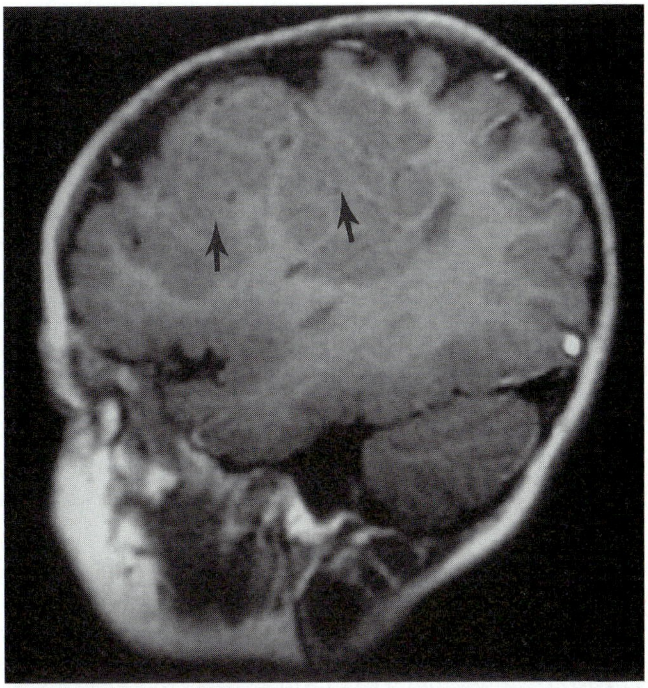

FIGURE 26-9

MRI of the brain showing cortical heterotopia (*arrows*).

uted to ischemic laminar necrosis occurring in the fifth month of gestation, later than that responsible for lissencephaly and pachygyria. Laminar necrosis in polymicrogyria occurs in layer V. Superficial to this necrotic cortical band, the cortex consists of normal layers I to IV.

The clinical presentation of patients with polymicrogyria varies with the extent of the malformation. Patients with diffuse polymicrogyria involving the entire cortex present with microcephaly, hypotonia, seizures, and developmental retardation, similar to the presentation in patients with lissencephaly. Patients with bilateral focal polymicrogyria usually are moderately developmentally delayed and spastic. Patients with unilateral focal polymicrogyria most often have congenital hemiplegia, mild to moderate developmental delay, and focal motor seizures.

Cortical Heterotopias

A cortical heterotopia (Fig. 26-9) is characterized by islands of gray matter along the route of neuroblast migration. The islands consist of a collection of normal neurons in abnormal locations secondary to an arrest of the radial migration of neuroblasts. The onset of the migration defect occurs no later than the latter part of the fifth month of gestation. Heterotopias have been associated with a wide

Heterotopia (Greek *heteros,* "other, different"; *topos,* "place"). Displacement of parts; the presence of tissue in an abnormal location. Neuronal heterotopia refers to the presence of gray matter within white matter as a result of abnormal neuronal migration during histogenesis.

KEY CONCEPTS

- Cortical heterotopias involve the presence of islands of gray matter within the white matter. Three types are recognized: subependymal (nodular), focal subcortical (laminar), and diffuse (band), also known as double cortex.

variety of genetic, vascular, and environmental causes. Heterotopias are clinically divided into three groups: (1) subependymal (nodular), (2) focal subcortical (laminar), and (3) diffuse (band) (double cortex). Subependymal (nodular) heterotopias are subependymal masses of gray matter which form clusters of rounded nodules that are well separated from the cortex by normally myelinated white matter. They usually are localized at the corners of the lateral ventricles. Focal subcortical (laminar) heterotopias are separated from both the cortex and the ventricles by thick layers of white matter. Diffuse (band) heterotopias (double cortex) consist of bilateral symmetric layers of heterotopic neurons between the lateral ventricles and the cerebral cortex. Patients with subependymal heterotopias tend to have normal development and mild clinical symptoms. The onset of seizures usually occurs in the second decade of life. Patients with focal subcortical heterotopias have variable symptoms and signs that depend on the extent of their heterotopias. Those with large heterotopias have moderate to severe developmental delay and hemiplegia, whereas those with smaller or thinner subcortical heterotopias may have normal development and motor function. Patients with diffuse band heterotopias (double cortex) have moderate or severe developmental delay and intractable seizures.

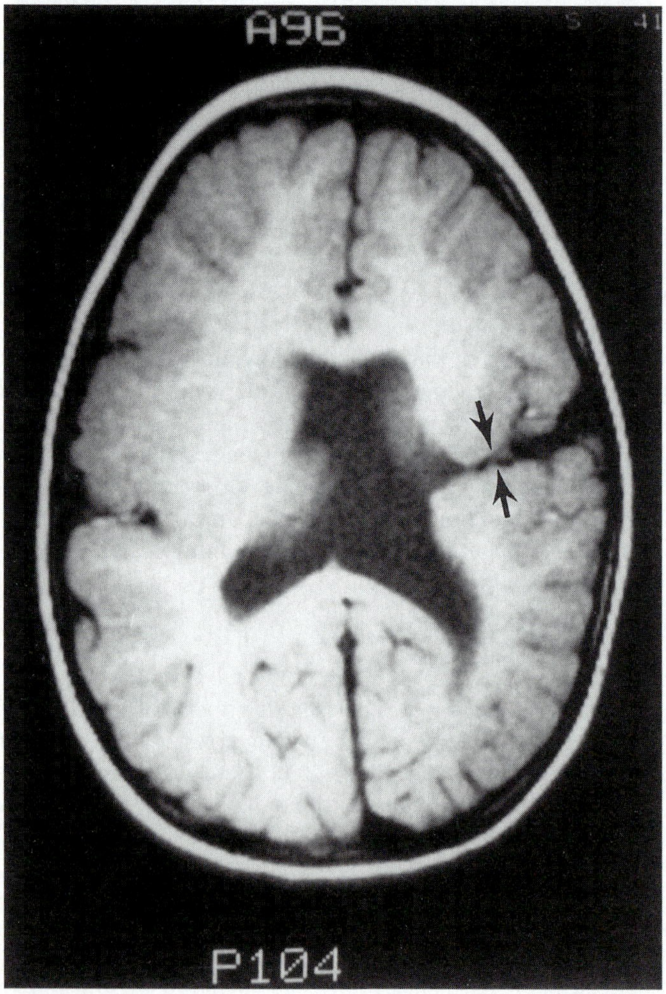

FIGURE 26-10

MRI of the brain showing schizencephalic cleft (*arrows*).

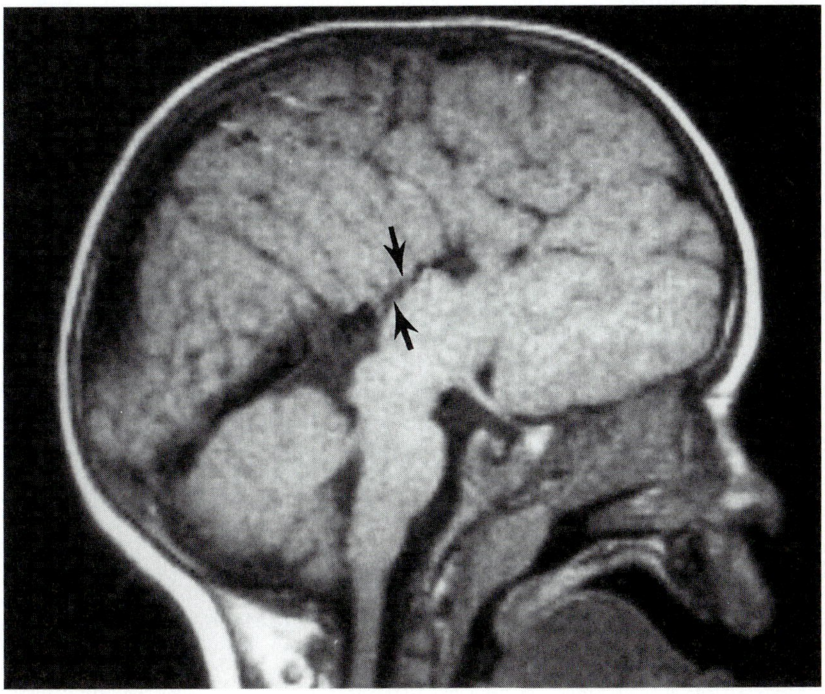

FIGURE 26-11

MRI of the brain showing agenesis of the corpus callosum (*arrows*).

Schizencephaly

Schizencephaly (Greek *schizein,* "to divide"; *enkephalos,* "brain"). A developmental brain anomaly characterized by the presence of unilateral or bilateral clefts in the cerebral hemisphere. A neuronal migration defect.

The term *schizencephaly* (Fig. 26-10) was coined by Yakovlev and Wadsworth in 1946 to describe gray matter–lined clefts in the cerebral hemispheres extending from the pia to the ependymal lining of the lateral ventricle. The walls of the clefts may be in apposition (closed lip, type I) or separated (open lip, type II). The onset of the malformation is considered to occur at 3 to 5 months of gestation. A focal watershed infarct in the cerebral mantle during early development has been proposed as a cause of schizencephaly. Familial occurrence raises the possibility of a genetic mechanism in the causation of this malformation. Previous reports of this malformation, derived primarily from pathologic specimens, suggested that this malformation was extremely rare, seen primarily in institutionalized patients with severe motor and intellectual deficits. The introduction of and improvements in imaging techniques such as computed axial tomography (CT) and magnetic resonance imaging (MRI) have enhanced awareness and increased recognition of the disorder. The clinical presentation varies with the extent of the malformation. Patients with bilateral malformations usually are developmentally delayed and have seizures. Patients with unilateral malformations may have only a motor deficit (hemiplegia) and seizures or may be developmentally delayed, depending on the extent of the malformation.

KEY CONCEPTS

- Schizencephaly refers to gray matter–lined clefts in the cerebral hemisphere. The clefts may be closed or open and unilateral or bilateral.

Agenesis of the Corpus Callosum

Corpus callosum malformations are commonly associated with other congenital brain malformations, suggesting a causal relationship. Both neurulation and migration defect malformations have been associated with agenesis of the corpus callosum (Fig. 26-11). Agenesis of the corpus callosum may be total or partial. In total absence of the corpus callosum, the medial surface of the hemisphere has an abnormal radial gyral pattern. The cingulate gyrus is poorly outlined, and most of the gyri extend perpendicularly to the roof of the third ventricle. The axons destined to form the corpus callosum instead turn parallel to the interhemispheric fissure and form the longitudinal callosal **bundles of Probst.** The bundle of Probst indents the superomedial borders of the lateral ventricles, giving them a characteristic crescent shape. In partial agenesis, the posterior portion (splenium) or the rostrum (late to develop) is missing. Absence of the corpus callosum may be an isolated anomaly with no clinical symptoms or may be associated with mental retardation and seizures. Sporadic as well as familial cases have been reported.

Bundle of Probst An anomalous bundle of nerve fibers associated with agenesis of the corpus callosum. Fibers destined to cross in the commissure instead course rostrocaudally in the superior medial part of the lateral ventricle parallel to the cingulate bundle.

KEY CONCEPTS

- Agenesis of the corpus callosum is commonly associated with other congenital brain malformations. It may be total or partial.

SUGGESTED READINGS

Altman N, et al: Advanced magnetic resonance imaging of disorders of neuronal migration and sulcation. *Int Pediatr* 1995; 10:16–25.

Barkovich AJ, et al: Formation, maturation, and disorders of brain neocortex. *AJNR* 1992; 13:423–446.

Barkovich AJ, Kjos BO: Schizencephaly: Correlation of clinical findings with MR characteristics. *AJNR* 1992; 13:85–94.

Barth PG: Disorders of neuronal migration. *Can J Neurol Sci* 1987; 14:1–16.

Bodensteiner J, et al: Hypoplasia of the corpus callosum: A study of 445 consecutive MRI scans. *J Child Neurol* 1994; 9:47–49.

Chamberlain MC, et al: Neonatal schizencephaly: Comparison of brain imaging. *Pediatr Neurol* 1990; 6: 382–387.

Gestaut H, et al: Lissencephaly (agyria-pachygyria): Clinical findings and serial EEG studies. *Dev Med Child Neurol* 1987; 29:167–180.

Hayward JC, et al: Lissencephaly-pachygyria associated with congenital cytomegalovirus infection. *J Child Neurol* 1991; 6:109–114.

Hoffman HJ: The tethered spinal cord. In Holtzman RNN, Stein BM (eds): *The Tethered Spinal Cord.* New York, Thieme-Stratton, 1985:91–98.

Larroche JC: Malformations of the nervous system. In Adams JH, et al (eds): *Greenfield's Neuropathology.* London, E. Arnold, 1984:385–450.

Larroche JC, Razavi-Encha F: Cytoarchitectonic abnormalities. In Vinken PJ, et al (eds): *Handbook of Clinical Neurology.* Amsterdam, Elsevier, 1987: 245–266.

Martin-Padilla M: The tethered cord syndrome: Developmental considerations: In Holtzman RNN, Stein BM (eds): *The Tethered Spinal Cord.* New York, Thieme Stratton, 1985:3–13.

Mathern GW, Peacock WJ: Diastematomyelia. In Park TS (ed): *Spinal Dysraphism.* Boston, Blackwell, 1992:91–103.

McLeod NA, et al: Normal and abnormal morphology of the corpus callosum. *Neurology* 1987; 37:1240–1242.

Miller GM, et al: Schizencephaly: A clinical and CT study. *Neurology* 1984; 34:997–1001.

Naidich TP: Congenital malformations of the brain. *Int Pediatr* 1990; 5:87–93.

Naidich TP, et al: Cephaloceles and related malformations. *AJNR* 1992; 13:655–690.

Norman MG, et al: *Congenital Malformations of the Brain: Pathological, Embryological, Clinical, Radiological, and Clinical Aspects.* New York, Oxford University Press, 1995.

Oakley GP: Folic acid-preventable spina bifida and anencephaly. *JAMA* 1993; 269:1292–1293.

Palmini A, et al: Stages and patterns of centrifugal arrest of diffuse neuronal migration disorders. *Dev Med Child Neurol* 1993; 35:331–339.

Rubenstein D, et al: Partial development of the corpus callosum. *AJNR* 1994; 15:869–875.

Snyder RD, et al: Anencephaly in the United States, 1968–1987: The declining incidence among white infants. *J Child Neurol* 1991; 6:304–305.

Storrs BB, et al: The tethered cord syndrome. *Int Pediatr* 1990; 5:99–103.

Van der Knaap MS, Valk J: Classification of congenital abnormalities of the CNS. *AJNR* 1988; 9:315–326.

Volpe JJ: Normal and abnormal human brain development. *Clin Perinatol* 1977; 4:3–30.

Williams RS: Cerebral malformations arising in the first half of gestation. In Evrard P, Minkowski (eds): *Developmental Neurobiology.* New York, Raven Press, 1989:11–20.

CHAPTER 27

CEREBRAL CIRCULATION

The constantly active brain requires a rich blood supply to sustain its ongoing activity. Irreversible brain damage (brain death) results if the blood supply to the brain is interrupted for more than a few minutes; consciousness is lost if the blood supply is interrupted for about 5 s. Lesions of the nervous system due to interruption of blood supply constitute the most common type of central nervous system disorders.

It is estimated that about 15 percent of cardiac output reaches the brain; about 20 percent of oxygen utilization of the body is consumed by the adult brain and as much as 50 percent by the infant brain. The blood flow through the human brain is estimated to be 800 ml/min, or approximately 50 ml/100 g of brain tissue per minute. This average value increases with an increase in functional activity of the brain or regions within it. The blood flow is markedly increased in the sensory motor area on vigorous exercise of the contralateral limb. Cerebral blood flow is faster in gray matter (70 to 80 ml/100 g per min) than in white matter (30 ml/100 g

KEY CONCEPTS

- Irreversible brain damage (brain death) occurs if blood supply to the brain is interrupted for more than a few minutes.

per min). Irreversible brain damage will occur if the cerebral blood flow is less than 15 ml/100 g per min.

SOURCES OF SUPPLY

Carotid (Greek *karotis,* "deep sleep"). The arteries of the neck are so called because it was known in ancient times that animals became sleepy when these vessels were compressed.

The brain receives its blood supply from four arterial trunks: two internal **carotid** arteries and two vertebral arteries. A knowledge of normal cerebral vascular anatomy is essential for understanding and localizing cerebrovascular disorders. This chapter will focus on blood supply of the cerebral cortex. Blood supplies of the spinal cord and brain stem are discussed in their respective chapters: Chap. 3, and Chaps. 5, 7, 9, 11, 13, and 15.

Internal Carotid Artery

Cavernous (Latin *cavernosus,* "containing caverns or hollow spaces").

The internal carotid arteries arise at the bifurcation of the common carotid arteries in the neck (Fig. 27-1), ascend in front of the transverse processes of the upper three cervical vertebrae, and enter the base of the skull through the carotid canal. Within the cranium, the internal carotid artery lies in the **cavernous** sinus. It then pierces the dura to begin its subarachnoid course. The internal carotid artery gives rise to the ophthalmic, anterior choroidal, anterior cerebral, middle cerebral, and posterior communicating branches. Within the cavernous sinus, the internal carotid artery lies close to the medial wall immediately adjacent to the abducens nerve (CN VI). Other cranial nerves in the sinus, situated along the lateral wall include the oculomotor (CN III), trochlear (CN IV), ophthalmic, and maxillary divisions of the trigeminal (CN V).

From its site of origin from the common carotid artery to its site of bifurcation into the anterior and middle cerebral arteries, the internal carotid artery is divided into four segments: (1) the cervical segment extends from the origin of the internal carotid artery from the common carotid to the site where it enters the carotid canal, (2) the intrapetrosal segment is the part of the artery as it courses through the petrous portion of the temporal bone, (3) the intracavernous segment courses through the cavernous sinus, and (4) the cerebral (supraclinoid) segment extends from the site of exit of the artery from the cavernous sinus to its bifurcation into the anterior and middle cerebral arteries. The intracavernous and cerebral segments are collectively known as the *carotid siphon* because of their characteristic S-shaped configuration. All the major branches of the internal carotid artery arise from the cerebral segment.

Ophthalmic Artery

The ophthalmic artery is the first intracranial branch of the internal carotid as it courses through the cavernous sinus. The ophthalmic artery supplies the optic nerve and gives rise to the central artery of the retina. Thus interruption of the blood supply from the internal carotid system may result in disturbances in visual acuity. The ophthalmic artery is also of importance because of its anastomotic connections

KEY CONCEPTS

- The brain receives its blood supply from four arterial trunks: two internal carotid arteries and two vertebral arteries.
- The internal carotid arteries provide blood supply to the rostral parts of the brain, whereas the vertebral arteries provide blood supply to the posterior parts of the brain.
- The ophthalmic branch of the internal carotid artery is an important anastomotic channel between the internal and external carotid circulations.

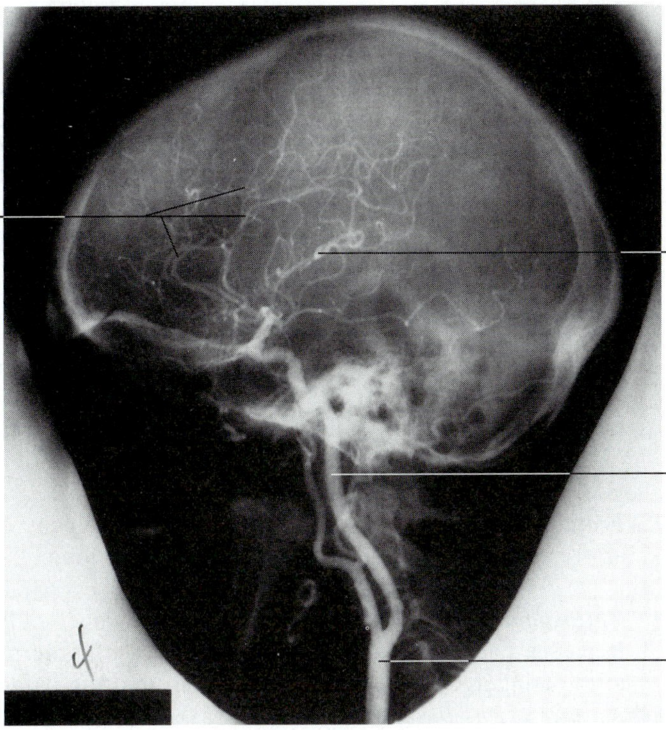

FIGURE 27-1

Lateral view of carotid arteriogram showing the distribution of anterior and middle cerebral arteries.

with branches of the external carotid system; this anastomotic relationship is essential in establishing collateral circulation when the internal carotid system is occluded in the neck.

Anterior Choroidal Artery

The anterior choroidal artery arises from the internal carotid artery after it emerges from the cavernous sinus. It passes ventral to the optic tract and supplies the optic tract, cerebral peduncles, lateral geniculate body, posterior part of the posterior limb of the internal capsule, tail of the caudate nucleus, uncus, amygdala, anterior hippocampus, choroid plexus of the temporal horn, and sometimes the globus pallidus. The anterior choroidal artery is prone to occlusion by thrombus because of its small caliber.

Anterior Cerebral Artery

The anterior cerebral artery (see Figs. 27-1 and 17-23) originates from the internal carotid artery lateral to the optic chiasm and courses dorsal to the optic nerve to reach the interhemispheric fissure, where it curves around the genu of the corpus callosum and continues as the pericallosal artery dorsal to the corpus callosum. As the two anterior cerebral arteries approach the interhemispheric fissure, they are joined by the anterior communicating artery. The anterior cerebral artery supplies

KEY CONCEPTS

- The anterior cerebral artery and its branches provide blood supply to the medial surface of the hemisphere as far back as the parieto-occipital fissure.

the medial aspect of the cerebral hemisphere as far back as the parieto-occipital fissure. The following are among its major branches.

Recurrent artery of Heubner. A branch of the anterior cerebral artery. Named after Otto Johann Leonhard Heubner, a German pediatrician.

Recurrent Artery of Heubner (Medial Striate Artery) This artery arises from the anterior cerebral artery either proximal or distal to the anterior communicating artery. It supplies the anterior limb and genu of the internal capsule and parts of the head of the caudate, rostral putamen, and globus pallidus. It also provides blood supply to the posterior portions of the gyrus rectus and orbitofrontal cortex. Thus occlusion of this artery will result in subcortical and cortical infarcts. The recurrent artery of Heubner varies in number from one to three.

Orbitofrontal Artery This branch arises distal to the anterior communicating artery and supplies the orbital gyri at the base of the frontal lobe and part of the septal area. The orbitofrontal artery or its branches may be displaced by subfrontal tumors, thus providing a clue, in cerebral angiograms, to the extracerebral location of the tumor (e.g., subfrontal meningioma).

Frontopolar Artery Arising at the level of the genu of the corpus callosum, this artery supplies most of the pole of the frontal lobe.

Callosomarginal Artery This is the major branch of the anterior cerebral artery. It passes backward and upward and gives off internal frontal branches before terminating in the paracentral branch around the paracentral lobule.

Pericallosal Artery This is the terminal branch of the anterior cerebral artery. It courses fairly close to the corpus callosum. It ordinarily gives rise to the paracentral artery, which also may be derived from the callosomarginal artery. The pericallosal artery terminates as the precuneal branch, which supplies the precuneus gyrus of the parietal lobe.

Occlusion of one anterior cerebral artery, in the absence of collateral circulation, will result in paralysis of the contralateral leg due to interruption of the blood supply to the leg area of the sensory motor cortex on the medial aspect of the hemisphere. Occlusion of both anterior cerebral arteries results in bilateral lower extremity paralysis and impaired sensations that mimic a spinal cord lesion.

Middle Cerebral Artery

The middle cerebral artery (see Figs. 27-1 and 17-24) is a continuation or the main branch of the internal carotid artery. It is divided into four segments: the M_1 (sphenoidal) segment courses posterior and parallel to the sphenoid ridge; the M_2 (insular) segment lies on the insula (island of Reil); the M_3 (opercular) segment courses over the frontal, parietal, and temporal opercula; and the M_4 (cortical) segment spreads over the cortical surface. It courses within the lateral (sylvian) fissure and divides into a number of branches that supply most of the lateral surface of the hemisphere. The middle cerebral artery territory does not reach the occipital or frontal poles or the upper margin of the hemisphere along the superior longitudinal fissure but does extend around the inferior margin of the cerebral hemisphere

KEY CONCEPTS

- Occlusion of the anterior cerebral artery results in contralateral paralysis and sensory deficit most marked in the lower extremity.
- The middle cerebral artery and its branches provide blood supply to most of the lateral surface of the hemisphere.

onto the inferior surfaces of the frontal and temporal lobes. The following are some of the more important branches.

Cortical Branches These include the rolandic (which supplies the primary sensory motor cortex), frontal, temporal, and parietal branches. The most rostral cortical division of the middle cerebral artery is known as the *candelabra branch* because of its division into two segments, simulating a candelabra.

Central (Perforating) Branches These include the lenticulostriate arteries, which supply the major parts of the caudate, putamen, globus pallidus, internal capsule, and thalamus. The perforating branches are involved in basal ganglia and internal capsule hemorrhages and infarcts. Charcot's artery, the artery of cerebral hemorrhage, is one of the perforating branches of the middle cerebral artery.

The middle cerebral artery thus supplies the following important neural structures: primary and association motor and somatosensory cortices, Broca's area of speech, prefrontal cortex, primary and association auditory cortices (including Wernicke's area), and the major association cortex (supramarginal and angular gyri). Occlusion of the middle cerebral artery results in contralateral paralysis (more marked in the upper extremity and face), contralateral loss of kinesthesia and discriminative touch, changes in mentation and personality, and aphasia when the left (dominant) hemisphere is involved.

Posterior Communicating Artery

The posterior communicating artery connects the internal carotid artery with the posterior cerebral artery. Some anatomists consider the posterior cerebral artery as a continuation of the posterior communicating artery. Branches of the posterior communicating artery supply the genu and anterior part of the posterior limb of the internal capsule, the anterior part of the thalamus, and parts of the hypothalamus and subthalamus.

Vertebral Artery

The vertebral artery arises from the subclavian artery near the thyrocervical trunk in the majority of cases and from the arch of the aorta in few cases. It ascends within the foramina of the transverse processes of the upper six cervical vertebrae (intraosseus segment), curves backward around the lateral mass of the atlas (atlantoaxial segment), and enters the cranium through the foramen magnum (intracranial segment). Within the cranium, the vertebral arteries lie on the inferior surface of the medulla oblongata. The two vertebral arteries join at the caudal end of the pons to form the basilar artery. The vertebral artery gives rise to the posterior spinal, anterior spinal, and posterior inferior cerebellar branches (Fig. 27-2). Meningeal branches supply the meninges of the posterior fossa, including the falx cerebelli.

The intraosseus segment is affected by osteoarthritis and atherosclerosis. The atlantoaxial segment is affected in fractures, dislocations, subluxations, birth trauma,

KEY CONCEPTS

- Occlusion of the middle cerebral artery results in contralateral paralysis and sensory deficit most marked in the upper extremity and face and aphasia if the left hemisphere is involved.
- The posterior communicating artery connects the internal carotid artery and the posterior cerebral arteries.
- The vertebral arteries join to form the basilar artery.

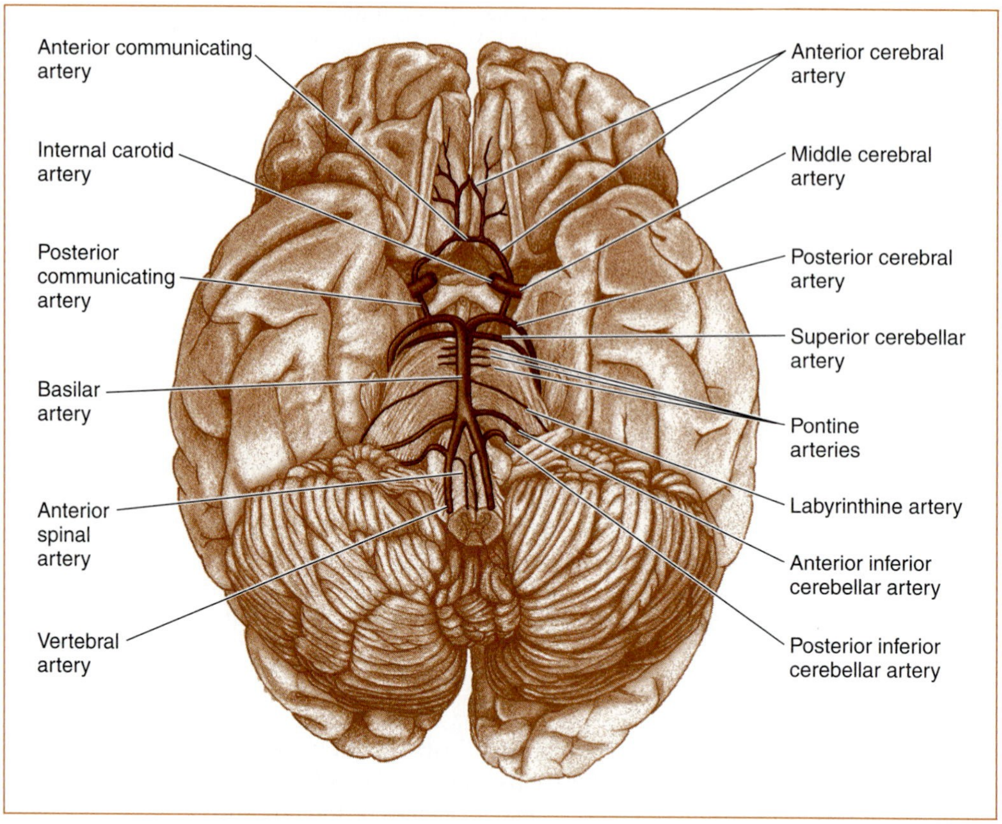

FIGURE 27-2

Schematic diagram of the major branches of the vertebral and basilar arteries and the Circle of Willis and arteries that contribute to the formation of the circle.

and chiropractic adjustments. The intracranial segment is involved more frequently than other segments in thrombotic occlusions.

Posterior Spinal Artery

The two posterior spinal arteries pass caudally over the medulla and the posterior surface of the spinal cord. They supply the posterior aspect of the medulla below the obex, as well as the posterior column and posterior horns of the spinal cord. One or both posterior spinal arteries may arise from the posterior inferior cerebellar arteries.

Anterior Spinal Artery

The anterior spinal artery starts as two vessels that join to form a single artery that descends on the ventral aspect of the medulla and into the anterior median fissure of the spinal cord. It supplies the medullary pyramids and the paramedian medullary structures, as well as the anterior two-thirds of the spinal cord. Occlusion of this artery in the spinal cord results in sudden onset of paralysis below the occlusion.

Posterior Inferior Cerebellar Artery (PICA)

Asymmetric in level of origin and diameter, these arteries follow an S-shaped course over the olive and inferior cerebellar peduncle to supply the inferior surface of the cerebellum, dorsolateral surface of the medulla oblongata, choroid plexus of the fourth ventricle, and part of the deep cerebellar nuclei. Occlusion of this artery gives rise to a characteristic group of signs and symptoms comprising the lateral medullary syndrome (Wallenberg's syndrome). The posterior inferior cerebellar artery may have common origin with the anterior inferior cerebellar artery from the basilar artery.

Basilar Artery

Formed by the union of the two vertebral arteries at the caudal end of the pons, the basilar artery (Fig. 27-2) runs in the pontine groove on the ventral aspect of the pons and terminates at the rostral end by dividing into the two posterior cerebral arteries. Branches include a series of paramedian (penetrating) arteries that supply the paramedian zone of the basilar portion of the pons (basis pontis) and the adjacent pontine tegmentum and a series of short and long circumferential arteries.

Paramedian Penetrating Arteries
These branches travel for variable distances caudally before penetrating the brain stem; hence a lesion in the brain stem may appear at levels more caudal than that of the occluded vessel.

Short Circumferential Arteries
These branches supply the anterolateral and posterolateral parts of the pons.

Long Circumferential Arteries
There are three long circumferential arteries.

Auditory (Labyrinthine) Artery This artery accompanies the facial (CN VII) and vestibulocochlear (CN VIII) cranial nerves and supplies the inner ear and root fibers of the facial nerve. Occlusion of this artery gives rise to deafness. It has variable origin from the basilar, anterior inferior cerebellar, and the posterior inferior cerebellar arteries.

Anterior Inferior Cerebellar Artery (AICA) This artery supplies the inferior surface of the cerebellum, the brachium pontis, and the restiform body, as well as the tegmentum of the lower pons and upper medulla. It may arise from a common stem with the auditory artery or the posterior inferior cerebellar artery.

Superior Cerebellar Artery This is the last branch of the basilar artery before its terminal bifurcation into the two posterior cerebral arteries, from which it is separated by the rootlets of the oculomotor nerve. It supplies the superior surface of the cerebellum, part of the dentate nucleus, the brachium pontis and conjunctivum, the tegmentum of the upper pons, and the inferior colliculus.

Posterior Cerebral Arteries (see Fig. 17-23)
These constitute the terminal branches of the basilar artery in 70 percent of cases, may arise from the carotid artery of one side in 20 to 25 percent of cases, and may arise on both sides in 5 to 10 percent of cases. They pass around the cerebral peduncle and supply the medial surfaces of the occipital lobe, including the primary and association visual cortices, temporal lobe, caudal parietal lobe, and the splenium of the corpus callosum.

Occlusion of one posterior cerebral artery results in contralateral loss of vision (homonymous hemianopia), with sparing of macular vision because of collateral

KEY CONCEPTS

- The posterior cerebral artery, the terminal branch of the basilar artery, supplies the medial surfaces of the occipital, temporal, and the caudal part of the parietal lobes.

circulation from the middle cerebral artery to the occipital pole, where macular vision is represented. Bilateral occlusion of the posterior cerebral artery results in prosopagnosia (loss of face recognition) and achromatopsia (loss of color vision). Perforating branches supply the cerebral peduncle, mamillary bodies, and the mesencephalon. Other branches include the thalamogeniculate artery, which supplies the lateral geniculate body and posterior thalamus, and the posterior choroidal artery, which supplies the choroid plexus of the third and lateral ventricles, tectum, and thalamus. Posterior cerebral artery branches also pass over the dorsal edge of the cerebral hemisphere to supply a small part of the lateral surface of the caudal parietal lobe and occipital lobe and the inferior temporal gyrus. The posterior cerebral artery may be compressed by herniation of the uncus in cases of increased intracranial pressure. As a consequence, the circulation of the visual cortex is impaired, resulting in cortical blindness.

CIRCLE OF WILLIS

The proximal portions of the anterior, middle, and posterior cerebral arteries connected by the anterior and posterior communicating arteries form a circle, the **circle of Willis** (Fig. 27-2), around the infundibulum of the pituitary and the optic chiasm. The circle constitutes an important anastomotic channel between the internal carotid and the vertebral basilar systems.

Circle of Willis. The anastomotic ring of arteries that encircles the pituitary stalk. It was first depicted by Johann Vesling in 1647 and further defined by Thomas Willis in 1664.

When either the internal carotid arteries (anterior circulation) or the vertebral basilar system (posterior circulation) becomes occluded, collateral circulation in the circle of Willis will provide blood to the area deprived of blood supply. The circle of Willis is complete in only 20 percent of individuals. In the majority of individuals, variation in size and/or origin of vessels is the rule.

CONDUCTING AND PENETRATING VESSELS

The arteries of the brain fall into two general types. The *conducting* or *superficial arteries* are those which run in the pia arachnoid and include the internal carotid and vertebral basilar systems and their branches. These vessels receive autonomic nerves and function as pressure-equalization reservoirs to maintain an adequate perfusion pressure for the penetrating arteries. It is estimated that the drop in the pressure head from large vessels to the penetrating arterioles does not exceed 10 to 15 percent. The *penetrating arterioles* supply the cortex and white matter and are organized in vertical and horizontal patterns. These are presumed to be the primary sites of regional autoregulation and do not receive a significant neural supply.

KEY CONCEPTS

- Occlusion of the posterior cerebral artery results in contralateral homonymous hemianopia with sparing of macular vision.
- The vertebral and basilar arteries provide blood supply to the spinal cord and brain stem.
- The circle of Willis is formed by the proximal portions of the anterior, middle, and posterior cerebral arteries connected by the anterior and posterior communicating arteries.

HISTOLOGY OF CEREBRAL VESSELS

Cerebral arteries differ from arteries elsewhere in the body in the following features:

1. Thinner walls
2. Absent external elastic laminae
3. Presence of astrocytic processes
4. Presence of a perivascular reticular sheath consisting of arachnoid trabeculae (the latter acquire an outer pial membrane when the vessel penetrates the brain substance).

Cerebral capillaries are structurally similar to capillaries elsewhere, except for being surrounded by perivascular glial (astrocytic) processes. Cerebral veins have thinner walls and are devoid of valves and muscle fibers. The absence of valves allows reversal of blood flow when occlusion of the lumen occurs in disease.

COLLATERAL CIRCULATION

Anastomotic channels are present in all parts of both the arterial and venous circulations. Their main purpose is to ensure a continuing blood flow to the brain in case of a major occlusion of a feeding vessel. Some of these channels, however, are not very effective in collateral circulation because of their small caliber. The following are the major sites of collateral circulation.

1. Extracranial anastomoses are found between cervical vessels, such as the vertebral and external carotids of the same side.
2. Extracranial-intracranial anastomoses occur between branches of the external carotid and the ophthalmic artery. This is a major site of communication between extracranial and intracranial circulations. Thus, when the internal carotid is obstructed proximal to the origin of the ophthalmic artery, flow is reversed in the ophthalmic artery. Another site of extracranial-intracranial anastomosis is through the rete mirabile, a group of small vessels that connect meningeal and ethmoidal branches of external carotid arteries with leptomeningeal branches of cerebral arteries.
3. Intracranial anastomoses occur in the circle of Willis. Under normal conditions, there is very little side flow or flow from posterior to anterior segments in the circle of Willis. In the presence of major occlusion, however, the communications across the anterior or posterior communicating artery become a very important channel for collateral circulation. Other sites of intracranial anastomoses include those among the superior cerebellar, anterior inferior cerebellar, and posterior inferior cerebellar in the cerebellum.

CEREBRAL VENOUS DRAINAGE

Cerebral venous drainage occurs through two systems, the superficial and the deep.

KEY CONCEPTS

- The circle of Willis comprises the major site of intracranial collateral circulation.
- Venous drainage of the cerebral hemisphere is via two systems: superficial and deep.

Superficial Venous System

The superficial system of veins (see Fig. 17-25) is divided into three groups.

Superior Cerebral Group
These veins drain the dorsolateral and dorsomedial surfaces of the hemisphere and enter the superior sagittal sinus at a forward angle against the flow of blood. Conventionally, the most prominent of these veins in the central sulcus is called the *superior anastomotic* ***vein of Tro!ard,*** which interconnects the superior and middle groups of veins.

Vein of Trolard. An anastomotic cerebral vein that interconnects the superior and middle groups of superficial cerebral veins. Named after Paulin Trolard, professor of anatomy in Algiers, who described the vein in his graduation thesis from the University of Paris in 1868.

Vein of Labbé. An anastomotic cerebral vein that crosses the temporal lobe about 5 cm behind its tip. This vein interconnects the middle and inferior groups of superficial cerebral veins. Named after Charles Labbé, the French anatomist.

Great cerebral vein of Galen. A major deep cerebral vein that drains into the straight sinus. Named after Claudius Galen, the Roman physician and founder of the galenical system of medicine.

Basal vein of Rosenthal. A deep cerebral vein that serves as a landmark for neuroradiologists in identifying pathology in deep cerebral structures. It was described by Friedrich Rosenthal, a German anatomist.

Middle Cerebral Group
These veins run along the sylvian fissure, drain the inferolateral surface of the hemisphere, and open into the cavernous sinus.

Inferior Cerebral Group
These veins drain the inferior surface of the hemisphere and open into the cavernous and transverse sinuses. The middle and inferior groups are interconnected by the inferior anastomotic **vein of Labbé,** which crosses the temporal lobe about 5 cm behind its tip. The medial surface of the hemisphere is drained by a number of veins that open into the superior and inferior sagittal sinuses, as well as into the basal vein and the **great cerebral vein of Galen.**

Deep Venous System

The deep venous system (Fig. 27-3) consists of a number of veins that drain into two main tributaries; these are the internal cerebral vein and the **basal vein (of Rosenthal)**. The two join beneath the splenium of the corpus callosum to form the great cerebral vein of Galen, which opens into the straight sinus.

Internal Cerebral Vein
This vein receives two tributaries.

Terminal Vein (Thalamostriate) Draining the caudate nucleus and possibly the thalamus, this vein passes forward in a groove between the caudate nucleus and thalamus in the body of the lateral ventricle and empties into the internal cerebral vein at the interventricular foramen of Monro.

Septal Vein This vein drains the septum pellucidum, the anterior end of the corpus callosum, and the head of the caudate nucleus and passes backward from the anterior column of the fornix to open at the interventricular foramen into the internal cerebral vein.

KEY CONCEPTS

- The superficial venous system consists of three groups of venous channels: superior, middle, and inferior.
- Two prominent superficial anastomotic venous channels are the anastomotic vein of Trolard and the inferior anastomotic vein of Labbé.
- The deep venous system drains via two main veins (the internal cerebral vein and the basal vein of Rosenthal) into the great cerebral vein of Galen.

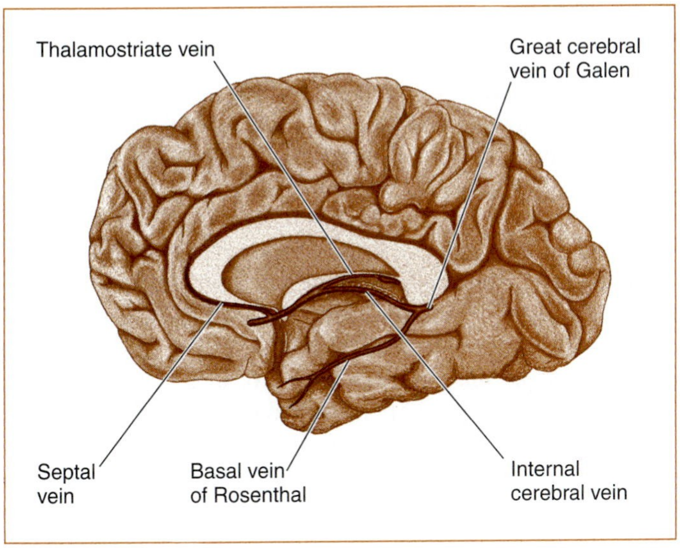

FIGURE 27-3

Schematic diagram of the deep system of venous drainage of the brain.

The internal cerebral vein of each side runs along the roof of the third ventricle in the velum interpositum. It extends from the region of the foramen of Monro rostrally to between the pineal body (below) and the splenium of the corpus callosum (above) caudally. The two internal cerebral veins join below the splenium of the corpus callosum to form the great vein of Galen.

Basal Vein of Rosenthal

This vein begins under the anterior perforated substance near the medial part of the anterior temporal lobe and runs backward to empty into the great cerebral vein. It drains blood from the base of the brain.

Visualization of the cerebral veins, particularly the deep group, is used during cerebral angiography in the localization of deep brain lesions.

Great Cerebral Vein (of Galen)

This vein receives the internal cerebral vein and the basal vein of Rosenthal and a number of other smaller veins (occipital, posterior callosal) and extends for a short distance under the splenium of the corpus callosum to empty into the straight sinus (rectus sinus).

CEREBELLAR VENOUS DRAINAGE

The cerebellum is drained by three groups of veins; these are the superior, anterior, and posterior groups.

1. The superior group drains the entire superior surface of the cerebellum and empties into the great cerebral vein or the straight sinus.
2. The anterior cerebellar vein (known to neurosurgeons as the *petrosal vein*) is a constant vein, draining the inferoanterior surface of the cerebellum and the pontine venous plexus. It opens into the superior petrosal sinus.
3. The posterior cerebellar vein empties into either the straight or the transverse sinus.

CEREBRAL DURAL VENOUS SINUSES

Cerebral dural venous sinuses are lined by endothelium and are devoid of valves. They lie between the periosteal and meningeal layers of the dura mater. They serve as low-pressure channels for venous blood flow back to the systemic circulation.

The *superior sagittal sinus* and the *inferior sagittal sinus* lie in the superior and inferior margins of the falx cerebri, respectively. The superficial cerebral veins drain into the superior and inferior sagittal sinuses. The superior sagittal sinus, in addition, drains cerebrospinal fluid from the subarachnoid space via arachnoid granulations, evaginations of the arachnoid matter (arachnoid villi), into the superior sagittal sinus. Caudally, the inferior sagittal sinus is joined by the great cerebral vein of Galen to form the *straight sinus* (*rectus sinus*) located at the junction of the falx cerebri and tentorium cerebelli. The straight sinus drains into the *confluence of sinuses.* The *two transverse sinuses* arise from the confluence of sinuses (**torcular Herophili**) and pass laterally and forward in a groove in the occipital bone. At the occipitopetrosal junction, they curve downward and backward as the *sigmoid sinus,* which drains into the internal jugular vein. The *occipital sinus* connects the confluence of sinuses (torcular Herophili) to the *marginal sinus* at the foramen magnum. The *superior petrosal sinus* lies in the dura at the anterior border of the tentorium cerebelli. It connects the petrosal vein and transverse sinus to the cavernous sinus. The *inferior petrosal sinus* joins the cavernous sinus to the jugular bulb and extends between the clivus and the petrous bone. The *cavernous sinus* lies on each side of the sphenoid sinus, the sella turcica, and the pituitary gland. The medial wall of the sinus contains the internal carotid artery and the abducens cranial nerve. The lateral wall contains the oculomotor and trochlear cranial nerves and the ophthalmic and maxillary divisions of the trigeminal cranial nerve. The two cavernous sinuses intercommunicate via the basilar venous plexuses and via venous channels anterior and posterior to the pituitary gland. Anteriorly, the ophthalmic vein drains into the cavernous sinus. Posteriorly, the cavernous sinus drains into the superior and inferior petrosal sinuses. Laterally, it joins the pterygoid plexus at the foramen ovale.

Torcular Herophili (Latin *torcula,* "wine press"). A cistern or well to collect the liquor from the wine press. Herophilus was the ancient Greek anatomist who described this region of the brain. The confluence of sinuses.

FACTORS REGULATING CEREBRAL CIRCULATION

Cerebral blood flow is a function of the pressure gradient and cerebral vascular resistance. The pressure gradient is determined primarily by arterial pressure. Resistance is a function of blood viscosity and size of cerebral vessels.

Extrinsic Factors

Systemic Blood Pressure

Arterial pressure is regulated by several circulatory reflexes, the most important of which are the baroreceptor reflexes. Baroreceptors in the aortic arch and carotid sinus are tonically active when arterial pressure is normal and vary their impulse

KEY CONCEPTS

- Cerebral dural venous sinuses lie within two layers of the dura mater and serve as low-pressure channels for venous blood flow back to the systemic circulation.
- The dural venous sinuses include the superior and inferior sagittal, straight, confluence, transverse, sigmoid, occipital, petrosal, and cavernous sinuses.

frequency directly with fluctuations in blood pressure. An increase in arterial pressure increases impulses from baroreceptors, with inhibition of sympathetic efferents to the cardiovascular system and stimulation of the cardiac vagus nerve, leading to a decrease in arterial pressure. The reverse occurs if the arterial pressure is decreased. Baroreceptor regulation of arterial pressure ceases when arterial pressure falls below 50 to 60 mmHg.

Fluctuations in systemic arterial blood pressure in the healthy young individual have very little, if any, effect on cerebral blood flow. Cerebral blood flow will be maintained with fluctuations in systolic blood pressure between 200 and 50 mmHg. A fall in systolic blood pressure below 50 mmHg may be accompanied by a reduction in cerebral blood flow; however, because more oxygen is extracted, consciousness is usually not impaired. Cerebral blood flow also may decrease if systolic pressure rises above 200 mmHg or diastolic pressure rises above 110 to 120 mmHg. The range of blood pressure fluctuations beyond which cerebral blood flow is affected is narrower in individuals with arteriosclerosis of cerebral vessels.

Blood Viscosity

Cerebral blood flow is inversely proportional to blood viscosity in humans. A major factor controlling blood viscosity is the concentration of red blood cells. A reduction in blood viscosity, as occurs in anemia, will increase cerebral blood flow. On the other hand, an increase in viscosity, as occurs in polycythemia, will decrease cerebral blood flow. Venesection in polycythemic patients have been shown to increase cerebral blood flow by 30 percent concomitant with a drop in viscosity and hematocrit.

Vessel Lumen

Minor reductions in the lumina of carotid and vertebral arteries are without effect on cerebral circulation. The vessel lumen must be reduced by 70 to 90 percent before a reduction in cerebral circulation occurs.

Intrinsic Factors

Autoregulation

The single most important factor controlling cerebral circulation is the phenomenon of *autoregulation,* by which smooth muscles in small cerebral arteries and arterioles can change their tension in response to intramural pressure to maintain a constant flow despite alterations in perfusion pressure. Thus cerebral blood vessels constrict in response to an increase in intraluminal pressure and dilate in response to a reduction in intraluminal pressure. This phenomenon is particularly useful in shunting blood from healthy regions where intraluminal pressure is higher to ischemic regions where a reduction in blood flow has occurred, resulting in a reduction in intraluminal pressure. Autoregulation operates independently of but synergistically with other intrinsic factors such as biochemical changes. The mechanism of autoregulation is poorly understood. In general, three theories have been proposed; these are the neurogenic, myogenic, and metabolic theories.

KEY CONCEPTS

- Extrinsic factors that regulate cerebral circulation include systemic blood pressure, blood viscosity, and vessel lumen.

Biochemical Factors

Several biochemical factors regulate cerebral circulation.

Carbon Dioxide Arterial P_{CO_2} is a major factor in the regulation of cerebral blood flow. Hypercapnia (high P_{CO_2}) produces marked vasodilatation and an increase in cerebral blood flow. The reverse occurs in hypocapnia (low P_{CO_2}). Thus inhalation of carbon dioxide increases cerebral blood flow, whereas hyperventilation decreases cerebral blood flow. Under normal conditions, it is estimated that a change of 1 mmHg in P_{CO_2} will induce a 5 percent change in cerebral blood flow.

The control of cerebral blood flow by carbon dioxide is mediated via the cerebrospinal fluid bathing cerebral arterioles. The pH of the cerebrospinal fluid (CSF) reflects the arterial P_{CO_2} and is also influenced by the level of bicarbonate in the CSF.

The effect of carbon dioxide on cerebral blood flow is important in dampening the effects of tissue P_{CO_2} in areas of brain ischemia. The increase in cerebral blood flow in such areas helps to wash out metabolically produced carbon dioxide and thus reestablishes homeostasis of brain pH.

Oxygen Moderate changes in arterial P_{O_2} do not alter cerebral blood flow. However, more marked changes in arterial P_{O_2} alter cerebral blood flow in a manner that is the reverse of that described for P_{CO_2}. Thus low P_{O_2} (below 50 mmHg) will increase cerebral blood flow, and high P_{O_2} will decrease cerebral blood flow. Although the exact mechanism of this effect is not known, it is believed to be independent of changes in P_{CO_2}.

pH Cerebral blood flow increases with the lowering of the pH and decreases in alkalosis.

Neural Factors

Sympathetic Supply

Sympathetic innervation of conducting vessels is amply documented from the cervical sympathetic chain. In contrast, very few, if any, penetrating vessels receive adrenergic nerves. Both myelinated preganglionic and unmyelinated postganglionic nerve plexuses have been demonstrated in the periadventitial tissue. Synaptic terminals also have been traced to the outer part of the muscular media. The number of nerve plexuses and terminals decreases with reduction in the caliber of the conducting vessel. Stimulation of the sympathetic system produces vasoconstriction and a decrease in cerebral blood flow. The effect is greater in the internal carotid artery system than in the vertebral basilar system.

Parasympathetic Supply

Although parasympathetic nerve fibers have been demonstrated in cerebral vessels of the conducting variety, a physiologic role for this system in the regulation of cerebral circulation is yet to be found. The vasoactive effects of sympathetic stimulation are counteracted by a minor change in pH. Thus neural factors in the regulation

KEY CONCEPTS

- Intrinsic factors that regulate cerebral circulation include autoregulation (the most effective) and biochemical alterations in carbon dioxide, oxygen, and pH.
- Among neural factors that regulate cerebral circulation, sympathetic supply is the more important.

of cerebral blood flow are believed to be of minor importance when compared with the biochemical factors.

Neuropeptides

Nerve fibers containing neuropeptide Y, vasoactive intestinal peptide (VIP), substance P (SP), and calcitonin gene–related peptide (CGRP) have been reported in adventitia or at the adventitia-media border of human cerebral arteries. In vitro studies reveal that neuropeptide Y causes vasoconstriction, whereas VIP, SP, and CGRP cause relaxation of precontracted vessels. The effect of neuropeptides on cerebral blood vessels is not mediated via adrenergic, cholinergic, or histaminergic receptors.

MEAN AND REGIONAL CEREBRAL BLOOD FLOW

Mean cerebral blood flow is rather constant during the performance of daily physiologic activities, such as muscular exercise, changes in posture, mental activity, and sleep. It is altered, however, in some pathologic conditions such as convulsions (increased), coma (decreased), anemia (increased), and cerebral vessel sclerosis (decreased). In contrast, regional cerebral blood flow is altered during the performance of physiologic activities; thus the regional blood flow in the occipital cortex is increased with visual activity and in the motor cortex during limb movement. Studies of regional cerebral blood flow in normal individuals have contributed significantly to a better understanding of the role of different brain regions in the performance of physiologic activities, such as reading, speaking, hearing, and movement. Determinations of regional cerebral blood flow also have elucidated regional derangements of distribution of blood flow in disease states, such as cerebral stroke.

Steal Syndrome

Ischemia of brain tissue, in which cerebral blood flow is below 20 ml/100 g per min, results in accumulation of lactic acid and secondary loss of tone of the regional blood vessels. These vessels are not capable of responding normally, in view of vasomotor paralysis, to factors that alter cerebral blood flow, such as carbon dioxide and oxygen. In such patients, administration of a vasodilator drug or induction of a state of hypercapnia dilates the normal vessels and increases blood flow in the brain regions supplied by such vessels at the expense of the ischemic region (steal syndrome). These agents should be used with great caution in such patients to avoid a serious and possibly fatal reduction in cerebral blood flow in the already ischemic region.

Autoregulation and Hypertension

Cerebral blood flow is normal in patients with moderate hypertension. Such patients therefore do not have cerebral symptoms. It has been found that the autoregulatory

KEY CONCEPTS

- Whereas mean cerebral blood flow is constant during performance of daily physiologic activities, regional cerebral blood flow is altered in the appropriate cerebral region during performance of physiologic activities.

mechanism in such patients is set at a higher threshold than that in normal individuals. However, if the blood pressure is increased acutely, then autoregulatory mechanisms break down and cerebral symptoms appear.

Cerebral Blood Flow in Epilepsy

During an epileptic attack, mean cerebral blood flow increases two- to threefold. This is a response to increased metabolic demands of brain tissues during such attacks.

Cerebral Blood Flow in Coma

The mean cerebral blood flow is severely reduced in states of unconsciousness. Attempts to correlate the degree of reduction of cerebral blood flow with the chances of recovery from the comatose state have not been successful.

KEY CONCEPTS

- Autoregulatory threshold is set at a higher level in moderately hypertensive patients in order to maintain constant cerebral blood flow.
- Mean cerebral blood flow is altered under abnormal states such as epilepsy (increased) and coma (decreased).

SUGGESTED READINGS

Brown MM, et al: Fundamental importance of arterial oxygen content in the regulation of cerebral blood flow in man. *Brain* 1985; 108:81–93.

Damasio H: A computed tomographic guide to the identification of cerebral vascular territories. *Arch Neurol* 1983; 40:138–142.

Edvinsson L, et al: Peptide-containing nerve fibers in human cerebral arteries: Immunocytochemistry, radioimmunoassay, and in vitro pharmacology. *Ann Neurol* 1987; 21:431–437.

Gibo H, et al: Microsurgical anatomy of the middle cerebral artery. *J Neurosurg* 1981; 54:151–169.

Glasberg MD, et al: Increase in both cerebral glucose utilization and blood flow during execution of a somatosensory task. *Ann Neurol* 1988; 23:152–160.

Ingvar DH, Schwartz MS: Blood flow patterns induced in the dominant hemisphere by speech and reading. *Brain* 1974; 97:273–288.

Lassen NA: Control of cerebral circulation in health and disease. *Circ Res* 1974; 34:749–760.

Lister JR, et al: Microsurgical anatomy of the posterior inferior cerebellar artery. *Neurosurgery* 1982; 10: 170–199.

Kuschinsky W, Wahl M: Local chemical and neurogenic regulation of cerebral vascular resistance. *Physiol Rev* 1978; 58:656–689.

Marinkovic SV, et al: Perforating branches of the middle cerebral artery: Microanatomy and clinical significance of their intracerebral segments. *Stroke* 1985; 16:1022–1029.

Marinkovic S, et al: Anatomical bases for surgical approach to the initial segment of the anterior cerebral artery: Microanatomy of Heubner's artery and perforating branches of the anterior cerebral artery. *Surg Radiol Anat* 1986; 8:7–18.

Marinkovic S, et al: Interpeduncular perforating branches of the posterior cerebral artery: Microsurgical anatomy of their extracerebral and intracerebral segments. *Surg Neurol* 1986; 26:349–359.

Marinkovic SV, et al: Distribution of the occipital branches of the posterior cerebral artery: Correlation with occipital lobe infarcts. *Stroke* 1987; 18:728–732.

Martin RG, et al: Microsurgical relationships of the anterior inferior cerebellar artery and the facial-vestibulocochlear nerve complex. *Neurosurgery* 1980; 6:483–507.

Soh K, et al: Regional cerebral blood flow in aphasia. *Arch Neurol* 1978; 35:625–632.

Waddington MM: *Atlas of Cerebral Angiography with Anatomic Correlation.* Boston, Little, Brown, 1974.

Wade JPH: Transport of oxygen to the brain in patients with elevated hematocrit values before and after venisection. *Brain* 1983; 106:513–523.

CHAPTER 28

CEREBRAL VASCULAR SYNDROMES

Cerebrovascular disorders (strokes) constitute the most common cause of brain lesions. The most common cerebrovascular disorders are cerebral **infarcts** resulting from occlusion of cerebral vessels by thrombosis or embolism. Less common is hemorrhage, usually from rupture of a congenitally abnormal sacculation of a cerebral blood vessel (aneurysm). Strokes are characterized by a relatively abrupt onset of a focal neurologic deficit. The conglomeration of sensory, motor, and behavioral clinical signs of the neurologic deficit usually reflects the affected vessel as well as the location and size of the cerebral lesion. Despite this predictable pattern of clinical signs with specific arterial territory, there is also sufficient variation in vascular patterns to produce perplexing clinicoanatomic and clinicopathologic syndromes.

Infarct (Latin *infarcire,* "to stuff or fill in"). Regional death of tissue caused by loss of blood supply. Originally described by Virchow.

KEY CONCEPTS

- Cerebrovascular disorders include cerebral infarcts (most common) and cerebral hemorrhages.
- Cerebral infarcts result from occlusion of a cerebral vessel by a thrombus or embolus.
- The clinical picture of cerebral infarcts reflects the affected vessel, the location, and the size of the lesion.

CEREBROVASCULAR OCCLUSION SYNDROMES

Middle Cerebral Artery Syndrome (Fig. 28-1)

This is the most frequently encountered stroke syndrome. The clinical picture varies according to the site of occlusion of the vessel and to the availability of collateral circulation. The conglomerate clinical signs and symptoms of this syndrome consist of

1. Contralateral hemiplegia or hemiparesis (complete or partial paralysis) affecting primarily the face and upper extremity and, to a lesser degree, the lower extremity. Weakness is greatest in the contralateral hand because more proximal limb and trunk muscles as well as facial muscles have greater representation in both hemispheres.
2. Contralateral sensory deficit, also more prominent in the face and upper extremity than in the lower extremity. Position, vibration, deep touch, two-point discrimination, and **stereognosis** are more affected than pain and temperature because the latter two sensory modalities may be perceived at the thalamic level.
3. Contralateral visual field deficit because of damage to the optic radiation, the tract that connects the lateral geniculate nucleus with the visual cortex. Depending on where the lesion in the optic tract is located, the visual field deficit may be a **homonymous hemianopia** (half-field deficit) or a quadrantanopia (quadrant-field deficit).
4. Contralateral conjugate gaze paralysis because of the involvement of the frontal eye field (area 8 of Brodmann). The gaze paralysis is usually transient for 1 to 2 days. The reason for this transient duration is not clear.

Stereognosis (Greek *stereos,* "solid"; *gnosis,* "know"). Three-dimensional tactile feeling.

Homonymous (Greek *homo,* "same"; *onoma,* "name"). Loss of vision in the same half field in each eye.

Hemianopia (Greek *hemi,* "half"; *an,* "negative"; *opia,* "vision"). Loss of vision in one-half the visual field.

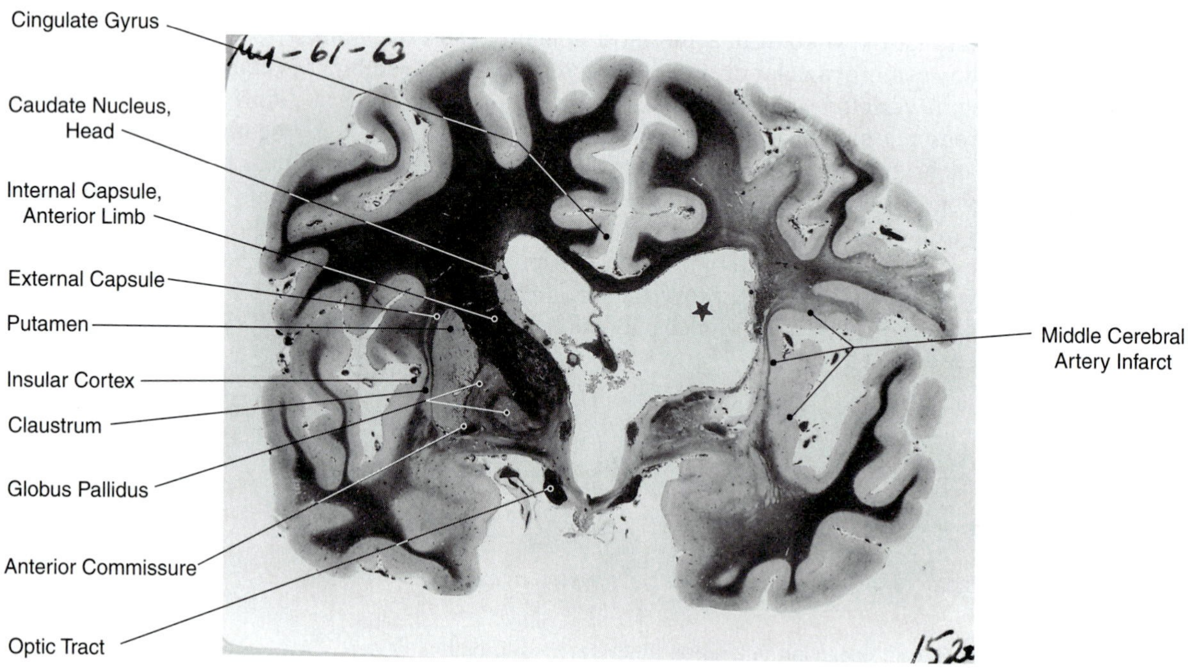
Cingulate Gyrus
Caudate Nucleus, Head
Internal Capsule, Anterior Limb
External Capsule
Putamen
Insular Cortex
Claustrum
Globus Pallidus
Anterior Commissure
Optic Tract
Middle Cerebral Artery Infarct

FIGURE 28-1

Coronal brain section showing middle cerebral artery territory infarct, and secondary enlargement of the lateral ventricle (*star*).

5. **Aphasia** (with impairment of repetition) if the dominant (left) hemisphere is involved. The aphasia may be of Broca's, Wernicke's, or global variety depending on the involved cortical region.
6. Inattention and neglect of the contralateral half of body or space and denial of illness if the nondominant (right) hemisphere is involved.
7. Spatial perception disorders if the right, nondominant hemisphere is involved. This includes such difficulties as copying simple pictures or diagrams (constructional **apraxia**), interpreting maps or finding one's way out (**topographagnosia**), and putting on clothes properly (dressing apraxia).
8. Gerstmann syndrome (finger agnosia, acalculia, right-left disorientation, and pure dysgraphia).

Language and spatial perception deficits tend to follow occlusion not of the proximal stem of the middle cerebral artery but of one of its several main branches. In such circumstances, other signs such as weakness or visual field defects may not be present. Similarly, occlusion of the rolandic branch of the middle cerebral artery produces motor and sensory deficits without disturbances of vision, language, or spatial perception. Hearing is unimpaired because of its bilateral representation.

Aphasia (Greek *a*, "negative"; *phasis*, "speech"). Impairment of language function, inability either to speak (motor aphasia) or to comprehend (sensory, receptive, aphasia).

Apraxia (Greek *a*, "negative"; *pratto*, "to do"). Inability to perform complex, purposeful movements, although muscles are not paralyzed.

Topographagnosia (Greek *topo*, "place"; *graphein*, "to write"; *gnosis*, "know"). Failure to localize a point on the body or read maps.

Lenticulostriate Artery Syndrome

Infarction in the territory of the lenticulostriate artery, a branch of the middle cerebral artery, is associated with pure motor hemiplegia because of involvement of the internal capsule.

Anterior Cerebral Artery Syndrome

The clinical manifestations of this syndrome vary according to the site of occlusion along the artery, the availability of collateral circulation, and whether there is unilateral or bilateral occlusion.

Unilateral Anterior Cerebral Artery Syndrome

Unilateral occlusion of the anterior cerebral artery is associated with the following clinical picture:

1. Contralateral hemiplegia or hemiparesis affecting primarily the lower extremity and to a lesser extent the upper extremity
2. Contralateral sensory deficit affecting primarily the lower extremity and to a lesser extent the upper extremity
3. Transcortical motor aphasia when the left (dominant) hemisphere is affected

Bilateral Anterior Cerebral Artery Syndrome (Fig. 28-2)

This syndrome occurs when both anterior cerebral arteries arise anomalously from a single trunk. In addition to the signs encountered in the unilateral syndrome, the following signs and symptoms occur in the bilateral syndrome due to involvement of orbitofrontal cortex, limbic structures, supplementary motor cortex, and cingulate gyrus:

1. Loss of initiative and spontaneity
2. Profound apathy
3. Memory and emotional disturbances
4. **Akinetic mutism** (complete unresponsiveness with open eyes only)
5. Disturbance in gait and posture
6. Grasp reflex
7. Disorder of sphincter control

Akinetic mutism (persistent vegetative state). The state in which patients appear awake and maintain a sleep-wake cycle but are unable to communicate in any way. The term was introduced by H. Cairns in 1941.

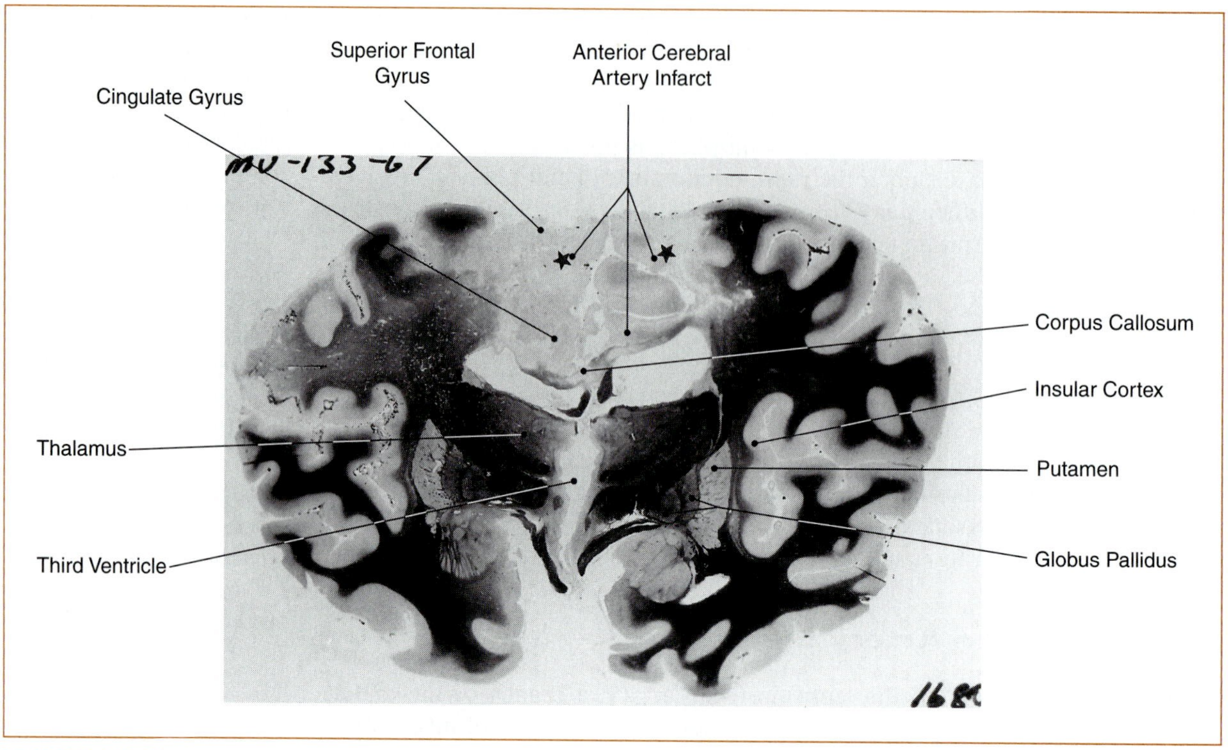

FIGURE 28-2

Coronal brain section showing bilateral anterior cerebral artery territory infarct (*star*).

The explanation for the occurrence of sphincter control disorder is not certain. It has been variably attributed to involvement of the motor and sensory cortices on the medial surface of the hemisphere (paracentral lobule) or to involvement of more anterior regions of the frontal lobe concerned with inhibition of bladder emptying.

Involvement of the anterior part of the corpus callosum may cause apraxia and tactile anomia of the left arm attributed to disconnection of the left (dominant) hemisphere language area from the right motor and sensory cortices.

Recurrent Artery of Heubner Syndrome

Infarction in the territory supplied by the recurrent artery of Heubner (medial striate artery), which is a branch of the anterior cerebral artery, results in the following signs:

1. Contralateral face and arm weakness without sensory loss
2. Behavioral and cognitive abnormalities, including abulia, agitation, neglect, and aphasia

The clinical signs reflect involvement of the anterior limb of the internal capsule, rostral basal ganglia (caudate nucleus and putamen), and the basal frontal lobe.

Internal Carotid Artery Syndrome

Amaurosis fugax (Greek *amaurosis,* "darkening"). Transient episode of monocular blindness. Used by Hippocrates for "a becoming dull of sight."

Occlusion of the internal carotid artery in the neck may be asymptomatic in the presence of adequate collateral circulation and slow occlusion or may result in the following clinical picture:

1. Transient monocular blindness (**amaurosis fugax**) due to involvement of the ophthalmic artery, the first intracranial branch of the internal carotid artery

2. Contralateral motor and sensory deficits equally severe in the face, upper extremity, and lower extremity
3. Contralateral visual field deficit (homonymous hemianopia)
4. Aphasia if the dominant hemisphere is involved
5. Perceptual deficits if the nondominant (right) hemisphere is involved

The internal carotid artery syndrome is thus a combination of the middle and anterior cerebral artery syndromes to which is added transient monocular blindness.

Anterior Choroidal Artery Syndrome (Fig. 28-3)

Occlusion of the anterior choroidal artery, a branch of the internal carotid artery, may be asymptomatic or may result in one or more of the following:

1. Contralateral motor deficit (hemiplegia) involving the face, arm, and leg due to involvement of the posterior part of the posterior limb of the internal capsule and the cerebral peduncle. This is the most consistent and persistent deficit.
2. Contralateral hemisensory deficit, usually transient, involving, in most cases, all sensory modalities (hemianesthesia) due to involvement of the sensory tracts within the posterior limb of the internal capsule.
3. Contralateral visual field defect (hemianopia or quadrantanopia) due to involvement of the retrolenticular part of the internal capsule (visual radiation) or the lateral geniculate nucleus. This is the most variable feature of the syndrome.

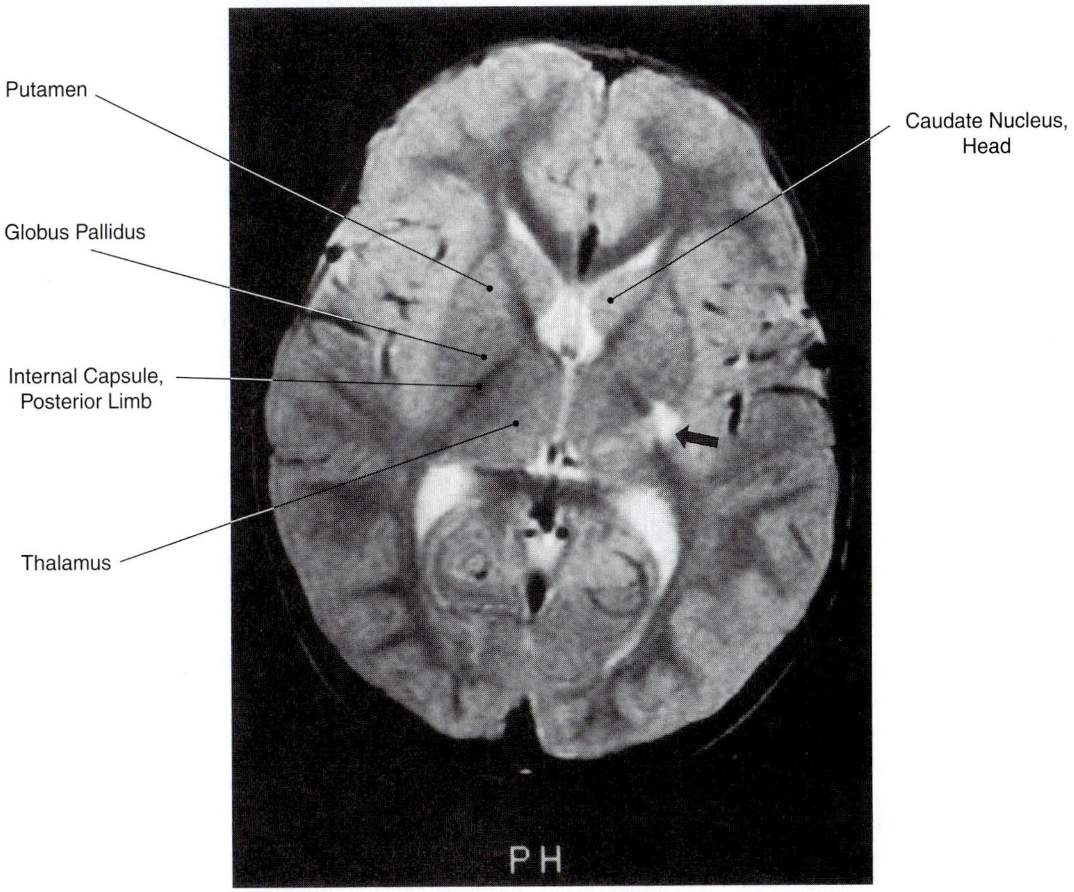

FIGURE 28-3

T2-weighted magnetic resonance image (MRI) showing bright signal intensity infarct (*arrow*) in the anterior choroidal artery territory.

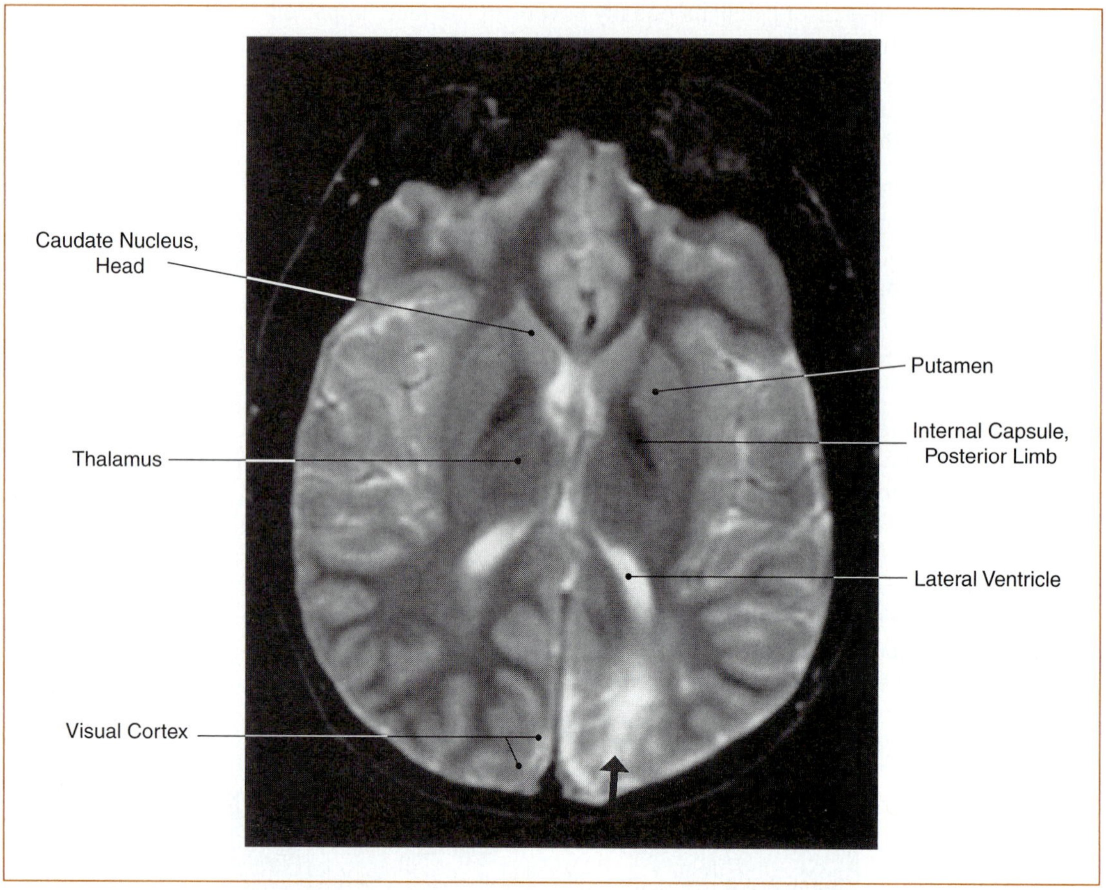
Caudate Nucleus,
Head
Thalamus
Visual Cortex
Putamen
Internal Capsule,
Posterior Limb
Lateral Ventricle

FIGURE 28-4

T2-weighted MRI showing bright signal intensity infarct (*arrow*) in the posterior cerebral artery territory.

Posterior Cerebral Artery Syndrome (Fig. 28-4)

The clinical picture of posterior cerebral artery occlusion is variable depending on whether it is unilateral or bilateral, the site of occlusion, and the availability of collateral circulation.

Unilateral Posterior Cerebral Artery Syndrome

Unilateral occlusion of the posterior cerebral artery is associated with the following:

1. Contralateral visual field deficit (hemianopia) due to involvement of the calcarine cortex. Macular (central) vision is usually spared because of macular representation in the occipital pole, which receives additional blood supply from the middle cerebral artery.
2. Visual and color agnosia, the inability to name a color or point to a color named by the examiner because of involvement of the inferiomesial aspect of the occipitotemporal lobe in the dominant hemisphere.
3. Contralateral sensory loss of all modalities with concomitant pain (thalamic syndrome) due to involvement of the ventral posterolateral and ventral posteromedial nuclei of the thalamus, which are supplied by deep penetrating branches of the posterior cerebral artery.
4. Pure **alexia** (alexia without **agraphia**) with a left-sided lesion affecting the posterior corpus callosum and the left visual cortex.

As a rule, the posterior cerebral artery syndrome is not associated with motor deficit. The hemiplegia reported occasionally in these patients is attributed to involvement of the midbrain by the infarct.

Alexia (Greek *a,* "negative"; *lexis,* "word"). Loss of the power to grasp the meaning of written or printed words.

Agraphia (Greek *a,* "negative"; *graphein,* "to write"). Inability to express thoughts in writing. The first modern descriptions were those of Jean Pitres in 1884 and Dejerine in 1891.

Bilateral Posterior Cerebral Artery Syndrome

This syndrome results from occlusion at the point of origin of both posterior cerebral arteries from the basilar artery. The syndrome is characterized by the following:

1. Cortical blindness, visual loss in both eyes in the presence of normal pupillary reactivity and normal fundus examination
2. Disturbance in facial recognition (**prosopagnosia**) due to bilateral involvement of the inferior occipitotemporal region (lingual and fusiform gyri)
3. Balint syndrome (**optic ataxia,** psychic paralysis of fixation), the inability to look to the peripheral field with disturbance of visual attention
4. **Anton's syndrome,** denial of blindness and confabulation of what the patient sees if the lesion extends to both parietal lobes
5. Agitated delirium and memory loss due to bilateral involvement of mesiotemporal territory

Syndromes of Penetrating Branches of Posterior Cerebral Artery

The clinical pictures associated with occlusion of penetrating branches of the posterior cerebral artery (thalamogeniculate and thalamoperforating) have been discussed in Chap. 12.

Prosopagnosia (Greek *prosopon,* "face"; *gnosia,* "to know"). Inability to recognize familiar faces.

Optic ataxia (Balint syndrome). Severe impairment of visually guided movements, such as when trying to reach for an object. Originally described by Rudolph Balint, a Hungarian neurologist, in 1909.

Anton's syndrome. Denial of blindness. Described by Gabriel Anton, an Austrian neurologist, in 1899. Although unable to see, patients with this syndrome deny their blindness and tend to confabulate about things seen.

Vertebral-Basilar Arteries Syndromes

Occlusion of the vertebral-basilar arterial system usually results in brain stem infarcts. The clinical picture varies according to the specific branch affected and the brain stem territory involved (e.g., lateral medullary syndrome, medial medullary syndrome, Benedikt syndrome, Weber's syndrome, etc.). Common to all vertebral-basilar artery syndromes are the following:

1. Bilateral long tract (motor and sensory) signs
2. Crossed motor and sensory signs (e.g., facial weakness or numbness combined with contralateral extremity weakness or numbness)
3. Cerebellar signs
4. Cranial nerve signs
5. Alteration in state of consciousness (stupor or coma)
6. Disconjugate eye movements

In general, the presence of "the four *D*s with crossed findings" suggests a brain stem stroke from vertebrobasilar occlusion. The four *D*s are diplopia, dysarthria, dysphagia, and dizziness.

Table 28-1 is a simplified comparison of the major signs and symptoms in internal carotid system and vertebrobasilar system occlusions.

Lacunar Syndromes

Lacunar syndromes result from occlusion of small penetrating end arteries (variably called *lenticulostriate, thalamogeniculate,* or *thalamoperforator*) from the proximal anterior cerebral, middle cerebral, posterior cerebral, and basilar arteries or the circle of Willis. They occur usually in patients with long-standing hypertension

KEY CONCEPTS

- Fairly consistent, though not absolute, anatomicoclinical correlations occur for each of the following vascular occlusion syndromes: middle cerebral artery, lenticulostriate artery, anterior cerebral artery, recurrent artery of Heubner, internal carotid artery, anterior choroidal artery, posterior cerebral artery, and vertebral-basilar arteries.

TABLE 28-1

Major Signs and Symptoms in Internal Carotid System and Vertebrobasilar System Occlusions

Symptom or Sign	Internal Carotid	Vertebrobasilar
Motor deficit	Contralateral	Bilateral, crossed
Sensory deficit	Contralateral	Bilateral, crossed
Visual deficit	Monocular blindness contralateral field defect	Bilateral, cortical blindness
Speech deficit (aphasia)	Present	Absent
Cranial nerve deficit	Absent	Present

and cerebral vessel atherosclerosis. Symptomatic lacunes most often involve the following brain regions: putamen, caudate nucleus, posterior limb of the internal capsule, thalamus, and basis pontis. Several discrete lacunar syndromes exist. The five well-recognized lacunar syndromes are

1. *Pure motor (hemiparesis) syndrome,* involving the contralateral face, arm, trunk, and leg due to a lacune (small infarct) in the corticospinal tract within the internal capsule or basis pontis. There are no sensory, speech, or visual deficits.
2. *Pure sensory syndrome,* involving the contralateral face, arm, trunk, and leg with loss or diminution of all sensory modalities (hemianesthesia) due to a lacuna in the sensory thalamic nuclei (ventral posterior lateral, ventral posterior medial). There are no motor, speech, or visual deficits.
3. *Ataxic hemiparesis syndrome,* characterized by weakness, pyramidal signs, and cerebellarlike ataxia involving the limbs on the same side due to a lacune in one of the following sites: (*a*) contralateral posterior limb of the internal capsule, (*b*) basis pontis, and (*c*) red nucleus with extension of the lesion to the adjcent cerebral peduncle. The internal capsule lesion involves the corticospinal (hemiparesis) and corticopontine fibers (cerebellarlike ataxia). The basis pontis lesion involves corticospinal (hemiplegia) and pontocerebellar (ataxia) fibers. The red nucleus lesion interrupts the cerebellothalamic fibers in the brachium conjunctivum (ataxia), and its extension into the cerebral peduncle explains the hemiparesis.
4. *Dysarthria–clumsy hand syndrome,* characterized by central (supranuclear) facial weakness, dysarthria, dysphagia, and hand paresis and clumsiness due to a lacuna in the basis pontis.
6. *État lacunaire syndrome.* This syndrome is associated with bilateral numerous lacunae in the frontal lobes. It is characterized by progressive dementia, shuffling gait, emotional lability (abrupt laughing and crying), and pseudobulbar palsy (hyperactive palate and gag reflex, lingual and pharyngeal paralysis, and difficulty swallowing).

KEY CONCEPTS

- Lacunar syndromes result from occlusion of small penetrating end arteries. Five well-defined lacunar syndromes occur: pure motor, pure sensory, ataxic hemiparesis, dysarthria–clumsy hand, and état lacunaire.

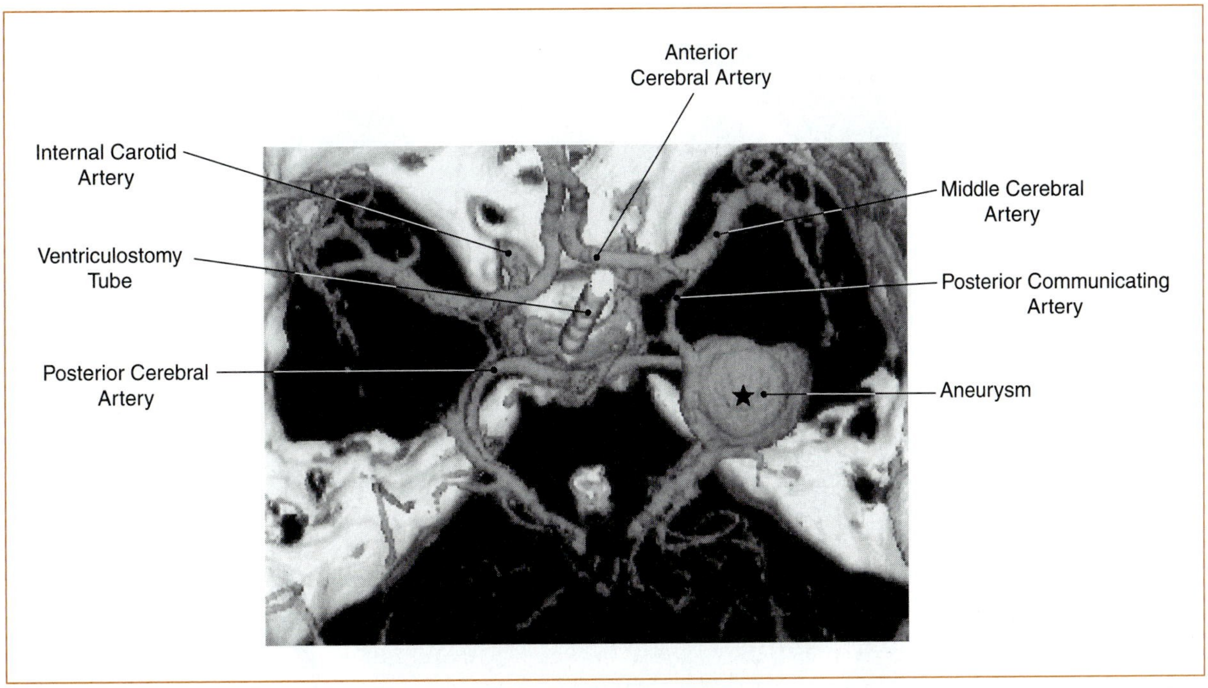
Anterior Cerebral Artery
Internal Carotid Artery
Ventriculostomy Tube
Posterior Cerebral Artery
Middle Cerebral Artery
Posterior Communicating Artery
Aneurysm

FIGURE 28-5

3-D computed tomography (CT) image showing an aneurysm (*star*).

CEREBRAL HEMORRHAGE SYNDROMES

Intracranial hemorrhage may result from (1) spontaneous rupture of an arterial wall because of long-standing hypertension, (2) rupture of a congenital saccular outpouching of a vessel wall (**aneurysm**) (Fig. 28-5), (3) rupture of an arteriovenous malformation (Fig. 28-6), (4) trauma to the head, or (5) a bleeding disorder. Hemor-

Aneurysm (Greek *aneurysma,* "a widening"). A widening, dilatation, or ballooning out of an artery due to weakness in its walls. The condition was known to Galen.

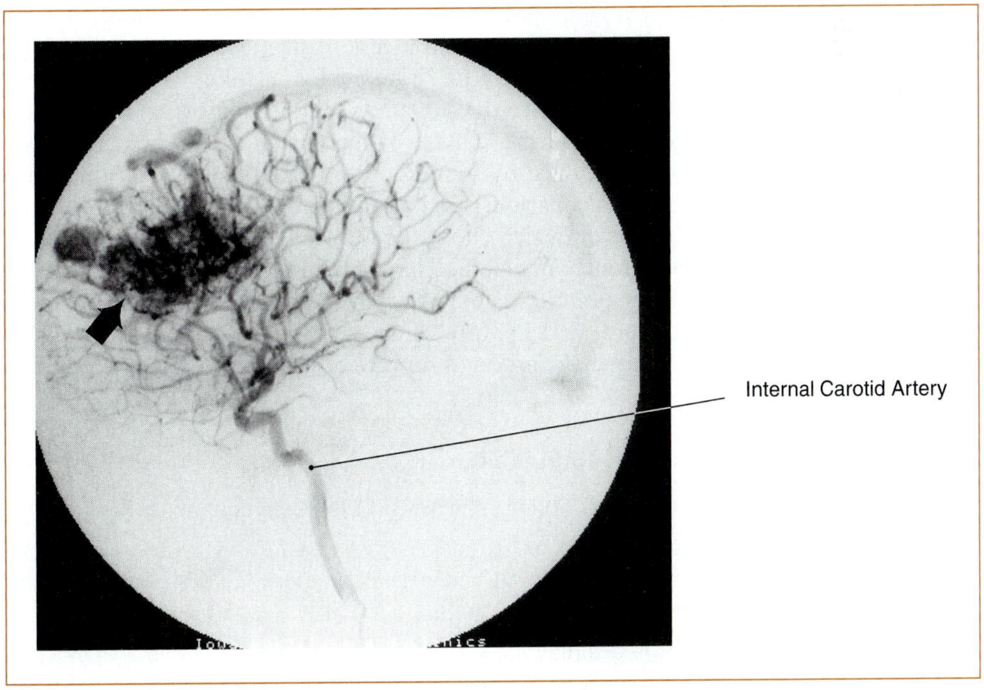
Internal Carotid Artery

FIGURE 28-6

Arteriogram showing an arteriovenous malformation (*arrow*).

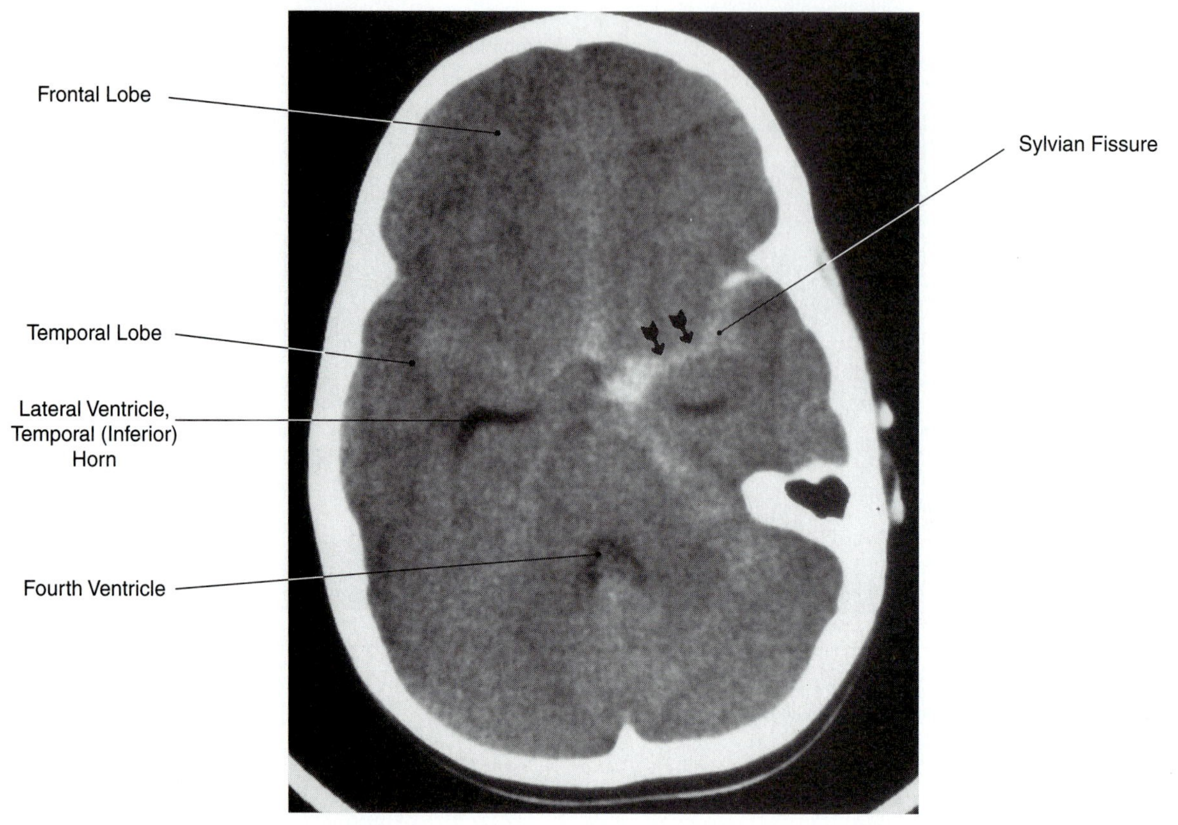
Frontal Lobe
Sylvian Fissure
Temporal Lobe
Lateral Ventricle, Temporal (Inferior) Horn
Fourth Ventricle

FIGURE 28-7

Computed Axial CT image showing blood (*arrows*) in the sylvian fissure.

rhage may occur (1) within the brain parenchyma, (2) into the ventricular system, or (3) into meningeal spaces (subarachnoid, subdural, epidural). The ensuing clinical picture varies depending on the location, size, cause, and rate of development of the hemorrhage. About 15 to 20 percent of strokes are due to hemorrhage, and roughly half of these are due to subarachnoid hemorrhage. Subarachnoid hemorrhage usually results from leakage or rupture of a congenital aneurysm. The clinical picture is characterized by sudden onset and includes severe headache, neck stiffness, and loss of consciousness. The diagnosis is established by computed tomographic (CT) scan, which shows dense areas of blood in the subarachnoid space (Fig. 28-7). Parenchymal hemorrhage is usually due to rupture of an arterial wall in hypertensive patients. In some cases, the hemorrhage may burst into the ventricular system. Subdural and epidural hemorrhages usually are associated with trauma. Subdural hemorrhage is due to rupture of bridging veins in the subdural space (Fig.

KEY CONCEPTS

- Cerebral hemorrhage constitutes 15 to 20 percent of strokes.
- Intracranial hemorrhage results from rupture of an arterial wall because of long-standing hypertension, congenital aneurysm, arteriovenous malformation, or trauma or a bleeding disorder.
- Hemorrhages may occur in one or more of the following spaces: cerebral parenchyma, ventricles, subarachnoid space, subdural space, and/or epidural space.

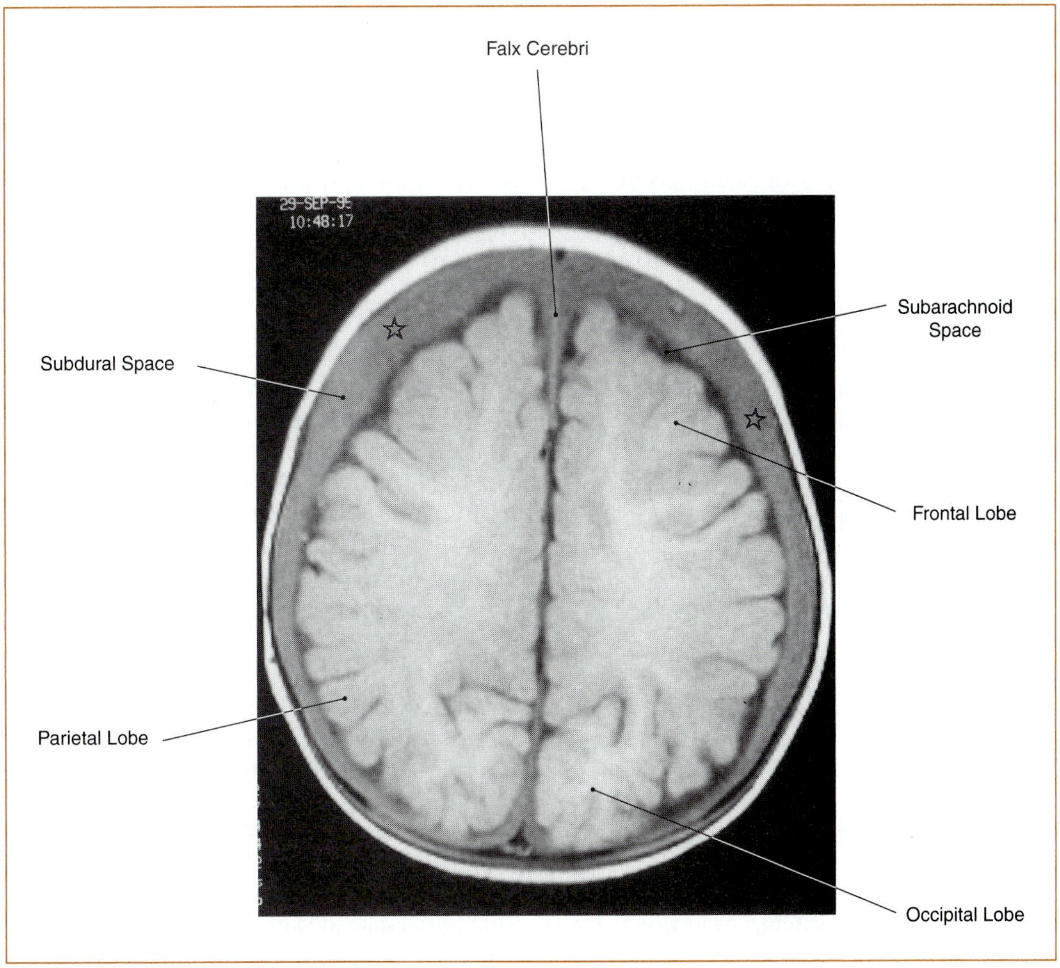
Falx Cerebri
29-SEP-95
10:48:17
Subarachnoid Space
Subdural Space
Frontal Lobe
Parietal Lobe
Occipital Lobe

FIGURE 28-8

MRI showing blood in the subdural space, subdural hematoma (*star*).

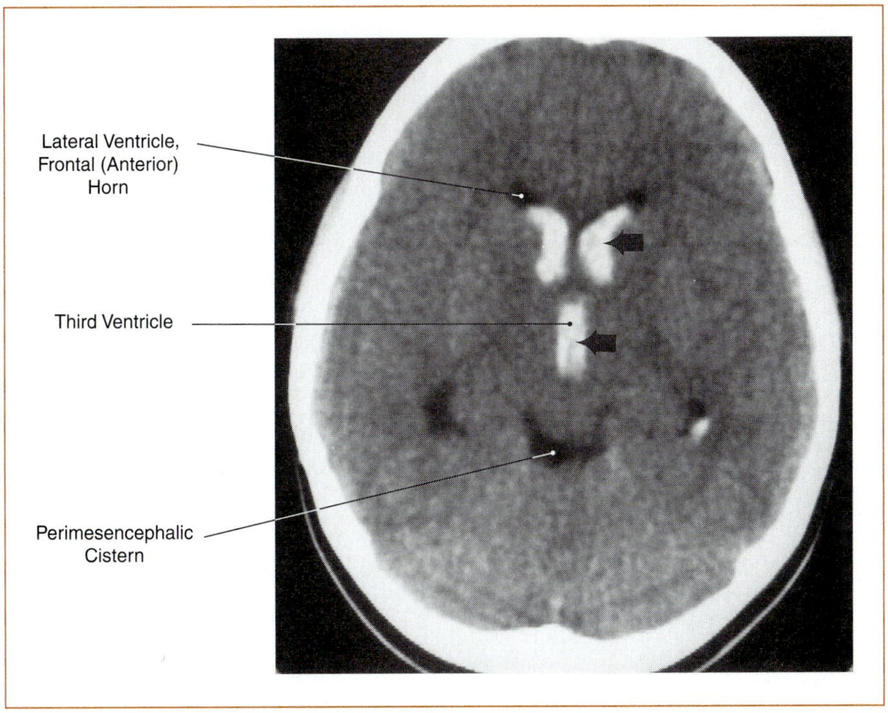
Lateral Ventricle, Frontal (Anterior) Horn
Third Ventricle
Perimesencephalic Cistern

FIGURE 28-9

CT image showing blood in the ventricular system (*arrow*).

28-8). Epidural hemorrhage, a life-threatening situation, is due to rupture of the middle meningeal artery in the epidural space. Bleeding from arteriovenous malformations may occur into the cerebral parenchyma, into the subarachnoid or subdural spaces, or into the ventricles (Fig. 28-9).

SUGGESTED READINGS

Archer C, Horenstein S: Basilar artery occlusion: Clinical and radiological correlation. *Stroke* 1977; 8:383–390.

Ausman JI, et al: Vertebrobasilar insufficiency: A review. *Arch Neurol* 1985; 42:803–808.

Biller J: Vascular syndromes of the cerebrum. In Brazis PW, et al (eds): *Localization of Clinical Neurology.* Boston, Little, Brown, 1985:362.

Caplan LR: Intracranial branch atheromatous disease: A neglected, understudied, and underused concept. *Neurology* 1989; 39:1246–1250.

Fisher CM: Lacunar strokes and infarcts: A review. *Neurology* 1982; 32:871–876.

Fisher CM: The posterior cerebral artery syndrome. *Can J Neurol Sci* 1986; 13:232–239.

Ghika J, et al: Infarcts in the territory of the deep perforators from the carotid system. *Neurology* 1989; 39:507–512.

Glass JD, et al: The dysarthria–clumsy hand syndrome: A distinct clinical entity related to pontine infarction. *Ann Neurol* 1990; 27:487–494.

Goodwin JA, et al: Symptoms of amaurosis fugax in atherosclerotic carotid artery disease. *Neurology* 1987; 37:829–832.

Helgason C, et al: Anterior choroidal artery-territory infarction: Report of cases and review. *Arch Neurol* 1986; 43:681–686.

Helweg-Larsen S, et al: Ataxic hemiparesis: Three different locations of lesions studied by MRI. *Neurology* 1988; 38:1322–1324.

Hommel M, et al: Hemiplegia in posterior cerebral artery occlusion. *Neurology* 1990; 40:1496–1499.

Hupperts RMM, et al: Infarcts in the anterior choroidal artery territory: Anatomical distribution, clinical syndromes, presumed pathogenesis, and early outcome. *Brain* 1994; 117:825–834.

Melo TP, et al: Pure motor stroke: A reappraisal. *Neurology* 1992; 42:789–798.

Nighoghossian N, et al: Pontine versus capsular pure motor hemiparesis. *Neurology* 1993; 43:2197–2201.

Wolfe N, et al: Frontal systems impairment following multiple lacunar infarcts. *Arch Neurol* 1990; 47:129–132.

CHAPTER 29

CEREBROSPINAL FLUID AND THE BARRIER SYSTEM

ANATOMY OF THE VENTRICULAR SYSTEM

The brain contains four ependyma-lined cavities known as *cerebral ventricles;* these are the right and left lateral ventricles, the third ventricle, and the fourth ventricle (Fig. 29-1). The four cavities communicate with each other and with the subarachnoid space: the lateral and third ventricles through the **foramen of Monro,** named after Alexander Monro, who described it in 1783 (Figs. 29-1 and 29-2), the third and fourth ventricles through the **aqueduct of Sylvius** (cerebral aqueduct or iter) (Fig. 29-2), and the fourth ventricle and the subarachnoid space through the **foramina of Magendie and Luschka.** The term *fifth ventricle* is sometimes used to refer

Foramen of Monro. Site of communication between the lateral and third ventricles. First described by Alexander Monro, the Scottish anatomist, in 1753. Before that time, it was assumed that the lateral and third ventricles communicated by a hole or passage at the upper end of the third ventricle called the *vulva* or by a place under the fornix called the *anus*.

KEY CONCEPTS

- The ventricular system is comprised of four interconnected spaces: two lateral ventricles, a third ventricle, and a fourth ventricle. The foramen of Monro connects the lateral and third ventricles. The aqueduct of Sylvius connects the third and fourth ventricles.
- The ventricular cavities communicate with the subarachnoid spaces around the brain and spinal cord via the foramen of Magendie and the two foramina of Luschka.

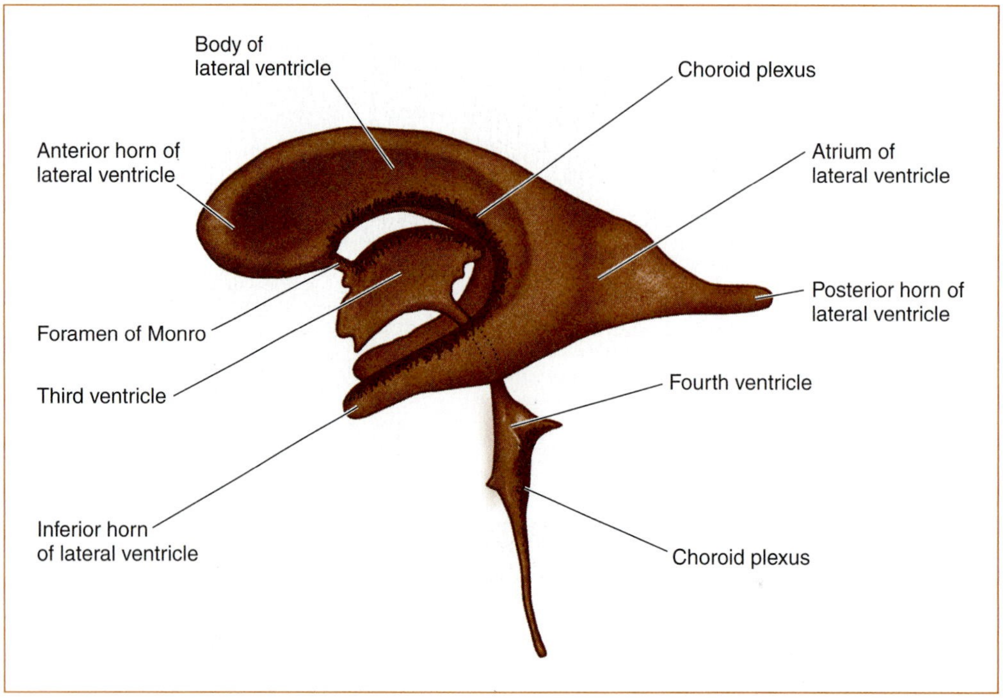

FIGURE 29-1

Schematic diagram in composite sagittal view showing the ventricular cavities of the brain with intraventricular sites of choroid plexus.

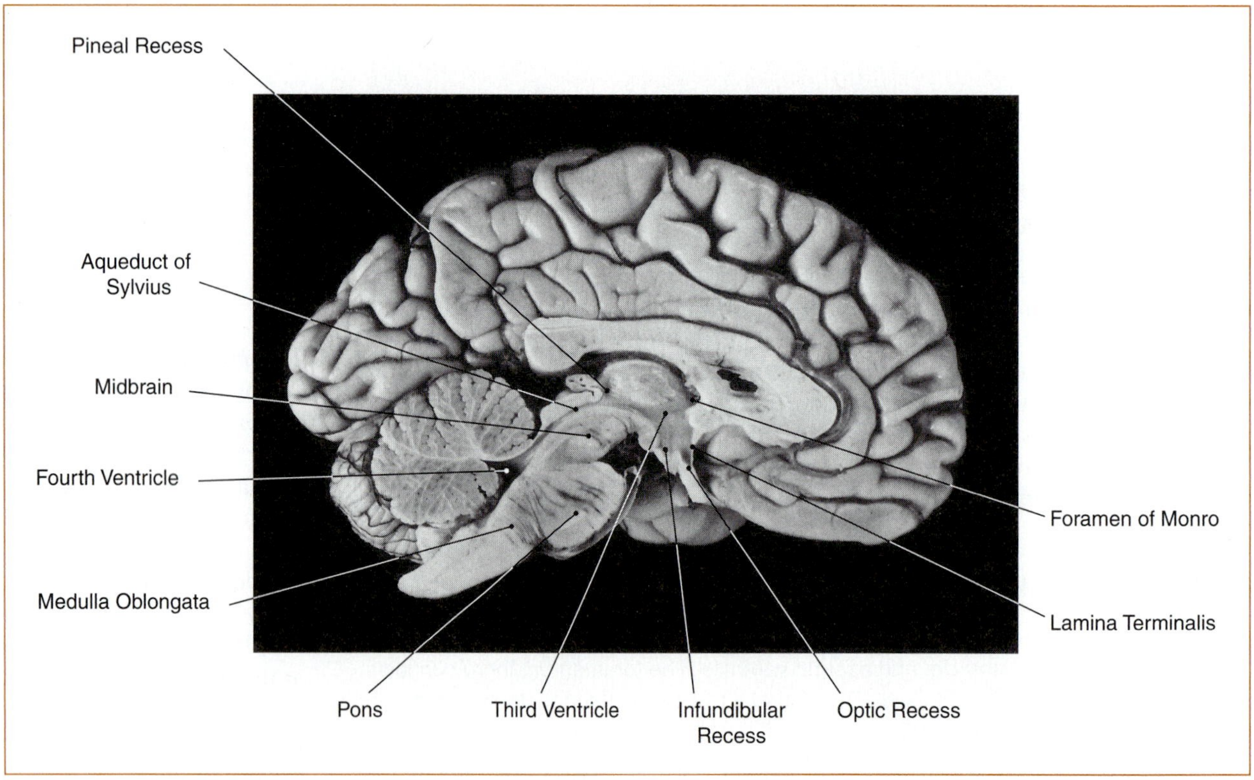

FIGURE 29-2

Midsagittal view of the brain showing the foramen of Monro, third ventricle, aqueduct of Sylvius, and fourth ventricle.

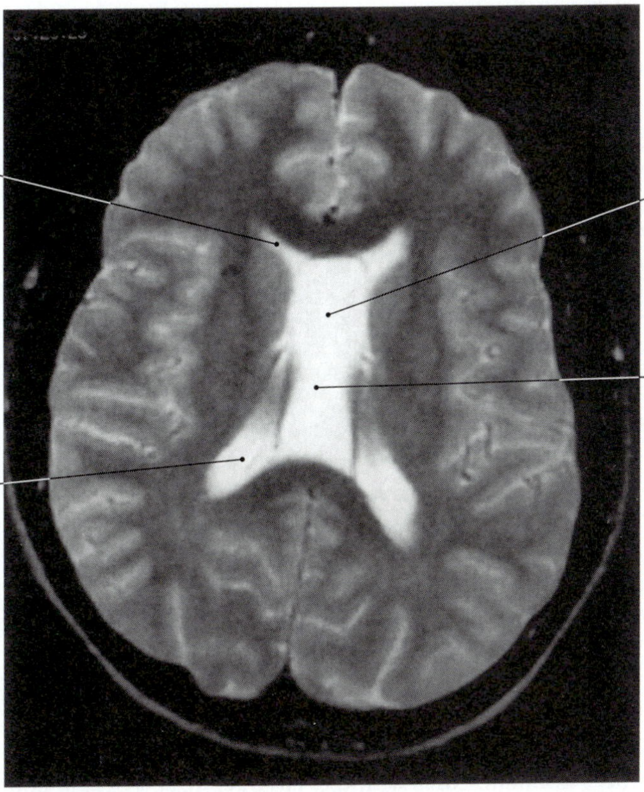

FIGURE 29-3

T2-weighted axial magnetic resonance image (MRI) showing cavum septum pellucidum and cavum vergae.

to the cavity (Figs. 29-3 and 29-4) that develops within the septum pellucidum (the cavum septum pellucidum). This, however, is a misnomer because the cavity is lined with astrocytes and does not have the ependymal lining characteristic of ventricular cavities, nor does it contain cerebrospinal fluid.

Cavum septum pellucidum is found in all premature newborns. It begins to close just before birth in full-term newborns and is frequently seen in brain images [computed tomographic (CT) scans and magnetic resonance imaging (MRI)] in neonates. Its incidence at 6 months of age and beyond falls to about 6 percent.

Posterior extension of the cavum septum pellucidum (Figs. 29-3 and 29-4) above the fornix and posterior to the foramen of Monro constitutes the **cavum vergae** (sixth ventricle), named after the Italian anatomist Andrea Verga, who described the cavum in 1851. It communicates with the cavum septi pelludici.

The cavum veli interpositi (interventricular cavum) is a triangular cavity located rostral to the superior (quadrigeminal) cistern below the fornix and above the thalamus and the roof of the third ventricle (Fig. 29-4). The cavity develops as a result of abnormal separation of the limbs of the fornix. The cavity tends to be

KEY CONCEPTS

- The cavum septum pellucidum and cavum vergae are intraventrical cavities within the septum pellucidum.
- The cavum velum interpositum communicates with the subarachnoid space.

Aqueduct of Sylvius. Narrow passage linking the third and fourth ventricles. Named after Franciscus de la Boe Sylvius, who described it in 1650.

Foramen of Magendie. Median aperture in the roof of the fourth ventricle connecting it with the cisterna magna. Named after François Magendie, the French physiologist, who described the foramen in 1842.

Foramen of Luschka. Paired openings in the lateral recesses of the fourth ventricle through which CSF from the fourth ventricle reaches the cisterna magna. Named after Hubert von Luschka, the German anatomist, in 1863.

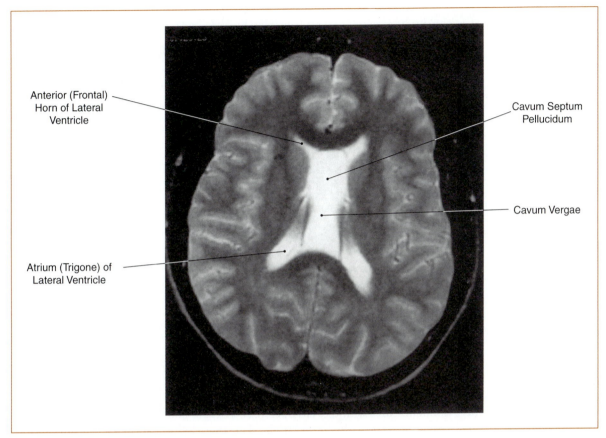

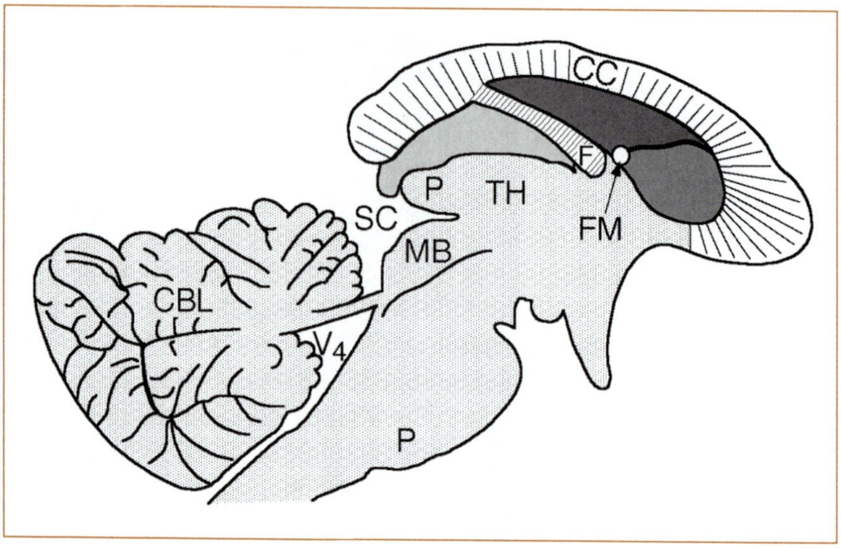

FIGURE 29-4

Schematic composite diagram showing the location and relationship, in midsagittal view, of the cavum septum pellucidum (medium gray), cavum vergae (dark gray), and cavum velum interpositum (light gray). CC, corpus callosum; TH, thalamus; FM, foramen of Monro; P, pineal gland; SC, superior cistern; MB, midbrain; P, pons; V_4, fourth ventricle; CBL, cerebellum.

Cavum vergae. Intraventricular cystic space in the body of the lateral ventricle and continuous with the cavum septum pellucidum. Named after Andrea Verga, the Italian anatomist who described it in 1851.

large in infants and becomes small beyond 2 years of age. The cavum veli interpositi communicates with the subarachnoid space, in contrast to the cavum vergae, which communicates with the ventricle. The two cavities also can be differentiated by their relationship to the fornix. The cavum vergae is located above the fornix, whereas the cavum interpositi is beneath the fornix. A composite schema of the cava septum pellucidum, vergae, and interpositum is shown in Fig. 29-4.

The lateral ventricles have an archlike configuration corresponding to the shape of the hemisphere. Each lateral ventricle is subdivided into five segments (Fig. 29-1):

1. Frontal (anterior) horn
2. Body
3. Atrium (trigone)
4. Occipital (posterior) horn
5. Temporal (inferior) horn

The frontal (anterior) horn is the part of the lateral ventricle rostral to the foramen of Monro (Figs. 29-1 and 29-2). In sections, this part of the ventricle has a butterfly configuration, with the corpus callosum forming its roof, the septum pellucidum and fornix constituting its medial wall, and the caudate nucleus bulging into the lateral wall. This characteristic bulge of the caudate nucleus into the lateral wall disappears in degenerative diseases of the brain involving the caudate nucleus such as in Huntington's chorea.

The body of the lateral ventricle (Fig. 29-1) extends from the foramen of Monro posteriorly to the trigone. The atrium or trigone (Fig. 29-1) is the area of confluence of the posterior part of the body with the occipital and temporal horns. The atrium is the most expanded subdivision of the ventricle and the site of early ventricular enlargement in degenerative diseases of the brain.

KEY CONCEPTS

- Each lateral ventricle is composed of an anterior (frontal) horn, body, atrium (trigone), posterior (occipital) horn, and inferior (temporal) horn.

The occipital (posterior) horn (Fig. 29-1) extends from the atrium backward toward the occipital pole. It is the most variable subdivision in shape and size, with the left usually larger than the right, and may be rudimentary or altogether absent. The calcarine fissure produces an impression in the medial wall of the occipital horn known as the *calcar avis.*

The temporal (inferior) horn (Fig. 29-1) extends from the atrium downward and forward into the temporal lobe and ends approximately 3 cm behind the temporal tip.

The lateral ventricles communicate with the third ventricle through the interventricular foramen of Monro (Fig. 29-1). The cavity of the third ventricle is enclosed between the two thalami and hypothalami. It is bounded anteriorly by the lamina terminalis (Fig. 29-2) and the anterior commissure, superiorly by ependyma fused with the overlying leptomeninges of the embryonic diencephalon (velum interpositum or tela choroidea) incorporating numerous blood vessels, posteriorly by the epithelamus, and inferiorly by hypothalamic structures (infundibular recess, tuber cinereum, and mamillary body).

The third ventricle has a number of recesses that are important in localizing lesions in the region of the third ventricle. These recesses include the pineal recess above the posterior commissure, the optic recess above the optic chiasma, and the infundibular recess into the infundibulum (Figs. 29-2 and 29-5).

The aqueduct of Sylvius (cerebral aqueduct or iter) is a narrow canal that connects the third and fourth ventricles through the midbrain (Fig. 29-2). It is about 1.5 to 2.0 cm long and 1 to 2 mm in diameter. Stenosis (narrowing) or complete obstruction of the aqueduct, which may occur congenitally or as a consequence of inflammatory processes, results in accumulation of cerebrospinal fluid, an increase in cerebrospinal pressure, and ventricular dilatation rostral to the site of obstruction.

The fourth ventricle lies between the anterior surface of the cerebellum and the posterior (dorsal) surfaces of the pons and medulla oblongata (Figs. 29-1 and 29-2). The fourth ventricle boundaries are discussed in the chapter on the medulla oblongata (Chap. 5). The fourth ventricle communicates with the subarachnoid space through three foramina in its roof. These are a midline foramen of Magendie and two lateral foramina of Luschka, which drain the lateral recesses of the fourth ventricle.

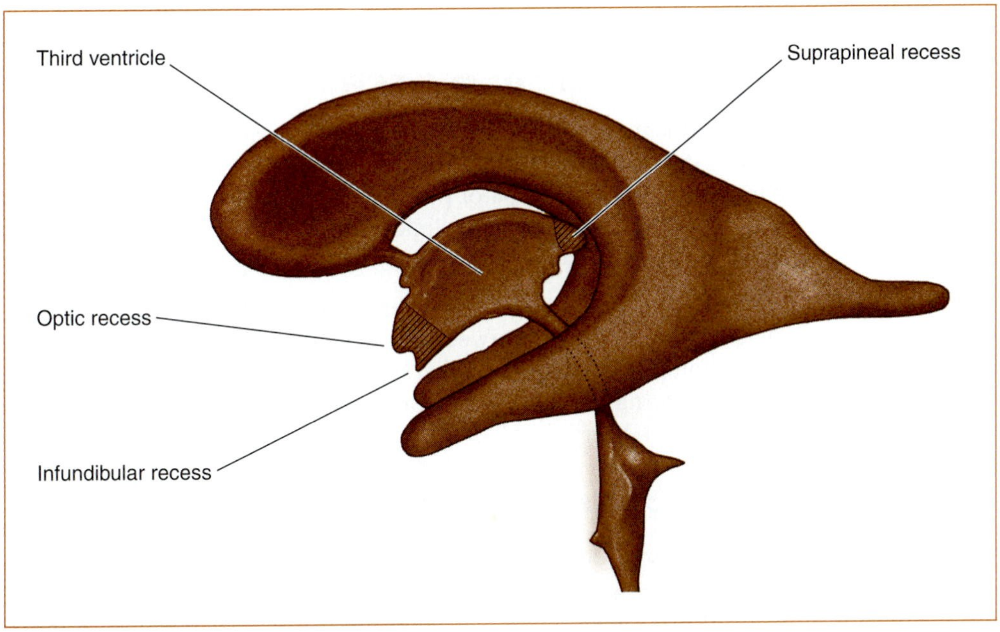

FIGURE 29-5

Schematic diagram of the ventricular system showing recesses of the third ventricle.

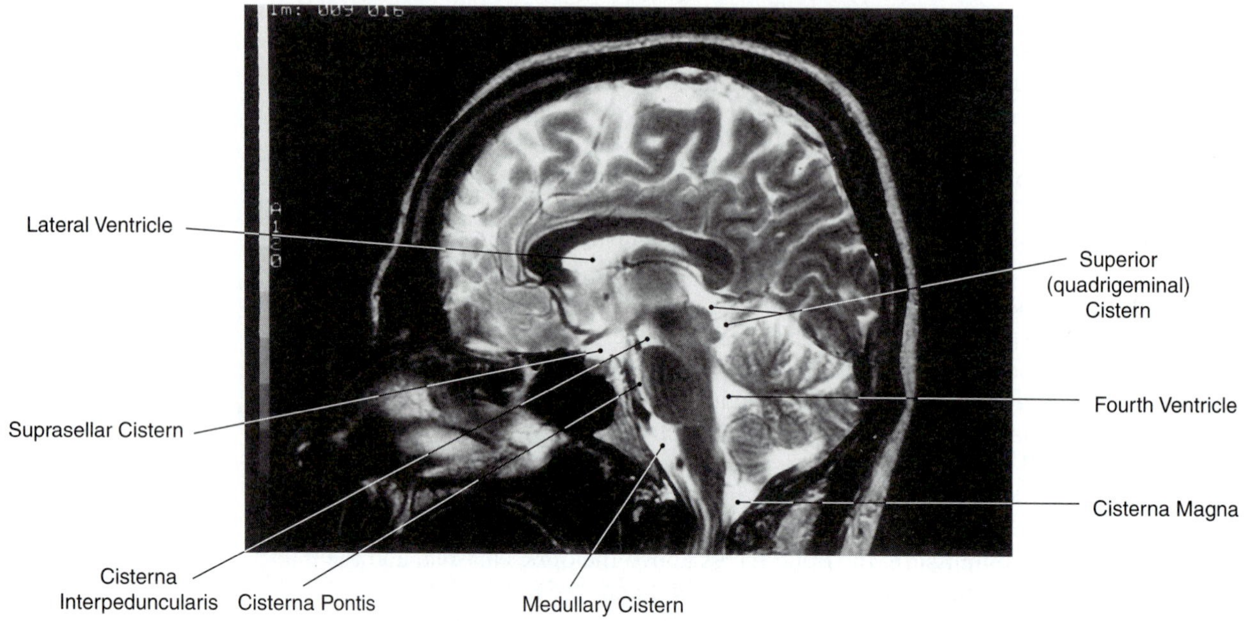

FIGURE 29-6

T2-weighted midsagittal magnetic resonance image (MRI) showing the major subarachnoid cisterns.

Ventricular cavities are lined by ependymal epithelium. In some specific sites, the ependymal lining is invaginated by a vascular pial fold known as the *choroid plexus.* Such choroid plexus sites are encountered in the body, atrium, inferior horn of the lateral ventricle, foramen of Monro, roof of the third ventricle, and posterior part of the roof of the fourth ventricle (Fig. 29-1). The choroid plexus achieves its largest size in the anterior part of the atrium (trigone), an area referred to as the *glomus*. The absence of choroid plexus from the anterior horn makes it an appropriate site for placement of shunt tubes for drainage of cerebrospinal fluid in hydrocephalus.

SUBARACHNOID CISTERNS

The subarachnoid cisterns are dilatations in the subarachnoid spaces located principally at the base of the brain. Radiologic visualization of the subarachnoid cisterns is important in localization of pathologic processes, especially those due to tumors in the base of the brain. The clinically relevant subarachnoid cisterns include the following (Fig. 29-6):

1. The cisterna magna (cisterna cerebellomedullaris), largest of the subarachnoid cisterns, is located between the medulla oblongata, the cerebellum, and the occipital bone (Fig. 29-6). Cerebrospinal fluid from the fourth ventricle reaches the cisterna magna via the foramina of Magendie and Luschka. The cisterna

KEY CONCEPTS

- Ventricular cavities are lined by ependyma and contain cerebrospinal fluid.
- Certain sites within the ventricular system contain choroid plexus. These include the body, trigone, and inferior horns of the lateral ventricle, the foramen of Monro, the roof of the third ventricle, and the posterior part of the roof of the fourth ventricle.

magna is continuous anteriorly with the cisterna pontis. The cisterna magna is occasionally accessed to obtain cerebrospinal fluid (**cisternal puncture**). A special needle for this purpose is inserted suboccipitally through the posterior atlanto-occipital membrane to the cisterna magna.

2. The medullary cistern lies ventral and lateral to the medulla oblongata (Fig. 29-6). The vertebral arteries are located in this cistern.
3. The cisterna pontis (Fig. 29-6) is located between the basis pontis and the clivus. It has a midline segment and two lateral extensions. The midline segment is important in localizing pathologic processes in the pontine area, whereas the lateral extensions are useful in localization of pathologic processes in the cerebellopontine angle. The basilar artery runs in the cisterna pontis.
4. The cisterna interpeduncularis (Fig. 29-6) extends between the cerebral peduncles and is helpful in localization of pathology in that region.
5. The suprasellar cistern (Fig. 29-6) is located dorsal to the sella turcica and communicates with the cisterna interpeduncularis. Some authors divide the suprasellar cistern into prechiasmatic and postchiasmatic parts. The former is located anterior to and above the optic chiasma, whereas the latter is located behind and below the optic chiasma. The suprasellar cistern is thus useful in localizing pathologic processes in or around the sella turcica and optic chiasma.
6. The superior (quadrigeminal) cistern (Fig. 29-6) is located dorsal to the midbrain. It contains the vein of Galen.

Cisternal puncture. Accessing CSF in the cisterna magna by inserting a needle in the suboccipital region through the atlanto-occipital membrane. The procedure was introduced by Oberga in 1908.

The interpeduncular and superior (quadrigeminal) cisterns are connected along the lateral surface of the midbrain by the ambient cistern (cisterna ambiens).

CHOROID PLEXUS

The choroid plexus is one of the sites for production of cerebrospinal fluid (CSF). It is composed of villi extending from the ventricular wall into the CSF. It is distributed in the body, trigone, and inferior horn of the lateral ventricle, foramen of Monro, roof of the third ventricle, and posterior part of the roof of the fourth ventricle (Fig. 29-1). Each villus is composed of an extensive network of fenestrated capillaries embedded in connective-tissue stroma (Fig. 29-7). Villi are lined by a single layer of choroidal cuboidal epithelium in continuity with the ependymal cell lining of the ventricular wall (Fig. 29-7). The apical surfaces of the choroidal epithelium in contact with CSF are specialized into microvilli that increase their ventricular surface. Choroidal epithelial cells are attached to each other by tight junctions that constitute an effective barrier to the free passage of substances from the blood vessels in the core of the villus into the CSF (blood-CSF barrier). Hydrostatic pressure within the fenestrated capillaries of choroid plexus forces water, solutes, and proteins out into the connective-tissue core of the villus. Macromolecular substances, however, are prevented from free passage to the CSF by the tight junctions between the lining choroidal epithelial cells.

CEREBROSPINAL FLUID

The classic concepts of formation, circulation, and absorption of cerebrospinal fluid elaborated early in this century have undergone major modifications in the last 25 years.

KEY CONCEPTS

- Subarachnoid cisterns are dilations within the subarachnoid space. They include the cisterna magna, medullary cistern, cisterna pontis, cisterna interpeduncularis, suprasellar cistern, superior cistern, and cisterna ambiens.

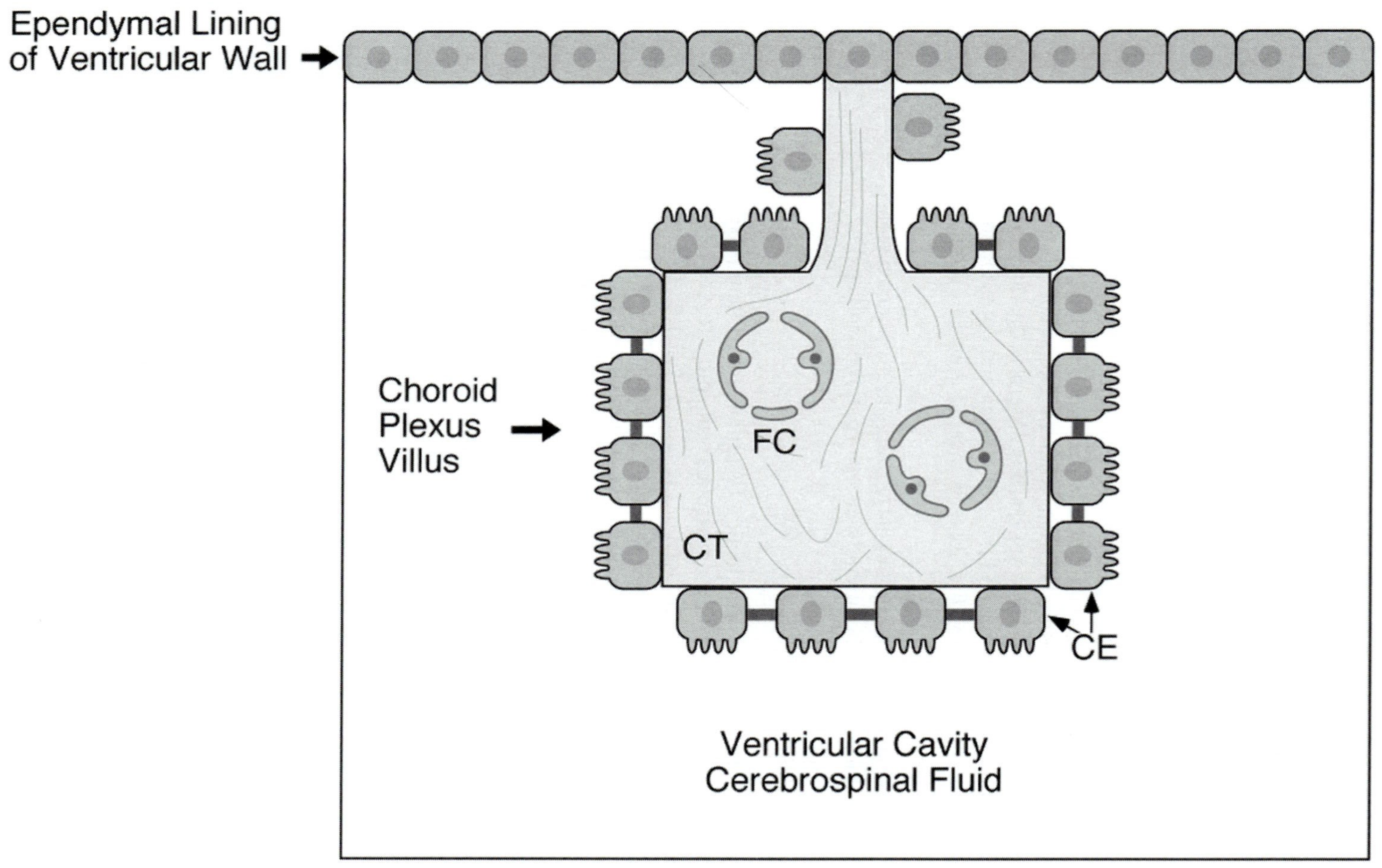

FIGURE 29-7

Schematic diagram of components of the choroid plexus. FC, fenestrated capillary; CT, connective tissue stroma; CE, choroidal epithelium with tight junctions.

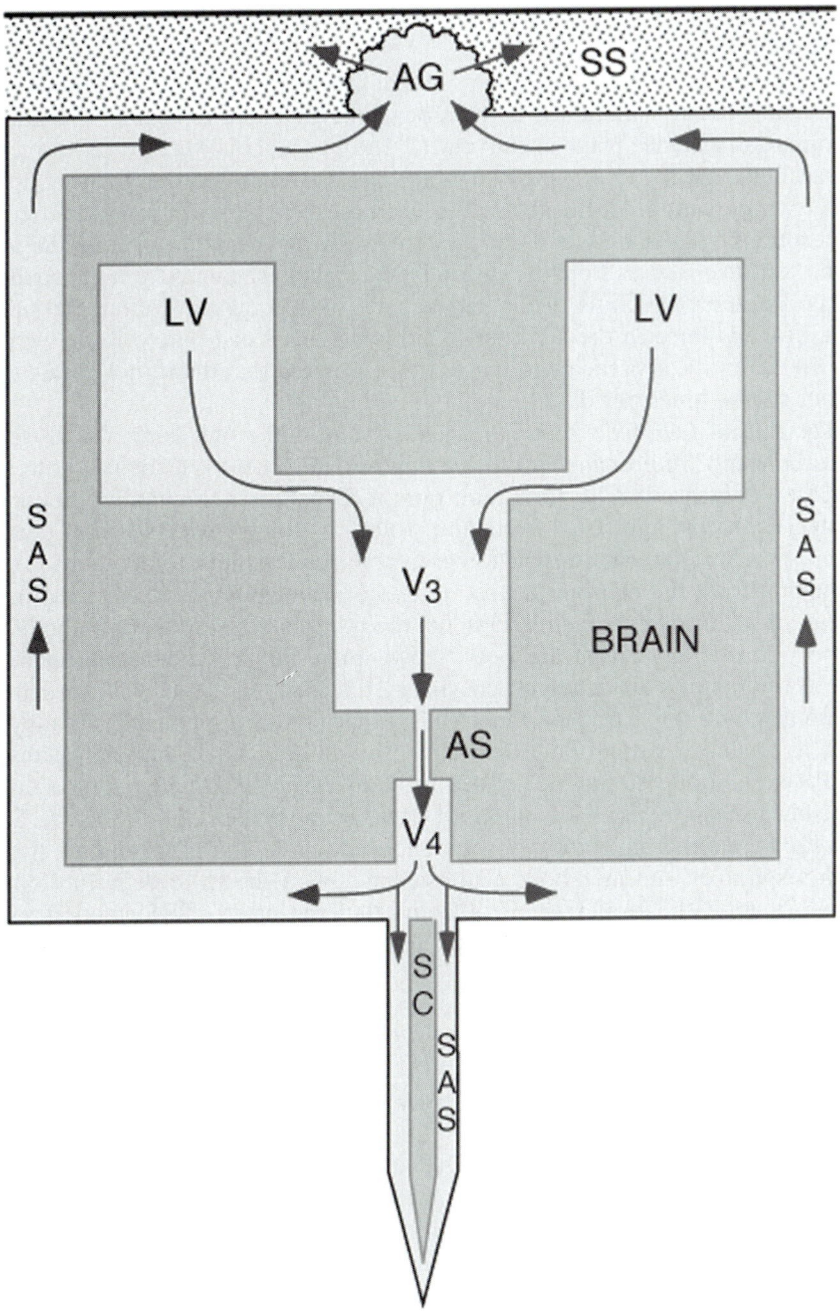

FIGURE 29-8

Schematic diagram showing by arrows the pattern of cerebrospinal fluid circulation from the lateral ventricles to the superior sagittal sinus. LV, lateral ventricle; V3, third ventricle; AS, aqueduct of Sylvius; V4, fourth ventricle; SC, spinal cord; SAS, subarachnoid space; AG, arachnoid granulations; SS, superior sagittal sinus.

Classic Concepts

According to the classic concepts elaborated by Cushing, Weed, and Dandy, the cerebrospinal fluid (CSF) is formed by the choroid plexus and circulates in the lateral ventricles, the foramen of Monro, the third ventricle, the aqueduct of Sylvius, and the fourth ventricle. It flows via the foramina of Magendie and Luschka to the cisterna magna and subarachnoid spaces, where it is finally absorbed through the arachnoid granulations in the superior sagittal sinus into the venous circulation (Fig. 29-8).

Current Concepts

Formation

Although the choroid plexus remains one of the major sites of CSF formation, CSF production can be maintained in the absence of the choroid plexus. Alternate sites of formation include (1) the ependyma, (2) the cerebral pial surface, (3) the cerebral extracellular spaces, and (4) the subarachnoid space. It is estimated that approximately 60 percent of CSF is formed in the lateral, third, and fourth ventricles and 40 percent is formed in the subarachnoid space. Approximately half the CSF formed in the ventricles comes from the choroid plexus; the rest comes from the ependymal lining. In humans, CSF is formed at the rate of 0.35 ml/min (about 500 ml/day). Its average volume in the adult is 130 ml, with 30 ml distributed in the ventricles and 100 ml in the subarachnoid space. It is estimated that the turnover rate of CSF is four to five times per day.

The rate of CSF formation is rather constant and is not generally affected by alterations in CSF pressure below 200 mm of CSF. There is evidence, however, to suggest a decrease in CSF formation rate in chronic, experimentally produced, or human hydrocephalus. CSF formation from the choroid plexus is also decreased with local arteriolar vasoconstriction or hypotension. Almost total cessation of CSF formation from the choroid plexus may result following vasoconstriction induced by low P_{CO_2} during hyperventilation. On the other hand, vasodilatation induced by carbon dioxide inhalation has been shown to result in a substantial increase in CSF formation. Drugs acting on enzyme systems may influence CSF formation by interfering with active transport mechanisms. Drugs that inhibit carbonic anhydrase, such as Diamox, can partially or completely inhibit CSF formation. Ouabain, an ATPase inhibitor, can produce effects similar to those of Diamox. Glucocorticoids have been shown to exert an inhibitory effect on the rate of CSF formation. Several diuretic agents also have been shown to reduce the rate of CSF formation. Although both respiratory and metabolic alkalosis have been shown to depress the rate of CSF formation, the former is more effective than the latter. CSF formation is known to increase with maturation; this may reflect the maturation of the enzyme systems involved in the secretory process.

CSF was considered to be an ultrafiltrate of plasma. Recent evidence seems to suggest, however, that CSF is formed by the following mechanisms.

Diffusion The rate of diffusion depends on particle size and the lipid solubility of the compound.

Active Transport Major cations that pass through the choroid plexus into the CSF are sodium and potassium. The concentration of sodium is higher in CSF than in plasma, whereas that of potassium is lower. Of all the cations in CSF, sodium is found in the greatest amount and is used to stabilize the pH and total cation concentration in CSF. Most of the sodium in CSF enters via the choroid plexus, and only a very small fraction traverses the brain capillaries and brain substance. The concentration of potassium in CSF is very stable and is not affected by fluctuations in

KEY CONCEPTS

- Besides the choroid plexus, the cerebrospinal fluid is formed in the ependyma, cerebral pial surface, cerebral extracellular space, and subarachnoid space.
- Cerebrospinal fluid is formed at the rate of 500 ml/day (0.35 ml/min), with an average turnover rate of four to five times per day.
- The volume of cerebrospinal fluid in the adult is 130 ml; the bulk (100 ml) of it is in the subarachnoid space.

blood or CSF pH. A proper balance between intracellular and extracellular potassium is critical to nerve cell function. Excess CSF potassium is quickly incorporated by neural tissue, whereas reduction in CSF potassium is compensated by movement of potassium from neural tissue to CSF. Chloride constitutes the major anion in CSF and seems to diffuse passively through the choroid plexus, although this passage is closely regulated by sodium and potassium transport.

Certain metabolic substances of low lipid solubility, such as glucose and some amino acids, reach CSF by means of specific carrier transport systems. The carrier systems for amino acids are independent of the glucose carriers.

Free Passage of Water Water moves freely across the blood-CSF barrier. Large molecules, such as plasma proteins, are almost completely blocked by the choroid plexus from entering CSF, although water movement is unrestricted. Studies utilizing perfusion techniques have shown that albumin transfer from blood to CSF is only partially dependent on bulk flow; a portion of the albumin probably enters CSF from surrounding neural tissue.

Circulation

CSF flows from the lateral ventricles through the foramen of Monro to the third ventricle and then through the aqueduct of Sylvius to the fourth ventricle, where it reaches the subarachnoid space of the brain and spinal cord through the foramina of Magendie and Luschka (Fig. 29-8).

Using isotope cisternography, CSF circulation can be followed from the lateral ventricles to the superior sagittal sinus, where it is resorbed. CSF reaches the basal cisterns in a few minutes, flowing from there into the rostral subarachnoid space and sylvian fissure and finally into the convexity of the brain. Isotopes injected into the lumbar subarachnoid space can be detected in basal cisterns within 1 h.

Three factors seem to facilitate CSF circulation.

Drift The drift of CSF from areas of positive balance to areas of negative balance facilitates circulation. Although CSF production and absorption are in almost perfect balance when the total CSF space is considered, any one point in the system may be at positive or negative balance. CSF will therefore drift from areas of positive balance to those of negative balance. This drift will contribute to CSF flow.

Oscillation CSF is also in a continuous state of oscillation, with a to-and-fro movement the amplitude of which increases as the fluid approaches the fourth ventricle. This oscillation contributes to the flow of CSF, and the increase in amplitude in the fourth ventricle facilitates the flow of CSF into the cisterna magna.

Pulsatile Movement Rhythmic movements synchronous with arterial pulse have been described in CSF. These pulsatile oscillations assume an upward and downward movement in the fourth ventricle and basal cisterns. The origin of these oscillations is believed to be the expansion of the cerebrum and its arteries during systole rather than choroid plexus pulsations, as previously assumed.

KEY CONCEPTS

- Cerebrospinal fluid (CSF) is formed by a variety of processes that include diffusion, active transport, and free passage of water.
- Circulation of CSF is facilitated by three processes: drift of CSF from areas of positive balance to areas of negative balance, oscillatory to and fro movement, and pulsatile movements synchronous with arterial pulse.

Resorption

The classic concept of CSF resorption states that the fluid is resorbed through the arachnoid granulations into the venous system of the superior sagittal sinus (Figs. 29-8 and 29-3). This concept was based on experiments in which CSF flow was studied after Prussian blue was injected intrathecally. Earlier studies on CSF resorption were hampered by the use of substances foreign to CSF, such as trypan blue and phenosulfophthaline, which do not occur naturally and to which the subarachnoid space is highly sensitive. With the advent of radioisotopic techniques, it was possible to study the behavior of substances that occur normally in CSF. Such studies have yielded the following observations:

1. Electrolytes are resorbed more slowly than water.
2. Electrolytes are resorbed more readily in the ventricles than in the subarachnoid space.
3. Albumin leaves the subarachnoid space more readily than it leaves the ventricles.
4. Albumin disappears more slowly than water or electrolytes.
5. Resorption occurs not only in arachnoid granulations but also in the ependyma of the ventricles.
6. Resorption in the subarachnoid space occurs by a fast component through the leptomeningeal vascular route and by a slow component into the perineural spaces.

Thus the present concepts of CSF resorption point to the following resorption sites:

1. Arachnoid granulations (main resorption site)
2. Leptomeningeal vessels
3. Perineural sheaths of cranial and spinal nerves
4. Ependyma of the ventricles

The controversy over reconciling the behavior of CSF outflow with its structural basis remains unresolved. Earlier studies suggest that substances varying widely in molecular weight and lipid solubility pass readily from CSF pathways to the blood. Such studies are at variance with ultrastructural observations of the arachnoid granulations, which show the presence of intact endothelium with tight junctions effectively separating CSF and blood compartments. More recent studies, however, may have resolved this controversy by suggesting a mechanism for CSF resorption in the arachnoid granulations similar to that described for drainage of ocular fluid in the canal of Schlemm. According to this hypothesis, exit of CSF via the arachnoid granulations is pressure-dependent. Endothelial cells of the arachnoid villus undergo vacuolation on the CSF side. Vacuoles increase in size because of the differential pressure gradient between CSF (higher) and blood compartments (lower) and ultimately reach the blood side of the endothelial cells, where they rupture and create a patent channel between CSF and blood. Such a hypothesis has been confirmed by electron microscopic observations of the behavior of arachnoid granulations.

In addition to this filtration route, it is believed that substances are resorbed by the two other routes of diffusion and active transport.

KEY CONCEPTS

- CSF is resorbed primarily through the arachnoid granulations into the superior sagittal sinus. Other sites include the leptomeningeal vessels, ependyma lining the ventricles, and sheaths of cranial and spinal nerves.

Function

CSF serves three principal functions:

1. It supports the weight of the brain within the skull. This buoyancy function is disturbed when CSF is withdrawn, resulting in headache because of more traction on vessels and nerves.
2. It acts as a buffer or cushion between the brain and adjacent dura and skull; it protects the brain from physical trauma during injury to the skull by dampening the effects of trauma.
3. It provides a stable chemical environment for the central nervous system. The chemical composition of CSF is rather stable even in the presence of major changes in the chemical composition of plasma.

Composition

CSF is a clear, colorless fluid composed of the following substances and elements:

Water Water is the major constituent of CSF.

Protein The value of protein in normal CSF is approximately 15 to 45 mg/dl. The lower value (15 mg/dl) reflects protein value in ventricular CSF; the higher value (45 mg/dl) reflects protein value in the lumbar subarachnoid space. Protein values increase in various disease states of the nervous system (infection, tumor, hemorrhage), as well as after obstruction of CSF pathways. Three proteins account for the bulk of CSF protein content: albumin and beta and gamma globulins. The presence of oligoclonal bands (electrophoretic bands in the immunoglobulin G region) and myelin basic proteins in the CSF suggest a demyelinating process such as multiple sclerosis.

Sugar The amount of glucose in normal CSF is approximately two-thirds that of the blood. Glucose value is slightly higher (75 mg/dl) in ventricular fluid than in lumbar subarachnoid space fluid (60 mg/dl). Ratio of CSF glucose to blood glucose is higher in newborns and premature infants, probably because of the immaturity of the blood-CSF barrier. The value decreases in meningitis and after meningeal infiltration by tumors.

Cells A normal sample of CSF contains up to three lymphocytes per cubic millimeter. An increase in the number of white cells in CSF occurs in infectious processes. In general, leukocytes predominate in bacterial infections (bacterial meningitis) and lymphocytes in viral infections (viral meningitis and encephalitis). Normal CSF contains no red blood cells (RBCs). The presence of RBCs in CSF occurs as a result of trauma during its collection or secondary to pathologic hemorrhage into the CSF. Traumatic RBCs are usually present in samples of CSF obtained early in the process of CSF collection and disappear in samples collected subsequently. RBCs from pathologic bleeding (e.g., subarachnoid hemorrhage) render the CSF grossly bloody and xanthochromic (yellow). The xanthochromia is due to release

KEY CONCEPTS

- CSF has three functions: buoyancy of the brain, physical buffer between brain and skull, and chemical buffer between the blood and brain.
- CSF contains water (major constituent), protein, glucose, electrolytes, and very few cells.
- Protein value in the CSF is much less than that in the blood. Ventricular CSF has less protein than lumbar CSF.

of bilirubin from the RBCs. Neoplastic cells may occur in some types of central nervous system neoplasms, particularly those associated with leptomeningeal dissemination.

Electrolytes CSF contains sodium, potassium, chloride, magnesium, and calcium. Sodium and potassium constitute the major cations, whereas chloride constitutes the major anion. The concentration of sodium, chloride, and magnesium ions is higher in CSF than in plasma, whereas the concentration of potassium and calcium ions is lower.

Physical Properties

Specific Gravity The specific gravity of normal CSF varies between 1.006 and 1.009. An increase in the protein content of the CSF raises its specific gravity.

Pressure Normal CSF pressure measured in the lumbar subarachnoid space varies between 50 and 200 mm of CSF (up to 8 mmHg), measured with the patient in the lateral recumbent position and relaxed. The normal pressure range is higher (200 to 300 mm of CSF) when measured in the upright seated position. CSF pressure is increased in central nervous system infections (meningitis), tumors, hemorrhage, thrombosis, and hydrocephalus.

Spinal (Lumbar), Cisternal, and Ventricular Taps (Punctures)

Lumbar puncture. A method of accessing CSF in the lumbar subarachnoid space by introducing a needle between the lumbar vertebrae. The procedure was introduced in 1891 by Heinrich Quinke, a German physician who obtained CSF for the first time from a living patient. William Gowers disapproved of the procedure and discouraged its use at the National Hospital in London until after his retirement.

The examination of CSF is of major value in neurologic diagnosis. Access to CSF for diagnosis dates back to 1891 when Quinke introduced the **lumbar puncture.** CSF can be obtained from three sites: (1) the spinal subarachnoid space (spinal or lumbar puncture), (2) the cisterna magna (cisternal puncture), and (3) the lateral ventricles (ventricular puncture). The first route is used most commonly. In this procedure (spinal or lumbar tap), a special needle is introduced using sterile techniques and local anesthesia in the L2-3, L3-4, or L4-5 vertebral space. The needle is gently eased into the subarachnoid space, and CSF is withdrawn. Since the conus medullaris of the spinal cord ends at the L-1 or L-2 vertebral level and the meninges extend to the S-1 or S-2 vertebral level, the space between L-2 and L-3 vertebrae constitutes a safe area into which to introduce the lumbar tap needle without the danger of injuring the spinal cord. The cisterna magna is accessed by a suboccipital route through the posterior atlanto-occipital membrane. The lateral ventricles are accessed through the brain substance. Withdrawal of CSF from the lumbar subarachnoid space is contraindicated in the presence of increased intracranial pressure. Spinal taps in such conditions may lead to herniation of the uncus of the temporal lobe through the tentorium or the cerebellar tonsils through the foramen magnum with resulting coma and death. The lumbar subarachnoid space, the cisternal space,

KEY CONCEPTS

- Glucose value in the CSF is about two-thirds that in blood.
- CSF normally contains no red cells and no more than three lymphocytes per cubic millimeter.
- CSF can be accessed at three sites: lumbar subarachnoid space, cisterna magna, and lateral ventricle.
- Access to the CSF via the lumbar subarachnoid space is contraindicated in states of increased intracranial pressure.

and the ventricles are entered not only to obtain CSF for examination but also to inject air, contrast material, or drugs for either diagnosis or treatment of neurologic disorders.

BRAIN BARRIER SYSTEM

The concept of a barrier system between blood and brain dates back to 1885, when it was found that intravenously injected acidic dyes stained all organs of the body except the brain. It was later observed that when these acidic dyes were injected into the CSF, the brain was stained. Thus a barrier was assumed to be located at the blood-brain interface that prevented entry of acidic dyes into the brain. It has since been discovered that these acidic dyes bind themselves to serum albumin and that the barrier to their entry to the brain is the low permeability of brain capillaries to the albumin to which the dyes are bound.

Although earlier studies conceived of only one barrier, at the blood-brain interface, studies dating back to the 1930s have elucidated the existence of other brain barrier sites. Consequently, the term *blood-brain barrier* has been replaced by the more useful term *brain barrier system.* Two separate barriers comprise this system: (1) the blood-brain barrier, located at the interface between the capillary wall and brain substance, and (2) the blood-CSF barrier, located in the choroid plexus. The blood-brain barrier is comprised of (1) capillary endothelial cells with tight junctions, (2) capillary basement membrane, and (3) perivascular glial processes abutting the capillary. The blood-brain barrier is the more extensive of the barriers. It separates blood within the capillaries from brain substance. In the blood-CSF barrier, tight junctions that join choroidal epithelial cells (Fig. 29-7) comprise the barrier at this site. The surface area of the blood-CSF barrier is only 0.02 percent of the surface area of the blood-brain barrier. The ependymal cells lining the ventricles are not joined together by tight junctions (Fig. 29-7) and thus do not constitute a barrier between the CSF and brain.

Studies on the mechanisms of the barrier system have shown that the anatomic substrates of the barrier (endothelial lining, basement membrane, glial processes, tight junctions) cannot account for all the observed phenomena of the barrier system. It is thus conceivable that other factors are operative in the barrier system. These factors include

1. *Protein binding.* Brain capillaries are essentially impermeable to albumin. Substances in plasma that are bound to protein will therefore have no access to the brain.
2. *Lipid solubility.* Substances with high lipid solubility enter the brain rather rapidly, whereas substances with low or no lipid solubility enter the brain very slowly or not at all.
3. *Blood flow.* This factor is operative in the entry to the brain of substances of

KEY CONCEPTS

- The brain barrier system has two components: blood-brain barrier and blood-CSF barrier.
- The blood-brain barrier is located at the interface between capillary walls and brain substance. It consists of capillary endothelium with tight junctions, capillary basement membrane, and astrocytic perivascular processes.
- The blood-CSF barrier is located in the choroid plexus and consists of tight junctions that join adjacent choroidal epithelial cells.
- Factors that play roles in the barrier system include protein binding and lipid solubility of the substance, blood flow, and metabolic requirements.

high lipid solubility. The rate of blood flow to a brain region will determine the amount of entry of such substances.

4. *Metabolic requirement.* The rate of entry of some substances into the brain seems to be dependent on the metabolic requirement of that region of the brain for the particular substance. Cholesterol, for example, is accumulated in the brain during myelin formation and decreases when myelination is completed.

The brain barrier system is more permeable in newborn infants than in adults. As the brain matures with age, the barrier system becomes less permeable. The brain of the newborn, for example, is permeable to bilirubin. A rise in bilirubin levels in the blood of a newborn is detrimental to brain function. In contrast, an excessive rise in serum bilirubin in the adult does not affect the brain.

Certain areas of the brain are devoid of a barrier system. These areas, known as *circumventricular organs,* include the area postrema of the medulla oblongata, neurohypophysis, pineal body, organ vasculosum of the lamina terminales, median eminence of hypothalamus, subcommissural organ, and subfornical organ. All these areas are characterized by rich vascularity, and some are secretory in function. Unlike vessels elsewhere in the brain, the endothelial lining of vessels in these areas is fenestrated.

KEY CONCEPTS

- Certain areas of the brain are devoid of brain barrier system. They include area postrema, neurohypophysis, pineal gland, organ vasculosum, median eminence, subcommissural organ, and subfornical organ. Collectively, these areas are known as the *circumventricular organs.*

SUGGESTED READINGS

Alami SY, Afifi AK: Cerebrospinal fluid examination. In Race GJ (ed): *Laboratory Medicine,* vol 4, chap 2. Hagerstown, Md, Harper & Row, 1973:1.

Bradbury M: The structure and function of the blood-brain barrier. *Fed Proc* 1984; 43:186–190.

Goldstein G, Betz A: The blood-brain barrier. *Sci Am* 1986; 255:74–83.

Gomez DG, et al: The spinal cerebrospinal fluid absorptive pathways. *Neuroradiology* 1974; 8:61–66.

Hughes RA, et al: Caves and cysts of the septum pellucidum. *Arch Neurol Psychiatry* 1955; 74:259–266.

Kempe LG, Busch E: Clinical significance of cisterna veli interpositi. *Acta Neurochir* 1967; 16:241–248.

Leech RW: Normal anatomy of ventricles, meninges, subarachnoid space, and venous system. In Leech RW, Brumback RA (eds): *Hydrocephalus: Current Clinical Concepts.* St Louis, Mosby–Year Book, 1991:18.

Leech RW: Normal physiology of cerebrospinal fluid. In Leech RW, Brumback RA (eds): *Hydrocephalus: Current Clinical Concepts.* St Louis, Mosby–Year Book, 1991:30.

Leslie W: Cyst of the cavum vergae. *Can Med Assoc J* 1940; 43:433–435.

Mori K: Subcallosal midline cysts in anomalies of the central nervous system. In Nadjmi M (ed): *Neuroradiologic Atlases.* New York, Thieme-Stratton, 1985:69.

Pryse-Phillips W: *Companion to Clinical Neurology.* Boston, Little, Brown, 1995.

Sage, MR, Wilson AJ: The blood-brain barrier: An important concept in neuroimaging. *AJNR* 1994; 15: 601–622.

Schwidde JT: Incidence of cavum septi pellucidi and cavum vergae in 1032 human brains. *Arch Neurol Psychiatry* 1952; 67:625–632.

Tyler HR, Tyler KL: Communication between lateral and third ventricle: First description. *Neurology* 1985; 35:1298.

Vastola EF: CSF formation and absorption estimates by constant flow infusion method. *Arch Neurol* 1980; 37:150–154.

Zellweger H, Van Epps EF: The cavus veli interpositi and its differentiation from cavum vergae. *AJR* 1959; 82:793–805.

C H A P T E R 30

CEREBROSPINAL FLUID AND THE BARRIER SYSTEM: CLINICAL CORRELATES

CEREBROSPINAL FLUID IN DISEASE

Cerebrospinal fluid (CSF) examination in patients with neurologic disorders can provide valuable information about the nature of the disease process. This is particularly true in infections (meningitis, encephalitis), autoimmune disorders (multiple sclerosis, Guillain-Barré polyneuritis), tumors, and hemorrhage.

Normal CSF obtained from the lumbar subarachnoid space is clear and colorless, is under 50 to 200 mm of CSF pressure in the recumbent relaxed state, and contains

TABLE 30-1

Cerebral Fluid Findings in Health and Disease

Condition	Color	Pressure, mmCSF	Cells/mm^3	Protein, mg/dl	Glucose, mg/dl	Other
Normal	Clear	50–200	0–3	15–45	60–80	—
Bacterial meningitis	Cloudy	↑	↑ (neutrophils)	↑	↓	Organism by gram stain and culture
Viral encephalitis	Clear	Normal or ↑	Normal or ↑ (lymphocytes)	Normal or ↑	Normal	Organism by culture
Multiple sclerosis	Clear	Normal	Normal or ↑	Normal or ↑ (increased gammaglobulins)	Normal	Oligoclonal and myelin basic proteins
Guillain-Barré syndrome	Clear	Normal	Normal	↑	Normal	Albuminocytologic dissociation
Brain tumor	Clear	↑	Normal or ↑	↑	Normal	Tumor cells in sediment
Spinal tumor	Yellow	Normal	Normal or ↑	↑	Normal	Tumor cells in sediment
Subarachnoid hemorrhage	Bloody	↑	↑ (red cells)	↑	↓	—

NOTE: ↑ = elevated; ↓ = decreased.

three cells (lymphocytes) or fewer per cubic millimeter, 15 to 45 mg of protein, and 60 to 80 mg/dl of glucose.

In bacterial meningitis the CSF is cloudy and turbid, is under considerably increased pressure (200 to 500 mm of CSF pressure), and contains an increased number of cells, almost all polymorphonuclear leukocytes (2000 to 10,000/mm^3), increased protein (100 to 1000 mg), and low glucose (below 20 mg/dl). Examination of fluid by Gram stain and culture reveals the organism responsible for the meningitis.

In viral encephalitis the CSF usually is clear, is under normal or slightly elevated pressure, and contains either a normal or a slightly increased number of cells (five to several hundred, mostly lymphocytes), normal or slightly increased protein (50 to 200 mg/dl), and normal glucose. Gram staining shows no bacteria. Culture of the CSF may reveal the viral agent involved.

In multiple sclerosis the CSF is clear, is under normal pressure, and contains a normal or an increased number (50 to 300) of cells, predominantly lymphocytes, normal or moderately increased protein including oligoclonal and myelin basic proteins, increased gamma globulins, and normal glucose.

KEY CONCEPTS

- Examination of cerebrospinal fluid (CSF) provides valuable information about the nature of neurologic disorders.

In **Guillain-Barré** the CSF is characterized by albuminocytologic dissociation in which protein is moderately to markedly elevated in the presence of normal cells. The fluid is clear, is under normal pressure, and contains a normal amount of glucose.

In brain tumors the CSF is clear, is under increased pressure, and contains a normal or increased number of cells, an increased amount of protein, and normal glucose. Spinning of the CSF may reveal the presence of tumor cells in the sediment. Seeding of tumor cells along the meninges is associated with an increase in cells and protein. Lumbar puncture is contraindicated in the presence of increased intracranial pressure to avoid herniation.

In spinal cord tumors the CSF may have a yellowish tinge as a result of the marked increase in protein, is under normal pressure, and contains a normal or slightly increased number of cells, a marked increase in protein, and normal glucose. Tumor cells may be found in the sediment.

In subarachnoid hemorrhage the CSF is bloody, is under markedly increased pressure, and contains a large number of red blood cells, a very high amount of protein (as a result of the presence of blood), and low glucose.

Table 30-1 summarizes CSF findings in health and disease.

Guillain-Barré syndrome. An acute inflammatory demyelinating polyneuropathy. Described by George Guillain, Jean Alexander Barré, and Andre Strohl, French physicians, in 1916.

VENTRICULOMEGALY

Enlargement of the ventricles (ventriculomegaly) usually is associated with one of the following conditions: (1) overproduction of CSF, as occurs in tumors of the choroid plexus (choroid plexus papilloma), (2) atrophy of the brain with secondary (compensatory) enlargement of the ventricles (**hydrocephalus ex vacuo**), as in **Alzheimer's disease,** (3) developmental failure of growth of the cerebral mantle (the brain beween the ventricle and the brain surface), as in the condition known as **colpocephaly,** or (4) obstruction of CSF flow or absorption, as in **hydrocephalus.**

The mechanism of ventriculomegaly in hypersecreting tumors of the choroid plexus (Fig. 30-1) is not clear. It may be due to overproduction of CSF in excess of resorption, overproduction of protein, or both.

Ventriculomegaly associated with brain atrophy may be focal (as in infarction) (Fig. 30-2) or generalized (as in Alzheimer's disease and hypoxic ischemic encephalopathy) and is a compensatory mechanism that fills the space created by the loss of brain substance. Hence, it is called hydrocephalus ex vacuo. It usually is associated with concomitant enlargement of the subarachnoid spaces.

Developmental ventriculomegaly is due to failure of growth of the cerebral mantle. In an 8-week-old embryo, the ventricles are large and the cerebral mantle is thin. With normal development, the cerebral mantle grows faster than do the ventricles so that by midgestation the ventricles become relatively small. If the cerebral mantle fails to grow normally, the ventricles remain relatively large, a

Hydrocephalus ex vacuo. An increase in the volume of cerebrospinal fluid and ventriculomegaly secondary to brain atrophy.

Alzheimer's disease. A type of cortical dementia named after Alois Alzheimer, the German neuropsychiatrist and pathologist who described the disease in 1906. The term *Alzheimer's disease* was coined by Ernst Kraepelin, a German psychiatrist, in 1910.

Colpocephaly. A developmental condition characterized by failure of development of the cerebral mantle and secondary ventriculomegaly with disproportionate enlargement of the occipital horns of the lateral ventricle. The term was coined by Yakovlev and Wadsworth in 1946.

Hydrocephalus (Greek *hydor,* "water"; *kephalé,* "head"). Dilatation of the cerebral ventricles. Known to Hippocrates, it was described accurately by Vesalius in 1550.

KEY CONCEPTS

- A characteristic CSF profile occurs in diverse neurologic disorders such as bacterial meningitis, viral encephalitis, multiple sclerosis, Guillain-Barré syndrome, brain tumors, spinal cord tumors, and subarachnoid hemorrhage.
- Ventriculomegaly is associated with overproduction of CSF, brain atrophy, developmental failure of growth of the cerebral mantle, and obstruction of CSF flow or absorption.
- The ventriculomegaly associated with brain atrophy is known as hydrocephalus ex vacuo.
- Colpocephaly refers to disproportionate ventriculomegaly of the posterior horn of the lateral ventricle caused by failure of normal development of the cerebral mantle.

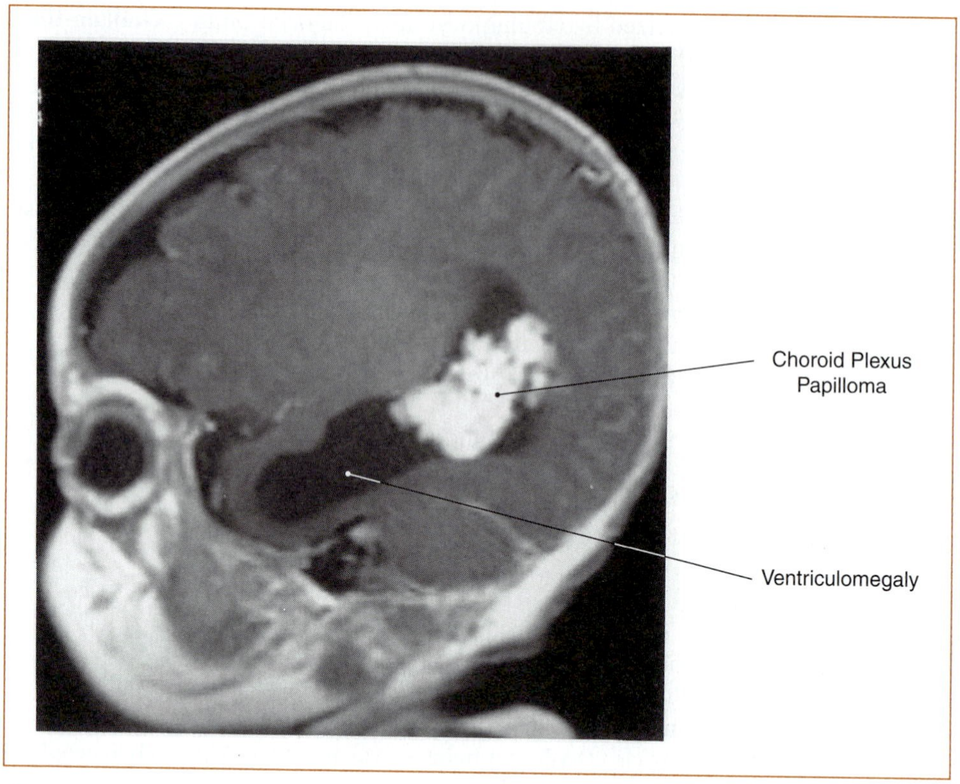

FIGURE 30-1

Parasagittal gadolinium enhanced magnetic resonance image (MRI) showing choroid plexus papilloma and ventriculomegaly.

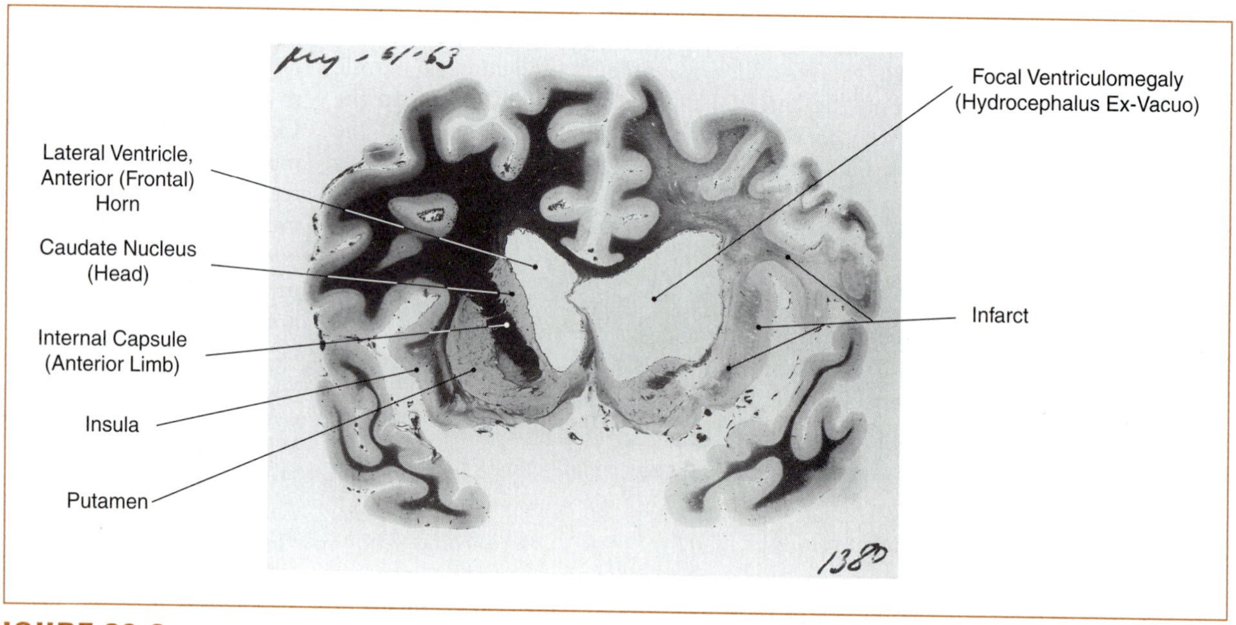

FIGURE 30-2

Coronal section of the brain showing cerebral infarct and secondary focal ventriculomegaly.

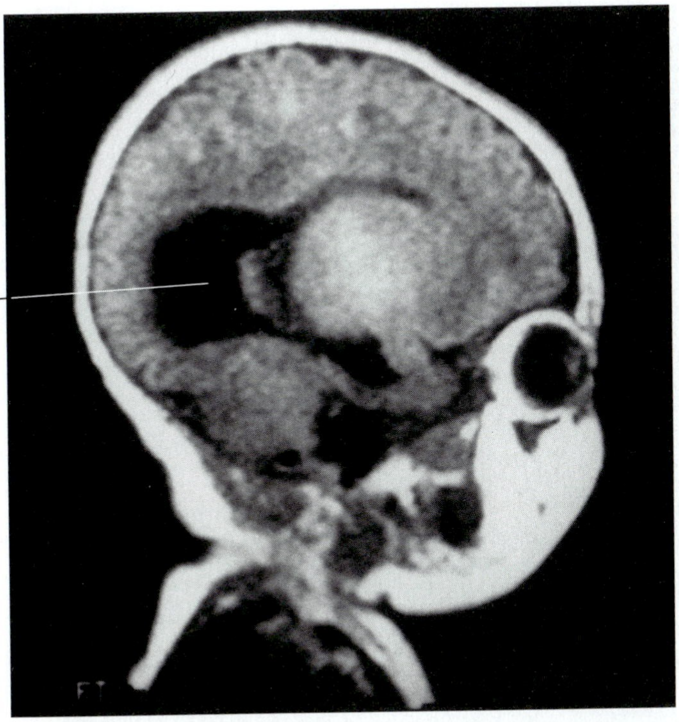

FIGURE 30-3

T1-weighted parasagittal magnetic resonance image (MRI) showing disproportionate enlargement of the occipital horn in colpocephaly.

condition known as colpocephaly (Fig. 30-3), a term coined by Yakovlev and Wadsworth in 1946 to refer to disproportionate enlargement of the occipital horns.

HYDROCEPHALUS

Hydrocephalus is a condition characterized by an increased amount of CSF in the ventricles (Fig. 30-4). Hippocrates was one of the first physicians to deal with hydrocephalus, advocating the use of laxatives and sneeze-inducing substances for its treatment. The surgical approach to the treatment of hydrocephalus, though suggested by Hippocrates and others, was not accepted as the most effective mode of treatment until the nineteenth century.

There are two types of hydrocephalus: communicating and noncommunicating. In **communicating hydrocephalus** there is free communication between the ventricles and the subarachnoid space. The obstruction to the flow of CSF in this type of hydrocephalus is usually distal to the ventricular system, in the subarachnoid

Communicating hydrocephalus. A type of hydrocephalus in which obstruction to CSF flow occurs between the roof of the fourth ventricle and the arachnoid granulations.

KEY CONCEPTS

- Hydrocephalus refers to an increasd amount of CSF in the ventricle, with or without a concomitant increase in CSF pressure.
- Hydrocephalus is classified into communicating and noncommunicating varieties.
- In communicating hydrocephalus the different ventricular cavities communicate with each other and with the subarachnoid spaces.

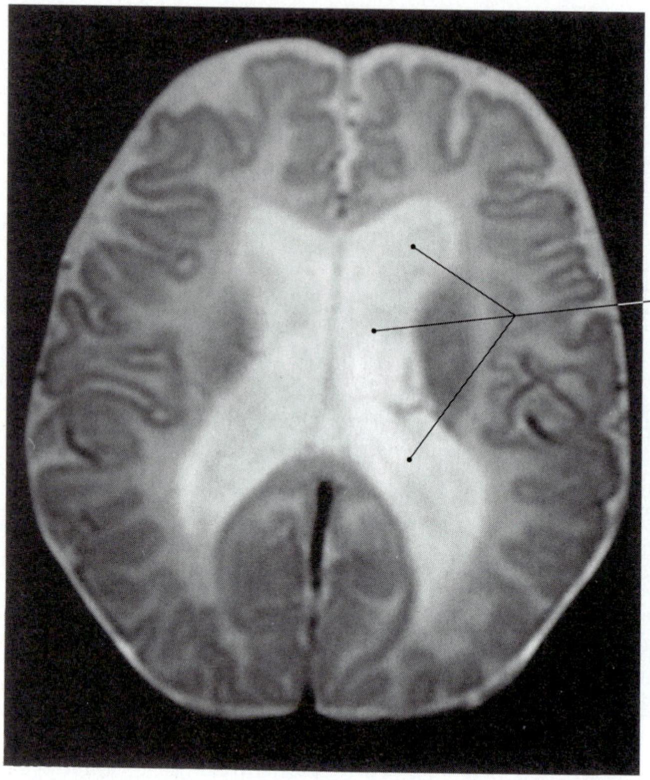

FIGURE 30-4

T2-weighted axial magnetic resonance image (MRI) showing enlarged ventricular cavities (ventriculomegaly) due to hydrocephalus.

Noncommunicating hydrocephalus. A type of hydrocephalus caused by obstruction of cerebrospinal fluid flow between the sites of its formation and the roof of the fourth ventricle.

Foramen of Monro. The site of communication between the lateral and third ventricles. Named after Alexander Monro, a Scottish anatomist who described it in 1753.

Aqueduct of Sylvius. A narrow passage linking the third and fourth ventricles. Named after Franciscus de la Boe Sylvius, who described it in 1650.

Foramen of Magendie. The median aperture in the roof of the fourth ventricle, connecting it with the cisterna magna. Named after François Magendie, a French physiologist who described it in 1842.

Foramen of Luschka. Paired openings in the lateral recesses of the fourth ventricle through which cerebrospinal fluid flows from the fourth ventricle to the cisterna magna. Named after Hubert von Luschka, a German anatomist, in 1863.

spaces (as a result of fibrosis from previous infection) or the arachnoid granulations (as a result of a lack of or abnormalities in those structures). This results in CSF accumulation and enlargement of all the ventricular cavities as well as the subarachnoid spaces.

In **noncommunicating hydrocephalus** CSF in the ventricular cavities cannot reach the subarachnoid spaces because of obstruction of CSF flow in the **foramen of Monro** (Fig. 30-5), the **aqueduct of Sylvius** (Fig. 30-6), or the **foramina of Magendie and Luschka.** Obstruction of the foramen of Monro—for example, by tumor—blocks the flow of CSF from the lateral ventricle to the third ventricle, resulting in an accumulation of CSF and enlargement of the lateral ventricle on the side of obstruction (Fig. 30-5). Obstruction of the aqueduct of Sylvius by tumor, inflammation, or congenital atresia results in accumulation of CSF and enlargement of the ventricular cavities draining into the aqueduct (third ventricle and both lateral ventricles) (Fig. 30-6). Obstruction at the foramina of Magendie and Luschka by

KEY CONCEPTS

- In noncommunicating hydrocephalus CSF within the ventricles cannot reach the subarachnoid spaces because of obstruction to CSF flow in the ventricular cavities (foramen of Monro, aqueduct of Sylvius) or the foramina of Magendie and Luschka.

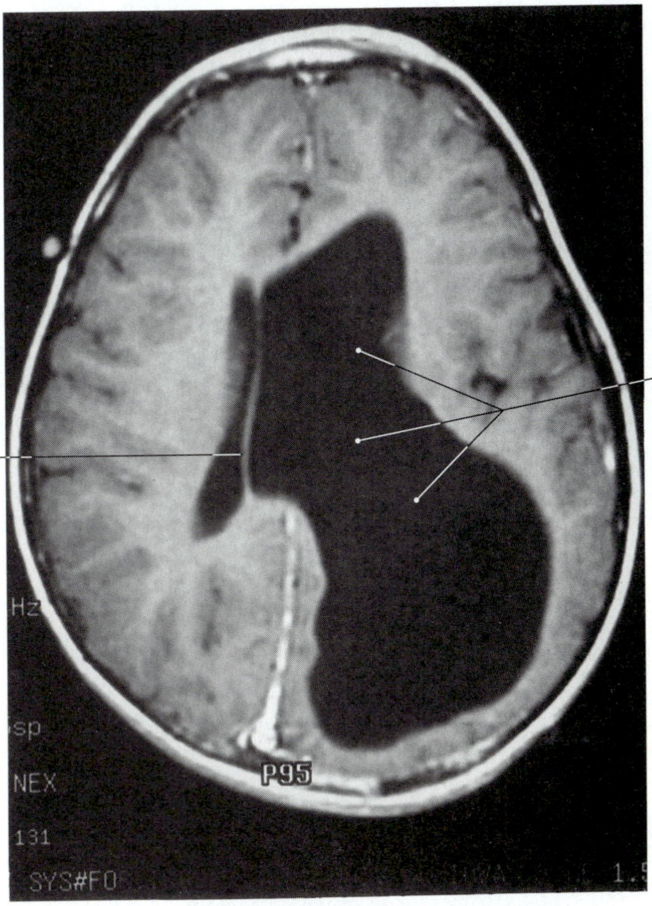

FIGURE 30-5

T1-weighted axial magnetic resonance image (MRI) showing unilateral enlargement of the lateral ventricle with displacement of the septum pellucidum across the midline due to obstruction of the foramen of Monro by atresia.

tumor, inflammation, or congenital atresia results in CSF accumulation and enlargement of the fourth, third, and both lateral ventricles.

In adults in whom the skull sutures have closed, hydrocephalus is associated with a marked increase in intracranial pressure. This is associated with headache, vomiting, dizziness, a decrease in the state of consciousness, and edema of the optic disks. In these patients, the lateral margins of the lateral ventricles become rounded and there is an outflow of CSF across the ependyma into the periventricular spaces (transependymal flow) (Fig. 30-7). Pressure exerted on the corticospinal fibers that

KEY CONCEPTS

- The site of obstruction in noncommunicating hydrocephalus determines which ventricular space or spaces are enlarged.
- Hydrocephalus in adults is associated with a marked increase in intracranial pressure.

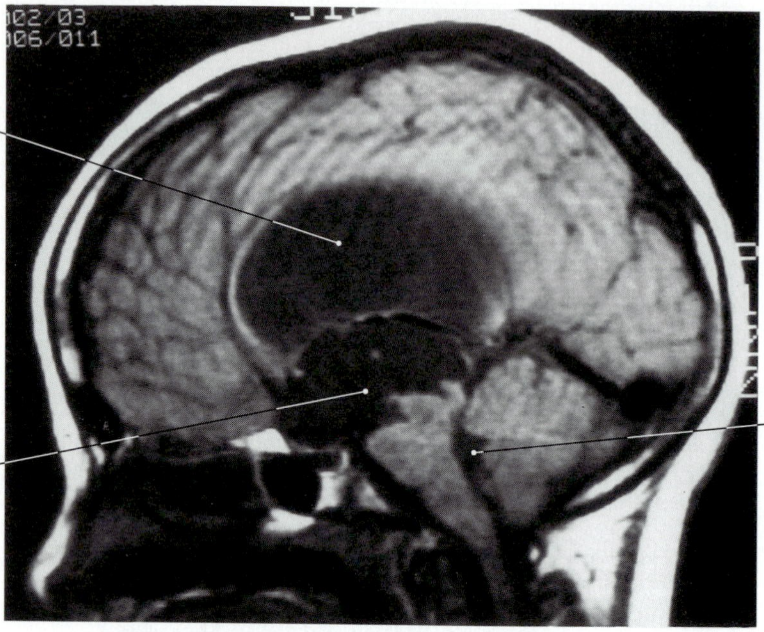

FIGURE 30-6

T1-weighted midsagittal magnetic resonance image (MRI) showing selective enlargement of the lateral and third ventricles due to aqueductal stenosis. The fourth ventricle is normal in size.

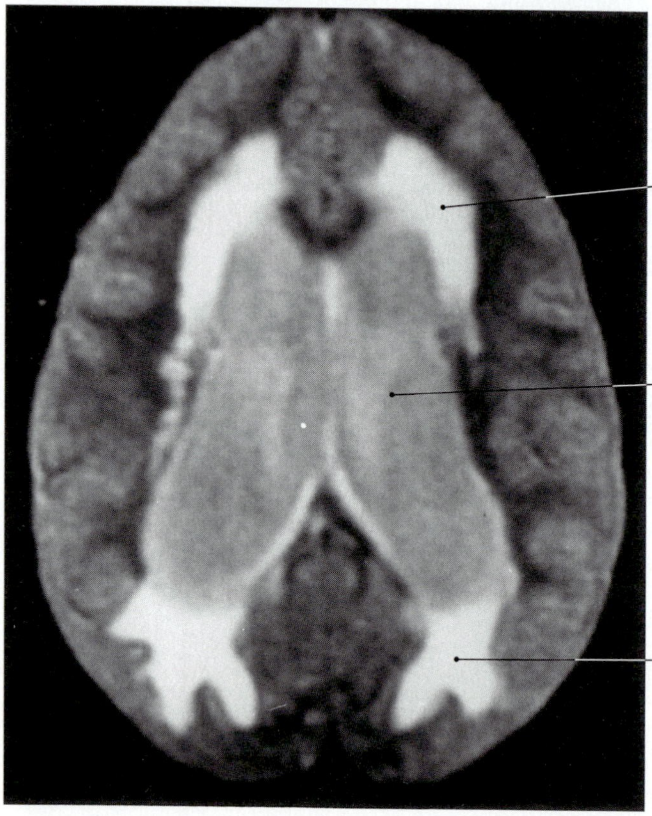

FIGURE 30-7

T2-weighted axial magnetic resonance image (MRI) showing transependymal flow of cerebrospinal fluid to the adjacent brain substance in hydrocephalus.

innervate the lower extremities, which travel in close proximity to the lateral ventricles, results in lower extremity weakness.

If hydrocephalus develops in early childhood, before closure of the skull sutures, the skull yields to the increased pressure by widening of the sutures and a progressive increase in head circumference. A rapid increase in intracranial pressure in these children may result in a decreased level of consciousness and alertness, vomiting, irritability, and the **"sun-setting" sign,** in which the upper lids are retracted and the globes are directed downward.

Sun-setting sign. Depression of the eyeball with failure of upward gaze and retraction of upper lid. Seen in children with hydrocephalus and pressure on the dorsal tectum.

Normal-Pressure Hydrocephalus

Normal-pressure hydrocephalus (a type of communicating hydrocephalus) is a disorder of the elderly characterized by uniform enlargement of the ventricular system without a concomitant increase in CSF pressure or intracranial pressure. The pathophysiology of normal-pressure hydrocephalus is poorly understood. Impaired resorption of CSF is believed to be the cause of CSF accumulation and ventricular enlargement. Clinically, the condition is characterized by dementia, urinary incontinence, and gait disturbance. These signs sometimes improve after shunting of the CSF to extracranial sites. Normal-pressure hydrocephalus is thus considered a treatable dementing disorder.

Benign External Hydrocephalus

Benign external hydrocephalus is a disorder of childhood characterized by the accumulation of CSF in the subarachnoid space over the brain surface, particularly over the frontal lobes and in the interhemispheric fissure, without significant involvement of the ventricular cavities (Fig. 30-8). The condition was first described in the eighteenth century by Underwood, who also observed its benign nature. The condition was rediscovered after the advent of newer imaging techniques. It is a self-limited condition which usually resolves spontaneously without sequelae.

KEY CONCEPTS

- In neuroimages, rounding of the lateral margins of the lateral ventricles and the presence of transependymal CSF flow indicate increased CSF pressure.
- Pressure exerted by the enlarged lateral ventricles on nearby corticospinal fibers that innervate the lower extremities results in lower extremity weakness.
- Hydrocephalus in early childhood before closure of the skull sutures results in suture widening and an increase in head circumference.
- The sun-setting sign in childhood hydrocephalus indicates increased intracranial pressure.
- Headache, vomiting, and a decreased state of consciousness and alertness are signs of increased intracranial pressure.
- Normal-pressure hydrocephalus refers to uniform enlargement of the ventricular system without a concomitant increase in CSF or intracranial pressure.
- Normal-pressure hydrocephalus is a treatable dementing disorder.
- Benign external hydrocephalus refers to the accumulation of CSF in the subarachnoid spaces around the brain without significant enlargement of the ventricular cavities.

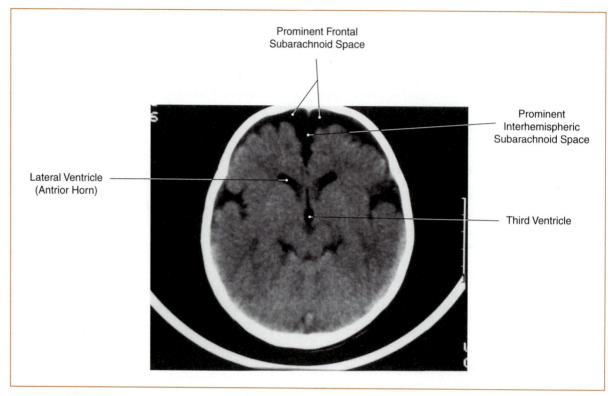

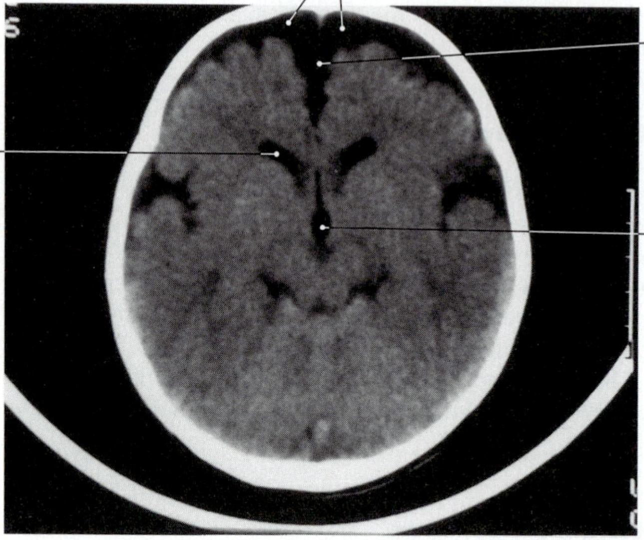
Prominent Frontal
Subarachnoid Space
Prominent
Interhemispheric
Subarachnoid Space
Lateral Ventricle
(Antrior Horn)
Third Ventricle

FIGURE 30-8

Computed axial tomography scan (CT) showing accumulation of cerebrospinal fluid in the subarachnoid space over the frontal lobe and in the interhemispheric fissure as seen in benign external hydrocephalus.

IDIOPATHIC INTRACRANIAL HYPERTENSION (PSEUDOTUMOR CEREBRI) AND BENIGN INTRACRANIAL HYPERTENSION

Idiopathic intracranial hypertension (IIH), which was described by Quincke in 1891, is a disorder characterized by increased intracranial pressure without hydrocephalus or brain tumor. It is more common in adult obese women of childbearing age and affects both sexes equally in childhood. These patients complain of headache, papilledema, and transient **visual obscuration.** Imaging studies usually show small ventricles. The condition responds to acetazolamide (Diamox), a carbonic anhydrase inhibitor, and to corticosteroids, both of which reduce or inhibit the formation of CSF. Studies of CSF hydrodynamics in **pseudotumor cerebri** differentiate two types: type I with normal CSF conductance and type II with very low conductance and high CSF pressure. Type I is believed to result from extracellular brain edema, and type II from impaired CSF resorption through the arachnoid granulations. CSF hydrodynamic studies suggest that patients with type II IIH share a common physiologic mechanism with patients who have normal-pressure hydrocephalus.

Visual obscuration. Transient dimming of vision caused by increased intracranial pressure.

Pseudotumor cerebri. A condition consisting of a rise in intracranial pressure in the absence of an intracranial mass or hydrocephalus. Known by other terms, including idiopathic intracranial hypertension, hydrops, serous meningitis, Julien-Marie-See syndrome, Dupré's syndrome, and Symonds syndrome. First described by Quincke in 1891.

KEY CONCEPTS

- Idiopathic intracranial hypertension is characterized by increased intracranial pressure without hydrocephalus or a brain tumor, small ventricular cavities, and a favorable response to acetazolamide or corticosteroids.

INTRAVENTRICULAR NEUROEPITHELIAL CYSTS

Intraventricular cysts are rare developmental cysts lined by neuroepithelium. The precise origin of these cysts is controversial. They are believed to arise from choroid plexus tissue derived from primitive neuroepithelium. They have been reported to occur in all the ventricular cavities, but most commonly in the third ventricle (colloid cysts of the third ventricle). A variety of names have been used to describe these cysts, including epithelial cysts, ependymal cysts, choroid plexus cysts, choroidal epithelial cysts, and subarachnoid ependymal cysts. The term *neuroepithelial cysts* was introduced by Fulton and Bailey in 1929. Intraventricular cysts contain a clear serous liquid resembling CSF with a mildly elevated protein content. The fluid in colloid cysts of the third ventricle is usually viscid with a gelatinous or mucinous appearance. Intraventricular cysts are clearly visible on magnetic resonance imaging (Fig. 30-9). They usually are asymptomatic and are found accidentally on neuroimaging studies. Some may enlarge and become symptomatic.

THE BOBBLE-HEAD DOLL SYNDROME

The **bobble-head doll syndrome** is a disorder of childhood characterized by a to-and-fro, 2- to 3-Hz rhythmic nodding of the head similar to that in a doll with a weighted head attached to a coil-spring neck. The movement disappears in the supine position and during sleep. This disorder was described by Benton in 1966. In the majority of cases the syndrome is associated with an intraventricular cyst in the region of the anterior third ventricle (Fig. 30-10) or an arachnoid cyst in the suprasellar region. The phenomenon results from intermittent obstruction of the foramen of Monro by the cyst. The head bobbing is believed to be a learned behavior which relieves the obstruction by means of posterior displacement of the cyst away from the foramen of Monro. The syndrome has less commonly been described in association with aqueductal stenosis and shunt obstruction. The syndrome is treated by shunting or fenestration of the cyst.

Bobble-head doll syndrome. A syndrome of to-and-fro rhythmic movement of the head associated with anterior third ventricle cysts or tumors. The movement is believed to be a learned behavior that relieves obstruction of the foramen of Monro.

DANDY-WALKER SYNDROME (MALFORMATION)

The Dandy-Walker malformation (Fig. 30-11) consists of the triad of (1) large cystic dilatation of the posterior part of the fourth ventricle, (2) complete or partial agenesis of the cerebellar vermis, and (3) enlargement of the posterior fossa with upward displacement of the tentorium, torcula, and transverse sinus. Hydrocephalus, though common, is not an essential feature of the syndrome. The syndrome

KEY CONCEPTS

- Intraventricular neuroepithelial cysts are developmental cysts lined by neuroepithelium. Most are asymptomatic.
- Intraventricular cysts may occur in any of the ventricular cavities but are most common in the third ventricle (colloid cysts of the third ventricle).
- The bobble-head doll syndrome is characterized by a to-and-fro rhythmic nodding of the head that resembles the movements of a doll with a weighted head attached to a coil-spring neck.
- Bobble-head doll syndrome is associated with third ventricular cysts and less commonly is associated with aqueductal stenosis and shunt obstruction.

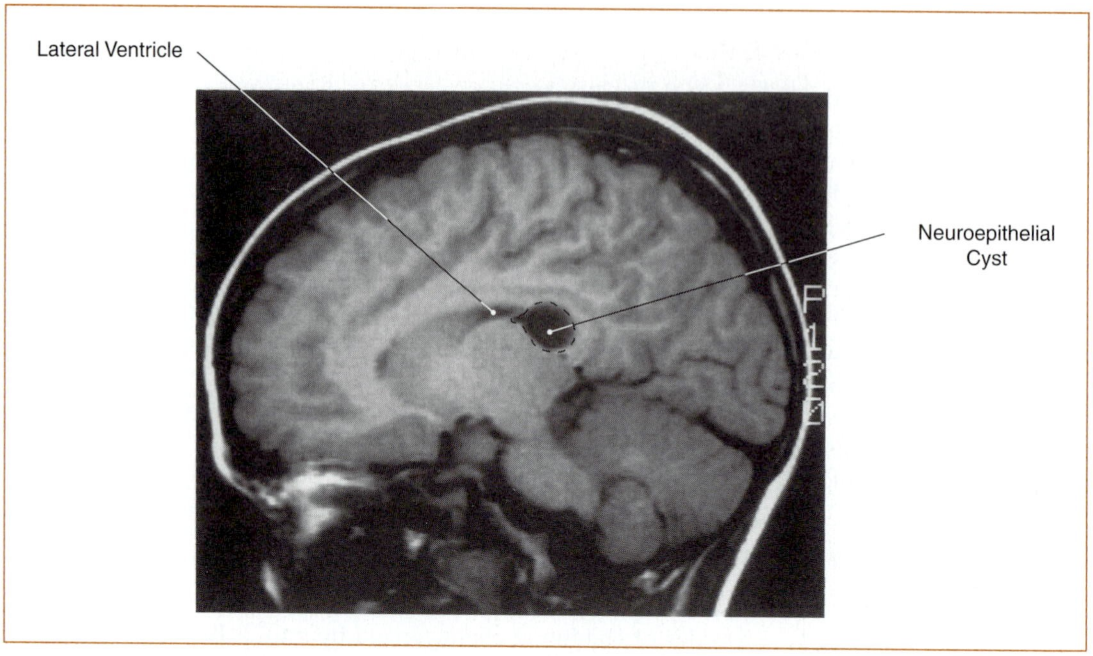

FIGURE 30-9

T1-weighted parasagittal magnetic resonance image (MRI) showing a neuroepithelial cyst in the posterior part of the lateral ventricle.

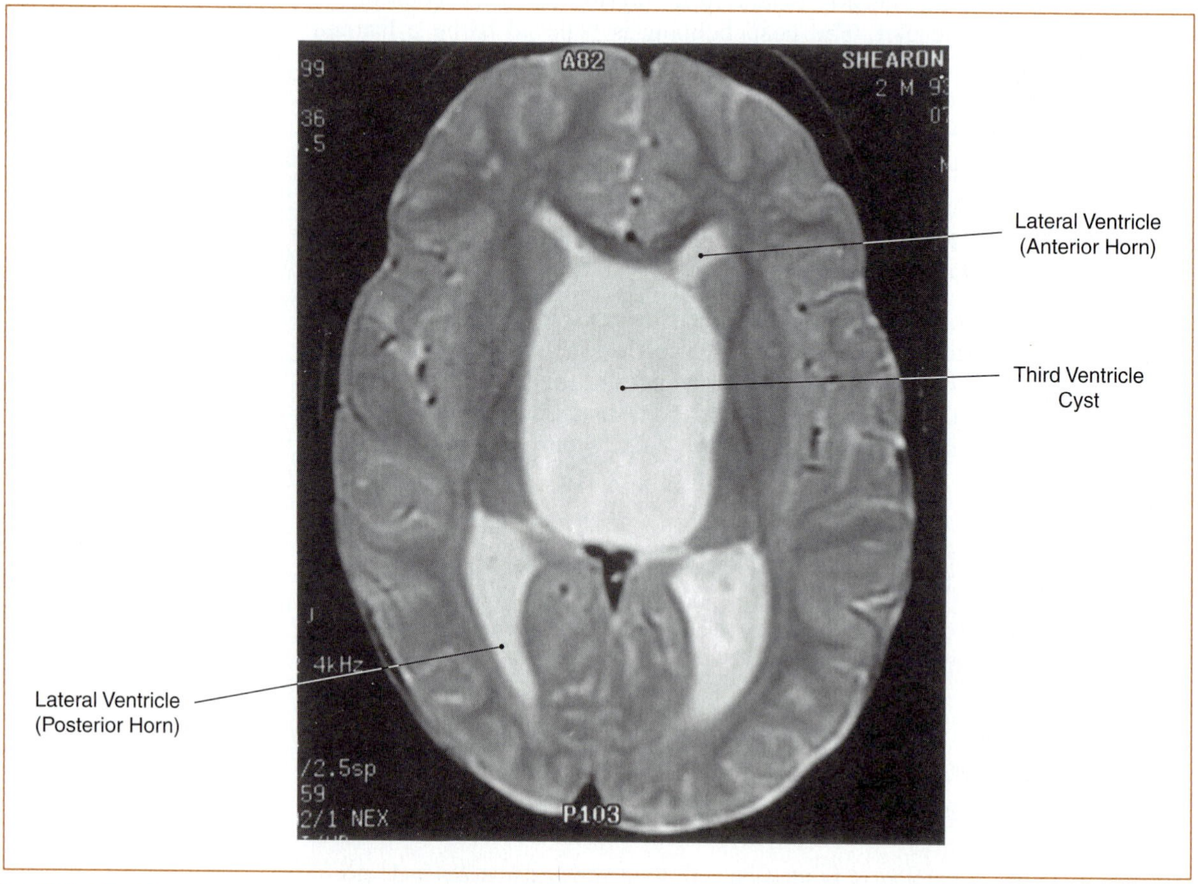

FIGURE 30-10

T2-weighted axial magnetic resonance image (MRI) showing a third ventricle cyst in the bobble-head doll syndrome.

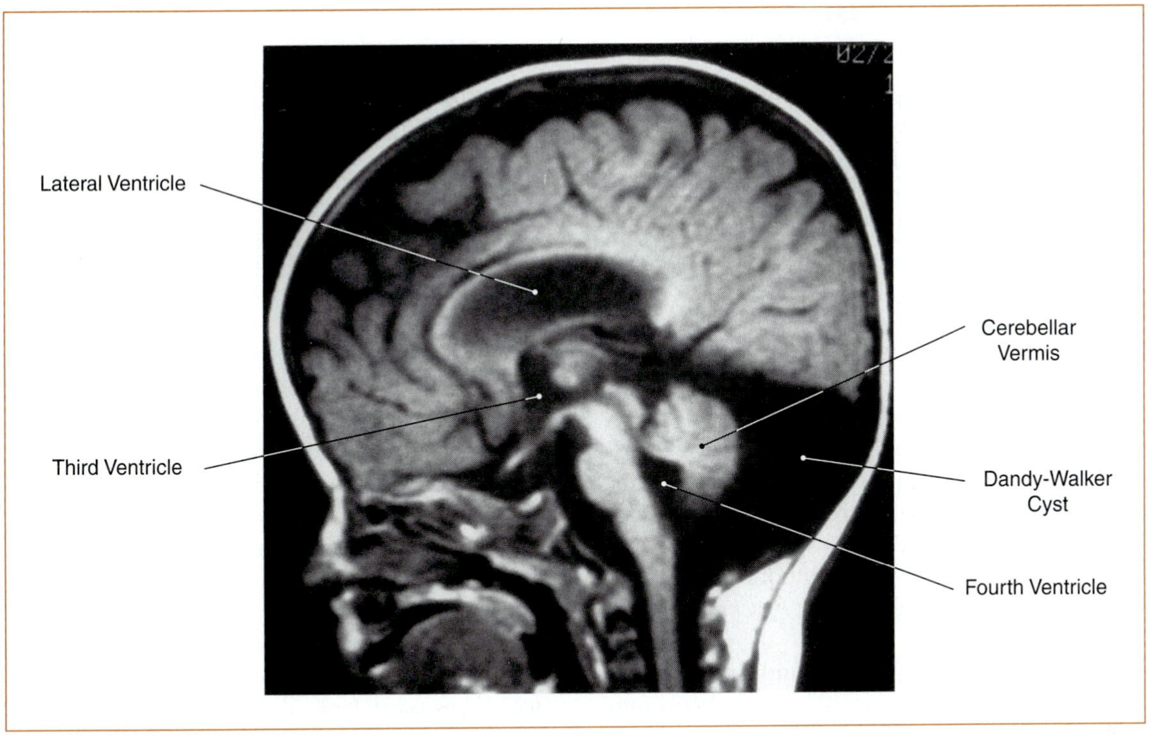

FIGURE 30-11

T1-weighted midsagittal magnetic resonance image (MRI) showing features of the Dandy-Walker syndrome.

was described by Sutton in 1887 and was recognized as a distinct entity in 1914 by Dandy and Blackfan, who attributed it to atresia of the foramina of Magendie and Luschka. In 1942 Taggart and Walker documented the entity and supported the proposed etiology of atresia. The term **Dandy-Walker syndrome** was proposed in 1954 by Benda, who recognized that atresia of the foramina of Magendie and Luschka is not an essential feature of the syndrome. The pathogenesis of the syndrome remains controversial. The syndrome arises early in gestation, at about 4 weeks, and involves multiple developmental defects of the central nervous system. Foraminal atresia may be a contributing factor in some cases. The cystic dilatation of the fourth ventricle is attributed to the persistence of the anterior membranous area that forms the roof of the fetal fourth ventricle, which ordinarily regresses and disappears as the choroid plexus and vermis develop.

Various treatment modalities have been tried with varying success, including ventriculoperitoneal shunting, opening of the fourth ventricle, and excision of the cyst membrane. Current treatment consists of shunting of the cyst to the peritoneum (cystoperitoneal shunt) combined with shunting of the lateral ventricles to the peritoneum (ventriculoperitoneal shunt).

Dandy-Walker syndrome. A developmental malformation characterized by large cystic dilatation of the fourth ventricle, agenesis of the cerebellar vermis, and upward displacement of the tentorium cerebelli, torcula, and transverse sinus. The condition was first described by J. B. Sutton in 1887 and was recognized as a distinct entity by Dandy and Blackfan in 1914 and by Taggert and Walker in 1942. The term *Dandy-Walker syndrome* was proposed by Benda in 1954.

KEY CONCEPTS

- Dandy-Walker syndrome is characterized by the triad of large cystic dilation of the fourth ventricle, agenesis of the cerebellar vermis, and enlargement of the posterior fossa.
- Atresia of the foramina of Magendie and Luschka or hydrocephalus may occur, but these entities are not essential to the diagnosis of Dandy-Walker syndrome.

SUGGESTED READINGS

Benda CE: The Dandy-Walker syndrome or the so-called atresia of the foramen of Magendie. *J Neuropathol Exp Neurol* 1954; 13:14–29.

Benson DF, et al: Diagnosis of normal pressure hydrocephalus. *N Engl J Med* 1970; 283:609–615.

Benton JW, et al: The bobble-head doll syndrome. *Neurology* 1966; 16:725–729.

Coker SB: Bobble-head doll syndrome due to trapped fourth ventricle and aqueduct. *Pediatr Neurol* 1986; 2:115–116.

Czervionke LF, et al: Neuroepithelial cysts of the lateral ventricle: MR appearance. *AJNR* 1987; 8:609–613.

Dandy WE, Blackfan KD: Internal hydrocephalus: An experimental, clinical, and pathological study. *Am J Dis Child* 1914; 8:406–482.

Dell S: Further observation on the "bobble-head doll syndrome." *J Neurol Neurosurg Psychiatry* 1981; 44:1046–1049.

Hart MN, et al: The Dandy-Walker syndrome: A clinicopathological study based on 28 cases. *Neurology* 1972; 22:771–780.

Herskowitz J, et al: Colpocephaly: Clinical, radiologic, and pathogenetic aspects. *Neurology* 1985; 35:1594–1598.

Leech RW, Goldstein E: Hydrocephalus: Classification and mechanisms. In Leech RW, Brumback RA (eds): *Hydrocephalus: Current Clinical Concepts.* St. Louis, Mosby 1991:45–70.

Norman MG, et al: Dandy Walker syndrome. In Norman MG, McGillivray BC, Kalousek DA, Hill A, Poskitt KJ (eds): *Congenital Malformations of the Brain: Pathological, Embryological, Clinical, Radiological, and Genetic Aspects.* New York, Oxford University Press, 1995:343–347.

Norman MG, et al: Hydrocephalus. In Norman MG, McGillivray BC, Kalousek DA, Hill A, Poskitt KJ (eds): *Congenital Malformations of the Brain: Pathological, Embryological, Clinical, Radiological, and Genetic Aspects.* New York, Oxford University Press, 1995:333–339.

New PFJ, Davis KR: Intraventricular noncolloid neuroepithelial cysts. *AJNR* 1981; 2:569–576.

Papazian O, et al: The history of hydrocephalus. *Int Pediatr* 1991; 6:233–235.

Pryse-Phillips W: *Companion to Clinical Neurology.* Boston, Little, Brown, 1995.

Puden RH: The surgical treatment of hydrocephalus: An historical review. *Surg Neurol* 1981; 15:15–26.

Sahar A, et al: Choroid plexus papilloma: Hydrocephalus and cerebrospinal fluid dynamics. *Surg Neurol* 1980; 13:476–478.

Sarnat HB: Dandy-Walker malformation. In Norman MG, McGillivray BC, Kalousek DA, Hill A, Poskitt KJ (eds): *Cerebral Dysgenesis: Embryology and Clinical Expression.* New York, Oxford University Press, 1992:305–316.

Sutton JB: The lateral recesses of the fourth ventricle: Their relation to certain cysts and tumors of the cerebellum and to occipital meningocele. *Brain* 1887; 9:352–361.

Taggart JK, Walker AE: Congenital atresia of the foramens of Luschka and Magendie. *Arch Neurol Psychiatr* 1942; 48:583–612.

Wiese JA, et al: Bobble-head doll syndrome: Review of the pathophysiology and CSF dynamics. *Pediatr Neurol* 1985; 1:361–366.

Williams MA, Razumovsky AY: Cerebrospinal fluid circulation, cerebral edema, and intracranial pressure. *Curr Opin Neurol* 1996; 6:847–853.

CHAPTER 31

MAJOR SENSORY AND MOTOR PATHWAYS

MAJOR SENSORY PATHWAYS

Pathway for Conscious Proprioception

The pathway for **kinesthesia** (position and vibration sense) and discriminative touch (well-localized touch and two-point discrimination) is the posterior column–medial lemniscus system (Fig. 31-1).

The **receptors** for this system are (1) cutaneous mechanoreceptors (hair follicles and touch pressure receptors) which convey the sensations of touch, vibration, hair movement, and pressure and (2) proprioceptive receptors (muscle spindle, **Golgi tendon organ,** and joint receptors). Muscle receptors (muscle spindles and Golgi tendon organs) are the primary receptors that convey position sense. Joint receptors may be concerned with signaling joint movement but not joint position.

Proprioception (Latin *proprius,* "one's own"; *perceptio,* "perception"). The sense of position and movement.

Kinesthesia (Greek *kinesis,* "motion"; *aisthesis,* "sensation"). The sense of perception of movement.

Receptor (Latin *recipere,* "to receive"). A sensory nerve ending or sensory organ that receives sensory stimuli.

Golgi tendon organ. Specialized stretch receptors in the tendons. Named after Camillo Golgi, an Italian anatomist.

KEY CONCEPTS

- The major sensory pathways include those for conscious proprioception (posterior column–medial lemniscus system), unconscious proprioception (dorsal and ventral spinocerebellar tracts), and pain and temperature (spinothalamic tract).
- The receptors for the posterior column–medial lemniscus system are cutaneous mechanoreceptors and proprioceptive receptors in muscles, tendons, and joints.

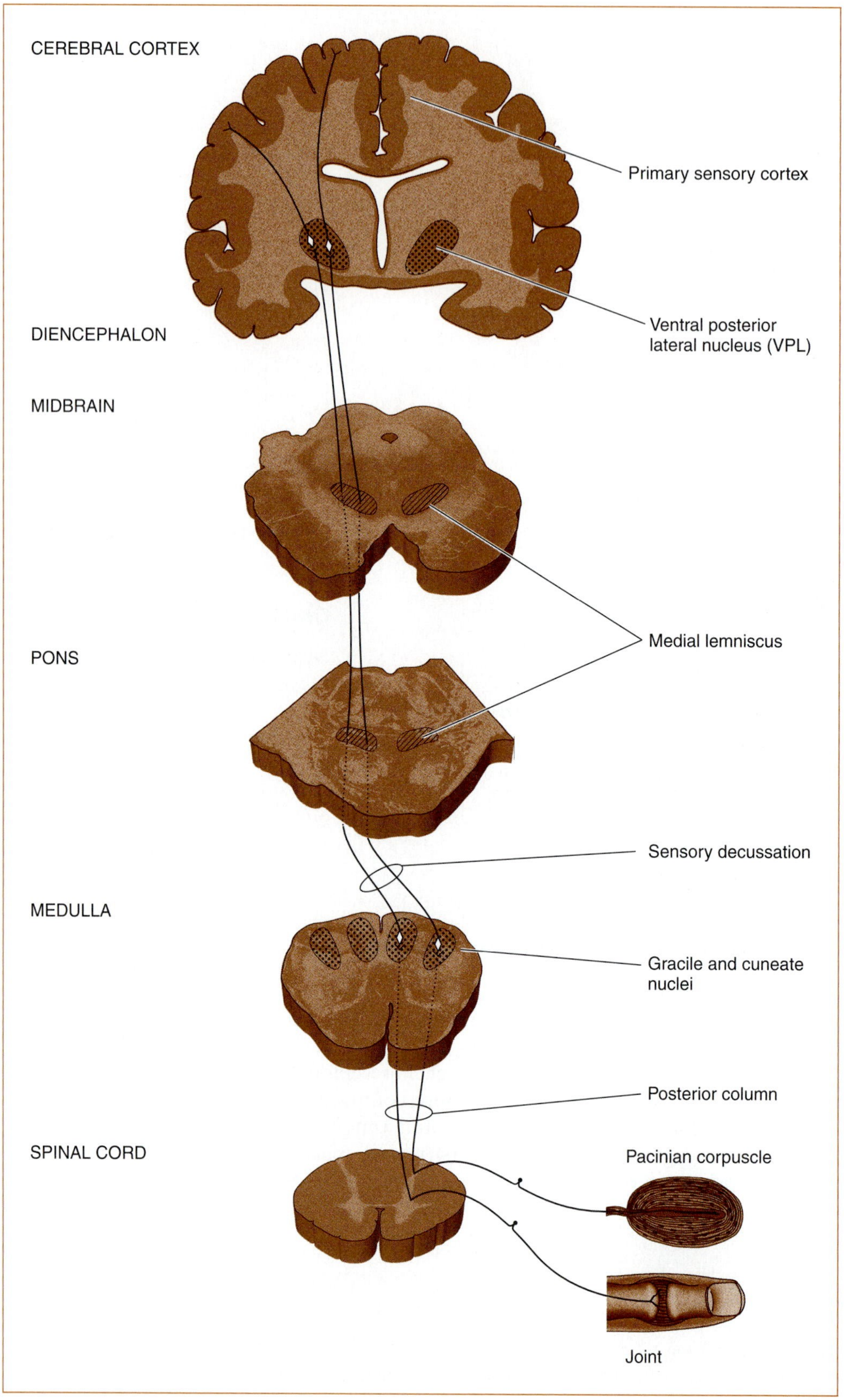
CEREBRAL CORTEX
Primary sensory cortex
DIENCEPHALON
Ventral posterior lateral nucleus (VPL)
MIDBRAIN
Medial lemniscus
PONS
Sensory decussation
MEDULLA
Gracile and cuneate nuclei
Posterior column
SPINAL CORD
Pacinian corpuscle
Joint

FIGURE 31-1

Schematic diagram of the pathway for kinesthesia and discriminative touch.

Impulses arising in the receptors travel via the thickly myelinated large nerve fibers that enter the spinal cord as the dorsolateral division of the posterior (dorsal) root and occupy the posterior **funiculus** of the spinal cord. Those arising below the sixth thoracic spinal segment form the medial part of the posterior funiculus (gracile tract). Those arising above the sixth thoracic segment form the lateral part of the posterior funiculus (cuneate tract). Fibers in the gracile and cuneate tracts project on neurons in the posterior column nuclei of the medulla oblongata (nuclei gracilis and cuneatus). Axons of neurons in the posterior column nuclei (second-order neurons, internal arcuate fibers) decussate in the tegmentum of the medulla oblongata (sensory, lemniscal **decussation**) to form the medial lemniscus, which ascends throughout the medulla oblongata, pons, and midbrain to terminate on neurons of the ventral posterolateral nucleus (VPL) of the thalamus. The axons of neurons in this thalamic nucleus (third-order neurons) project on the terminal station of this pathway in the somesthetic (primary sensory) cortex of the parietal lobe.

Funiculus (Latin *funis,* "cord"). A bundle of white matter containing one or more tracts.

Gracilis (Latin, "slender, thin"). The fasciculus or tractus gracilis is so named because it is slender.

Cuneatus (Latin, "wedge"). The fasciculus cuneatus is so named because of its wedge shape.

Decussation (Latin *decussare,* "to cross like an X"). X-shaped crossing of nerve fiber tracts in the midline, as in the motor (pyramidal) and sensory (lemniscal) decussations.

Lesions in the posterior column–medial lemniscus system are manifested clinically by the following signs:

1. Inability to identify the position of a limb in space with the eyes closed. These patients are unable to tell whether a joint is in a position of flexion or one of extension.
2. Inability to identify objects placed in the hands, such as keys and coins, from their shape, size, and texture with the eyes closed.
3. Loss of two-point discrimination. These patients are unable to recognize two stimuli simultaneously applied to the skin when the stimuli are separated by the minimal necessary distance for their proper identification as two stimuli.
4. Inability to perceive vibration when a vibrating tuning fork is applied to a bony prominence.
5. Inability to maintain a steady standing posture when the eyes are closed and the feet are placed close together (**Romberg test**). These patients begin to sway and may fall when they close their eyes, eliminating visual compensation.

Romberg test. A test for conscious proprioception. The inability to maintain a steady standing posture when the eyes are closed and the feet are placed close together. Named after Moritz Heinrich Romberg, a German physician who described the test in 1840.

Some of the fibers in the posterior funiculus send collateral branches that terminate on neurons in the gray matter of the posterior horn. These collaterals give the posterior column system a role in modifying sensory activity in the posterior horn. This role is inhibitory to pain impulses. Thus, lesions in the posterior funiculus decrease the threshold to painful stimuli. Nonpainful stimuli become painful, and painful stimuli are triggered by lower stimulation thresholds.

In addition to its classical role in sensory transmission, the dorsal column plays a role in certain types of motor control. The dorsal column transmits to the motor

KEY CONCEPTS

- The posterior column is somatotopically organized into the gracile tract and the cuneate tract. Gracile fibers are those entering the spinal cord below the sixth thoracic segment and include lower extremity fibers. Cuneate fibers are those entering above the sixth thoracic segment and include upper extremity fibers.
- Posterior column fibers ascend ipsilateral to their side of entry into the spinal cord and synapse on the nuclei gracilis and cuneatus in the medulla oblongata.
- Second-order fibers from the nuclei gracilis and cuneatus cross in the medulla oblongata (sensory, lemniscal decussation) to form the medial lemniscus.
- Medial lemniscal fibers terminate on neurons in the ventral posterior lateral nucleus of the thalamus.

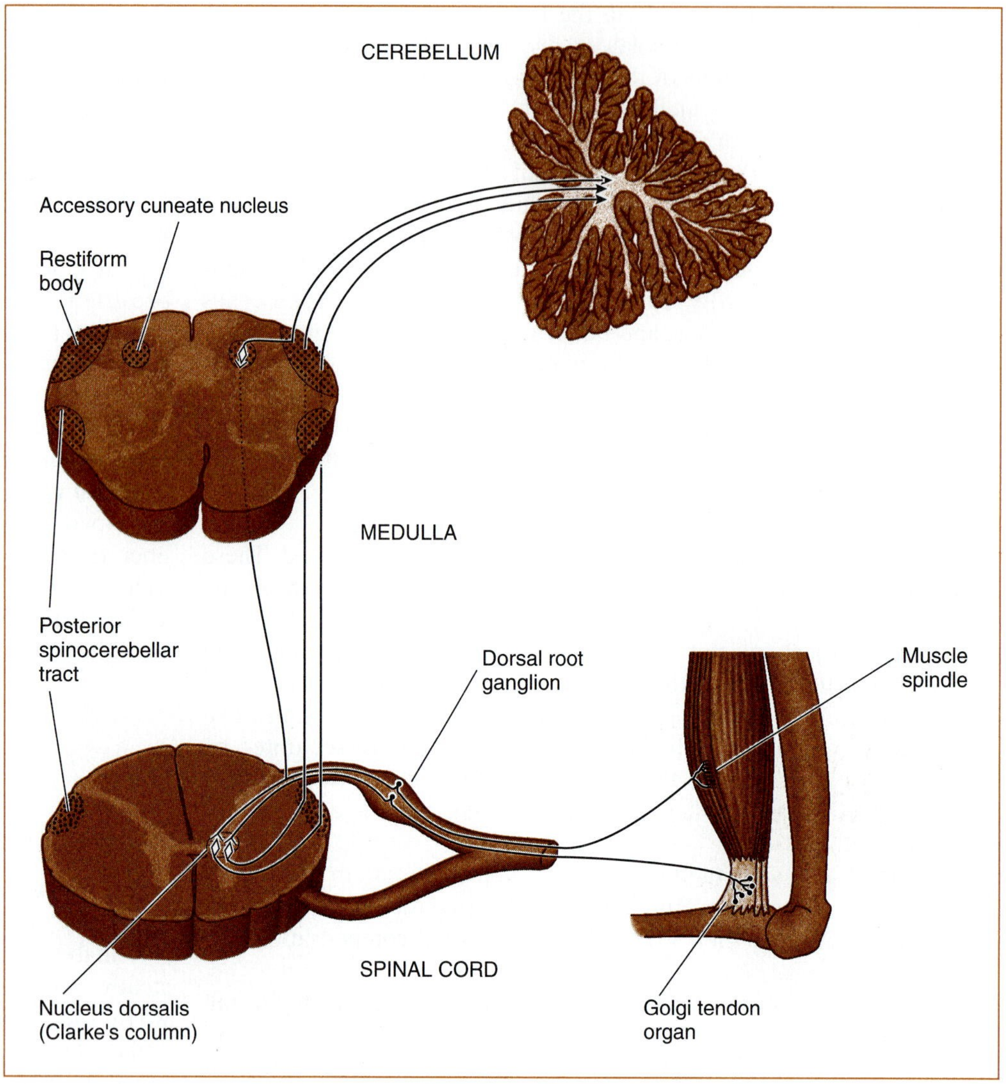
CEREBELLUM
Accessory cuneate nucleus
Restiform body
MEDULLA
Posterior spinocerebellar tract
Dorsal root ganglion
Muscle spindle
SPINAL CORD
Nucleus dorsalis (Clarke's column)
Golgi tendon organ

FIGURE 31-2

Schematic diagram of the posterior spinocerebellar pathway.

cortex sensory information from muscle spindles, joint receptors, and cutaneous receptors that is necessary in planning, initiating, programming, and monitoring tasks that involve manipulative movements by the digits.

Pathways for Nonconscious Proprioception

Nucleus dorsalis (Clarke's nucleus). A nucleus in the intermediate zone of the spinal cord gray matter that gives rise to the dorsal spinocerebellar tract. Named after Jacob Augustus Lockhart Clarke, an English anatomist who described this nucleus in 1851.

Nonconscious proprioception is mediated via the two spinocerebellar tracts (Figs. 31-2 and 31-3), the posterior (dorsal) and the anterior (ventral).

The posterior spinocerebellar tract conveys impulses from the muscle spindle and the Golgi tendon organ. Such impulses travel via groups Ia, Ib, and II nerve fibers; enter the spinal cord in the dorsolateral, thickly myelinated, large-diameter fiber portion of the posterior root; and project on the ipsilateral **nucleus dorsalis** (Clarke's nucleus) and the accessory cuneate nucleus. Axons of neurons in the nucleus dorsalis (second-order neurons) form the posterior spinocerebellar tract, which ascends in the lateral funiculus of the spinal cord and the medulla oblongata

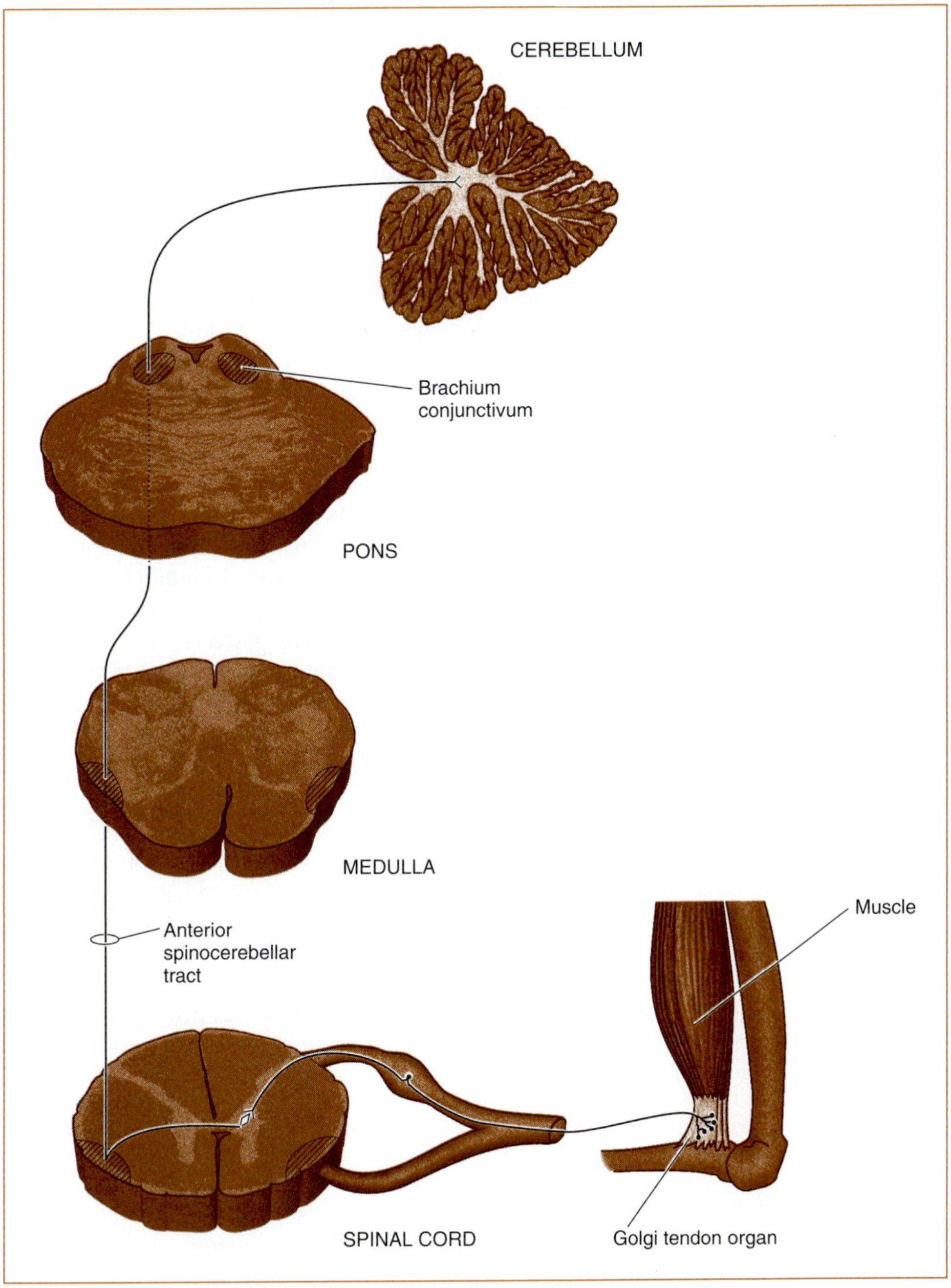

FIGURE 31-3

Schematic diagram of the anterior spinocerebellar pathway.

to reach the cerebellum via the inferior cerebellar peduncle (**restiform body**). Axons of neurons in the accessory cuneate nucleus form the cuneocerebellar tract, which reaches the cerebellum via the restiform body. Information relayed to the cerebellum via the posterior spinocerebellar tract and the cuneocerebellar tract relates to muscle contraction, including the phase, rate, and strength of contraction.

Restiform body (Latin *restis,* "a rope"; *forma,* "form" or "shape"). The restiform body (inferior cerebellar peduncle) is a compact bundle of nerve fibers connecting the medulla oblongata and the cerebellum. It was described and named by Humphrey Ridley, an English anatomist, in 1695.

KEY CONCEPTS

- Receptors for the posterior (dorsal) spinocerebellar tract are in the muscle spindle and Golgi tendon organ.

The anterior spinocerebellar tract conveys impulses from the Golgi tendon organ via Ib afferents. Incoming fibers project on neurons in the posterior horn of the spinal cord (laminae V to VII). Axons of neurons in these laminae decussate to the contralateral lateral funiculus to form the anterior spinocerebellar tract, which ascends throughout the spinal cord, medulla oblongata, and pons; loops backward to join the superior cerebellar peduncle (brachium conjunctivum); and enters the cerebellum. The anterior spinocerebellar tract conveys to the cerebellum information related to interneuronal activity and the effectiveness of descending pathways.

Lesions in the spinocerebellar pathways (such as those which occur in hereditary spinocerebellar degeneration) result in incoordinate movement. These patients tend to walk with a wide base, stagger, and frequently fall.

Pathway for Pain and Temperature

Small-diameter, unmyelinated, or thinly myelinated fibers (C fibers and A delta fibers) that convey pain and thermal sensations (Fig. 31-4) enter the spinal cord via the ventrolateral division of the dorsal (posterior) root. Within the spinal cord they ascend for one or two segments and project on neurons in several laminae (I to VI) in the posterior horn. From tract neurons in laminae I and V to VII, axons cross in the anterior white commissure and form the lateral spinothalamic tract in the lateral funiculus. Sacral fibers are laterally placed in the tract, and cervical fibers are more medially placed. The spinothalamic tract ascends throughout the spinal cord and brain stem to project on neurons in the VPL of the thalamus. Axons of VPL neurons project to the somesthetic cortex.

Lesions of the spinothalamic tract result in diminution or loss of pain and thermal sense contralateral to the lesion. When the tract is affected in the spinal cord, the sensory deficit begins one or two segments below the level of the lesion.

The spinothalamic tract may be sectioned surgically (cordotomy) to relieve intractable pain.

Trigeminal Pathways

Exteroceptive (Latin, "to take outside"). Received from outside. Exteroceptive receptors receive impulses from the outside.

The trigeminal pathways convey **exteroceptive** and proprioceptive sensations from the face to the thalamus. They thus correspond to the spinothalamic and posterior

KEY CONCEPTS

- The cuneocerebellar tract is homologous to the dorsal spinocerebellar tract
- Cells of origin of the dorsal spinocerebellar and cuneocerebellar tracts are in the nucleus dorsalis (Clarke's nucleus) and the accessory cuneate nucleus, respectively.
- Receptors for the anterior (ventral) spinocerebellar tract are in the Golgi tendon organ.
- Cells of origin of the ventral spinocerebellar tract are in laminae V to VII of the dorsal horn.
- The dorsal spinocerebellar tract reaches the cerebellum via the restiform body. The ventral spinocerebellar tract reaches the cerebellum via the brachium conjunctivum.
- Cells of origin of the spinothalamic tract are in laminae I and V to VII of the dorsal horn.
- The spinothalamic fibers are somatotopically organized so that sacral originating fibers are lateral in the tract and cervical originating fibers are medial in the tract.
- Spinothalamic fibers terminate on neurons in the ventral posterior lateral nucleus of the thalamus.

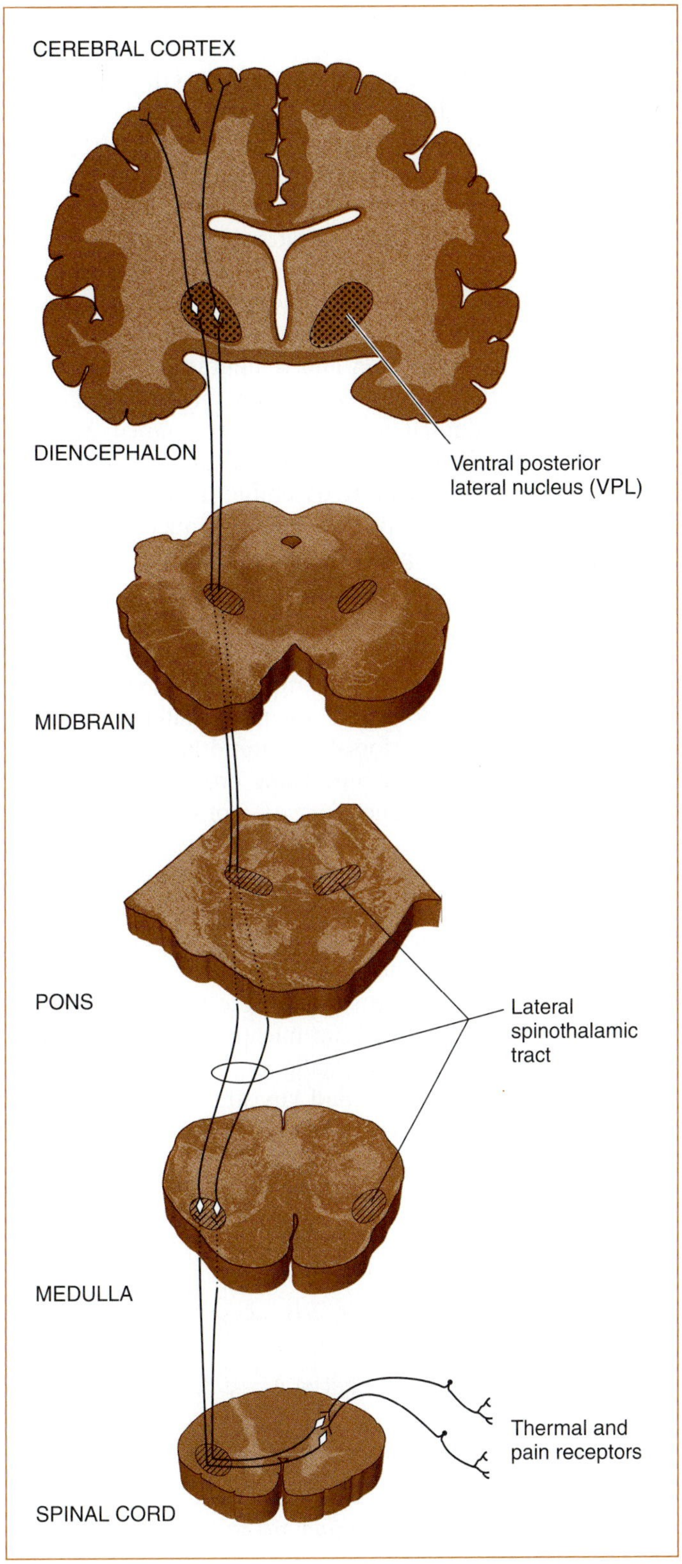
CEREBRAL CORTEX
DIENCEPHALON
Ventral posterior
lateral nucleus (VPL)
MIDBRAIN
PONS
Lateral
spinothalamic
tract
MEDULLA
Thermal and
pain receptors
SPINAL CORD

FIGURE 31-4

Schematic diagram of the pathway for specific pain and temperature sensations.

column–medial lemniscus pathways, which convey similar sensations from the rest of the body.

Exteroceptive fibers are general somatic sensory fibers that convey pain, temperature, and touch sensations from the face and the anterior aspect of the head. Neurons of origin of these fibers are located in the semilunar (gasserian) **ganglion** (see Fig. 7-18). Peripheral processes of neurons in the ganglion are distributed in the three divisions of the trigeminal nerve: ophthalmic, maxillary, and mandibular. Central processes of these unipolar neurons enter the lateral aspect of the pons and distribute themselves as follows.

Ganglion (Greek, "swelling, knot"). A collection of nerve cells outside the central nervous system, as in the gasserian (trigeminal) ganglion.

Some of these fibers descend in the pons and the medulla and down to the level of the second or third cervical spinal segment as the descending (spinal) tract of the trigeminal nerve. They convey pain and temperature sensations. Throughout their caudal course these fibers project on neurons in the adjacent nucleus of the descending tract of the trigeminal nerve (spinal trigeminal nucleus). Axons of neurons in the spinal trigeminal nucleus cross the midline and form the ventral secondary ascending trigeminal (ventral trigeminothalamic) tract, which courses rostrally to terminate in the ventral posterior medial nucleus of the thalamus.

Other incoming fibers of the trigeminal nerve bifurcate on entry into the pons into ascending and descending branches. These fibers convey touch sensation. The descending branches join the spinal tract of the trigeminal nerve and follow the course that was outlined above. The shorter ascending branches project on the main (principal) sensory nucleus of the trigeminal nerve (see Fig. 7-18). From the main sensory nucleus, second-order fibers ascend ipsilaterally and contralaterally as the dorsal ascending trigeminal (dorsal trigeminothalamic) tract to the ventral posterior medial nucleus of the thalamus. Some crossed fibers also travel in the ventral ascending trigeminal tract. Once formed, both secondary trigeminal tracts (dorsal and ventral) lie lateral to the medial lemniscus between it and the spinothalamic tract. A schematic summary of the afferent and efferent trigeminal roots and their nuclei is shown in Fig. 7-19. Recent studies of trigeminothalamic fibers have revealed that the bulk of these fibers arise from the main sensory nucleus and the interpolaris segment of the spinal nucleus.

Proprioceptive fibers from deep structures of the face are peripheral processes of unipolar neurons in the mesencephalic nucleus of the trigeminal located at the rostral pontine and caudal mesencephalic levels. Proprioceptive fibers to the mesencephalic nucleus convey pressure and kinesthesia from the teeth, periodontium, hard palate, and joint capsules as well as impulses from stretch receptors in the muscles of mastication. The output from the mesencephalic nucleus is destined for the cerebellum, the thalamus, the motor nuclei of the brain stem, and the

KEY CONCEPTS

- Trigeminal pathways convey exteroceptive and proprioceptive sensations from the face.
- Exteroceptive fibers that convey pain and temperature from the face terminate on neurons in the spinal trigeminal nucleus.
- Exteroceptive fibers that convey touch from the face terminate on the spinal and main (principal) trigeminal nuclei.
- Proprioceptive fibers are peripheral processes of pseudounipolar neurons in the mesencephalic trigeminal nucleus.
- Second-order neurons of the spinal and main trigeminal nuclei constitute the ventral and dorsal secondary ascending trigeminal tracts, respectively. Both tracts terminate on neurons in the ventral posterior medial nucleus of the thalamus.

reticular formation. The mesencephalic nucleus is concerned with mechanisms that control the force of the bite.

MAJOR MOTOR PATHWAYS

Cortical Origin

Corticospinal (Pyramidal) Tract

The corticospinal tract (see Fig. 17-4) is the most important descending tract. From its origin in the cerebral cortex it descends through all levels of the neuraxis except the cerebellum. It arises primarily from the motor (area 4) and premotor (area 6) cortices and passes through the internal capsule, the cerebral peduncle, the basis pontis, and the pyramids of the medulla oblongata. In the caudal medulla, about 75 to 90 percent of the fibers decussate through the motor or pyramidal decussation to form the lateral corticospinal tract in the lateral funiculus of the spinal cord. About 8 percent of pyramidal fibers remain uncrossed and form the anterior corticospinal tract (Türck's bundle) in the anterior funiculus of the spinal cord. Fibers in the anterior corticospinal tract decussate at segmental spinal levels. In the final analysis, therefore, roughly about 98 percent of fibers in the pyramidal tract are crossed. The remaining 2 percent remain ipsilateral and form the tract of Barnes. Pyramidal tract fibers influence alpha motorneurons directly or via interneurons. They facilitate flexor motor neurons and inhibit extensor motor neurons. Lateral corticospinal tract fibers terminate on motor neurons in the lateral part of the ventral horn that supply the distal limb musculature. Anterior corticospinal tract fibers terminate on motor neurons in the medial part of the ventral horn that supply the neck, the trunk, and the proximal limb musculature.

The corticospinal tract is essential for skill and precision in movement and the execution of discrete fine finger movements. However, it cannot initiate these movements by itself; other corticofugal (cortically originating) fibers are needed for this. The corticospinal tract also regulates sensory relay processes and the selection of the sensory modality that reaches the cortex. The selection function is achieved via terminations of corticospinal tract fibers on primary afferent fibers and sensory relay neurons in the posterior (dorsal) horn of the spinal cord.

Lesions in this tract result in **paralysis**. If the lesion is above the level of the motor decussation, the paralysis is contralateral to the site of the lesion. In lesions of the pyramidal tract below the decussation, the paralysis is ipsilateral to the site of the lesion. In addition to paralysis, lesions in the corticospinal tract result in a conglomerate of neurologic signs, including (1) spasticity, (2) hyperactive myotatic reflexes (hyperreflexia), (3) Babinski's sign, and (4) clonus. Collectively, this conglomerate of signs is referred to as upper motor neuron signs.

Paralysis (Greek *para,* "beside"; *lyein,* "to loosen"). Loss of voluntary movement.

Corticopontocerebellar Tract

The corticopontocerebellar tract (see Fig. 17-5) constitutes by far the largest component of the cortically originating descending fiber system. It has been estimated to

KEY CONCEPTS

- Major motor pathways are of cortical and subcortical origin.
- Corticospinal fibers originate principally from the motor and premotor areas, descend throughout the neuraxis, mostly decussate in the medulla oblongata (motor decussation), and terminate on interneurons or alpha motorneurons in the spinal cord.

contain approximately 19 million fibers, in contrast to the pyramidal tract, which contains approximately 1 million. The tract originates from wide areas of the cerebral cortex, but primarily from the primary sensory and motor cortices, and descends in the internal capsule, cerebral peduncle, and basis pontis, from which its fibers project on pontine nuclei. Second-order neurons from pontine nuclei cross to the contralateral side of the basis pontis, enter the middle cerebellar peduncle (brachium pontis), and project on the cerebellum.

Although the pontocerebellar projection is primarily crossed, it has been estimated that 30 percent of the pontine projection to the cerebellar vermis and 10 percent of the projection to the cerebellar hemisphere are ipsilateral. The density of projection to the cerebellar hemisphere is three times that to the vermis. The corticopontocerebellar tract is somatotopically organized. The primary motor cortex projects to the medial pontine nuclei, the primary sensory cortex projects to the lateral pontine nuclei, the arm area of the sensory motor cortex projects to the dorsal pontine nuclei and the leg area projects to the ventral pontine nuclei, the caudal pontine nuclei project to the anterior lobe of the cerebellum, and the rostral pontine nuclei project to the posterior lobe of the cerebellum. The corticopontocerebellar tract is one of several pathways by which the cerebral cortex influences the cerebellum; it plays a role in the rapid correction of movement. Lesions of the corticopontocerebellar pathway result in **ataxia**. The ataxia that occurs contralateral to frontal or temporal lobe pathology is explained by interruption of the corticopontine pathway.

Somatotopic (Greek *soma,* "body"; *topos,* "place"). Representation of parts of the body in corresponding parts of the brain or spinal cord.

Ataxia (Greek *taxis,* "order"). Lack of order. Lack of coordination with unsteadiness of movement.

Corticobulbar Tract

Corticobulbar fibers (Fig. 31-5) originate from the face areas of the cerebral cortex. They descend in the genu of the internal capsule, the cerebral peduncle (where they occupy a dorsolateral corner of the corticospinal segment of the peduncle as well as a small area in the medial part of the base of the peduncle), and the basis pontis (where they intermix with corticospinal fibers) and pyramid but do not reach the spinal cord. At different levels of the neuraxis, they project on cranial nerve nuclei. Some corticobulbar fibers project directly on cranial nerve nuclei (trigeminal, facial, and hypoglossal); the majority, however, project on reticular nuclei before reaching the cranial nerve nuclei. This system is known as the corticoreticulobulbar tract. The majority of cranial nerve nuclei receive bilateral cortical input. Bilateral interruption of the corticobulbar or corticoreticulobulbar fiber system results in **paresis** (weakness) of the muscles supplied by the corresponding cranial nerve nucleus. This condition is known as pseudobulbar palsy.

Paresis (Greek *parienai,* "to relax, to let go"). Slight or incomplete paralysis.

Other Corticofugal Tracts

Other corticofugal tracts include the corticothalamic, corticostriate, and corticohypothalamic tracts, which serve as feedback mechanisms from the cortex to these sites.

Corticothalamic fibers arise from cortical areas that receive thalamic projections. They descend in the internal capsule and enter the thalamus via the thalamic radiation, which also includes reciprocal thalamocortical fibers.

KEY CONCEPTS

- Corticopontocerebellar fibers constitute the largest component of corticofugal fibers. They originate principally from primary sensory and motor cortices and synapse on pontine nuclei. Second-order neurons from the pontine nuclei terminate in the cerebellum.
- Corticobulbar fibers originate from the face areas of the cerebral cortex and terminate directly or indirectly (via reticular neurons) on cranial nerve nuclei. Most cranial nerve nuclei receive bilateral corticobulbar fibers.

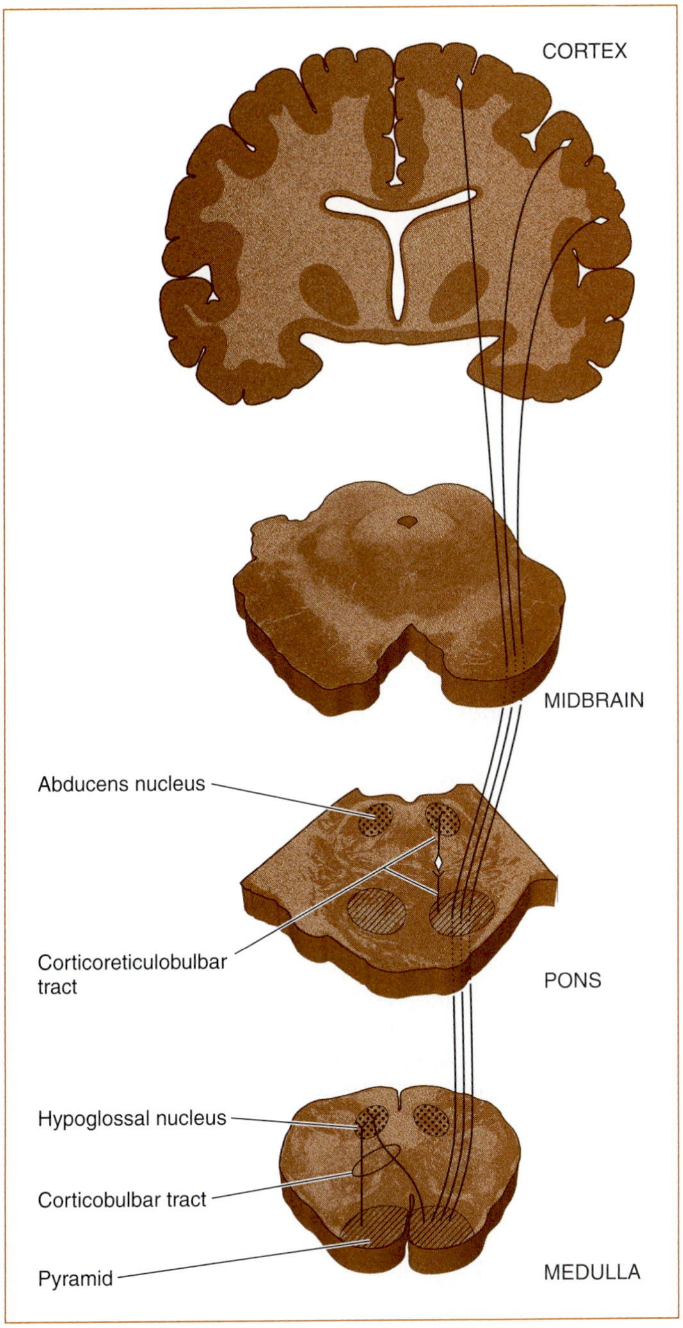

FIGURE 31-5

Schematic diagram of the corticobulbar pathway.

Corticostriate fibers can be direct or indirect. Direct corticostriate projections reach the neostriatum via the internal and external capsules. Indirect corticostriate pathways include the corticothalamostriate and the collaterals of the cortico-olivary and corticopontine pathways. Almost all cortical area contribute to the corticostriate

KEY CONCEPTS

- Corticothalamic fibers originate from cortical areas that receive thalamic projections and serve a feedback mechanism.

projections. Corticostriate pathways are somatotopically organized so that cortical association areas project preferentially to the caudate nucleus, whereas sensorimotor cortical areas preferentially project to the putamen.

Corticohypothalamic fibers arise from the prefrontal cortex, cingulate gyrus, olfactory cortex, hippocampus, and septal area. They reach the hypothalamus via the internal capsule.

Subcortical Origin

Tracts of subcortical origin arise from the midbrain, pons, and medulla oblongata.

Midbrain

Rubro (Latin, *ruber,* "red"). The rubrospinal tract originates from the red nucleus.

The major motor pathway from the midbrain is the **rubro**spinal tract (see Fig. 9-14). This tract originates from neurons in the caudal (magnicellular) part of the red nucleus, crosses in the ventral tegmental decussation of the midbrain, and descends in the midbrain, pons, medulla, and spinal cord, where it occupies a position in the lateral funiculus in close proximity to the lateral corticospinal tract. The rubrospinal tract is considered an indirect corticospinal tract. Like the corticospinal tract, the rubrospinal tract facilitates flexor motor neurons and inhibits extensor motor neurons. In most mammals the rubrospinal tract is the major output of the red nucleus. With evolution the output of the red nucleus to the spinal cord decreased, and in humans the red nucleus sends its major output to the inferior olive, which in turn projects to the cerebellum.

Pons

The major motor pathways emanating from the pons are the lateral and medial vestibulospinal and pontine reticulospinal tracts.

Lateral Vestibulospinal Tract The lateral vestibulospinal tract (see Fig. 7-9) originates from the lateral vestibular nucleus and descends ipsilaterally in the pons, medulla, and spinal cord, where it occupies a position in the lateral funiculus. The lateral vestibulospinal tract terminates on interneurons in laminae VII and VIII, with some direct terminations on alpha motorneuron dendrites in the same laminae. The lateral vestibulospinal tract facilitates extensor motor neurons and inhibits flexor motor neurons.

KEY CONCEPTS

- Corticostriate fibers originate from wide areas of the cortex. Cortical association areas project preferentially on the caudate nucleus, whereas sensorimotor cortical areas project on the putamen.
- Corticohypothalamic fibers arise from the prefrontal cortex, cingulate gyrus, olfactory cortex, hippocampus, and septal area.
- Cortically originating (cortifugal) motor pathways include the corticospinal (pyramidal), corticopontocerebellar, corticobulbar, corticothalamic, corticostriate, and corticohypothalamic tracts.
- The rubrospinal tract originates from the caudal (magnicellular) part of the red nucleus, crosses in the midbrain, and terminates in the gray matter of the spinal cord.
- In humans most efferent fibers of the red nucleus terminate on neurons in the inferior olive.

Medial Vestibulospinal Tract The neurons of origin of the medial vestibulospinal tract are located in the medial vestibular nucleus. From their neurons of origin, fibers join the ipsilateral and contralateral medial longitudinal fasciculus, descend in the anterior funiculus of the cervical cord segments, and terminate on neurons in laminae VII and VIII. They exert a facilitatory effect on flexor motor neurons. This tract plays a role in controlling head position.

Pontine Reticulospinal Tract The pontine reticulospinal tract arises mainly from the medial group of pontine reticular nuclei (nuclei reticularis pontis caudalis and oralis), descends primarily ipsilaterally through the pons and medulla oblongata, and occupies a position in the anterior funiculus of the spinal cord. It facilitates extensor motor neurons and inhibits flexor motor neurons.

Medulla Oblongata The major descending pathway from the medulla oblongata is the medullary reticulospinal tract. It arises mainly from the medial (central) group of medullary reticular nuclei (nucleus reticularis gigantocellularis), descends primarily ipsilateral to its site of origin, and occupies a position in the lateral funiculus of the spinal cord. It facilitates flexor motor neurons and inhibits extensor motor neurons.

KEY CONCEPTS

- The lateral vestibulospinal tract originates from the lateral vestibular nucleus and descends ipsilaterally to terminate on interneurons and dendrites of motor neurons in laminae VII and VIII of the spinal cord.
- The medial vestibulospinal tract originates from the medial vestibular nucleus and descends ipsilaterally and contralaterally as a component of the medial longitudinal fasciculus to terminate on neurons in laminae VII and VIII of the cervical spinal cord.
- Reticulospinal tracts originate from reticular nuclei in the pons and medulla oblongata and descend primarily ipsilaterally but also contralaterally to terminate on laminae VII and VIII of the spinal cord.
- Subcortically originating fibers include the rubrospinal, vestibulospinal, and reticulospinal tracts.

SUGGESTED READINGS

Brodal P: The corticopontine projection in the Rhesus monkey: Origin and principles of organization. *Brain* 1978; 101:251–283.

Brodal P: The pontocerebellar projection in the Rhesus monkey: An experimental study with retrograde axonal transport of horseradish peroxidase. *Neuroscience* 1979; 4:193–208.

Cherubini E, et al: Caudate neuronal responses evoked by cortical stimulation: Contribution of an indirect corticothalamic pathway. *Brain Res* 1979; 173:331–336.

Davidoff RA: The dorsal column. *Neurology* 1989; 39: 1377–1385.

Davidoff RA: The pyramidal tract. *Neurology* 1990; 40:332–339.

Iwatsubo T, et al: Corticofugal projections to the motor nuclei of the brainstem and spinal cord in humans. *Neurology* 1990; 40:309–312.

Matsushita M, et al: Anatomical organization of the spinocerebellar system in the cat as studied by retrograde transport of horseradish peroxidase. *J Comp Neurol* 1979; 184:81–106.

Nathan PW, et al: The corticospinal tract in man: Course and location of fibers at different segmental levels. *Brain* 1990; 113:303–324.

Smith MC, Deacon P: Topographical anatomy of the

posterior column of the spinal cord in man: The long ascending fibers. *Brain* 1984; 107:671–698.

Wiesendanger R, et al: An anatomical investigation of the corticopontine projection in the primate (Macaca fascicularis and Saimiri sciureus): II. The projection from frontal and parietal association areas. *Neuroscience* 1979; 4:747–765.

Willis WD: Studies of the spinothalamic tract. *Tex Rep Biol Med* 1979; 38:1–45.

Yeterian EH, VanHoesen GW: Cortico-striate projections in the Rhesus monkey: The organization of certain cortico-caudate connections. *Brain Res* 1978; 139:43–63.

PART TWO

ATLAS

SECTIONAL ANATOMY

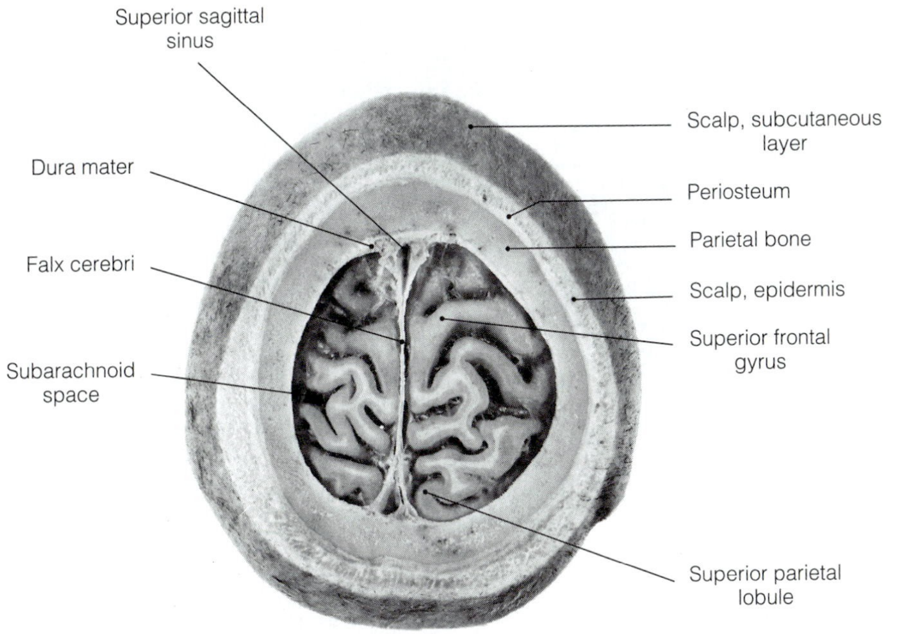
Superior sagittal sinus
Dura mater
Falx cerebri
Subarachnoid space
Scalp, subcutaneous layer
Periosteum
Parietal bone
Scalp, epidermis
Superior frontal gyrus
Superior parietal lobule

FIGURE A1-1

Axial section through the upper part of the cerebral hemispheres showing parts of the frontal and parietal lobes separated by the falx cerebri.

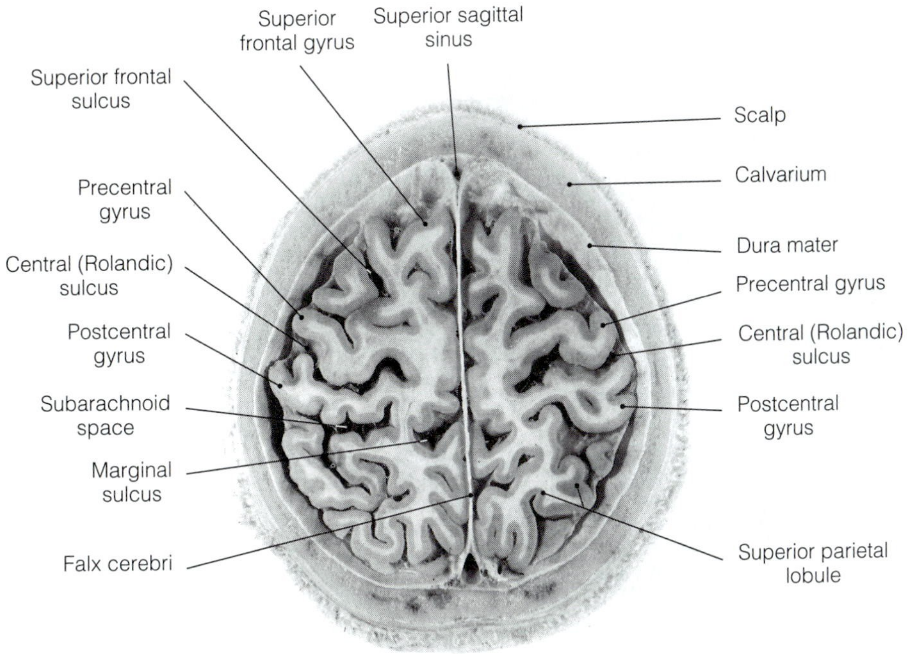
Superior frontal gyrus
Superior sagittal sinus
Superior frontal sulcus
Precentral gyrus
Central (Rolandic) sulcus
Postcentral gyrus
Subarachnoid space
Marginal sulcus
Falx cerebri
Scalp
Calvarium
Dura mater
Precentral gyrus
Central (Rolandic) sulcus
Postcentral gyrus
Superior parietal lobule

FIGURE A1-2

Superficial axial section through the pre- and postcentral gyri.

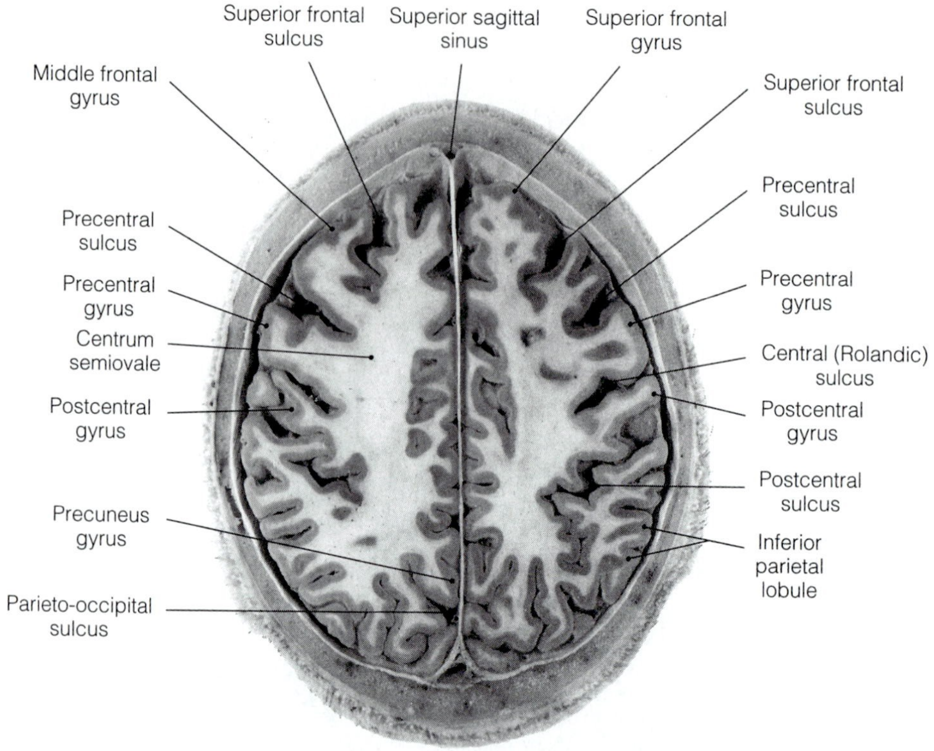

FIGURE A1-3

Axial section through the centrum semiovale in a plane above the lateral ventricles.

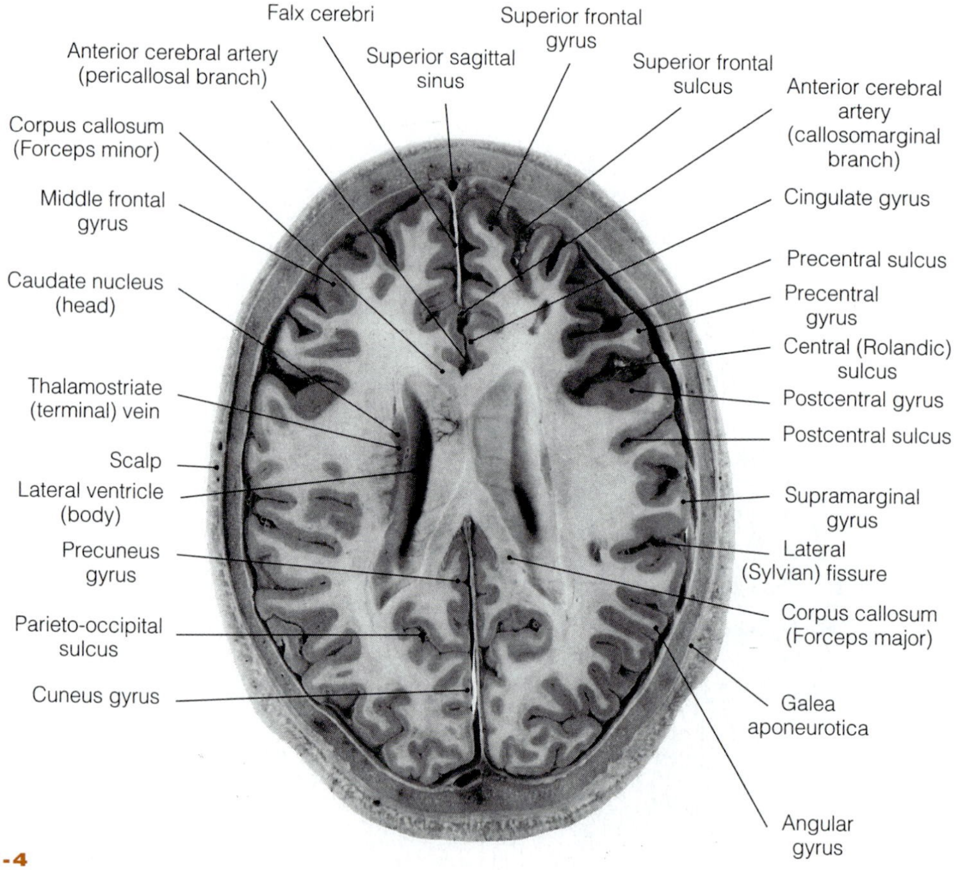

FIGURE A1-4

Axial section through the body of the lateral ventricles and the forceps minor and major.

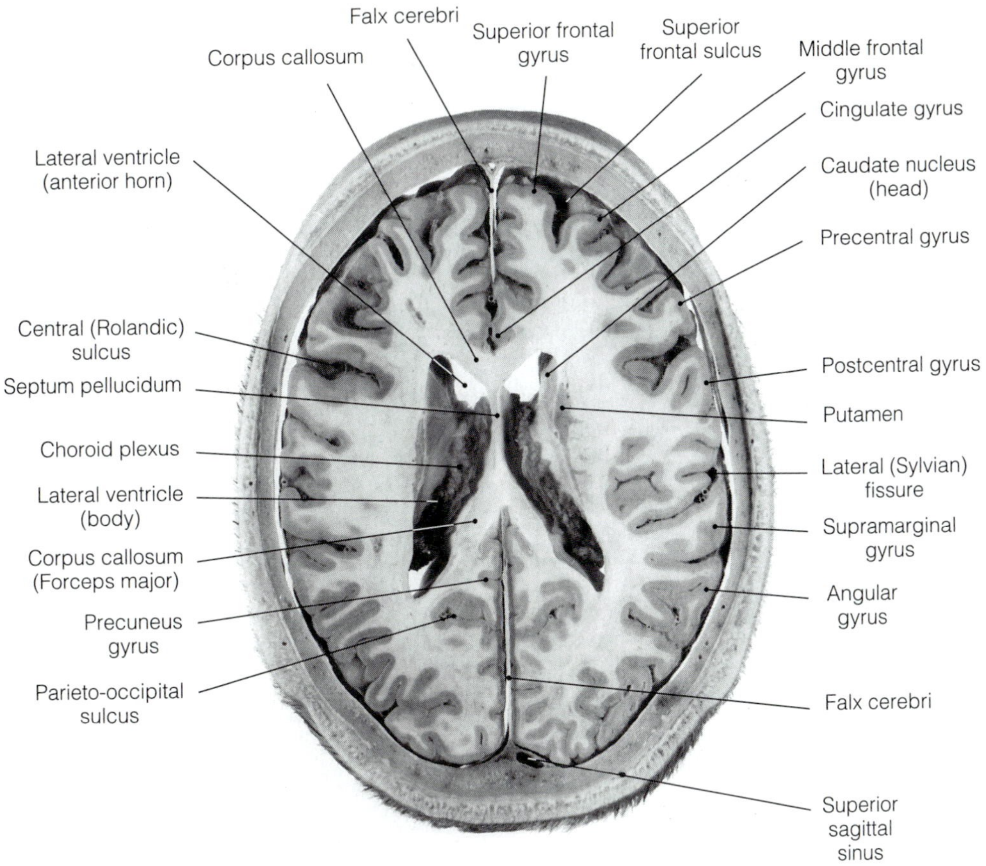
Falx cerebri
Corpus callosum
Superior frontal gyrus
Superior frontal sulcus
Middle frontal gyrus
Cingulate gyrus
Lateral ventricle (anterior horn)
Caudate nucleus (head)
Precentral gyrus
Central (Rolandic) sulcus
Septum pellucidum
Postcentral gyrus
Putamen
Choroid plexus
Lateral (Sylvian) fissure
Lateral ventricle (body)
Supramarginal gyrus
Corpus callosum (Forceps major)
Angular gyrus
Precuneus gyrus
Parieto-occipital sulcus
Falx cerebri
Superior sagittal sinus

FIGURE A1-5

Axial section through the body and anterior horn of the lateral ventricle.

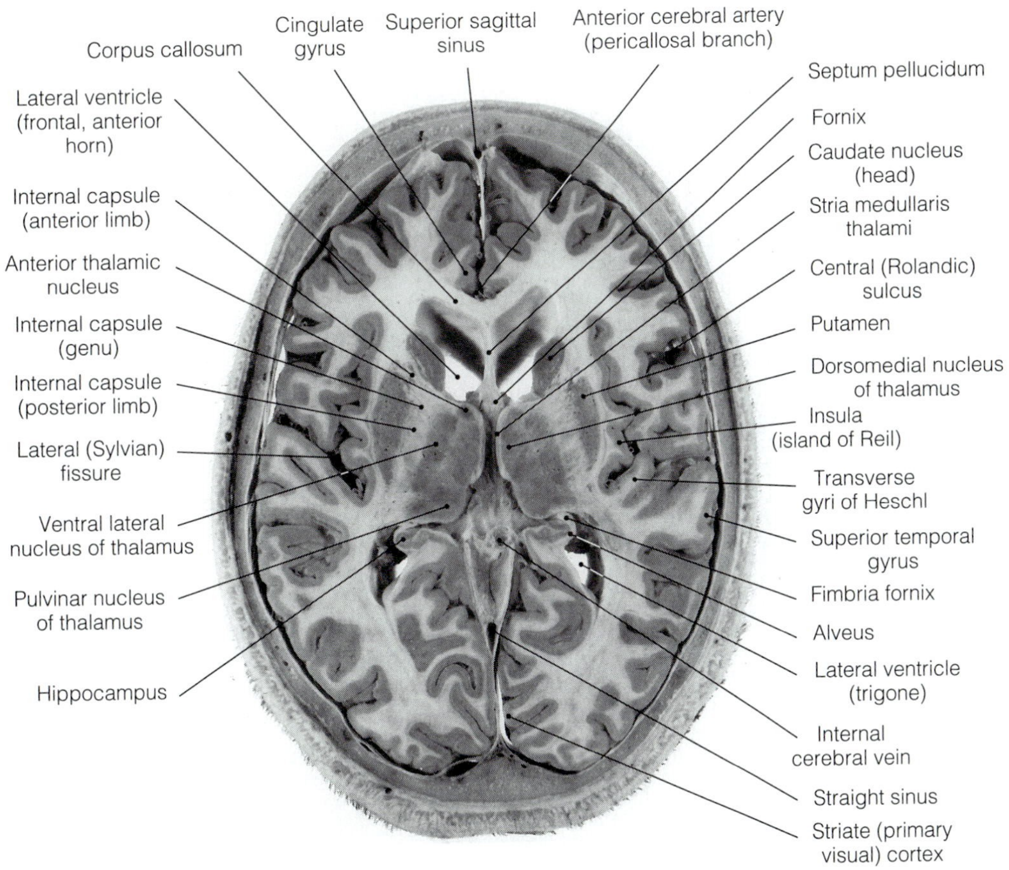
Corpus callosum
Cingulate gyrus
Superior sagittal sinus
Anterior cerebral artery (pericallosal branch)
Septum pellucidum
Lateral ventricle (frontal, anterior horn)
Fornix
Caudate nucleus (head)
Internal capsule (anterior limb)
Stria medullaris thalami
Anterior thalamic nucleus
Central (Rolandic) sulcus
Putamen
Internal capsule (genu)
Dorsomedial nucleus of thalamus
Internal capsule (posterior limb)
Insula (island of Reil)
Lateral (Sylvian) fissure
Transverse gyri of Heschl
Ventral lateral nucleus of thalamus
Superior temporal gyrus
Fimbria fornix
Pulvinar nucleus of thalamus
Alveus
Lateral ventricle (trigone)
Hippocampus
Internal cerebral vein
Straight sinus
Striate (primary visual) cortex

FIGURE A1-6

Axial section through the thalamus and basal ganglia.

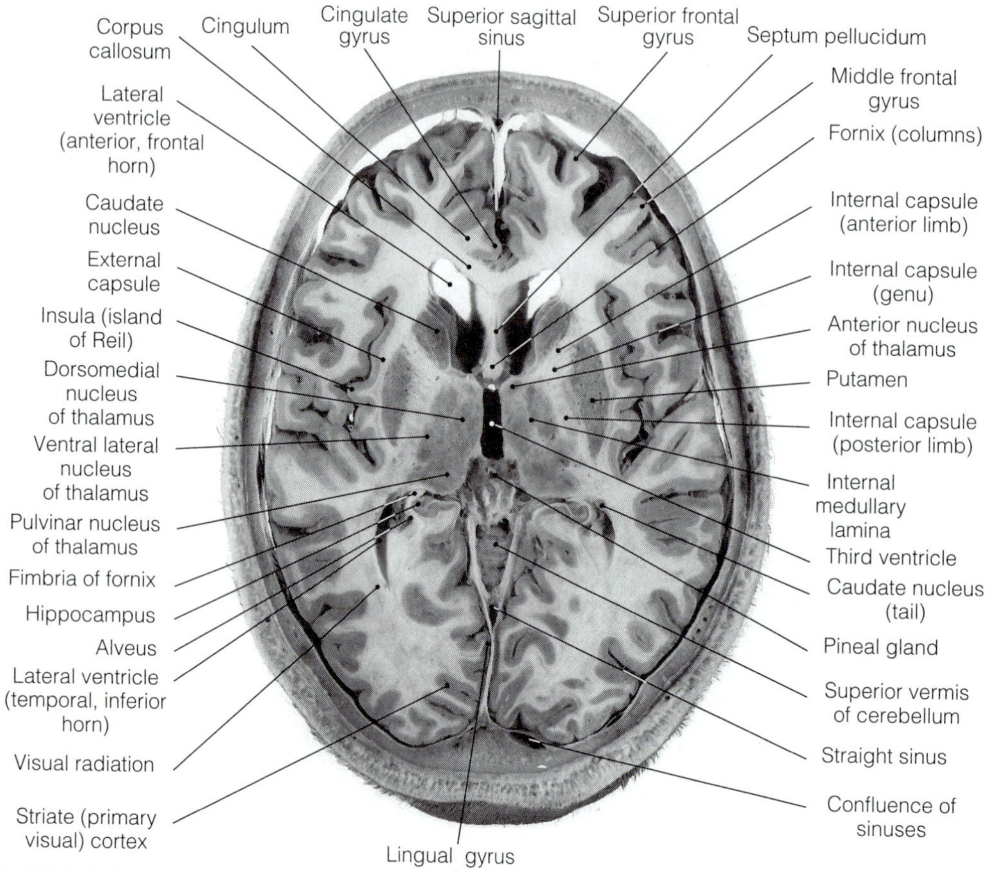
Corpus callosum
Cingulum
Cingulate gyrus
Superior sagittal sinus
Superior frontal gyrus
Septum pellucidum
Middle frontal gyrus
Fornix (columns)
Lateral ventricle (anterior, frontal horn)
Caudate nucleus
External capsule
Insula (island of Reil)
Dorsomedial nucleus of thalamus
Ventral lateral nucleus of thalamus
Pulvinar nucleus of thalamus
Fimbria of fornix
Hippocampus
Alveus
Lateral ventricle (temporal, inferior horn)
Visual radiation
Striate (primary visual) cortex
Lingual gyrus
Internal capsule (anterior limb)
Internal capsule (genu)
Anterior nucleus of thalamus
Putamen
Internal capsule (posterior limb)
Internal medullary lamina
Third ventricle
Caudate nucleus (tail)
Pineal gland
Superior vermis of cerebellum
Straight sinus
Confluence of sinuses

FIGURE A1-7

Axial section through the thalamus and basal ganglia.

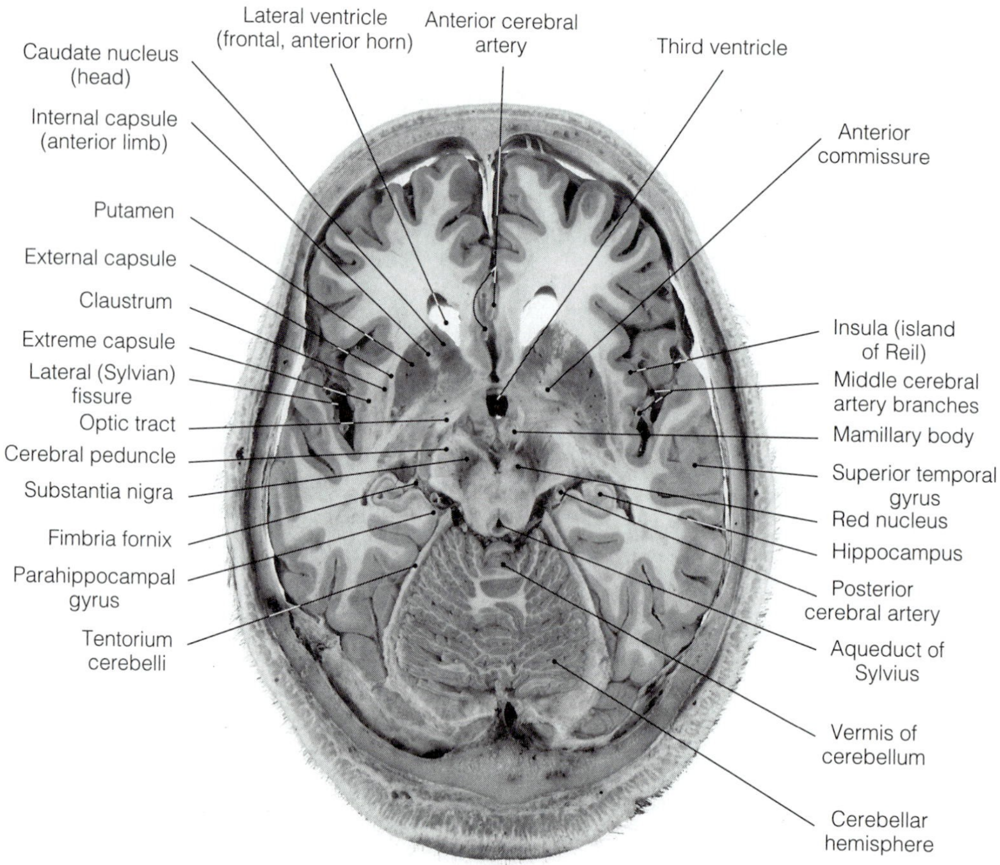
Caudate nucleus (head)
Lateral ventricle (frontal, anterior horn)
Anterior cerebral artery
Third ventricle
Anterior commissure
Internal capsule (anterior limb)
Putamen
External capsule
Claustrum
Extreme capsule
Lateral (Sylvian) fissure
Optic tract
Cerebral peduncle
Substantia nigra
Fimbria fornix
Parahippocampal gyrus
Tentorium cerebelli
Insula (island of Reil)
Middle cerebral artery branches
Mamillary body
Superior temporal gyrus
Red nucleus
Hippocampus
Posterior cerebral artery
Aqueduct of Sylvius
Vermis of cerebellum
Cerebellar hemisphere

FIGURE A1-8

Axial section through the basal ganglia, midbrain, and cerebellum.

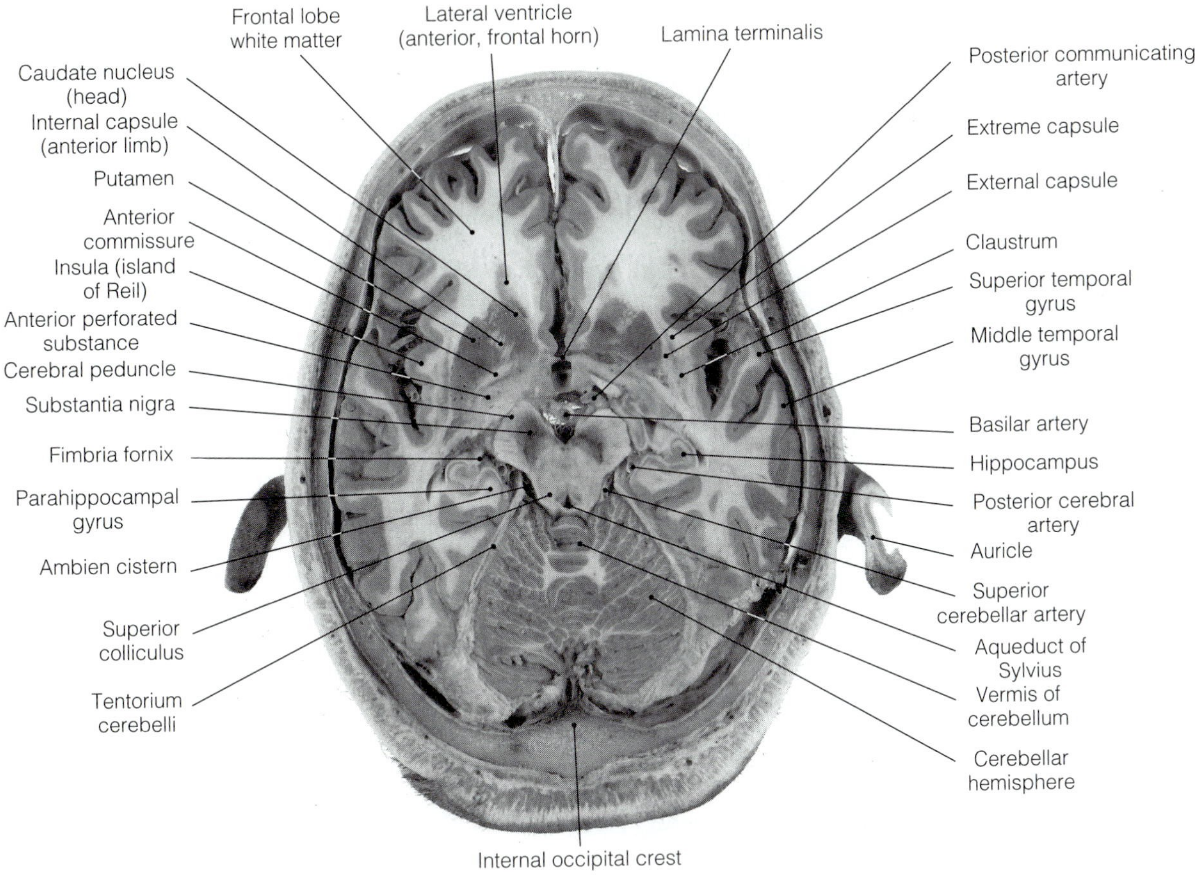

Frontal lobe white matter
Lateral ventricle (anterior, frontal horn)
Lamina terminalis
Caudate nucleus (head)
Internal capsule (anterior limb)
Putamen
Anterior commissure
Insula (island of Reil)
Anterior perforated substance
Cerebral peduncle
Substantia nigra
Fimbria fornix
Parahippocampal gyrus
Ambien cistern
Superior colliculus
Tentorium cerebelli
Posterior communicating artery
Extreme capsule
External capsule
Claustrum
Superior temporal gyrus
Middle temporal gyrus
Basilar artery
Hippocampus
Posterior cerebral artery
Auricle
Superior cerebellar artery
Aqueduct of Sylvius
Vermis of cerebellum
Cerebellar hemisphere
Internal occipital crest

FIGURE A1-9

Axial section through the anterior commissure, basal ganglia, midbrain, and cerebellum.

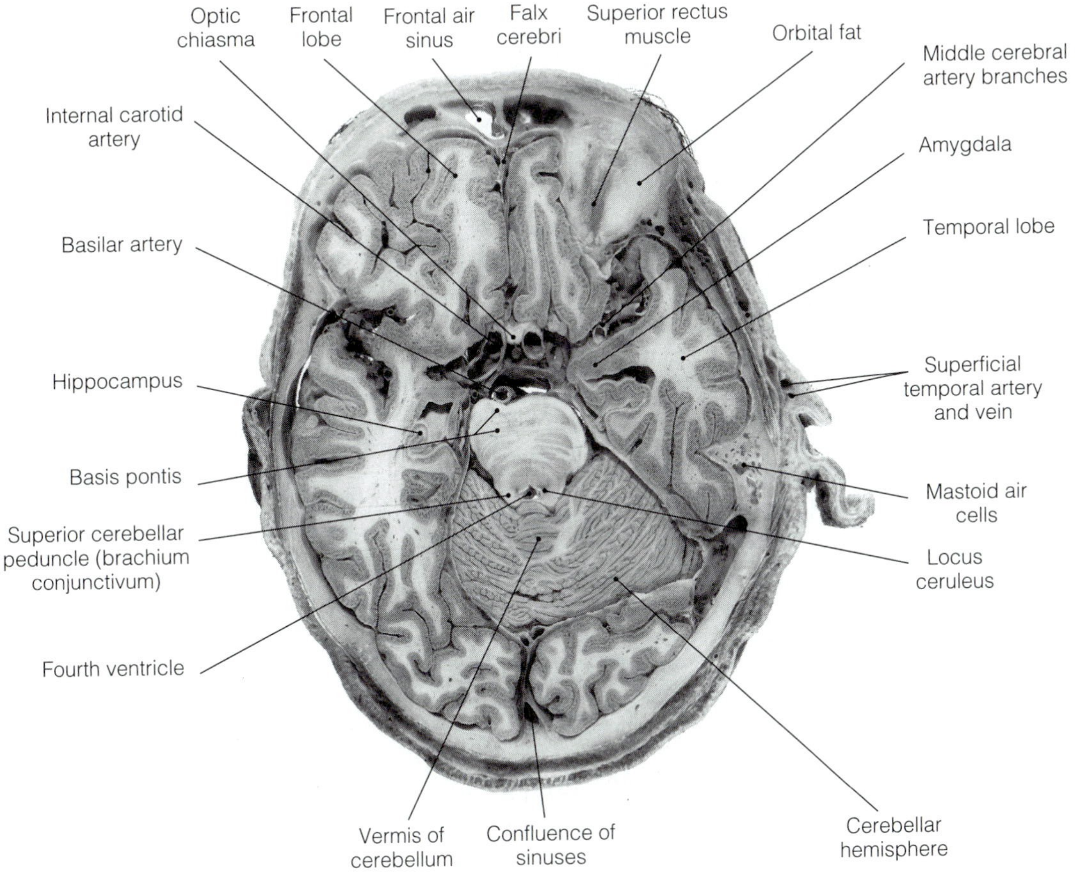

Optic chiasma
Frontal lobe
Frontal air sinus
Falx cerebri
Superior rectus muscle
Orbital fat
Middle cerebral artery branches
Internal carotid artery
Amygdala
Temporal lobe
Basilar artery
Superficial temporal artery and vein
Hippocampus
Basis pontis
Mastoid air cells
Superior cerebellar peduncle (brachium conjunctivum)
Locus ceruleus
Fourth ventricle
Vermis of cerebellum
Confluence of sinuses
Cerebellar hemisphere

FIGURE A1-10

Axial section through the pons and cerebellum.

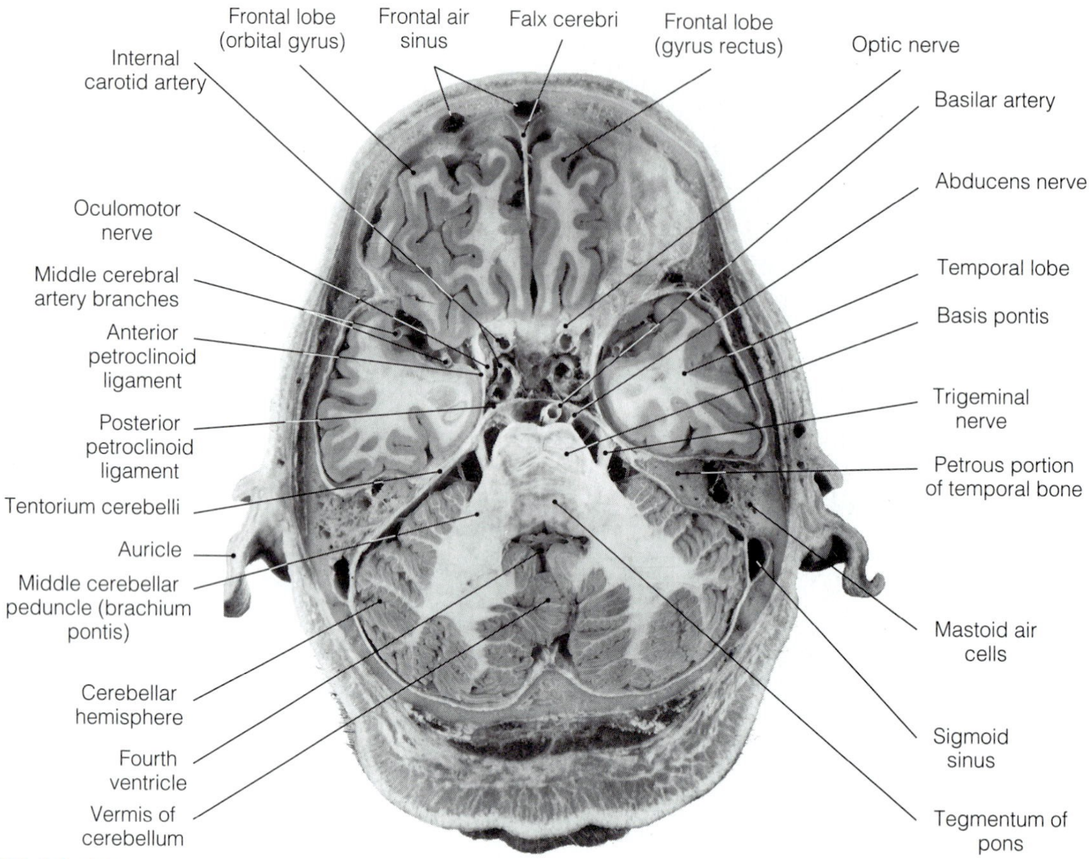

Frontal lobe (orbital gyrus)
Frontal air sinus
Falx cerebri
Frontal lobe (gyrus rectus)
Internal carotid artery
Optic nerve
Basilar artery
Abducens nerve
Oculomotor nerve
Middle cerebral artery branches
Temporal lobe
Basis pontis
Anterior petroclinoid ligament
Trigeminal nerve
Posterior petroclinoid ligament
Petrous portion of temporal bone
Tentorium cerebelli
Auricle
Middle cerebellar peduncle (brachium pontis)
Mastoid air cells
Cerebellar hemisphere
Sigmoid sinus
Fourth ventricle
Vermis of cerebellum
Tegmentum of pons

FIGURE A1-11

Axial section through the middle cerebellar peduncle (brachium pontis).

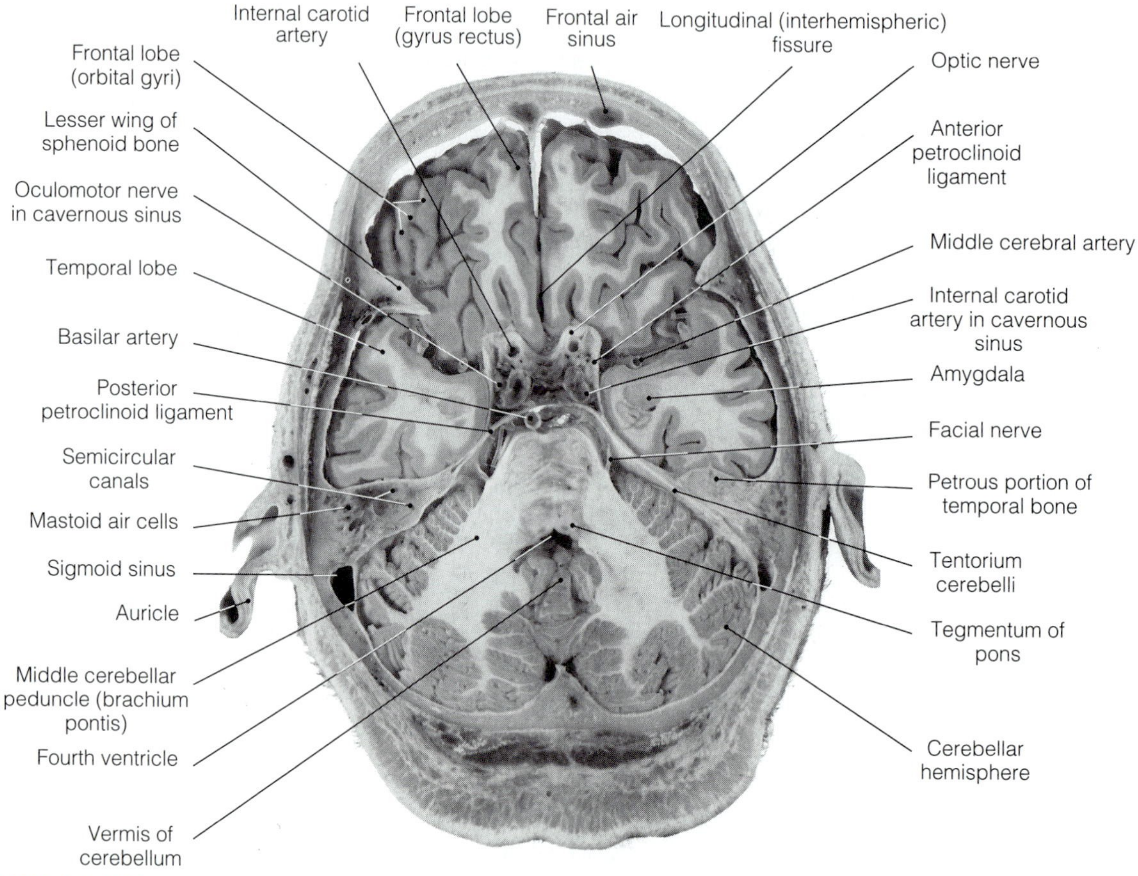

Internal carotid artery
Frontal lobe (gyrus rectus)
Frontal air sinus
Longitudinal (interhemispheric) fissure
Frontal lobe (orbital gyri)
Optic nerve
Lesser wing of sphenoid bone
Anterior petroclinoid ligament
Oculomotor nerve in cavernous sinus
Temporal lobe
Middle cerebral artery
Internal carotid artery in cavernous sinus
Basilar artery
Amygdala
Posterior petroclinoid ligament
Facial nerve
Semicircular canals
Petrous portion of temporal bone
Mastoid air cells
Tentorium cerebelli
Sigmoid sinus
Auricle
Tegmentum of pons
Middle cerebellar peduncle (brachium pontis)
Fourth ventricle
Cerebellar hemisphere
Vermis of cerebellum

FIGURE A1-12

Axial section through the pons and cerebellum.

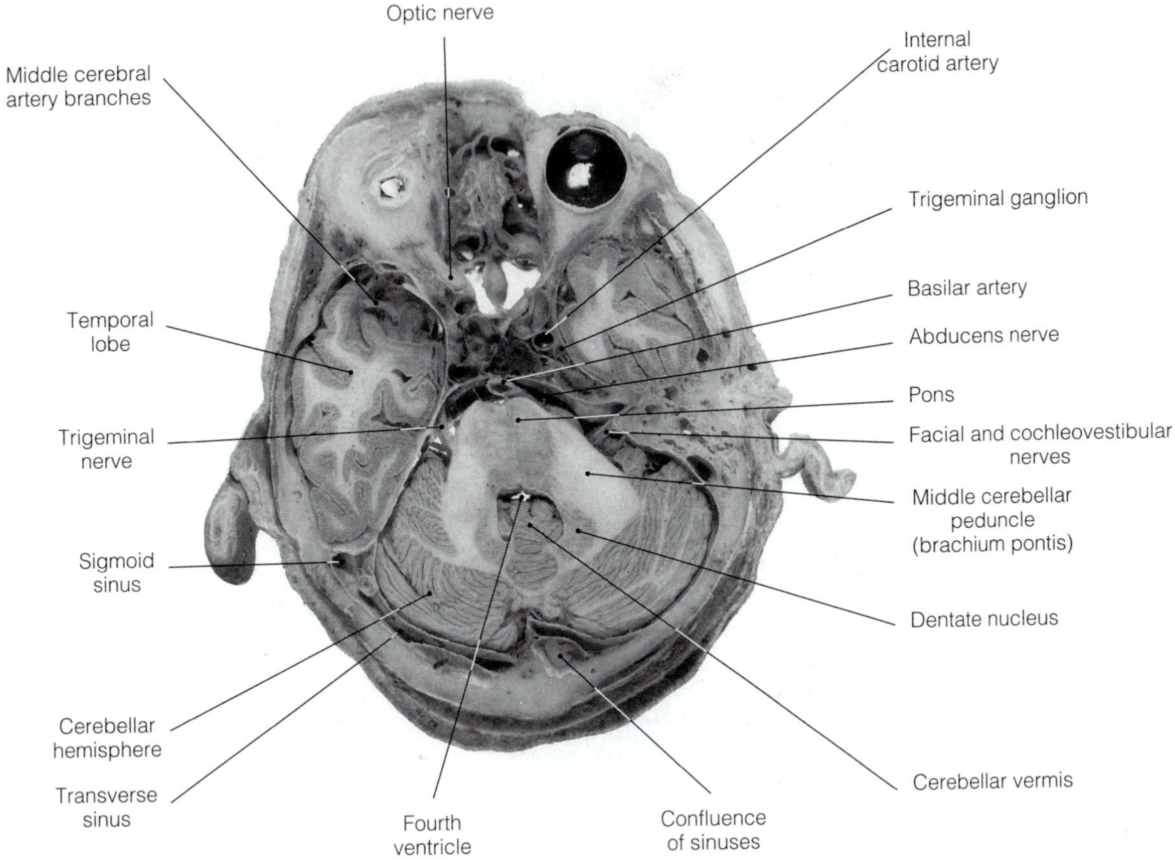

Optic nerve
Middle cerebral artery branches
Internal carotid artery
Trigeminal ganglion
Basilar artery
Abducens nerve
Temporal lobe
Pons
Trigeminal nerve
Facial and cochleovestibular nerves
Middle cerebellar peduncle (brachium pontis)
Sigmoid sinus
Dentate nucleus
Cerebellar hemisphere
Cerebellar vermis
Transverse sinus
Fourth ventricle
Confluence of sinuses

FIGURE A1-13

Axial section through the temporal lobes and cerebellum.

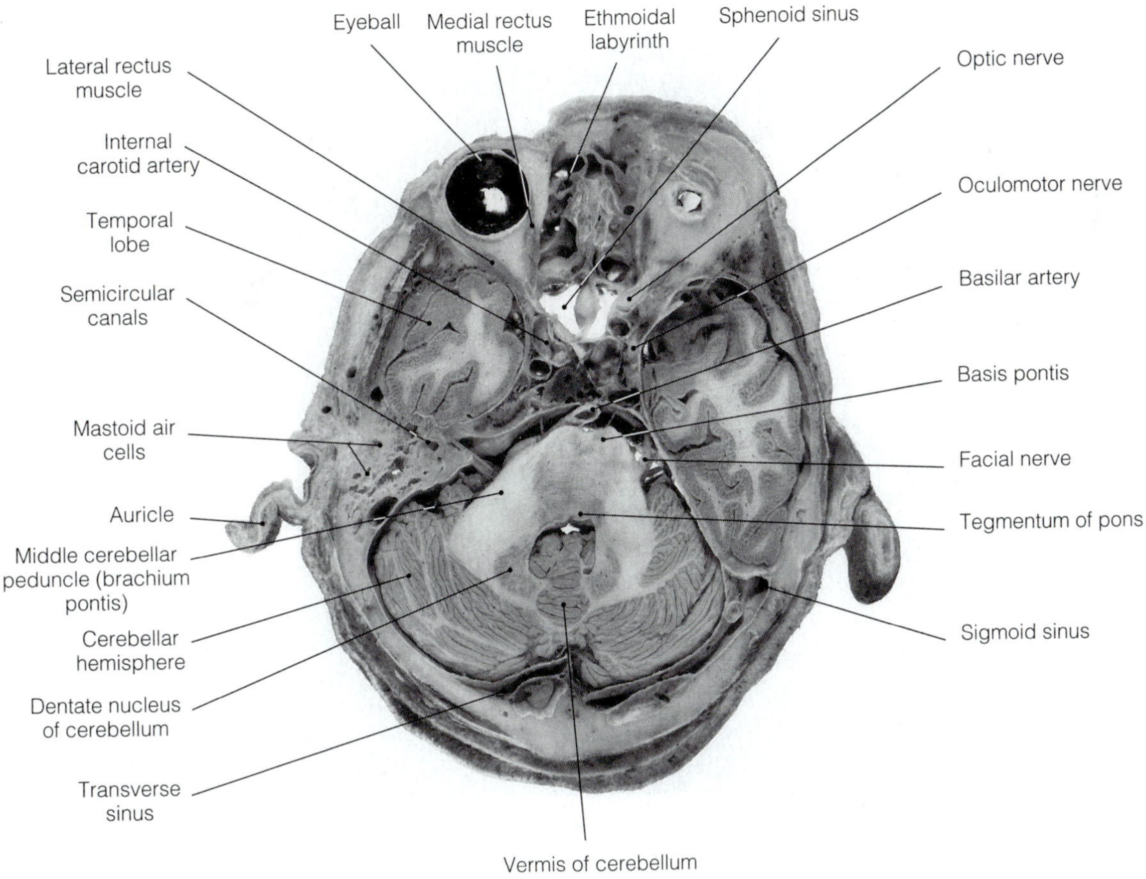

Eyeball
Medial rectus muscle
Ethmoidal labyrinth
Sphenoid sinus
Lateral rectus muscle
Optic nerve
Internal carotid artery
Oculomotor nerve
Temporal lobe
Basilar artery
Semicircular canals
Basis pontis
Mastoid air cells
Facial nerve
Auricle
Tegmentum of pons
Middle cerebellar peduncle (brachium pontis)
Sigmoid sinus
Cerebellar hemisphere
Dentate nucleus of cerebellum
Transverse sinus
Vermis of cerebellum

FIGURE A1-14

Axial section through the temporal lobe and brain stem.

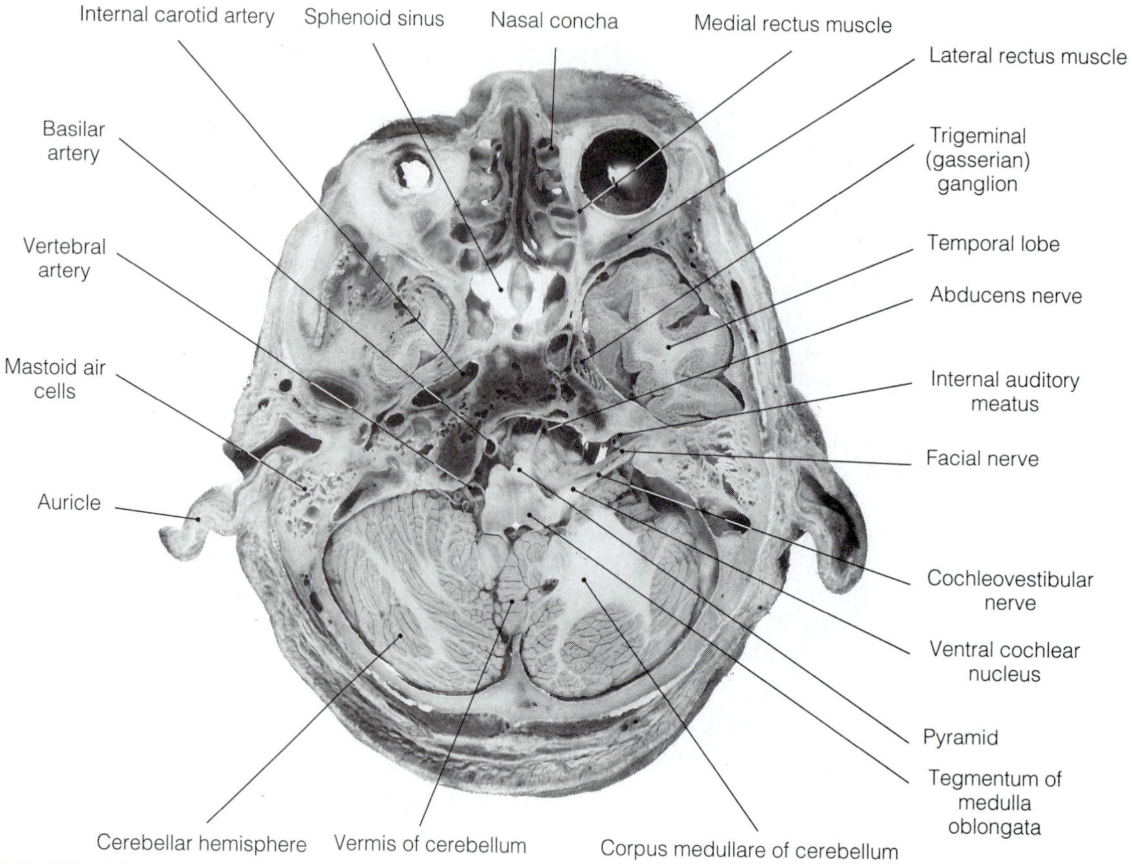

Internal carotid artery
Sphenoid sinus
Nasal concha
Medial rectus muscle
Lateral rectus muscle
Basilar artery
Trigeminal (gasserian) ganglion
Vertebral artery
Temporal lobe
Abducens nerve
Mastoid air cells
Internal auditory meatus
Facial nerve
Auricle
Cochleovestibular nerve
Ventral cochlear nucleus
Pyramid
Tegmentum of medulla oblongata
Cerebellar hemisphere
Vermis of cerebellum
Corpus medullare of cerebellum

FIGURE A1-15

Axial section through the temporal lobe, medulla oblongata, and cerebellum.

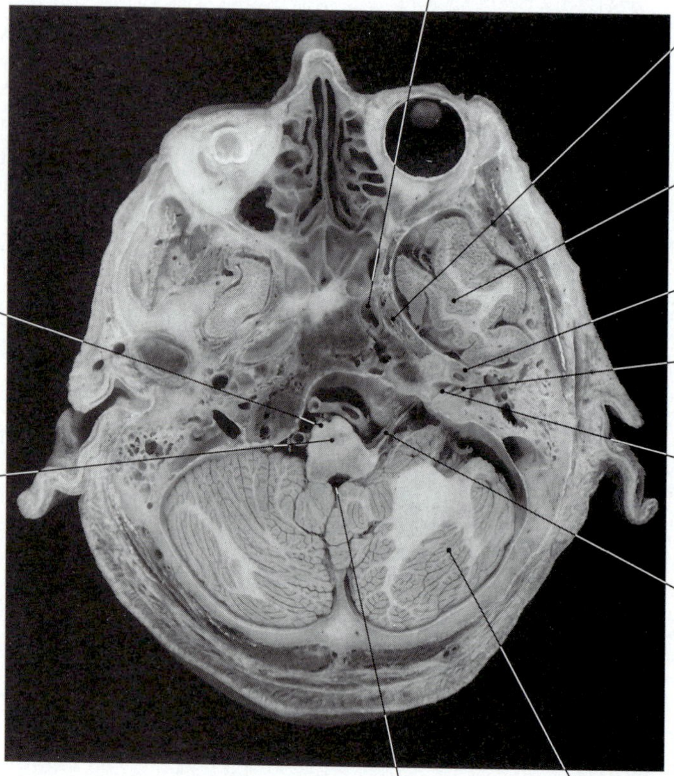

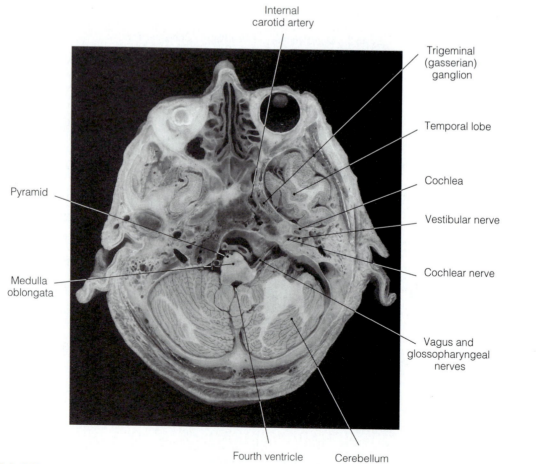

Internal carotid artery
Trigeminal (gasserian) ganglion
Temporal lobe
Cochlea
Pyramid
Vestibular nerve
Medulla oblongata
Cochlear nerve
Vagus and glossopharyngeal nerves
Fourth ventricle
Cerebellum

FIGURE A1-16

Axial section through the temporal lobe, medulla oblongata, and cerebellum.

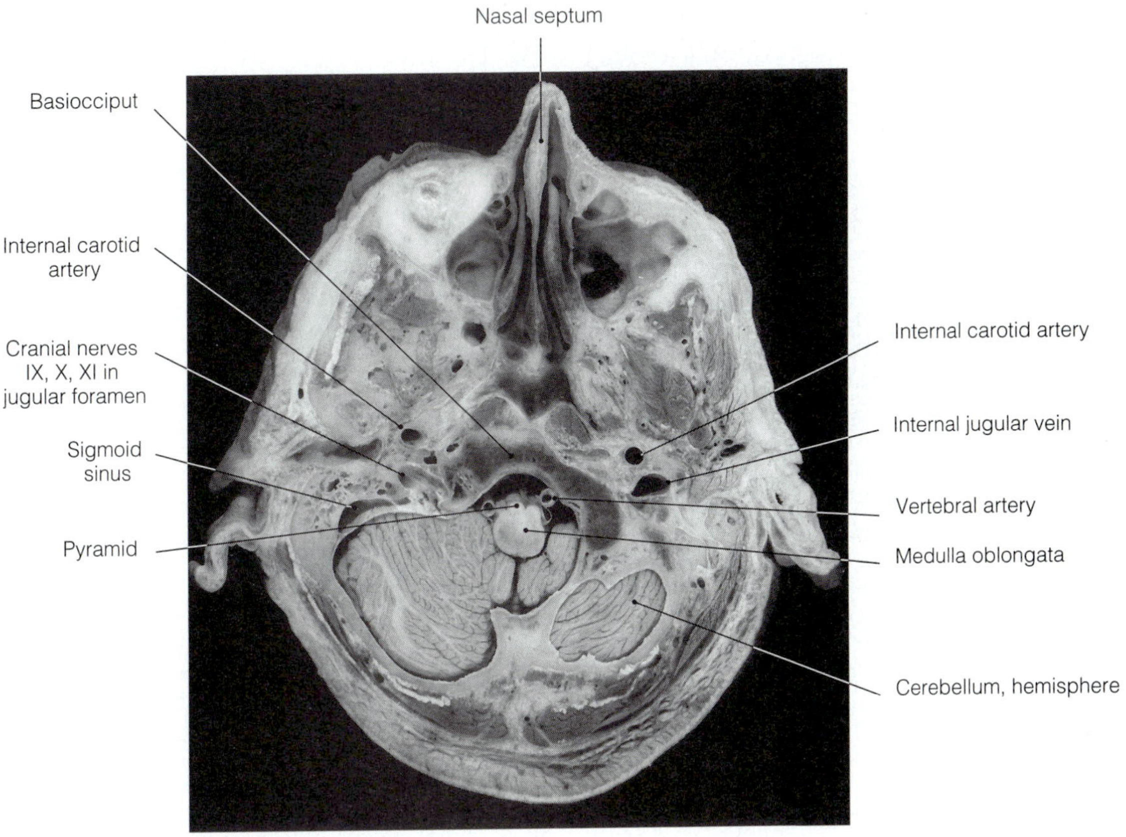
Nasal septum
Basiocciput
Internal carotid artery
Cranial nerves IX, X, XI in jugular foramen
Sigmoid sinus
Pyramid
Internal carotid artery
Internal jugular vein
Vertebral artery
Medulla oblongata
Cerebellum, hemisphere

FIGURE A1-17

Axial section through the lower medulla oblongata and cerebellum.

SAGITTAL YAKOVLEV

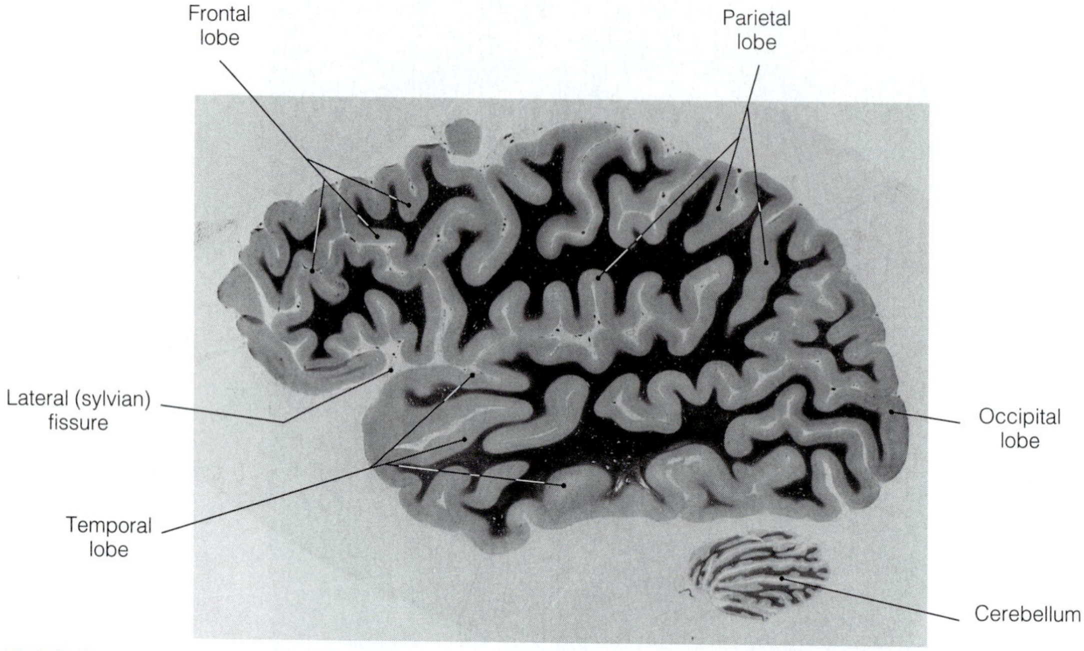
Frontal lobe
Parietal lobe
Lateral (sylvian) fissure
Occipital lobe
Temporal lobe
Cerebellum

FIGURE A2-1

Parasagittal brain section just superficial to the insula.

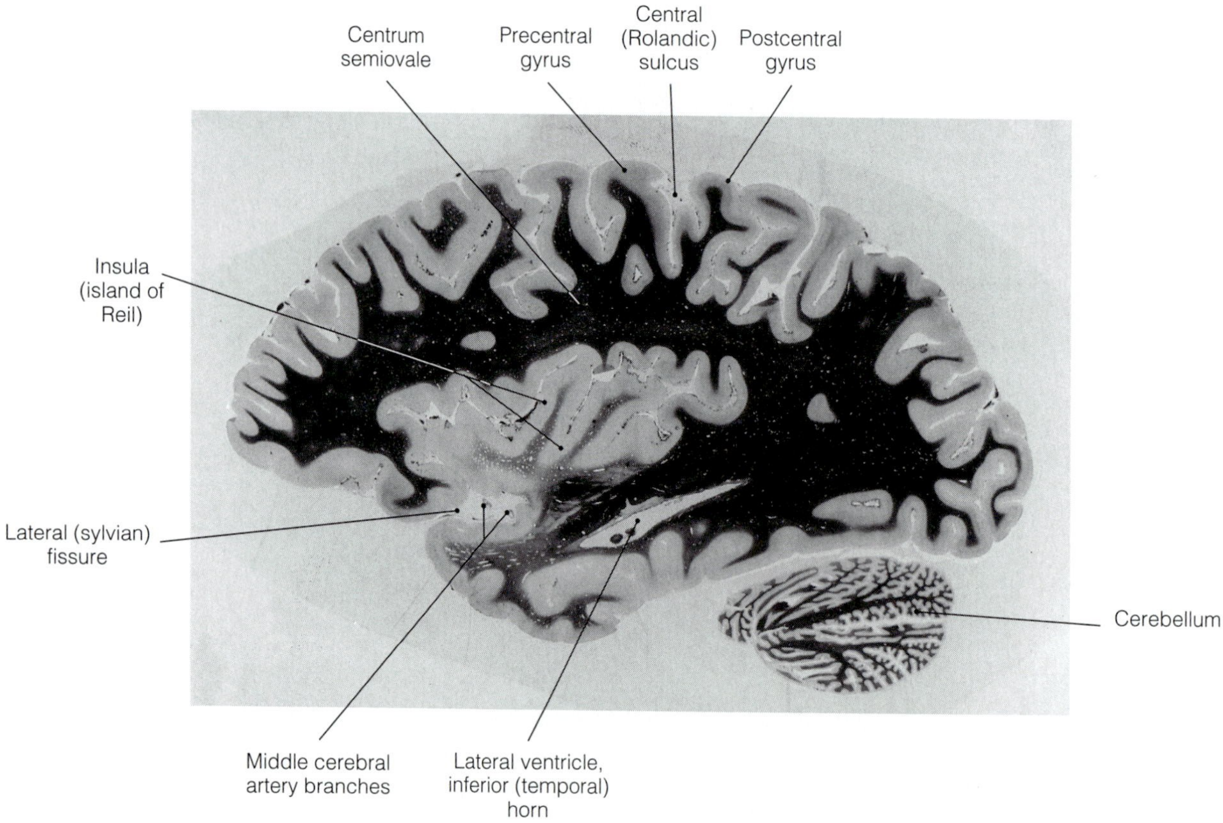
Centrum semiovale
Precentral gyrus
Central (Rolandic) sulcus
Postcentral gyrus
Insula (island of Reil)
Lateral (sylvian) fissure
Cerebellum
Middle cerebral artery branches
Lateral ventricle, inferior (temporal) horn

FIGURE A2-2

Parasagittal brain section through the insula.

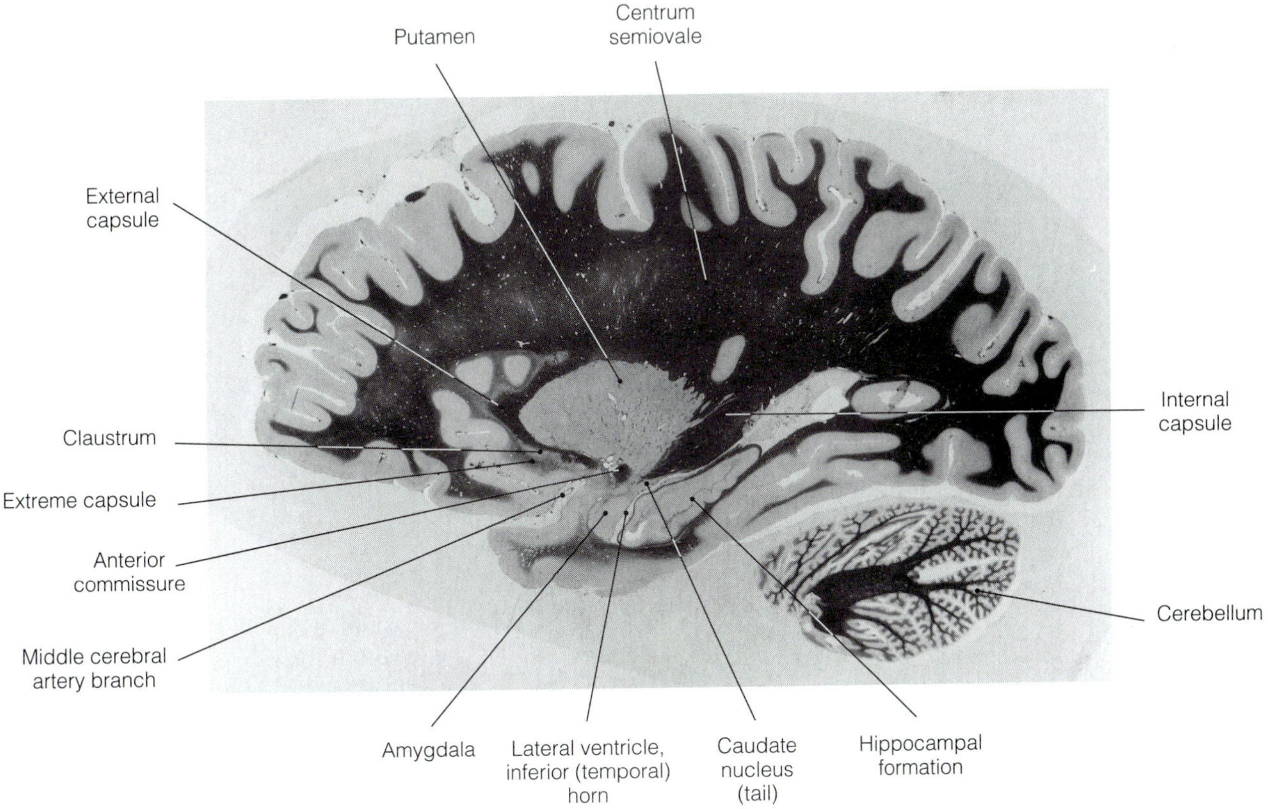

FIGURE A2-3

Parasagittal brain section through the putamen.

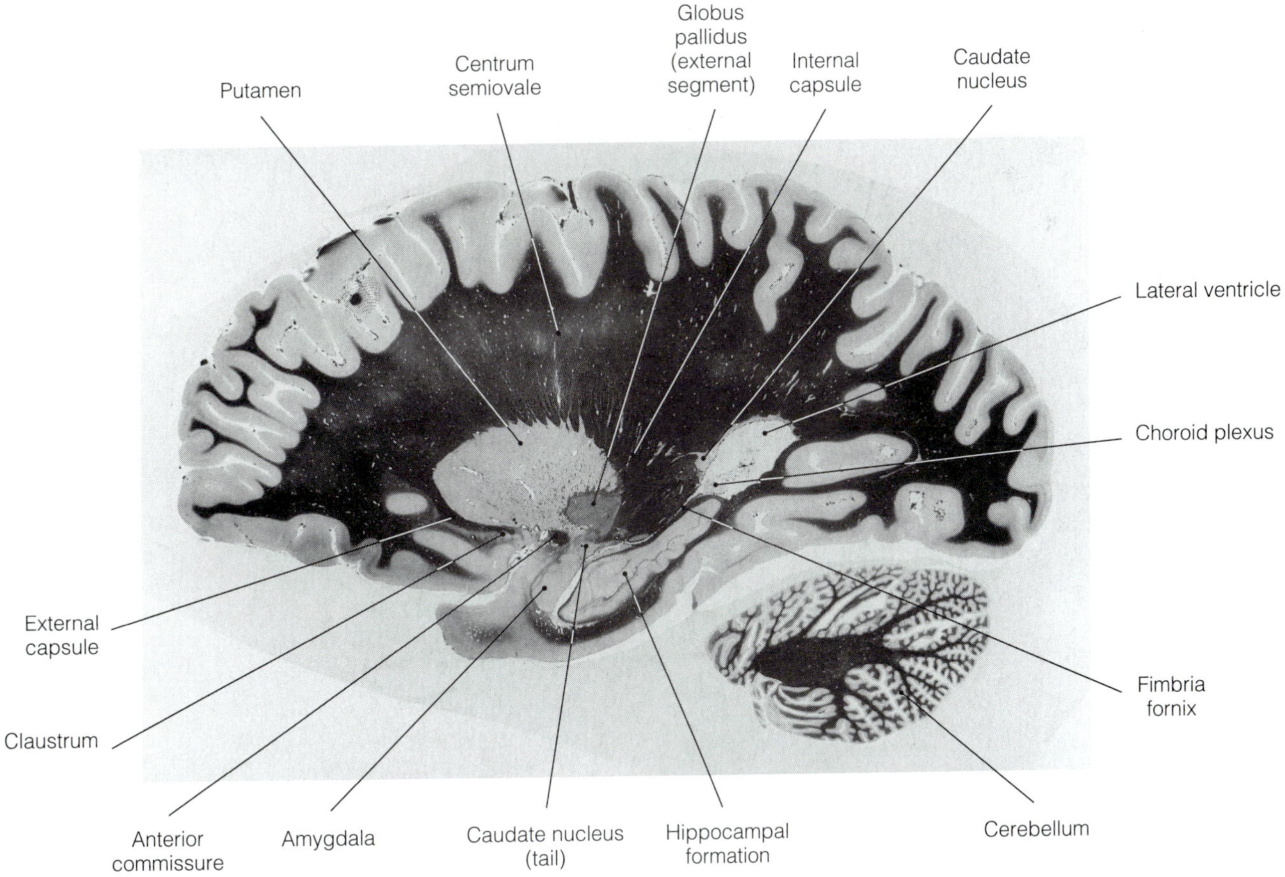

FIGURE A2-4

Parasagittal brain section through the lenticular nucleus.

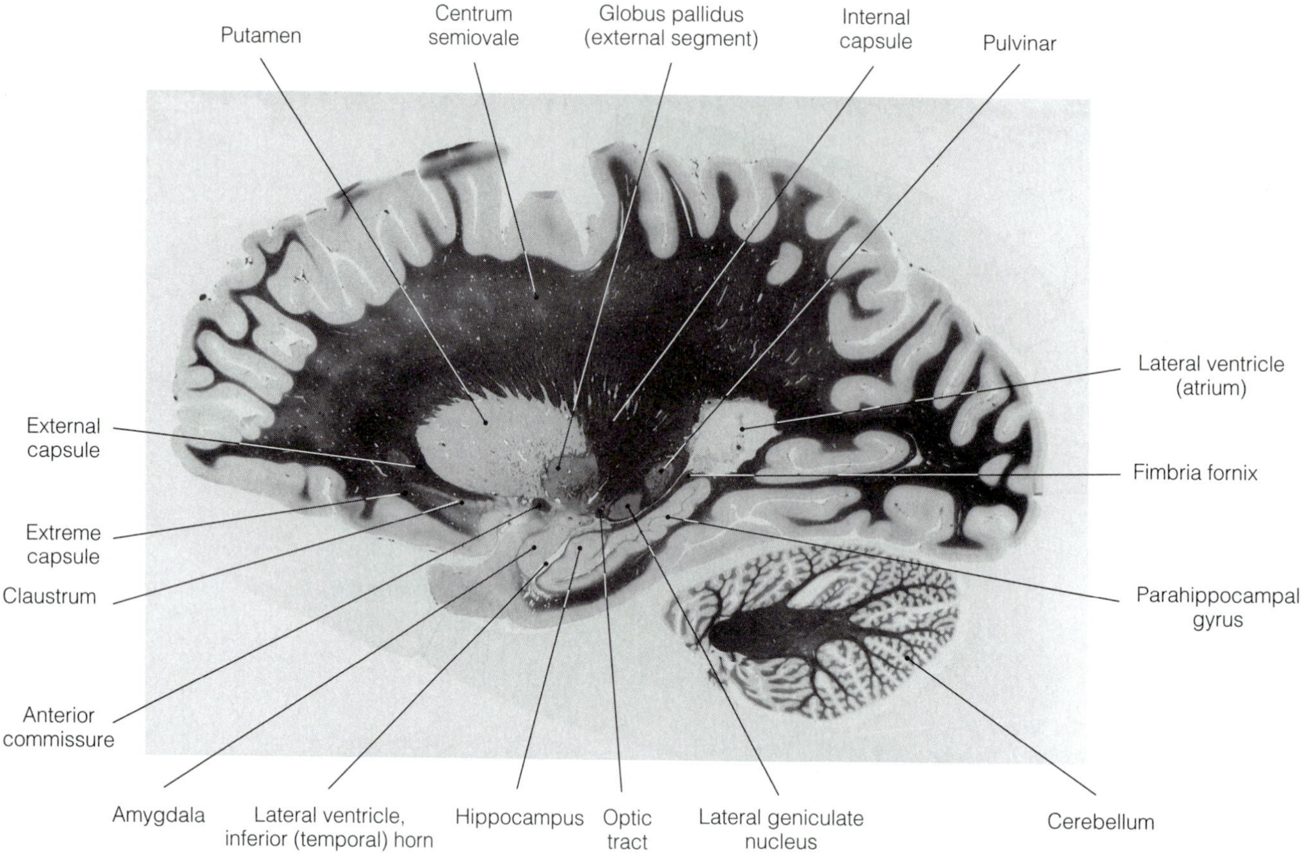
Putamen
Centrum semiovale
Globus pallidus (external segment)
Internal capsule
Pulvinar
Lateral ventricle (atrium)
External capsule
Fimbria fornix
Extreme capsule
Claustrum
Parahippocampal gyrus
Anterior commissure
Amygdala
Lateral ventricle, inferior (temporal) horn
Hippocampus
Optic tract
Lateral geniculate nucleus
Cerebellum

FIGURE A2-5

Parasagittal brain section through the lenticular nucleus and lateral geniculate nucleus.

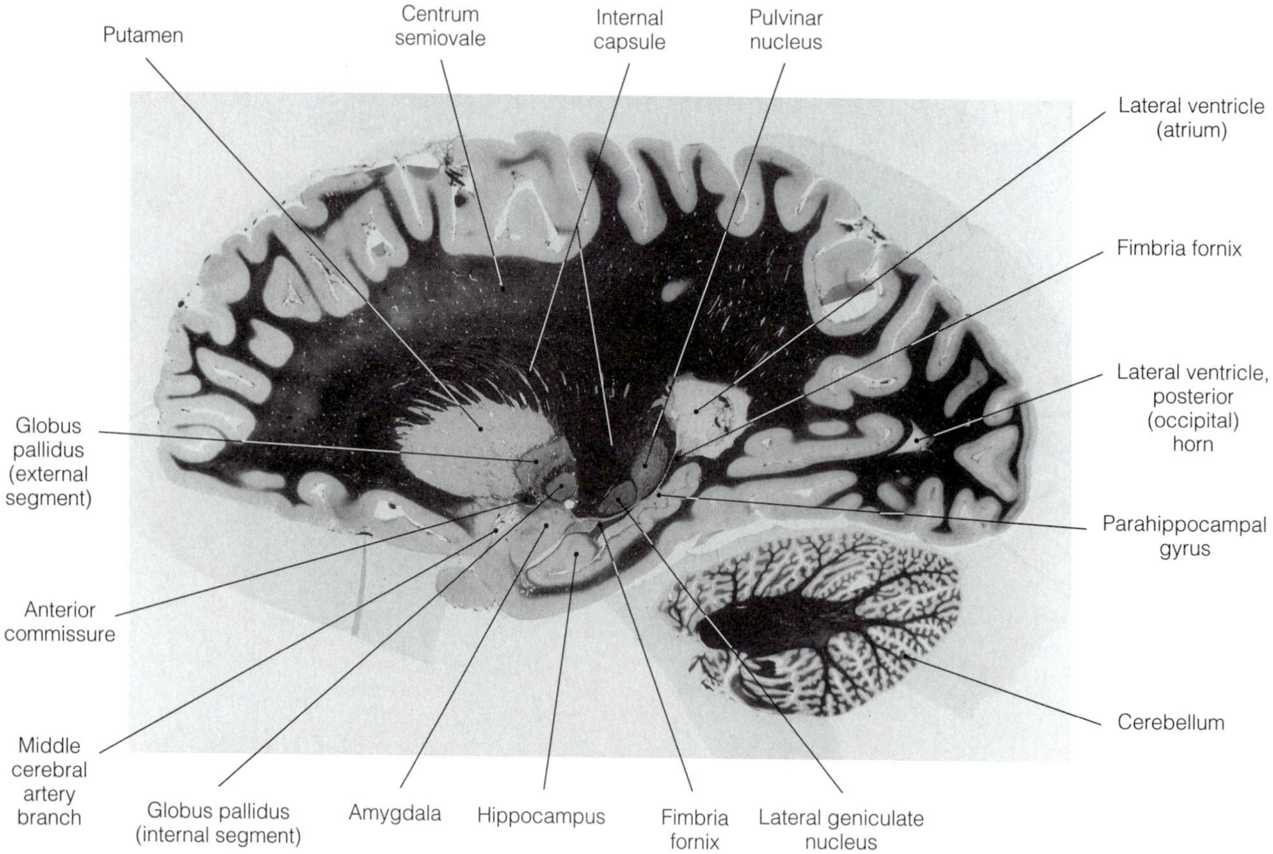
Putamen
Centrum semiovale
Internal capsule
Pulvinar nucleus
Lateral ventricle (atrium)
Fimbria fornix
Lateral ventricle, posterior (occipital) horn
Globus pallidus (external segment)
Parahippocampal gyrus
Anterior commissure
Cerebellum
Middle cerebral artery branch
Globus pallidus (internal segment)
Amygdala
Hippocampus
Fimbria fornix
Lateral geniculate nucleus

FIGURE A2-6

Parasagittal brain section through the lateral geniculate nucleus, amygdala, and hippocampus.

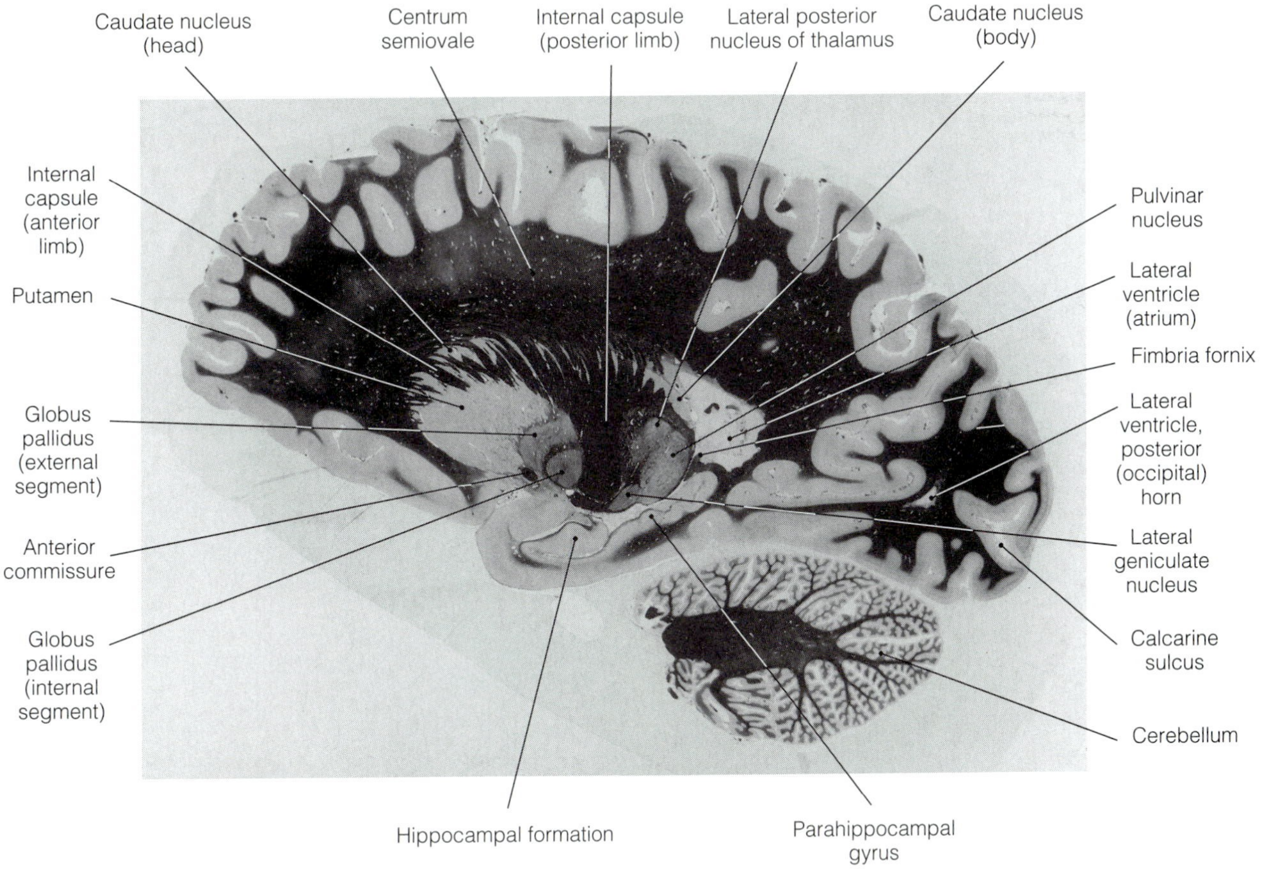
Caudate nucleus (head)
Centrum semiovale
Internal capsule (posterior limb)
Lateral posterior nucleus of thalamus
Caudate nucleus (body)
Internal capsule (anterior limb)
Putamen
Globus pallidus (external segment)
Anterior commissure
Globus pallidus (internal segment)
Pulvinar nucleus
Lateral ventricle (atrium)
Fimbria fornix
Lateral ventricle, posterior (occipital) horn
Lateral geniculate nucleus
Calcarine sulcus
Cerebellum
Hippocampal formation
Parahippocampal gyrus

FIGURE A2-7

Parasagittal brain section through the neostriatum and pulvinar nucleus.

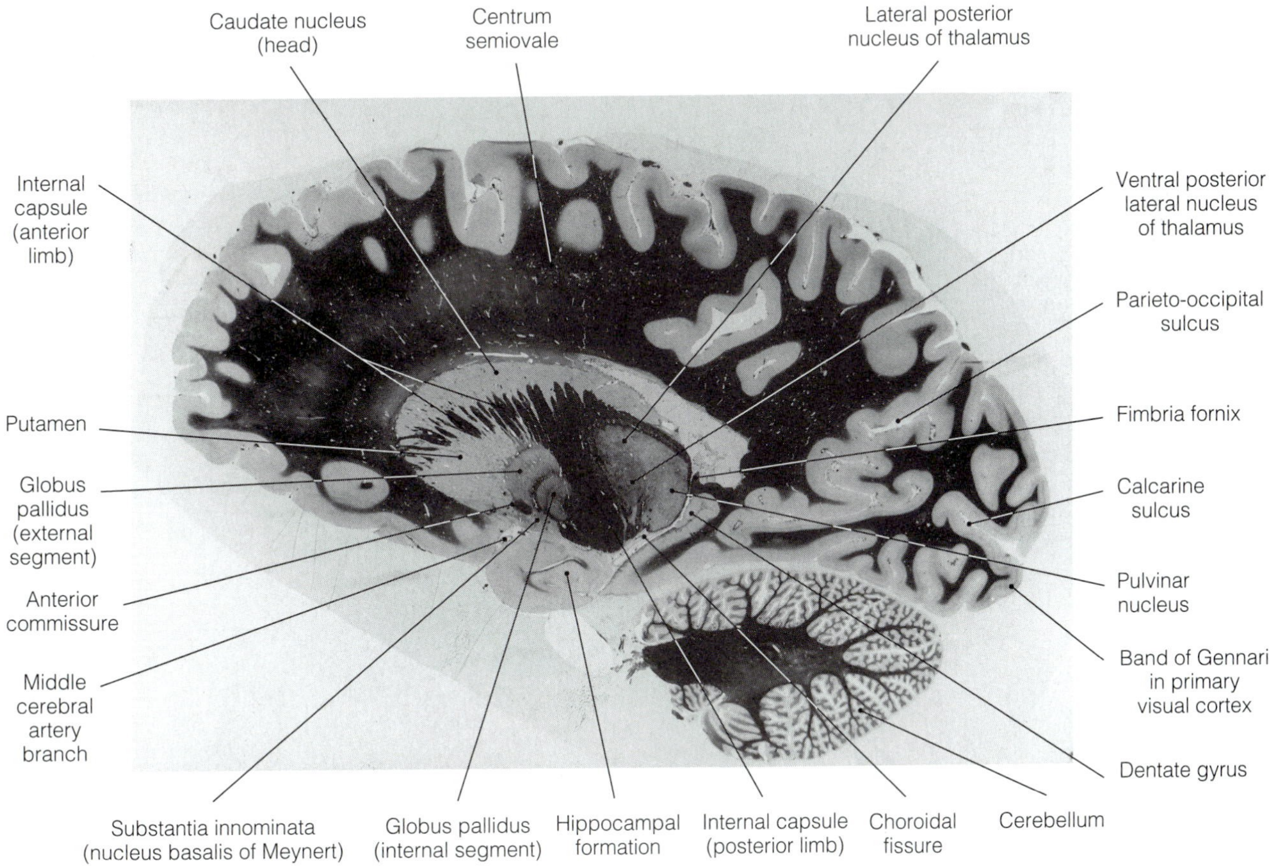
Caudate nucleus (head)
Centrum semiovale
Lateral posterior nucleus of thalamus
Internal capsule (anterior limb)
Putamen
Globus pallidus (external segment)
Anterior commissure
Middle cerebral artery branch
Ventral posterior lateral nucleus of thalamus
Parieto-occipital sulcus
Fimbria fornix
Calcarine sulcus
Pulvinar nucleus
Band of Gennari in primary visual cortex
Dentate gyrus
Substantia innominata (nucleus basalis of Meynert)
Globus pallidus (internal segment)
Hippocampal formation
Internal capsule (posterior limb)
Choroidal fissure
Cerebellum

FIGURE A2-8

Parasagittal brain section through the corpus striatum.

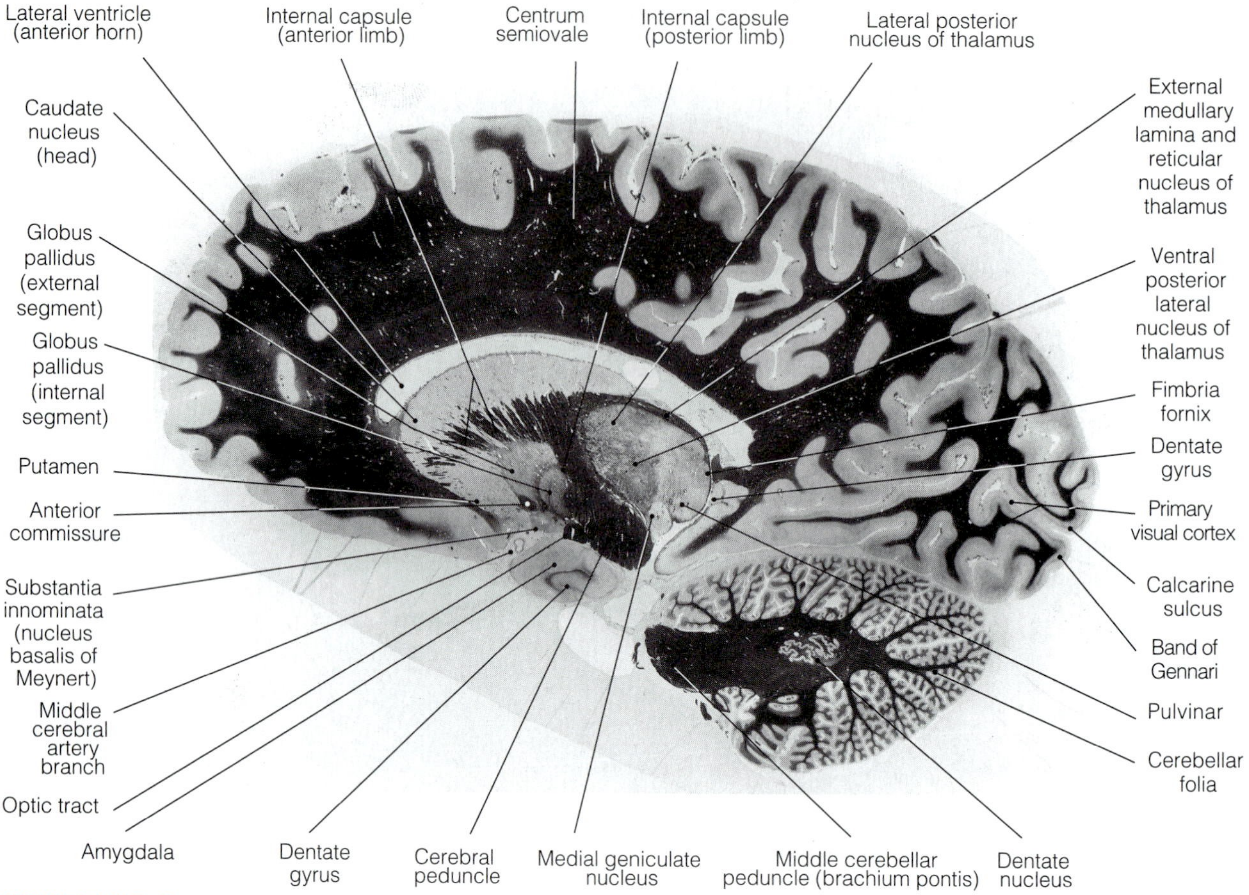
Lateral ventricle (anterior horn)
Internal capsule (anterior limb)
Centrum semiovale
Internal capsule (posterior limb)
Lateral posterior nucleus of thalamus
Caudate nucleus (head)
External medullary lamina and reticular nucleus of thalamus
Globus pallidus (external segment)
Ventral posterior lateral nucleus of thalamus
Globus pallidus (internal segment)
Fimbria fornix
Dentate gyrus
Putamen
Anterior commissure
Primary visual cortex
Substantia innominata (nucleus basalis of Meynert)
Calcarine sulcus
Band of Gennari
Middle cerebral artery branch
Pulvinar
Cerebellar folia
Optic tract
Amygdala
Dentate gyrus
Cerebral peduncle
Medial geniculate nucleus
Middle cerebellar peduncle (brachium pontis)
Dentate nucleus

FIGURE A2-9

Parasagittal brain section through the lateral thalamus.

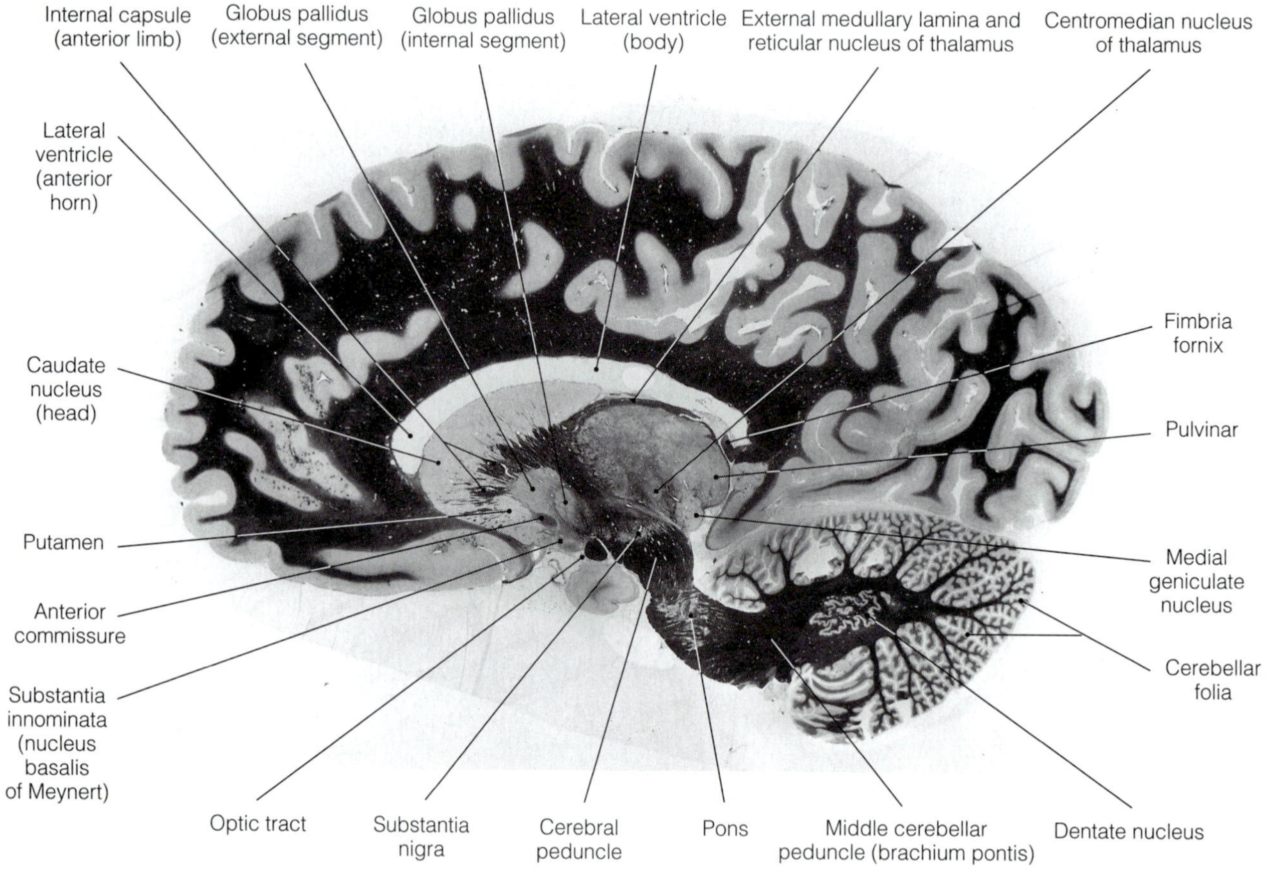
Internal capsule (anterior limb)
Globus pallidus (external segment)
Globus pallidus (internal segment)
Lateral ventricle (body)
External medullary lamina and reticular nucleus of thalamus
Centromedian nucleus of thalamus
Lateral ventricle (anterior horn)
Fimbria fornix
Caudate nucleus (head)
Pulvinar
Putamen
Medial geniculate nucleus
Anterior commissure
Cerebellar folia
Substantia innominata (nucleus basalis of Meynert)
Optic tract
Substantia nigra
Cerebral peduncle
Pons
Middle cerebellar peduncle (brachium pontis)
Dentate nucleus

FIGURE A2-10

Parasagittal brain section through the centromedian nucleus of the thalamus.

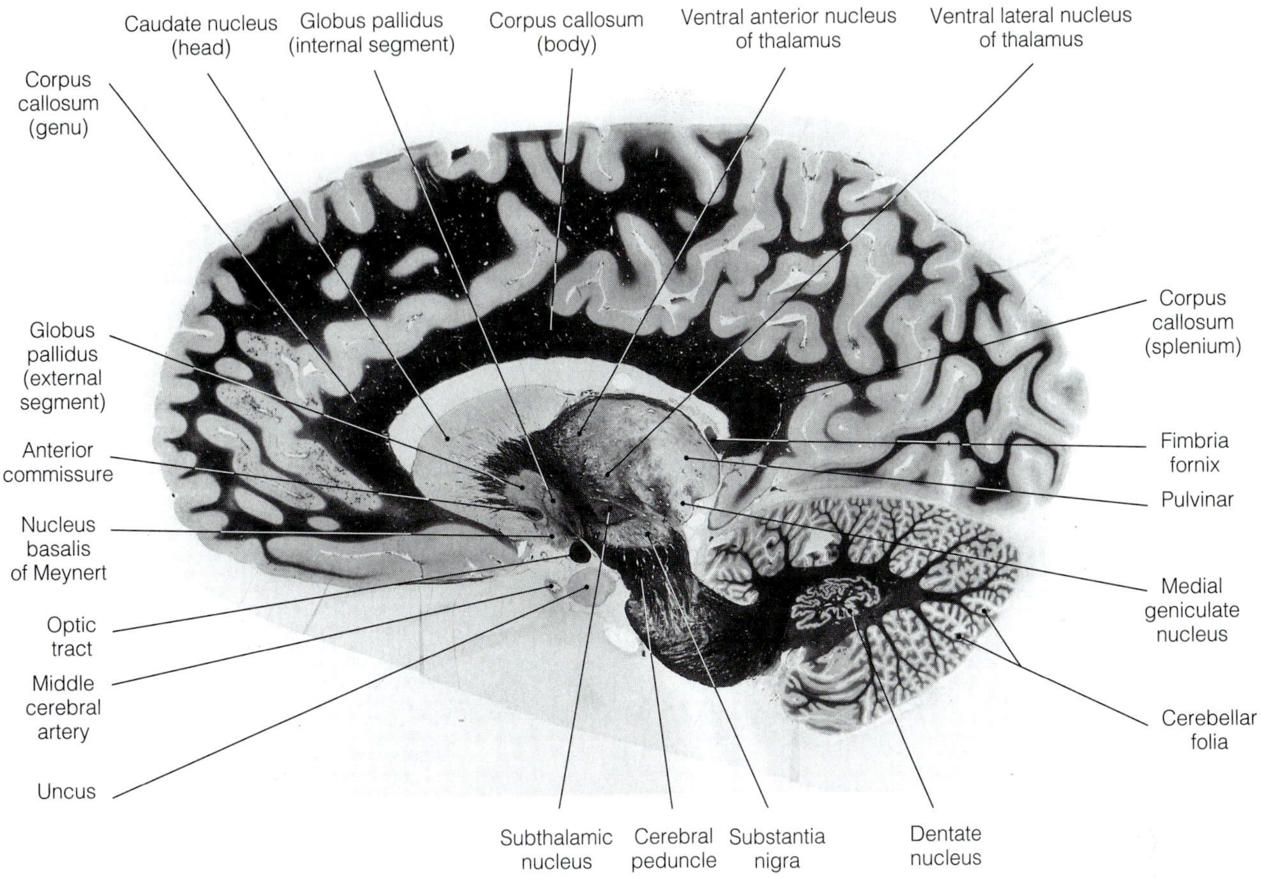
Caudate nucleus (head)
Globus pallidus (internal segment)
Corpus callosum (body)
Ventral anterior nucleus of thalamus
Ventral lateral nucleus of thalamus
Corpus callosum (genu)
Globus pallidus (external segment)
Anterior commissure
Nucleus basalis of Meynert
Optic tract
Middle cerebral artery
Uncus
Corpus callosum (splenium)
Fimbria fornix
Pulvinar
Medial geniculate nucleus
Cerebellar folia
Subthalamic nucleus
Cerebral peduncle
Substantia nigra
Dentate nucleus

FIGURE A2-11

Parasagittal brain section through the substantia nigra and cerebral peduncle.

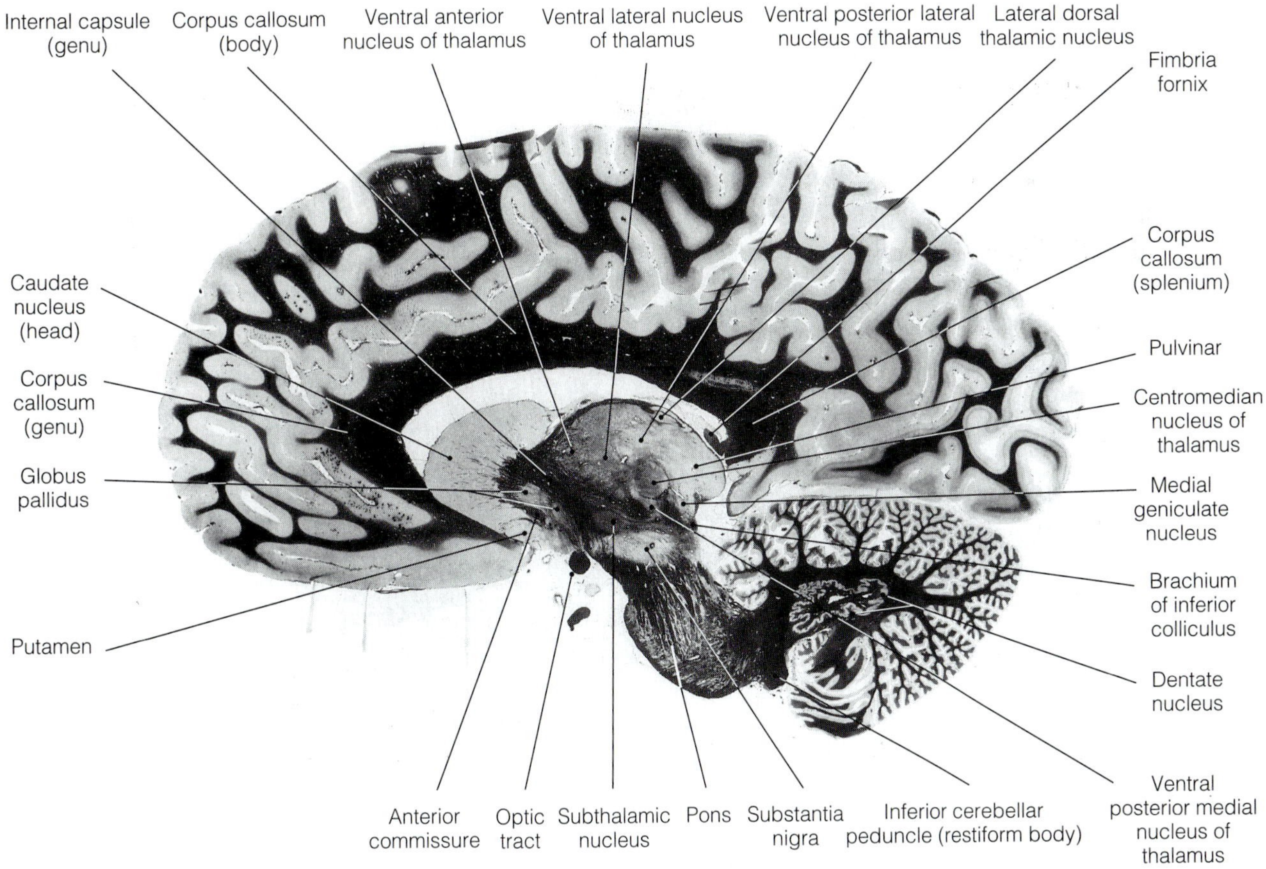
Internal capsule (genu)
Corpus callosum (body)
Ventral anterior nucleus of thalamus
Ventral lateral nucleus of thalamus
Ventral posterior lateral nucleus of thalamus
Lateral dorsal thalamic nucleus
Fimbria fornix
Caudate nucleus (head)
Corpus callosum (genu)
Globus pallidus
Putamen
Corpus callosum (splenium)
Pulvinar
Centromedian nucleus of thalamus
Medial geniculate nucleus
Brachium of inferior colliculus
Dentate nucleus
Ventral posterior medial nucleus of thalamus
Anterior commissure
Optic tract
Subthalamic nucleus
Pons
Substantia nigra
Inferior cerebellar peduncle (restiform body)

FIGURE A2-12

Parasagittal brain section through the centromedian nucleus of thalamus and subthalamic nucleus.

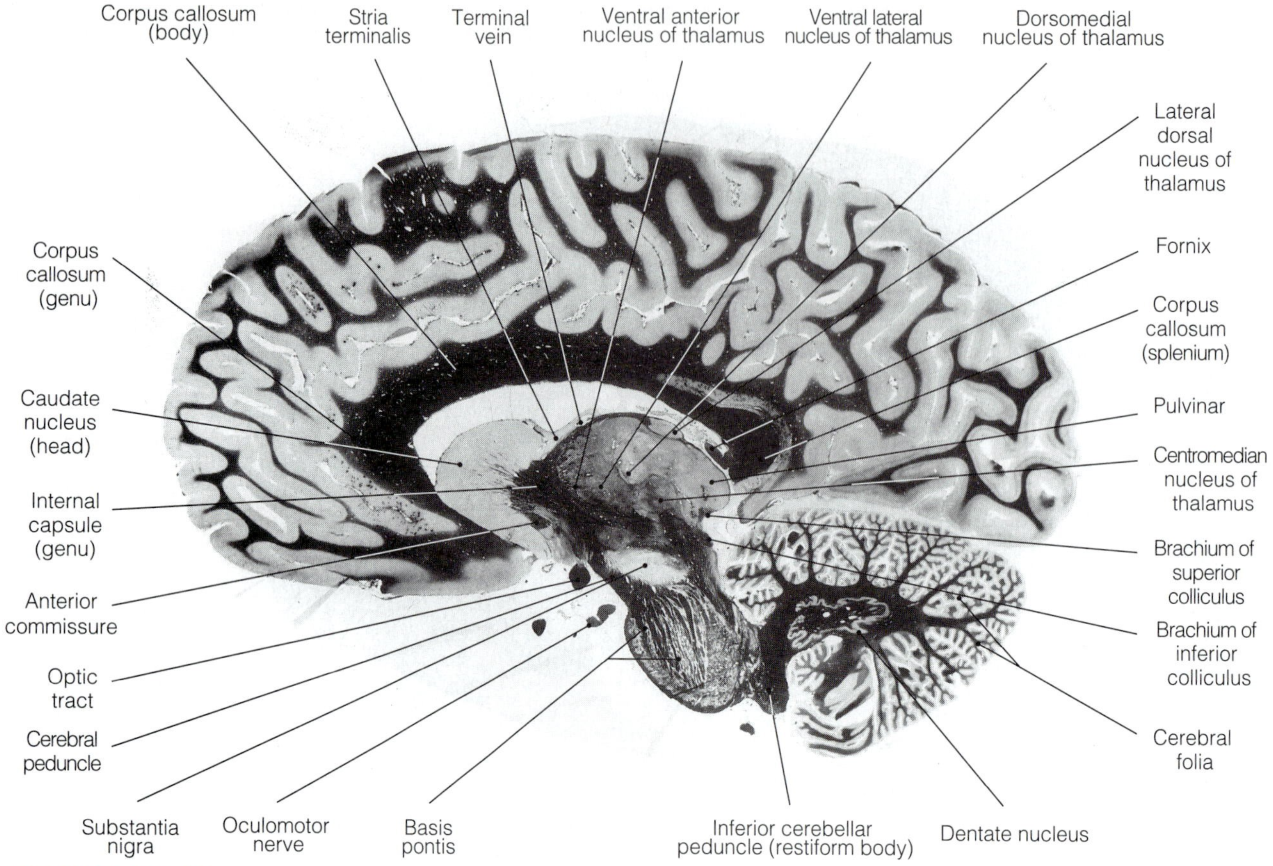

Corpus callosum (body)
Stria terminalis
Terminal vein
Ventral anterior nucleus of thalamus
Ventral lateral nucleus of thalamus
Dorsomedial nucleus of thalamus
Lateral dorsal nucleus of thalamus
Fornix
Corpus callosum (splenium)
Pulvinar
Centromedian nucleus of thalamus
Brachium of superior colliculus
Brachium of inferior colliculus
Cerebral folia
Corpus callosum (genu)
Caudate nucleus (head)
Internal capsule (genu)
Anterior commissure
Optic tract
Cerebral peduncle
Substantia nigra
Oculomotor nerve
Basis pontis
Inferior cerebellar peduncle (restiform body)
Dentate nucleus

FIGURE A2-13

Parasagittal brain section through the dorsomedial nucleus of the thalamus and oculomotor nerve.

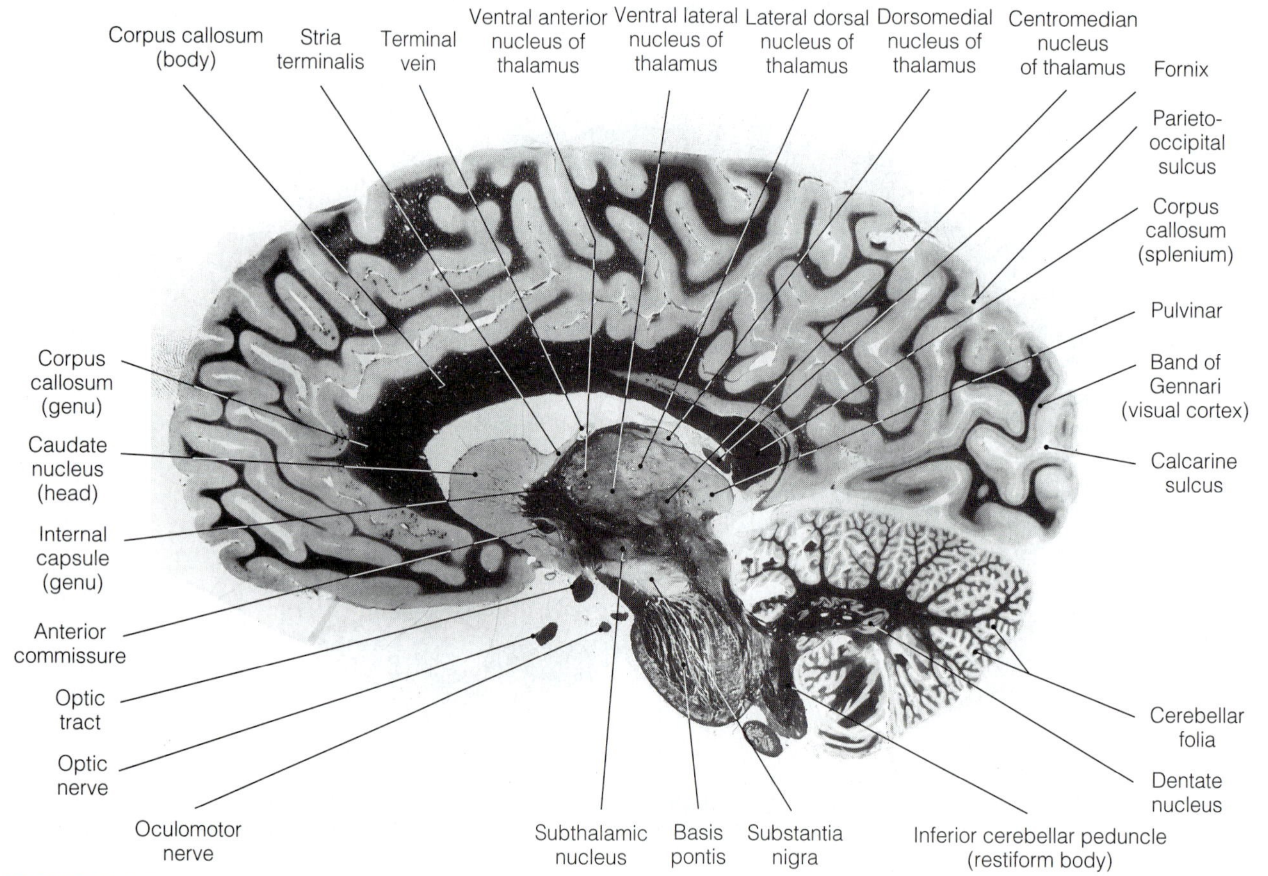

Corpus callosum (body)
Stria terminalis
Terminal vein
Ventral anterior nucleus of thalamus
Ventral lateral nucleus of thalamus
Lateral dorsal nucleus of thalamus
Dorsomedial nucleus of thalamus
Centromedian nucleus of thalamus
Fornix
Parieto-occipital sulcus
Corpus callosum (splenium)
Pulvinar
Band of Gennari (visual cortex)
Calcarine sulcus
Corpus callosum (genu)
Caudate nucleus (head)
Internal capsule (genu)
Anterior commissure
Optic tract
Optic nerve
Oculomotor nerve
Subthalamic nucleus
Basis pontis
Substantia nigra
Inferior cerebellar peduncle (restiform body)
Cerebellar folia
Dentate nucleus

FIGURE A2-14

Parasagittal brain section through the medial thalamus.

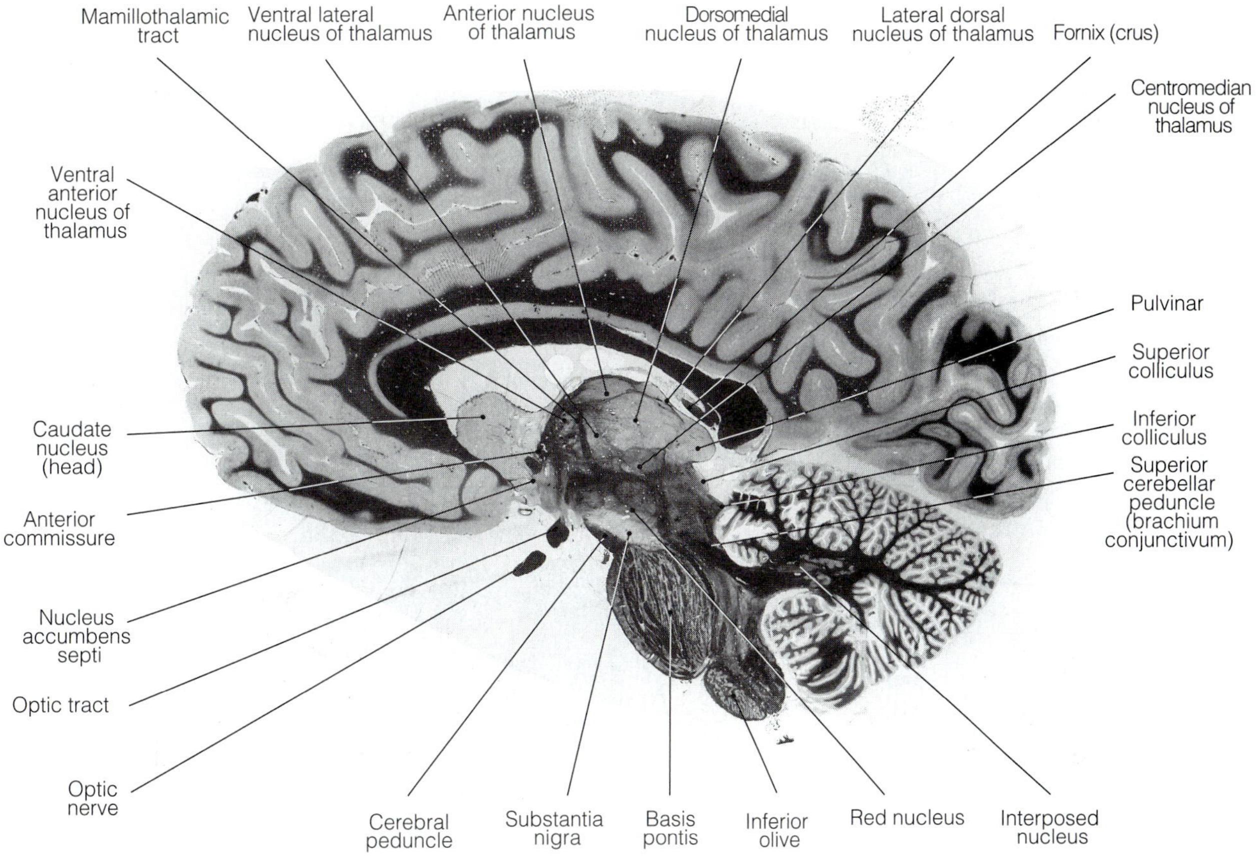
Mamillothalamic tract
Ventral lateral nucleus of thalamus
Anterior nucleus of thalamus
Dorsomedial nucleus of thalamus
Lateral dorsal nucleus of thalamus
Fornix (crus)
Centromedian nucleus of thalamus
Ventral anterior nucleus of thalamus
Pulvinar
Superior colliculus
Inferior colliculus
Superior cerebellar peduncle (brachium conjunctivum)
Caudate nucleus (head)
Anterior commissure
Nucleus accumbens septi
Optic tract
Optic nerve
Cerebral peduncle
Substantia nigra
Basis pontis
Inferior olive
Red nucleus
Interposed nucleus

FIGURE A2-15

Parasagittal brain section through the inferior olive and oculomotor nerve rootlets.

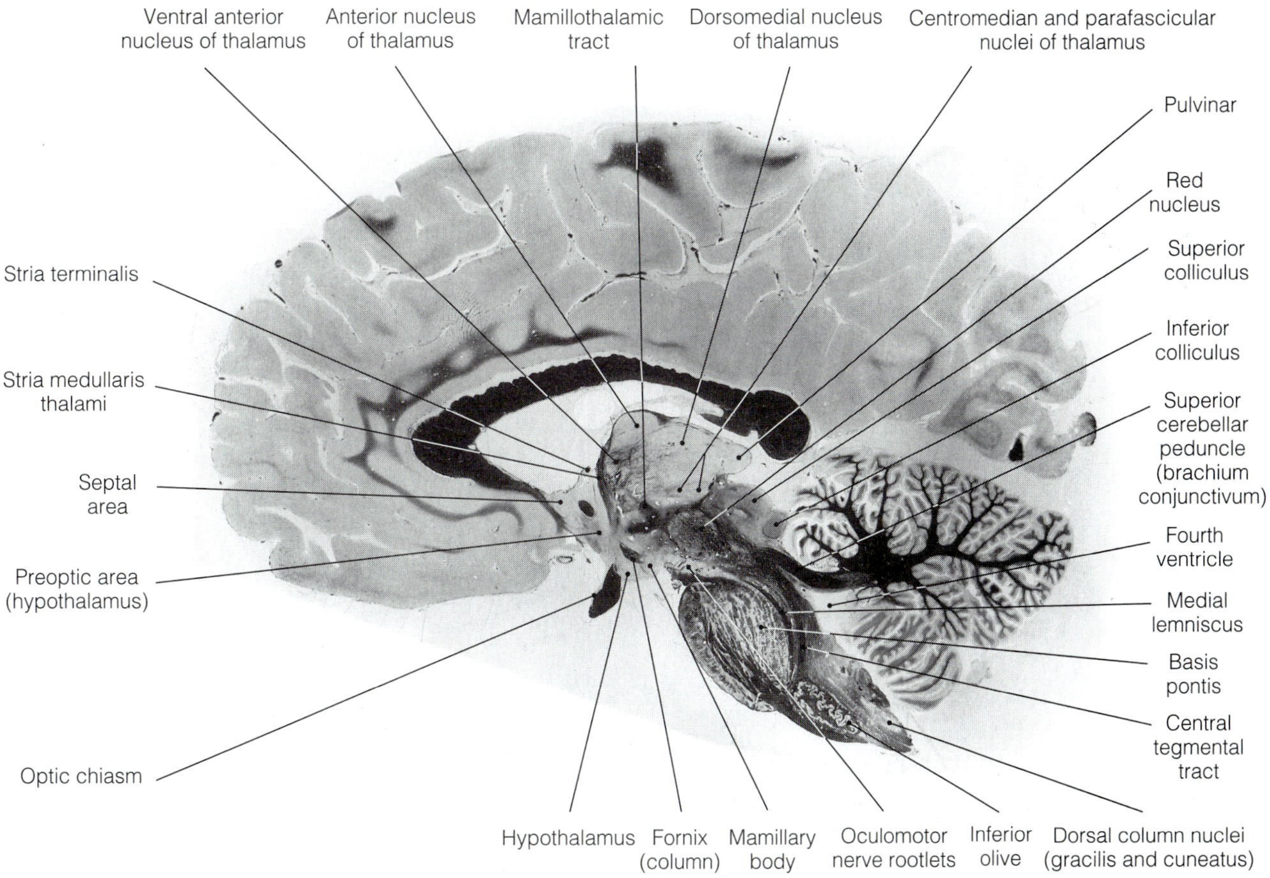
Ventral anterior nucleus of thalamus
Anterior nucleus of thalamus
Mamillothalamic tract
Dorsomedial nucleus of thalamus
Centromedian and parafascicular nuclei of thalamus
Pulvinar
Red nucleus
Superior colliculus
Inferior colliculus
Superior cerebellar peduncle (brachium conjunctivum)
Fourth ventricle
Medial lemniscus
Basis pontis
Central tegmental tract
Stria terminalis
Stria medullaris thalami
Septal area
Preoptic area (hypothalamus)
Optic chiasm
Hypothalamus
Fornix (column)
Mamillary body
Oculomotor nerve rootlets
Inferior olive
Dorsal column nuclei (gracilis and cuneatus)

FIGURE A2-16

Parasagittal brain section through the red nucleus and optic chiasma.

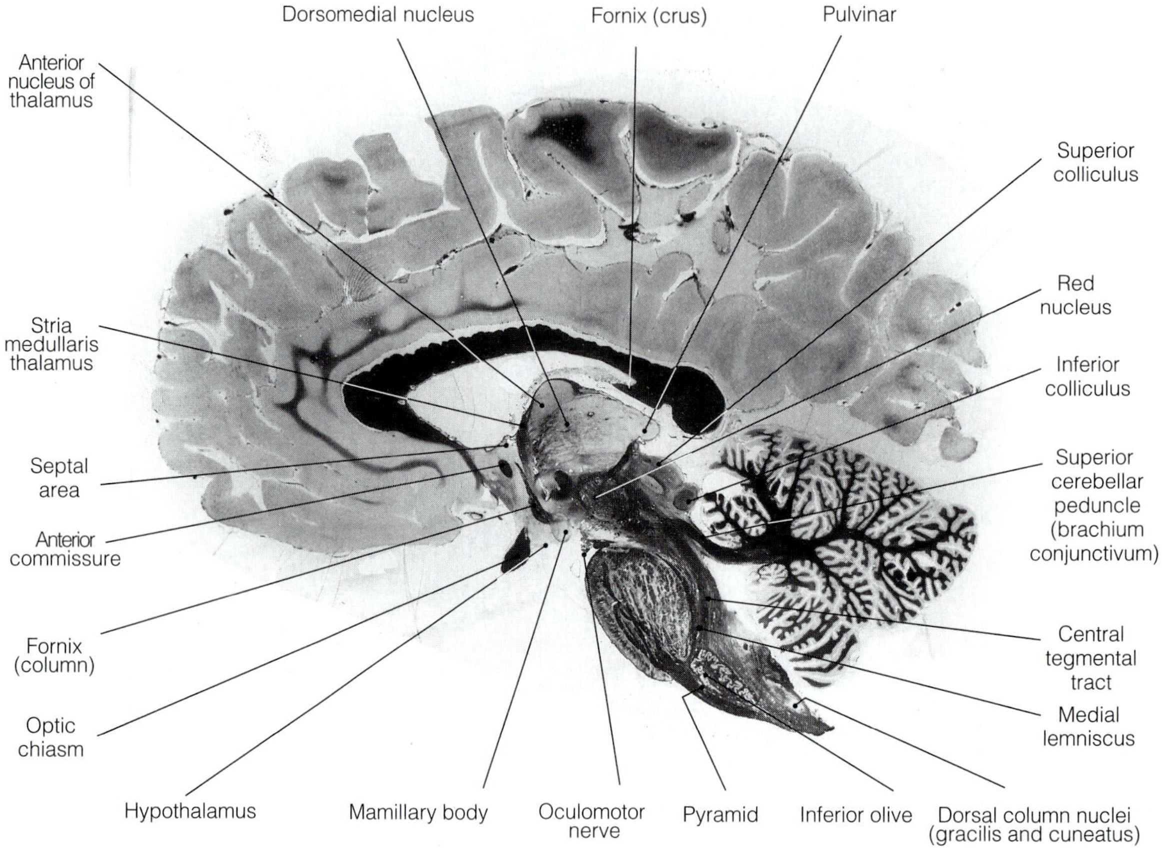
Dorsomedial nucleus
Fornix (crus)
Pulvinar
Anterior nucleus of thalamus
Superior colliculus
Red nucleus
Stria medullaris thalamus
Inferior colliculus
Septal area
Superior cerebellar peduncle (brachium conjunctivum)
Anterior commissure
Fornix (column)
Central tegmental tract
Optic chiasm
Medial lemniscus
Hypothalamus
Mamillary body
Oculomotor nerve
Pyramid
Inferior olive
Dorsal column nuclei (gracilis and cuneatus)

FIGURE A2-17

Parasagittal brain section through the crus and columns of the fornix.

AXIAL YAKOVLEV

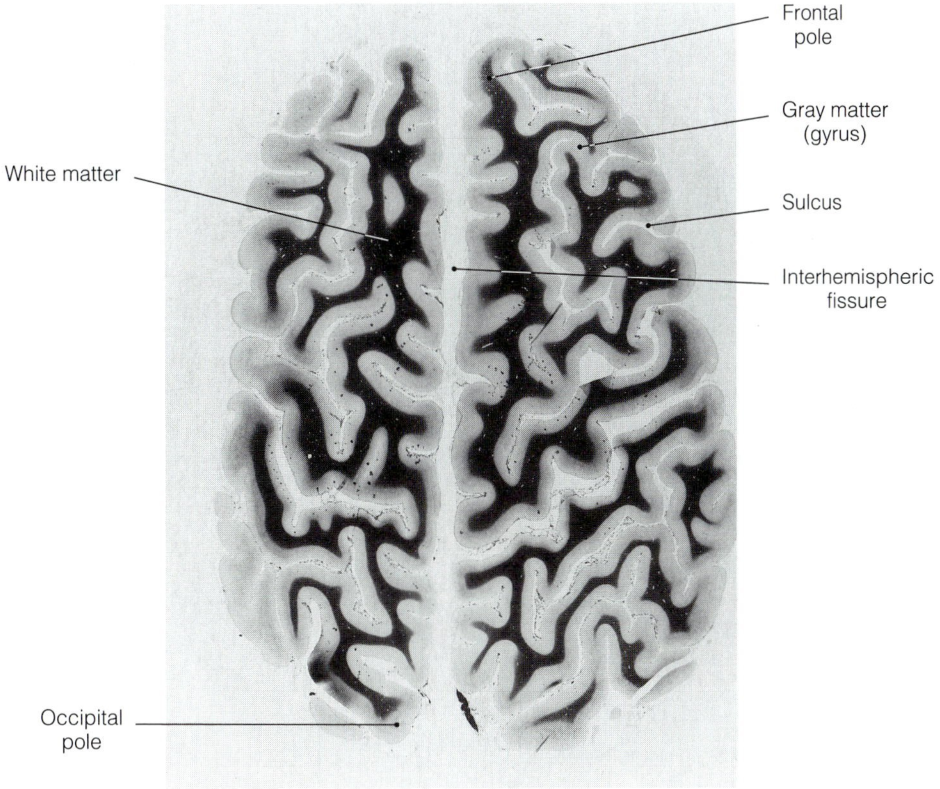
Frontal
pole
Gray matter
(gyrus)
White matter
Sulcus
Interhemispheric
fissure
Occipital
pole

FIGURE A3-1

Axial section of the brain through the frontal and occipital poles.

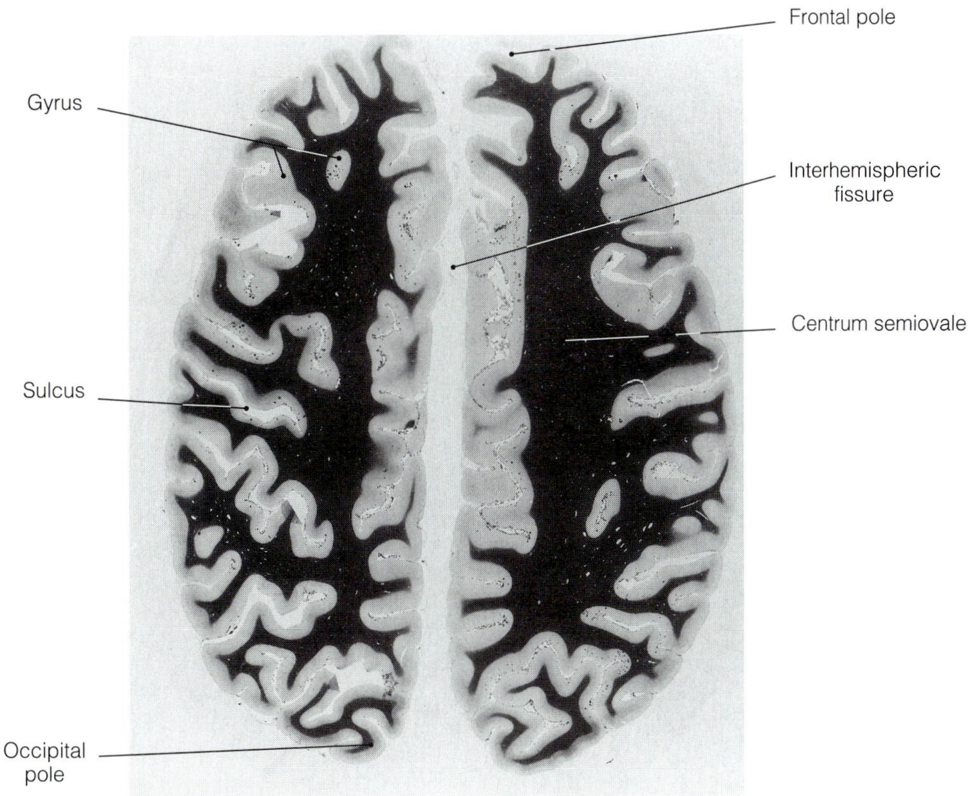
Frontal pole
Gyrus
Interhemispheric
fissure
Centrum semiovale
Sulcus
Occipital
pole

FIGURE A3-2

Axial section of the brain through the centrum semiovale.

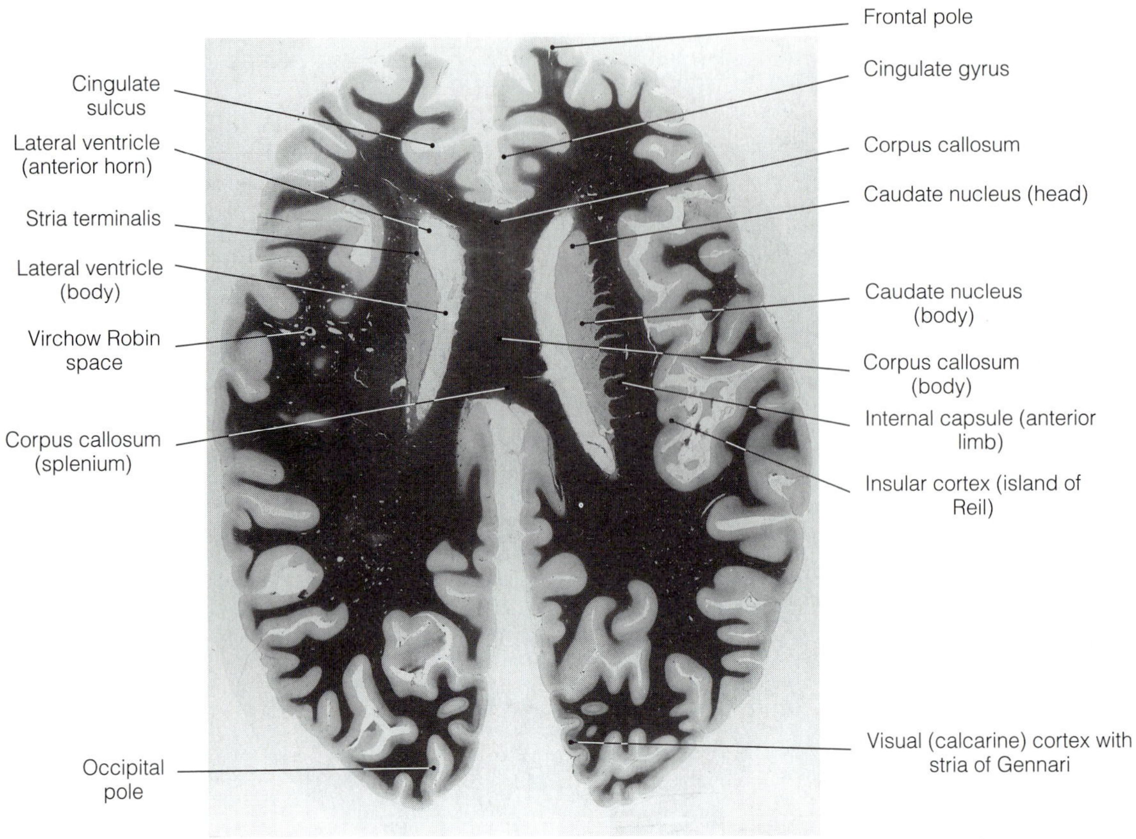
Frontal pole
Cingulate sulcus
Cingulate gyrus
Lateral ventricle (anterior horn)
Corpus callosum
Caudate nucleus (head)
Stria terminalis
Lateral ventricle (body)
Caudate nucleus (body)
Virchow Robin space
Corpus callosum (body)
Corpus callosum (splenium)
Internal capsule (anterior limb)
Insular cortex (island of Reil)
Occipital pole
Visual (calcarine) cortex with stria of Gennari

FIGURE A3-3

Axial section of the brain through the body of the corpus callosum.

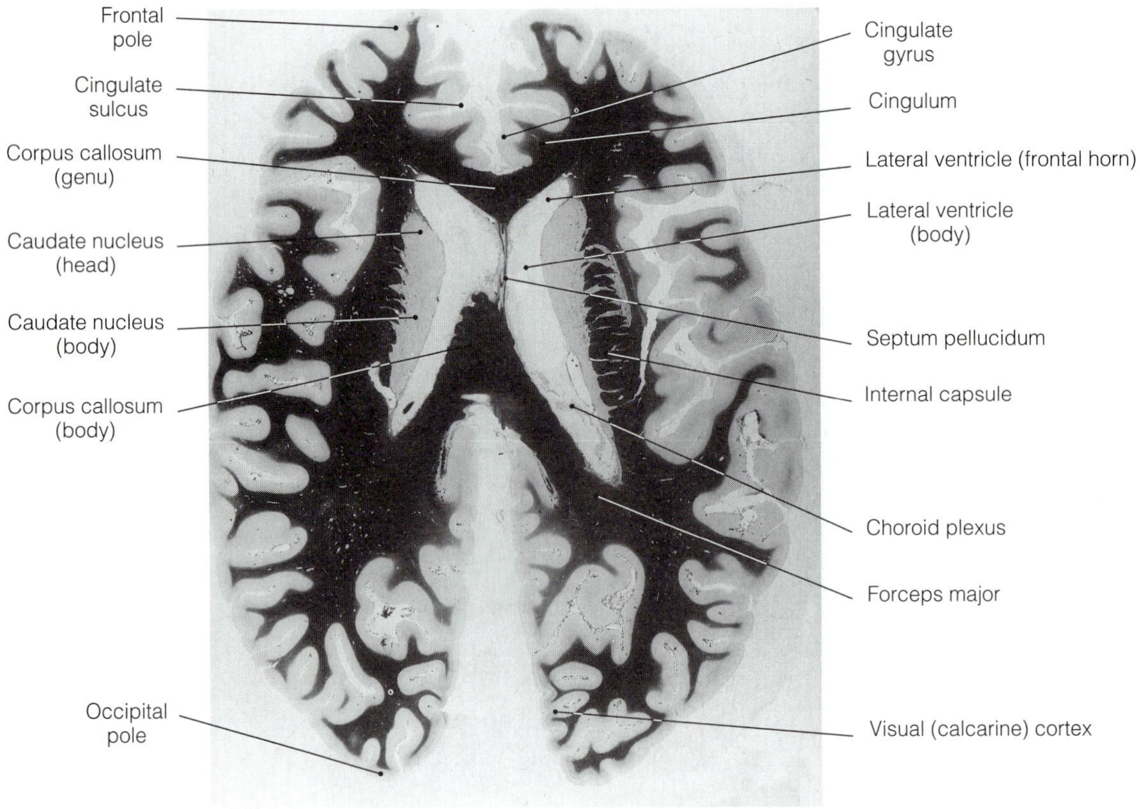
Frontal pole
Cingulate gyrus
Cingulate sulcus
Cingulum
Corpus callosum (genu)
Lateral ventricle (frontal horn)
Lateral ventricle (body)
Caudate nucleus (head)
Septum pellucidum
Caudate nucleus (body)
Internal capsule
Corpus callosum (body)
Choroid plexus
Forceps major
Occipital pole
Visual (calcarine) cortex

FIGURE A3-4

Axial section of the brain through the body and frontal horn of the lateral ventricle.

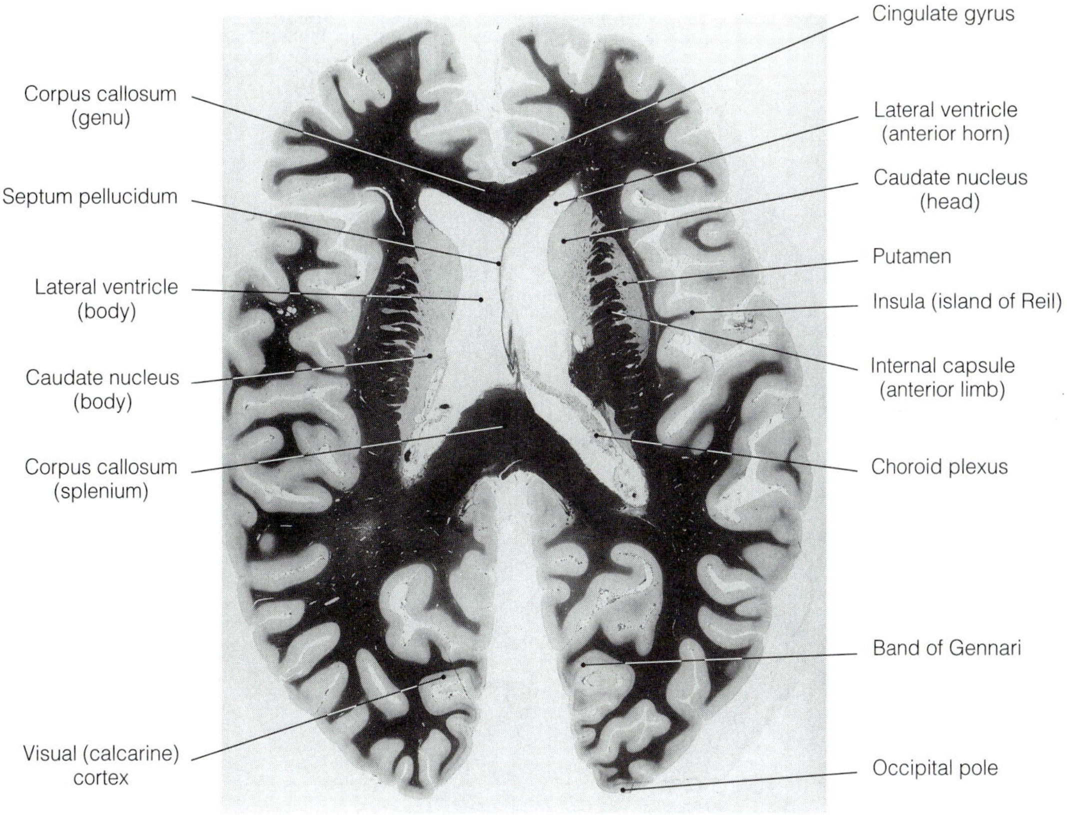
Corpus callosum
(genu)
Septum pellucidum
Lateral ventricle
(body)
Caudate nucleus
(body)
Corpus callosum
(splenium)
Visual (calcarine)
cortex
Cingulate gyrus
Lateral ventricle
(anterior horn)
Caudate nucleus
(head)
Putamen
Insula (island of Reil)
Internal capsule
(anterior limb)
Choroid plexus
Band of Gennari
Occipital pole

FIGURE A3-5

Axial section of the brain through the genu and splenium of the corpus callosum.

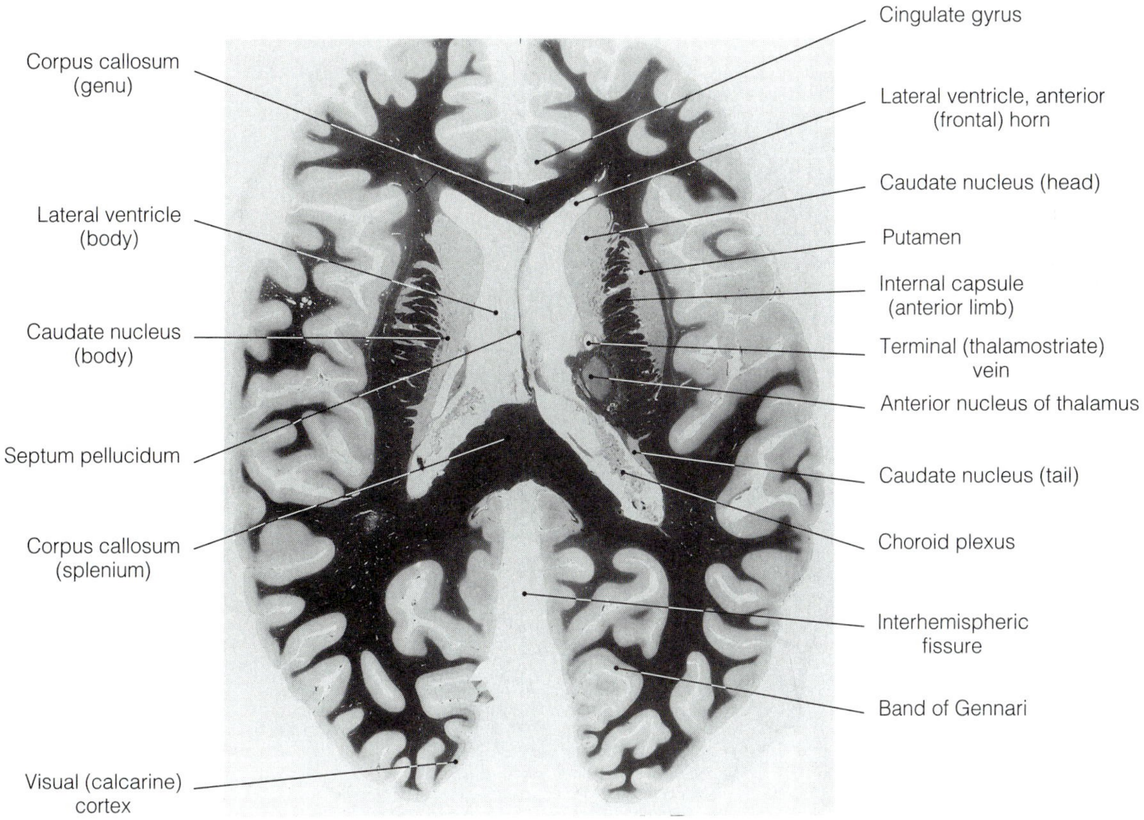
Corpus callosum
(genu)
Lateral ventricle
(body)
Caudate nucleus
(body)
Septum pellucidum
Corpus callosum
(splenium)
Visual (calcarine)
cortex
Cingulate gyrus
Lateral ventricle, anterior
(frontal) horn
Caudate nucleus (head)
Putamen
Internal capsule
(anterior limb)
Terminal (thalamostriate)
vein
Anterior nucleus of thalamus
Caudate nucleus (tail)
Choroid plexus
Interhemispheric
fissure
Band of Gennari

FIGURE A3-6

Axial section of the brain through the superior thalamus.

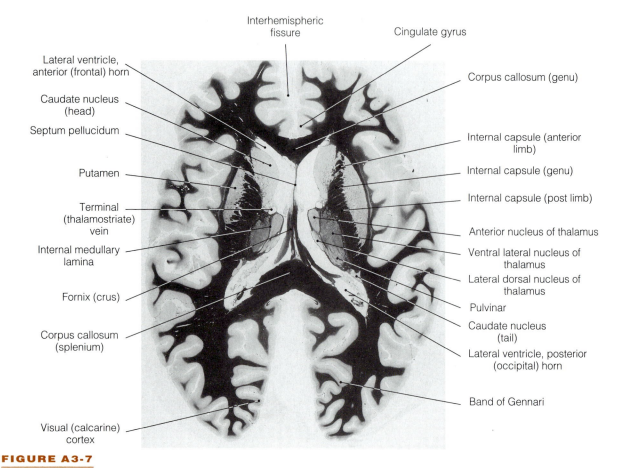

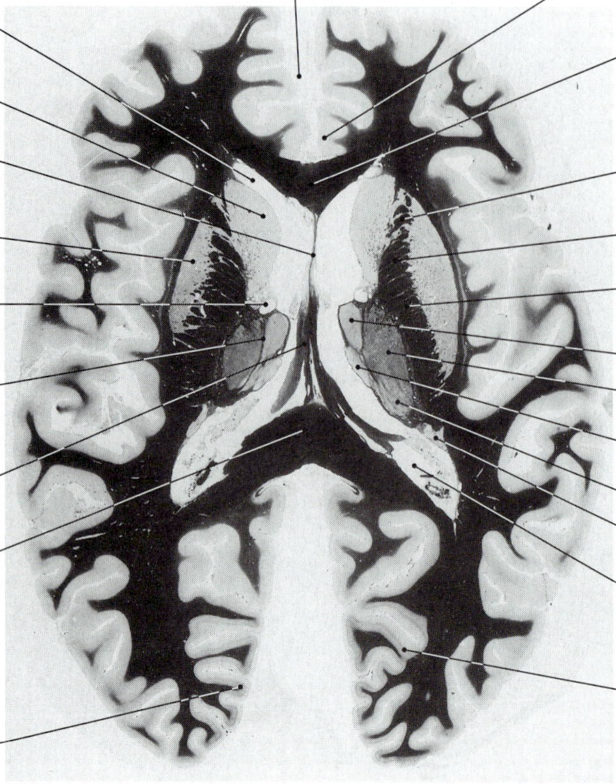
Interhemispheric fissure
Cingulate gyrus
Lateral ventricle, anterior (frontal) horn
Corpus callosum (genu)
Caudate nucleus (head)
Septum pellucidum
Internal capsule (anterior limb)
Internal capsule (genu)
Putamen
Internal capsule (post limb)
Terminal (thalamostriate) vein
Anterior nucleus of thalamus
Internal medullary lamina
Ventral lateral nucleus of thalamus
Lateral dorsal nucleus of thalamus
Fornix (crus)
Pulvinar
Caudate nucleus (tail)
Corpus callosum (splenium)
Lateral ventricle, posterior (occipital) horn
Band of Gennari
Visual (calcarine) cortex

FIGURE A3-7

Axial section of the brain through the crus of the fornix and dorsal thalamus.

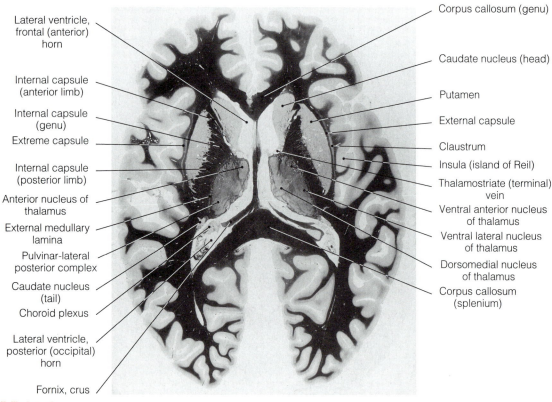

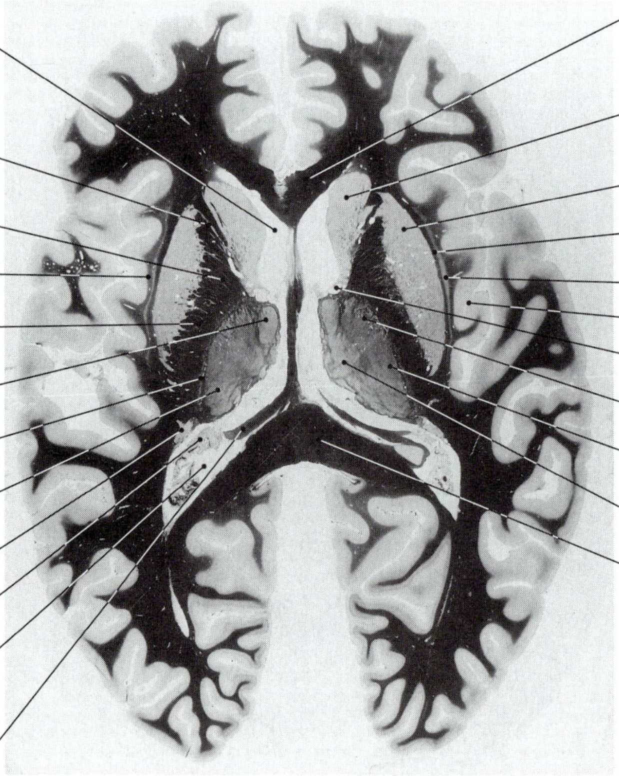
Corpus callosum (genu)
Lateral ventricle, frontal (anterior) horn
Caudate nucleus (head)
Internal capsule (anterior limb)
Putamen
Internal capsule (genu)
External capsule
Extreme capsule
Claustrum
Insula (island of Reil)
Internal capsule (posterior limb)
Thalamostriate (terminal) vein
Anterior nucleus of thalamus
Ventral anterior nucleus of thalamus
External medullary lamina
Ventral lateral nucleus of thalamus
Pulvinar-lateral posterior complex
Dorsomedial nucleus of thalamus
Caudate nucleus (tail)
Corpus callosum (splenium)
Choroid plexus
Lateral ventricle, posterior (occipital) horn
Fornix, crus

FIGURE A3-8

Axial section the brain through the frontal and occipital horns of the lateral ventricle.

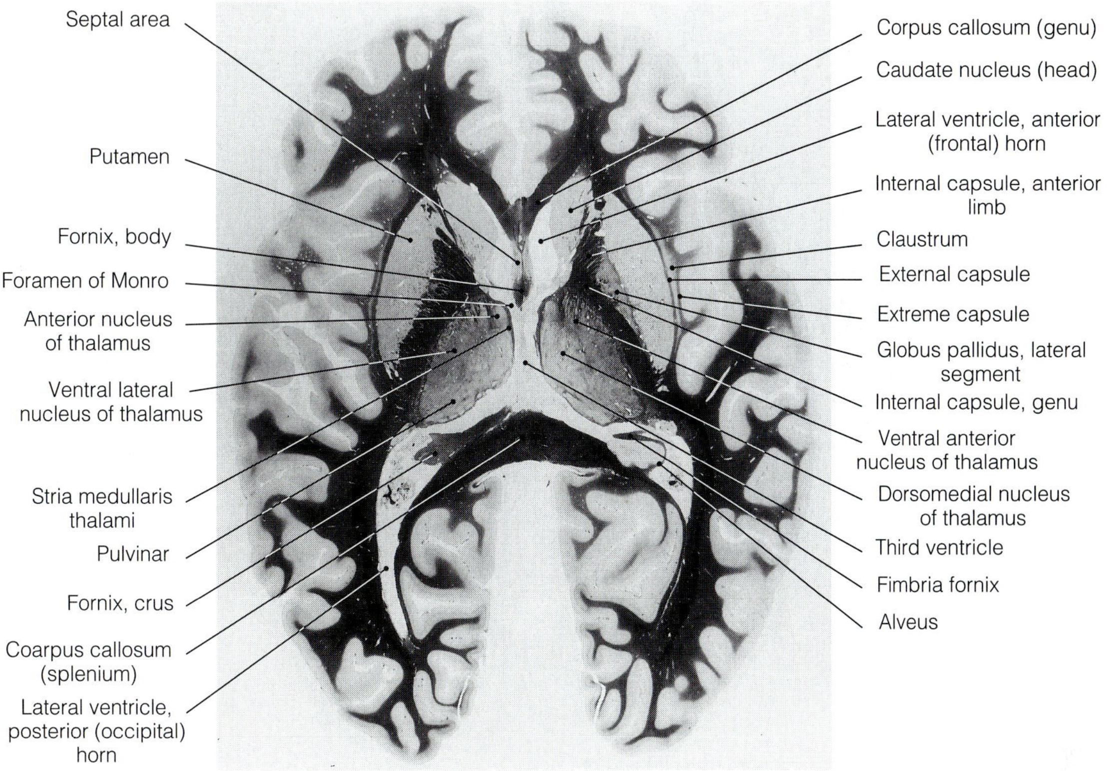
Septal area
Putamen
Fornix, body
Foramen of Monro
Anterior nucleus of thalamus
Ventral lateral nucleus of thalamus
Stria medullaris thalami
Pulvinar
Fornix, crus
Coarpus callosum (splenium)
Lateral ventricle, posterior (occipital) horn
Corpus callosum (genu)
Caudate nucleus (head)
Lateral ventricle, anterior (frontal) horn
Internal capsule, anterior limb
Claustrum
External capsule
Extreme capsule
Globus pallidus, lateral segment
Internal capsule, genu
Ventral anterior nucleus of thalamus
Dorsomedial nucleus of thalamus
Third ventricle
Fimbria fornix
Alveus

FIGURE A3-9

Axial section of the brain through the foramen of Monro.

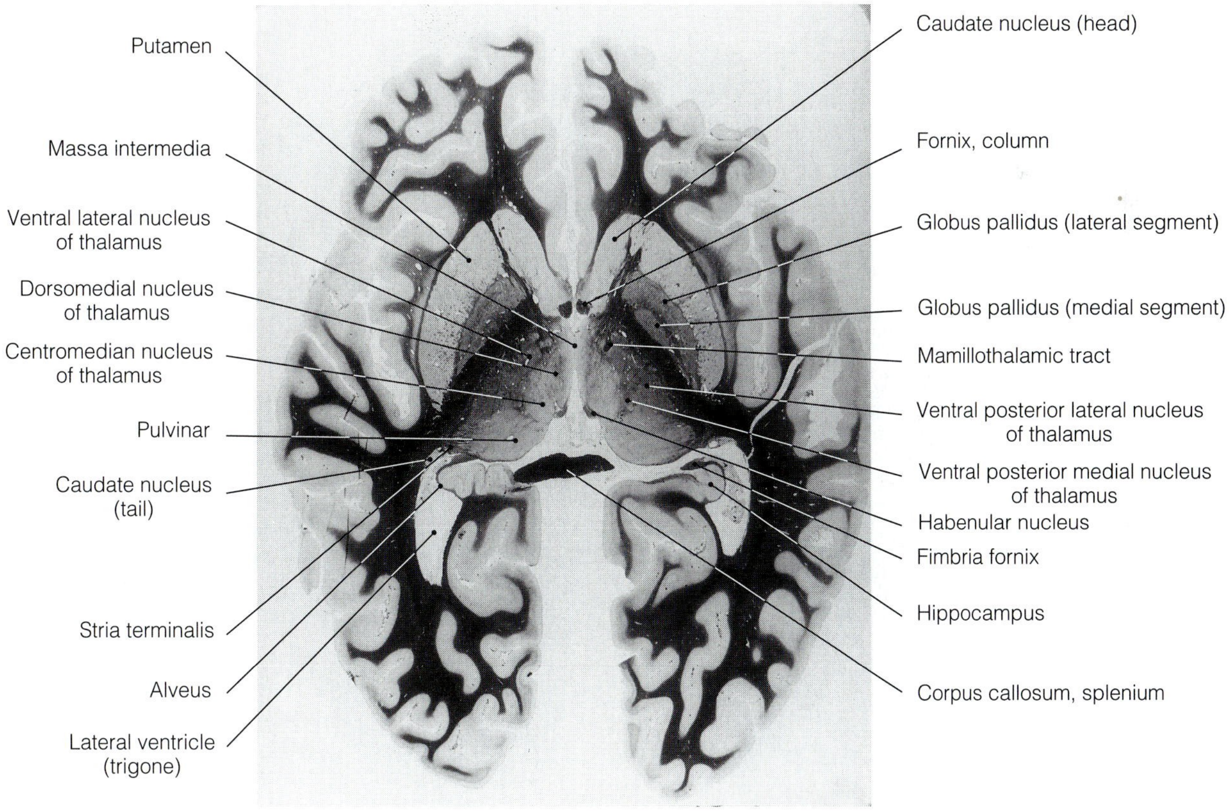
Putamen
Massa intermedia
Ventral lateral nucleus of thalamus
Dorsomedial nucleus of thalamus
Centromedian nucleus of thalamus
Pulvinar
Caudate nucleus (tail)
Stria terminalis
Alveus
Lateral ventricle (trigone)
Caudate nucleus (head)
Fornix, column
Globus pallidus (lateral segment)
Globus pallidus (medial segment)
Mamillothalamic tract
Ventral posterior lateral nucleus of thalamus
Ventral posterior medial nucleus of thalamus
Habenular nucleus
Fimbria fornix
Hippocampus
Corpus callosum, splenium

FIGURE A3-10

Axial section of the brain through the trigone of the lateral ventricle.

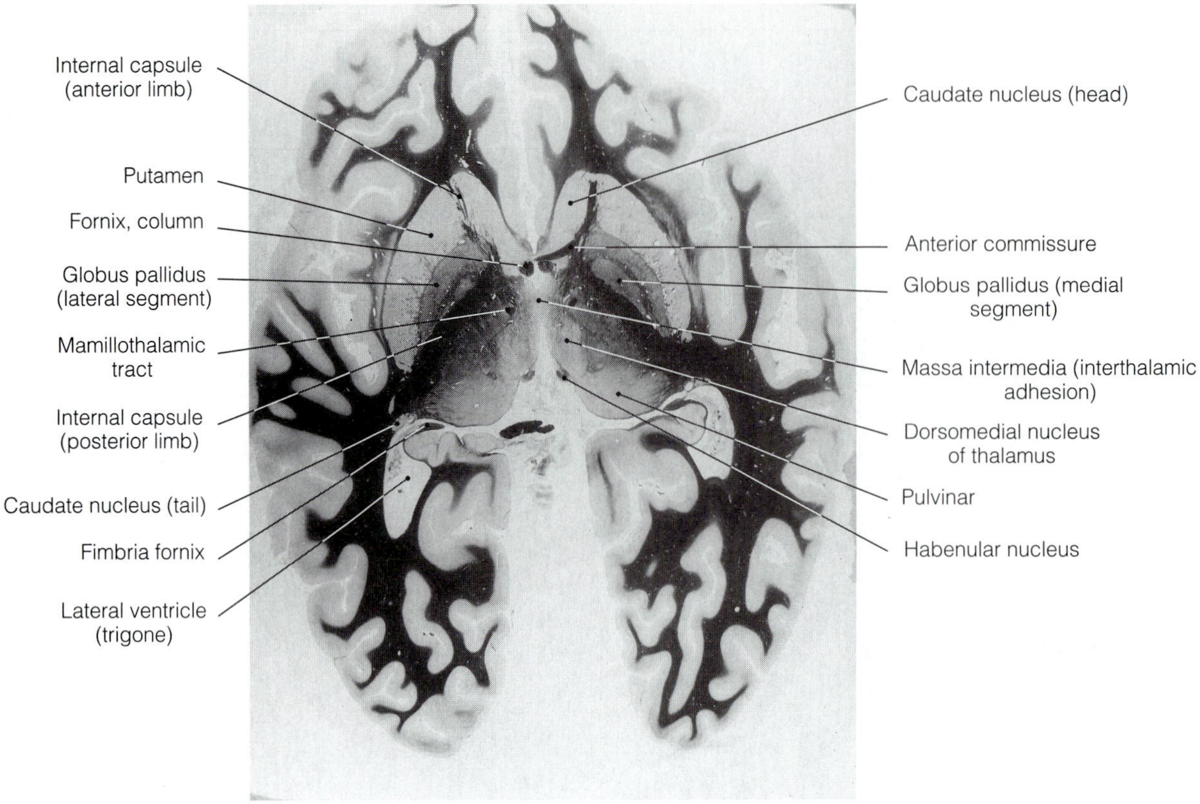
Internal capsule
(anterior limb)
Putamen
Fornix, column
Globus pallidus
(lateral segment)
Mamillothalamic
tract
Internal capsule
(posterior limb)
Caudate nucleus (tail)
Fimbria fornix
Lateral ventricle
(trigone)
Caudate nucleus (head)
Anterior commissure
Globus pallidus (medial
segment)
Massa intermedia (interthalamic
adhesion)
Dorsomedial nucleus
of thalamus
Pulvinar
Habenular nucleus

FIGURE A3-11

Axial section of the brain through the anterior commissure and massa intermedia.

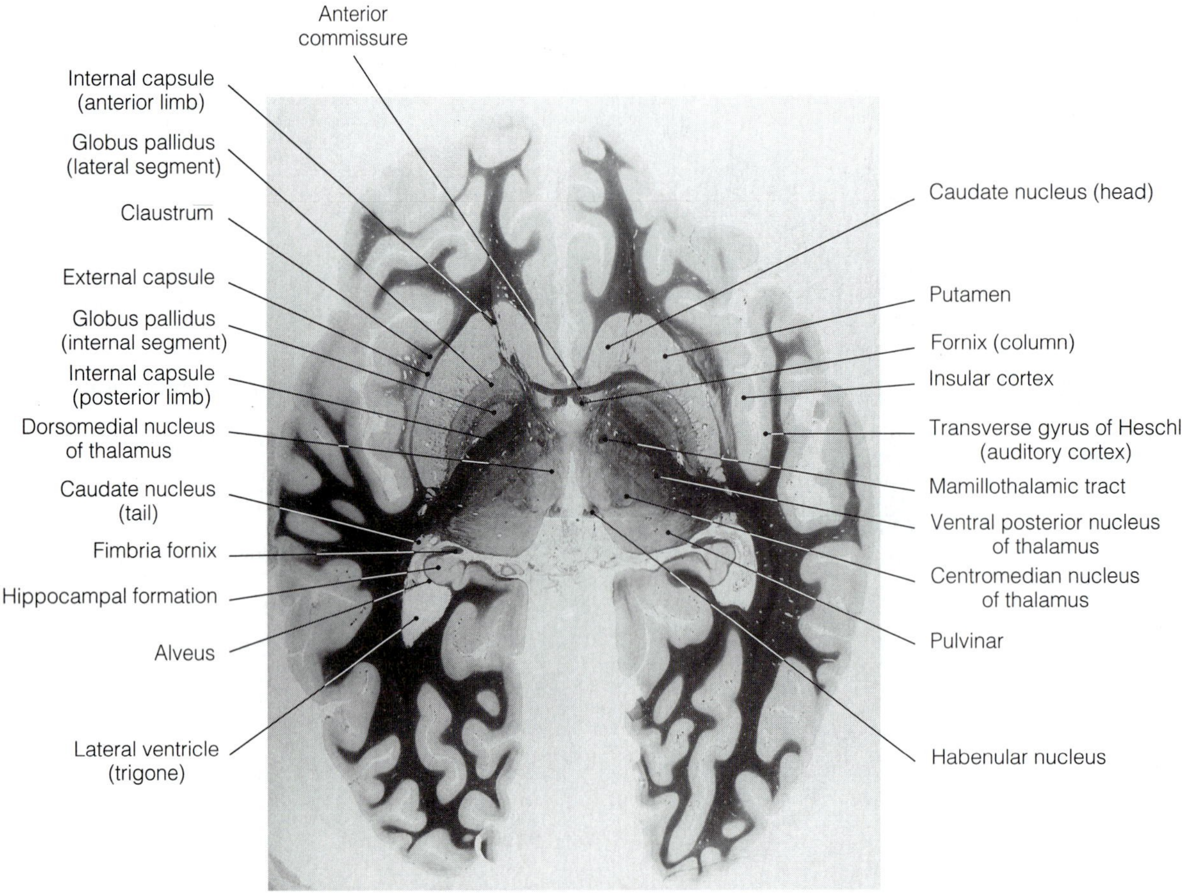
Anterior
commissure
Internal capsule
(anterior limb)
Globus pallidus
(lateral segment)
Claustrum
External capsule
Globus pallidus
(internal segment)
Internal capsule
(posterior limb)
Dorsomedial nucleus
of thalamus
Caudate nucleus
(tail)
Fimbria fornix
Hippocampal formation
Alveus
Lateral ventricle
(trigone)
Caudate nucleus (head)
Putamen
Fornix (column)
Insular cortex
Transverse gyrus of Heschl
(auditory cortex)
Mamillothalamic tract
Ventral posterior nucleus
of thalamus
Centromedian nucleus
of thalamus
Pulvinar
Habenular nucleus

FIGURE A3-12

Axial section of the brain through the anterior commissure and habenular nucleus.

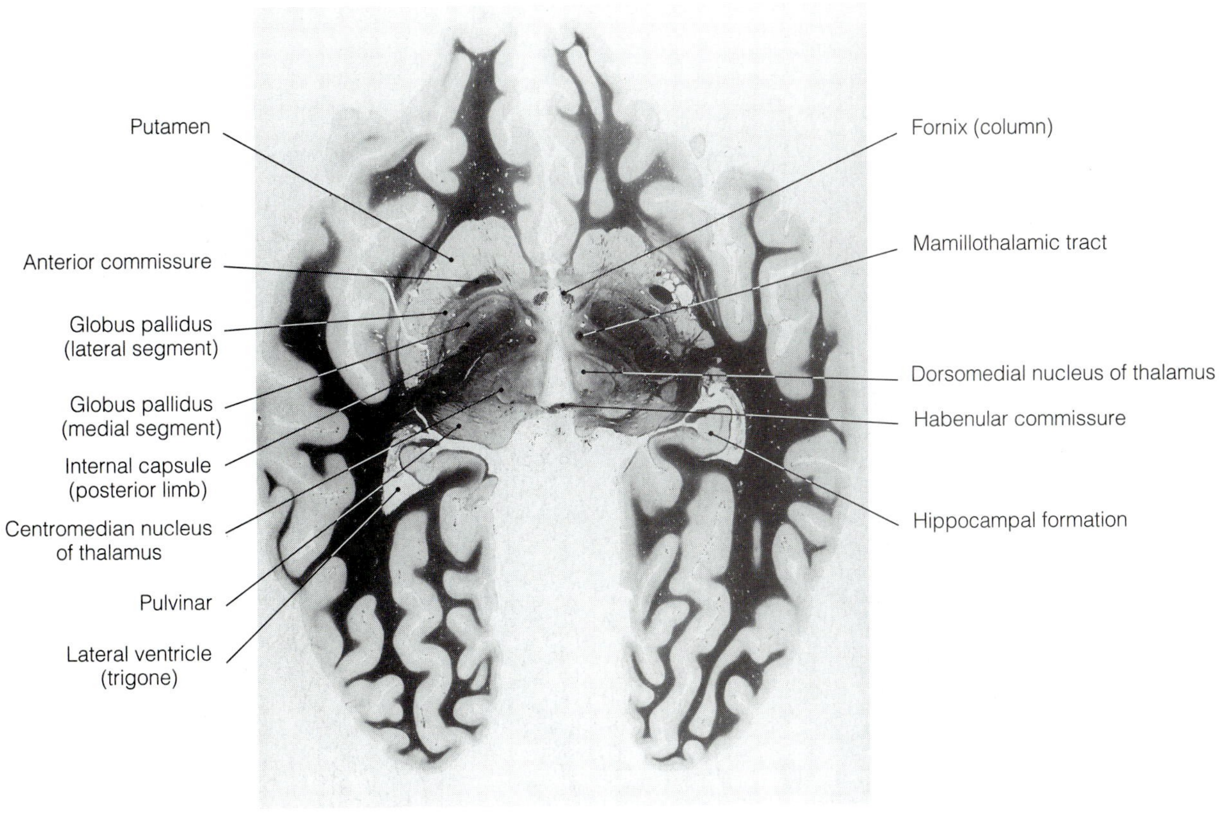

Putamen
Anterior commissure
Globus pallidus
(lateral segment)
Globus pallidus
(medial segment)
Internal capsule
(posterior limb)
Centromedian nucleus
of thalamus
Pulvinar
Lateral ventricle
(trigone)
Fornix (column)
Mamillothalamic tract
Dorsomedial nucleus of thalamus
Habenular commissure
Hippocampal formation

FIGURE A3-13

Axial section of the brain through the habenular commissure.

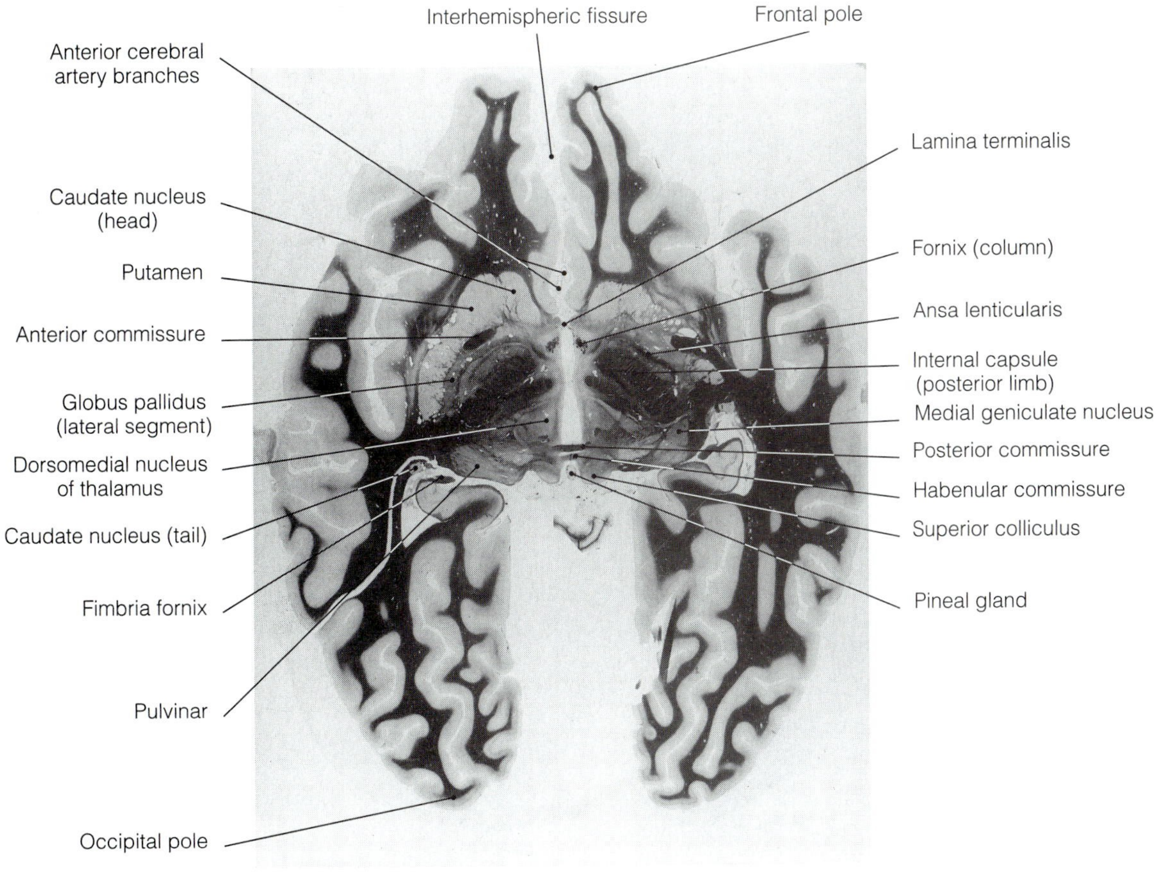

Interhemispheric fissure
Frontal pole
Anterior cerebral
artery branches
Caudate nucleus
(head)
Putamen
Anterior commissure
Globus pallidus
(lateral segment)
Dorsomedial nucleus
of thalamus
Caudate nucleus (tail)
Fimbria fornix
Pulvinar
Occipital pole
Lamina terminalis
Fornix (column)
Ansa lenticularis
Internal capsule
(posterior limb)
Medial geniculate nucleus
Posterior commissure
Habenular commissure
Superior colliculus
Pineal gland

FIGURE A3-14

Axial section of the brain through the habenular and posterior commissures.

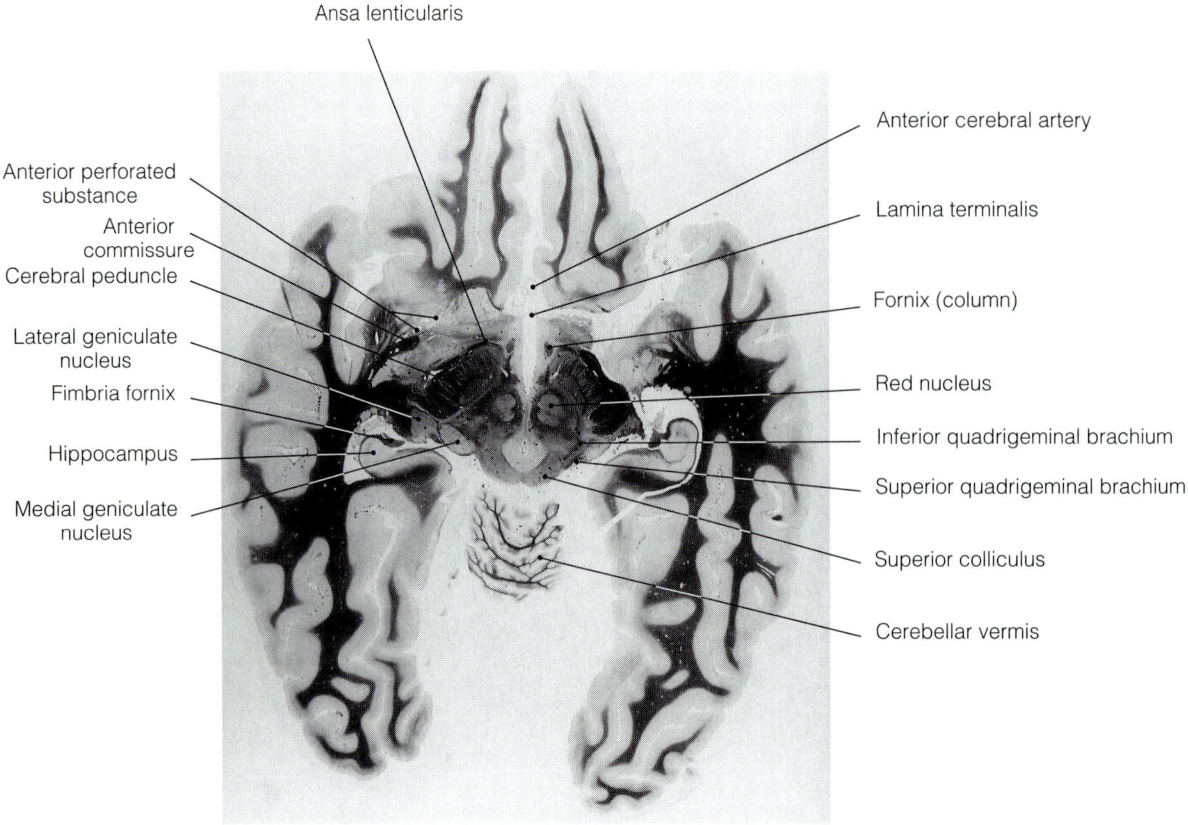
Ansa lenticularis
Anterior perforated substance
Anterior commissure
Cerebral peduncle
Lateral geniculate nucleus
Fimbria fornix
Hippocampus
Medial geniculate nucleus
Anterior cerebral artery
Lamina terminalis
Fornix (column)
Red nucleus
Inferior quadrigeminal brachium
Superior quadrigeminal brachium
Superior colliculus
Cerebellar vermis

FIGURE A3-15

Axial section of the brain through the anterior perforated substance.

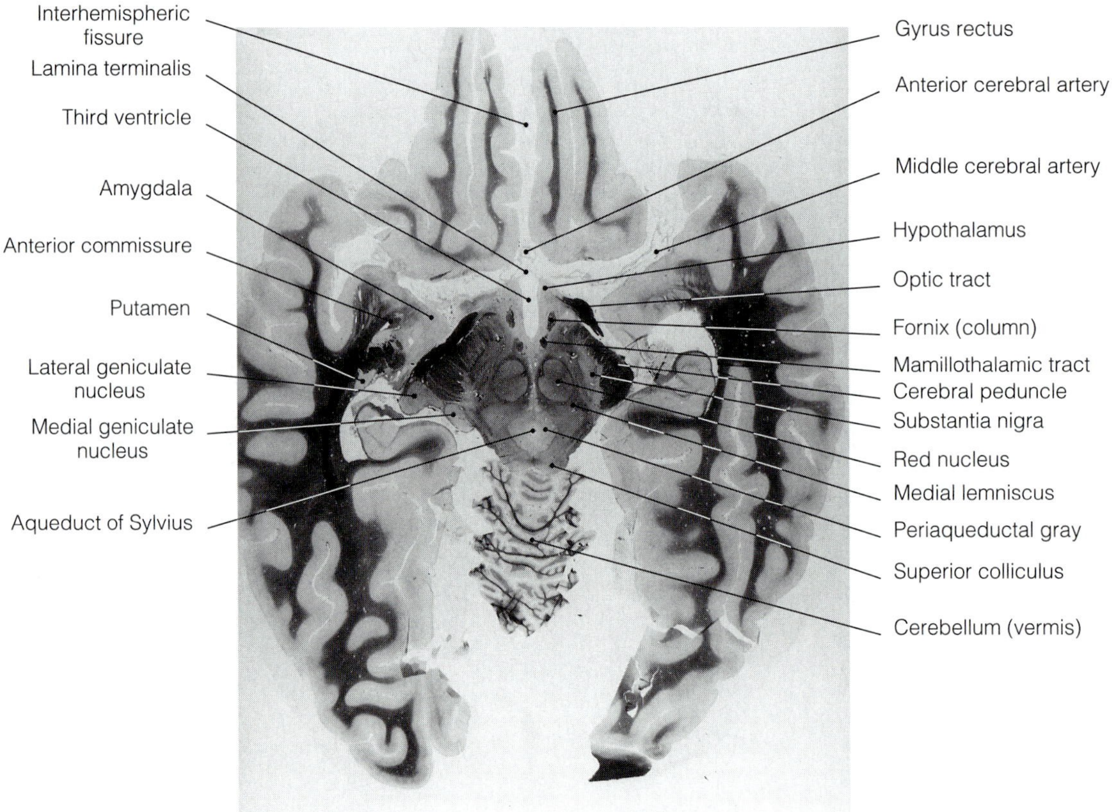
Interhemispheric fissure
Lamina terminalis
Third ventricle
Amygdala
Anterior commissure
Putamen
Lateral geniculate nucleus
Medial geniculate nucleus
Aqueduct of Sylvius
Gyrus rectus
Anterior cerebral artery
Middle cerebral artery
Hypothalamus
Optic tract
Fornix (column)
Mamillothalamic tract
Cerebral peduncle
Substantia nigra
Red nucleus
Medial lemniscus
Periaqueductal gray
Superior colliculus
Cerebellum (vermis)

FIGURE A3-16

Axial section of the brain through the dorsal midbrain.

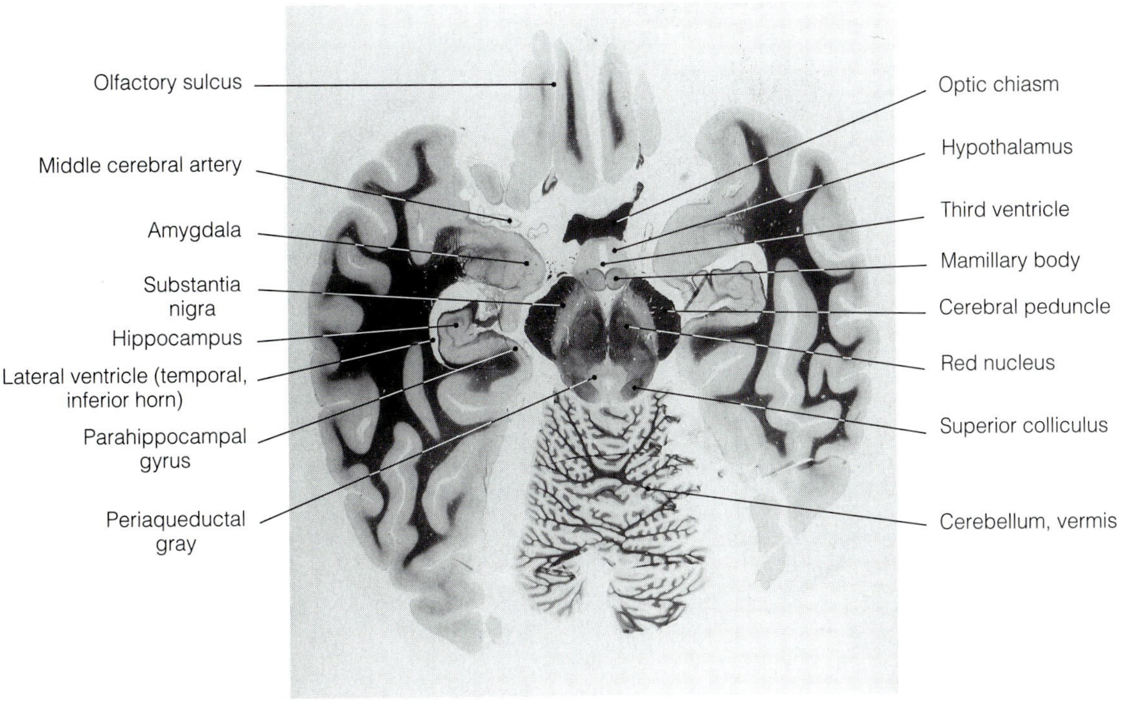
Olfactory sulcus
Middle cerebral artery
Amygdala
Substantia nigra
Hippocampus
Lateral ventricle (temporal, inferior horn)
Parahippocampal gyrus
Periaqueductal gray
Optic chiasm
Hypothalamus
Third ventricle
Mamillary body
Cerebral peduncle
Red nucleus
Superior colliculus
Cerebellum, vermis

FIGURE A3-17

Axial section of the brain through the mamillary body and optic chiasma.

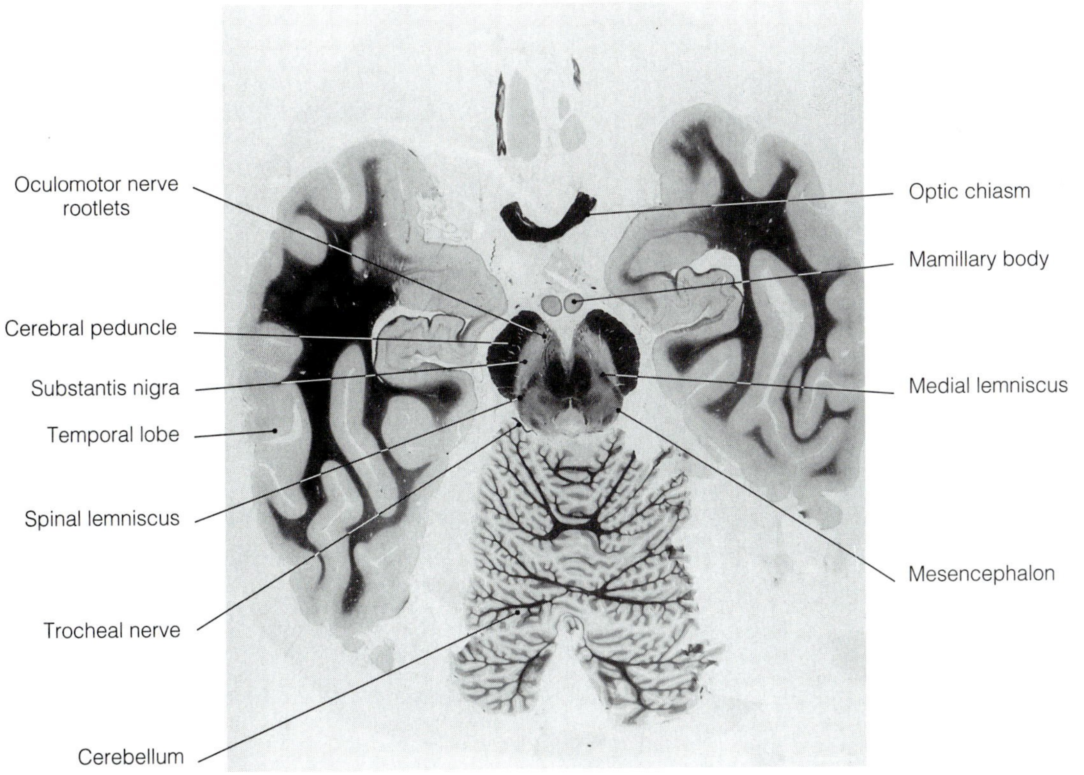
Oculomotor nerve rootlets
Cerebral peduncle
Substantis nigra
Temporal lobe
Spinal lemniscus
Trocheal nerve
Cerebellum
Optic chiasm
Mamillary body
Medial lemniscus
Mesencephalon

FIGURE A3-18

Axial section of the brain through the mamillary body and optic chiasma.

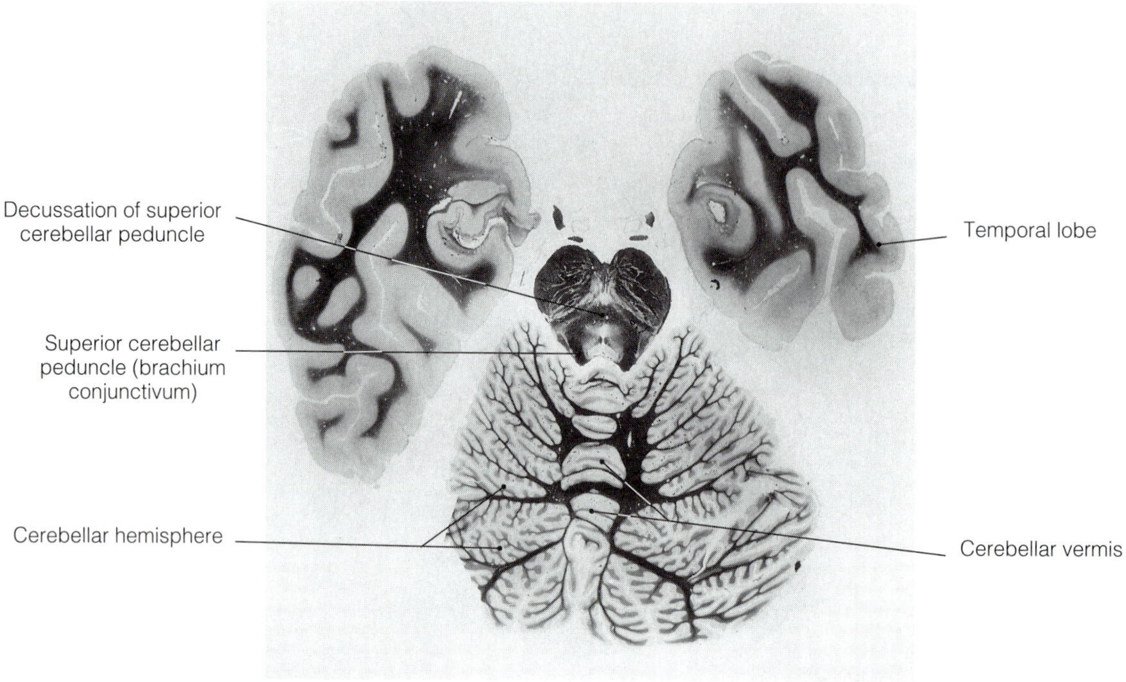
Decussation of superior cerebellar peduncle
Superior cerebellar peduncle (brachium conjunctivum)
Cerebellar hemisphere
Temporal lobe
Cerebellar vermis

FIGURE A3-19

Axial section of the brain through the caudal midbrain.

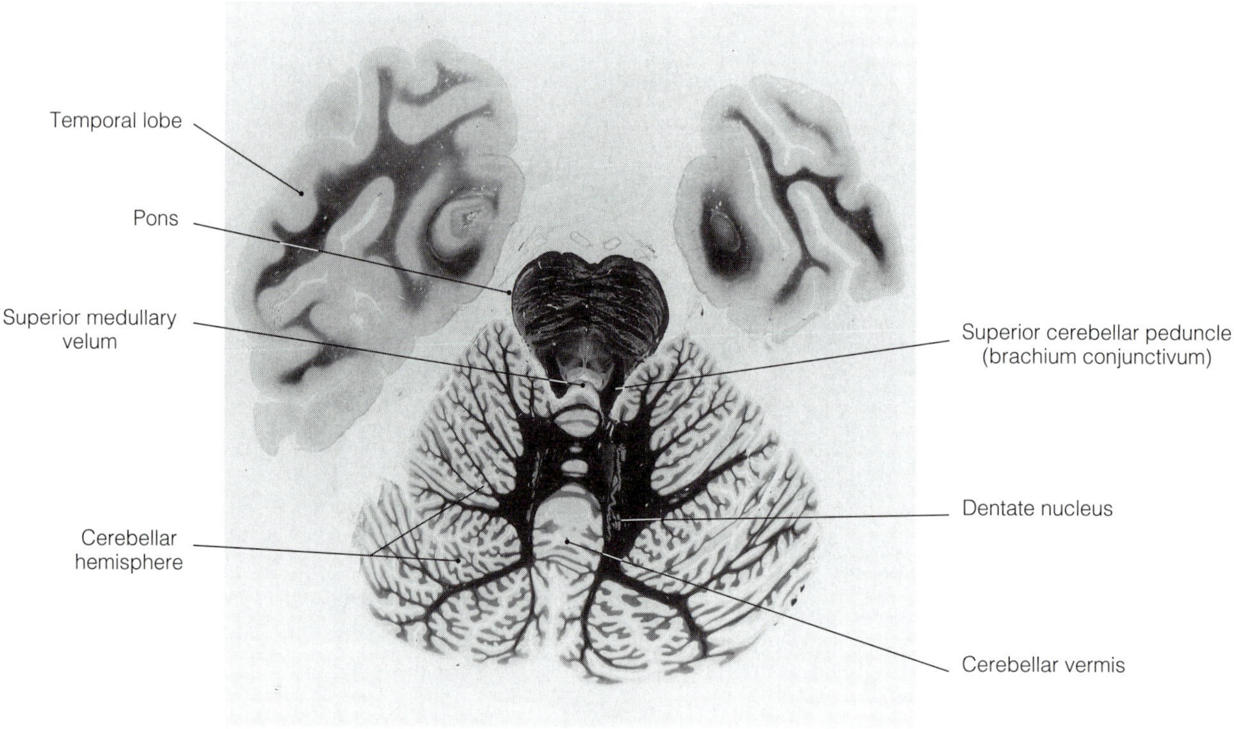
Temporal lobe
Pons
Superior medullary velum
Cerebellar hemisphere
Superior cerebellar peduncle (brachium conjunctivum)
Dentate nucleus
Cerebellar vermis

FIGURE A3-20

Axial section of the brain through the pons.

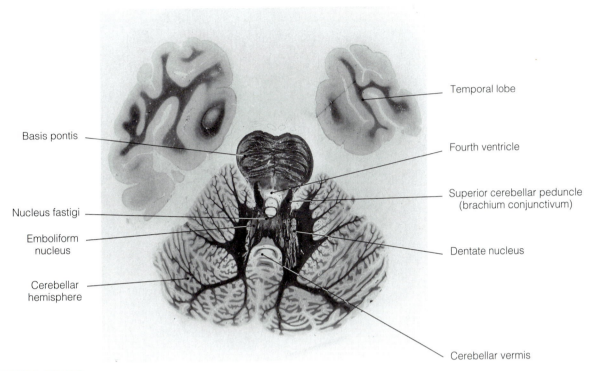

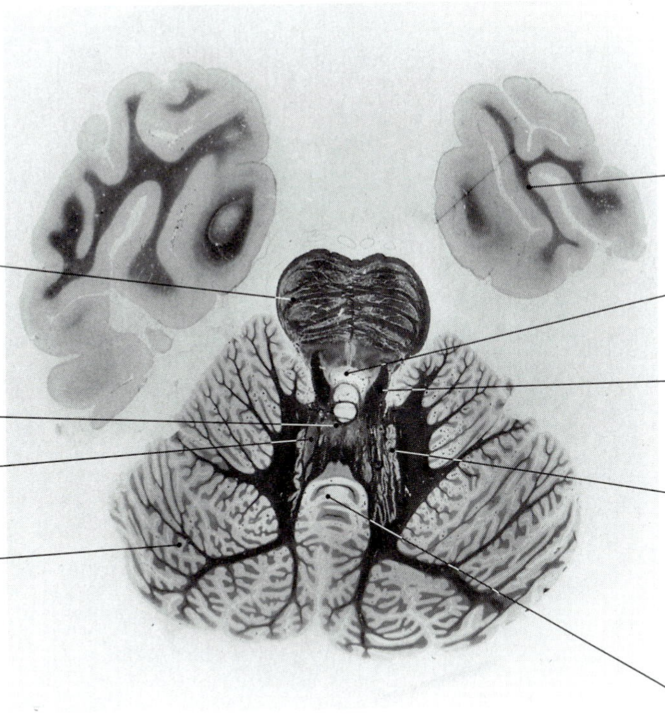
Temporal lobe
Basis pontis
Fourth ventricle
Superior cerebellar peduncle
(brachium conjunctivum)
Nucleus fastigi
Emboliform
nucleus
Dentate nucleus
Cerebellar
hemisphere
Cerebellar vermis

FIGURE A3-21

Axial section of the brain through the deep cerebellar nuclei.

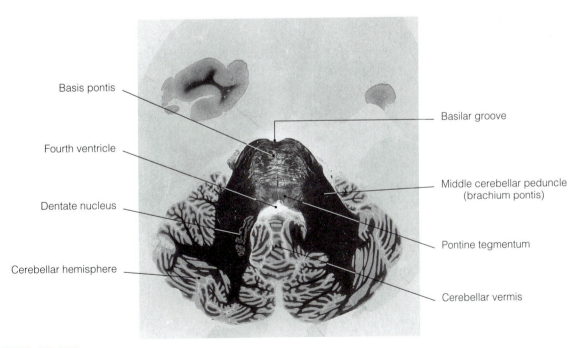

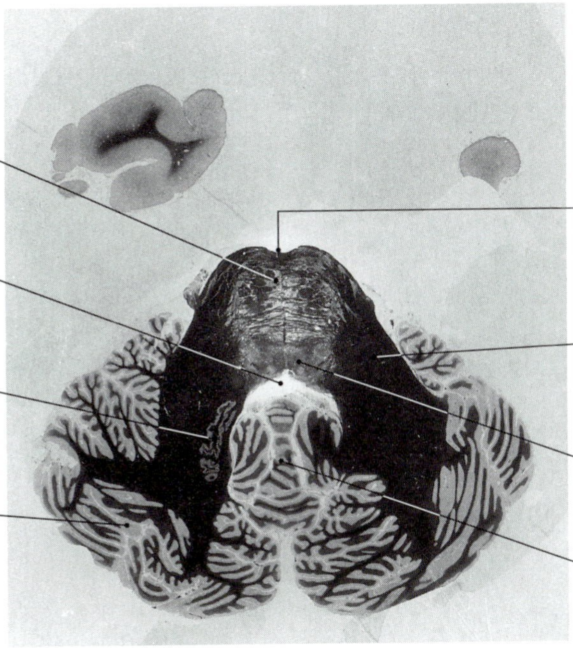
Basis pontis
Basilar groove
Fourth ventricle
Middle cerebellar peduncle
(brachium pontis)
Dentate nucleus
Pontine tegmentum
Cerebellar hemisphere
Cerebellar vermis

FIGURE A3-22

Axial section of the brain stem through the middle cerebellar peduncle.

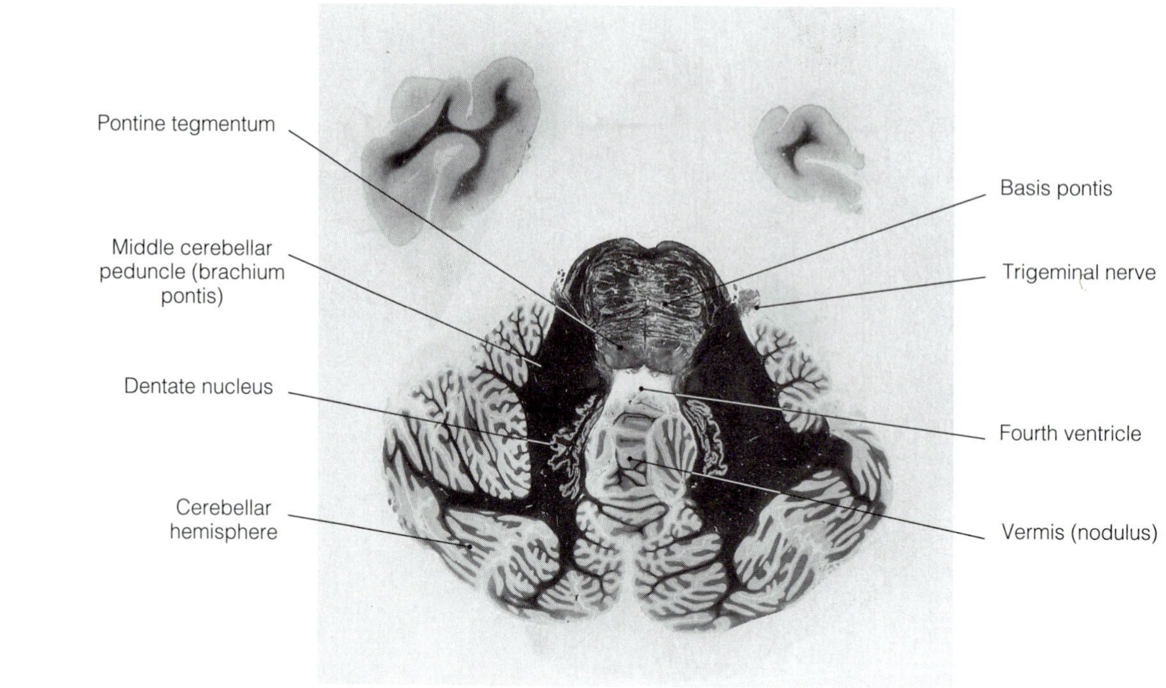
Pontine tegmentum
Middle cerebellar peduncle (brachium pontis)
Dentate nucleus
Cerebellar hemisphere
Basis pontis
Trigeminal nerve
Fourth ventricle
Vermis (nodulus)

FIGURE A3-23

Axial section of the brain stem at the level of the trigeminal nerve.

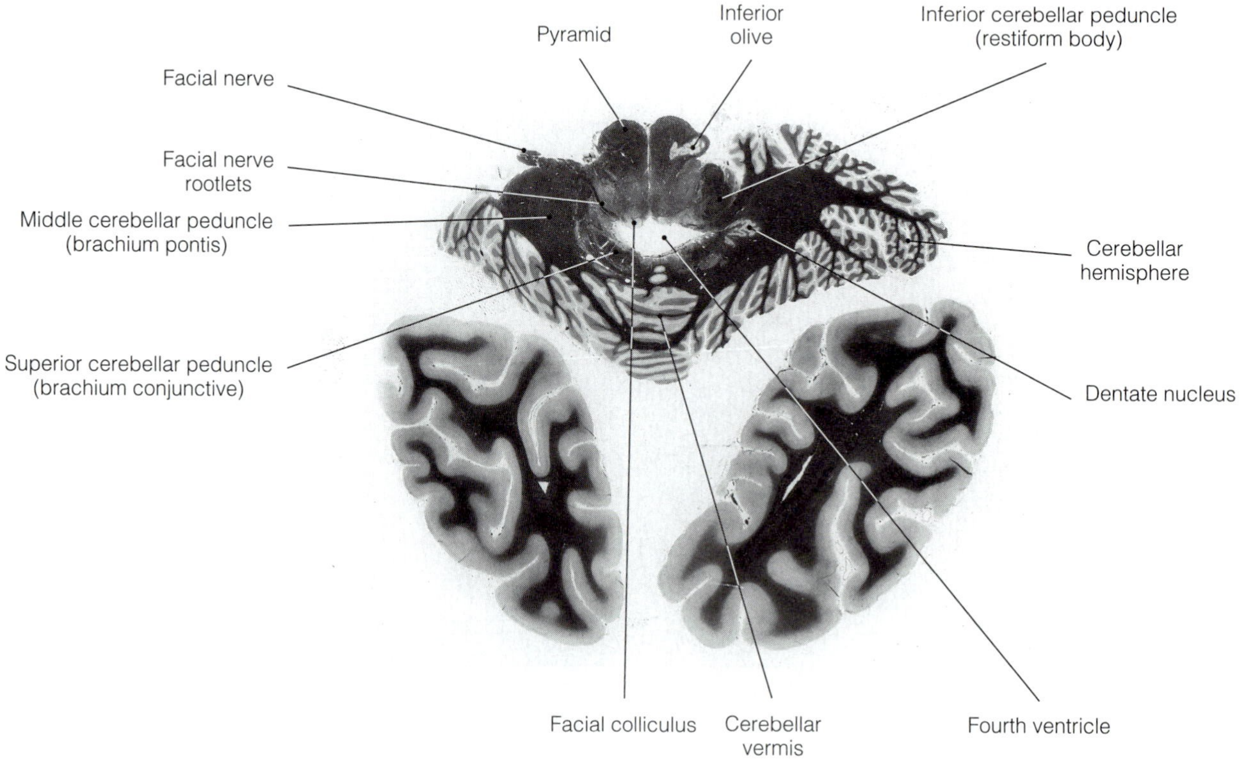
Pyramid
Inferior olive
Inferior cerebellar peduncle (restiform body)
Facial nerve
Facial nerve rootlets
Middle cerebellar peduncle (brachium pontis)
Superior cerebellar peduncle (brachium conjunctive)
Cerebellar hemisphere
Dentate nucleus
Facial colliculus
Cerebellar vermis
Fourth ventricle

FIGURE A3-24

Axial section of the barin through the ponto-medullary junction.

CORONAL YAKOVLEV

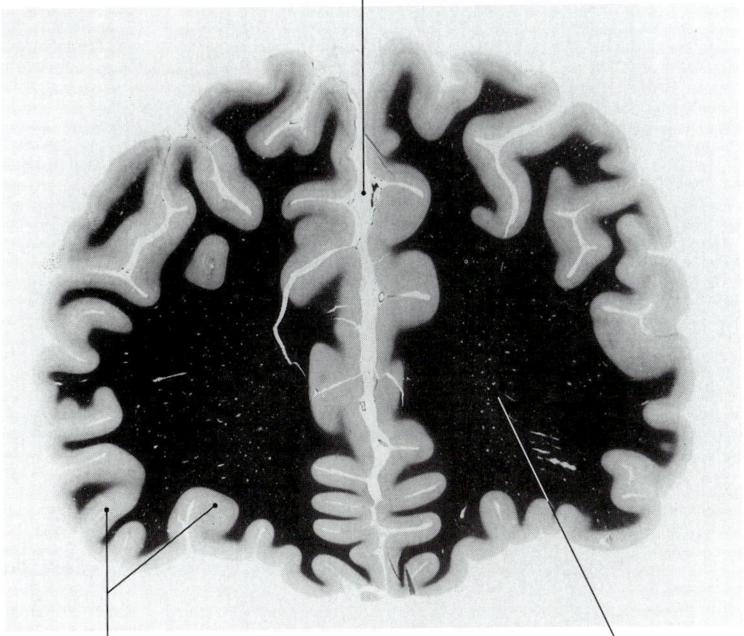

Interhemispheric fissure
Cortical gyri
Centrum semiovale

FIGURE A4-1

Coronal section of the frontal lobe rostral to the genu of the corpus callosum.

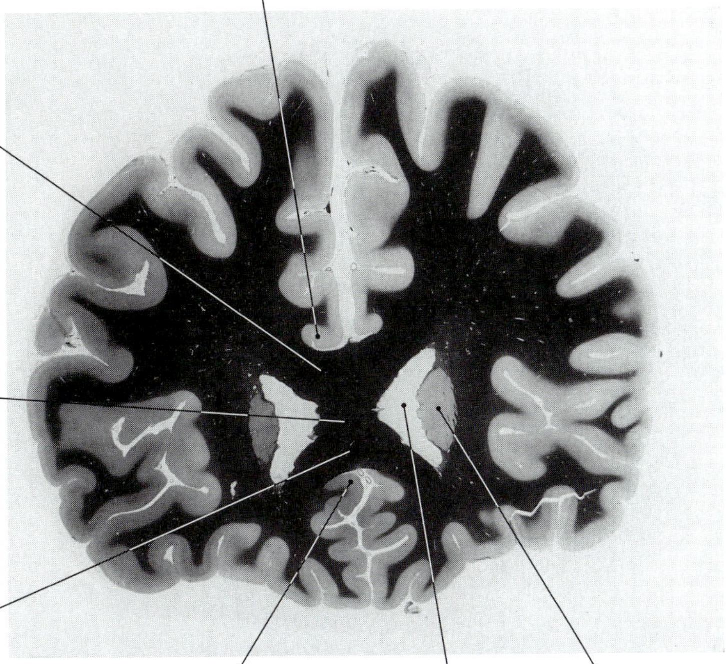

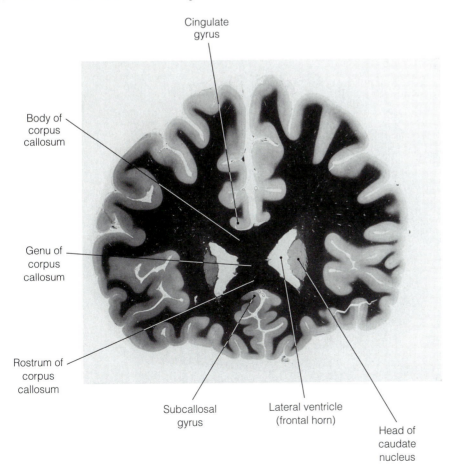

Cingulate gyrus
Body of corpus callosum
Genu of corpus callosum
Rostrum of corpus callosum
Subcallosal gyrus
Lateral ventricle (frontal horn)
Head of caudate nucleus

FIGURE A4-2

Coronal section of the brain through the genu and rostrum of the corpus callosum.

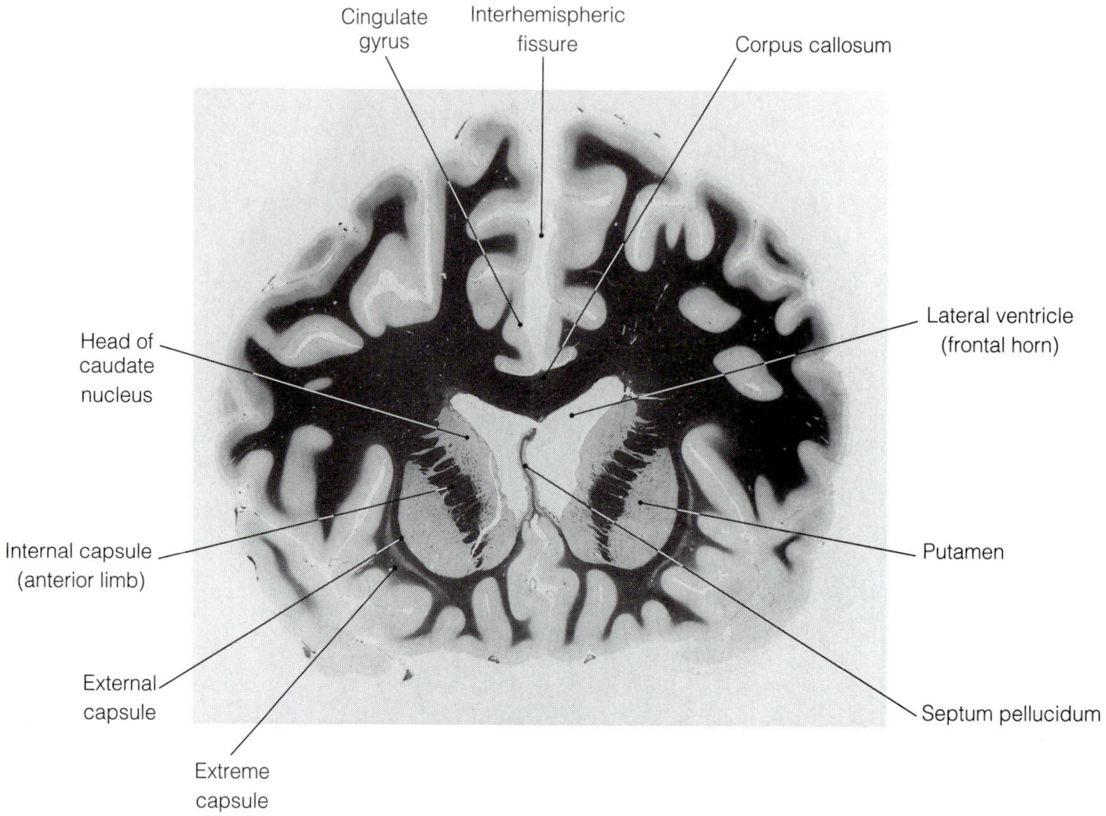

Cingulate gyrus
Interhemispheric fissure
Corpus callosum
Lateral ventricle (frontal horn)
Head of caudate nucleus
Internal capsule (anterior limb)
Putamen
External capsule
Septum pellucidum
Extreme capsule

FIGURE A4-3

Coronal section of the brain through the rostral striatum (neostriatum).

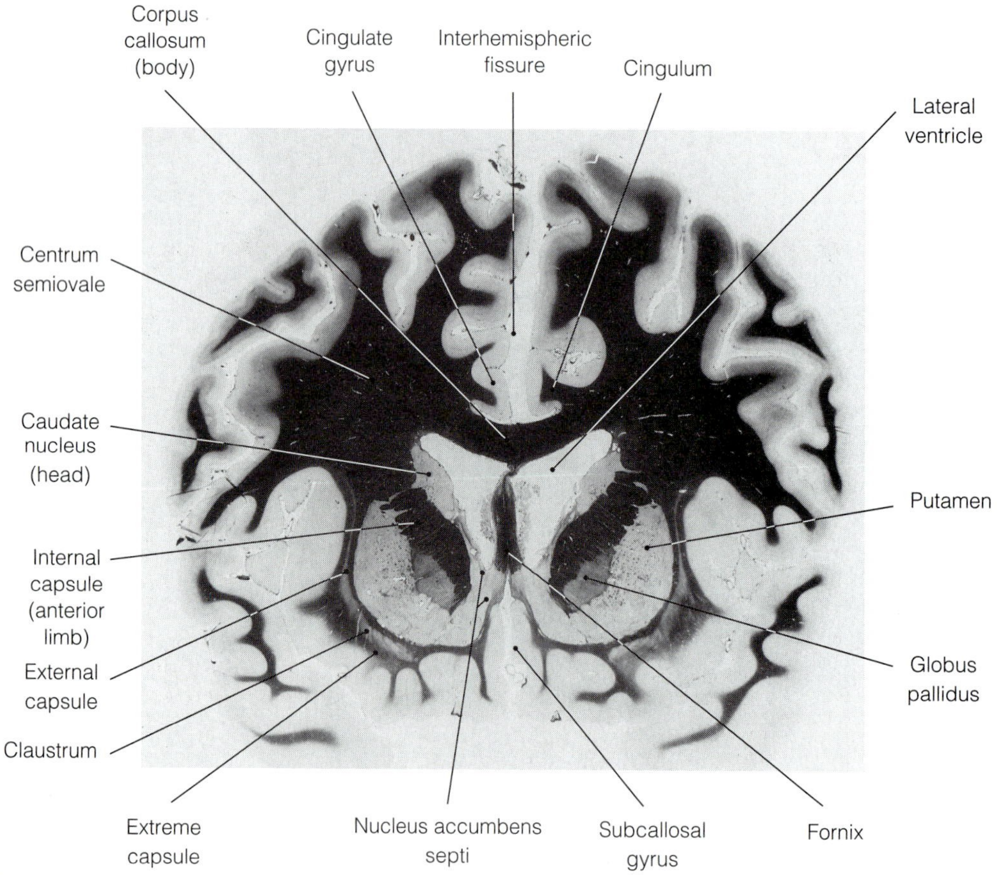

Corpus callosum (body)
Cingulate gyrus
Interhemispheric fissure
Cingulum
Lateral ventricle
Centrum semiovale
Caudate nucleus (head)
Putamen
Internal capsule (anterior limb)
External capsule
Globus pallidus
Claustrum
Extreme capsule
Nucleus accumbens septi
Subcallosal gyrus
Fornix

FIGURE A4-4

Coronal section of the brain through the corpus striatum.

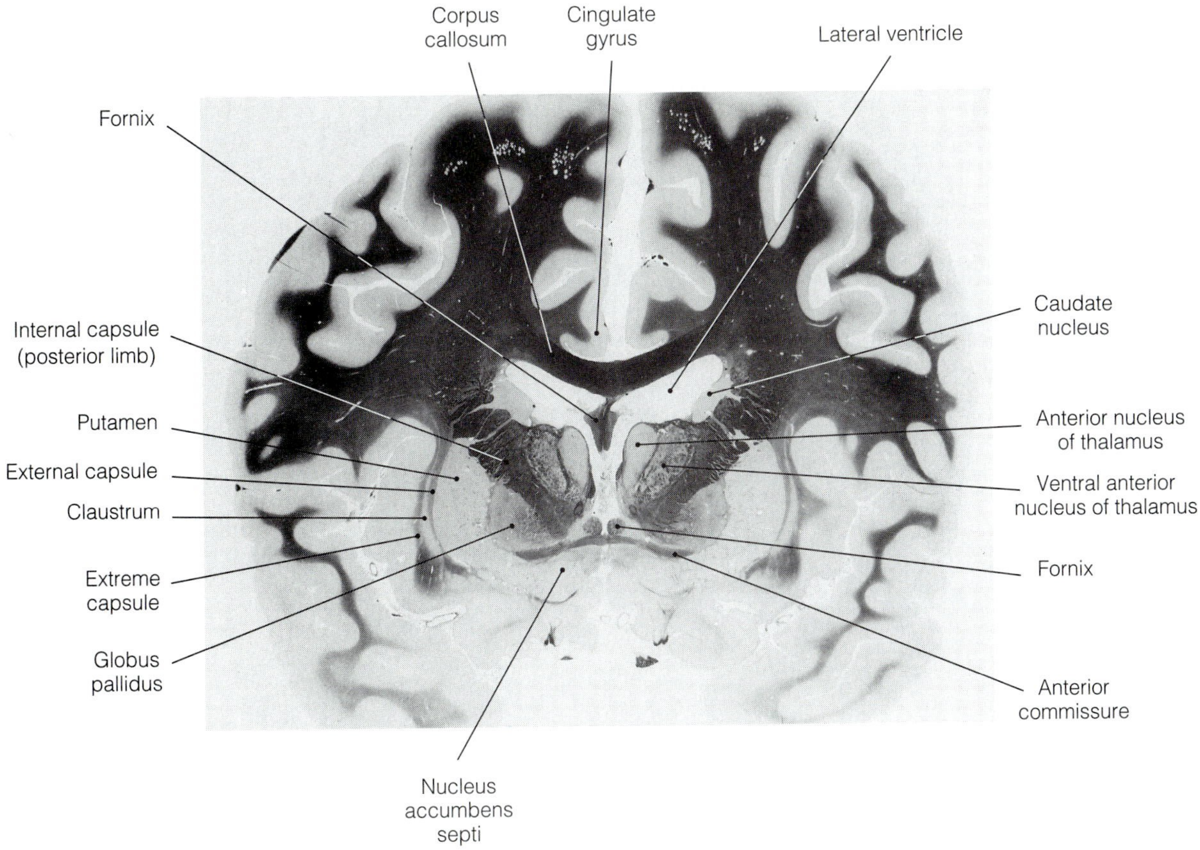
Corpus callosum
Cingulate gyrus
Lateral ventricle
Fornix
Caudate nucleus
Internal capsule (posterior limb)
Putamen
Anterior nucleus of thalamus
External capsule
Ventral anterior nucleus of thalamus
Claustrum
Fornix
Extreme capsule
Globus pallidus
Anterior commissure
Nucleus accumbens septi

FIGURE A4-5

Coronal section of the brain through the anterior commissure.

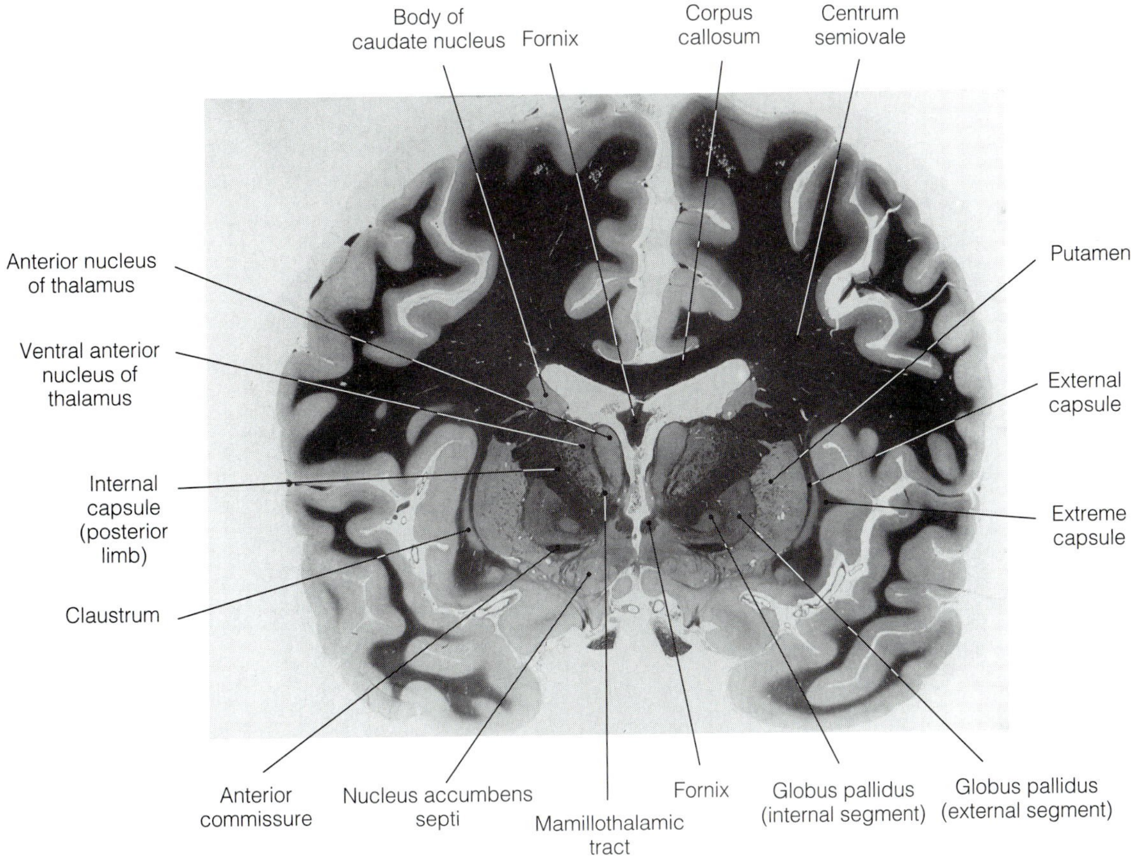
Body of caudate nucleus
Fornix
Corpus callosum
Centrum semiovale
Anterior nucleus of thalamus
Putamen
Ventral anterior nucleus of thalamus
External capsule
Internal capsule (posterior limb)
Extreme capsule
Claustrum
Anterior commissure
Nucleus accumbens septi
Mamillothalamic tract
Fornix
Globus pallidus (internal segment)
Globus pallidus (external segment)

FIGURE A4-6

Coronal section of the brain through the rostral thalamus.

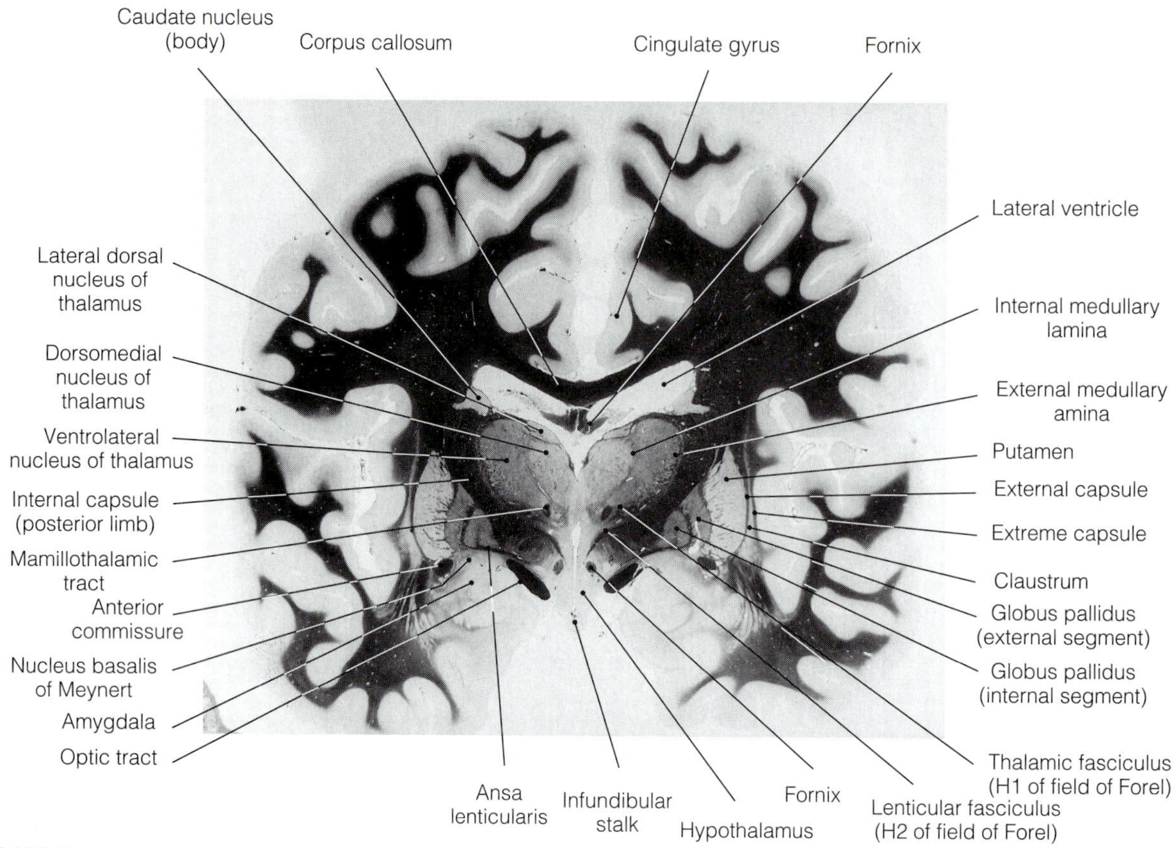
Caudate nucleus (body)
Corpus callosum
Cingulate gyrus
Fornix
Lateral ventricle
Lateral dorsal nucleus of thalamus
Internal medullary lamina
Dorsomedial nucleus of thalamus
External medullary amina
Ventrolateral nucleus of thalamus
Putamen
External capsule
Internal capsule (posterior limb)
Extreme capsule
Mamillothalamic tract
Claustrum
Anterior commissure
Globus pallidus (external segment)
Nucleus basalis of Meynert
Globus pallidus (internal segment)
Amygdala
Optic tract
Thalamic fasciculus (H1 of field of Forel)
Ansa lenticularis
Infundibular stalk
Hypothalamus
Fornix
Lenticular fasciculus (H2 of field of Forel)

FIGURE A4-7

Coronal section of the brain through the midthalamus.

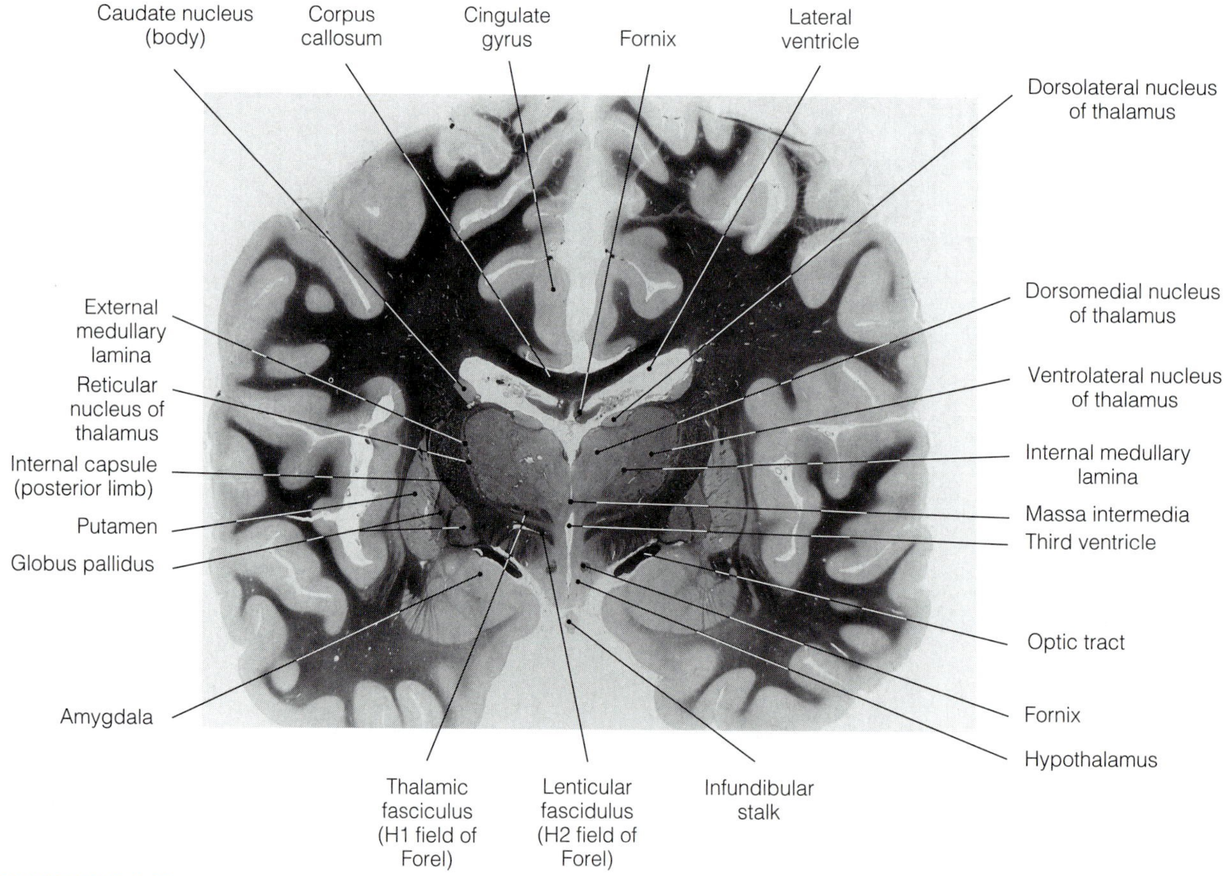
Caudate nucleus (body)
Corpus callosum
Cingulate gyrus
Fornix
Lateral ventricle
Dorsolateral nucleus of thalamus
External medullary lamina
Dorsomedial nucleus of thalamus
Reticular nucleus of thalamus
Ventrolateral nucleus of thalamus
Internal capsule (posterior limb)
Internal medullary lamina
Putamen
Massa intermedia
Globus pallidus
Third ventricle
Optic tract
Amygdala
Fornix
Hypothalamus
Thalamic fasciculus (H1 field of Forel)
Lenticular fascidulus (H2 field of Forel)
Infundibular stalk

FIGURE A4-8

Coronal section of the brain through the fields of Forel.

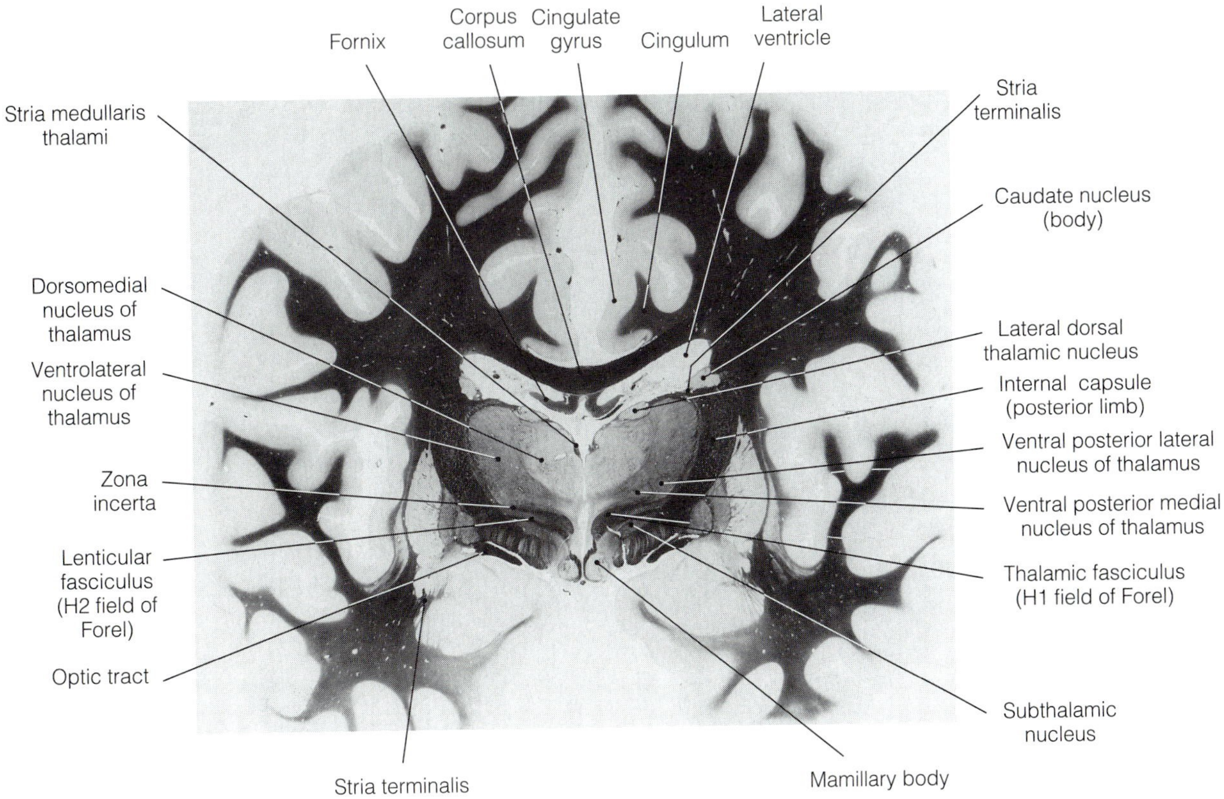
Fornix
Corpus callosum
Cingulate gyrus
Cingulum
Lateral ventricle
Stria medullaris thalami
Stria terminalis
Caudate nucleus (body)
Dorsomedial nucleus of thalamus
Lateral dorsal thalamic nucleus
Ventrolateral nucleus of thalamus
Internal capsule (posterior limb)
Ventral posterior lateral nucleus of thalamus
Zona incerta
Ventral posterior medial nucleus of thalamus
Lenticular fasciculus (H2 field of Forel)
Thalamic fasciculus (H1 field of Forel)
Optic tract
Subthalamic nucleus
Stria terminalis
Mamillary body

FIGURE A4-9

Coronal section of the brain through the mamillary body and subthalamus.

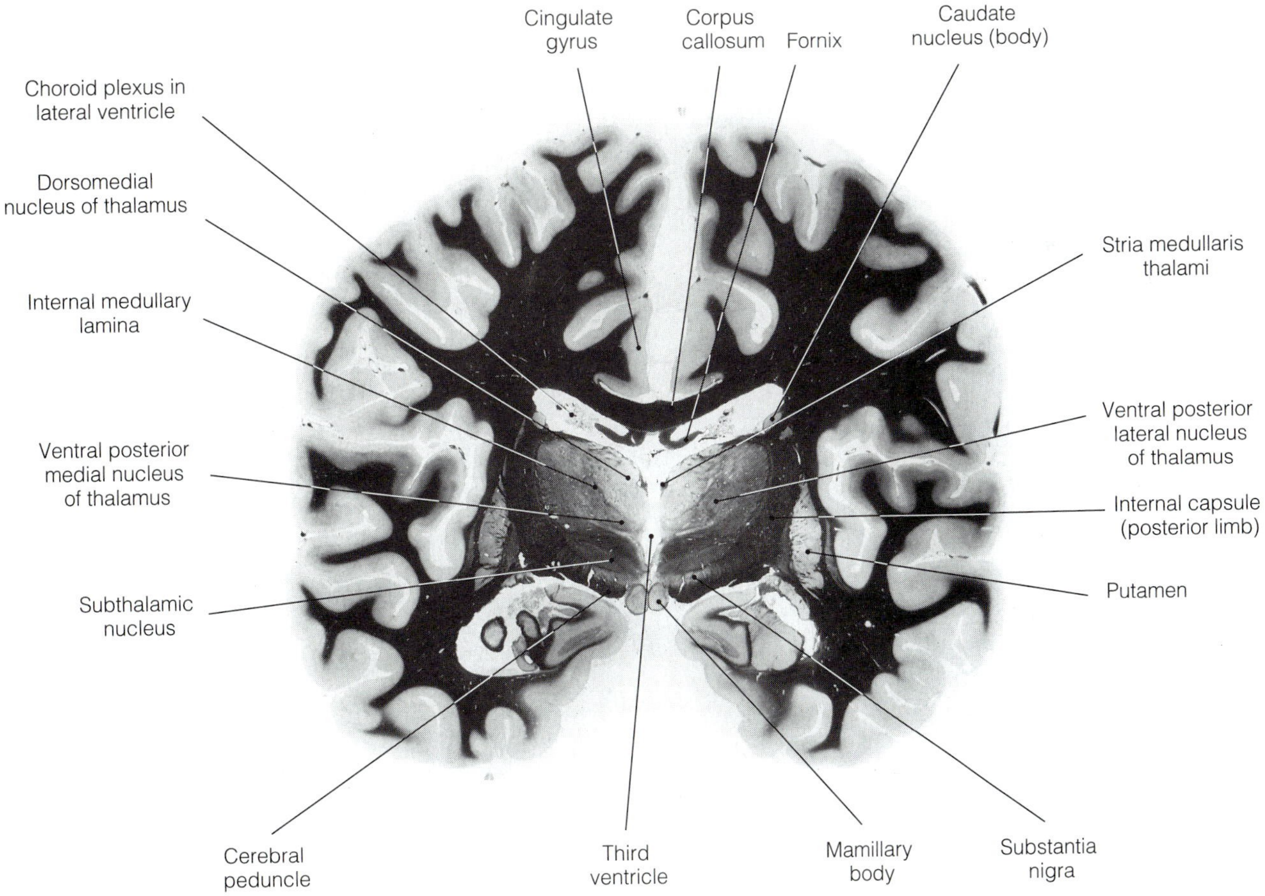
Cingulate gyrus
Corpus callosum
Fornix
Caudate nucleus (body)
Choroid plexus in lateral ventricle
Dorsomedial nucleus of thalamus
Stria medullaris thalami
Internal medullary lamina
Ventral posterior medial nucleus of thalamus
Ventral posterior lateral nucleus of thalamus
Internal capsule (posterior limb)
Putamen
Subthalamic nucleus
Cerebral peduncle
Third ventricle
Mamillary body
Substantia nigra

FIGURE A4-10

Coronal section of the brain through the caudal thalamus.

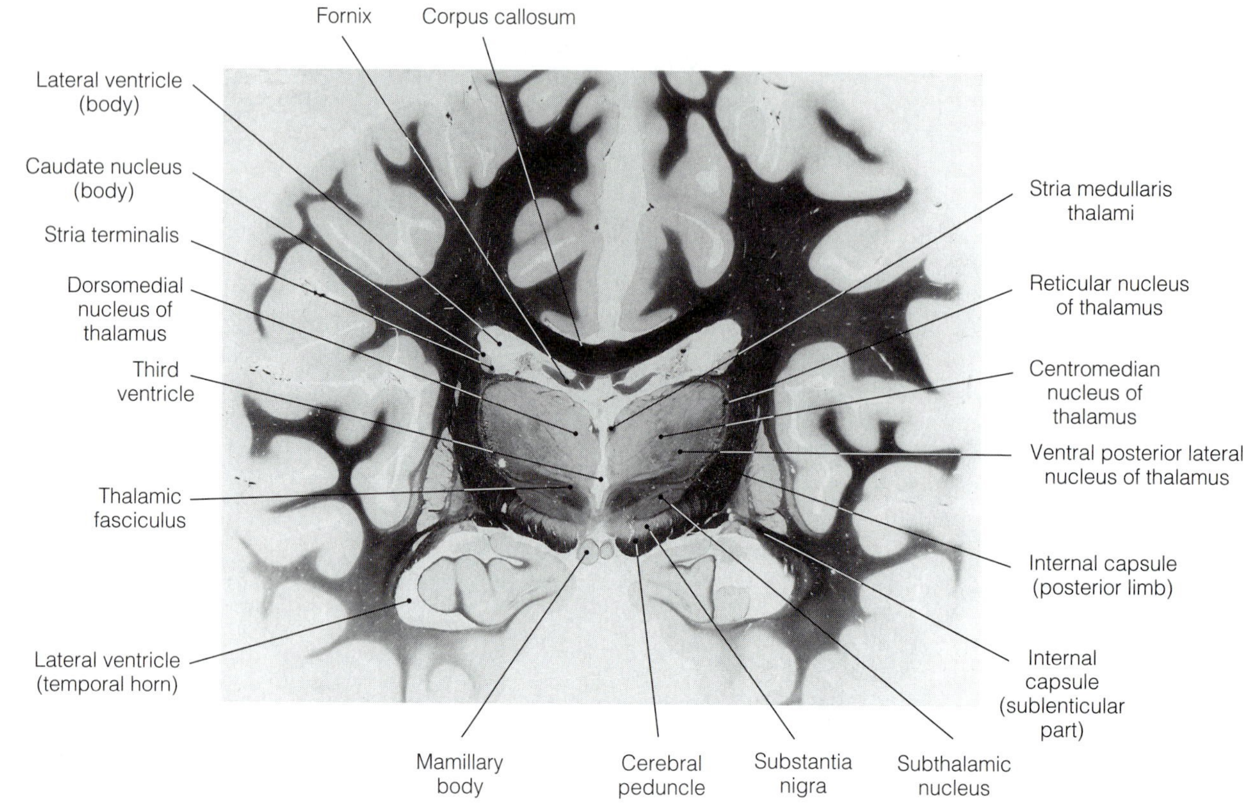

FIGURE A4-11

Coronal section of the brain through the subthalamic region.

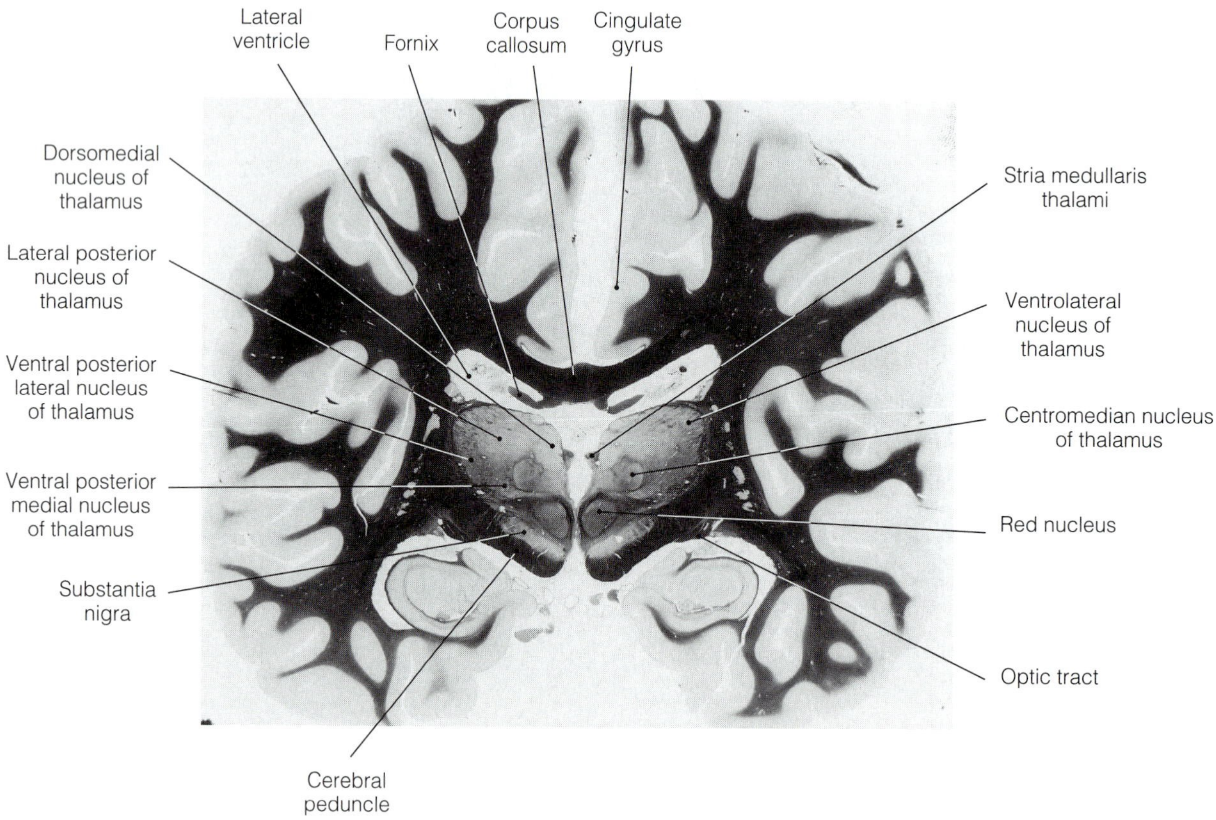

FIGURE A4-12

Coronal section of the brain through the diencephalic-mesencephalic junction.

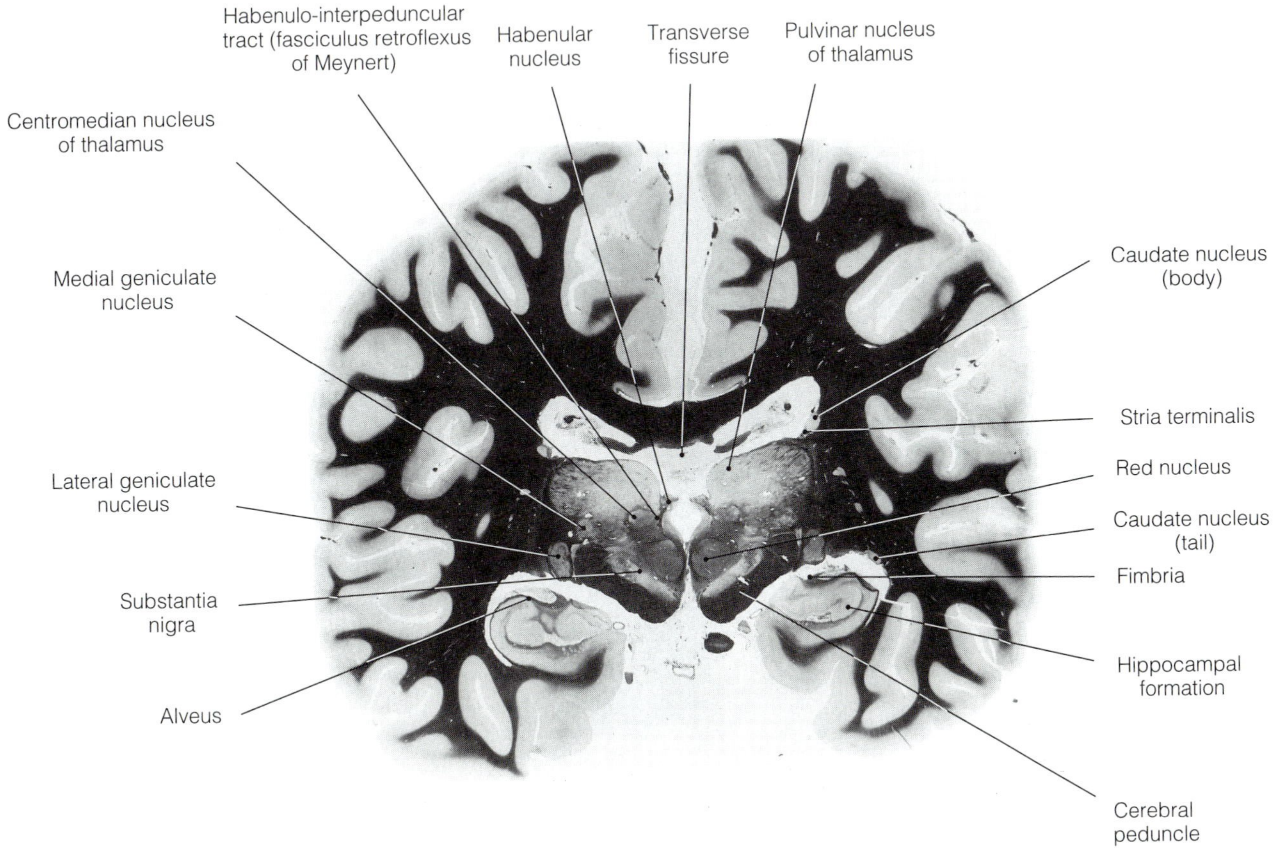

Habenulo-interpeduncular tract (fasciculus retroflexus of Meynert)
Habenular nucleus
Transverse fissure
Pulvinar nucleus of thalamus
Centromedian nucleus of thalamus
Medial geniculate nucleus
Lateral geniculate nucleus
Substantia nigra
Alveus
Caudate nucleus (body)
Stria terminalis
Red nucleus
Caudate nucleus (tail)
Fimbria
Hippocampal formation
Cerebral peduncle

FIGURE A4-13

Coronal section of the brain through the habenula and lateral geniculate nucleus.

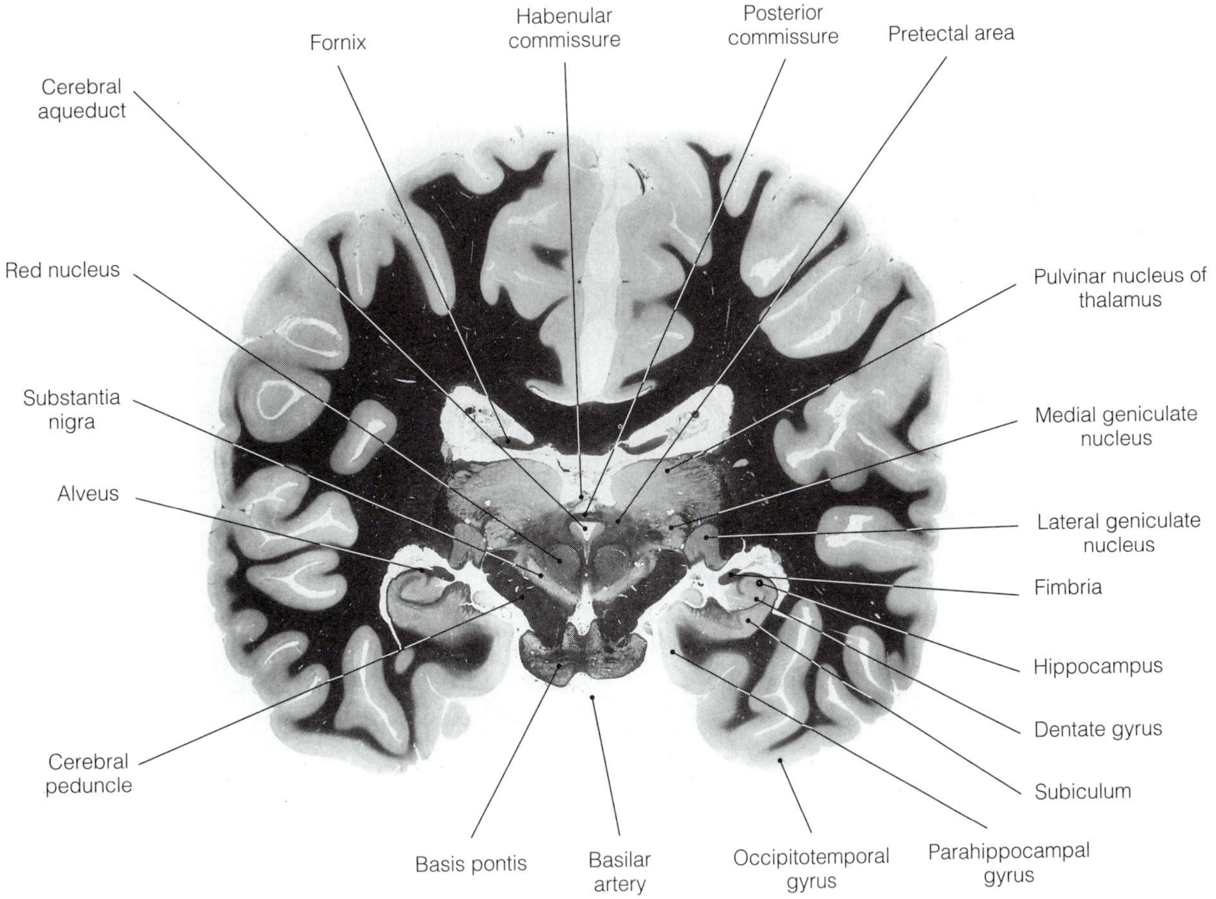

Fornix
Habenular commissure
Posterior commissure
Pretectal area
Cerebral aqueduct
Red nucleus
Substantia nigra
Alveus
Cerebral peduncle
Pulvinar nucleus of thalamus
Medial geniculate nucleus
Lateral geniculate nucleus
Fimbria
Hippocampus
Dentate gyrus
Subiculum
Basis pontis
Basilar artery
Occipitotemporal gyrus
Parahippocampal gyrus

FIGURE A4-14

Coronal section of the brain through the pretectal area.

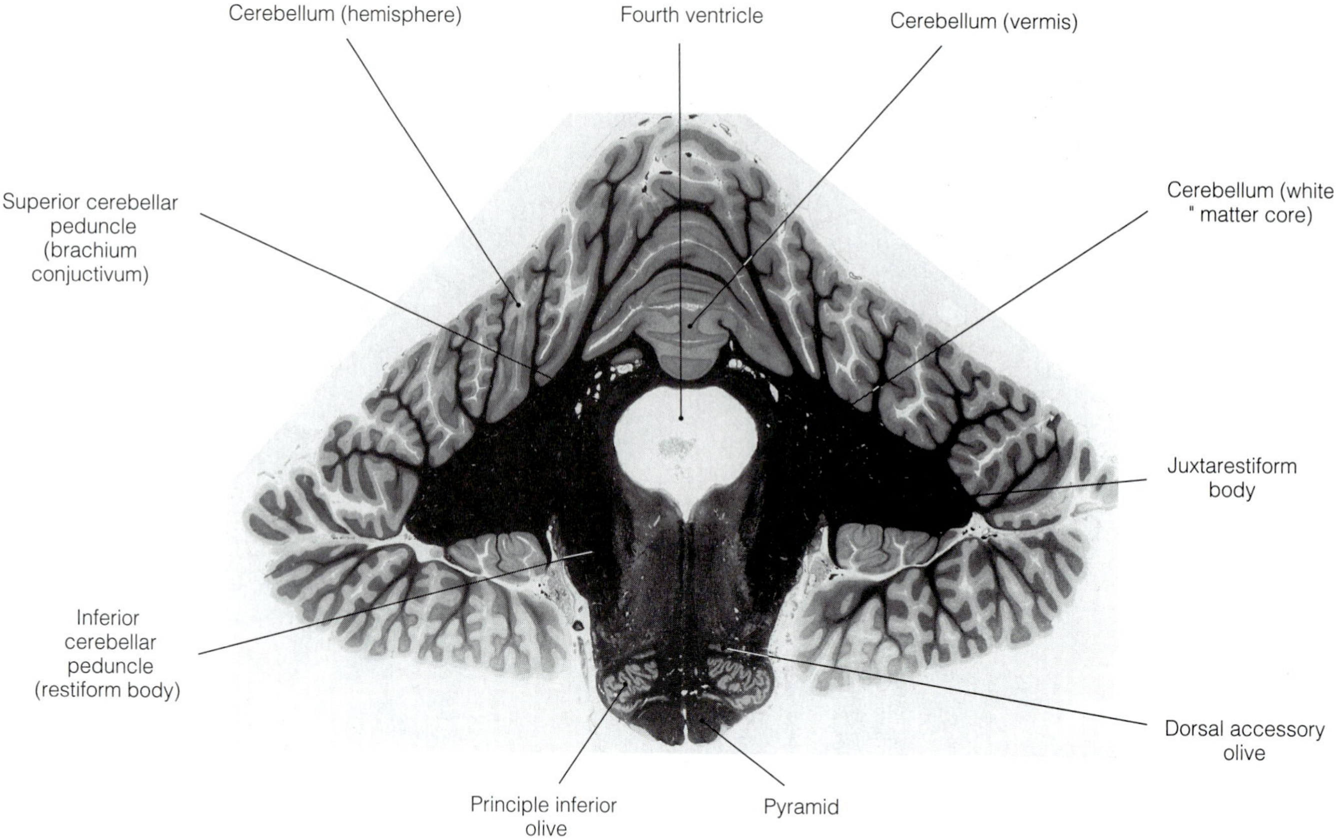
Cerebellum (hemisphere)
Fourth ventricle
Cerebellum (vermis)
Superior cerebellar peduncle (brachium conjuctivum)
Cerebellum (white " matter core)
Juxtarestiform body
Inferior cerebellar peduncle (restiform body)
Dorsal accessory olive
Principle inferior olive
Pyramid

FIGURE A4-15

Coronal section of the brain through the medulla oblongata.

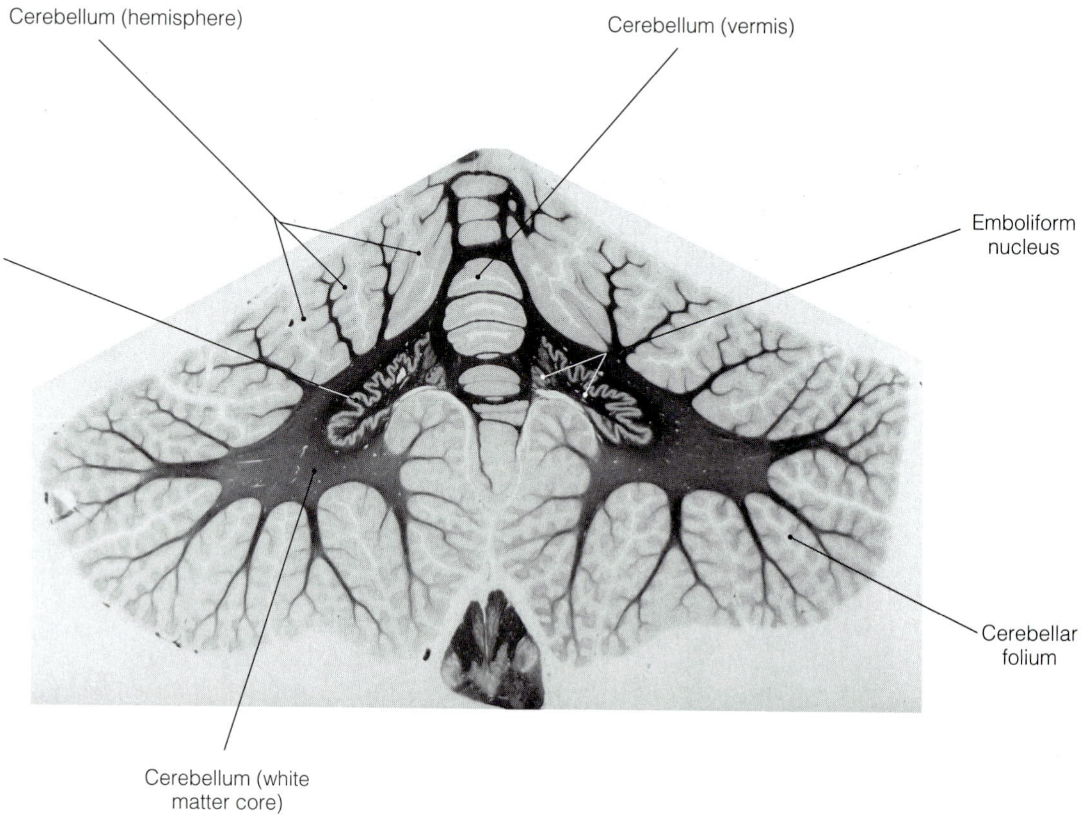
Cerebellum (hemisphere)
Cerebellum (vermis)
Dentate nucleus
Emboliform nucleus
Cerebellar folium
Cerebellum (white matter core)

FIGURE A4-16

Coronal section of the brain through the dentate nucleus of the cerebellum.

BRAIN STEM

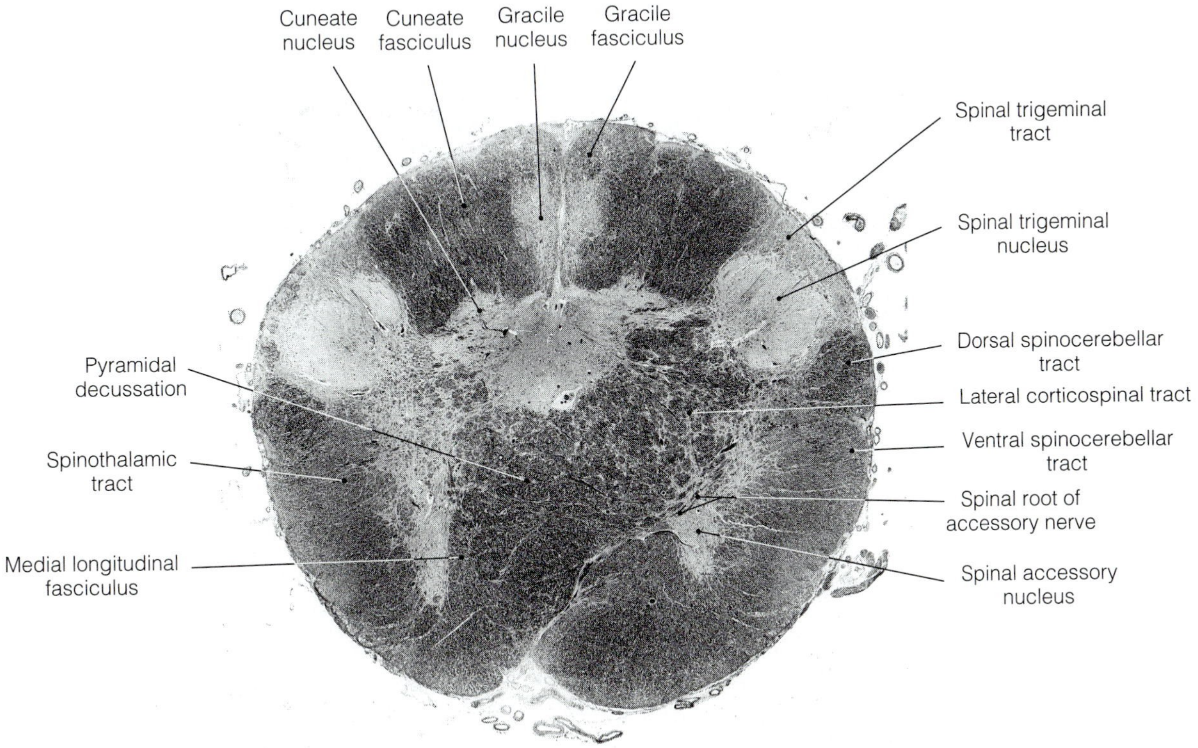
Cuneate nucleus
Cuneate fasciculus
Gracile nucleus
Gracile fasciculus
Spinal trigeminal tract
Spinal trigeminal nucleus
Dorsal spinocerebellar tract
Lateral corticospinal tract
Ventral spinocerebellar tract
Spinal root of accessory nerve
Spinal accessory nucleus
Pyramidal decussation
Spinothalamic tract
Medial longitudinal fasciculus

FIGURE A5-1

Coronal section of the brain stem through the medulla oblongata at the level of the motor (pyramidal) decussation.

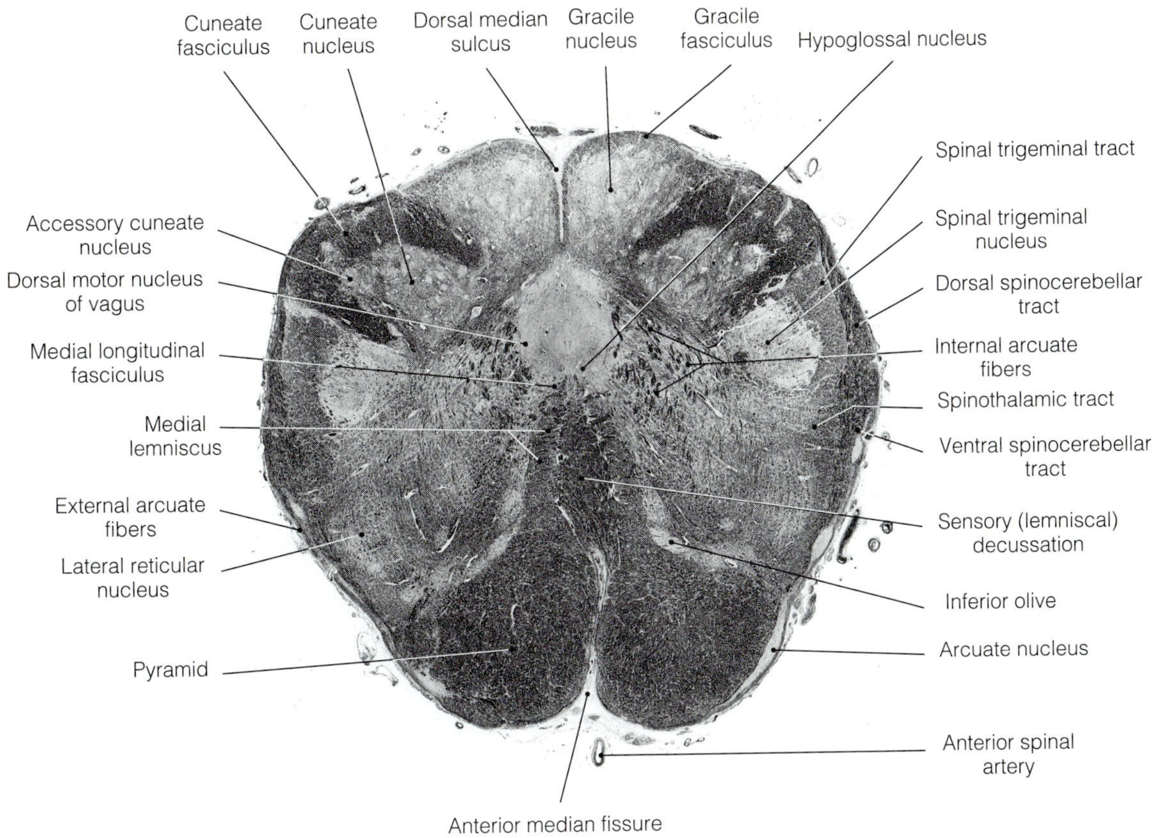
Cuneate fasciculus
Cuneate nucleus
Dorsal median sulcus
Gracile nucleus
Gracile fasciculus
Hypoglossal nucleus
Spinal trigeminal tract
Spinal trigeminal nucleus
Dorsal spinocerebellar tract
Internal arcuate fibers
Spinothalamic tract
Ventral spinocerebellar tract
Sensory (lemniscal) decussation
Inferior olive
Arcuate nucleus
Anterior spinal artery
Anterior median fissure
Accessory cuneate nucleus
Dorsal motor nucleus of vagus
Medial longitudinal fasciculus
Medial lemniscus
External arcuate fibers
Lateral reticular nucleus
Pyramid

FIGURE A5-2

Coronal section of the brain stem through the medulla oblongata at the level of the sensory (lemniscal) decussation.

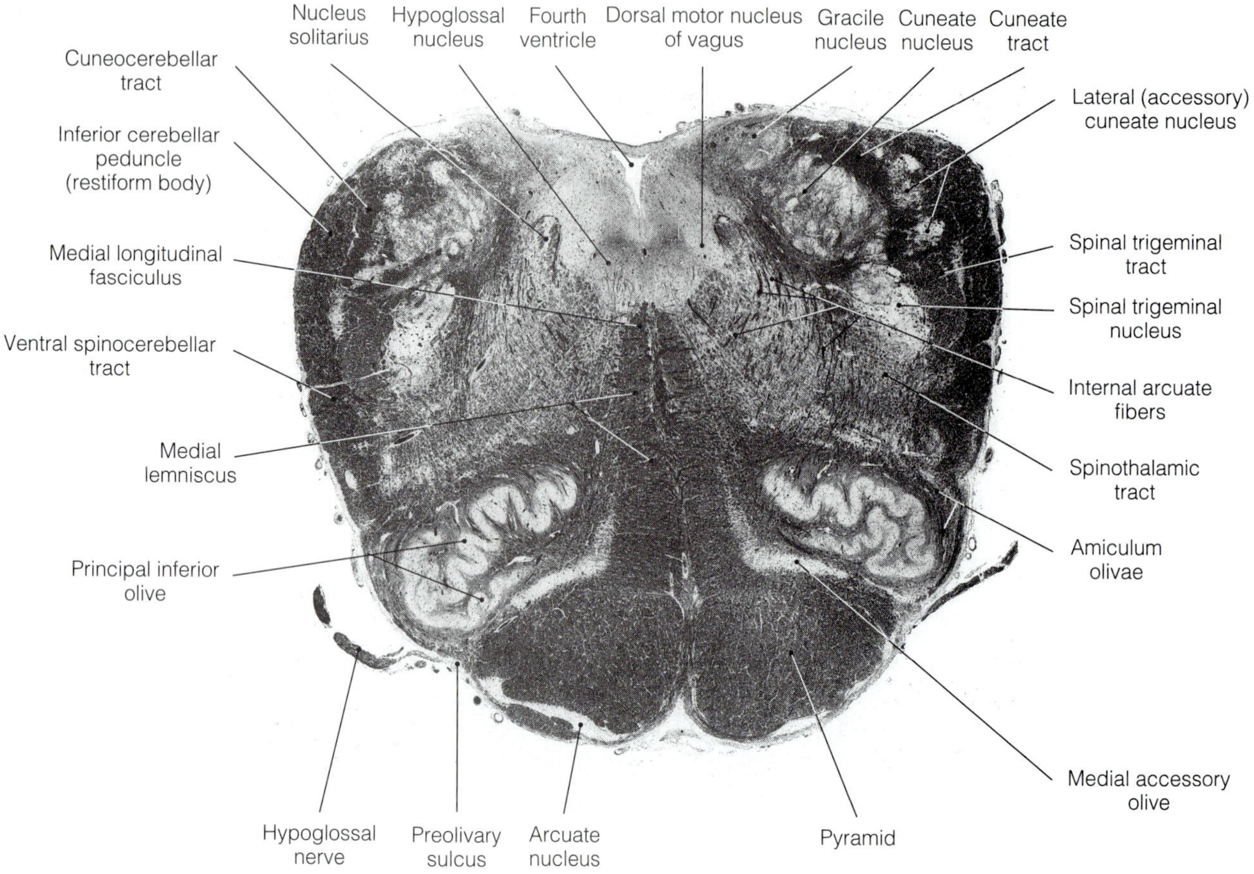

FIGURE A5-3

Coronal section of the brain stem through the medulla oblongata at the level of the obex.

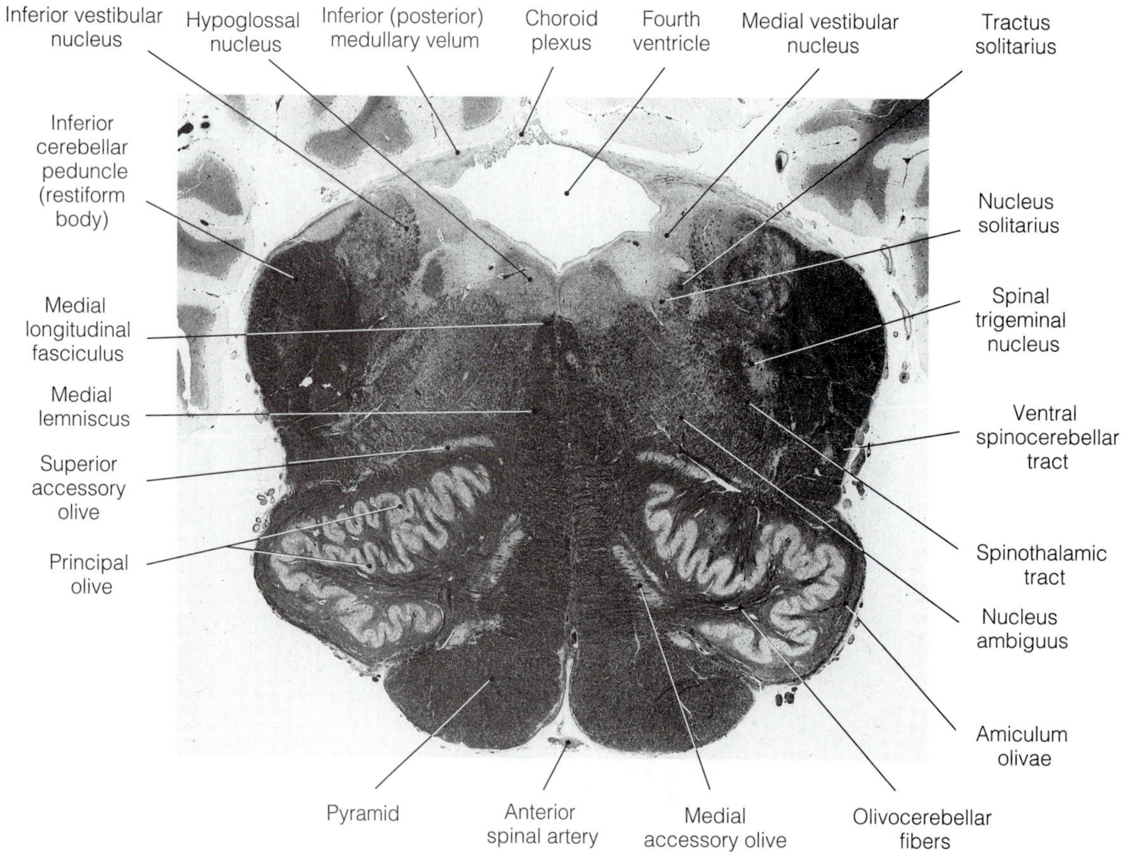

FIGURE A5-4

Coronal section of the brain stem through the medulla oblongata at the level of the middle inferior olivary complex.

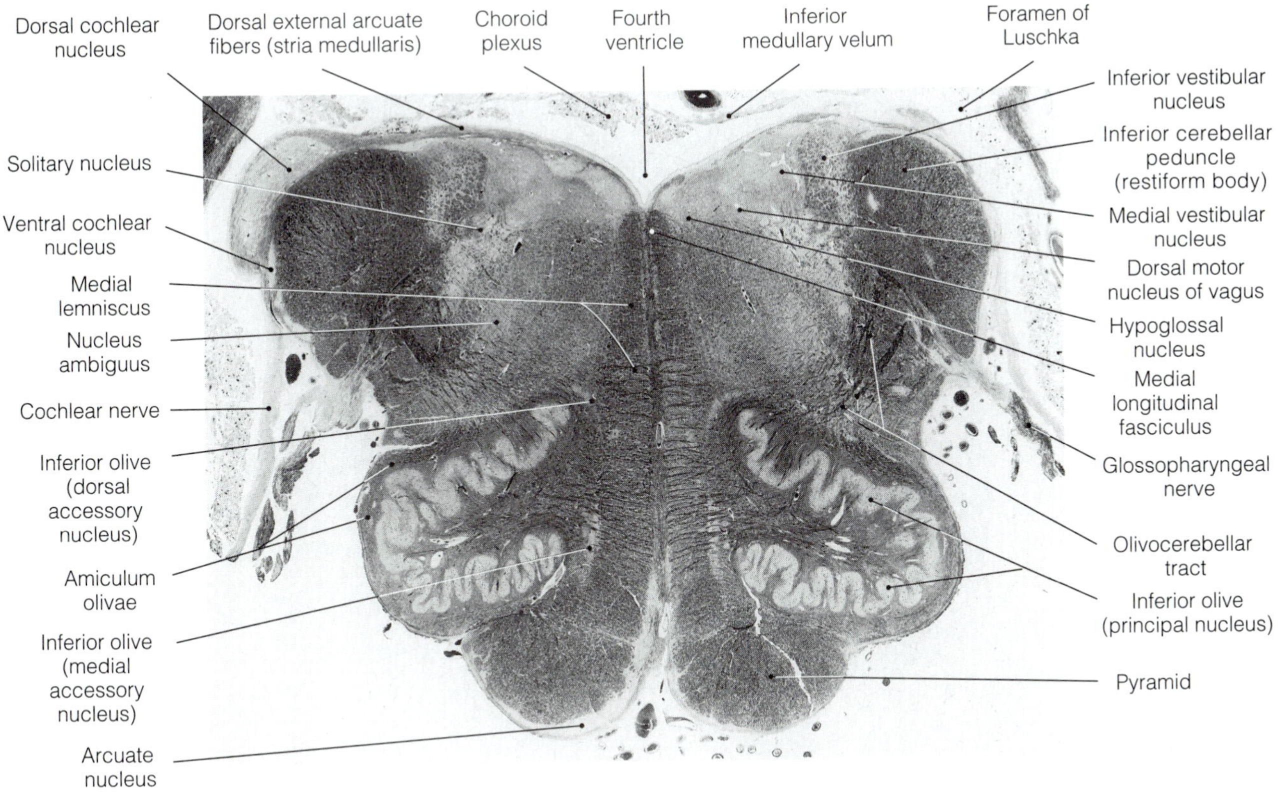
Dorsal cochlear nucleus
Dorsal external arcuate fibers (stria medullaris)
Choroid plexus
Fourth ventricle
Inferior medullary velum
Foramen of Luschka
Inferior vestibular nucleus
Inferior cerebellar peduncle (restiform body)
Medial vestibular nucleus
Dorsal motor nucleus of vagus
Hypoglossal nucleus
Medial longitudinal fasciculus
Glossopharyngeal nerve
Olivocerebellar tract
Inferior olive (principal nucleus)
Pyramid
Solitary nucleus
Ventral cochlear nucleus
Medial lemniscus
Nucleus ambiguus
Cochlear nerve
Inferior olive (dorsal accessory nucleus)
Amiculum olivae
Inferior olive (medial accessory nucleus)
Arcuate nucleus

FIGURE A5-5

Coronal section of the brain stem through the medulla oblongata at the level of cochlear nuclei and glossopharyngeal nerve.

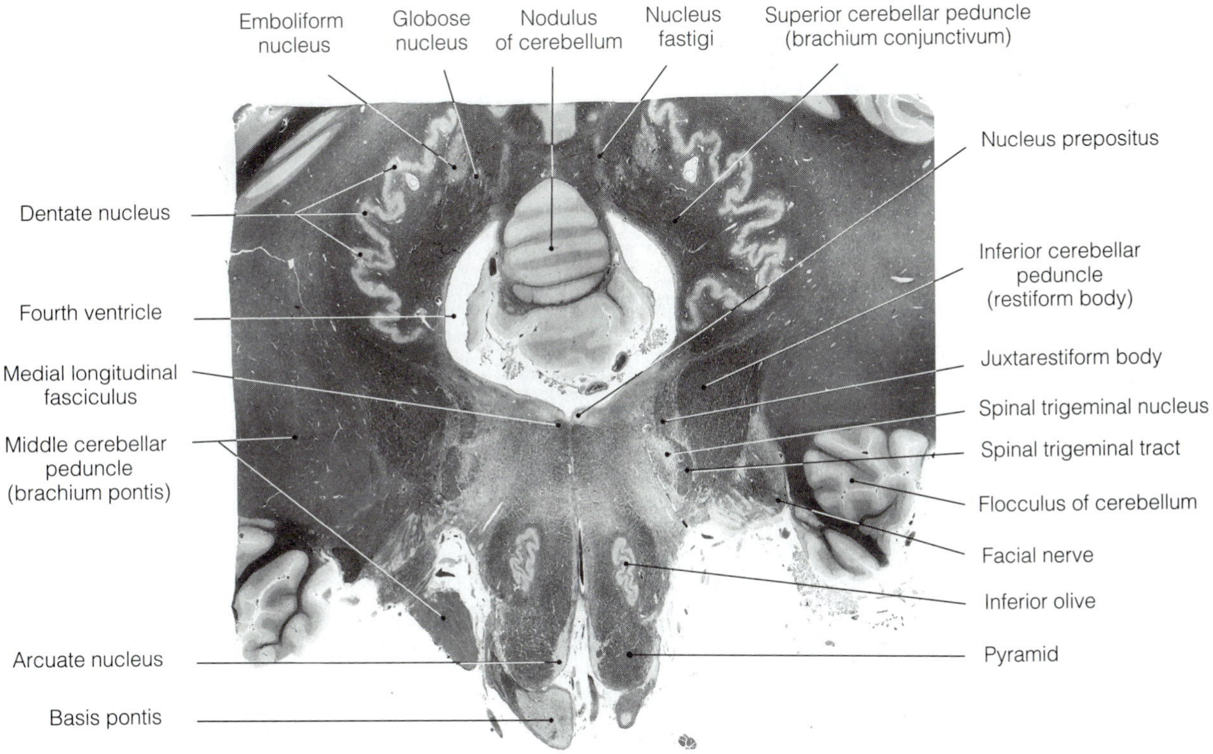
Emboliform nucleus
Globose nucleus
Nodulus of cerebellum
Nucleus fastigi
Superior cerebellar peduncle (brachium conjunctivum)
Nucleus prepositus
Inferior cerebellar peduncle (restiform body)
Juxtarestiform body
Spinal trigeminal nucleus
Spinal trigeminal tract
Flocculus of cerebellum
Facial nerve
Inferior olive
Pyramid
Dentate nucleus
Fourth ventricle
Medial longitudinal fasciculus
Middle cerebellar peduncle (brachium pontis)
Arcuate nucleus
Basis pontis

FIGURE A5-6

Coronal section of the brain stem through the pontomedullary junction.

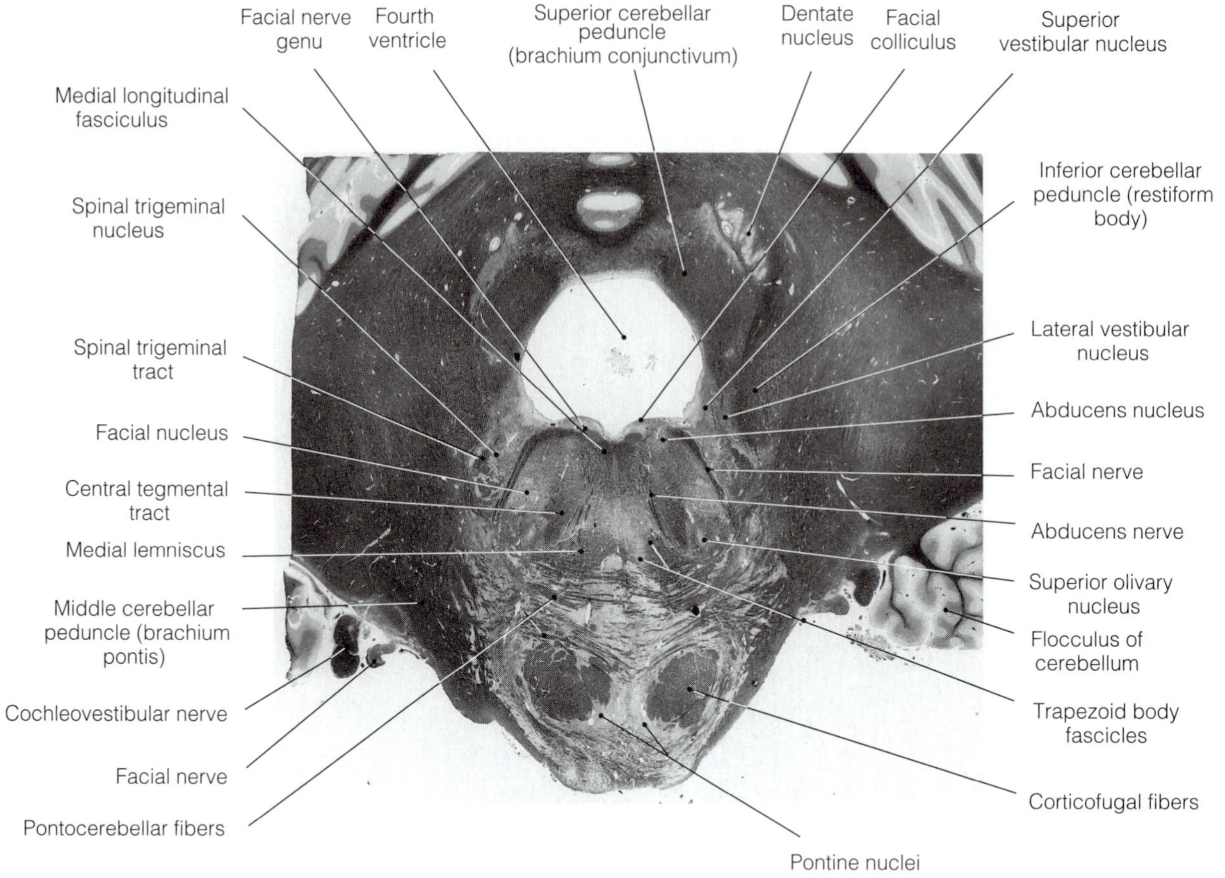
Facial nerve genu
Fourth ventricle
Superior cerebellar peduncle (brachium conjunctivum)
Dentate nucleus
Facial colliculus
Superior vestibular nucleus
Medial longitudinal fasciculus
Spinal trigeminal nucleus
Inferior cerebellar peduncle (restiform body)
Spinal trigeminal tract
Lateral vestibular nucleus
Abducens nucleus
Facial nucleus
Facial nerve
Central tegmental tract
Abducens nerve
Medial lemniscus
Superior olivary nucleus
Middle cerebellar peduncle (brachium pontis)
Flocculus of cerebellum
Cochleovestibular nerve
Trapezoid body fascicles
Facial nerve
Corticofugal fibers
Pontocerebellar fibers
Pontine nuclei

FIGURE A5-7

Coronal section of the brain stem through the pons at the level of the abducens and facial nerves.

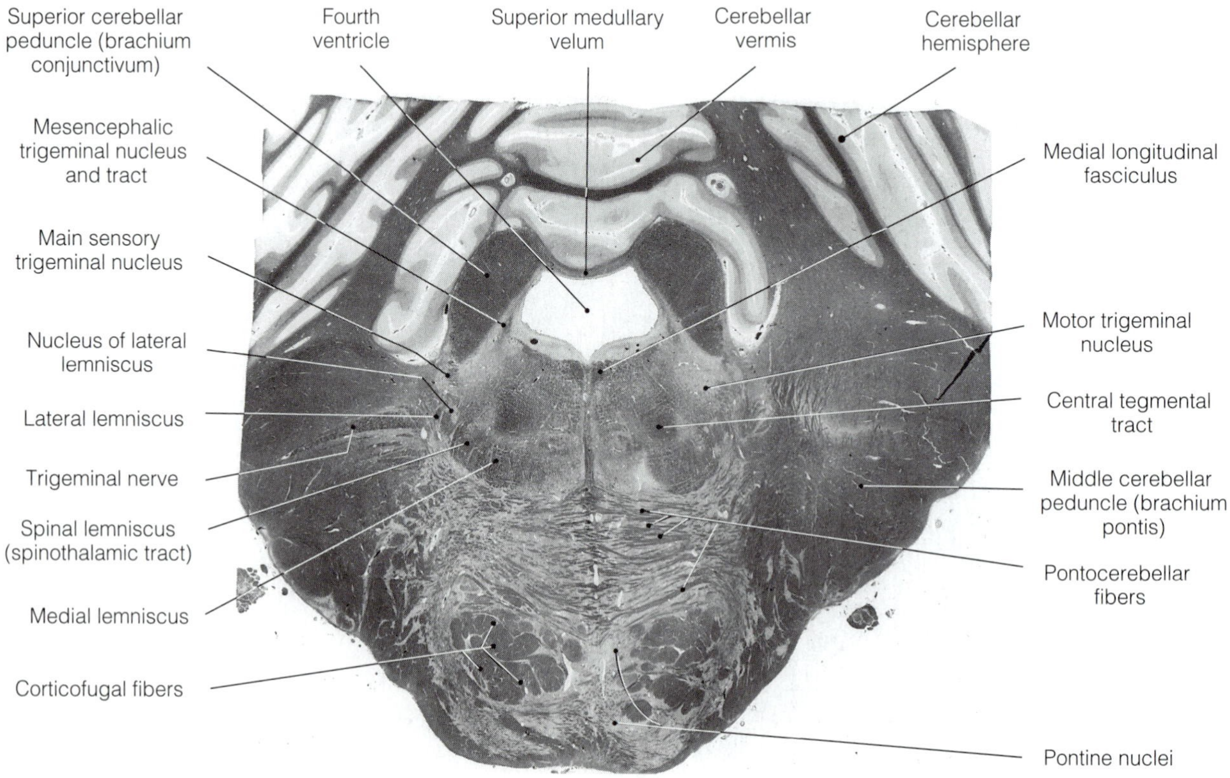
Superior cerebellar peduncle (brachium conjunctivum)
Fourth ventricle
Superior medullary velum
Cerebellar vermis
Cerebellar hemisphere
Mesencephalic trigeminal nucleus and tract
Medial longitudinal fasciculus
Main sensory trigeminal nucleus
Nucleus of lateral lemniscus
Motor trigeminal nucleus
Lateral lemniscus
Central tegmental tract
Trigeminal nerve
Middle cerebellar peduncle (brachium pontis)
Spinal lemniscus (spinothalamic tract)
Pontocerebellar fibers
Medial lemniscus
Corticofugal fibers
Pontine nuclei

FIGURE A5-8

Coronal section of the brain stem through the midpons at the level of sensory and motor nuclei of the trigeminal nerve.

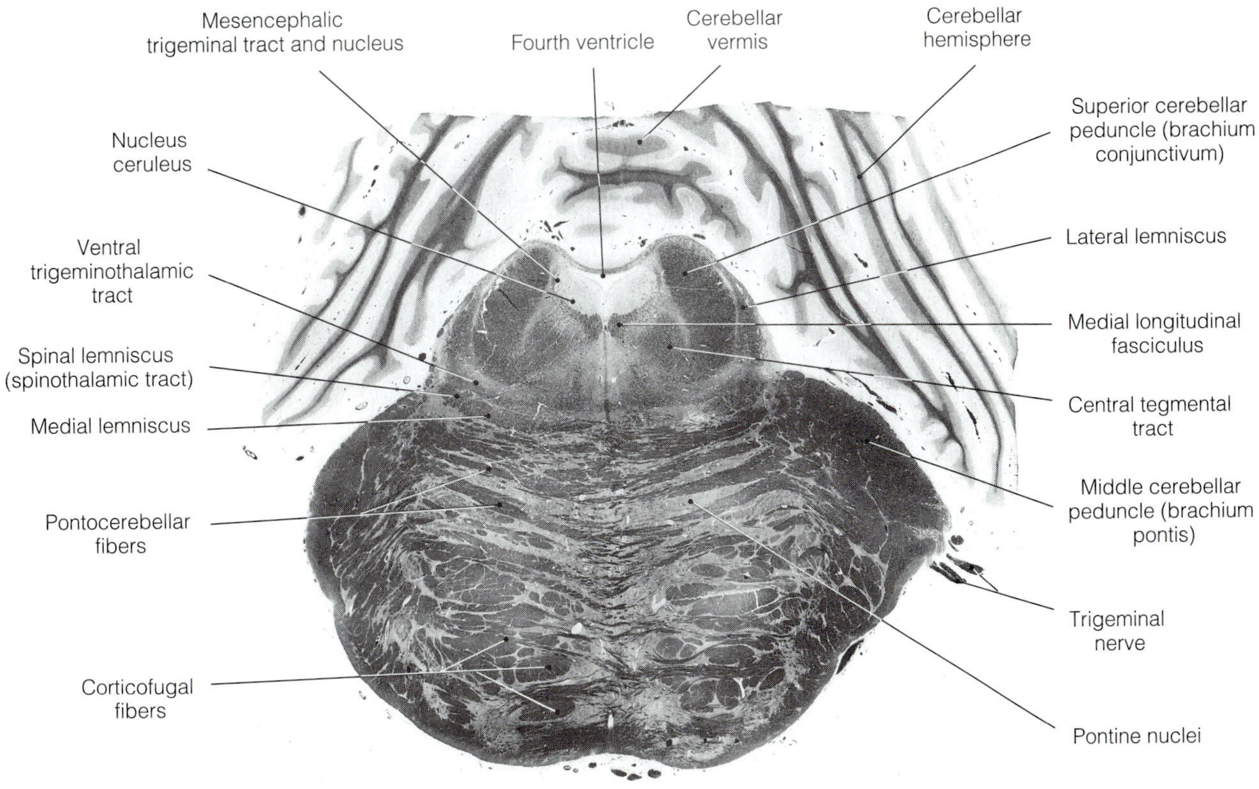

FIGURE A5-9

Coronal section of the brain stem through the rostral pons at the level of the isthmus.

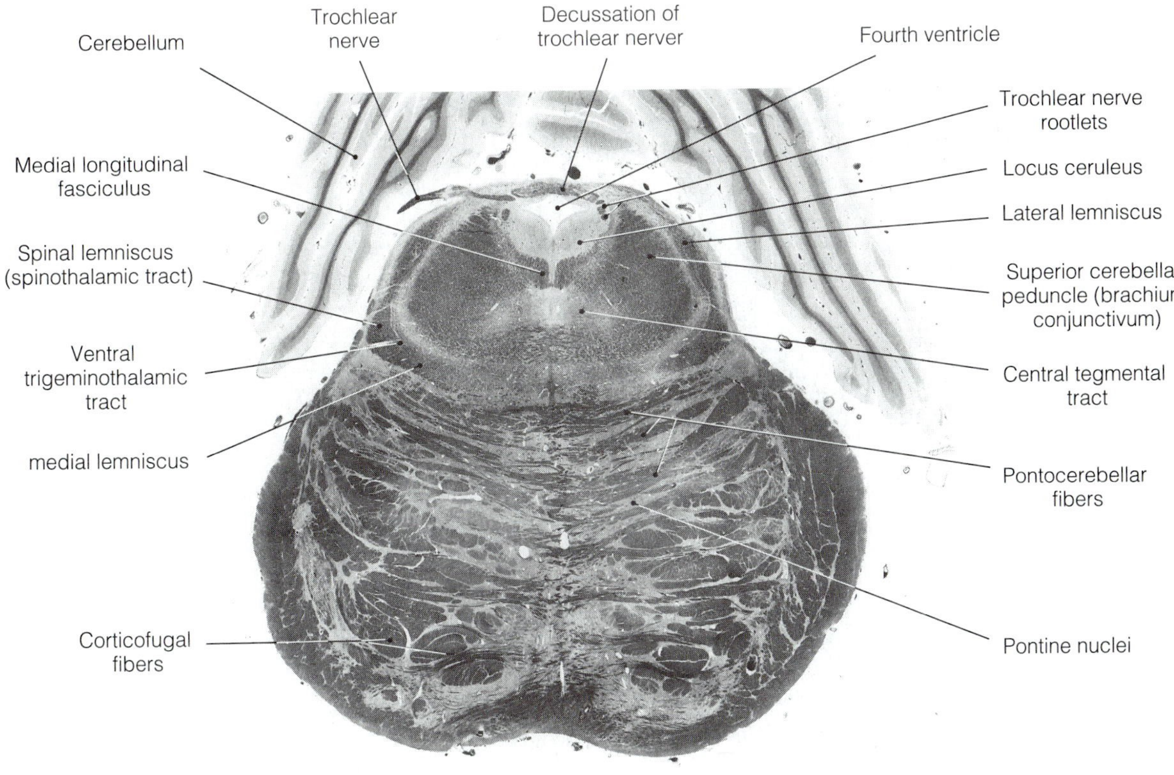

FIGURE A5-10

Coronal section of the brain stem through the rostral pons at the level of the trochlear nerve.

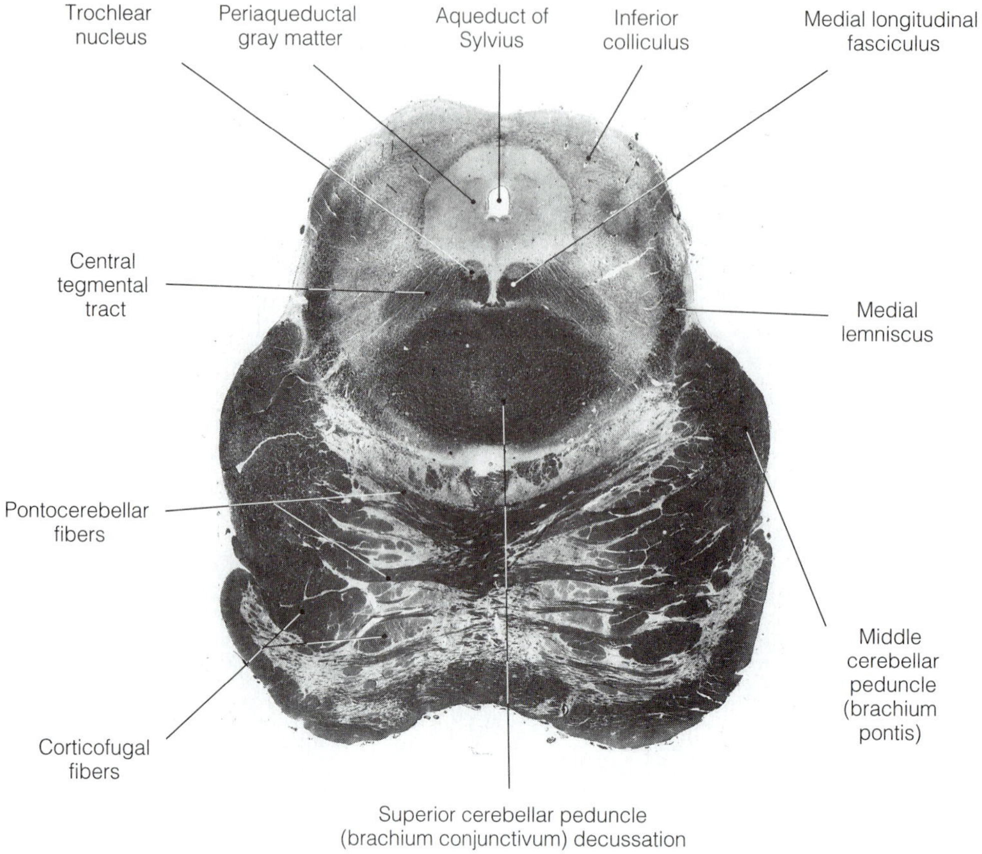
Trochlear nucleus
Periaqueductal gray matter
Aqueduct of Sylvius
Inferior colliculus
Medial longitudinal fasciculus
Central tegmental tract
Medial lemniscus
Pontocerebellar fibers
Middle cerebellar peduncle (brachium pontis)
Corticofugal fibers
Superior cerebellar peduncle (brachium conjunctivum) decussation

FIGURE A5-11

Coronal section of the brain stem through the midbrain at the level of the caudal inferior colliculus and trochlear nucleus.

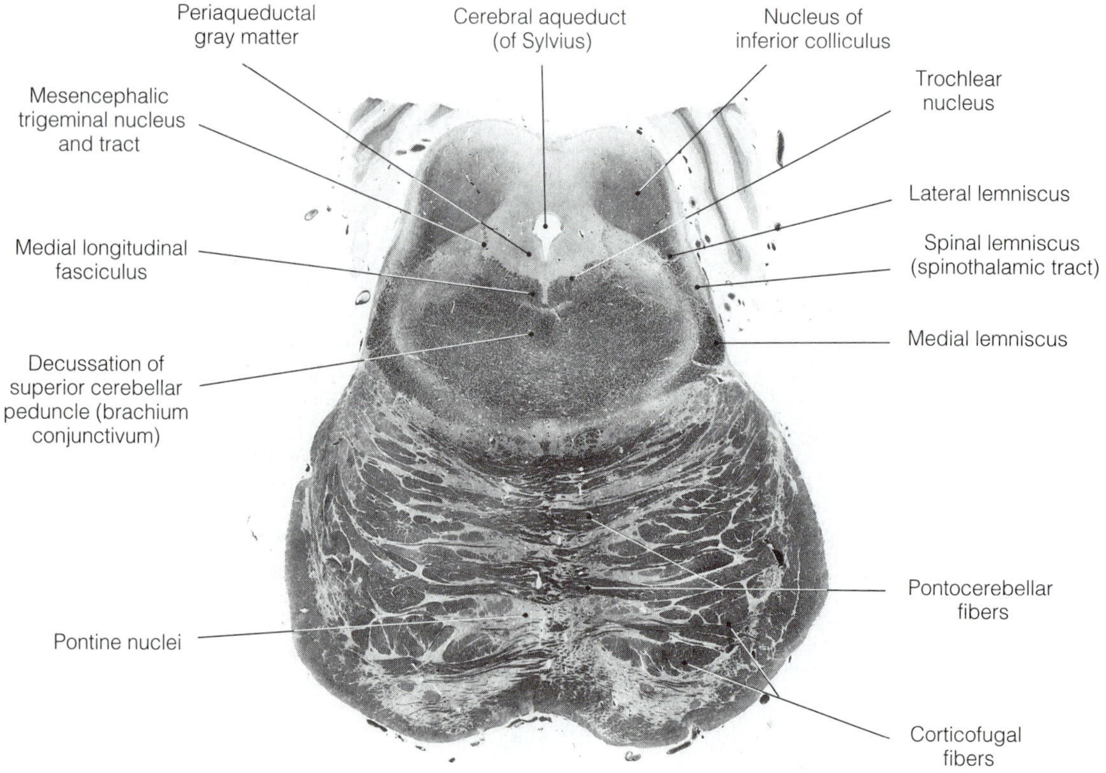
Periaqueductal gray matter
Cerebral aqueduct (of Sylvius)
Nucleus of inferior colliculus
Mesencephalic trigeminal nucleus and tract
Trochlear nucleus
Lateral lemniscus
Medial longitudinal fasciculus
Spinal lemniscus (spinothalamic tract)
Medial lemniscus
Decussation of superior cerebellar peduncle (brachium conjunctivum)
Pontocerebellar fibers
Pontine nuclei
Corticofugal fibers

FIGURE A5-12

Coronal section of the brain stem through the midbrain at the level of the inferior colliculus.

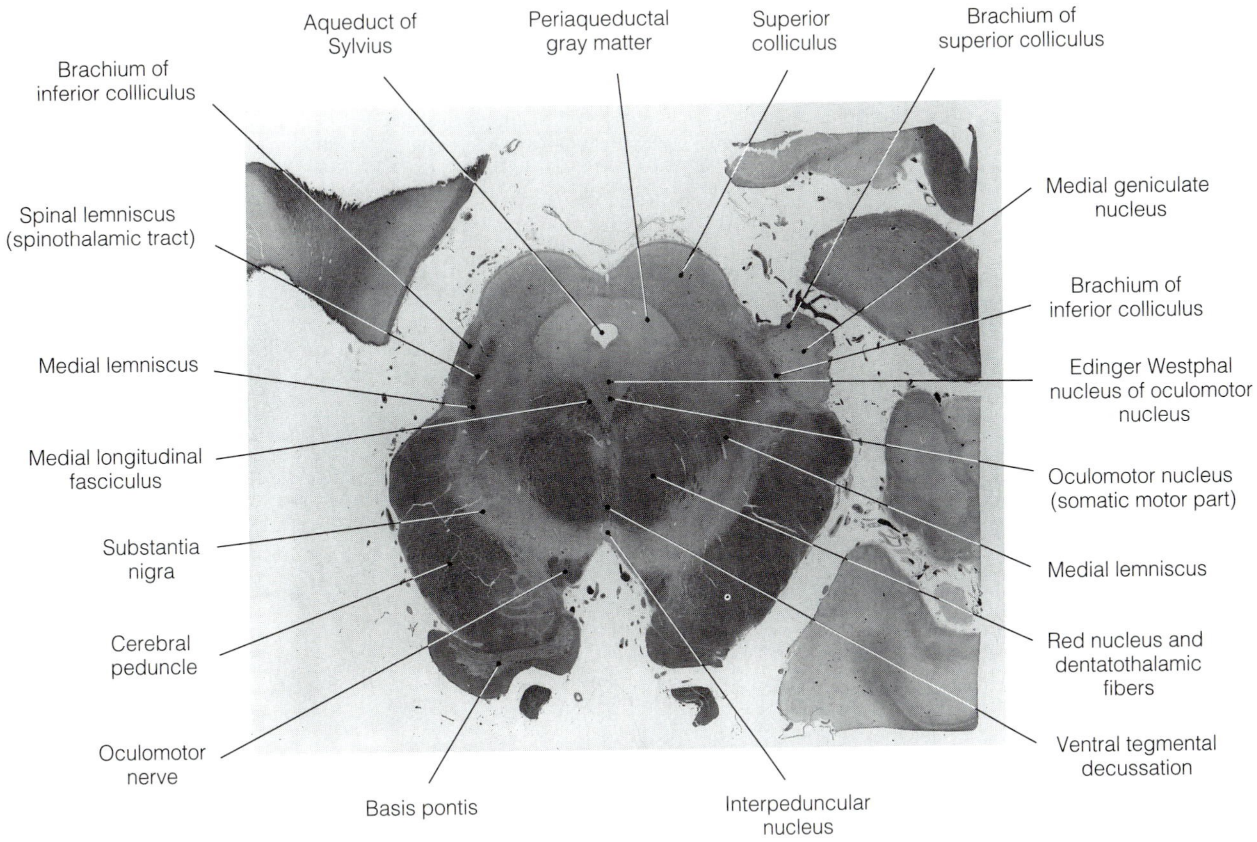
Aqueduct of Sylvius
Periaqueductal gray matter
Superior colliculus
Brachium of superior colliculus
Brachium of inferior collliculus
Spinal lemniscus (spinothalamic tract)
Medial lemniscus
Medial longitudinal fasciculus
Substantia nigra
Cerebral peduncle
Oculomotor nerve
Basis pontis
Interpeduncular nucleus
Medial geniculate nucleus
Brachium of inferior colliculus
Edinger Westphal nucleus of oculomotor nucleus
Oculomotor nucleus (somatic motor part)
Medial lemniscus
Red nucleus and dentatothalamic fibers
Ventral tegmental decussation

FIGURE A5-13

Coronal section of the brain stem through the midbrain at the level of the superior colliculus.

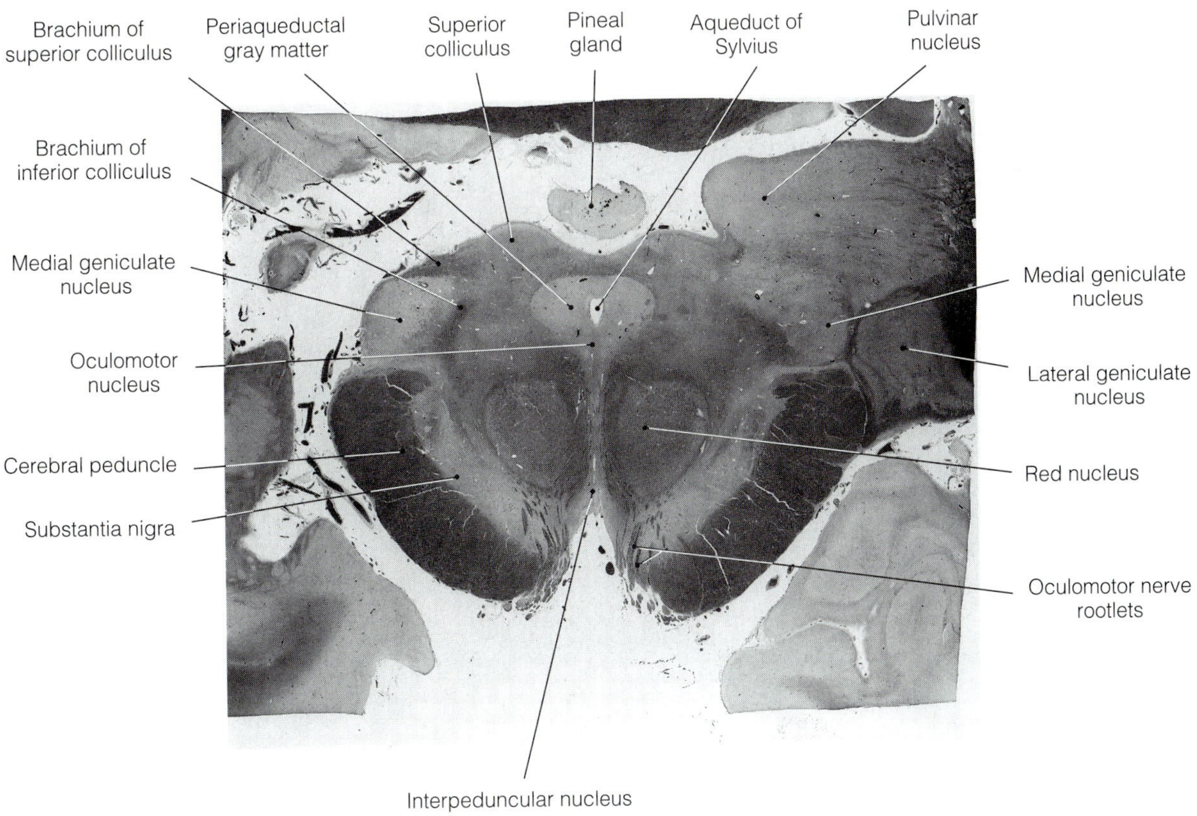
Brachium of superior colliculus
Periaqueductal gray matter
Superior colliculus
Pineal gland
Aqueduct of Sylvius
Pulvinar nucleus
Brachium of inferior colliculus
Medial geniculate nucleus
Oculomotor nucleus
Cerebral peduncle
Substantia nigra
Medial geniculate nucleus
Lateral geniculate nucleus
Red nucleus
Oculomotor nerve rootlets
Interpeduncular nucleus

FIGURE A5-14

Coronal section of the brain stem through the midbrain at the level of the rostral superior colliculus.

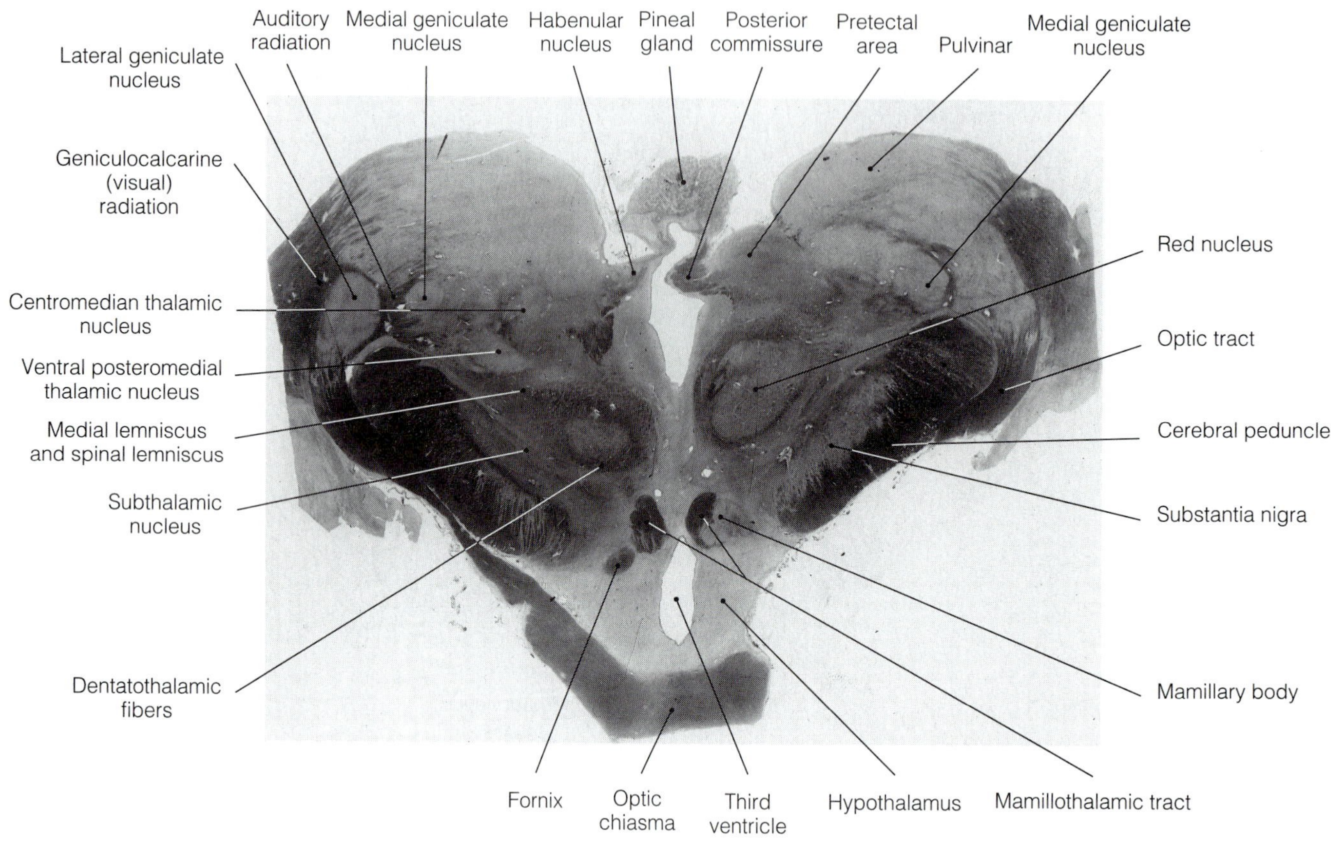

FIGURE A5-15

Coronal section of the brain stem throughthe midbrain-diencephalic junction.

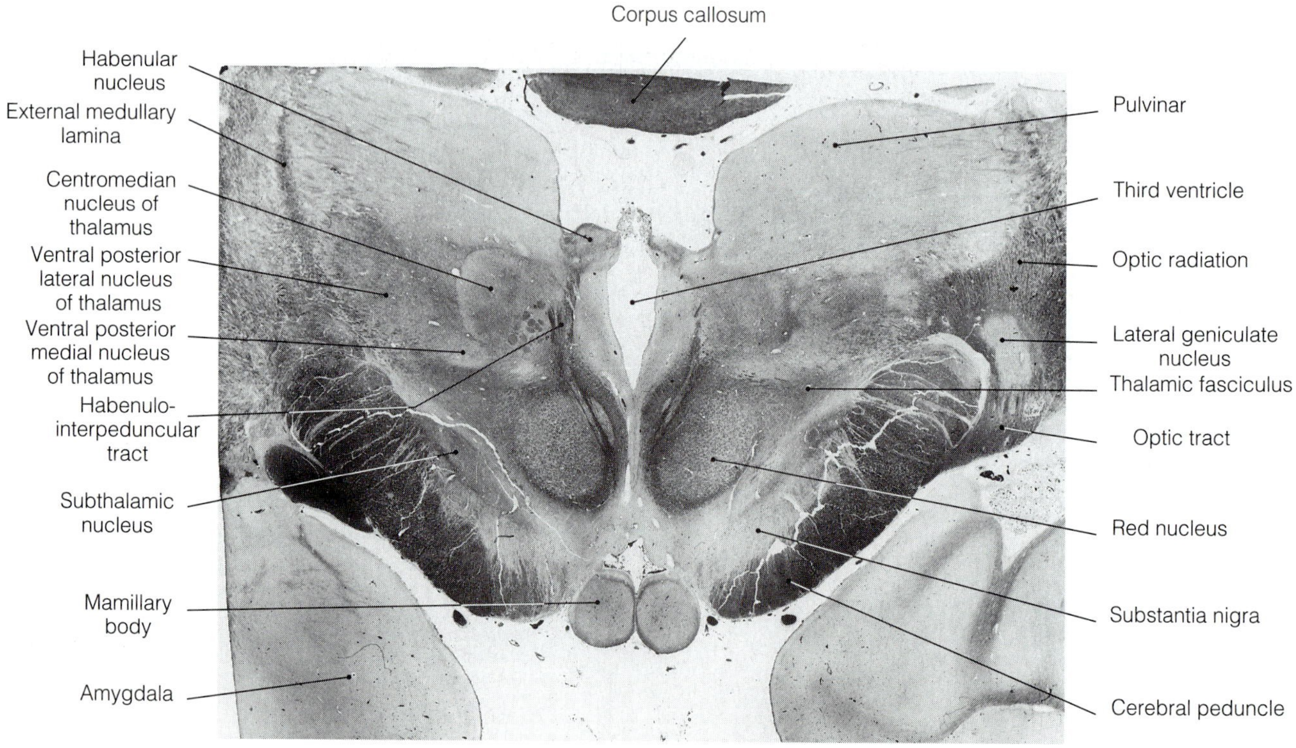

FIGURE A5-16

Coronal section of the brain stem through the caudal diencephalon at the level of the habenular nuclei and mamillary bodies.

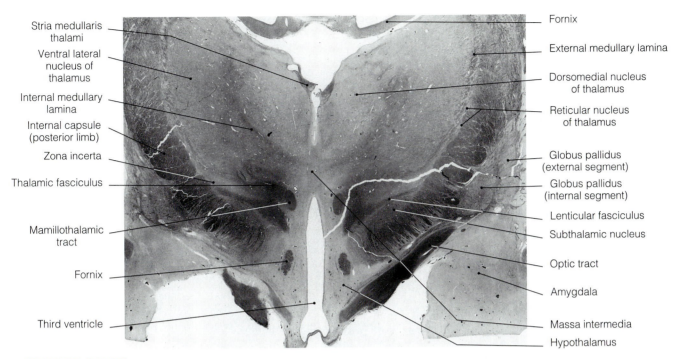

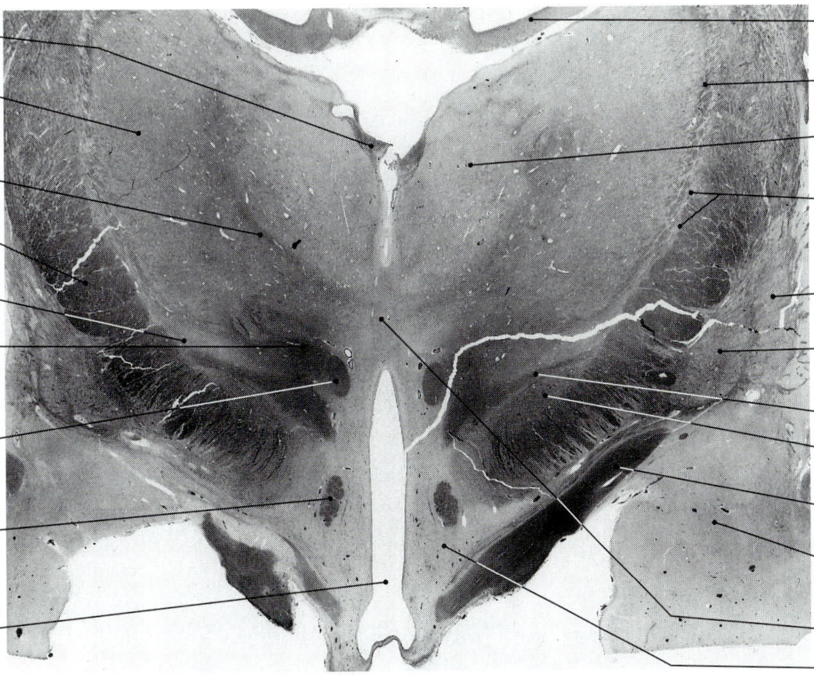
Stria medullaris thalami
Ventral lateral nucleus of thalamus
Internal medullary lamina
Internal capsule (posterior limb)
Zona incerta
Thalamic fasciculus
Mamillothalamic tract
Fornix
Third ventricle
Fornix
External medullary lamina
Dorsomedial nucleus of thalamus
Reticular nucleus of thalamus
Globus pallidus (external segment)
Globus pallidus (internal segment)
Lenticular fasciculus
Subthalamic nucleus
Optic tract
Amygdala
Massa intermedia
Hypothalamus

FIGURE A5-17

Coronal section of the brain stem through the middiencephalon at the level of the ventral lateral nucleus of the thalamus.

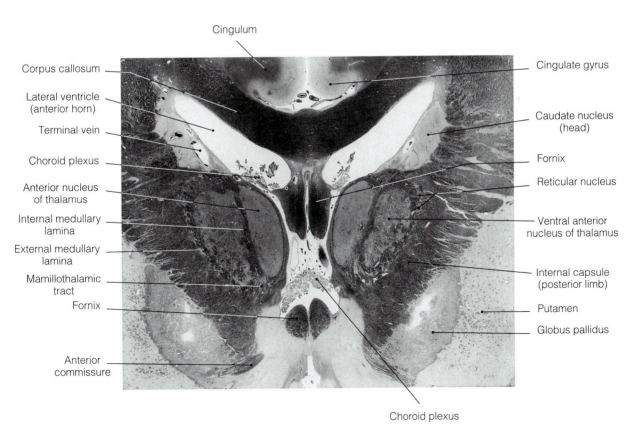

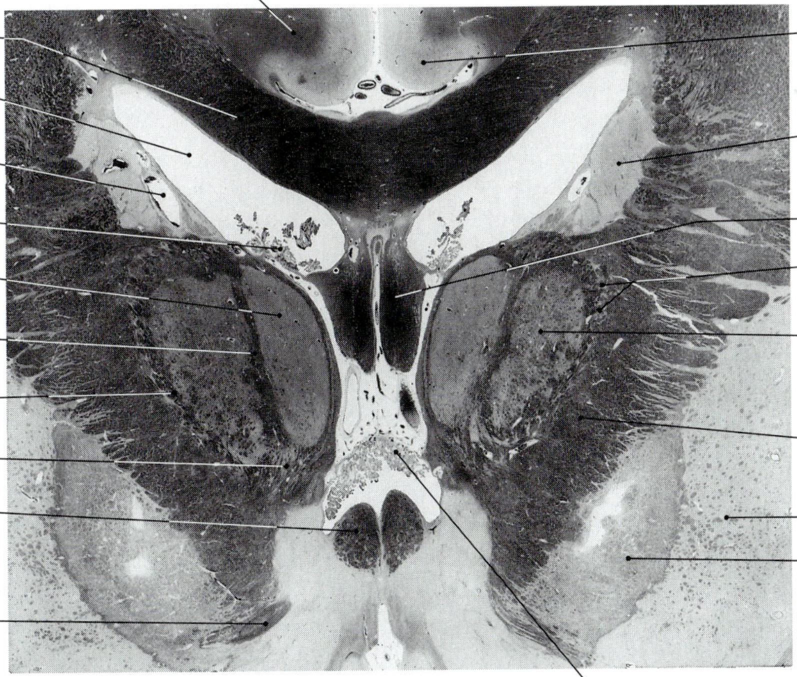
Cingulum
Corpus callosum
Lateral ventricle (anterior horn)
Terminal vein
Choroid plexus
Anterior nucleus of thalamus
Internal medullary lamina
External medullary lamina
Mamillothalamic tract
Fornix
Anterior commissure
Cingulate gyrus
Caudate nucleus (head)
Fornix
Reticular nucleus
Ventral anterior nucleus of thalamus
Internal capsule (posterior limb)
Putamen
Globus pallidus
Choroid plexus

FIGURE A5-18

Coronal section of the brain stem through the rostral diencephalon at the level of the ventral anterior thalamic nucleus.

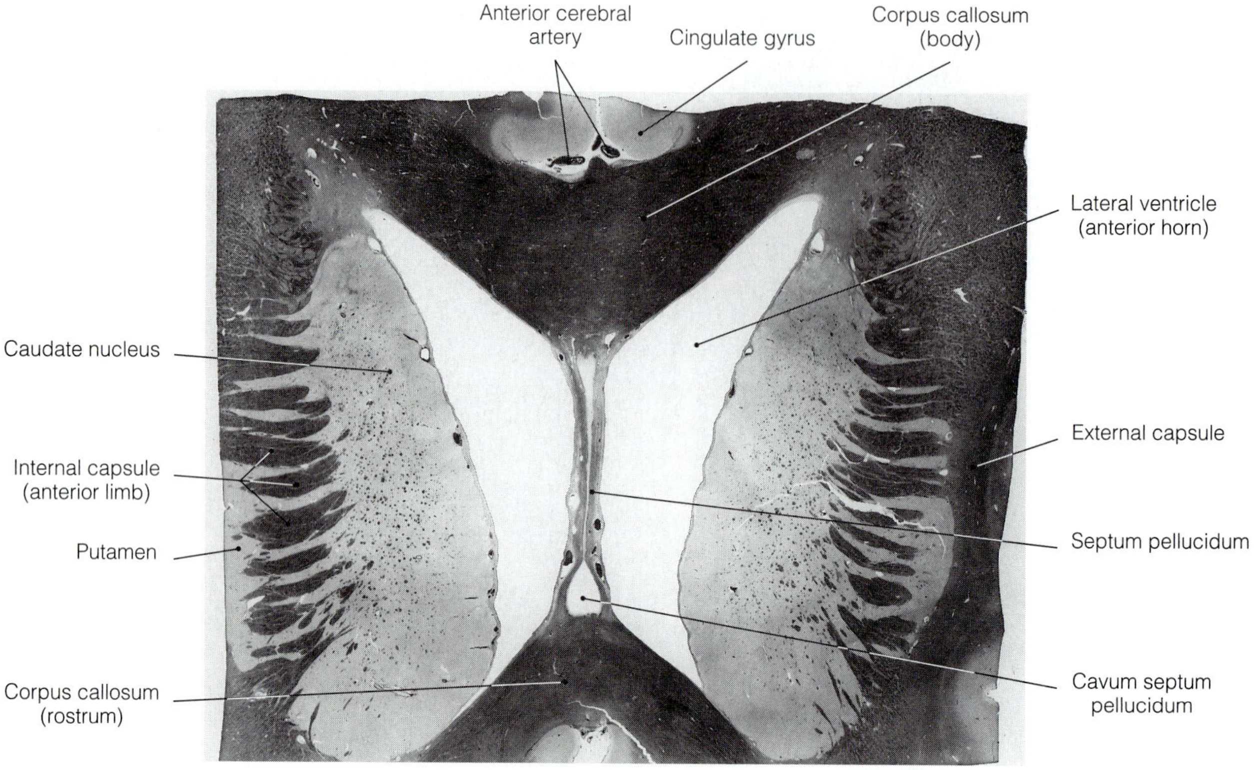
Anterior cerebral artery
Cingulate gyrus
Corpus callosum (body)
Lateral ventricle (anterior horn)
Caudate nucleus
External capsule
Internal capsule (anterior limb)
Septum pellucidum
Putamen
Corpus callosum (rostrum)
Cavum septum pellucidum

FIGURE A5-19

Coronal section of the brain stem through the basal ganglia at the level of the head of the caudate nucleus and the putamen.

SPINAL CORD

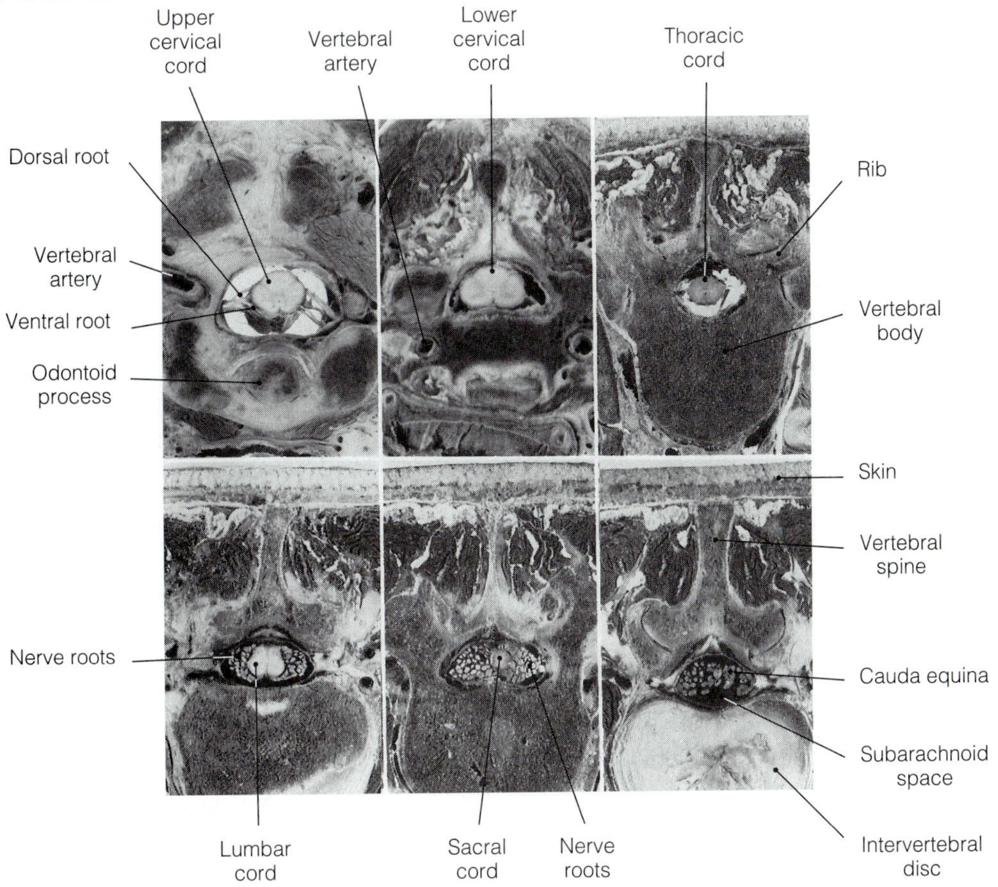

Upper cervical cord
Vertebral artery
Lower cervical cord
Thoracic cord
Dorsal root
Vertebral artery
Ventral root
Odontoid process
Rib
Vertebral body
Skin
Vertebral spine
Nerve roots
Cauda equina
Subarachnoid space
Intervertebral disc
Lumbar cord
Sacral cord
Nerve roots

FIGURE A6-1

Composite coronal sections of spinal cord at different levels.

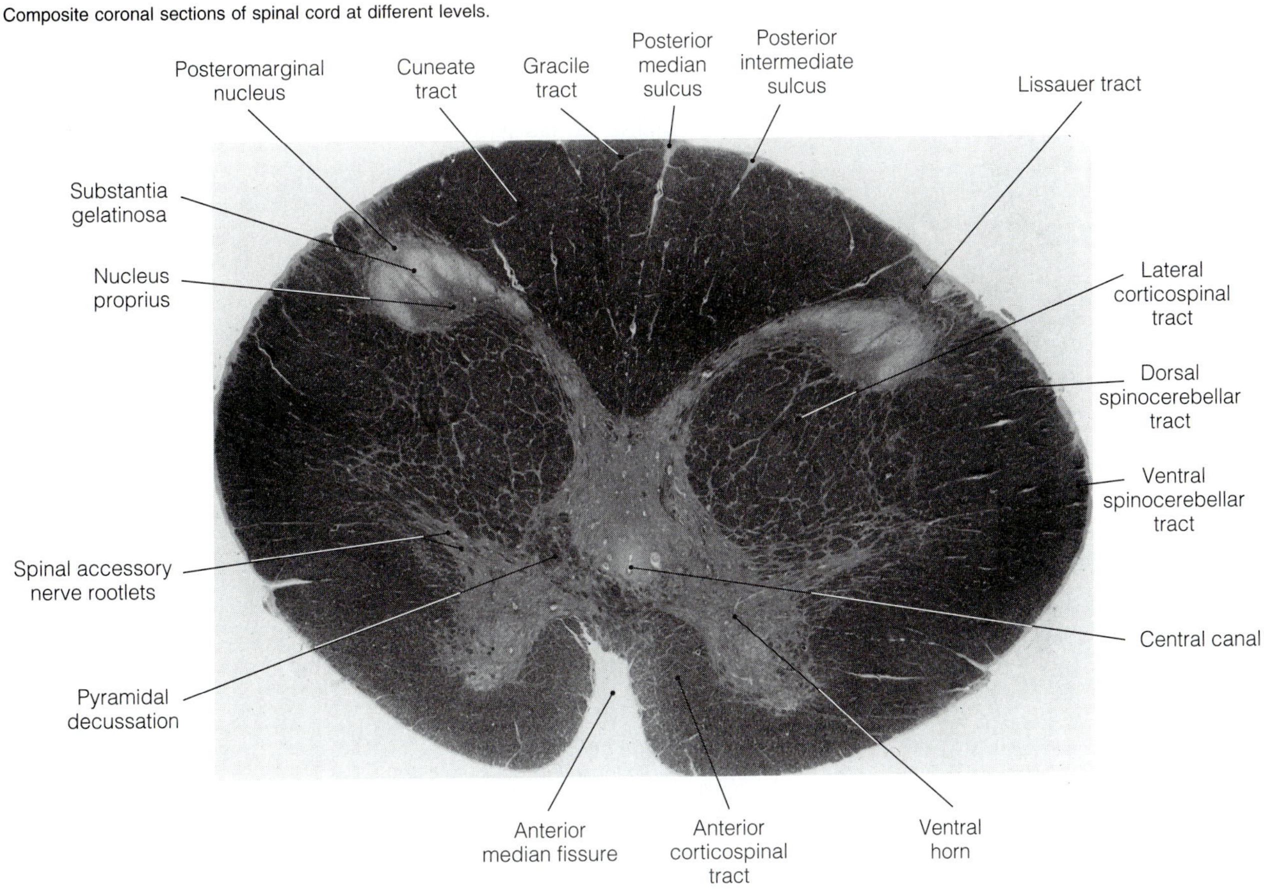

Posteromarginal nucleus
Cuneate tract
Gracile tract
Posterior median sulcus
Posterior intermediate sulcus
Lissauer tract
Substantia gelatinosa
Nucleus proprius
Lateral corticospinal tract
Dorsal spinocerebellar tract
Ventral spinocerebellar tract
Spinal accessory nerve rootlets
Central canal
Pyramidal decussation
Anterior median fissure
Anterior corticospinal tract
Ventral horn

FIGURE A6-2

Coronal section of the spinal cord at the upper cervical (C_1–C_2) level.

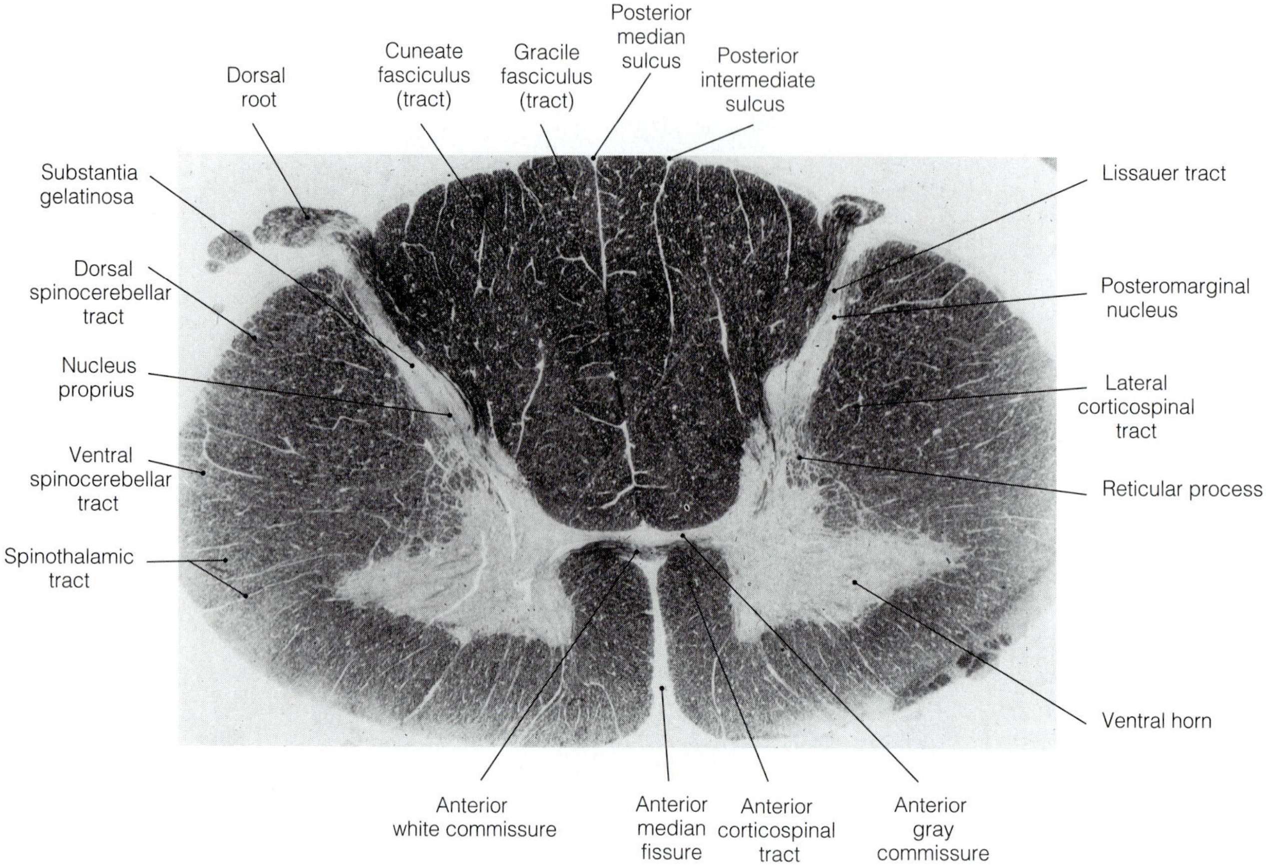
Posterior median sulcus
Cuneate fasciculus (tract)
Gracile fasciculus (tract)
Posterior intermediate sulcus
Dorsal root
Substantia gelatinosa
Lissauer tract
Dorsal spinocerebellar tract
Posteromarginal nucleus
Nucleus proprius
Lateral corticospinal tract
Ventral spinocerebellar tract
Reticular process
Spinothalamic tract
Ventral horn
Anterior white commissure
Anterior median fissure
Anterior corticospinal tract
Anterior gray commissure

FIGURE A6-3

Coronal section of the spinal cord at the lower cervical (C_8) level.

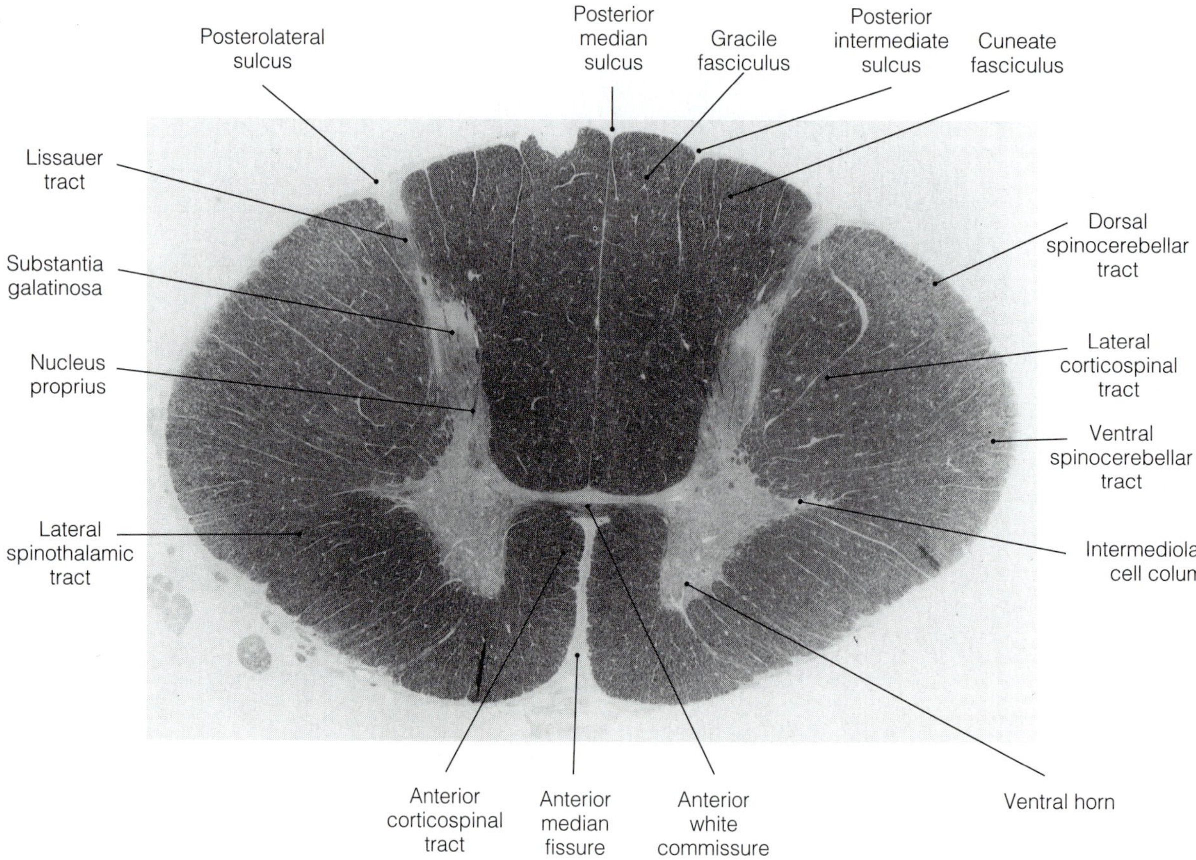
Posterolateral sulcus
Posterior median sulcus
Gracile fasciculus
Posterior intermediate sulcus
Cuneate fasciculus
Lissauer tract
Dorsal spinocerebellar tract
Substantia galatinosa
Nucleus proprius
Lateral corticospinal tract
Ventral spinocerebellar tract
Lateral spinothalamic tract
Intermediolateral cell column
Anterior corticospinal tract
Anterior median fissure
Anterior white commissure
Ventral horn

FIGURE A6-4

Coronal section of the spinal cord at the upper thoracic (T_2–T_4) level.

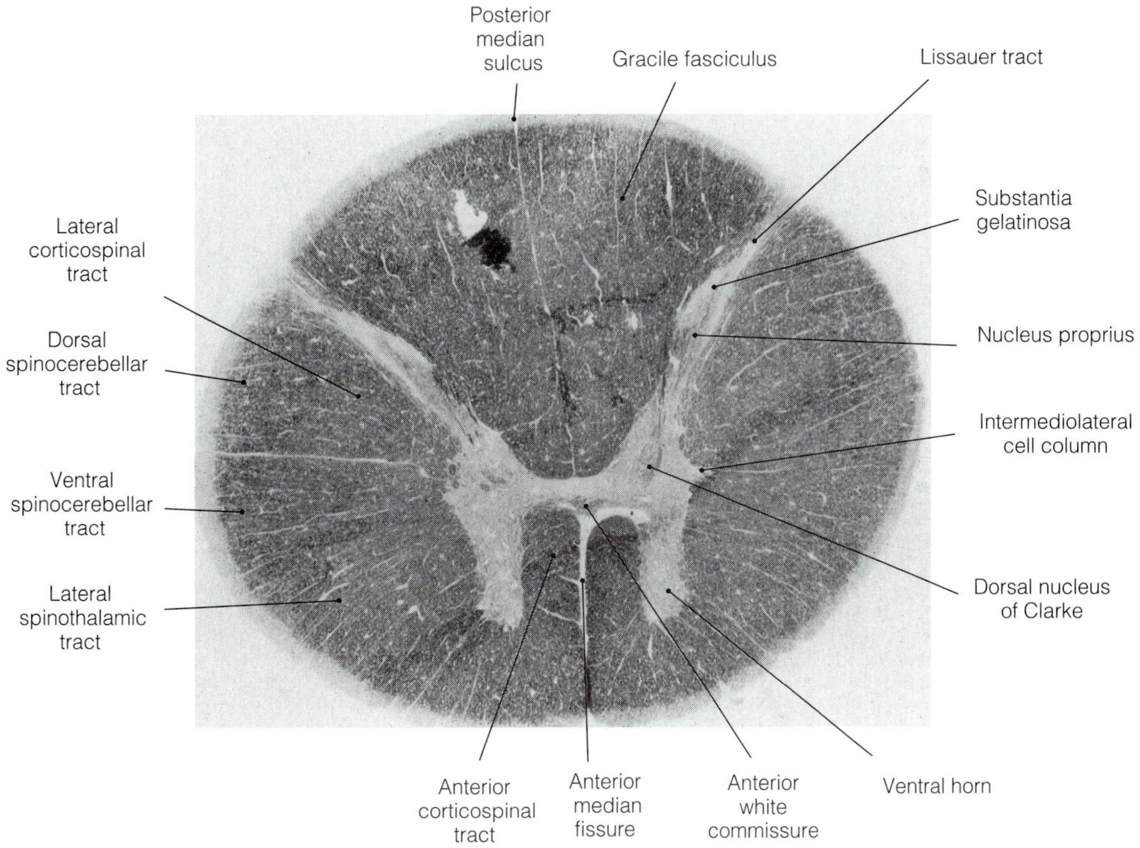

FIGURE A6-5

Coronal section of the spinal cord at the lower thoracic (T_7–T_8) level.

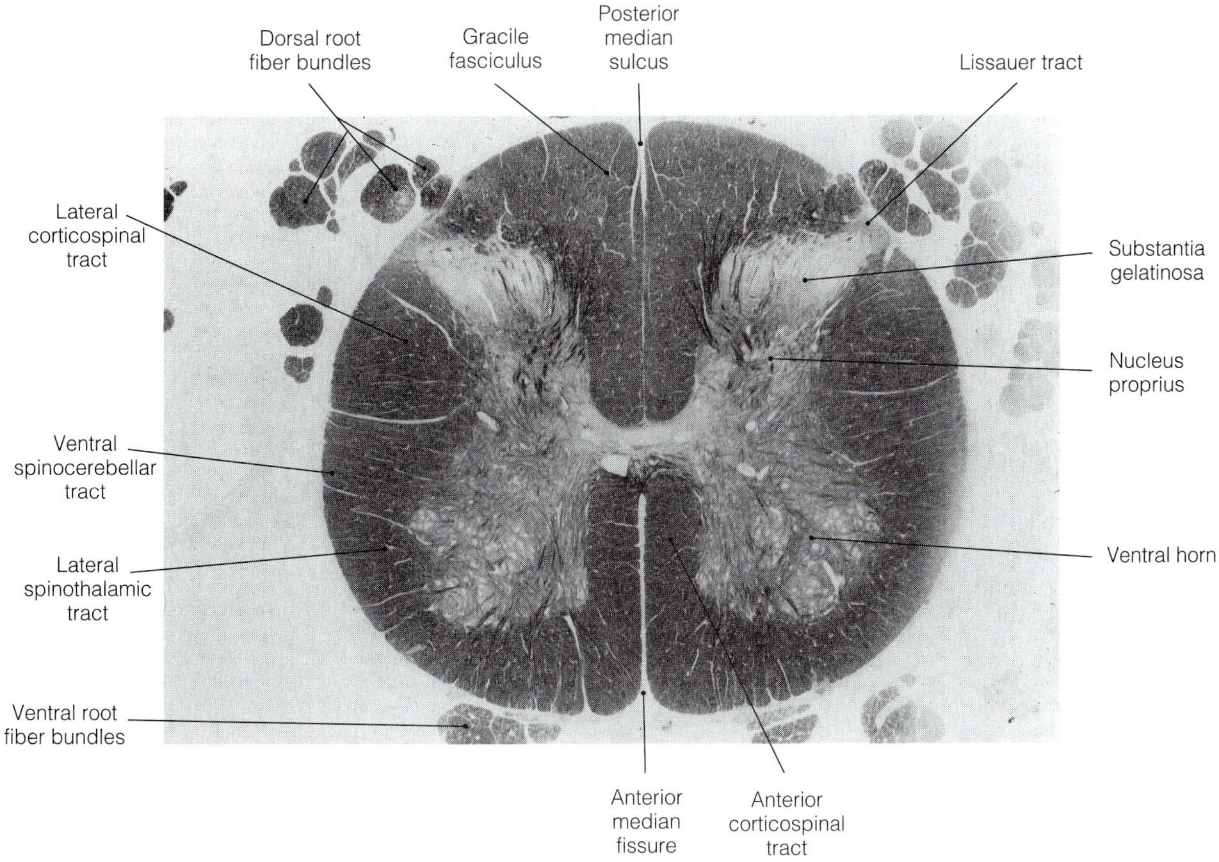

FIGURE A6-6

Coronal section of the spinal cord at the lower lumbar (L_3–L_4) level.

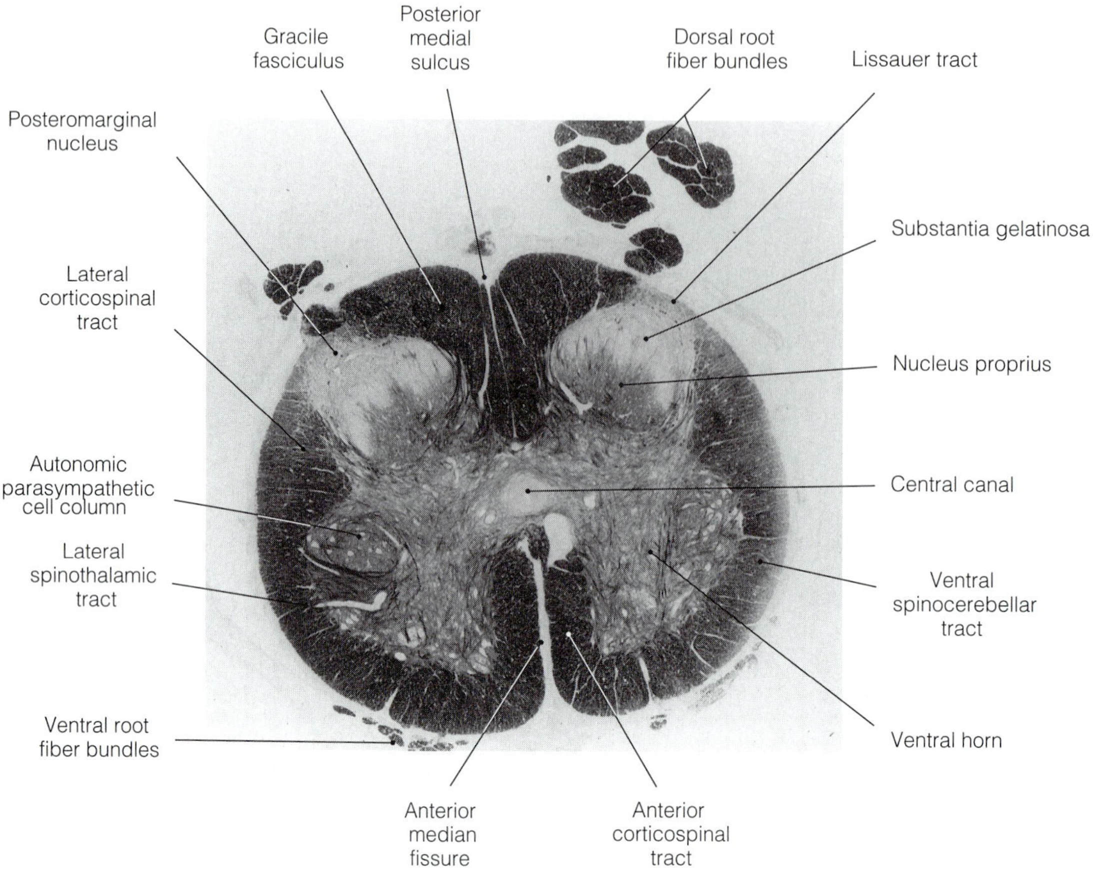

Gracile fasciculus
Posterior medial sulcus
Dorsal root fiber bundles
Lissauer tract
Posteromarginal nucleus
Substantia gelatinosa
Lateral corticospinal tract
Nucleus proprius
Autonomic parasympathetic cell column
Central canal
Lateral spinothalamic tract
Ventral spinocerebellar tract
Ventral root fiber bundles
Ventral horn
Anterior median fissure
Anterior corticospinal tract

FIGURE A6-7

Coronal section of the spinal cord at the level of the third sacral (S_3) segment.

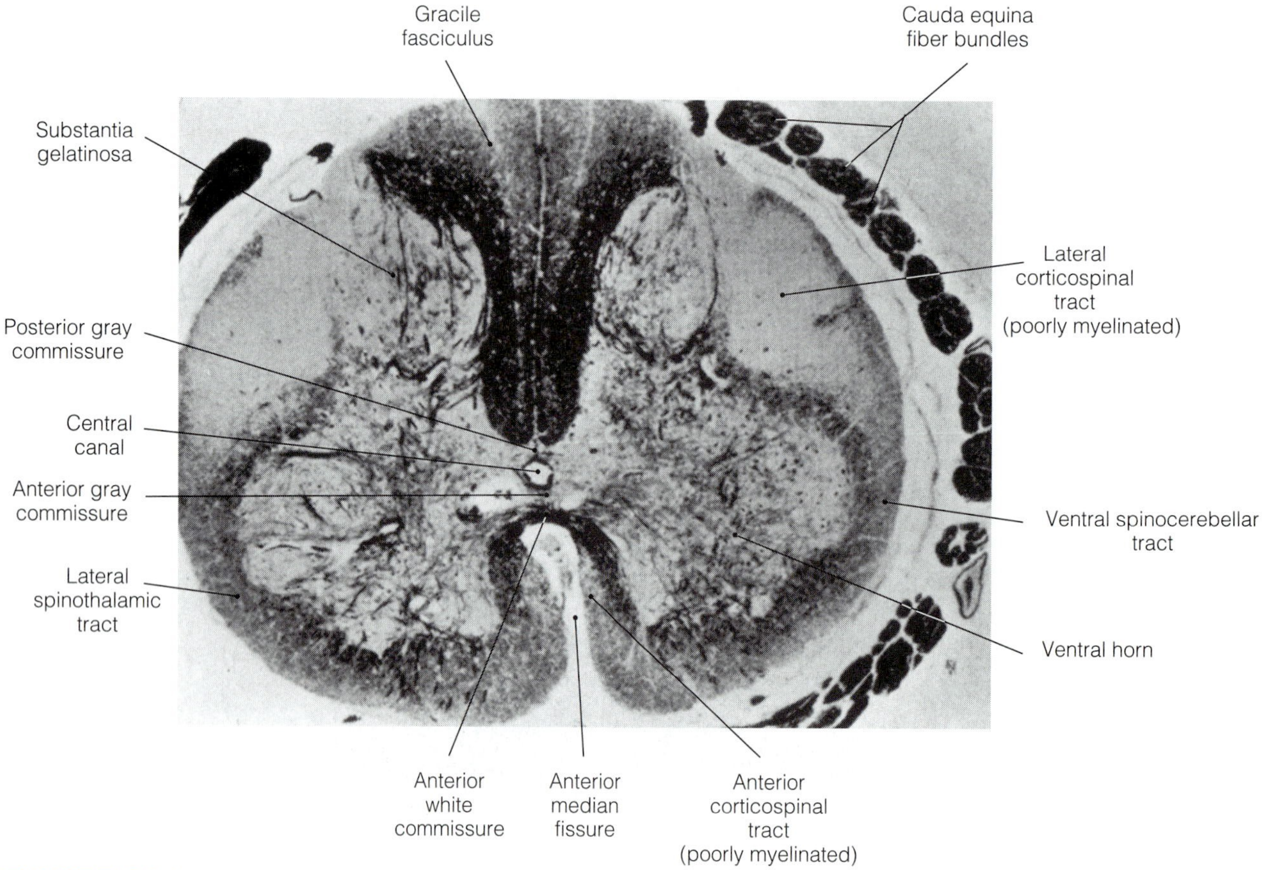

Gracile fasciculus
Cauda equina fiber bundles
Substantia gelatinosa
Lateral corticospinal tract (poorly myelinated)
Posterior gray commissure
Central canal
Anterior gray commissure
Ventral spinocerebellar tract
Lateral spinothalamic tract
Ventral horn
Anterior white commissure
Anterior median fissure
Anterior corticospinal tract (poorly myelinated)

FIGURE A6-8

Coronal section of the spinal cord of a term stillborn infant at the lower lumbar (L_5) level showing variation in degree of myelination of different tracts.

SAGITTAL MRI

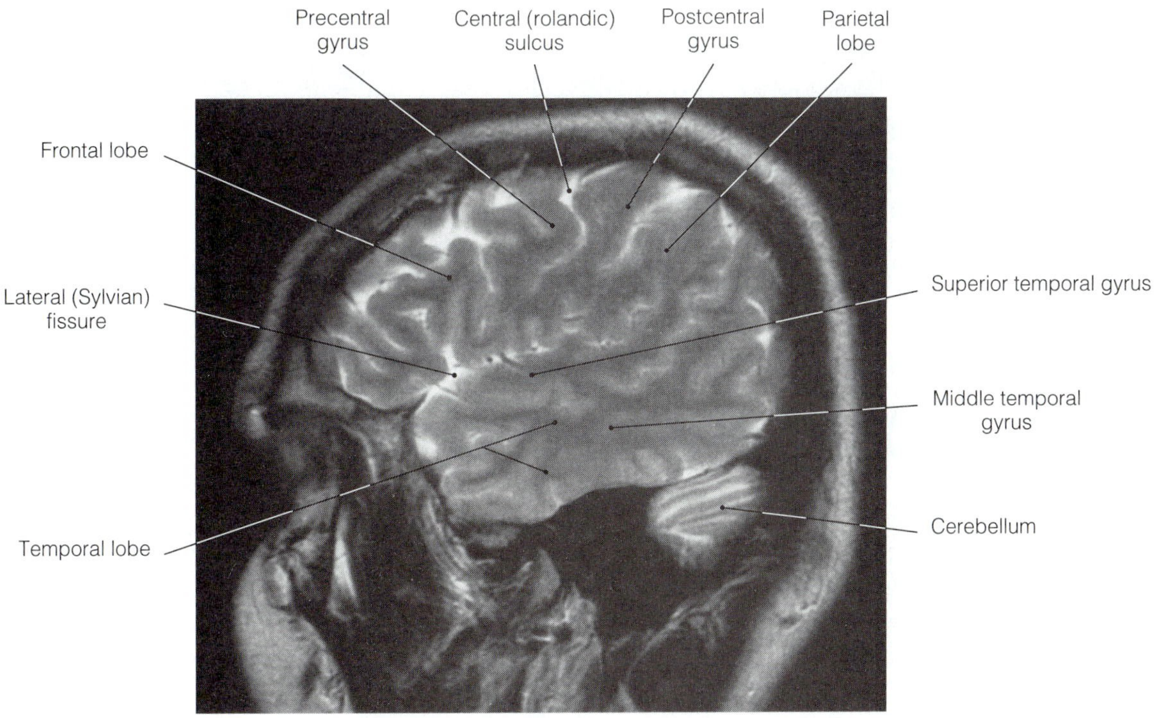
Precentral gyrus
Central (rolandic) sulcus
Postcentral gyrus
Parietal lobe
Frontal lobe
Lateral (Sylvian) fissure
Temporal lobe
Superior temporal gyrus
Middle temporal gyrus
Cerebellum

FIGURE A7-1

T2-weighted parasagittal section of the brain showing the frontal, parietal, and temporal lobes.

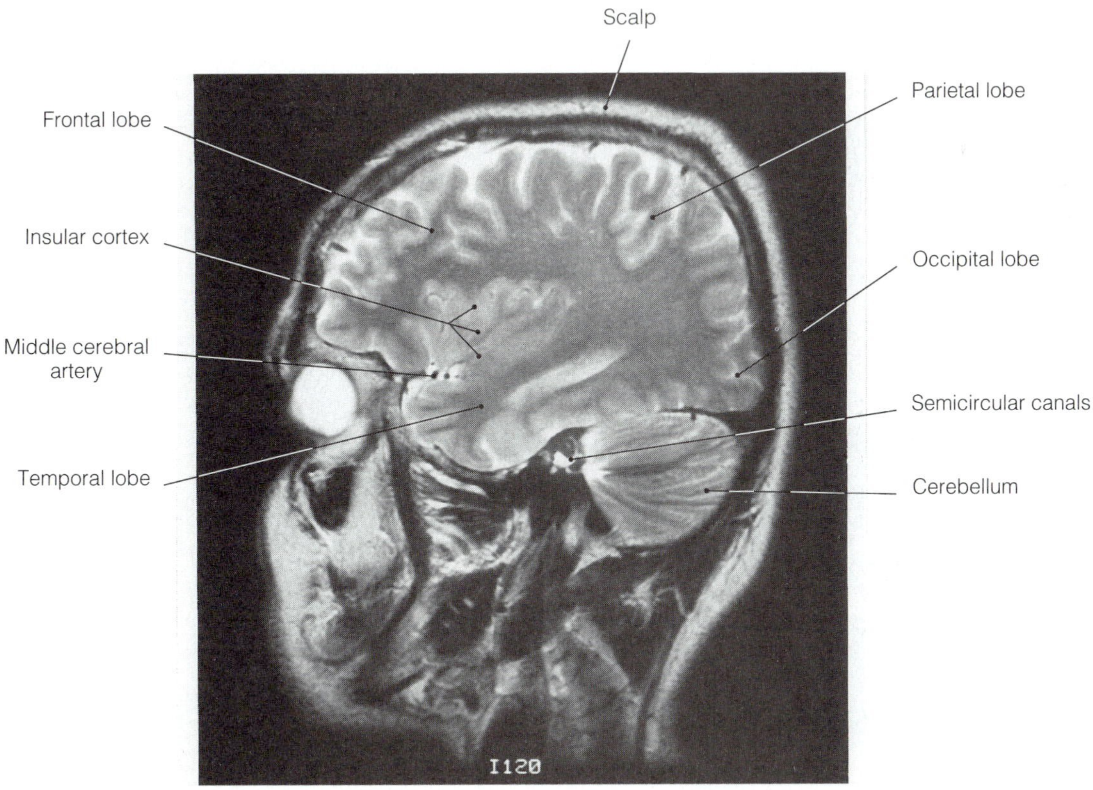
Scalp
Frontal lobe
Insular cortex
Middle cerebral artery
Temporal lobe
Parietal lobe
Occipital lobe
Semicircular canals
Cerebellum
I120

FIGURE A7-2

T2-weighted parasagittal section of the brain through the insular cortex.

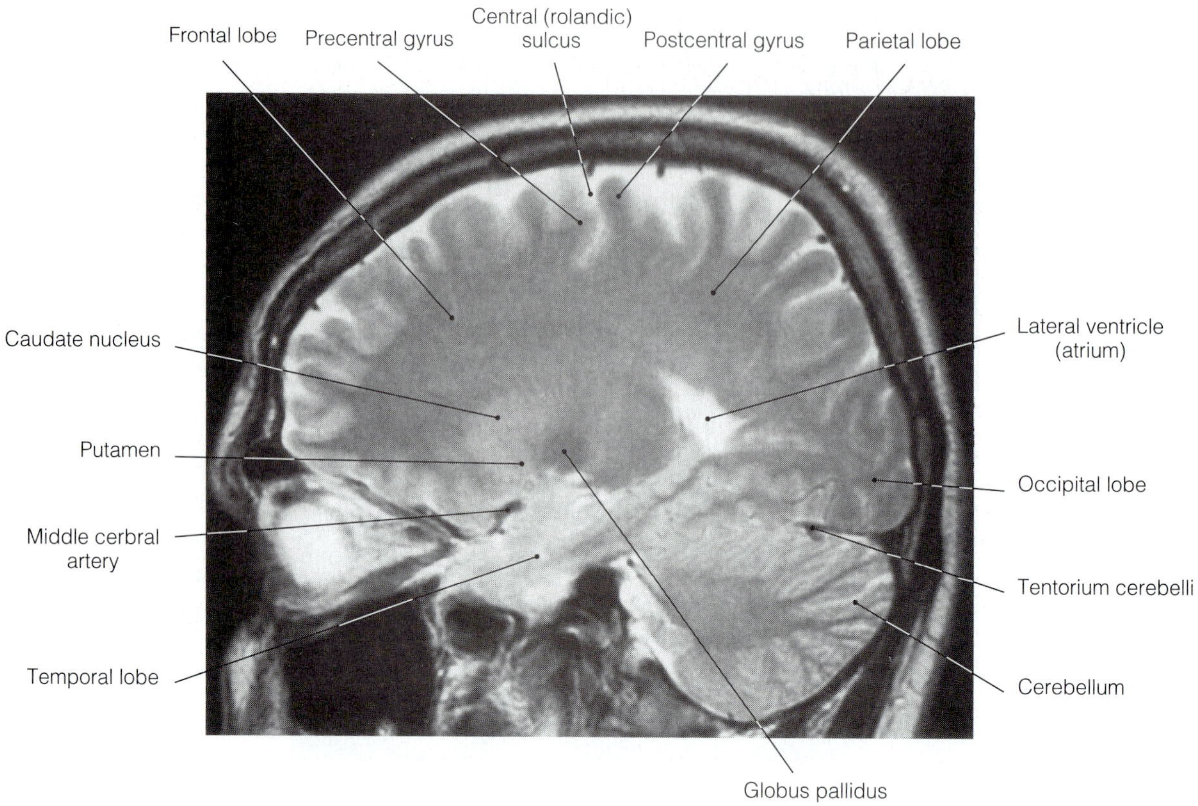
Frontal lobe
Precentral gyrus
Central (rolandic) sulcus
Postcentral gyrus
Parietal lobe
Caudate nucleus
Lateral ventricle (atrium)
Putamen
Occipital lobe
Middle cerbral artery
Tentorium cerebelli
Temporal lobe
Cerebellum
Globus pallidus

FIGURE A7-3

T2-weighted parasagittal section of the brain through the basal ganglia.

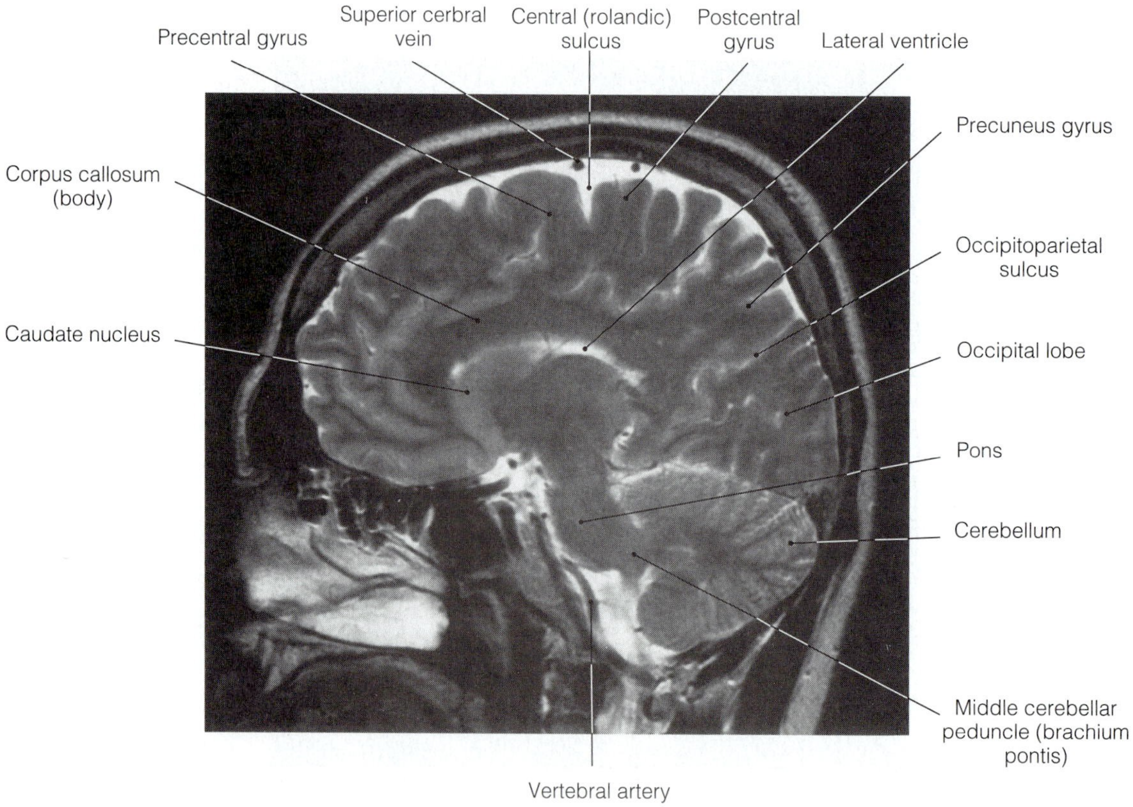
Precentral gyrus
Superior cerbral vein
Central (rolandic) sulcus
Postcentral gyrus
Lateral ventricle
Precuneus gyrus
Corpus callosum (body)
Occipitoparietal sulcus
Caudate nucleus
Occipital lobe
Pons
Cerebellum
Middle cerebellar peduncle (brachium pontis)
Vertebral artery

FIGURE A7-4

T2-weighted parasagittal section of the brain close to the midline through the brain stem.

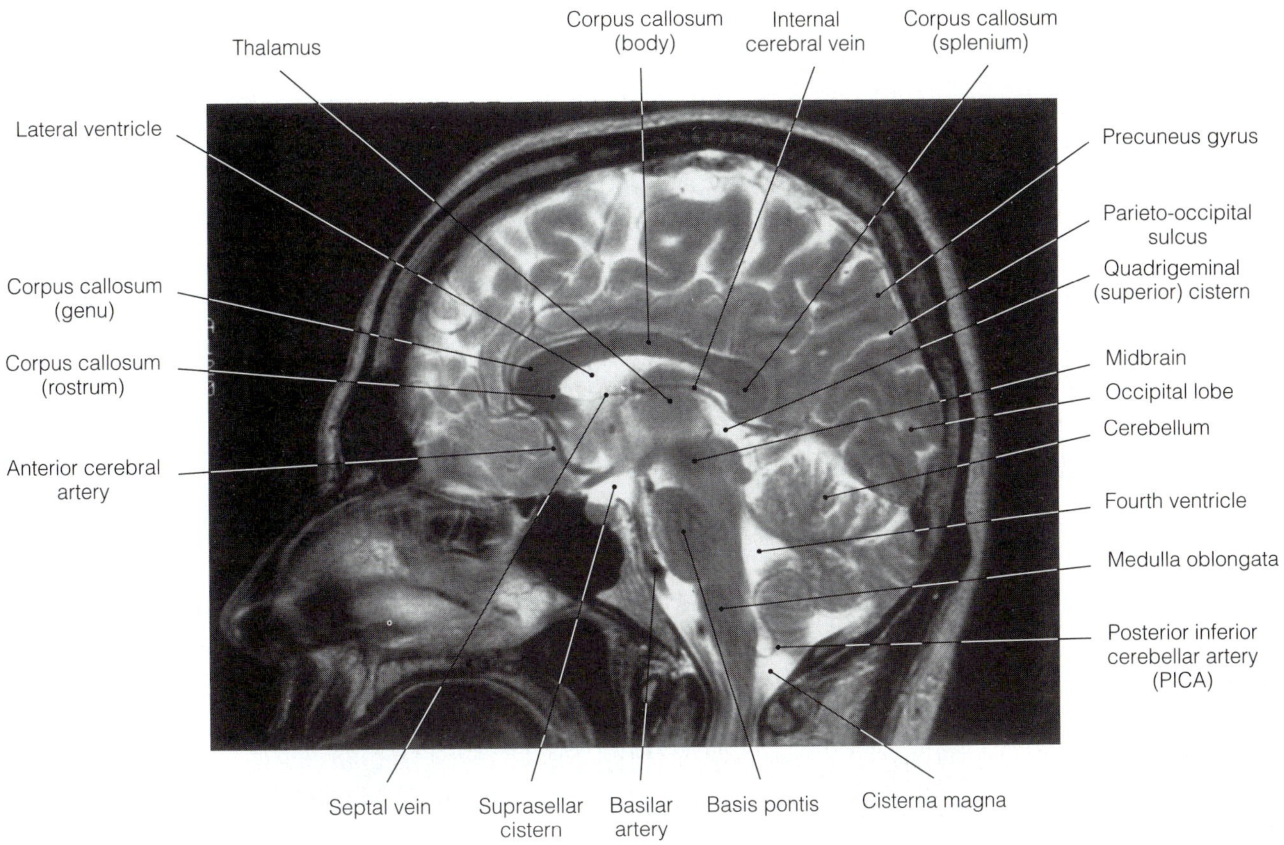

FIGURE A7-5

T2-weighted midsagittal section of the brain through the corpus callosum and thalamus.

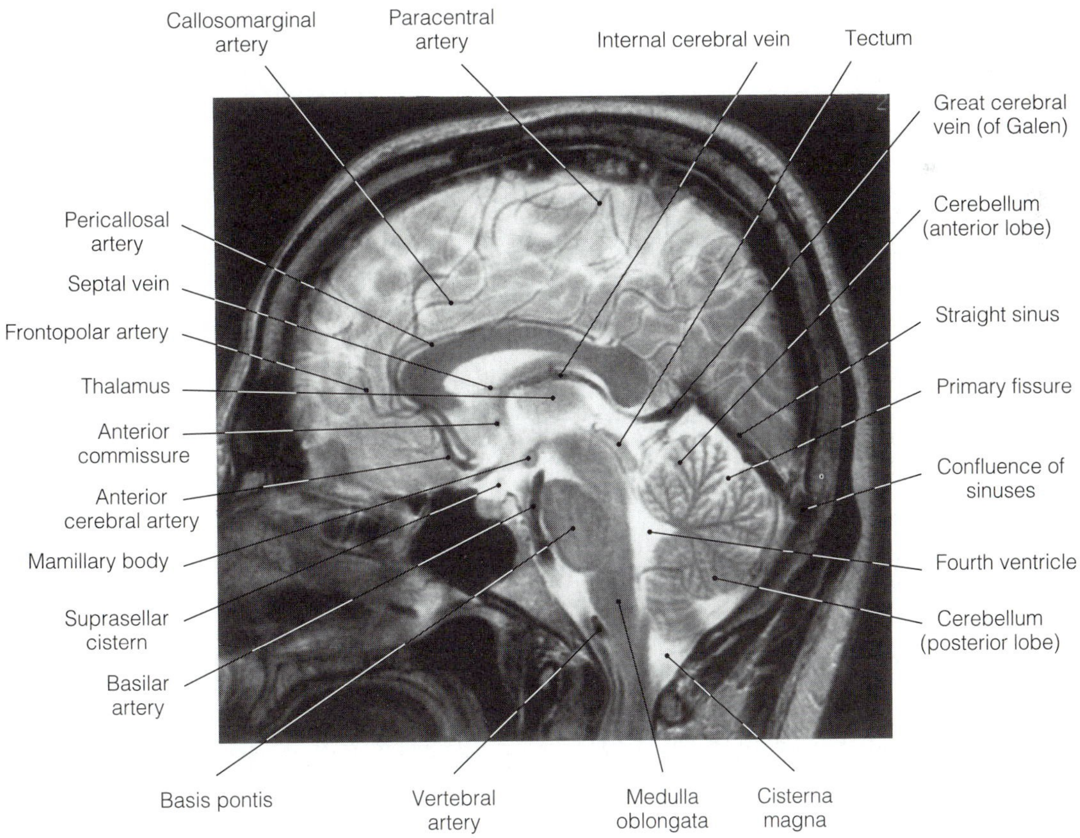

FIGURE A7-6

T2-weighted midsagittal section of the brain through the corpus callosum and brain stem.

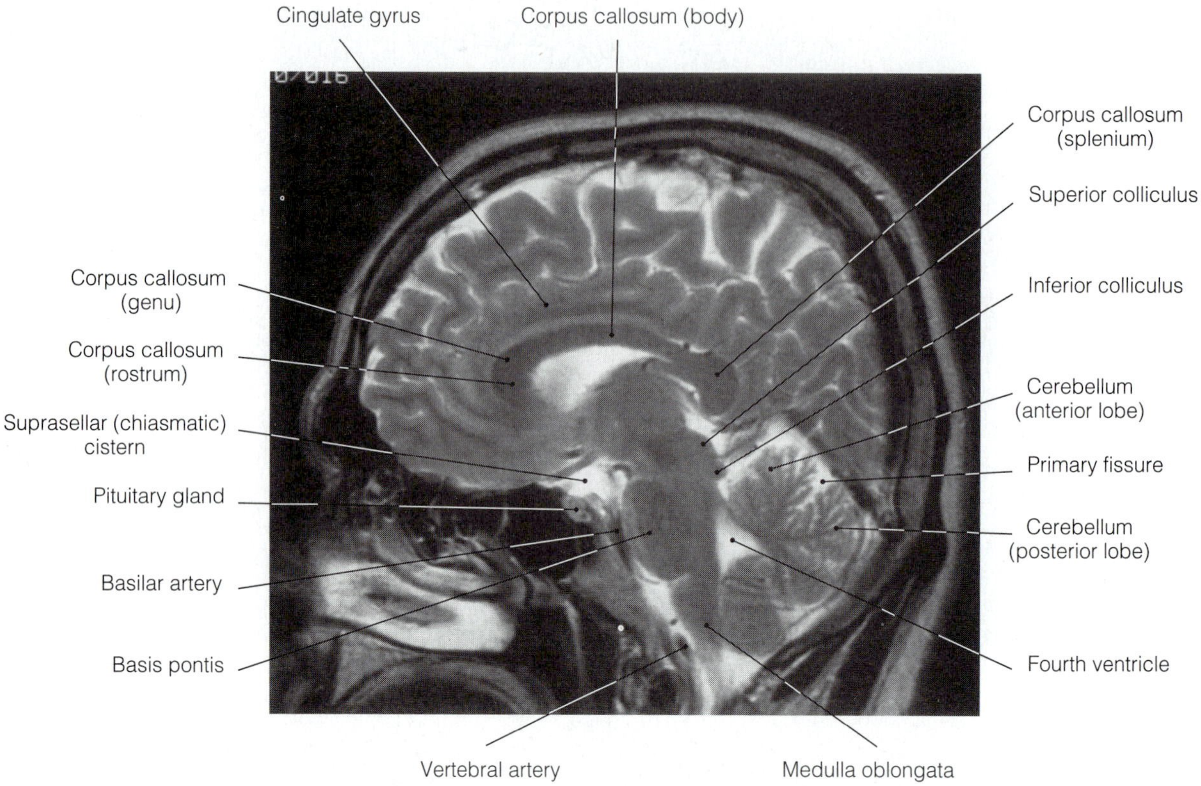
Cingulate gyrus
Corpus callosum (body)
Corpus callosum (splenium)
Superior colliculus
Inferior colliculus
Cerebellum (anterior lobe)
Primary fissure
Cerebellum (posterior lobe)
Fourth ventricle
Corpus callosum (genu)
Corpus callosum (rostrum)
Suprasellar (chiasmatic) cistern
Pituitary gland
Basilar artery
Basis pontis
Vertebral artery
Medulla oblongata

FIGURE A7-7

T2-weighted midsagittal section of the brain through the corpus callosum and brain stem.

AXIAL MRI

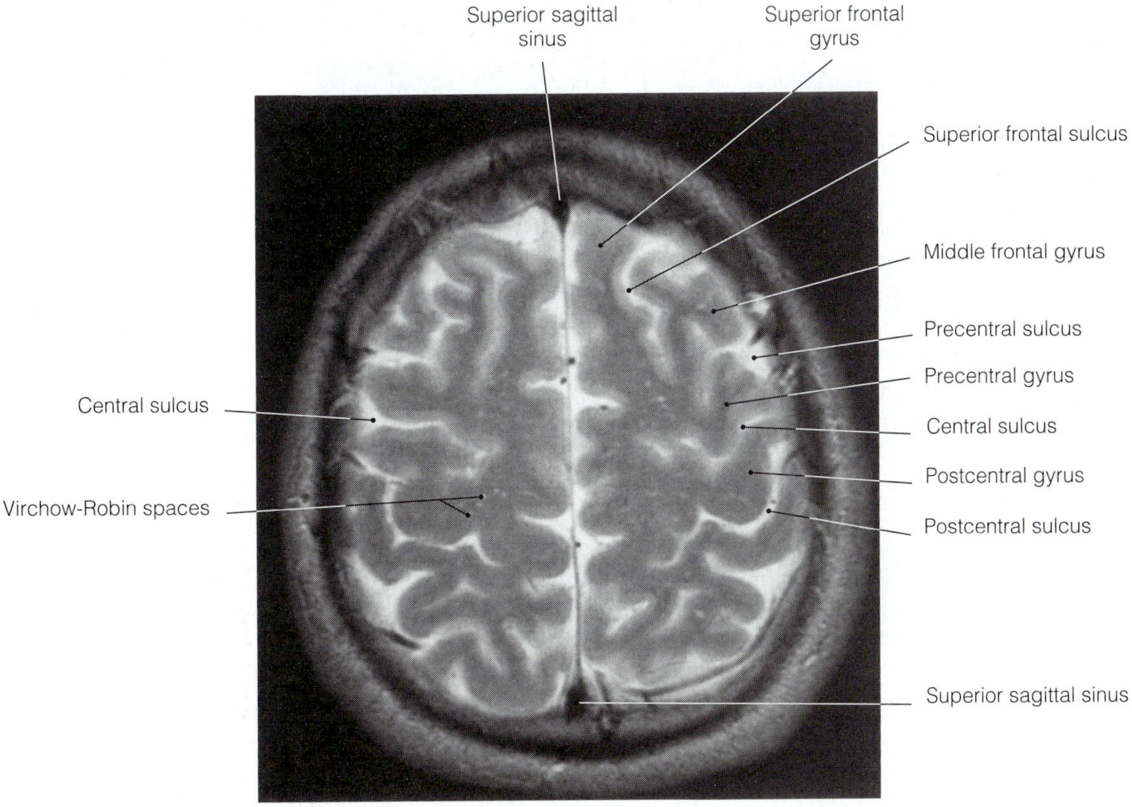
Superior sagittal sinus
Superior frontal gyrus
Superior frontal sulcus
Middle frontal gyrus
Precentral sulcus
Precentral gyrus
Central sulcus
Postcentral gyrus
Postcentral sulcus
Superior sagittal sinus
Central sulcus
Virchow-Robin spaces

FIGURE A8-1

T2-weighted axial section of the upper part of the brain through the frontal and parietal lobes.

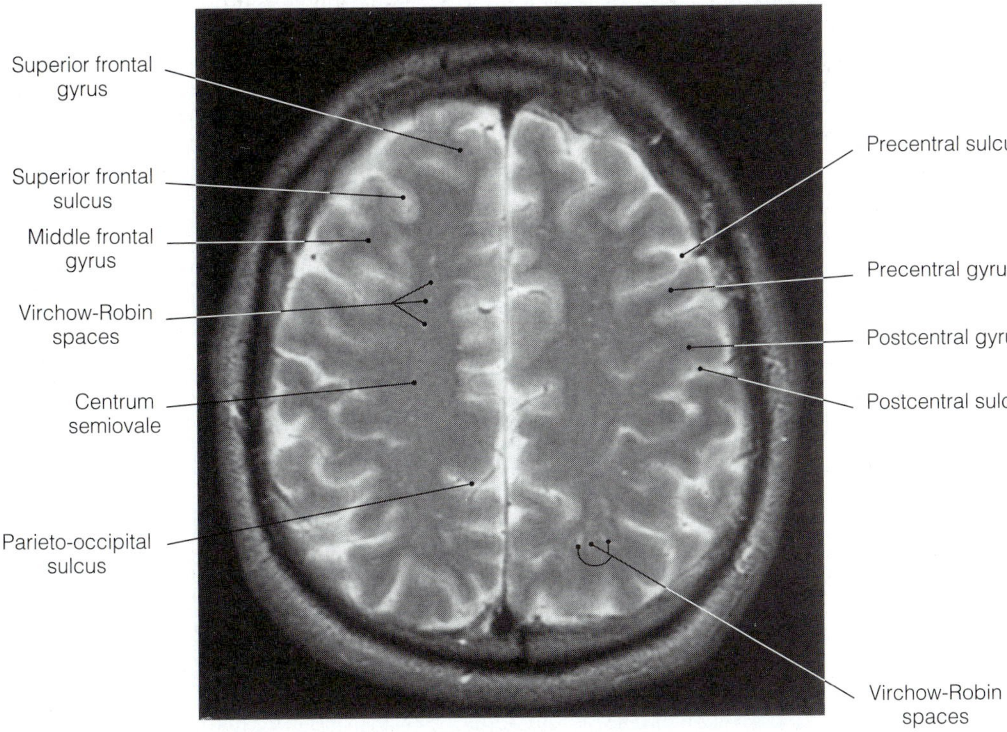
Superior frontal gyrus
Superior frontal sulcus
Middle frontal gyrus
Virchow-Robin spaces
Centrum semiovale
Parieto-occipital sulcus
Precentral sulcus
Precentral gyrus
Postcentral gyrus
Postcentral sulcus
Virchow-Robin spaces

FIGURE A8-2

T2-weighted axial section of the upper part of the brain through the centrum semiovale of the frontal and parietal lobes.

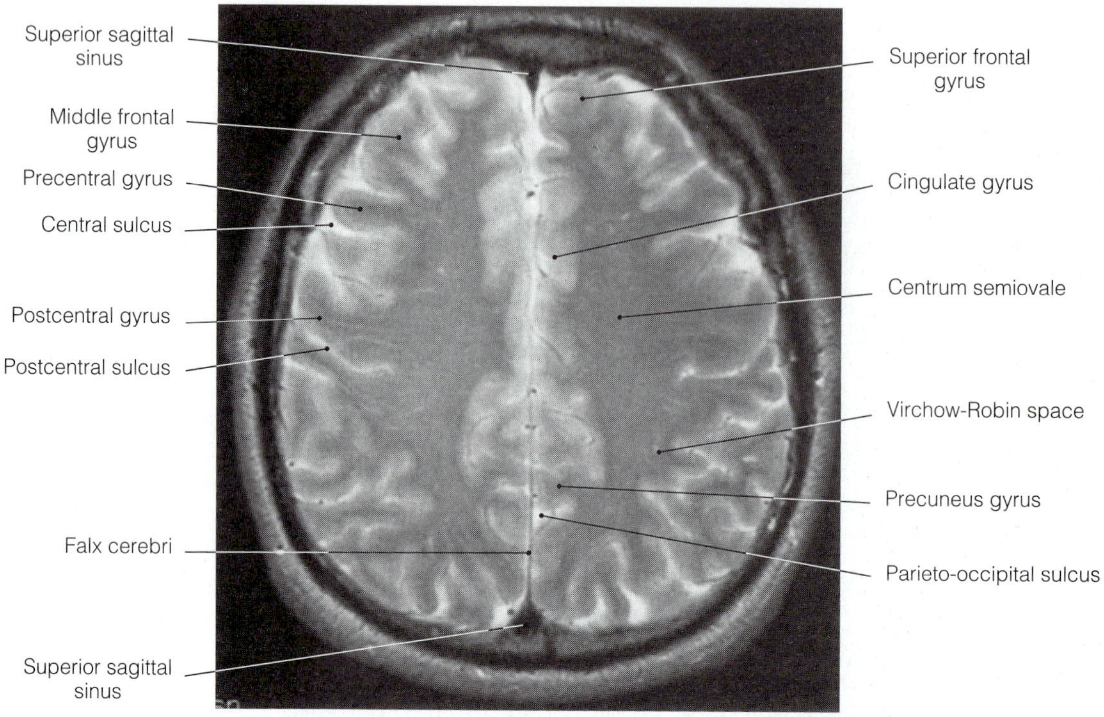
Superior sagittal sinus
Middle frontal gyrus
Precentral gyrus
Central sulcus
Postcentral gyrus
Postcentral sulcus
Falx cerebri
Superior sagittal sinus
Superior frontal gyrus
Cingulate gyrus
Centrum semiovale
Virchow-Robin space
Precuneus gyrus
Parieto-occipital sulcus

FIGURE A8-3

T2-weighted axial section of the brain through the centrum semiovale of the frontal and parietal lobes.

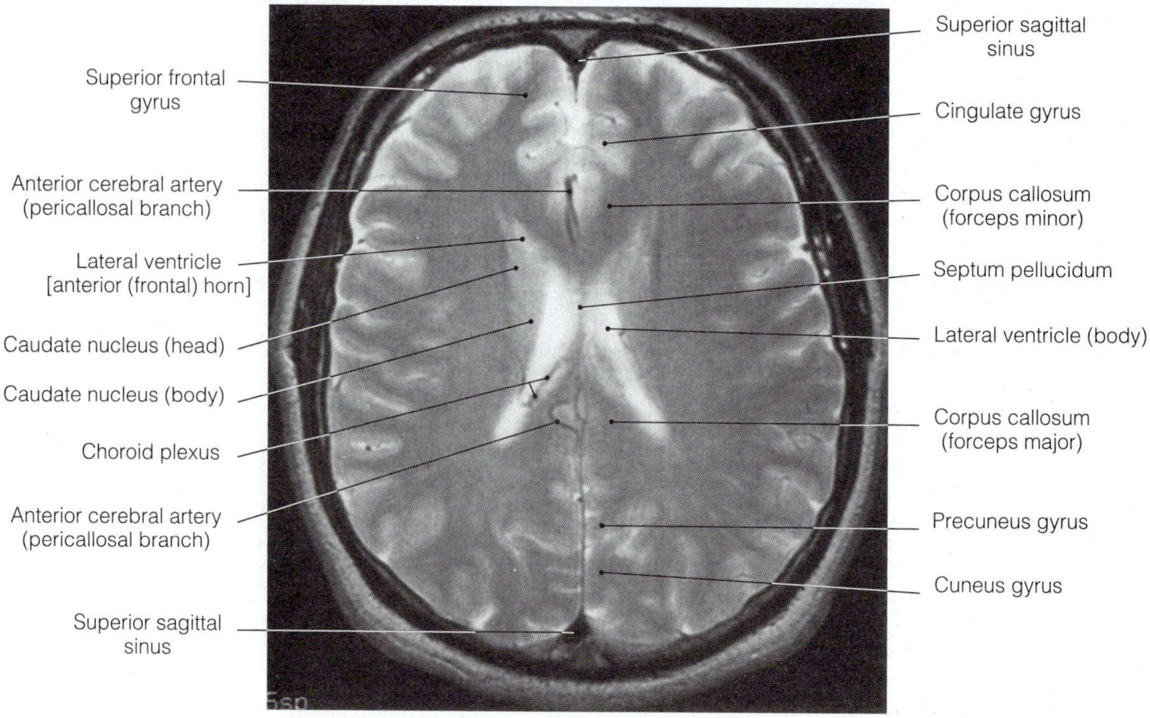
Superior frontal gyrus
Anterior cerebral artery (pericallosal branch)
Lateral ventricle [anterior (frontal) horn]
Caudate nucleus (head)
Caudate nucleus (body)
Choroid plexus
Anterior cerebral artery (pericallosal branch)
Superior sagittal sinus
Superior sagittal sinus
Cingulate gyrus
Corpus callosum (forceps minor)
Septum pellucidum
Lateral ventricle (body)
Corpus callosum (forceps major)
Precuneus gyrus
Cuneus gyrus

FIGURE A8-4

T2-weighted axial section of the brain through the body of the lateral ventricle.

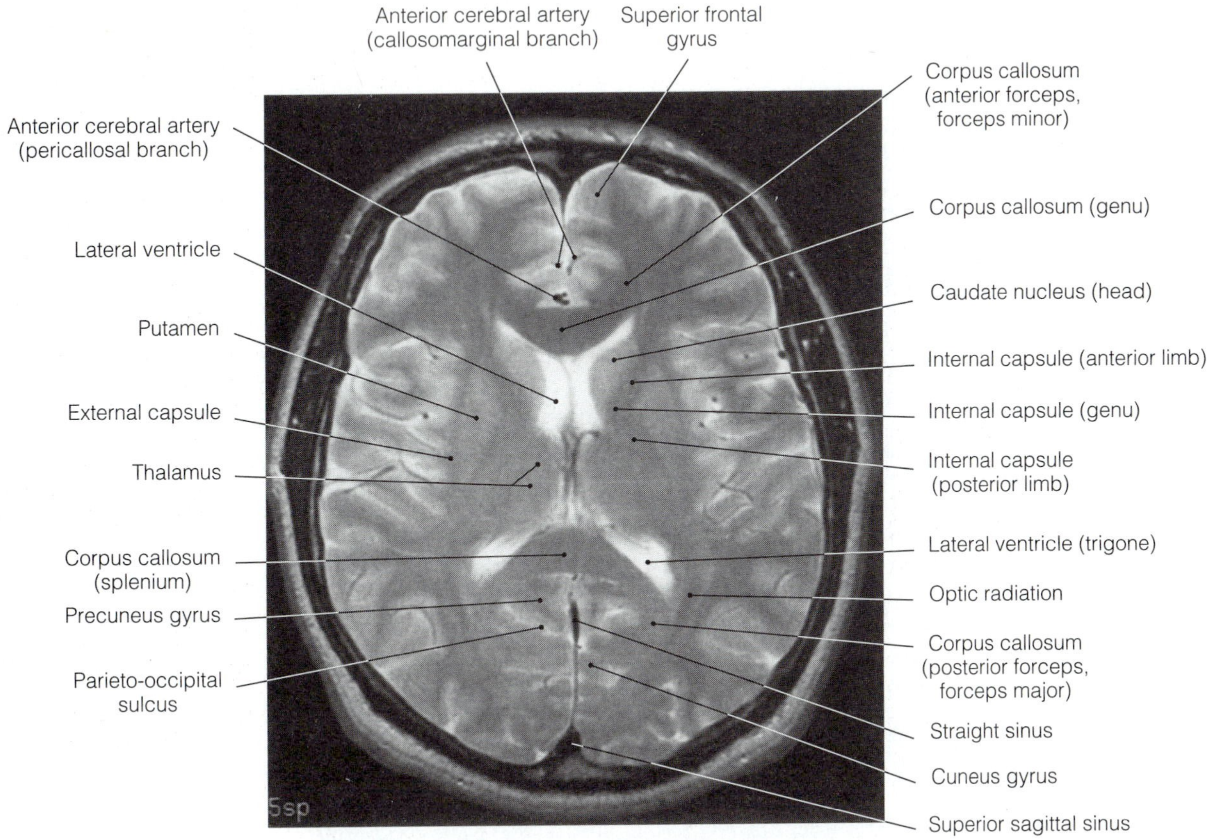
Anterior cerebral artery (callosomarginal branch)
Superior frontal gyrus
Anterior cerebral artery (pericallosal branch)
Lateral ventricle
Putamen
External capsule
Thalamus
Corpus callosum (splenium)
Precuneus gyrus
Parieto-occipital sulcus
Corpus callosum (anterior forceps, forceps minor)
Corpus callosum (genu)
Caudate nucleus (head)
Internal capsule (anterior limb)
Internal capsule (genu)
Internal capsule (posterior limb)
Lateral ventricle (trigone)
Optic radiation
Corpus callosum (posterior forceps, forceps major)
Straight sinus
Cuneus gyrus
Superior sagittal sinus
5sp

FIGURE A8-5

T2-weighted axial section of the brain through the genu and splenium of the corpus callosum.

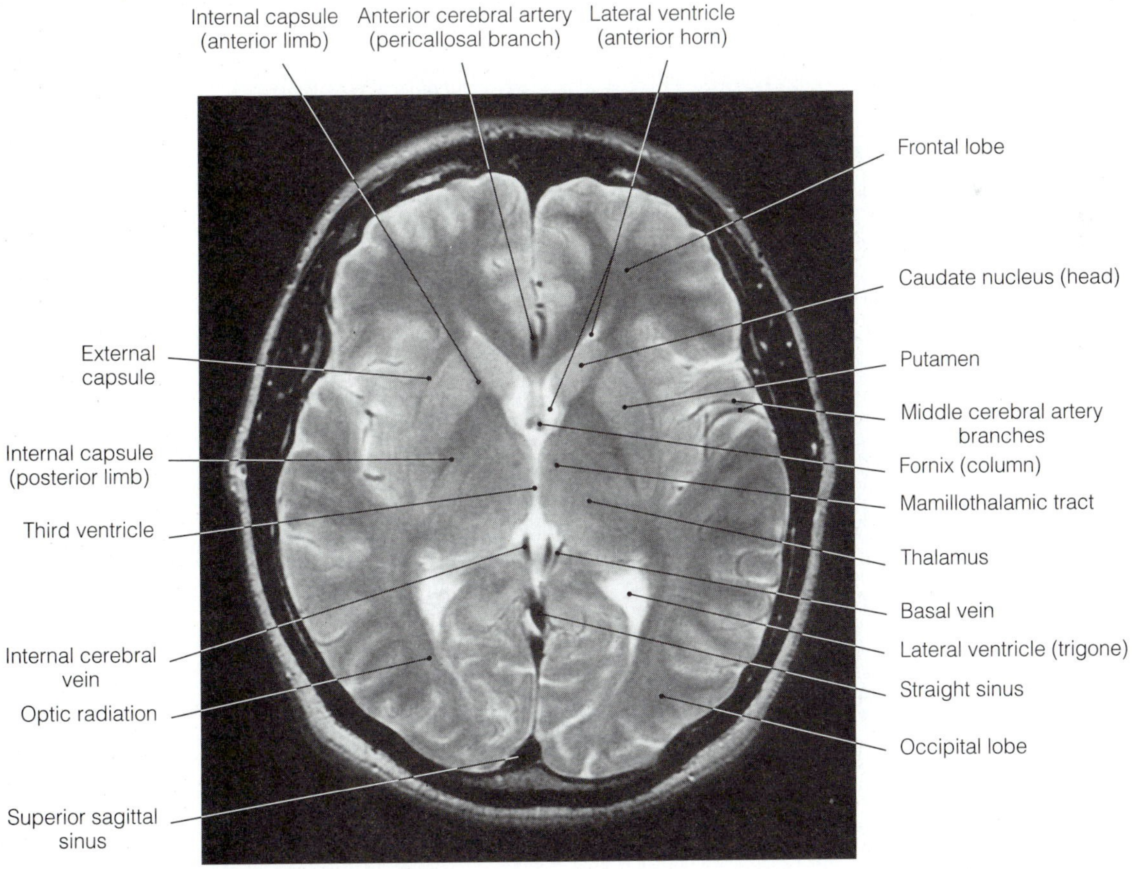
Internal capsule (anterior limb)
Anterior cerebral artery (pericallosal branch)
Lateral ventricle (anterior horn)
External capsule
Internal capsule (posterior limb)
Third ventricle
Internal cerebral vein
Optic radiation
Superior sagittal sinus
Frontal lobe
Caudate nucleus (head)
Putamen
Middle cerebral artery branches
Fornix (column)
Mamillothalamic tract
Thalamus
Basal vein
Lateral ventricle (trigone)
Straight sinus
Occipital lobe

FIGURE A8-6

T2-weighted axial section of the brain through the thalamus.

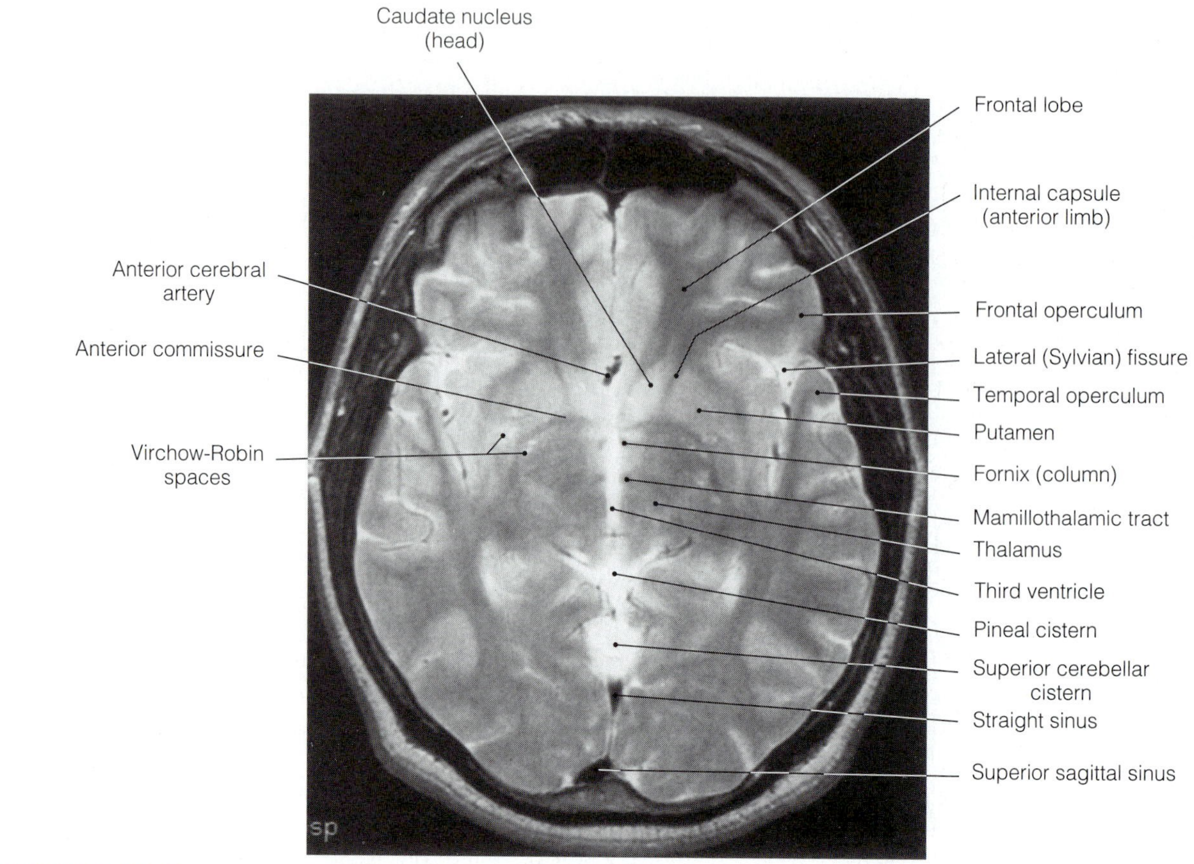
Caudate nucleus (head)
Frontal lobe
Internal capsule (anterior limb)
Anterior cerebral artery
Frontal operculum
Anterior commissure
Lateral (Sylvian) fissure
Temporal operculum
Putamen
Virchow-Robin spaces
Fornix (column)
Mamillothalamic tract
Thalamus
Third ventricle
Pineal cistern
Superior cerebellar cistern
Straight sinus
Superior sagittal sinus
sp

FIGURE A8-7

T2-weighted axial section of the brain through the anterior commissure and the thalamus.

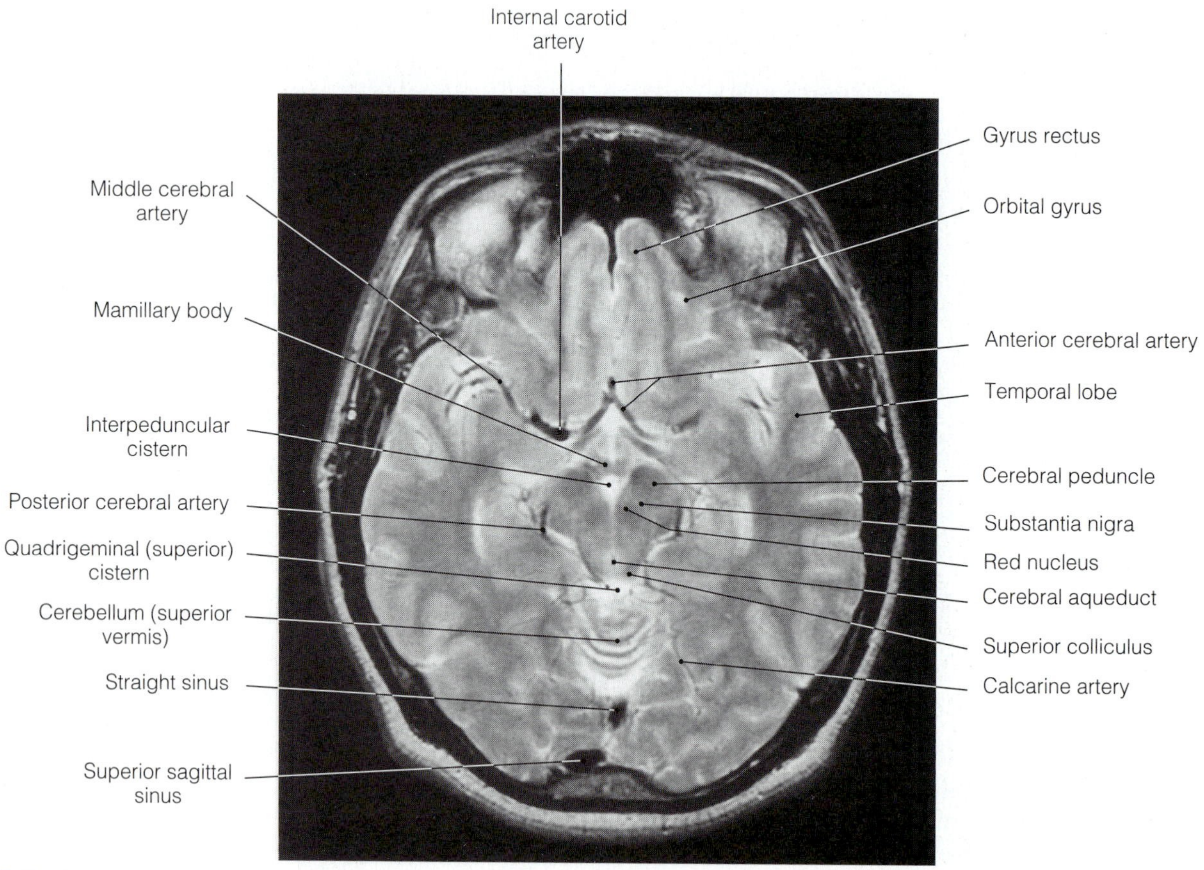
Internal carotid artery
Gyrus rectus
Middle cerebral artery
Orbital gyrus
Mamillary body
Anterior cerebral artery
Temporal lobe
Interpeduncular cistern
Cerebral peduncle
Posterior cerebral artery
Substantia nigra
Quadrigeminal (superior) cistern
Red nucleus
Cerebral aqueduct
Cerebellum (superior vermis)
Superior colliculus
Calcarine artery
Straight sinus
Superior sagittal sinus

FIGURE A8-8

T2-weighted axial section of the brain through the rostral midbrain.

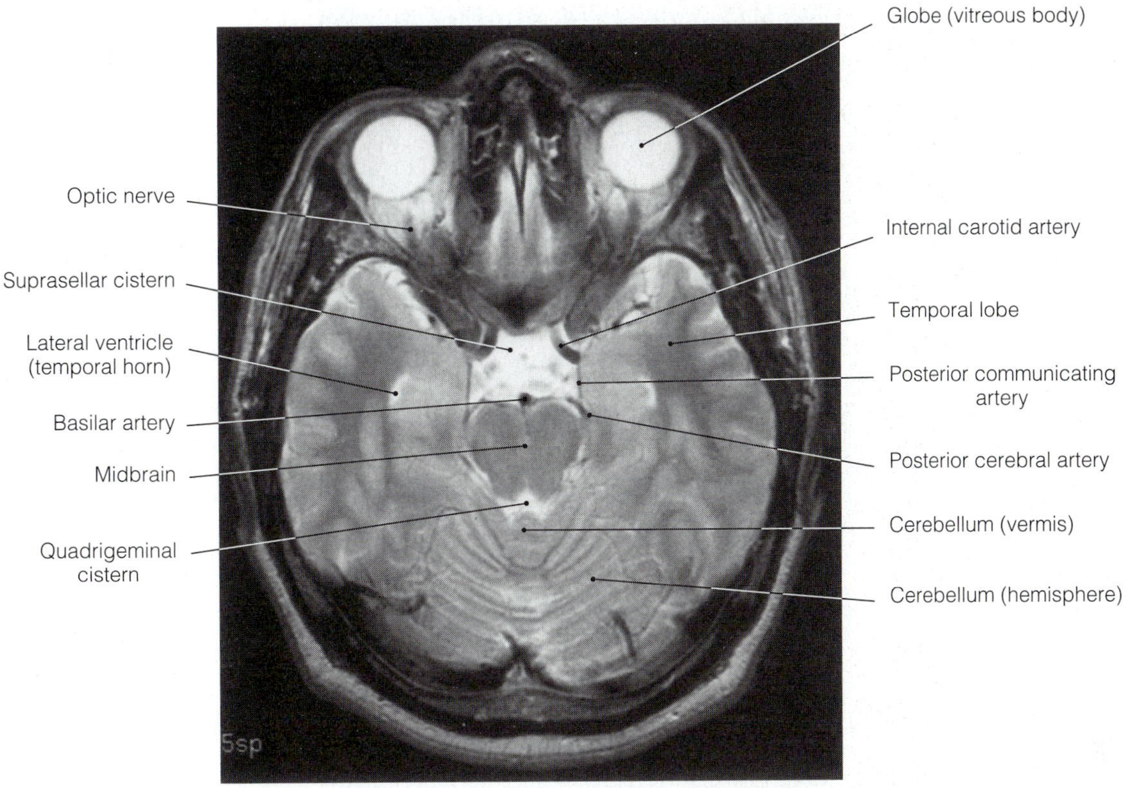
Globe (vitreous body)
Optic nerve
Internal carotid artery
Suprasellar cistern
Temporal lobe
Lateral ventricle (temporal horn)
Posterior communicating artery
Basilar artery
Midbrain
Posterior cerebral artery
Cerebellum (vermis)
Quadrigeminal cistern
Cerebellum (hemisphere)
5sp

FIGURE A8-9

T2-weighted axial section of the brain through the caudal midbrain.

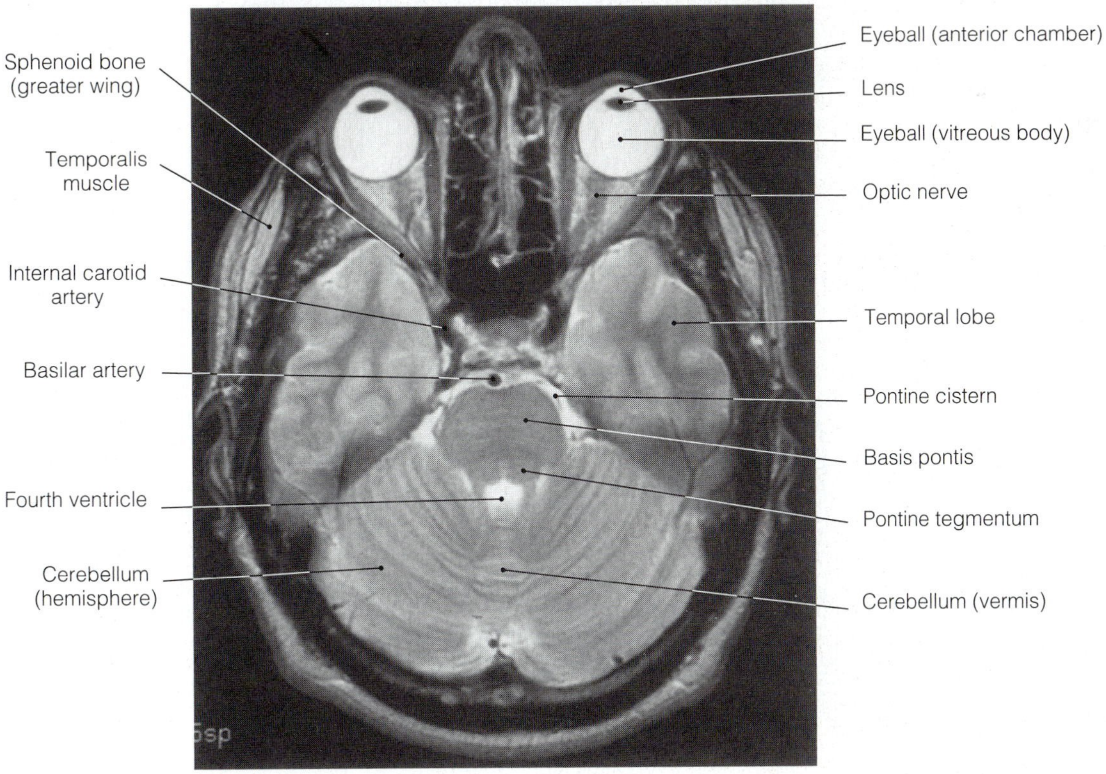
Eyeball (anterior chamber)
Sphenoid bone (greater wing)
Lens
Eyeball (vitreous body)
Temporalis muscle
Optic nerve
Internal carotid artery
Temporal lobe
Basilar artery
Pontine cistern
Basis pontis
Fourth ventricle
Pontine tegmentum
Cerebellum (hemisphere)
Cerebellum (vermis)
5sp

FIGURE A8-10

T2-weighted axial section of the brain through the pons and cerebellum.

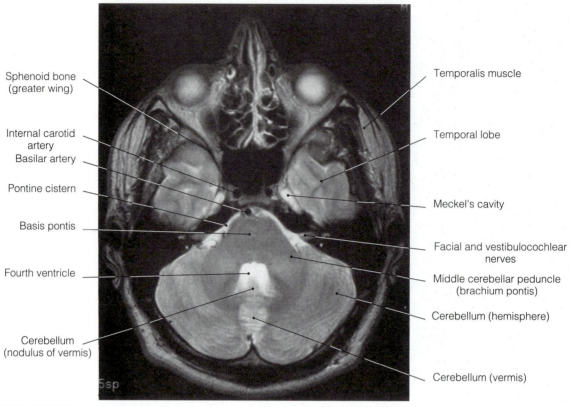

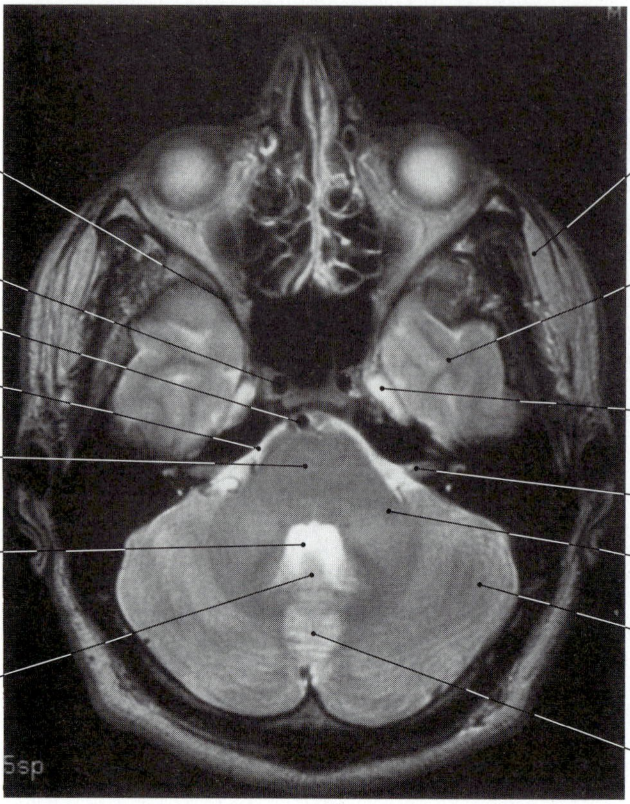
Sphenoid bone (greater wing)
Internal carotid artery
Basilar artery
Pontine cistern
Basis pontis
Fourth ventricle
Cerebellum (nodulus of vermis)
Temporalis muscle
Temporal lobe
Meckel's cavity
Facial and vestibulocochlear nerves
Middle cerebellar peduncle (brachium pontis)
Cerebellum (hemisphere)
Cerebellum (vermis)
5sp

FIGURE A8-11

T2-weighted axial section of the brain through the middle cerebellar peduncle and cerebellum.

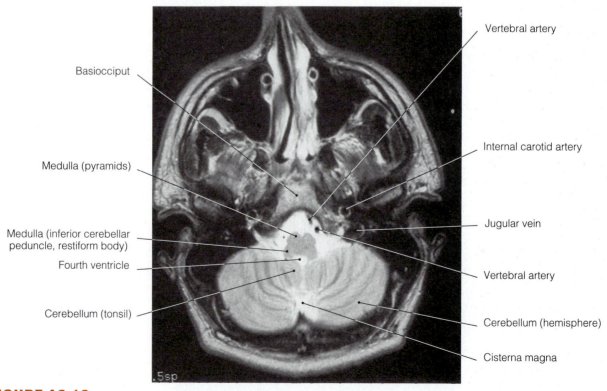

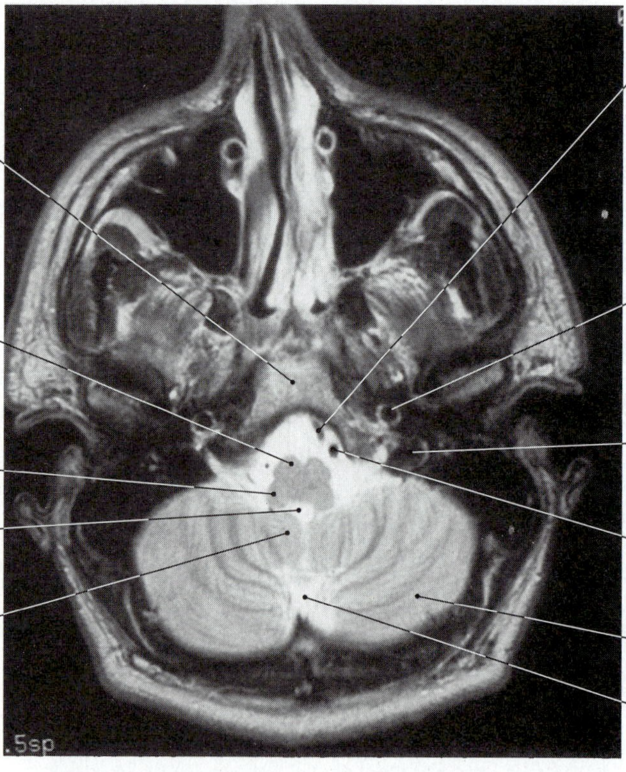
Basiocciput
Medulla (pyramids)
Medulla (inferior cerebellar peduncle, restiform body)
Fourth ventricle
Cerebellum (tonsil)
Vertebral artery
Internal carotid artery
Jugular vein
Vertebral artery
Cerebellum (hemisphere)
Cisterna magna
5sp

FIGURE A8-12

T2-weighted axial section of the brain through the medulla oblongata and cerebellum.

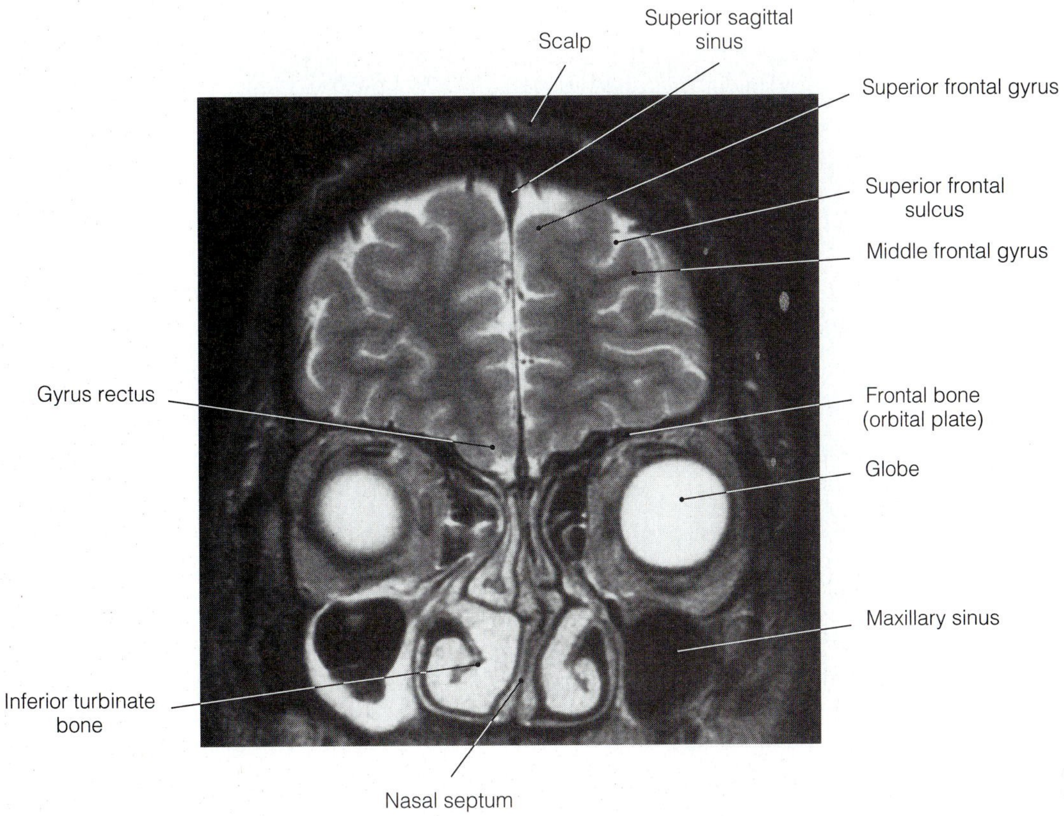
Scalp
Superior sagittal sinus
Superior frontal gyrus
Superior frontal sulcus
Middle frontal gyrus
Gyrus rectus
Frontal bone (orbital plate)
Globe
Maxillary sinus
Inferior turbinate bone
Nasal septum

FIGURE A9-1

T2-weighted coronal section of the brain at the level of the frontal pole.

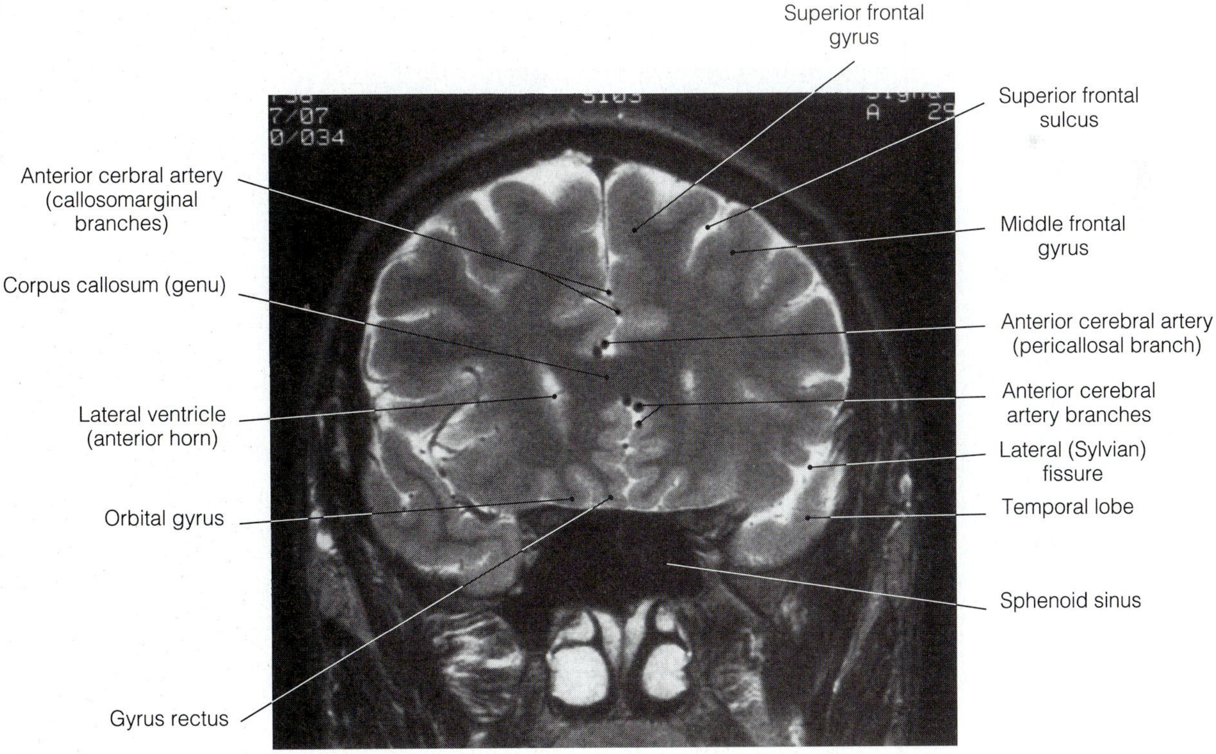
Superior frontal gyrus
Superior frontal sulcus
Anterior cerebral artery (callosomarginal branches)
Middle frontal gyrus
Corpus callosum (genu)
Anterior cerebral artery (pericallosal branch)
Lateral ventricle (anterior horn)
Anterior cerebral artery branches
Lateral (Sylvian) fissure
Orbital gyrus
Temporal lobe
Sphenoid sinus
Gyrus rectus

FIGURE A9-2

T2-weighted coronal section of the brain at the level of the rostral frontal lobe and tip of the anterior horn of the lateral ventricle.

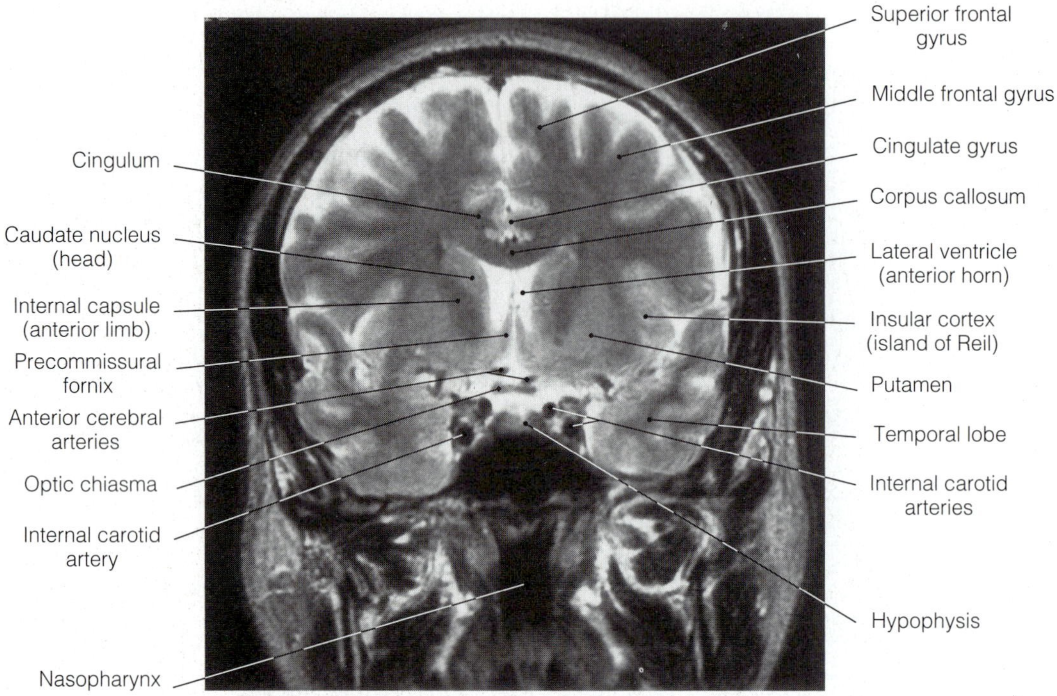
Superior frontal gyrus
Middle frontal gyrus
Cingulate gyrus
Corpus callosum
Lateral ventricle (anterior horn)
Insular cortex (island of Reil)
Putamen
Temporal lobe
Internal carotid arteries
Hypophysis
Cingulum
Caudate nucleus (head)
Internal capsule (anterior limb)
Precommissural fornix
Anterior cerebral arteries
Optic chiasma
Internal carotid artery
Nasopharynx

FIGURE A9-3

T2-weighted coronal section of the brain at the level of the neostriatum.

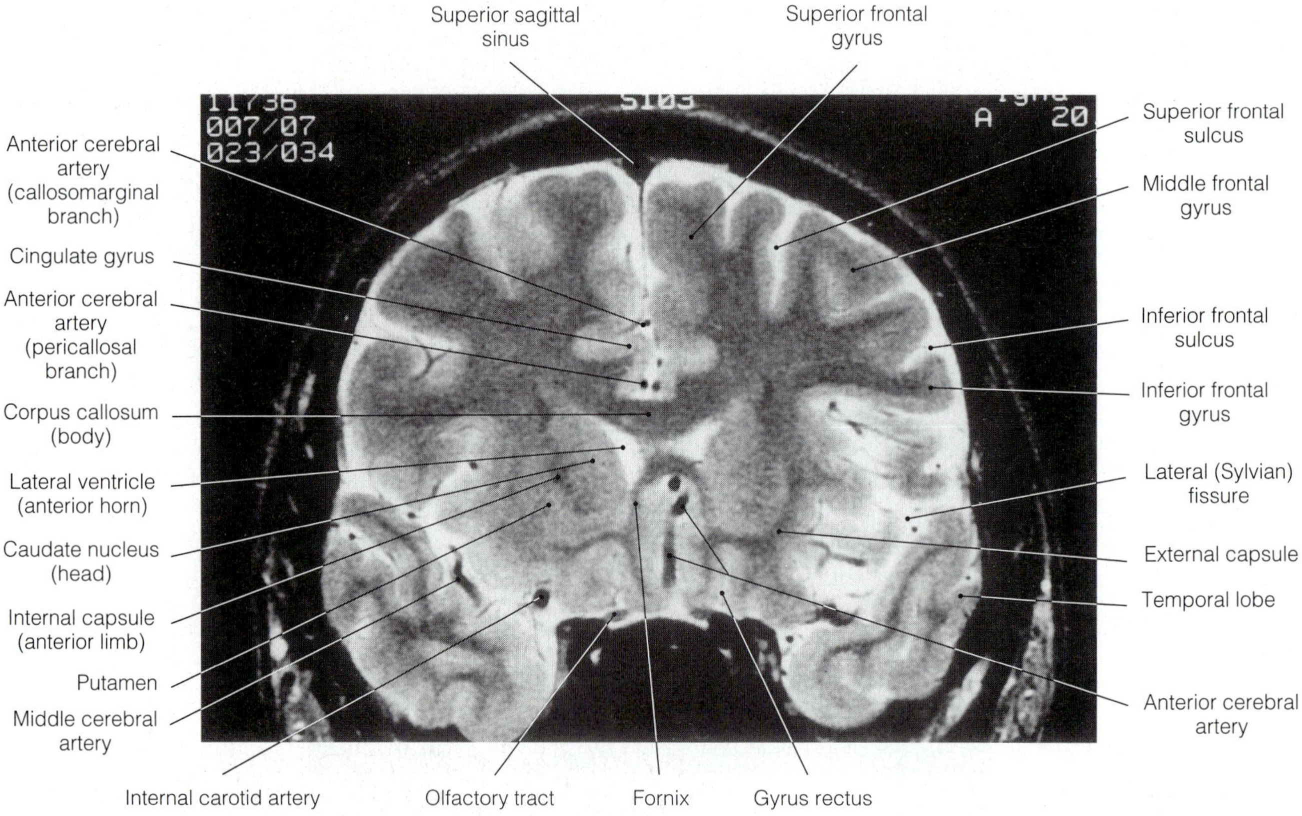
Superior sagittal sinus
Superior frontal gyrus
007/07
023/034
Superior frontal sulcus
Middle frontal gyrus
Inferior frontal sulcus
Inferior frontal gyrus
Lateral (Sylvian) fissure
External capsule
Temporal lobe
Anterior cerebral artery
Anterior cerebral artery (callosomarginal branch)
Cingulate gyrus
Anterior cerebral artery (pericallosal branch)
Corpus callosum (body)
Lateral ventricle (anterior horn)
Caudate nucleus (head)
Internal capsule (anterior limb)
Putamen
Middle cerebral artery
Internal carotid artery
Olfactory tract
Fornix
Gyrus rectus

FIGURE A9-4

T2-weighted coronal section of the brain at the level of the neostriatum.

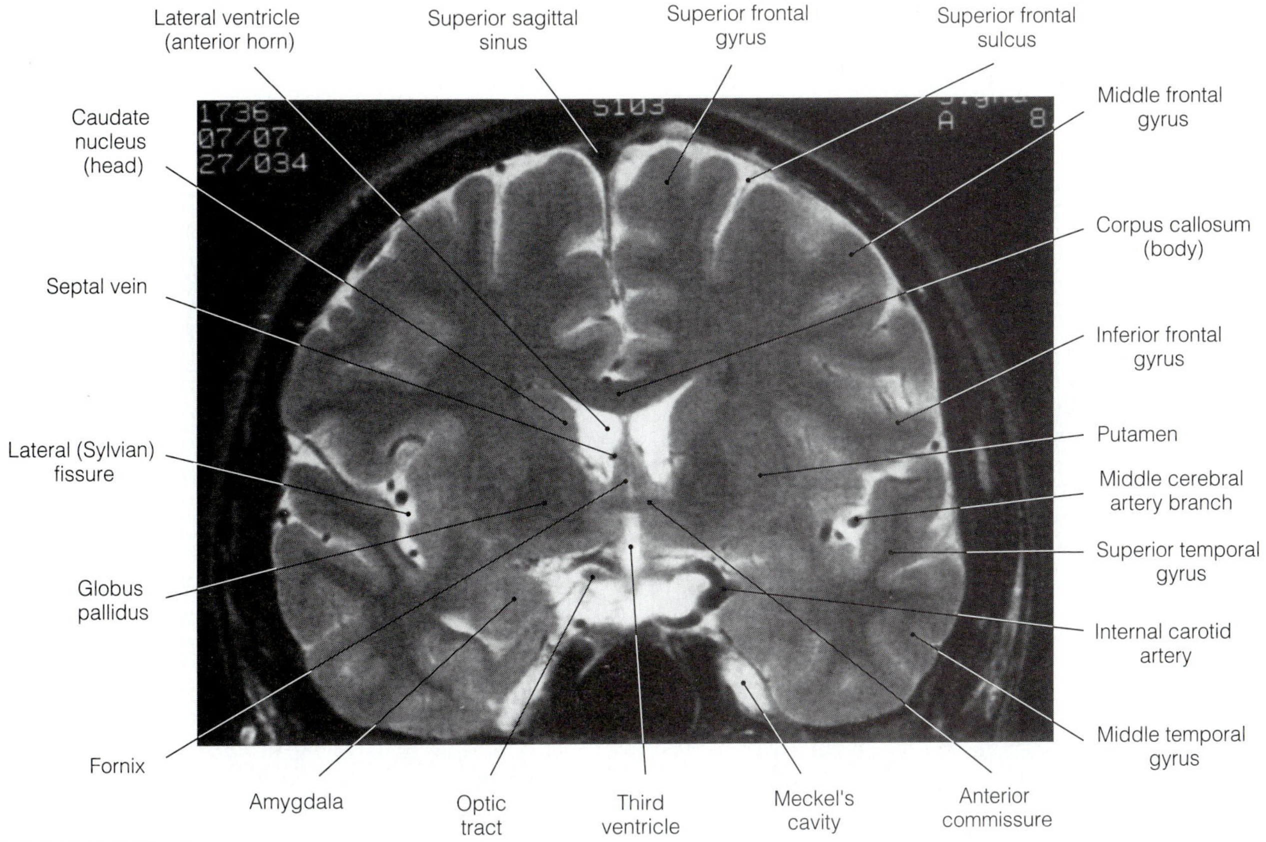
Lateral ventricle (anterior horn)
Superior sagittal sinus
Superior frontal gyrus
Superior frontal sulcus
Caudate nucleus (head)
Middle frontal gyrus
Corpus callosum (body)
Septal vein
Inferior frontal gyrus
Putamen
Lateral (Sylvian) fissure
Middle cerebral artery branch
Superior temporal gyrus
Globus pallidus
Internal carotid artery
Middle temporal gyrus
Fornix
Amygdala
Optic tract
Third ventricle
Meckel's cavity
Anterior commissure

FIGURE A9-5

T2-weighted coronal section of the brain at the level of the amygdaloid nucleus and corpus striatum.

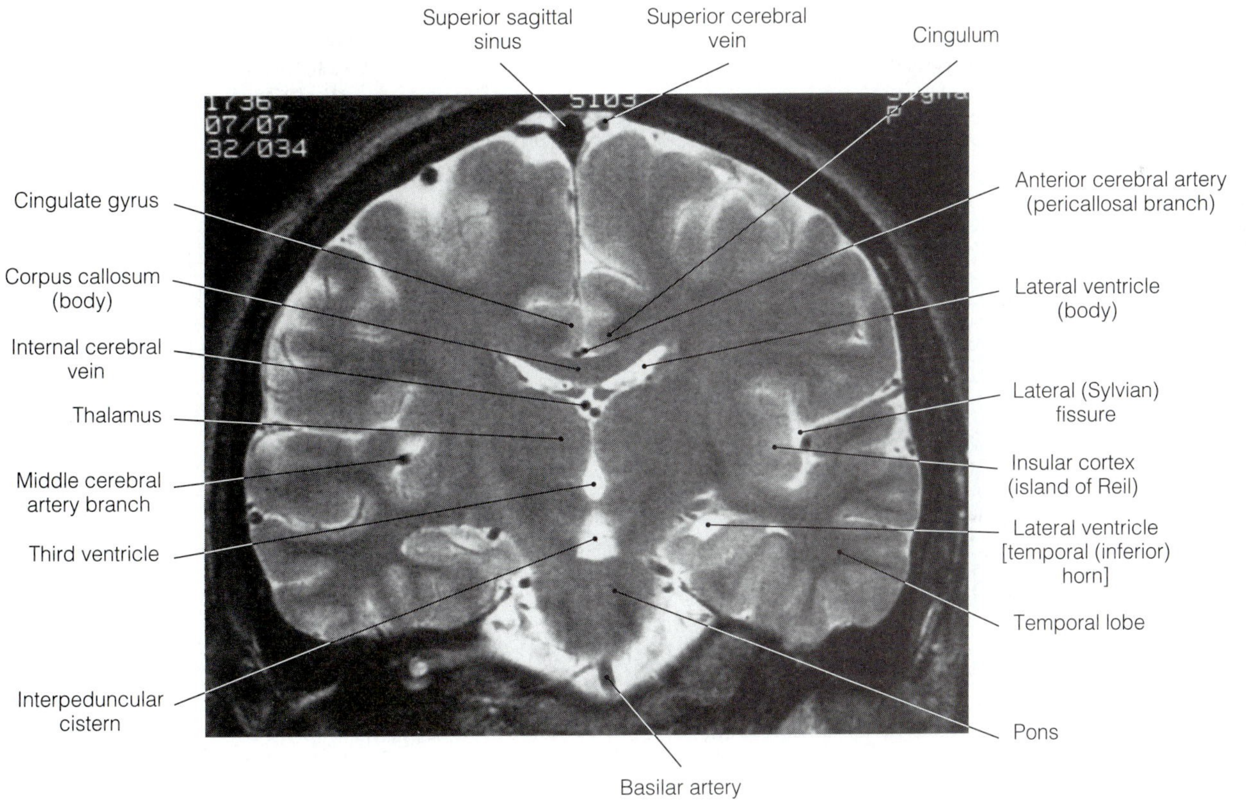
Superior sagittal sinus
Superior cerebral vein
Cingulum
Anterior cerebral artery (pericallosal branch)
Cingulate gyrus
Corpus callosum (body)
Lateral ventricle (body)
Internal cerebral vein
Lateral (Sylvian) fissure
Thalamus
Insular cortex (island of Reil)
Middle cerebral artery branch
Lateral ventricle [temporal (inferior) horn]
Third ventricle
Temporal lobe
Interpeduncular cistern
Pons
Basilar artery

FIGURE A9-6

T2-weighted coronal section of the brain at the level of the thalamus and third ventricle.

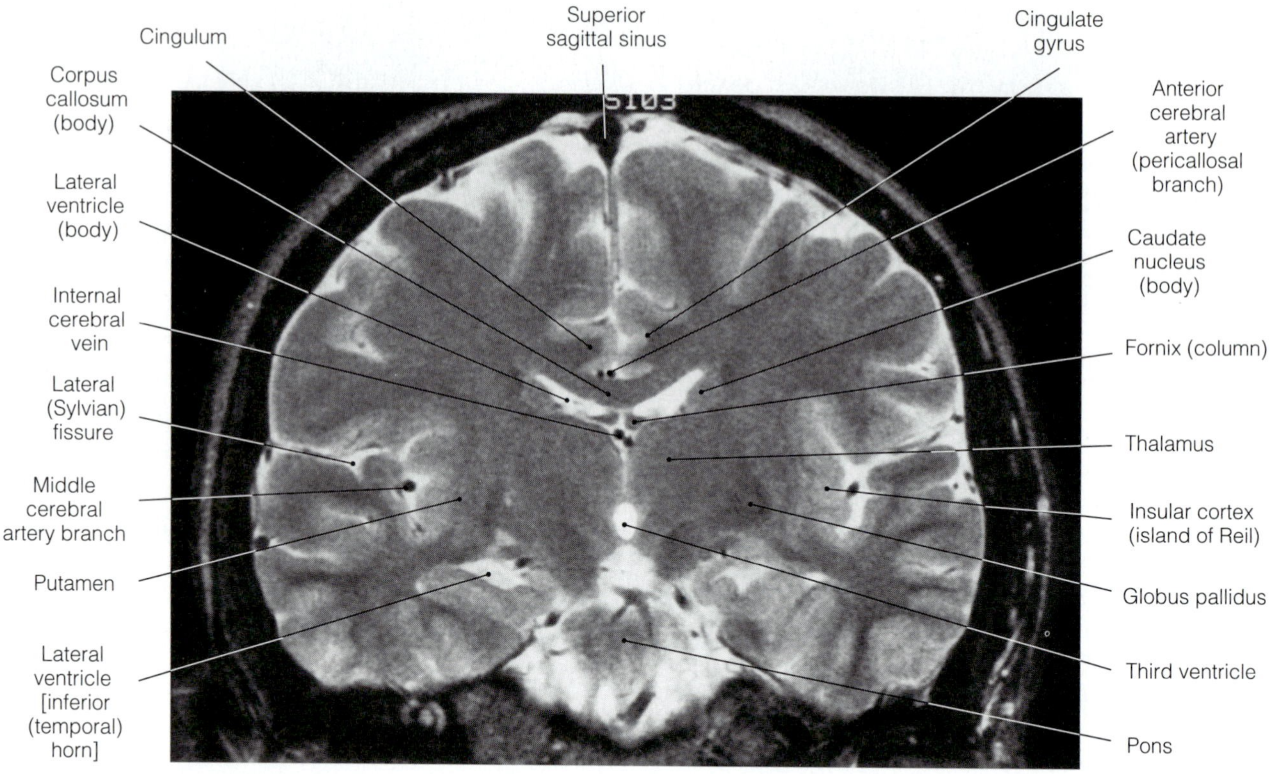

FIGURE A9-7

T2-weighted coronal section of the brain at the level of the thalamus and third ventricle.

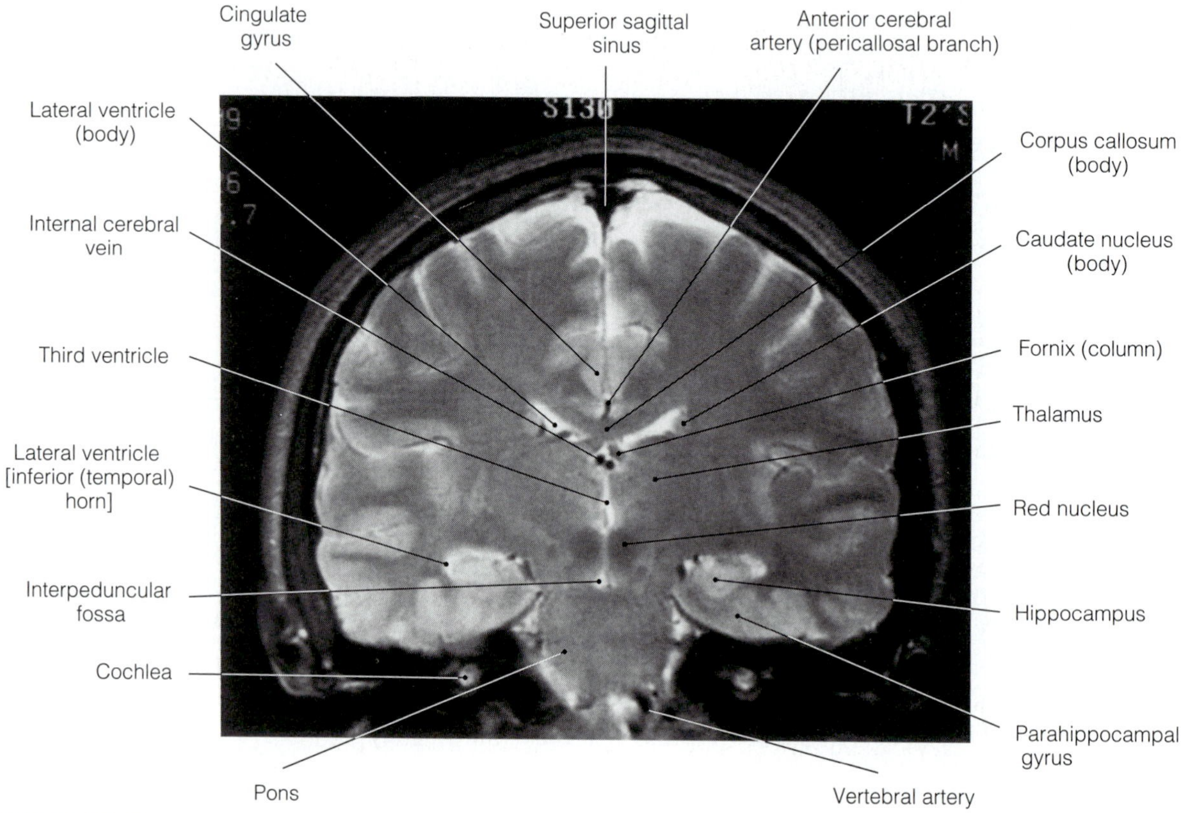

FIGURE A9-8

T2-weighted coronal section of the brain at the level of the caudal thalamus.

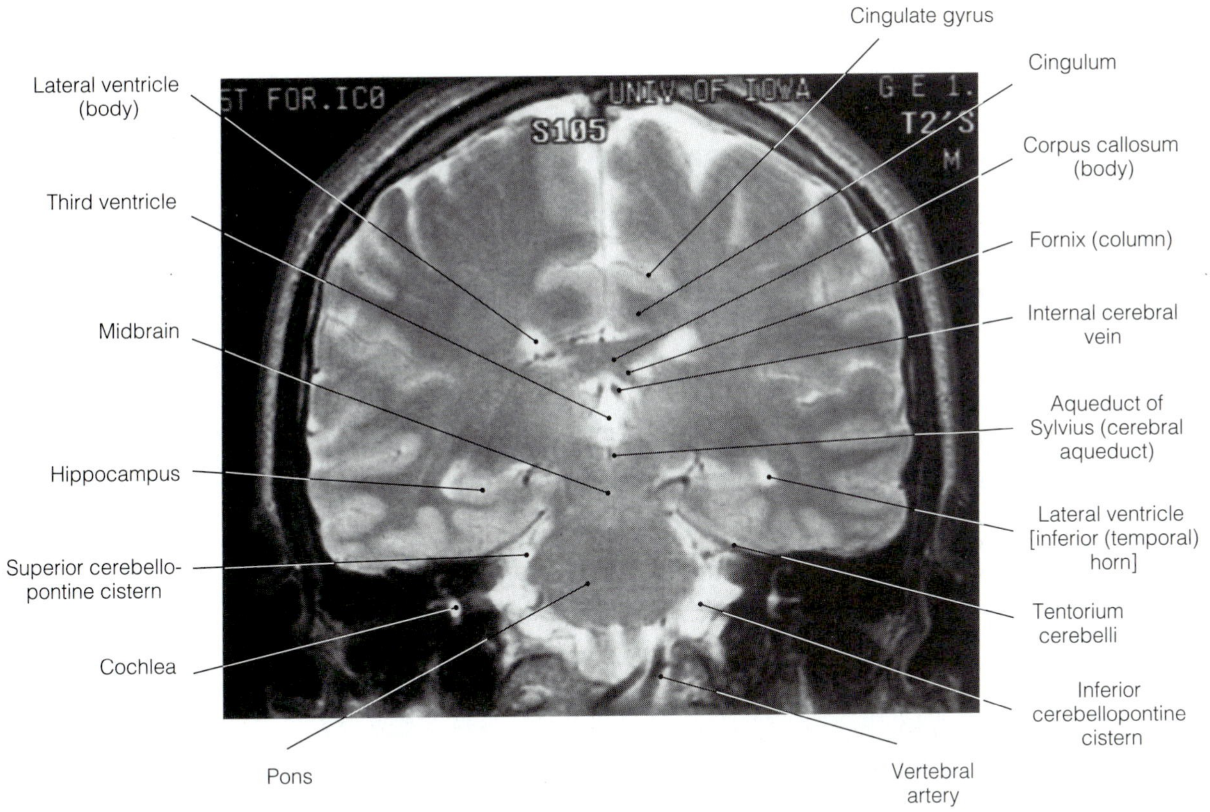
Cingulate gyrus
Cingulum
Lateral ventricle (body)
Corpus callosum (body)
Third ventricle
Fornix (column)
Internal cerebral vein
Midbrain
Aqueduct of Sylvius (cerebral aqueduct)
Hippocampus
Lateral ventricle [inferior (temporal) horn]
Superior cerebello-pontine cistern
Tentorium cerebelli
Cochlea
Inferior cerebellopontine cistern
Pons
Vertebral artery

FIGURE A9-9

T2-weighted coronal section of the brain at the level of the caudal thalamus, midbrain, and pons.

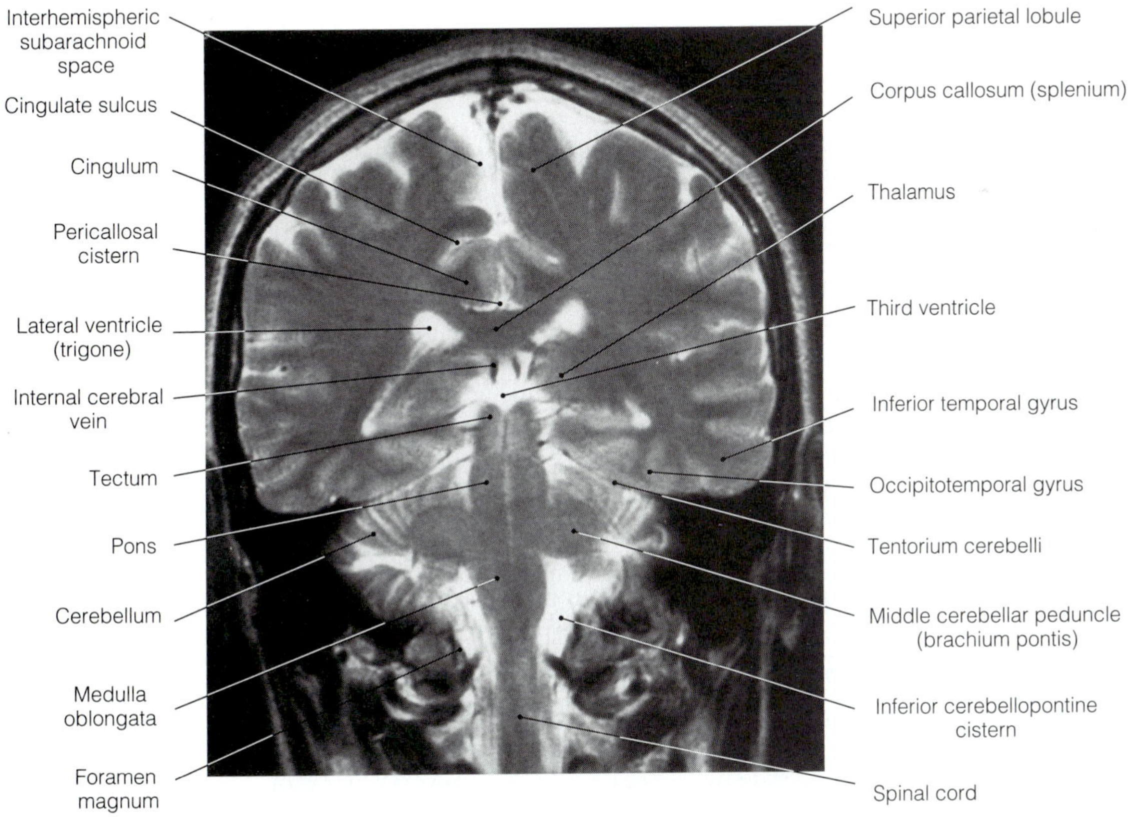
Interhemispheric subarachnoid space
Superior parietal lobule
Cingulate sulcus
Corpus callosum (splenium)
Cingulum
Thalamus
Pericallosal cistern
Lateral ventricle (trigone)
Third ventricle
Internal cerebral vein
Inferior temporal gyrus
Tectum
Occipitotemporal gyrus
Pons
Tentorium cerebelli
Cerebellum
Middle cerebellar peduncle (brachium pontis)
Medulla oblongata
Inferior cerebellopontine cistern
Foramen magnum
Spinal cord

FIGURE A9-10

T2-weighted coronal section of the brain through the cerebral hemisheres and brain stem.

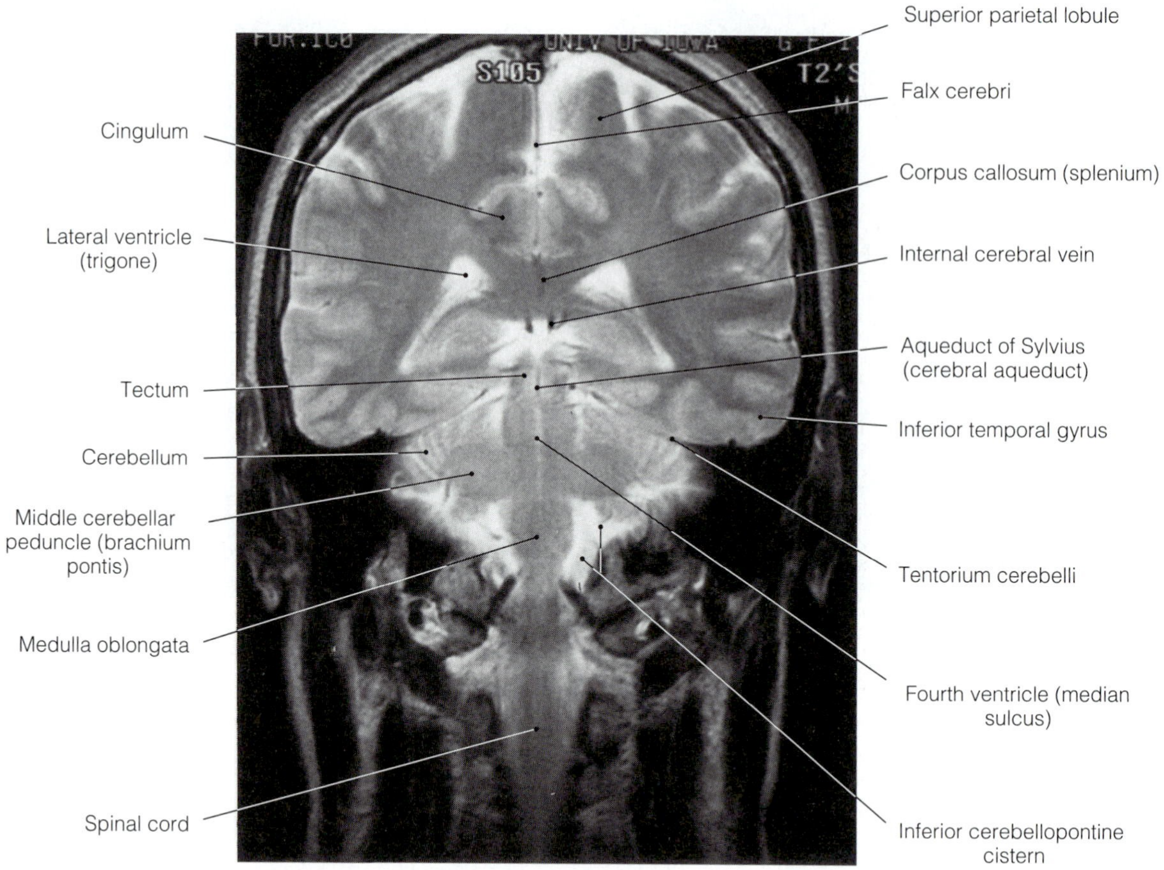
S105
Superior parietal lobule
Falx cerebri
Corpus callosum (splenium)
Internal cerebral vein
Aqueduct of Sylvius (cerebral aqueduct)
Inferior temporal gyrus
Tentorium cerebelli
Fourth ventricle (median sulcus)
Inferior cerebellopontine cistern
Cingulum
Lateral ventricle (trigone)
Tectum
Cerebellum
Middle cerebellar peduncle (brachium pontis)
Medulla oblongata
Spinal cord

FIGURE A9-11

T2-weighted coronal section of the brain through the cerebral hemispheres and brain stem.

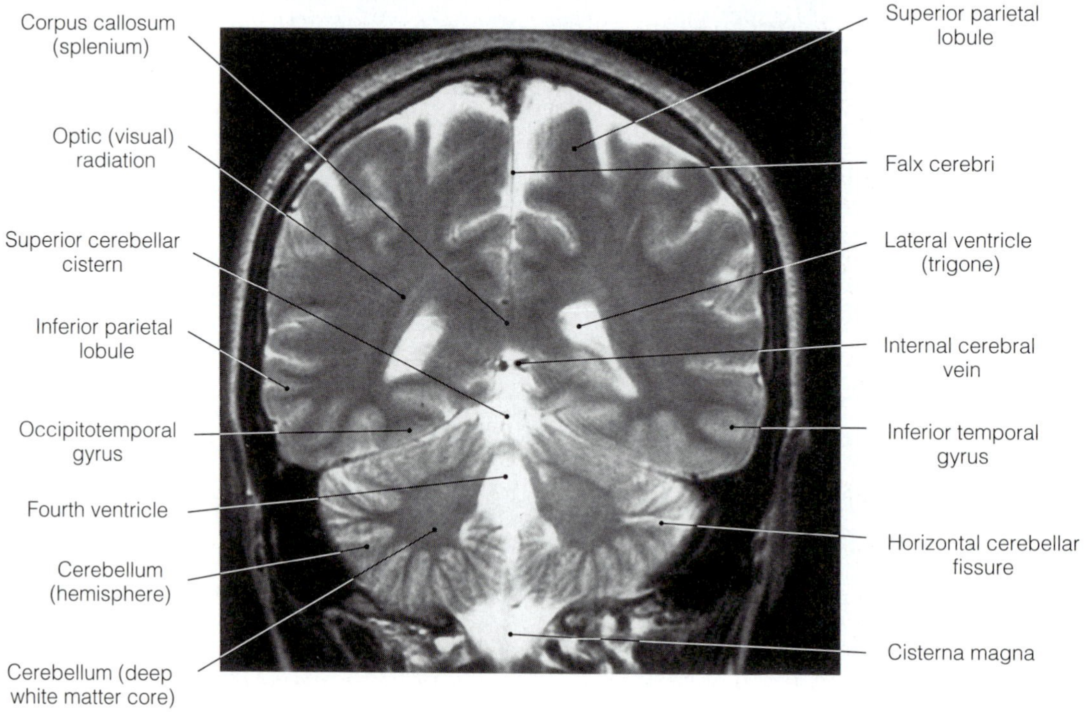
Corpus callosum (splenium)
Optic (visual) radiation
Superior cerebellar cistern
Inferior parietal lobule
Occipitotemporal gyrus
Fourth ventricle
Cerebellum (hemisphere)
Cerebellum (deep white matter core)
Superior parietal lobule
Falx cerebri
Lateral ventricle (trigone)
Internal cerebral vein
Inferior temporal gyrus
Horizontal cerebellar fissure
Cisterna magna

FIGURE A9-12

T2-weighted coronal section of the brain at the level of the parietotemporal lobes and cerebellum.

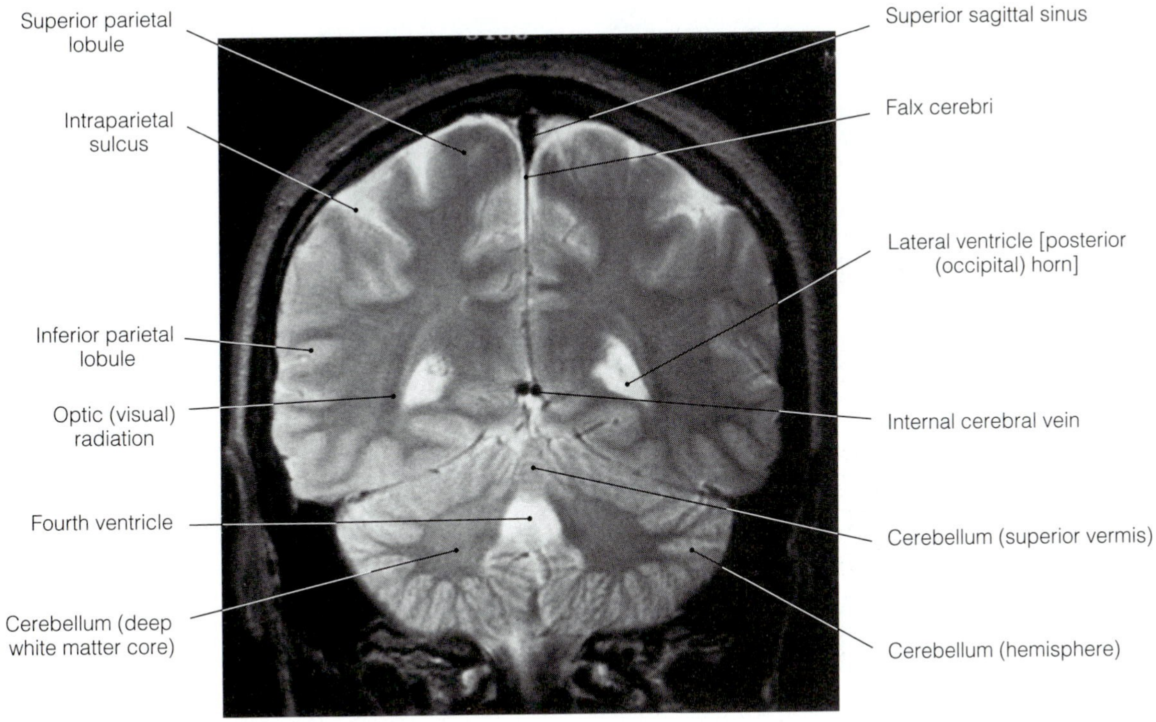
Superior parietal lobule
Intraparietal sulcus
Inferior parietal lobule
Optic (visual) radiation
Fourth ventricle
Cerebellum (deep white matter core)
Superior sagittal sinus
Falx cerebri
Lateral ventricle [posterior (occipital) horn]
Internal cerebral vein
Cerebellum (superior vermis)
Cerebellum (hemisphere)

FIGURE A9-13

T2-weighted coronal section of the brain at the level of the occipital horn of the lateral ventricle.

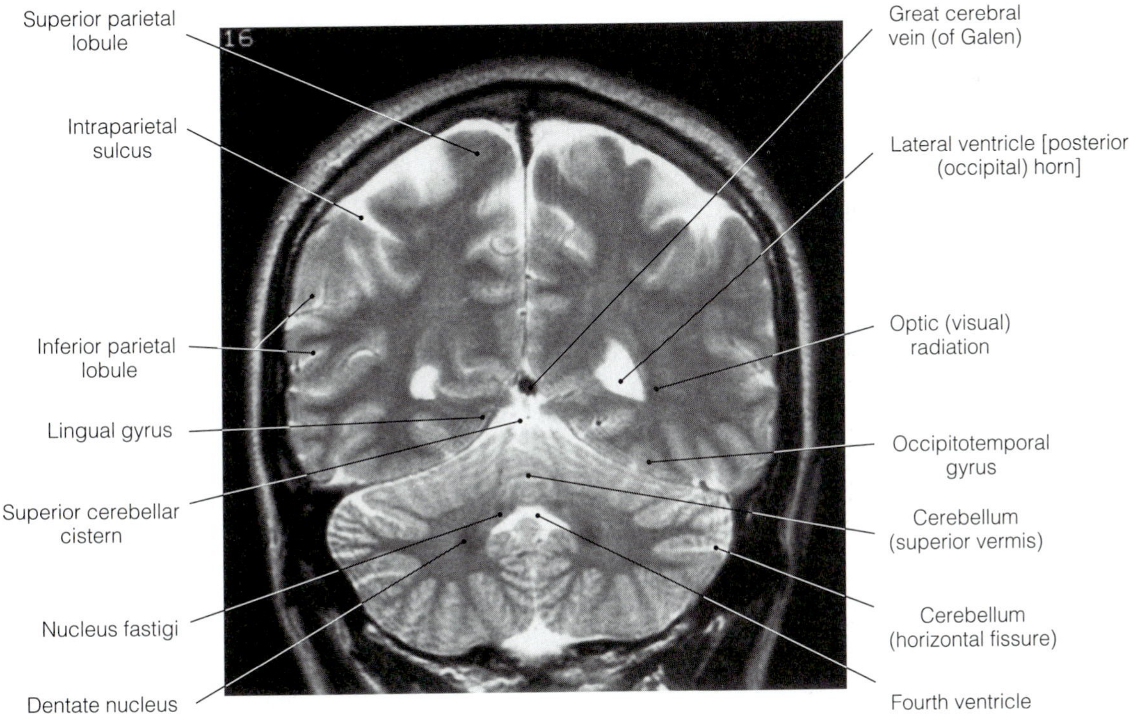
16
Superior parietal lobule
Intraparietal sulcus
Inferior parietal lobule
Lingual gyrus
Superior cerebellar cistern
Nucleus fastigi
Dentate nucleus
Great cerebral vein (of Galen)
Lateral ventricle [posterior (occipital) horn]
Optic (visual) radiation
Occipitotemporal gyrus
Cerebellum (superior vermis)
Cerebellum (horizontal fissure)
Fourth ventricle

FIGURE A9-14

T2-weighted coronal section of the brain at the level of the occipital horn of the lateral ventricle.

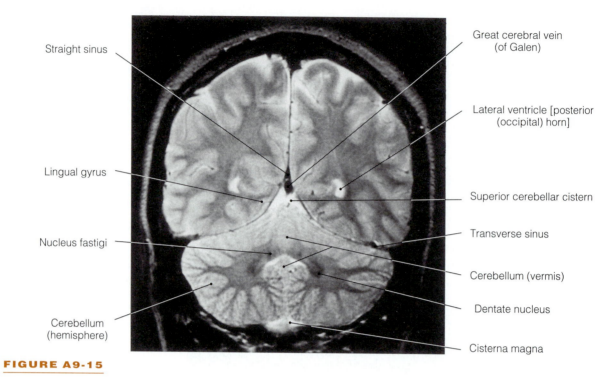

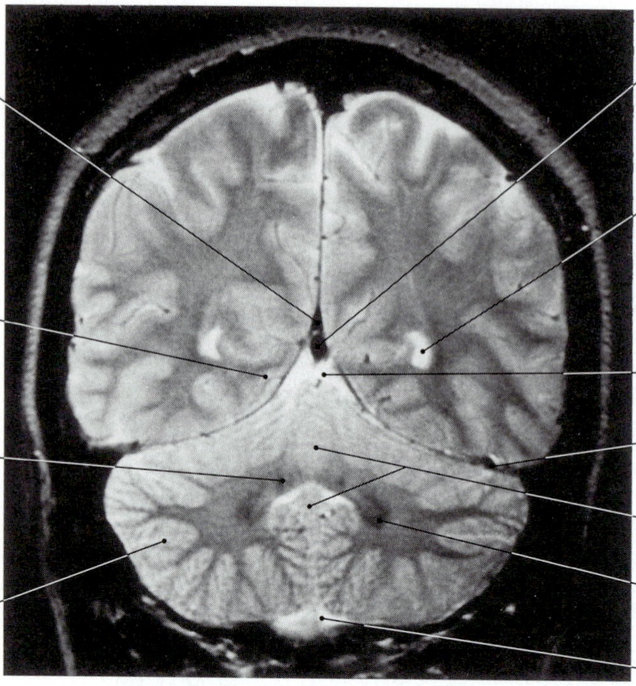
Straight sinus
Lingual gyrus
Nucleus fastigi
Cerebellum
(hemisphere)
Great cerebral vein
(of Galen)
Lateral ventricle [posterior
(occipital) horn]
Superior cerebellar cistern
Transverse sinus
Cerebellum (vermis)
Dentate nucleus
Cisterna magna

FIGURE A9-15

T2-weighted coronal section of the brain at the level of the occipital lobe and cerebellum.

BIBLIOGRAPHY

Afifi AK, Bergman RA: *Basic Neuroscience: A Structural and Functional Approach*, 2d ed. Baltimore, Urban & Schwarzenberg, 1986.

Angevine JB, Cotman CW: *Principles of Neuroanatomy*. New York, Oxford University Press, 1981.

Barr ML, Kiernan JA: *The Human Nervous System: An Anatomical Viewpoint*, 6th ed. Philadelphia, Lippincott, 1993.

Bergman RA, Afifi AK, Heidger PM: *Histology*. Philadelphia, Saunders, 1996

Bergman RA, Afifi AK, Heidger PM: *Atlas of Microscopic Anatomy. A Functional Approach: Companion to Histology and Neuroanatomy*, 2d ed. Philadelphia, Saunders, 1989.

Brazis PW, Masdeu JC, Biller J: *Localization in Clinical Neurology*. Boston, Little Brown, 1985.

Brodal P: *The Central Nervous System: Structure and Function*. New York, Oxford University Press, 1992.

Brodal A: *Neurological Anatomy in Relation to Clinical Medicine*, 3d ed. London, Oxford University Press, 1981.

Carpenter MB: *Core Text of Neuroanatomy*, 4th ed. Baltimore, Williams & Wilkins, 1991.

Clarke E, Dewhurst K: *An Illustrated History of Brain Function: Imaging the Brain from Antiquity to the Present*, 2d ed. San Francisco, Norman Publishing, 1996.

Conn PM: *Neuroscience in Medicine*. Philadelphia, Lippincott, 1995.

Damasio H: *Human Brain Anatomy in Computerized Images*. New York, Oxford University Press, 1995.

DeArmond SJ, Fusco MM, Dewey MM: *Structure of the Human Brain: A Photographic Atlas*, 3d ed. New York, Oxford University Press, 1989.

Dorland's Illustrated Medical Dictionary, 27th ed. Philadelphia, Saunders, 1988.

Dunkerley GB: *A Basic Atlas of the Human Nervous System*. Philadelphia, F. A. Davis, 1975.

Duus P: *Topical Diagnosis in Neurology: Anatomy, Physiology, Signs, Symptoms*, 2d ed. New York, Thieme, 1989.

Fitzgerald MJT: *Neuroanatomy: Basic and Clinical*, 2d ed. London, Bailliere Tindall, 1992.

Fix JD: *Atlas of the Human Brain and Spinal Cord*. Rockville, MD, Aspen Publishing, 1987.

Fix JD, Punte CS: *Atlas of the Human Brain Stem and Spinal Cord*. Baltimore, University Park Press, 1981.

Gluhbegovic N, Williams TH: *The Human Brain: A Photographic Guide*. Hagerstown, MD, Harper & Row, 1980.

Haines DE: *Fundamental Neuroscience.* New York, Churchill Livingstone, 1997.

Heimer L: *The Human Brain and Spinal Cord: Functional Neuroanatomy and Dissection Guide*, 2d ed. New York, Springer-Verlag, 1995.

Martin JH: *Neuroanatomy: Text and Atlas*, 2d ed. Stamford, CT, Appleton & Lange, 1996.

Montgomery EB, Wall M, Henderson VW: *Principles of Neurologic Diagnosis.* Boston, Little Brown, 1986.

Montemuro DG, Bruni JE: *The Human Brain in Dissection*, 2d ed. New York, Oxford University Press, 1988.

Noback CR, Strominger NL, Demarest RJ: *The Human Nervous System: Structure and Function*, 5th ed. Baltimore, Williams & Wilkins, 1996.

Nolte J, Angevine JB: *The Human Brain: In Photographs and Diagrams.* St. Louis, Mosby, 1995.

Pryse-Phillips W: *Companion to Clinical Neurology.* Boston, Little Brown, 1995.

Roberts M, Hanaway J: *Atlas of the Human Brain in Sections.* Philadelphia, Lea & Febiger, 1970.

Schnitzlein HN, Reed Murtagh F: *Imaging Anatomy of the Head and Spine: A Photographic Color Atlas of MRI, CT, Gross and Microscopic Anatomy in Axial, Coronal, and Sagittal Planes.* Baltimore, Urban & Schwarzenberg, 1985.

Skinner HA: *The Origin of Medical Terms*, 2d ed. Baltimore, Williams & Wilkins, 1961.

Smith CG: *Serial Dissection of the Human Brain.* Baltimore, Urban & Schwarzenberg, 1981.

Waxman SG: *Correlative Neuroanatomy*, 23d ed. Stamford, CT, Appleton & Lange, 1996.

Wilson-Pauwels L, Akesson EJ, Stewart PA: *Cranial Nerves: Anatomy and Clinical Comments.* Toronto, B.C. Decker, 1988.

Young PA, Young PH: *Basic Clinical Neuroanatomy.* Baltimore, Williams & Wilkins, 1997.

Yuh WTC, Tali ET, Afifi AK, et al: *MRI of Head and Neck Anatomy.* New York, Churchill Livingston, 1994.

Zuleger S, Staubesand J: *Atlas of the Central Nervous System in Sectional Planes: Selected Myelin Stained Sections of the Human Brain and Spinal Cord.* Baltimore, Urban & Schwarzenberg, 1977.

INDEX

The letter *t* or *f* following a page number indicates that either a table or a figure is being referenced.

ISBN 0-07-001589-9
90000
9 780070 015890
AFIFI: FUNC. NEURO (U.S.)